Advanced Biophotonics

SERIES IN OPTICS AND OPTOELECTRONICS

Recent titles in the series

Advanced Biophotonics: Tissue Optical Sectioning
Ruikang K Wang and Valery V Tuchin (Eds.)

Handbook of Silicon Photonics
Laurent Vivien and Lorenzo Pavesi (Eds.)

Microlenses: Properties, Fabrication and Liquid Lenses
Hongrui Jiang and Xuefeng Zeng

Laser-Based Measurements for Time and Frequency Domain Applications: A Handbook
Pasquale Maddaloni, Marco Bellini, and Paolo De Natale

Handbook of 3D Machine Vision: Optical Metrology and Imaging
Song Zhang (Ed.)

Handbook of Optical Dimensional Metrology
Kevin Harding (Ed.)

Biomimetics in Photonics
Olaf Karthaus (Ed.)

Optical Properties of Photonic Structures: Interplay of Order and Disorder
Mikhail F Limonov and Richard De La Rue (Eds.)

Nitride Phosphors and Solid-State Lighting
Rong-Jun Xie, Yuan Qiang Li, Naoto Hirosaki, and Hajime Yamamoto

Molded Optics: Design and Manufacture
Michael Schaub, Jim Schwiegerling, Eric Fest, R Hamilton Shepard, and Alan Symmons

An Introduction to Quantum Optics: Photon and Biphoton Physics
Yanhua Shih

Principles of Adaptive Optics, Third Edition
Robert Tyson

Optical Tweezers: Methods and Applications
Miles J Padgett, Justin Molloy, and David McGloin (Eds.)

Thin-Film Optical Filters, Fourth Edition
H Angus Macleod

Laser Induced Damage of Optical Materials
R M Wood

Advanced Biophotonics

Tissue Optical Sectioning

Edited by

Ruikang K. Wang
Valery V. Tuchin

CRC Press
Taylor & Francis Group
Boca Raton London New York

CRC Press is an imprint of the
Taylor & Francis Group, an **informa** business
A TAYLOR & FRANCIS BOOK

Taylor & Francis
Taylor & Francis Group
6000 Broken Sound Parkway NW, Suite 300
Boca Raton, FL 33487-2742

First issued in paperback 2018

ISBN-13: 978-1-4398-9581-8 (hbk)
ISBN-13: 978-1-138-38218-3 (pbk)

Library of Congress Cataloging-in-Publication Data

Advanced biophotonics : tissue optical sectioning / editor, Ruikang K. Wang, Valery V. Tuchin.
pages cm. -- (Series in optics and optoelectronics ; 19)
Summary: "This reference provides an overview of optical imaging and manipulation technologies in biophotonics, covering both basic and advanced optical imaging techniques. It reviews the principles and fundamentals of bioimaging and molecular imaging/manipulation techniques. It also presents an overview of instrumentation, basic algorithms, and data processing methods. Accessible to students and researchers, the book discusses a range of application areas, including established and newer methodologies in biotechnology, biomedical engineering, biophysics, medicine, and pharmacology"-- Provided by publisher.
Includes bibliographical references and index.
ISBN 978-1-4398-9581-8 (hardback)
1. Imaging systems in medicine. 2. Imaging systems in biology. 3. Optical tomography. 4. Photonics. I. Wang, Ruikang K. II. Tuchin, V. V. (Valerii Viktorovich)

R857.O6A353 2013
616.07'545--dc23 2013018225

Visit the Taylor & Francis Web site at
http://www.taylorandfrancis.com

and the CRC Press Web site at
http://www.crcpress.com

Contents

Preface

Photonics is the science and technology of generation, manipulation, and detection of light. The field uses the quantum-like particles of light, i.e., the photons, instead of electrons to transmit, process, and store information. Biophotonics is recently emerged from the applications of photonics in the fields of biology and medicine. The invention of lasers in the 1960s revolutionized photonics, and made rapid technological advancements that produced useful tools, such as bar code scanners, CD players and laser pointers that are already playing an important part in our daily life. The fluorescence microscope is the first taste of the power of biophotonics that brought us the important molecular information within cells in almost all biological laboratories. Today, biophotonics is widely regarded as the key science upon which the next generation of clinical tools and biomedical research instrumentation will be based. Although nature has used the principle of biophotonics to harness light for photosynthesis, it wasn't until about 10 years ago that a substantial translation of photonics technologies to biological applications began to transform medical and life sciences.

The knowledge of biophotonics essentially includes the fundamentals of many interdisciplinary fields and how they are uniquely related to each other. Researchers and students who are interested in biophotonics should have a solid understanding of the physics of light, and the engineering of devices and instruments that are used to generate, modify, and manipulate light. On the other hand, they must also understand the fundamentals of biology and medicine, such as the molecular and cellular processes that occur in living systems to properly and meaningfully utilize the biophotonics techniques to address their biological questions. Healthy and diseased tissues have differing biological processes in different states; thus, it is also important to have a fundamental understanding of pathophysiology, and common disease states such as cancer, cardiovascular disease, neurodegenerative disease, and infectious disease, to name just a few.

Although still "young," biophotonics is now steadily becoming an important discipline that investigates fundamental principles and develops new optical technology for the interaction of light or photons with biological organisms, tissues, cells, and molecules. One of the most important elements in this discipline is the rapid developments of innovative bio-imaging technologies that brought us the opportunities to visualize tissue organization, biochemical compositions, and functional information about tissue without any harm to its native state. The light with wavelengths between visible and near-infrared ranges is highly scattered within a turbid medium, such as biological tissue. Therefore, the bio-imaging methods that attempt to form images from light passing through tissue can be classified into two categories—ballistic (minimally scattered) optical microscopy and diffuse (multiply scattered) optical tomography. The former provides fine resolution but with a shallow imaging depth in tissue—up to about 1–2 mm, as defined by the optical diffusion limit. The representative technologies in this category include confocal microscopy, multiphoton microscopy, optical coherence tomography, and others.

When incident photons reach their diffusion limit, most of them have undergone tens of scattering events, making the ability to focus the light extremely difficult. Fortunately, diffuse optical tomography can effectively utilize the multiply scattering photons to provide an image that represents information centimeters into tissue, albeit with poor spatial resolution—roughly about one-third of the imaging depth. However, randomized paths of the diffuse photons render the image reconstruction mathematically ill-posed. It still remains a challenge for pure optical imaging to attain fine spatial resolution at depths beyond the optical diffusion limit. Until recently, photoacoustic imaging has been developed to break this limitation, in which the researchers innovatively use photon-absorption in tissue that can be converted into ultrasonic waves, which are scattered much less. For this, we have seen impressive progress over just the last few years that has manifested the power of photoacoustic imaging to investigate the molecular and cellular processes that occur in living systems.

Currently, there are a number of professional books (including edited) that were published by different publishers, which describe methods and techniques of biophotonics imaging for medical diagnostics and therapy. Many of them are devoted to specific topics of biomedical optics such as tissue optics, confocal, nonlinear microscopy (including multiphoton microscopy), optical coherence tomography, and others. There is still a lack of a comprehensive imaging book that describes advanced biophotonics imaging methods and techniques intensively developed in recent years, a gap that this current book tries to address. We believe that this assembled book is the next step in presenting contemporary advances in biophotonics imaging and will allow researchers, bioengineers, and medical doctors to be acquainted with major recent bioimaging technologies that apply biophotonics science and technology, which are dispersed in numerous journals of physical, chemical, biophysical, and biomedical profiles.

It is, however, impossible to present all imaging techniques that use the photonics science and technology to address biological and medical questions, particularly when this field is still rapidly evolving and novel imaging methods are constantly conceptualized. The editors hope that this book will be useful for researchers, practitioners, and professionals in the field of biophotonics, and can be used by scientists or professionals in other disciplines, such as laser physics and technology, fiber optics, spectroscopy, materials science, biology, and medicine. Graduate and also undergraduate students specializing in biomedical physics and engineering, biomedical optics and biophotonics will also find this book a useful resource.

This book represents a valuable contribution by well-known experts in the field of biomedical optics and biophotonics with their particular interest in a variety of "hot" biophotonics problems. We greatly appreciate the cooperation and contributions of all authors in the book, who have done great work in the preparation of their chapters.

We would like to thank all those authors and publishers who freely granted permissions to reproduce their copyrighted works. We are grateful to Dr. John Navas, Senior Editor, Physics, of Taylor & Francis/CRC Press, for his idea to publish such a book, valuable suggestions, and help on preparation of the manuscript. We are also very much thankful to Professor Vladimir L. Derbov, Saratov State University, for preparation of the camera-ready manuscript and help in the technical editing of the book.

Ruikang K. Wang

Valery V. Tuchin

The Editors

Ruikang K. Wang, PhD, is Professor of Bioengineering with the University of Washington, Seattle. After two years postdoctoral research training at Glasgow, Scotland, he joined as a Lecturer, and then, Senior Lecturer in Bioimaging Science with Keele Medical School, England. In 2002, he became a chair professor in Biomedical Optics at Cranfield University, England, where he created and directed the Biophotonics and Imaging Laboratory. In 2005, he joined Oregon Health and Science University, Oregon, where he was Professor of Biomedical Engineering and the Director of the Biophotonics and Imaging Laboratory. He is author and co-author of more than 200 peer-reviewed journal articles, one monograph in optical information processing, as well as 12 book chapters. He is a fellow of the Optical Society of America and a fellow of the International Society for Optics and Photonics (SPIE). His current research interests include biophotonics and imaging, optical coherence tomography, optical microangiography, and their applications in neurology, ophthalmology, dermatology and cancer.

Valery V. Tuchin, PhD, holds the Optics and Biophotonics Chair and is a Director of Research-Educational Institute of Optics and Biophotonics at Saratov State University, Head of Laboratory on Laser Diagnostics of Technical and Living Systems, Inst. of Precise Mechanics and Control, RAS, and FiDiPro Professor (Finland Distinguished Professor) of Optoelectronics and Measurement Techniques Laboratory, University of Oulu, Finland. His research interests include biophotonics, biomedical optics and laser medicine, physics of optical and laser measurements. He has authored more than 300 peer-reviewed papers and books, including his latest, *Tissue Optics: Light Scattering Methods and Instrumentation for Medical Diagnosis* (PM166, SPIE Press, second edition, 2007), *Dictionary of Biomedical Optics and Biophotonics* (PM217, SPIE Press, Bellingham, WA, 2012), and three volume *Handbook of Biophotonics* (Wiley-VCH Verlag GmbH & Co. KGaA, Weinheim, 2011-2012. Eds.: J. Popp, V.V. Tuchin, A. Chiou, and S.H. Heinemann). He has been awarded Honored Science Worker of the Russian Federation and SPIE Fellow, and is a Vice-President of the Russian Photobiology Society. In 2007 he was awarded the SPIE Educator Award.

The Editors

List of Contributors

Jennifer Kehlet Barton
Department of Biomedical Engineering, The University of Arizona, Tucson, Arizona

Chao-Wei Chen
Department of Electrical and Computer Engineering, University of Maryland, College Park, Maryland

Yu Chen
Fischell Department of Bioengineering, University of Maryland, College Park, Maryland

Kenny F. Chou
Department of Bioengineering and Human Photonics Lab, University of Washington, Seattle, Washington

Riccardo Cicchi
National Institute of Optics - National Research Council (INO-CNR), Florence, Italy; European Laboratory for Non-Linear Spectroscopy (LENS), University of Florence, Sesto Fiorentino, Italy

Ryan L. Coe
Department of Bioengineering and Human Photonics Lab, University of Washington, Seattle, Washington

David J. Cuccia
Modulated Imaging Inc., Irvine, California

Andrea Curatolo
Optical+Biomedical Engineering Laboratory (OBEL), School of Electrical, Electronic and Computer Engineering, The University of Western Australia, Crawley, Western Australia, Australia

Susan M. Daly
Department of Physics & Energy, University of Limerick, Ireland

Alexander Doronin
The Jack Dodd Centre for Quantum Technology, Department of Physics, University of Otago, New Zealand

Jacque Duncan
Department of Ophthalmology, University of California, San Francisco, California

Anthony J. Durkin
Beckman Laser Institute and Medical Clinic, University of California, Irvine, California

Nirmalya Ghosh
Department of Physical Sciences, Indian Institute of Science Education and Research (IISER), Kolkata, Mohanpur, West Bengal, India

Christopher A. Girkin
Department of Ophthalmology, University of Alabama at Birmingham, Birmingham, Alabama

Zijian Guo
Optical Imaging Laboratory, Department of Biomedical Engineering, Washington University in St. Louis, St. Louis, Missouri

Timothy R. Hillman
Former address: Optical+Biomedical Engineering Laboratory (OBEL), School of Electrical, Electronic and Computer Engineering, The University of Western Australia, Crawley, Western Australia, Australia

Shuliang Jiao
Department of Ophthalmology, University of Southern California, Los Angeles, California

Brendan F. Kennedy
Optical+Biomedical Engineering Laboratory (OBEL), School of Electrical, Electronic and Computer Engineering, The University of Western Australia, Crawley, Western Australia, Australia

David Layden
Department of Physics and Astronomy, University of Waterloo, Waterloo, Ontario, Canada

Martin J. Leahy
Tissue Optics and Microcirculation Imaging Group, School of Physics, National University of Ireland, Galway, Ireland

Qingming Luo
Britton Chance Center for Biomedical Photonics, Wuhan National Laboratory for Optoelectronics, Huazhong University of Science and Technology, Wuhan, China; Key Laboratory of Biomedical Photonics of Ministry of Education, Huazhong University of Science and Technology, Wuhan, China

Amaan Mazhar
Beckman Laser Institute and Medical Clinic, University of California, Irvine, California

Igor Meglinski
The Jack Dodd Centre for Quantum Technology, Department of Physics, University of Otago, New Zealand

Michael G. Meyer
VisionGate Inc., Phoenix, Arizona

Qin Miao
Department of Bioengineering and Human Photonics Lab, University of Washington, Seattle, Washington

Vasilis Ntziachristos
Institute for Biological and Medical Imaging and Chair for Biological Imaging, Helmholtz Zentrum München and Technische Universität München Ingolstädter Neuherberg, Germany

Francesco S. Pavone
European Laboratory for Non-Linear Spectroscopy (LENS), University of Florence, Sesto Fiorentino, Italy; Department of Physics, University of Florence, Sesto Fiorentino, Italy

Austin Roorda
School of Optometry, University of California, Berkeley, California

Leonardo Sacconi
National Institute of Optics - National Research Council (INO-CNR), Florence, Italy; European Laboratory for Non-Linear Spectroscopy (LENS), University of Florence, Sesto Fiorentino, Italy

David D. Sampson
Optical+Biomedical Engineering Laboratory (OBEL), School of Electrical, Electronic and Computer Engineering, The University of Western Australia, Crawley, Western Australia, Australia

Eric J. Seibel
Department of Mechanical Engineering and Human Photonics Lab, University of Washington, Seattle, Washington

Liang Song
Institute of Biomedical and Health Engineering, Shenzhen Institutes of Advanced Technology, Chinese Academy of Sciences, Shenzhen, China

Hrebesh M. Subhash
Division of Biomedical Engineering, School of Medicine, Oregon Health and Science University, Portland, Oregon

Adrian Taruttis
Institute for Biological and Medical Imaging and Chair for Biological Imaging, Helmholtz Zentrum München and Technische Universität München Ingolstädter Landstr. 1, Neuherberg, Germany

Bruce J. Tromberg
Beckman Laser Institute and Medical Clinic, University of California, Irvine, California

Valery V. Tuchin
Saratov State University, Russian Federation; Institute of Precise Mechanics and Control of RAS, Saratov, Russian Federation; University of Oulu, Finland

Alex Vitkin
Division of Biophysics and Bioimaging, Ontario Cancer Institute; Department of Medical Biophysics and Radiation Oncology, University of Toronto, Toronto, Ontario, Canada

Lihong V. Wang
Optical Imaging Laboratory, Department of Biomedical Engineering, Washington University in St. Louis, St. Louis, Missouri

Ruikang K. Wang
Biophotonics and Imaging Laboratory, Department of Bioengineering, University of Washington, Seattle, Washington

Xin-Cheng Yao
Department of Biomedical Engineering, Vision Sciences Research Center, University of Alabama at Birmingham, Birmingham, Alabama

Hao F. Zhang
Department of Biomedical Engineering, Northwestern University, Evanston, Illinois

Yuhua Zhang
Department of Ophthalmology, University of Alabama at Birmingham, Birmingham, Alabama

Dan Zhu
Britton Chance Center for Biomedical Photonics, Wuhan National Laboratory for Optoelectronics, Huazhong University of Science and Technology, Wuhan, China; Key Laboratory of Biomedical Photonics of Ministry of Education, Huazhong University of Science and Technology, Wuhan, China

1

Monte Carlo Modeling of Photon Migration for the Needs of Biomedical Optics and Biophotonics

Igor Meglinski and Alexander Doronin

The Jack Dodd Centre for Quantum Technology, Department of Physics, University of Otago, New Zealand

Key words: optical diagnostics, Monte Carlo simulation, biotissue imaging

1.1 Introduction

Nowadays optical diagnostics (OD) and photonics-based imaging techniques strongly influence a number of fields including biomedicine, environmental, automotive, combustion, material and life science, etc. [1–3]. OD as well as x-ray, computer tomography, ultrasound imaging, and magnetic resonance are the examples of technologies that have emerged from physics and engineering and have had a significant impact on medical diagnostics and clinical practice [4, 5]. OD encompasses a range of modalities, all of which rely on detecting and analyzing the changes of laser/optical radiation due to interaction with the matter/biological tissues. OD systems and experimental photonics technologies have been significantly improved with the new developments in fiber optics, laser delivery/detection systems [6], Charge Coupled Device (CCD), and therefore become available for various medical and biological applications [2, 5, 7]. Thus, nowadays a number of new OD technologies successfully contribute to healthcare in many medical specialties: dermatology, ophthalmology, oncology, gynecology, gastroenterology, neonatology, etc. [2, 8].

Modern research trends are focused on making medical diagnostics cheaper, faster and consequently more productive by applying new optical techniques incorporated with fast computer algorithms to process and analyze the data in real time. Conceptual design, further optimization and/or modification of the particular experimental OD systems requires careful selection of multiple technical parameters, including intensity, laser beam profile, coherence, polarization, wavelength of incident laser/optical radiation; size, position, numerical aperture, sensitivity of the detector. An

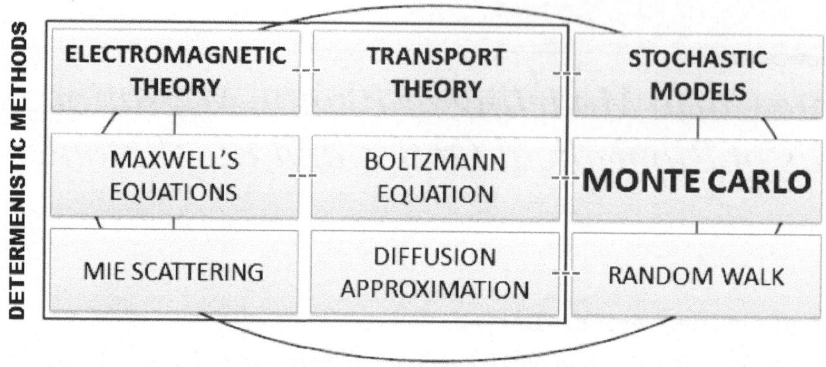

Figure 1.1: Schematic presentation of the major models used to describe optical radiation transfer in turbid media [9–22]. Dashed lines show the relations between different approaches.

estimation of how the spatial and temporal structural alterations in biological tissues can be distinguished by variations of these parameters is also required.

Various aspects of optical radiation propagation within highly scattering randomly inhomogeneous media have been extensively covered in numerous modeling and theoretical studies. These models are tightly related to the structure of the medium and can be separated into two basic categories: stochastic computational and deterministic models (Fig. 1.1).

In **Electromagnetic Theory** propagation of electromagnetic waves through a spatially varying medium, such as tissue, are described by Maxwell's equations [14, 23, 24]. Maxwell's equations are part of fundamental laws of physics and rigorously treat the radiation transfer or transfer of energy of electromagnetic waves.

The description of multiple scattering of optical radiation in the framework of electromagnetic theory employs continuous and discrete models of tissue (Fig. 1.2). In the continuous model, tissue is considered as a random medium whose permittivity $\varepsilon(\mathbf{r},t)$ fluctuates randomly as $\varepsilon_2(\mathbf{r},t)$ with the position about a mean value ε_1, i.e. $\varepsilon(\mathbf{r},t) = \varepsilon_1 + \varepsilon_2(\mathbf{r},t)$. Continuous model combined with electromagnetic theory based on Maxwell's equations could be very effective to study light propagation in biological tissue. However, due to the complex and highly disordered structure of tissues, the defining $\varepsilon(\mathbf{r},t)$ becomes extremely complicated. There have been a number of non-successful attempts to apply this model in the field of tissue optics, except a possibility of determination of refractive indices of various tissues [25]. Therefore, the relevance of electromagnetic theory within tissue optics lies mainly in the study of influence of morphological features of tissue components on distribution of scattered light.

Another modeling approach is based on presenting tissues as an ensemble of discrete scattering and absorbing particles (see Fig. 1.2 b). In this approach, each local center of scattering and absorption corresponds to a statistical average over physically small volume that is a statistical average over several acts of scattering and absorption in cell micro-structure. This theoretical model is well suited for description of light propagation in suspensions of scattering particles (e.g., microspheres). The spatial distribution of light is then obtained by adding the fields, by employing an idea of field perturbation, as a first approximation to the unperturbed single scattering theory [14]. This approach, however, does not lead to solvable equations for practical problems.

Mie computations are mainly realistically performed in order to compute the scattering properties of calibration suspensions of latex spheres [26] and tissue phantoms [26, 27], rather than defining the scattering properties of tissues. Mie theory has serious limitations when applied to describe multiple light scattering by a group of cells in tissue. Perhaps scattering of light in diluted blood samples is

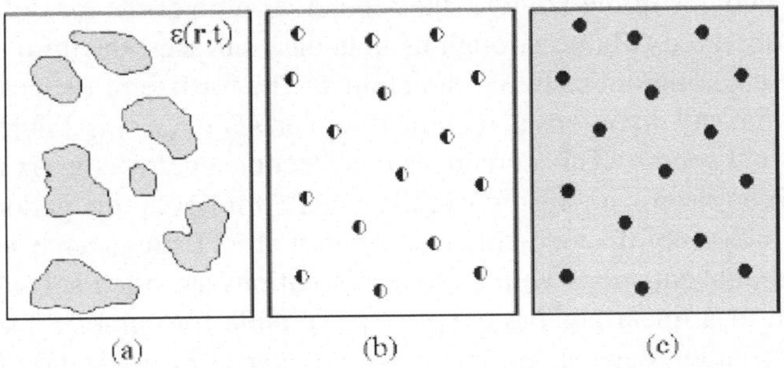

Figure 1.2: Schematic presentation of different tissue models of biological tissues: (a) with random spatial and/or temporal fluctuations of refractive index, (b) an ensemble of randomly distributed scattering and absorbing centers and (c) an ensemble of scattering centers in an absorbing continuum.

one of the few exceptions [2, 28]. Alternative techniques used for simulation of scattering of light on a single particle, e.g., red blood cell [2] are the T-matrix or the extended boundary method based on expansion into spherical harmonics with various boundary conditions, i.e. expressed in terms of integrals over the particle surface of electric and magnetic currents, the method of moments, WKB (Wentzel, Kramers, Brillouin) [14] and RGD approximations.

Radiative transfer is a model describing photon transport in a random scattering medium. The uses of transport theory span across a number of disciplines, including atmospheric and ocean radiative transfer, astrophysics, geophysics and others. The central equation, the radiative transfer equation (RTE) (1.1), mathematically expresses a macroscopic energy balance and describes the statistical average transport of photons and their energy through the turbid medium [14, 29].

$$\underbrace{\left[\frac{1}{v}\frac{\partial}{\partial t}\right.}_{1} + \underbrace{\mathbf{s}\cdot\nabla}_{2} + \underbrace{\left.(\mu_s+\mu_a)\right]}_{3} L(\mathbf{r},\mathbf{s},t) = \underbrace{\mu_s \oint_{4\pi} p\left(\mathbf{s},\mathbf{s}'\right) L\left(\mathbf{r},\mathbf{s}',t\right) d\Omega'}_{4} + \underbrace{Q\left(\mathbf{r},\mathbf{s},t\right)}_{5}, \tag{1.1}$$

where $L(\mathbf{r},\mathbf{s},t)$ is the radiance (the average power flux density at point $\mathbf{r}$ in the direction $\mathbf{s}$ within a unit solid angle at time t), μ_s and μ_a are the optical scattering and absorption coefficients, $p(\mathbf{s},\mathbf{s}')$ is the scattering phase function, $Q(\mathbf{r},\mathbf{s},t)$ is the radiant source function, and v is the speed of light propagation in the medium.

RTE is the equivalent to the equation of Boltzmann's kinetic theory of gases and to the equation of neutron transport theory [30]. The theory is heuristically derived by considering the energy balance of incoming, outgoing, absorbed, scattered, and emitted light of an infinitesimal volume element. It deals with the description of intensity propagation through a scattering medium. The medium is assumed to be homogeneous with constant characteristics of scattering and absorption and containing discrete, bounded regions of absorption and scattering inhomogeneities (see Fig. 1.2 b). Light propagation is envisioned as a stream of photons. A fundamental peculiarity of radiative transfer theory is that intensity of light is only considered, and the method simply ignores the wave phenomena. To enable the correlation between the radiometric, measurable quantities provided by the transport theory and the field characteristics given by electromagnetic theory, it has been proved that RTE can be regarded as an approximate reformulation of Maxwell's equations for a random medium under certain premises [14, 31].

The left-hand and the right-hand sides of (1.1) accounts for photon leaving and entering a small volume element of a medium. In order of appearance, the first term describes the time variation in a number of photons in the volume, the second term gives the loss of photons in the direction $\mathbf{s}$, escaping the observed volume through its boundary surfaces, the third term accounts for photon absorption and scattering out of initial direction $\mathbf{s}$. The forth term defines photons gained by scattering process from any directions $\mathbf{s}'$ into the direction $\mathbf{s}$. $Q(\mathbf{r}, \mathbf{s}, t)$ is a number of photons produced by an external light source. This concludes macroscopic energy conservation for a small medium volume. There is a growing interest in validity of RTE for light propagation in biological media and comprehensive reviews of the mathematical solution of RTE are given elsewhere [30, 32, 33].

Integro-differential equations with analytical solutions are often solved numerically by conversion to a system of a linear algebraic equations suitable for numerical solution [2, 14, 34]. The accuracy of the solution depends on the actual number of discretization terms considered. To do this, the radiance $L(\mathbf{r}, \mathbf{s})$ (time-dependence is omitted here for brevity) is represented only by its value at discrete values of independent variables. The integration and differentiation operators are replaced by their discrete counterparts, differences and summation. For example, to approximate the angular distribution of the specific intensity, the direction variable is discretized at N values in the RTE. The set of directions is determined by the selected quadrature method. Historically this was not rigorously derived from the transport equation, but was derived using heuristic arguments. Two-flux, or so-called Kubelka-Munk theory [35, 36], and four-flux theories have been used extensively for this purpose. The two-flux theory relates the propagation of opposing light fluxes to scattering and absorption coefficients of a medium. The two-flux model is inadequate for describing a collimated beam incident to a tissue surface. In this case, the four-flux model is utilized, where the fluxes separate into collimated flux (forward and backward) and a diffuse flux (forward and backward). A further refinement of the four-flux theory can be obtained by considering fluxes in more directions. To take into account the effect of finite collimated beam, two more radial fluxes are added, one directed inwards and the other outwards from the main axes of the collimated beam. An example of using the discrete ordinate method for imaging reconstruction in optical diffuse tomography is given in [37].

Alternatively, the discretization can be performed in terms of N small solid angles (cones) qualified by cosine of angles between the initial direction of photon packets and direction of scattering, $\mu_i = \cos(\mathbf{s} \cdot \mathbf{s}')$. The phase function is then substituted by a redistribution matrix with elements, $h(\mu_i, \mu_j)$, corresponding to the fraction of incident light in a cone μ_i, which is scattered into a cone μ_j.

The adding-doubling method is based on this discretization for a slab of tissue, thin along the z-axis and of infinite extent in the xy-plane [38]. The thickness of the slab should be also small so that the integration of the radiance along z-axis can be approximated by its average at the top and bottom of the layer. This is imperative to be able to solve the discrete, azimuthally averaged transport equation:

$$\mu_i \frac{\partial L(z, \mu_i)}{\partial z} + (\mu_s + \mu_a) L(z, \mu_i) = \\ = \mu_s \sum_{j=1}^{N} \varpi_j \left[h(\mu_i, \mu_j) L(z, \mu_j) + h(\mu_i, -\mu_j) L(z, -\mu_j) \right]. \quad (1.2)$$

Here, the weighting factors ϖ_j are determined by a selected integration procedure. The equation (1.2) can be solved via integration over the thickness, $z_1 - z_0 = \Delta z$, of a thin slab:

$$\mu_i \left[L(z_1, \mu_i) - L(z_0, \mu_i) \right] + (\mu_s + \mu_a) \Delta z L_{1/2}(\mu_i) = \\ = \mu_s \Delta z \sum_{j=1}^{N} \varpi_j \left[h(\mu_i, \mu_j) L_{1/2}(\mu_j) + h(\mu_i, -\mu_j) L_{1/2}(-\mu_j) \right], \quad (1.3)$$

where $L_{1/2}(\mu_i) = 1/2 \left(L(z_0, \mu_i) + L(z_1, \mu_i) \right)$ is the average of radiance at the top and the bottom of the slab. The results are expression dependent on the radiance at the top z_0 and bottom z_1, of the slab, which consequently are the only parameters to be determined. The adding-doubling method is thus mainly used to compute the reflectance and transmittance rather than the fluence inside. The results for a slab, which is twice as thick as the initial slab, are obtained by adding the contributions from each individual slab. This is repeated until the actual physical thickness is reached. The method provides a fast way to go from thin to very thick samples. It applies to problems with inhomogeneous layers and anisotropic scattering.

A formal method to solve a differential equation is to find the solution to its homogeneous part and expand the general solution in terms of the homogeneous solution obtained [30]. This eigenvector - eigenvalue problem has for the transport equation been treated, but has never really been applied to tissue optics. A simpler approach than using the rather complex eigenfunctions, would be to expand the radiance using a well-known appropriate function series. Considering the angular distribution of diffusely scattered light, a realistic choice of orthogonal expansion functions for the diffuse radiance are spherical harmonics. For example, the HG phase function only depends on angle θ or rather $\cos\theta$. An expansion of the phase function into spherical-harmonic function reduces to an expansion into Legendre polynomials:

$$p_{\mathrm{HG}}(\cos\theta) = \frac{1}{4\pi}\frac{1-g^2}{(1+g^2-2g\cos\theta)^{3/2}} = \sum_{n=0}^{N}\frac{2n+1}{4\pi}g^n P_n(\cos\theta), \tag{1.4}$$

where g is the anisotropy and the first Legendre polynomials defined as [39]:

$$\begin{aligned} P_0(x) &= 1, & P_1(x) &= x, \\ P_2(x) &= \frac{1}{2}\left(3x^2-1\right), & P_3(x) &= \frac{1}{2}\left(5x^3-3x\right). \end{aligned} \tag{1.5}$$

A general expression for the phase function can be formulated as an expansion series in Legendre polynomials $P_n(\mathbf{s},\mathbf{s}')$:

$$p(\mathbf{s},\mathbf{s}') = \sum_{n=0}^{\infty}\frac{2n+1}{4\pi}b_n P_n(\mathbf{s},\mathbf{s}'), \tag{1.6}$$

where b_n are the expansion coefficients given by

$$b_n = \oint_{4\pi} p(\mathbf{s},\mathbf{s}')\, P_n(\mathbf{s},\mathbf{s}')\, d\Omega'. \tag{1.7}$$

Legendre polynomials $P_n(\cos\theta)$ have proven to be well-suited to axial-symmetric tissue geometry [30, 40]. This implies that the radiance must first be separated into one primary, collimated part, L_c, and one scattered (diffuse) part, L_d:

$$L(\mathbf{r},\mathbf{s}) = L_c(\mathbf{r},\mathbf{s}) + L_d(\mathbf{r},\mathbf{s}). \tag{1.8}$$

Note, that collimated radiance L_c is the collimated light that has not been scattered by the medium. Thus, the collimated part fulfills Beer-Lambert's law:

$$\frac{\partial L_c(\mathbf{r},\mathbf{s})}{\partial s} = -\mu_t L_c(\mathbf{r},\mathbf{s}). \tag{1.9}$$

The diffuse radiance L_d is the part of light that has been scattered at least once. Its angular distribution can be approximated by a truncated series of spherical-harmonic function (Legendre polynomials). For L_d an equation of transfer is only different from the general transfer equation (1.1) in its source term [40]. As collimated light is not scattered, its equation of transfer is equal to:

$$\left[\mathbf{s}\cdot\nabla + (\mu_s+\mu_a)\right] L_c(\mathbf{r},\mathbf{s}) = Q_c(\mathbf{r},\mathbf{s}), \tag{1.10}$$

where $Q_c(\mathbf{r},\mathbf{s})$ is the collimated part of a light source $Q(\mathbf{r},\mathbf{s})$. Typically, in major OD applications, the light source is located at the surface of the medium (tissue). Thus, it is convenient to introduce the boundary conditions: $Q_c(\mathbf{r},\mathbf{s}) = 0$.

The general RTE for the diffuse radiance L_d is found by substitution of (1.8) into equation of transfer (1.1), and subtraction of (1.10) from the result:

$$[\mathbf{s}\cdot\nabla + (\mu_s+\mu_a)]L_d(\mathbf{r},\mathbf{s},t) = \mu_s \oint_{4\pi} p(\mathbf{s},\mathbf{s}')L_d(\mathbf{r},\mathbf{s}')\,d\Omega' + $$

$$+ Q_d(\mathbf{r},\mathbf{s}) + \mu_s \oint_{4\pi} p(\mathbf{s},\mathbf{s}')L_c(\mathbf{r},\mathbf{s}')\,d\Omega', \quad (1.11)$$

$L_c(\mathbf{r},\mathbf{s}')$ is defined by (1.9), that makes the equation an analogue of the RTE for the total radiance L (1.1) with an extra source term.

The angular distribution of the diffuse radiance L_d can be approximated by a truncated series of Legendre polynomials. Expanding $L_d(\mathbf{r},\mathbf{s})$ into Legendre series with the expansion coefficients $L_n(\mathbf{r})$ similar as it has been done to the phase function (1.6) and (1.7) and substituting it into the (1.1) leads to

$$\sum_{i=0}^{\infty}[\mathbf{s}\cdot\nabla + (\mu_s+\mu_a)](2i+1)L_i(\mathbf{r})P_i(\mathbf{s}) = \frac{\mu_s}{4\pi}\sum_{j=0}^{\infty}\sum_{k=0}^{\infty}(2j+1)L_j(\mathbf{r})(2k+1)b_k \times$$

$$\times \oint_{4\pi} \underline{P_j(\mathbf{s}')P_k(\mathbf{s}')d\Omega'} + Q_d(\mathbf{r},\mathbf{s}) + \mu_s \oint_{4\pi} p(\mathbf{s},\mathbf{s}')L_c(\mathbf{r},\mathbf{s}')\,d\Omega'. \quad (1.12)$$

The Legendre polynomials are orthogonal over $(-1,1)$ with weighting function 1 and satisfy

$$\int_{-1}^{1} P_i(x)P_j(x)dx = \frac{2}{2i+1}\delta_{ij}. \quad (1.13)$$

Thus, in (1.12) the integral over $d\Omega'$ vanishes, when $j \neq k$:

$$\sum_{i=0}^{\infty}[\mathbf{s}\cdot\nabla + (\mu_s+\mu_a-\mu_s b_i)](2i+1)L_i(\mathbf{r})P_i(\mathbf{s}) = Q_d(\mathbf{r},\mathbf{s}) +$$

$$+ \mu_s \oint_{4\pi} p(\mathbf{s},\mathbf{s}')L_c(\mathbf{r},\mathbf{s}')\,d\Omega', \quad (1.14)$$

and a set of differential equations is finally obtained by multiplying (1.14) by $P_n(\mathbf{s})$. This is followed by another integration over $d\Omega'$. Subsequently, the addition theorem for Legendre polynomials is employed. In the P_N approximation, only N first terms of Legendre polynomial series are taken into account that gives a system of $N+1$ coupled first-order differential equations [14, 29, 30, 34, 40]. The systems can be reduced to a system of coupled second-order differential equations. Finally, the solution for unknowns $L_n(\mathbf{r})$ can be found with the use of a finite-difference or finite-element code.

Diffusion approximation (also known as the P_1 approximation of RTE solution) is an analytical closed-form solution which is suitable for a number of particular problems in various OD applications. With additional assumption of negligible anisotropy in the source, the result is the pair of coupled (time-dependent) equations [12, 14, 18, 34, 41]:

$$\begin{cases} \frac{1}{v}\frac{\partial\phi(\mathbf{r},t)}{\partial t} + \nabla\cdot\mathbf{J}(\mathbf{r},t) + \mu_a\phi(\mathbf{r},t) = S(\mathbf{r},t), \\ \frac{1}{v}\frac{\partial\mathbf{J}(\mathbf{r},t)}{\partial t} + \frac{1}{3}\nabla\phi(\mathbf{r},t) + \mu_{tr}\mathbf{J}(\mathbf{r},t) = 0, \end{cases} \quad (1.15)$$

where $\phi(\mathbf{r},t)$ and $\mathbf{J}(\mathbf{r},t)$ are the fluence rate and flux at $(\mathbf{r},t)$, and $S(\mathbf{r},t)$ is the photon source:

$$\phi(\mathbf{r},t) = \oint\limits_{4\pi} L(\mathbf{r},\mathbf{s}',t)d\Omega', \quad \mathbf{J}(\mathbf{r},t) = \oint\limits_{4\pi} \mathbf{s}'L(\mathbf{r},\mathbf{s}',t)d\Omega',$$

$$S(\mathbf{r},t) = \oint\limits_{4\pi} Q(\mathbf{r},\mathbf{s}',t)d\Omega'. \tag{1.16}$$

The transport coefficient is defined as $\mu_{tr} = \mu_s' + \mu_a$, where $\mu_s' = \mu_s(1-g)$ refers to the reduced scattering coefficient. The diffusion equation is obtained by eliminating $\mathbf{J}$ between two equations (1.15):

$$\left(\frac{1}{v}\frac{\partial}{\partial t} - D\nabla^2 + \mu_a\right)\phi(\mathbf{r},t) = S(\mathbf{r},t), \tag{1.17}$$

where D is the diffusion coefficient, defined as $D = 1/3\mu_{tr}$.

The radiance in diffusion approximation is expressed as

$$L(\mathbf{r},\mathbf{s},t) = \frac{1}{4\pi}\phi(\mathbf{r},t) + \frac{3}{4\pi}\mathbf{J}(\mathbf{r},t)\cdot\mathbf{s}, \tag{1.18}$$

whereas in most practical diagnostics problems the measurable quantity $R(\rho,t)$ is the number of photons that reach the unit area of a surface in a unit time at given source-detector separation ρ and at given time t. $R(\rho,t)$ defines the diffuse reflectance and is calculated as a current of detected photons across the medium boundary [34, 41]:

$$R_f(\rho,t) = -D\nabla\phi(\rho,z,t)\cdot(-\mathbf{z})|_{z=0}. \tag{1.19}$$

The diffusion equation is a second-order differential equation and its solution is commonly considered for the partial-current boundary conditions, the zero-boundary conditions, and the extrapolated boundary conditions [42, 43, 44]. It has been demonstrated that the solution is more accurate when applied to the reflectance as the integral of the radiance over the backward hemisphere [42, 43]:

$$R(\rho,t) = \iint\limits_{2\pi}\left(\phi(\rho,z,t) + 3D\frac{\partial\phi(\rho,z,t)}{\partial z}\right)\bigg|_{z=0}(1-R_{Fres}(\theta))\frac{d\Omega}{4\pi}, \tag{1.20}$$

where $R_{Fres}(\theta)$ is the Fresnel reflection coefficient for incident light at angle θ relative to the normal to the medium boundary. For the extrapolated boundary condition and having employed the method of image sources to solve the diffusion equation for fluence rate ϕ within the medium lead to [45]:

$$\phi(\rho,z,t) = \frac{v}{(4\pi Dvt)^{3/2}}\exp(-\mu_a vt)\left\{\exp\left[-\frac{(z-z_0)^2+\rho^2}{4Dvt}\right] - \right.$$
$$\left. - \exp\left[-\frac{(z+z_0+2z_b)^2+\rho^2}{4Dvt}\right]\right\}. \tag{1.21}$$

The first term is due to a point source at $z_0 = (\mu_{tr})^{-1}$ that results from the perpendicularly incident collimated light, and the second one is due to a negative image source at $-z_0 - 2z_b$. The fluence rate is set to zero at the extrapolated boundary located at z_b

$$z_b = \frac{1+R_{eff}}{1-R_{eff}}2D. \tag{1.22}$$

Here, R_{eff} represents the fraction of photons that have been internally diffusely reflected at the medium boundary.

According to [42]:

$$R_{eff} \equiv \frac{R_\phi + R_j}{2 - R_\phi + R_j}.$$

$$R_\phi \equiv \int_0^{\pi/2} 2\sin\theta\cos\theta R_{Fres}(\theta)d\theta, \quad R_j \equiv \int_0^{\pi/2} 3\sin\theta\cos^2\theta R_{Fres}(\theta)d\theta. \tag{1.23}$$

It is possible to regroup (1.20) and express it in terms of conventional expression for ϕ (1.21) and $R_f(\rho,t)$ (1.19) [42, 43]:

$$R(\rho,t) = \underbrace{\frac{1}{2}\left(\frac{1}{2} - \frac{R_\phi}{2}\right)}_{C_\phi} \phi(\rho,t) + \underbrace{\frac{1}{2}(1 - R_j)}_{C_j} R_f(\rho,t). \tag{1.24}$$

The derivation of the diffusion equation as it has been shown above is not unique. Some other approaches, all assuming isotropic scattering, such as a random walk, elementary kinetic theory (e.g. [46]) are known. These approaches do not necessarily provide the same expression for the diffusion coefficient D. There is a number of studies discussing an exact expression for D [41, 46, 47] as well as a number of models have been proposed, trading off accuracy for computational ease [2]. The main limitation of the diffusion approximation is that the distance between sources and detectors should be much greater than the mean transport length so that enough scattering events occur to generate a diffuse field [48, 49]. Additionally, the source and detector sizes must be small enough as compared to the distance of their separation. The diffusion approximation is also not valid for photons with short arrival time ("snake" or low-order scattering photons) to the detector [50].

Stochastic models are an alternative to deterministic models and have been developed to model light transport in biological tissues [34, 51]. Stochastic methods proceed in a very different way from deterministic methods. These methods involve modeling of individual photon interactions either implicitly, i.e. by deriving the probability density functions for photons transitions. The problem of light transport through a scattering medium like a biological tissue is considered to be probabilistic in nature for two reasons. Firstly, at the level of individual photons, light scattering is a probabilistic phenomenon governed by the laws of quantum mechanics. Secondly, considering light intensities averaged over a larger number of photons, the nature of the scattering medium itself is random due to the large variety in distribution, shape and orientation of the scattering centers.

Random walk theory (RWT) describes the statistical behavior of light propagation in scattering medium, constrained along the elements of a discrete lattice. RWT is based on two assumptions: the tissues continuum is replaced by a cubic lattice with a step size inversely proportional to the scattering coefficient, and that photons move isotropically between adjacent lattice points which significantly restricts the number of possible photon directions [52, 53]. The derived functions are the joint probabilities that a photon emerges at distance ρ on surface after n lattice steps, where ρ measures the axial distance from the point of insertion to the point of re-emission. For a finite slab, one can derive the joint probabilities in reflection and transmission after taking into account appropriate boundary and initial conditions. Time-dependent expressions have been derived for a homogeneous scattering medium and are in a good agreement with the results of diffusion theory. Anisotropy for the case of continuous-wave and time-resolved measurements for both reflectance and transmission modes was introduced in [54]. The advantage of RWT is the ability to produce relatively simple mathematical expressions for various quantities of interest such as diffuse reflectance and transmittance. The disadvantage includes a constant lattice step, that makes difficult an application of the model of a layered medium. All resulting restrictions, similar to those for the diffusion approximation, are also valid for RWT.

Photon path-integral formalism The RTE describing light propagation can be interpreted as a collection of photon paths taken by radiation as it travels in the medium, $\mathbf{r}(t)$. Thus, a path integral (PI) $P[\mathbf{r}(t)]$ is an integral over all such possible paths traveled by photons. Optical fields are described using the concept of an ensemble of effective optical paths of partial contributions [55, 56, 57]. PI methods analytically find the most important paths and develop quantitative estimates based on them. The multiple scattering contributions are only computed along the most probable paths and the rest of the paths are dealt with implicitly via analytic integration of multiple scattering. This technique has been experimentally verified [58]. The great virtue of the PI approach is the huge computational saving it affords by making systematic, rather than random, searches through photon histories. Hence, the PI formalism offers analytic solutions to the RTE without using the diffusion approximation, and it is well suited to describing the propagation of both early-arriving and fully-diffused photons. The number of studies on this subject is still quite limited [59, 60] and practical implementations are confined to a few publications [55, 58].

1.2 Monte Carlo Method

The Monte Carlo (MC) method is a prominent example of stochastic methods that stand alone when analytic approaches have difficulties in giving a satisfactory solution. In this probabilistic technique, the trajectories of individual multiple scattered photons are traced through the media, each interaction being governed by random processes of scattering and absorption. Due to the lack of intrinsic constraints, facing the problem of combining computation complexity of light propagation model and ability to cope with the optical parameters of biological tissues, which are anticipated to vary spatially and temporally as well as individually, MC technique is chosen as a primary tool for modeling of optical radiation propagation in biological tissues by many researchers [2, 38, 61–69].

The basic assumption of MC is that the process of photon migration is considered as a sequence of random non-correlated events or Markov process [61, 71, 72]. In case of light propagation this means that the probability that a photon will change from its present state to another state is independent of its previous states, i.e. it has no awareness of its previous history. For scattering, for this to be true, the scattering particles will have to be distributed non-periodically (a regular lattice would produce a diffraction pattern), and the light should be non-coherent so that interference effects are typically ignored.

In case of radiative transfer in biological tissue, the MC method is a method to estimate the exact solution of RTE. This is done by sampling the set of all possible paths of photon packets (or photons) through the tissue. In a simple case the random paths of a large number of photon packets are simulated. The expected value of a random or stochastic variable can be seen as the integral over all possible values of that variable multiplied by their probabilities. Estimation of an expected value using the MC method is thus a form of a numerical quadrature. Indeed, the RTE (stationary form in a homogeneous medium) can be written as an integral equation [30]:

$$L(\mathbf{r},\mathbf{s}) = \int_{\mathrm{R}=0}^{\infty} \exp(-\mu_{tr}\mathrm{R})\,\mu_s \int_{4\pi} p\left(\mathbf{s},\mathbf{s}'\right) L(\mathbf{r}-\mathrm{R}\mathbf{s},\mathbf{s}')d\Omega' d\mathrm{R} + \int_{\mathrm{R}=0}^{\infty} \exp(-\mu_{tr}\mathrm{R})\,Q(\mathbf{r}-\mathrm{R}\mathbf{s},\mathbf{s})d\mathrm{R}. \quad (1.25)$$

Here, the radiance L at position $\mathbf{r}$ in direction $\mathbf{s}$ originates from the light source and from the radiance scattered elsewhere into direction $\mathbf{s}$; R is a path length. The second term defines light in direction $\mathbf{s}$ that originates from source Q at positions $\mathbf{r}-\mathrm{R}\mathbf{s}$, that survives the transfer from positions $\mathbf{r}-\mathrm{R}\mathbf{s}$ to position $\mathbf{r}$, by factor $\exp(-\mu_{tr}\mathrm{R})$. The first integral term represents light that has been

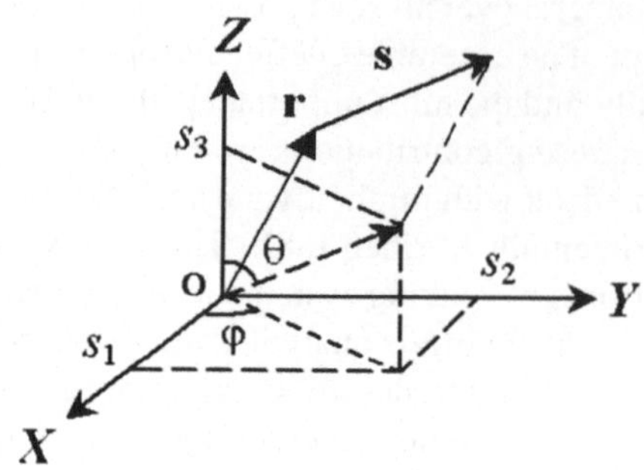

Figure 1.3: The Cartesian coordinate system (XYZ) is employed to specify the position **r** of a photon in the modeling medium: angles θ and φ are the polar and azimuth angles which define s, the direction of photon packet propagation. s_1, s_2, s_3 are the direction cosines.

scattered at positions $\mathbf{r}-R\mathbf{s}$, from direction $\mathbf{s}'$ into direction **s**, that also reached position **r**.

1.2.1 Implementation of Monte Carlo simulation

Photon packets propagate through scattering matter. The points where interactions with the matter occur are described by *probability density function* (pdf). If x is a variable that characterizes the interaction (e.g. scattering angle or distance), its pdf $p(x)$ is defined as:

$$\int_{-\infty}^{\infty} p(x)dx \equiv 1 \qquad\qquad F(x) = P(x \leq a) \equiv \int_{-\infty}^{a} p(x)dx, \tag{1.26}$$

where $F(x)$, $0 \leq F(x) \leq 1$ is the cumulative probability function (cpdf). $F(x)$ is equal to a probability $P(x \leq a)$ that a random variable x is less than a. By taking the inverse, F^{-1} the random samples can then be obtained from this function by the use of random numbers ξ uniformly distributed between 0 and 1 according to [71]:

$$\xi = \int_{-\infty}^{x} p(x)dx \qquad \rightarrow \qquad x = F^{-1}(\xi). \tag{1.27}$$

There are also other techniques such as rejection sampling or table-lookup method that can be used for the same purpose [71].

The photon's phase space $\{\mathbf{r},\mathbf{s}\}$ is the collection of dynamic variables that describe the photon's absolute location in the medium referred to the coordinate system, **r**, and its direction, **s**, referred back to fixed set of axes in the same coordinate system (Fig. 1.3). The coordinate system is usually the one where the fixed components of the experiment resides. **r** represents the 3-component vector $\mathbf{r} = (x,y,z)$, and **s** represents the 3-component vector $\mathbf{s} = (s_1,s_2,s_3)$. The direction of incident photons is specified by the initial polar angle θ and azimuthal angle φ and the components of the vector **s** are often referred to the direction cosines, $\{s_1,s_2,s_3\} = \{\sin\theta\cos\varphi, \sin\theta\sin\varphi, \cos\theta\}$.

A photon packet phase space can be supplemented with other variables, such as intensity, polarization, etc. In simple MC simulation statistic weight of a photon packet is introduced into the phase space to characterize the photon packet contribution to the variable of interest, e.g. reflectance or transmittance.

In its phase space the photon packet is represented by the pdf, which is dependent on space coordinates, direction cosines, and the statistical weight. The simulation is based on the modeling

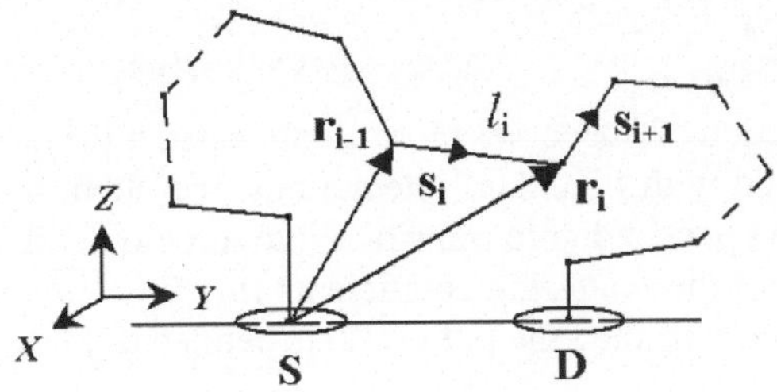

Figure 1.4: Schematic presentation of a photon packet propagation in a scattering medium. l_i is the photon packet path length between $i-1$-th and i-th scattering centers located at $\mathbf{r}_{i-1}$ and $\mathbf{r}_i$. Unit vectors $\mathbf{s}_i$ and $\mathbf{s}_{i+1}$ define the direction of photon packet propagation prior to and straight after the scattering event.

of a large number of possible trajectories of the photon packets from the site of the photons' injection into the medium (source) to the site, where the photons leave the medium (detector) (Fig. 1.4).

The pdf can be factorized as a product of three independent pdfs, i.e. the pdf of position, the pdf of scattering, the pdf of importance, reflecting the physical fact that the spatial, directional and importance distributions are *mutually independent* from each other. Hence, an individual trajectory of a photon packet is modeled as a sequence of the following elementary simulations: i) generation of photon path lengths, ii) simulation of scattering event, iii) reflections/refractions on the medium boundaries, iv) absorption events, v) fluorescence events, vi) an act of Raman scattering, etc. for particular OD applications. The initial and final states of the photons are entirely determined by the source and the detector geometries and numerical apertures.

1.2.2 Transfer of a photon packet in the medium

Assume the trajectory of a photon packet consists of i points with coordinates given by $\mathbf{r}_k$, $k=\overline{1..i}$. Given that a photon packet has a direction $\mathbf{s}_i$ and a distance l_i to travel, the new position $\mathbf{r}_i$ is given by:

$$\mathbf{r}_i = \mathbf{r}_{i-1} + \mathbf{s}_i l_i. \tag{1.28}$$

The distance l_i (or l for brevity) is referred to a free path length, and is determined according to the corresponding pdf.

$$l = -\frac{\ln \xi}{\mu_s}, \tag{1.29}$$

where ξ is a uniformly distributed random number between 0 and 1.

Path length distribution $p(l)$ can take on any positive values [72]:

$$p(l) = \mu_t \exp(-\mu_t l) = \mu_s \exp(-\mu_s l)\exp(-\mu_a l) + \mu_a \exp(-\mu_a l)\exp(-\mu_s l), \tag{1.30}$$

where $\mu_t = \mu_s + \mu_a$ is the extinction coefficient. The first term in (1.30) describes photon scattering, along with its reduction due to the absorption in a medium, $\exp(-\mu_a l)$. The second term determines photon absorption in the medium. For the major OD applications, the main interest lies in the detection of photon packets by a particular detector, rather than calculating the fraction of the incident photons that have been absorbed in a medium. Factorizing the first term into the product of the pdf of scattering, $p_s(l)$ and attenuation factor, $\exp(-\mu_a l)$, it is seen that the acts of scattering and absorption can be modeled independently, i.e.:

$$p(l) = p_s(l)\exp(-\mu_a l) \tag{1.31}$$

and

$$p_s(l) = \mu_s \exp(-\mu_s l). \tag{1.32}$$

The procedure of selection of l becomes more complicated if the medium is heterogeneous. Leaving the problems associated with boundary interactions, the attention is drawn to variation of a free path length of a photon packet due to transition into a region with different scattering coefficients. Consider n regions with the scattering coefficients μ_{sk}, $k = \overline{1..n}$. If the photon packet crosses the distances l_k, in these regions, then the pdf (1.32) is defined as [71]:

$$p_s(l) = \mu_{sj} \exp\left[-\left(\sum_{k=1}^{j-1} \mu_{sk} l_k\right) - \mu_{sj}\left(l - \sum_{k=1}^{j-1} l_k\right)\right],$$
$$\text{provided that} \quad \sum_{k=1}^{j-1} l_k \leq l \leq \sum_{k=1}^{j} l_k. \tag{1.33}$$

Note that l_j is a maximum possible distance that a packet can cross in the j-th region. Thus, the path length selection can be carried out by determining j from the inequalities:

$$\sum_{k=1}^{j-1} \mu_{sk} l_k \leq -\ln \xi \leq \sum_{k=1}^{j} \mu_{sk} l_k \tag{1.34}$$

and then calculating

$$l = \sum_{k=1}^{j-1} l_k + \frac{1}{\mu_{sj}}\left(-\ln \xi - \sum_{k=1}^{j-1} \mu_{sk} l_k\right). \tag{1.35}$$

The implementation of (1.35) is not straightforward as the distances l_k are not known. Instead of this, a step-by-step procedure is applied [69]. If a boundary demarcating a region of space with different scattering coefficients the path length that the packet has traveled in the region $k-1$ is subtracted from the total path length l, i.e. $l^* = l - l_{k-1}$. Based on (1.35), the remaining step l^* to be traveled in region k has to be converted in accordance with the new scattering coefficient:

$$l^{**} = l^* \frac{\mu_{s(k-1)}}{\mu_{sk}}. \tag{1.36}$$

This procedure repeats until the path length l^{**} is not long enough to intersect the interface of the adjacent layer. If a void region, i.e. $\mu_{sk} = 0$, is encountered in the course of propagation, the photon packet is moved directly to the next adjacent boundary following its direction.

The photon packet path length l to next interaction can be sampled by considering the medium as uniform in terms of the local scattering coefficient. If the medium consists of inhomogeneities with different scattering coefficients the photon packet is stopped at that boundary and its path length l is truncated at that boundary. The next free path is taken from that boundary point with the scattering coefficient being that of the region beyond the boundary. Other possible techniques can be found in [71].

1.2.3 Scattering

Variations of refractive index are responsible for light scattering in tissues. The refraction variations are determined by the biochemical makeup of the tissue and will influence the amplitude of the scattered light. In terms of tissue morphology, the relative size of organelles and cells with respect to the wavelength of incident light affects the angular distribution of the scattered light. Increasing difference in the index of refraction between the cell components and surrounding result in an increasing scattering of the medium [2]. Mammalian cells range from 10 to 30 μm in diameter, and

TABLE 1.1: The average cellular constituents and their scattering properties, collected from [2] and references within.

Structure	Diameter, μm	n	Shape	Scattering properties
Red Blood Cell	8.5	1.40	disk	Mie
Mitochondria	1	1.38-1.41	cylindrical	Mie
Nucleus	7	1.39-1.47	spherical	Mie
Lysosomes	0.25-0.8		spherical	Mie
Endoplasmic reticulum	few		folded sheets	Mie + Rayleigh
Microtubules & filaments		1.5		Rayleigh
Golgi apparatus		1.5		Rayleigh
Cytosol		1.354		

their internal organelles appear in a broad assortment of shapes and sizes. Table 1.1 lists the most common cellular organelles inside mammalian cells.

Although the cytoplasmic components such as Golgi apparatus, lysosomes, endoplasmic reticulum, mitochondria, etc., appear to be greatly different in their structure and organization [73, 74], a few generalizations can be made: a) most of cytoplasmic organelles and inclusions are smaller than 1 μm in size; b) they are not homogeneous bodies but rather complex structures. Typical nuclei size ranges from 5 to 10 μm and like other cell organelles, nuclei are not a uniform object and have a complex internal structure. The cell mainly contains an aqueous solution of electrolytes and proteins, the cytoplasm, with an effective refractive index of approximately 1.38, while the cell membrane and cell organelles are composed of phospholipid layers and proteins with refractive indices in the range of 1.43-1.51 [25]. However, since the fraction of these higher refractive index components is rather small, i.e. in the order of 5%, the effective cellular refractive index can be estimated to $\sim$ 1.40. When studying the spatial variations in the refractive index over a microscopic scale such as the inside of a cell using a phase microscope, it is found that the cell membrane and the nucleus are the components which are the dominant contributions to the cellular effective refractive index; these are far more important than, for example, the mitochondria. This does not mean, however, that the membrane and the nucleus are the main scatterers in tissue. Apart from the refractive index, parameters such as structure, size and concentration of the scattering object must also be taken into account. For instance, the cell membrane has a thickness of only 5-10 nm and thus has a relatively insignificant effect on the total light scattering from the cell, despite its high refractive index. Instead, a high correlation between the reduced scattering coefficient and the mitochondrial content has been found [75]. Tissues of high mitochondrial content exhibit high scattering coefficients. Light scattering from tissues with high concentrations of mitochondria such as liver tissue, can to large extent (but far from completely) be attributed to this organelle despite its low refractive index. The basic lipid bilayer membrane is about 9 nm in width. The refractive index mismatch between lipid and the surrounding aqueous medium causes strong scattering of light. Folding of lipid membranes presents larger size lipid structures which affect longer wavelengths of light. The density of lipid/water interfaces within the mitochondria make them especially strong scatterers of light. Lipid droplets inside the cells of adipose tissue have been shown to be a major contributor to the cellular scattering, due to their high refractive index and high volume fraction (88%) in the cell [75]. The strong scattering characteristics of lipid particles is further confirmed by the high correlation found between the lipid content of liver tissue and the reduced scattering coefficient [76], when the influence of the mitochondrial content has been compensated for.

Apart from cellular components, connective tissue fibers are found to be responsible for scattering [77, 78]. It was shown that scattering in neonatal skin is mostly dominated by Mie scattering from cylindrical collagen fibers [79]. The refractive index of collagen has been measured to be between 1.46 and 1.55 [80]. Rayleigh scattering was also presented emerging mostly from collagen fibrils, which are much smaller and do not bundle. S. Jacques [78] has attributed scattering of soft tissues in the near-infrared region to membraneous structures that were modelled as spherical Mie scatterers in 0.2–2 μm diameter range. Table 1.1 gives some insight into the nature of scattering from cellular constituents.

Detailed theoretical information on the light scattering from specific cells and their organelles can be obtained by utilizing the various methods based on electromagnetic theory [2, 81]. The general results for such computations show that small scatterers, compared to wavelength, yield essentially isotropic scattering, whereas particles of greater size exhibit more pronounced forward scattering. Mie computations utilizing a cylindrical-particle model can also be applied to investigate the influence of the size of an elongated scattering object such as collagen fibers on the light scattering [79]. Correspondingly, thin (compared to wavelength) fibers yield scattering with isotropic character, whereas enlargement, as observed for instance due to maturity of collagen fibers in neonatal skin, increases the anisotropy and the scattering cross section.

Although contribution to the total cellular scattering from the nucleus is relatively small, changes in its size and refractive index influences the angular distribution of the scattered light. RGD computation of a layered sphere model with a particle size in the order of a lymphocyte (a type of white blood cell) ($\sim$ 8-10 μm), reveals that an increased nucleus diameter, at constant total cell size, increases the forward scattering. This is supported by results of finite-difference time-domain computations [82], however, the decrease of refractive index of either nucleus or the surrounding cytoplasm causes a decrease in the forward scattering [82].

Experimental evidence supports the hypothesis that light scattering in biological tissues is anisotropic with significant forward scattering, $g \simeq 0.7$–0.97 [83]. Goniometer measurements of a number of animal model tissues indicate that g as a function of wavelength is approximately 0.9 with a tendency to increase with wavelength. Similar values of the anisotropy factor g in the range of 0.7–0.95 for skin tissue in the visible spectral range have been reported in [84]. Forward-peaked scattering functions for human stratum corneum and epidermis at ultraviolet and visible wavelengths has been demonstrated in [85]. Values of g between 0.71 at 300 nm and 0.78 at 540 nm, varying linearly with wavelength have been presented in [86]. With the full thickness epidermis, the distribution of the transmitted light also peak, although less strongly than with stratum corneum.

It has been shown in [86] that a least squares fit identifies the Henyey-Greenstein (HG) phase function as a good choice for describing scattering behavior in the stratum corneum. The HG scattering phase function, an empirical approximation for Mie scattering from particles with a distribution of sizes [87], is defined as

$$p_{HG}(\cos\theta) = \frac{1}{4\pi}\frac{1-g^2}{\left(1+g^2-2g\cos\theta\right)^{3/2}} \tag{1.37}$$

where θ is the scattering angle.

It should be pointed out that since the epidermis is very thin and because its micro-structure composed of keratin fibers is analogous to the collagen fibers of the dermis, dermal scattering can be used to approximate skin scattering. The refractive index ratio between stratum corneum and air is about 1.51 [88–90]. This gives rise to surface scattering, which follows the Fresnel's equations [24] and is affected by the presence of folds in stratum corneum. The influence of stratum corneum fold structure on the detected optical signal localization in biological tissues has been discussed in [91].

The photon packet is scattered at the scattering center and a new direction of the packet is determined relative to the origin of photon direction (Figure 1.5). The coordinate system (XYZ) contains

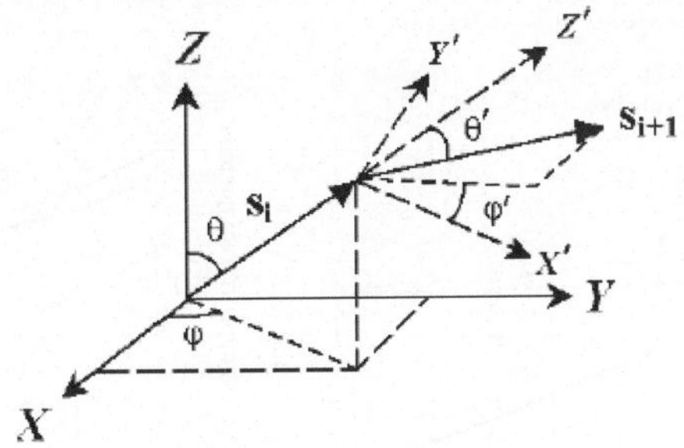

Figure 1.5: A new direction defined in local coordinate system $(X'Y'Z')$ by the deviations in the polar angle θ' and azimuthal angle φ' in terms of the coordinate system (XYZ). Unit vectors $\mathbf{s}_i$ and $\mathbf{s}_{i+1}$ define the direction of photon packet propagation prior to and straight after scattering.

the absolute initial direction $\mathbf{s}_i$. New direction $\mathbf{s}_{i+1}$ is originally defined in local coordinate system $(X'Y'Z')$ by the deviations in the polar angle θ' and azimuthal angle φ', relative to the previous direction. In the coordinate system $(X'Y'Z')$ a new direction $\mathbf{s}_{i+1}$ is given by the direction cosines $\{\sin\theta'\cos\varphi', \sin\theta'\sin\varphi', \cos\theta'\}$. In XYZ a new direction $\mathbf{s}_{i+1}$ and the corresponding direction cosines $\{s_{1i+1}, s_{2i+1}, s_{3i+1}\}$ are defined as [61, 70, 92–94]:

$$\begin{pmatrix} s_1 \\ s_2 \\ s_3 \end{pmatrix}_{i+1} = \begin{bmatrix} \dfrac{s_{1i}s_{3i}}{\sqrt{1-s_{3i}^2}} & -\dfrac{s_{2i}}{\sqrt{1-s_{3i}^2}} & s_{1i} \\ \dfrac{s_{2i}s_{3i}}{\sqrt{1-s_{3i}^2}} & \dfrac{s_{1i}}{\sqrt{1-s_{3i}^2}} & s_{2i} \\ -\sqrt{1-s_{3i}^2} & 0 & s_{3i} \end{bmatrix} \begin{pmatrix} \sin\theta'\cos\varphi' \\ \sin\theta'\sin\varphi' \\ \cos\theta' \end{pmatrix}, \tag{1.38}$$

where $\mathbf{s}_i = \{s_{1i}, s_{2i}, s_{3i}\}$ are the direction cosines before the i-th scattering. If $|s_{3i}|$ is too close to 1, the photon is assumed not to deflect, and

$$\begin{pmatrix} s_1 \\ s_2 \\ s_3 \end{pmatrix}_{i+1} = \begin{pmatrix} \sin\theta'\cos\varphi' \\ \sin\theta'\sin\varphi' \\ \dfrac{s_{3i}}{|s_{3i}|}\cos\theta' \end{pmatrix}. \tag{1.39}$$

The values of deviations are determined from the corresponding cpdfs: $\theta' = F_{\theta'}^{-1}(\xi)$ and $\varphi' = F_{\varphi'}^{-1}(\xi)$ (see 1.27). The HG scattering phase function p_{HG} is typically used. The phase function is effectively the pdf of scattering and fulfills all requirements for pdf (1.27). p_{HG} is factorized as follows:

$$p_{HG} = p_{\theta'}(\theta')p_{\varphi'}(\varphi'),$$
$$p_{\theta'}(\cos\theta') = \frac{1}{2}\frac{1-g^2}{(1+g^2-2g\cos\theta')^{3/2}}, \quad p_{\varphi'}(\varphi') = \frac{1}{2\pi}. \tag{1.40}$$

The cpdf of $p_{\theta'}(\cos\theta')$, $F_{\theta'}(\cos\theta')$, is given by

$$F_{\theta'}(\cos\theta') = \frac{1}{2g}\left(\frac{1-g^2}{\sqrt{1+g^2-2g\cos\theta'}} - (1-g)\right) \tag{1.41}$$

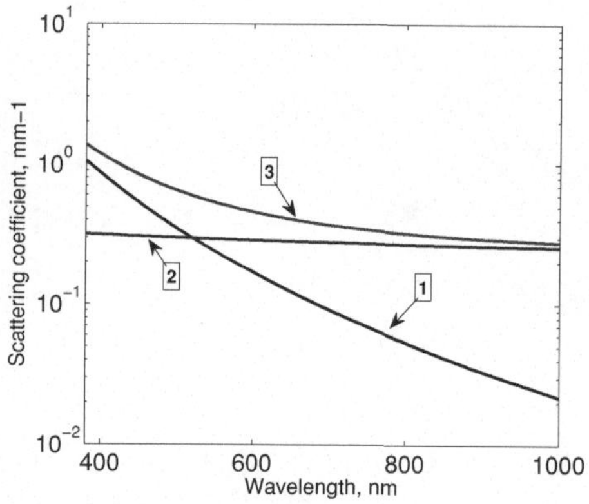

(a)

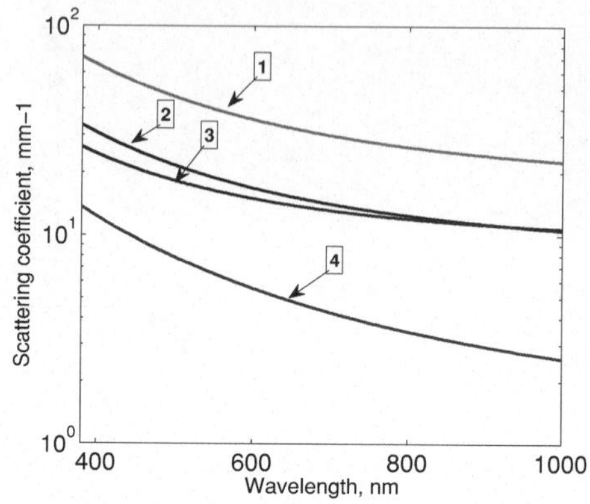

(b)

Figure 1.6: Reduced scattering coefficient of human skin (a) suggested in [79], where: 1 - Rayleigh scattering, 2 - Mie scattering by collagen fibers, 3 - the combined Rayleigh and Mie scattering; scattering properties of tissues used in the simulation (b), where: 1 - stratum corneum; 2 - living epidermis; 3 - papillary dermis; 4 - upper blood net dermis; 5 - reticular dermis; 6 - deep blood net dermis; 7 - subcutaneous fat.

Applying transformation (1.27), the choice for $\cos\theta'$ and φ' can be expressed as follows:

$$\cos\theta' = \begin{cases} \dfrac{1}{2g}\left(1+g^2-\left[\dfrac{1-g^2}{1-g+2g\xi}\right]^2\right), & \text{if } g>0 \\ 2\xi-1, & \text{if } g=0. \end{cases}$$
$$\varphi' = 2\pi\xi. \tag{1.42}$$

Note, any other scattering phase function can be used, instead of the HG function. If analytical inversion, see (1.27) and (1.41), is not possible, then the table lookup method is invoked [71, 95, 96]. According to this method, points within equally probable intervals of the variable to be selected are picked up randomly from a pre-calculated table of the inversed cpdf of the variable similar to (1.26). The cpdf for the scattering angle θ' or rather $\cos\theta'$ can be numerically constructed:

$$F(\cos\theta') = \int_{-1}^{\cos\theta'} p(\cos\theta)d\cos\theta, \quad F(1)=1. \tag{1.43}$$

The inverted cpdf, $icpdf = F^{-1}(\cos\theta')$, containing values of $\cos\theta'$, can be calculated and stored in the array $icpdf[k]$, $k = 1..\max(k)$. For all k the two values, $cpdf[k-1]\cdot\max(k)$ and $cpdf[k]\cdot\max(k)$ that most closely correspond to the index value k are looked up in the array $cpdf[k]$. Notice that $\max(cpdf[k]) = 1$ and $\min(cpdf[k]) = 0$ (1.26). Lagrange polynomial or any other and appropriate interpolation technique is performed to find the best approximate value. Finally, the array $icpdf[k]$ filled with equally probable values of $\cos\theta'$ obeying the assumed pdf, is constructed. The usage of the table is straightforward.

A generated random number ξ is re-scaled to span over the entire array $icpdf[k]$, i.e. simply multiplied by $\max(k)$, and is used to find corresponding index k^*, such that $k^*-1 \le \max(k)\xi \le k^*$. Again, Lagrange interpolating polynomials are used to find the value $\cos\theta'$ corresponding to $\max(k)\xi$.

The approximated scattering coefficients of human skin layers based on a combination of Mie and Rayleigh theories are presented in Fig. 1.6 and were obtained from a number of sources ([2, 78, 79, 97, 98, 99]).

1.2.4 Absorption

There are two major assumptions which are used in the modeling of tissue absorption. The first assumption is that absorption occurs at discrete sites corresponding to the position of scattering and absorbing centers (see Fig. 1.2 b). The advantage of this method is that it is relatively easy to keep the track of the absorbed dose in the tissue [63, 64, 69, 100]. Absorption is modeled by terminating a photon packet in an unbiased way by comparing a random number with a single scattering albedo, $\frac{\mu_s}{\mu_s+\mu_a}$. If a random number is less than albedo, scattering occurs, otherwise absorption takes place [66]. However, this will result in a rapid death of a packet, and consequently long computational time. To avoid this a photon packet is attributed with the statistical weight W [71]. During the course of photon packet propagation, the weight W will be decreasing, that is understood as the absorption.

We consider the model when absorption takes place along the path of the photon packet. This approach corresponds to the tissues model presented by an ensemble of scattering centers in an absorbing continuum. The same assumption has been favored in a number of studies, where the optical radiation detected on the surface of the medium is of interest [67, 101, 102, 103, 104]. A combination of both methods can be used to account absorption of discrete particles and absorbing background [105]. The implication of this approach is that for the photons that have passed through a heterogeneous medium with regions of different absorption coefficients, μ_{ak}, $k = \overline{1..n}$.

Absorption is modeled in the similar manner (1.31), by attenuation of the statistical weight of a photon packet:

$$W_d = W_0 \exp\left(-\sum_k \mu_{ak} l_k\right), \tag{1.44}$$

where W_d is the weight of the detected photon packet, and W_0 is the initial weight of the photon packet, typically equal to 1. Intensity of the exiting radiation is given by:

$$I_d = I_{in} \exp\left(-\sum_k \mu_{ak} l_k\right), \tag{1.45}$$

where I_d is the intensity observed at detector, and I_{in} is the intensity of incident radiation, l_k is the total path length in the k-th region in the medium.

Thus, the photon packet represents a group of many photons, and is a part of photons initially injected into the medium. At each point of the trajectory the weight of the group of photons is equal to the number of unabsorbed photons which represents the probability to reach this point along the trajectory. The statistical weight W_d of each stored photon is counted by:

$$W_d = W_0 (1 - R_{in}) \left[\prod_{p=1}^{M} R^*\right] (1 - R_{out}) \exp\left(-\sum_k \mu_{ak} l_k\right). \tag{1.46}$$

Notice that the absorption μ_{ak} does not influence the photon histories. The separate simulation of the scattering and absorption agrees with the Beer-Lambert law and allows the rapid recalculation of the probing radiation intensity on the detector domain for a set of the medium absorption coefficients without re-calculation of trajectories of photon packets.

Two major tissue layers are conventionally recognized as comprising human skin, i.e. epidermis and dermis (Figure 1.7). The outer, most superficial, layer is the epidermis that varies relatively little in thickness over most of the body, between 75 and 150 μm, apart from on the palms and foot

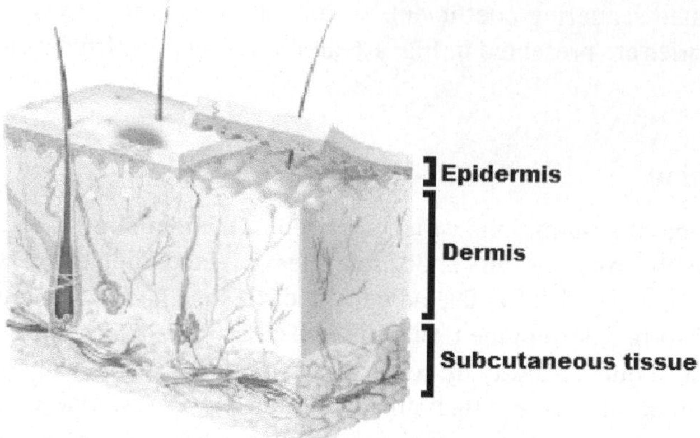

Figure 1.7: Schematic presentation of human skin structure.

soles, where the thickness can be 0.5 mm [106]. The dermis lying beneath the epidermis is a dense elastic connective tissue that constitutes the principal mass of the skin. There is a considerable variation in the thickness of the dermis, an average thickness is 1–2 mm [107]. Underlying the skin is subcutaneous (under-the-skin) tissue, or hypodermis, an average thickness is 1–2 mm.

For MC simulations the extended multi-layer skin model developed in [108] is used. Table 1.2 presents a summary of the typical optical properties of skin tissue layers collected from a number of sources [68, 72, 84, 86, 88–90, 97, 99, 107, 109–116].

TABLE 1.2: Typical optical properties of human skin.

	Skin layer	μ_s, mm^{-1}	μ_a, mm^{-1}	g	n	t, μm.
1	Stratum corneum	80-100	0.1	0.8-0.9	1.5-1.55	10-20
2	Living epidermis	35-60	0.15	0.8-0.85	1.34-1.4	80-100
3	Papillary dermis	30-35	0.068	0.8-0.9	1.39	150-200
4	Upper blood net dermis	25-27	0.095	0.9-0.95	1.4	80-100
5	Reticular dermis	20-25	0.073	0.76-0.8	1.39-1.4	1150-1500
6	Deep blood net dermis	30-35	0.118	0.95	1.38-1.4	80-120
7	Subcutaneous fat	5-15	0.068	0.75-0.8	1.44	5000-6000

The absorption of skin layers takes into account concentration of blood (C_{blood}) in various vascular beds, oxygen saturation (S), water content (C_{H2O}), melanin fraction (C_{mel}), and is defined as [108]:

$$\mu_a^{Strat.corneum}(\lambda) = (1 - C_{H_2O})\mu_a^{baseline}(\lambda) + C_{H_2O}\mu_a^{water}(\lambda) \tag{1.47}$$

$$\mu_a^{Living\,epidermis}(\lambda) = (1 - C_{H_2O})\left[C_{mel}(B_{mel}\mu_a^{mel}(\lambda) + (1 - B_{mel})\mu_a^{ph.mel}(\lambda)) + (1 - C_{mel})\mu_a^{baseline}(\lambda)\right] + \\ + C_{H_2O}\mu_a^{water}(\lambda) \tag{1.48}$$

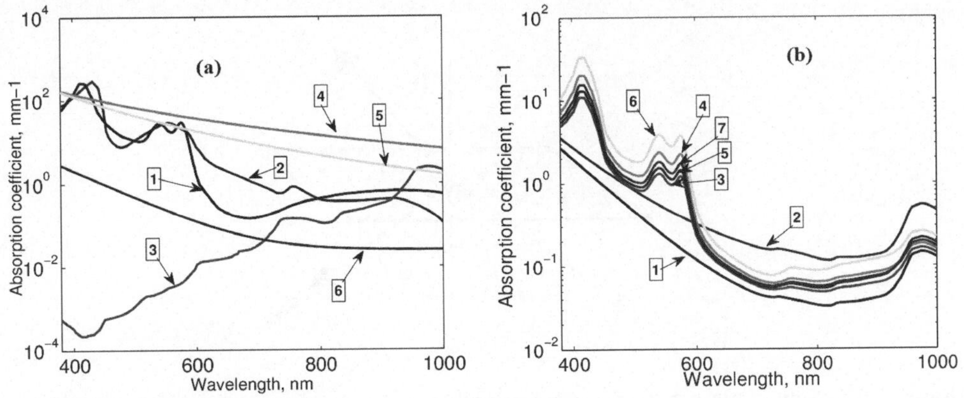

Figure 1.8: Absorption coefficients of key skin tissues chromophores (a), where: 1 - oxy-hemoglobin, 2 - deoxy-hemoglobin, 3 - water, 4 - eumelanin, 5 - pheomelanin, 6 - baseline; Absorption coefficients of the human skin layers (b) counted by equations (1.47), (1.48), (1.49).

$$\begin{aligned}\mu_a^{Dermis}(\lambda) = (1 - C_{H_2O})\left[(C_{blood}F_{Hb}F_{RBC}Ht)(S\mu_a^{oxy}(\lambda) + (1-S)\mu_a^{deoxy}(\lambda))\right] + \\ +(1-C_{H_2O})\left[(1 - C_{blood}F_{Hb}F_{RBC}Ht)\mu_a^{baseline}(\lambda)\right] + \\ +C_{H_2O}\mu_a^{water}(\lambda)\end{aligned} \quad (1.49)$$

Here ${\mu_a}^{mel}(\lambda)$ is the absorption coefficient of eumelanin, ${\mu_a}^{ph.mel}(\lambda)$ is the absorption coefficient of pheomelanin, B_{mel} is the volume fraction of the blend between two melanin types, ${\mu_a}^{oxy}(\lambda)$ is the absorption coefficient of oxy-hemoglobin, ${\mu_a}^{deoxy}(\lambda)$ is the absorption coefficient of deoxy-hemoglobin, ${\mu_a}^{baseline}(\lambda)$ is the absorption coefficient of other water-free tissues, Ht is the hematocrit, F_{Hb} is the volume fraction of hemoglobin, F_{RBC} is the volume fraction of erythrocytes. The absorption of the main skin chromophores and skin layers are summarized in Figure 1.8.

Blood and water content in the layers of human skin is presented in Table 1.3 and is collected from a wide range of literature [72, 77, 107, 117–121].

Total hemoglobin volume fraction in blood γ is calculated assuming that hemoglobin is contained in the erythrocytes only, i.e. $\gamma = F_{Hb}F_{RBC}Ht$. Here $Ht = 0.45$ is the hematocrit, the volume fraction of packed red blood cells in the whole blood, $F_{RBC} = 0.25$ is the volume fraction of erythrocytes in the total volume of all blood cells, $F_{Hb} = 0.99$ is the volume fraction of hemoglobin in erythrocytes, and oxygen saturation $SO_2 = 0.6$ [99, 108].

TABLE 1.3: Volume fraction of blood C_{blood} and water C_{H_2O} in the dermal layers of human skin.

	Skin layer	C_{blood}	C_{H_2O}
1	Papillary dermis	0.04	0.5
2	Upper blood net dermis	0.3	0.6
3	Reticular dermis	0.04	0.7
4	Deep blood net dermis	0.1	0.7
5	Subcutaneous fat	0.05	0.7

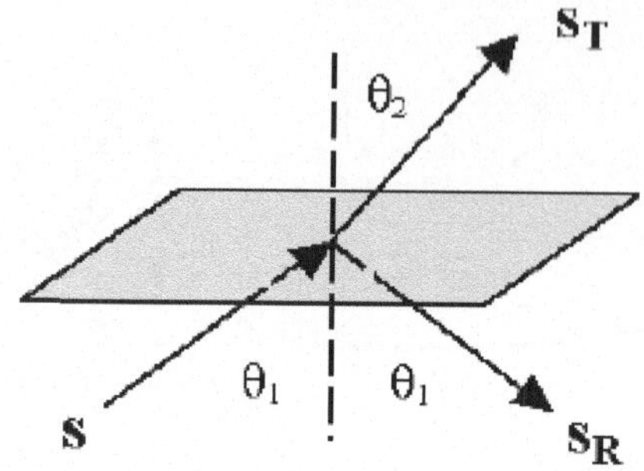

Figure 1.9: Schematic presentation of reflection and refraction of the photon packet at a planar boundary: **s** is a direction unit vector of an incident photon packet, $\mathbf{s}_R$ is a direction unit vector of the reflected photon packet, $\mathbf{s}_T$ is a direction unit vector of the transmitted/refracted photon packet.

1.2.5 Reflection and refraction

Fresnel reflection at the surface of an organ can be thought of as a macroscopic scattering, which is *dependent* on the direction of incoming light relative to the tissue surface normal. The refractive indices of a number of tissues have been measured and estimated to be in the range from 1.38 to 1.41 at 633 nm with an approximate decrease of 1% per 100 nm in the visible part of the spectrum [88, 122]. However, subcutaneous tissue is an exception having a refractive index of approximately 1.44.

For light incident at small to intermediate angles on air-tissue and water-tissue interfaces, the refractive indices of this order of magnitude result in Fresnel reflection in the order of about 4% and less than 1%, respectively. However, for small source-detector separations the total effect is considerable.

Therefore, on the media surface, a photon packet undergoes specular reflection and refraction [24], which are taken into account by splitting the photon packet into the reflected and the transmitted parts, the weights of which are attenuated as:

$$W = W_0 (1 - R_{in}) \left[\prod_{p=1}^{M} \Re(\xi) \right] (1 - R_{out}), \tag{1.50}$$

where W_0 is the initial weight of the photon packet, M is the number of the photon packet reflections/refractions at the internal boundary interfaces, including total internal reflection from the outer boundaries, R_{in} and R_{out} account for reflections on the medium/air boundary, when the photon packet enters and leaves the medium respectively. Internal boundaries are treated differently from the surface between the two scattering regions of media. The photon packet is kept as a whole and in an unbiased manner decides if all of the photon packets are either reflected or transmitted. $\Re(\xi)$ is the Fresnel reflection coefficient $\Re(\xi) = R$, when the packet is reflected, which occurs if $\xi \leq R$, or $\Re(\xi) = 1 - R$, if it is transmitted into the medium 2, when $\xi > R$. R is defined as follows (Fig. 1.9):

$$R = \begin{cases} \dfrac{(n_2 - n_1)^2}{(n_2 + n_1)^2} & \text{if } \theta_1 = 0 \\ \dfrac{1}{2}\left[\dfrac{\sin^2(\theta_1 - \theta_2)}{\sin^2(\theta_1 + \theta_2)} + \dfrac{\tan^2(\theta_1 - \theta_2)}{\tan^2(\theta_1 + \theta_2)}\right] & \text{if } 0 < \theta_1 < \theta_{cr} \\ 1 & \text{if } \theta_{cr} \leq \theta_1 < \dfrac{\pi}{2} \end{cases} \tag{1.51}$$

Either reflected or transmitted/refracted, the photon packet changes its direction that is accounted for by Snell's law [24]. Since the azimuthal angle φ (Figure 1.9) does not change under either reflection or refraction, in terms of the direction cosines transmission/refraction from a medium 1 into a medium 2 is equivalent to

$$\begin{pmatrix} s_1 \\ s_2 \\ s_3 \end{pmatrix}_T = \begin{pmatrix} s_1 \frac{n_1}{n_2} \\ s_2 \frac{n_1}{n_2} \\ \begin{cases} +\sqrt{1-(1-s_3^2)(\frac{n_1}{n_2})^2}, & \text{if } s_3 \geq 0 \\ -\sqrt{1-(1-s_3^2)(\frac{n_1}{n_2})^2}, & \text{if } s_3 < 0 \end{cases} \end{pmatrix}, \tag{1.52}$$

and reflection is equivalent to

$$\begin{pmatrix} s_1 \\ s_2 \\ s_3 \end{pmatrix}_R = \begin{pmatrix} s_1 \\ s_2 \\ -s_3 \end{pmatrix}. \tag{1.53}$$

where $\mathbf{s} = \{s_1, s_2, s_3\}$ is a direction unit vector of an incident photon packet, $\mathbf{s}_T$ is a direction unit vector of transmitted photon packet, $\mathbf{s}_R$ is a direction unit vector of reflected photon packet. Note that angles θ_1 and θ_2 are found from Snell's law: $n_1 \sin\theta_1 = n_2 \sin\theta_2$, where n_1 and n_2 are the refractive indices of the media 1 and 2, respectively. In transition from a medium with a higher refractive index to one with a lower refractive index, total internal reflection occurs for angles larger than the critical angle $\theta_{cr} = \sin^{-1}\frac{n_2}{n_1}$.

Thus, given a photon packet position $\mathbf{r}_i$, its direction $\mathbf{s}_i$ and the proposed path length distance l_i, the distance to the bounding interface is calculated from basic knowledge of geometry. A simple plane interface only is considered in this chapter. However, the same approach can be applied for almost any surface, including rough interfaces; see for example [93, 94].

The general equation for a plane of arbitrary orientation is:

$$\mathbf{n} \cdot (\mathbf{r} - \mathbf{P}_0) = 0, \tag{1.54}$$

where $\mathbf{n}$ is the unit normal to the plane, and $\mathbf{P}_0$ is a radius-vector of any point on the surface of the plane. Inserting (1.28) in (1.54) and solving for l_i gives:

$$l_i^* = -\frac{\mathbf{n} \cdot (\mathbf{r}_i - \mathbf{P}_0)}{\mathbf{n} \cdot \mathbf{s}_i}, \tag{1.55}$$

Thus, instead of the full distance l_i, the packet travels the distance l_i^* to the interface or boundary, where reflection or transmission occurs. Then the distance to the interface is subtracted from the path length $l_i^{**} = l_i - l_i^*$. If the photon packet is reflected, it continues to move with the path length l_i^{**} in the direction given by $\mathbf{s}_R$, (1.53). Otherwise, it is transmitted in the direction given by $\mathbf{s}_T$, (1.52), with the path length l_i^{**} that is scaled following the difference of scattering coefficients, see (1.36).

An example of specular reflection and refraction simulated by MC for a semi-infinite medium with the scattering coefficient $\mu_s = 30$ mm^{-1} and a zero absorption, $g = 0.9$, $n = 1.5$ are presented in Figure 1.10. All photon packets are injected perpendicularly into a homogeneous semi-infinite medium at point $(0,0,0)$. The statistical weight of *singly-refracted* photon packets were collected as a function of the angle of exit, θ_t. Thus, W_1 denotes the weight of refracted photon packets, $W_1 = (1-R_0)(1-R(\theta_i))$, where $\theta_i = \cos^{-1} s_3$. R_0 is the external specular reflection coefficient for light incident normally at the medium/air interface from air. $R(\theta_i)$ is the internal specular reflection coefficient for light incident at the medium/air interface. The excellent agreement is seen between the calculated value of the Fresnel reflectance and the value produced by the MC simulation (see Figure 1.10).

The discrete structure of the MC results is the result of a discrete representation of the Fresnel reflection/refraction coefficients.

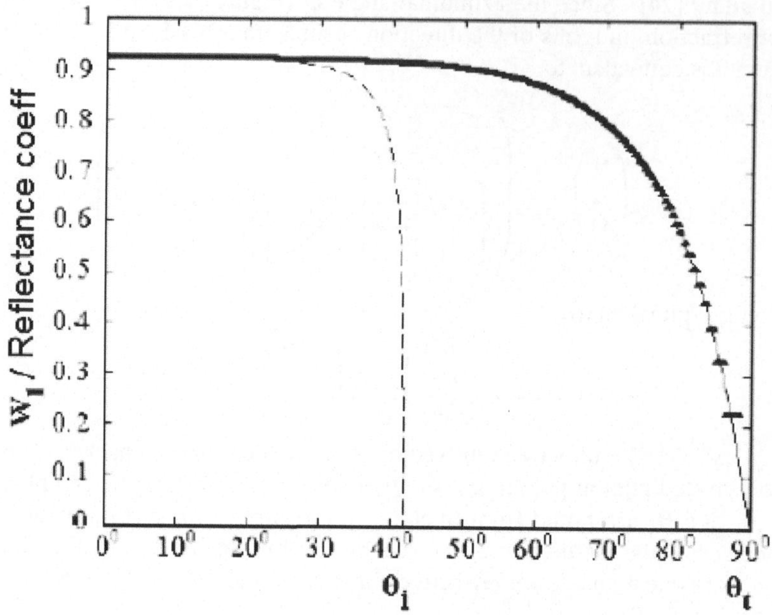

Figure 1.10: Angular distribution of the weight of photon packets emerging from the medium ($n_1 = 1.5$) to another medium ($n_2 = 1.0$). The triangles present the angular distribution of W_1 (MC). The solid and dashed lines are the Fresnel reflectance coefficients $(1-R_0)(1-R(\theta_i))$ as a function of the exit angle θ_t and the angle of incidence θ_i, respectively. Total internal reflection at the critical angle $\theta_{cr} = \sin^{-1}\frac{n_2}{n_1} = 41.8°$ is clearly observed.

The refractive index mismatching at the external boundary results in Fresnel refraction and reflection [123]. To study the effect of mismatching, all the detected photons are grouped into three categories with respect to the number of the photon packet interactions (reflections/refractions) at the outer boundary. The first group, W_1, is a fraction of the detected photon packets that are free of boundary reflections (but may have possible total internal reflections), i.e. these photons have been detected once they crossed the boundary (Figure 1.11). W_2 is a fraction of the detected photons that have been reflected off the boundary once before being detected. The third group, W_3, consists of all the other detected photon packets, i.e. those packets that have reflected off the boundary more than once. The statistical weights of these photon packets are represented by W_1, W_2, and W_3:

$$
\begin{aligned}
W_1 &= W_0'(1-R(\theta_i)),\\
W_2 &= W_0'(1-R(\theta_i))R(\theta_i),\\
W_3 &= W_0'\sum_{k=3}^{M}(1-R_k(\theta_i))\prod_{j=1}^{k-1}R_j(\theta_i).
\end{aligned}
\tag{1.56}
$$

where $W_0' = W_0(1-R_{in})$ and W_0 is the initial weight of the photon packet, M is the number of the photon packet reflections/refractions at the internal medium interfaces, including total internal reflection from the outer boundaries, and R_{in} accounts for reflection, when the photon packet enters the medium. Note that for W_3 $M \geq 3$ (see Eq. 1.50).

Spatial photon weight distributions W_1, W_2, W_3 versus radius of the detector area (r_D) are demonstrated in Figure 1.12 for a non-absorbing and absorbing media. The discrete structure of the sta-

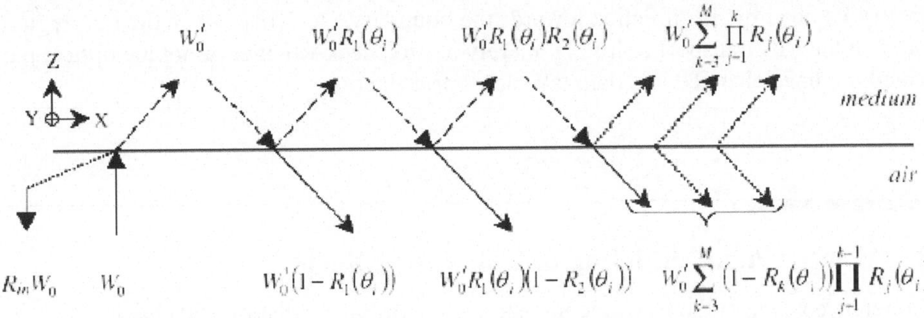

Figure 1.11: Schematic of reflections and refractions of photon packet interactions at the outer boundary of a medium. W_0 is the initial weight of a photon packet, R_{in} is the Fresnel coefficient of the initial specular reflection. $W_0^{'} = (1 - R_{in})W_0$ is the photon packet weight after initial specular reflection. $R(\theta_i)$ is the Fresnel reflection coefficient, and θ_i is the angle of incidence. W_1 is a fraction of the detected photon packets that are free of boundary reflections (except possible total internal reflections), i.e. these photons are detected once they have crossed the boundary. W_2 is a fraction of the detected photons that have been reflected once off the boundary before being detected. W_3 consists of all the other detected photon packets, i.e. those packets that have reflected off the boundary more than once.

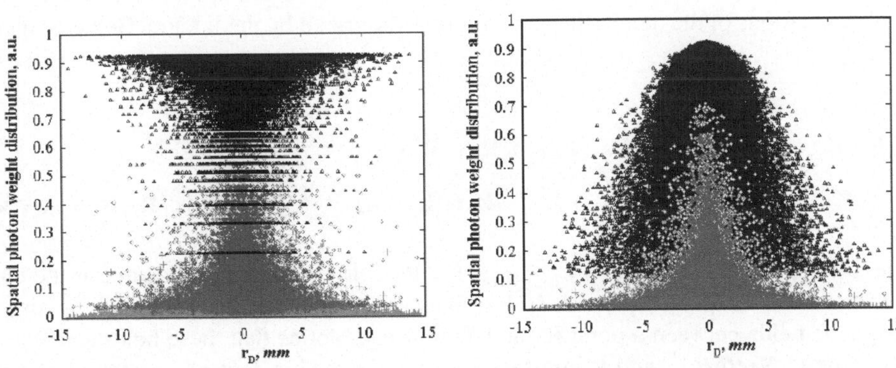

Figure 1.12: Spatial photon weight distribution versus radius of the detector area (r_D): (a) a non-absorbing medium (b) an absorbing medium, $\mu_a = 0.01$ mm^{-1}. The triangles (▲) specify the weight of the photon packets which have experienced one reflection/refraction event on the air-medium boundary, diamonds (◇) represent the weight of the photon packets having acted on the medium boundary twice, crosses (+) show the weight of the high order photon packets reflected/refracted on the air-medium boundary. The optical properties of a semi-infinite highly scattering medium are: $\mu_s = 30$ mm^{-1}, $g = 0.9$, $n = 1.5$.

tistical weight distribution has resulted from a discretization of the Fresnel reflection coefficient, is clearly seen in Figure 1.12 (a), and is completely masked by absorption in Figure 1.12 (b).

Thus, the inclusion of boundaries/interfaces permits the development of applications in complex multi-layered media with inclusions of inhomogeneities. These objects can be very simple, such as a planar interface between two semi-infinite media or a collection of objects such as a complex radiation source or detector. The technique to address both of these problems is essentially the same. The position of a photon packet within the medium is identified by a region number (e.g. number of layer), its position, its direction towards the boundary, etc. Thus, when the new region number is defined in the MC transport routine, it merely has to check whether or not the optical parameters of the medium have changed and then take appropriate action.

1.3 Monte Carlo Modeling of Coherent Effects

Coherence is one of the fundamental parameters of laser radiation and characterizes the degree to which the oscillating electromagnetic laser radiation maintains a near-constant phase shift in space and time. Despite multiple scattering, coherent effects such as the coherent backscattering (CBS) and spatial and temporal intensity correlations are observed due to the wave nature of light in various dielectric media, such as colloid suspensions, liquid crystals and biological tissues [124–126]. This has triggered active research in the field of optics during the past decades [11, 20, 127–131].

The stochastic MC techniques are widely employed in the studies of coherent effects in multiple scattering randomly inhomogeneous media [127, 129–135].

1.3.1 Field correlation transfer

Let a medium occupy a half space $z > 0$, where z is the Cartesian coordinate normal to the boundary. Field correlation transfer in a randomly inhomogeneous medium with temporal and spatial fluctuations of the dielectric permittivity is described by the integral Bethe-Salpeter equation [19, 136]:

$$\widehat{\Gamma}(\mathbf{R}_2,\mathbf{R}_1,t\,|\,\mathbf{k}_s,\mathbf{k}_i) = k_0^4\widetilde{G}(\mathbf{k}_s-\mathbf{k}_i,t)\delta(\mathbf{R}_2-\mathbf{R}_1)\widehat{I}+ \\ +k_0^4\int d\mathbf{R}_3\widetilde{G}(\mathbf{k}_s-\mathbf{k}_{23},t)\widehat{\Lambda}(\mathbf{R}_2-\mathbf{R}_3)\widehat{\Gamma}(\mathbf{R}_3,\mathbf{R}_1,t\,|\,\mathbf{k}_{23},\mathbf{k}_i), \quad (1.57)$$

where the fourth-rank tensor $\widehat{\Gamma} = \Gamma_{\beta_1\beta_2\alpha_1\alpha_2}(\mathbf{R}_2,\mathbf{R}_1,t\,|\,\mathbf{k}_s,\mathbf{k}_i)$ is the propagator or the Green's function of the Bethe-Salpeter equation. It describes the propagation of two complex-conjugated electromagnetic fields between a point $\mathbf{R}_1$ and a point $\mathbf{R}_2$. Notice that these fields arrive at $\mathbf{R}_2$ delayed by the time t. Vectors $\mathbf{k}_i$ and $\mathbf{k}_s$ are the wave-vectors of incident and scattered plane waves, indices $\alpha_1\alpha_2$ and $\beta_1\beta_2$ being polarization indices of the incident and scattered fields. $|\mathbf{k}_i| = |\mathbf{k}_s| = k = k_0 n$, $k_0 = 2\pi/\lambda$ is the wave-number, λ is the wavelength, and $n = n_1 + in_2$ is the refractive index of the medium. The real part n_1 determines the reflectivity mismatch at the medium boundary. The imaginary part of n determines the photon mean free path length $(2n_2k_0)^{-1} = l$. Vector $\mathbf{k}_{ij} = k(\mathbf{R}_i-\mathbf{R}_j)|\mathbf{R}_i-\mathbf{R}_j|^{-1}$ determines the wave-vector between $\mathbf{R}_i$ and $\mathbf{R}_j$.

The fourth-rank tensor $\widehat{\Lambda}(\mathbf{R})$

$$\Lambda_{\alpha\beta\mu\nu}(\mathbf{R}) = \left(\widehat{I}-\frac{\mathbf{R}\otimes\mathbf{R}}{R^2}\right)_{\alpha\mu}\left(\widehat{I}-\frac{\mathbf{R}\otimes\mathbf{R}}{R^2}\right)_{\beta\nu}\frac{\exp(-R/l)}{R^2} \quad (1.58)$$

is a direct product of the conjugated pair of the Green's functions of Maxwell's equations in a far-field zone. It describes a transformation of a pair of fields with polarization μ and ν into a pair of fields with polarization α and β as a result of a single scattering.

In a weak scattering limit $\lambda \ll l$, which usually fulfills in the dielectric media, $\widetilde{G}(\mathbf{q},t)$ is a Fourier transform of the permittivity correlation function:

$$\widetilde{G}(\mathbf{q},t) = \frac{1}{(4\pi)^2}\int d\mathbf{r}\langle\delta\varepsilon(0,0)\delta\varepsilon(\mathbf{r},t)\rangle\exp(-i\mathbf{qr}). \quad (1.59)$$

An important statement in the multiple scattering problems, the so-called optical theorem relates the single scattering cross section and the scattering length $l_s = \mu_s^{-1}$. In the Born approximation for electromagnetic field the optical theorem takes the form:

$$l_s^{-1} = \Gamma_R^{-1} k_0^4 \int d\Omega_s \widetilde{G}_0(\mathbf{k}_s - \mathbf{k}_i), \tag{1.60}$$

where $\widetilde{G}_0(\mathbf{k}_s - \mathbf{k}_i)$ is the Fourier transform of the statistical correlator of the dielectric permittivity fluctuations, $\Gamma_R = 2(1 + \overline{\cos^2\theta})^{-1}$ is a Rayleigh factor, $\overline{\cos^2\theta}$ is the square cosine of the scattering angle θ between vectors $\mathbf{k}_i$ and $\mathbf{k}_s$ weighted by the single scattering cross section:

$$\overline{\cos^2\theta} = \frac{\int d\Omega_s \widetilde{G}_0(\mathbf{k}_s - \mathbf{k}_i)\cos^2\theta_s}{\int d\Omega_s \widetilde{G}_0(\mathbf{k}_s - \mathbf{k}_i)}. \tag{1.61}$$

Photon MFP l is given by

$$\frac{1}{l} = \frac{1}{l_s} + \frac{1}{l_a}, \tag{1.62}$$

where l_a is the characteristic length absorption induced by inelastic scattering. For media investigated l_a is much greater than l and, consequently, l/l_s is close to 1.

The normalized correlation function of dielectric permittivity fluctuations is defined as:

$$p(\mathbf{k}_i - \mathbf{k}_s, t) = \frac{\widetilde{G}(\mathbf{k}_i - \mathbf{k}_s, t)}{\int \widetilde{G}(\mathbf{k}_i - \mathbf{k}_s, 0) d\Omega_s}. \tag{1.63}$$

For $t = 0$, $p(\mathbf{k}_i - \mathbf{k}_s, t)$ transforms into the scattering phase function $p_0(\mathbf{k}_i - \mathbf{k}_s) = p(\mathbf{k}_i - \mathbf{k}_s, 0)$, which describes the single scattering cross section.

Iterating the Bethe-Salpeter equation (1.57) and bearing in mind the optical theorem (1.60), one obtains the series of scattering orders

$$\begin{aligned}\widehat{\Gamma}(\mathbf{R}_2, \mathbf{R}_1, t|\mathbf{k}_s, \mathbf{k}_i) &= \Gamma_R l_s^{-1} p(\mathbf{k}_i - \mathbf{k}_s, t)\delta(\mathbf{R}_2 - \mathbf{R}_1)\widehat{I} + \Gamma_R^2 l_s^{-2} p(\mathbf{k}_s - \mathbf{k}_{21}, t)\times \\ &\widehat{\Lambda}(\mathbf{R}_{21}) p(\mathbf{k}_{21} - \mathbf{k}_i, t) + \Gamma_R^3 l_s^{-3} \int d\mathbf{R}_3 p(\mathbf{k}_s - \mathbf{k}_{23}, t)\widehat{\Lambda}(\mathbf{R}_{23}) p(\mathbf{k}_{23} - \mathbf{k}_{31}, t)\times \\ &\widehat{\Lambda}(\mathbf{R}_{31}) p(\mathbf{k}_{31} - \mathbf{k}_i, t) + \ldots,\end{aligned} \tag{1.64}$$

which is usually illustrated by ladder diagrams [137].

In the far-field zone the temporal field correlation function of the scattered radiation can be expressed as the sum of the non-coherent and interference components:

$$\widehat{C}^E(t\,|\,\mathbf{k}_s, \mathbf{k}_i) = \widehat{C}^{(L)}(t\,|\,\mathbf{k}_s, \mathbf{k}_i) + \widehat{C}^{(V)}(t\,|\,\mathbf{k}_s, \mathbf{k}_i), \tag{1.65}$$

where $\widehat{C}^{(L)}(t\,|\,\mathbf{k}_s, \mathbf{k}_i)$ represents the contribution of the ladder diagrams, which describe the non-coherent component, and $\widehat{C}^{(V)}(t\,|\,\mathbf{k}_s, \mathbf{k}_i)$ is the interferential component observed in the backscattering direction.

For normal incidence and almost backscattering direction, ladder and interferential components of the temporal correlation function have the forms [138, 139]:

$$\begin{aligned}C^{(L)}_{\beta_1\beta_2\alpha_1\alpha_2}(t\,|\,\mathbf{k}_s, \mathbf{k}_i) = \int d\mathbf{R}_1 d\mathbf{R}_2 \Gamma_{\beta_1\beta_2\alpha_1\alpha_2}(\mathbf{R}_2, \mathbf{R}_1, t\,|\,\mathbf{k}_s, \mathbf{k}_i)\times \\ \times \exp\left(-\frac{z_1 + z_2}{l}\right),\end{aligned} \tag{1.66}$$

and

$$C^{(V)}_{\beta_1\beta_2\alpha_1\alpha_2}(t\,|\,\mathbf{k}_s,\mathbf{k}_i) = \int d\mathbf{R}_1 d\mathbf{R}_2 \left[\Gamma_{\beta_1\alpha_2\alpha_1\beta_2}\left(\mathbf{R}_2,\mathbf{R}_1,t \,\middle|\, \frac{\mathbf{k}_s-\mathbf{k}_i}{2}, \frac{\mathbf{k}_i-\mathbf{k}_s}{2}\right) - \right.$$

$$\left. - k_0^4 \widetilde{G}(\mathbf{k}_s-\mathbf{k}_i,t)\delta(\mathbf{R}_2-\mathbf{R}_1)\delta_{\alpha_1\beta_1}\delta_{\alpha_2\beta_2}\right] \exp\left(-\frac{z_1+z_2}{l} + i(\mathbf{k}_s+\mathbf{k}_i)_\perp \cdot (\mathbf{R}_2-\mathbf{R}_1)_\perp\right), \quad (1.67)$$

where subscript $\perp$ denotes the component perpendicular to the normal to the medium boundary. Clearly, for exact backscattering $\mathbf{k}_s = -\mathbf{k}_i$, the polarized component of the interferential contribution $\widehat{C}^{(V)}(t\,|\,\mathbf{k}_s,\mathbf{k}_i)$ exactly equals the polarized component of the main, non-coherent contribution $\widehat{C}^{(L)}(t\,|\,\mathbf{k}_s,\mathbf{k}_i)$ prior to subtracting the single scattering contribution. Depolarized components are not equal.

The methods using light to study motions by means of speckle fluctuations have appeared with numerous names over the years [140–146]. For particles that are undergoing random relative motion, e.g., Brownian motion, the phases of the individual scattered waves are changing randomly and independently of the other scattered waves. The intensity at the detector will thus fluctuate. The time scale of the intensity fluctuations is related to the rate at which the phase of the scattered waves is changing and thus depends on the motion of the scattering particles and on the momentum transfer $\mathbf{q}$. The intensity fluctuations are more rapid at larger scattering angles and for faster moving particles. The field correlation function is explicitly related to the motions within the sample under study.

The non-coherent component defines the temporal field correlation function:

$$g_1(t) = \frac{C^{(L)}(t\,|-\mathbf{k}_i,\,\mathbf{k}_i)}{C^{(L)}(0\,|-\mathbf{k}_i,\,\mathbf{k}_i)}. \quad (1.68)$$

CBS is an interferential enhancement of the average scattered intensity reflected off a disordered scattering medium [138]. It originates from a two-wave constructive interference near exact backscattering between waves traveling along a given scattering path and its time-reversed counterpart. Physically, it is obvious that the effect will dephase rapidly away from backscattering. For classical scatterers, bearing on general symmetry arguments valid in the absence of any magnetic field, the CBS interfering amplitudes have been shown to have equal weights at exact backscattering in the so-called parallel polarization channels [147]. In the linear-linear channel the incoming and detected light fields have the same linear polarization. In the perpendicular channels, nothing ensures the equality of the two interfering amplitudes, and the contrast of the interference is decreased. Notice that single scattering events require a separate treatment as direct and reversed paths coincide in the backward direction and do not contribute to the CBS enhancement.

The interferential component (1.67) at $t = 0$ describes the CBS intensity peak:

$$I^{CBS}(\theta_s) = \frac{C^{(V)}(0\,|\,\mathbf{k}_s,\,\mathbf{k}_i)}{C^{(V)}(0\,|-\mathbf{k}_i,\,\mathbf{k}_i)} \quad (1.69)$$

and its angular dependence.

1.3.2 Scalar field

As mentioned above, in the Born approximation the Bethe-Salpeter equation can be represented as a series of scattering orders, which is equivalent to a series of the ladder diagrams. To develop a general stochastic method for coherent effects modeling, a relation will be established between the analytical procedure of the summation of successive terms of a ladder-diagram series and the conventional MC technique.

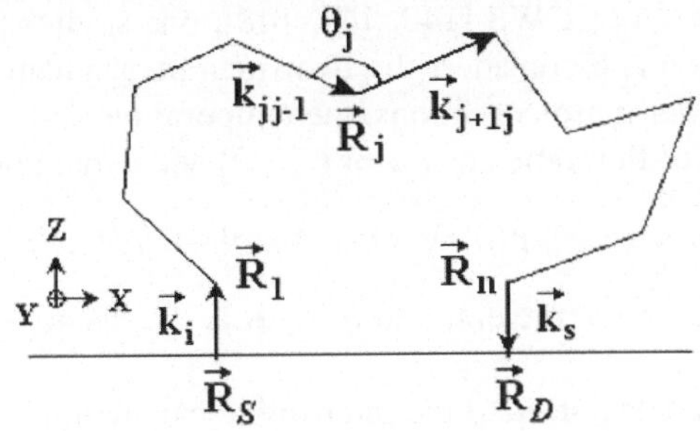

Figure 1.13: Stochastic trajectory of a photon between a point of source $\mathbf{R}_S$ and a point of detector $\mathbf{R}_D$. $\mathbf{R}_1$ and $\mathbf{R}_n$ are the points of the first and final scattering events. Vectors $\mathbf{k}_{jj-1}$ and $\mathbf{k}_{j+1j}$ are wave-vectors before and after the j-th scattering event at $\mathbf{R}_j$, θ_j is the angle between them.

First, let's consider scalar fields. For a scalar field, a tensor $\widehat{\Lambda}(\mathbf{R})$ is transformed into a scalar function $\Lambda_0(R)$=$R^{-2}\exp(-R/l)$, and the Rayleigh factor Γ_R becomes equal to 1. The first term of an iterative series (1.64) describes single scattering, second term – double scattering, etc.

The conventional MC method describes the propagation of optical radiation as a stochastic process, which consists of one, two, ... n scattering events. The difference between iterative solution (1.64) and conventional radiative transfer equation (1.1) is just a matter of how one writes them. Indeed, in terms of numerical simulation, an extra term $\widehat{\Lambda}(R_{jj-1})p_0(\mathbf{k}_j-\mathbf{k}_{j-1})$ in eq. (1.64) is equivalent to simulation of photon transport for a distance $R=|\mathbf{R}_j-\mathbf{R}_{j-1}|$ in a direction $\mathbf{k}_j$. It is very similar to how the conventional MC method works. Indeed, as a results of the MC simulation a stochastic trajectory of a photon appears. It has the origin at a point $\mathbf{R}_0=\mathbf{R}_S$ followed by n sequent points $\mathbf{R}_1$, $\mathbf{R}_2$, $\mathbf{R}_3$,..., $\mathbf{R}_n$, which represents n scattering events, and a point $\mathbf{R}_D$, where the photon packet is detected (Figure 1.13).

The difficulties associated with the iterative solution to the Bethe-Salpeter equation are that the integrals over $\mathbf{R}_i$ cannot be factorized, i.e. integration over particular $\mathbf{R}_i$ cannot be performed independently from the rest or at least some of $\mathbf{R}_i$. In numerical MC modeling a direction and the length of the next photon step are determined in an unbiased way that helps to make this kind of factorization.

Due to the way the phase function is defined, i.e.

$$\int p_0(\mathbf{k}_i-\mathbf{k}_s)d\Omega=1 \tag{1.70}$$

the statistical weight of a photon packet does not change after scattering. In theoretical description, this is granted by the optical theorem. Indeed, $\int\Lambda_0(R)d\mathbf{R}=4\pi l$, hence, the expansion parameter of eq. (1.64) is equal to

$$l_s^{-1}\int d\Omega_n\int d\mathbf{R}_{j+1}\Lambda_0(\mathbf{R}_{j+1}-\mathbf{R}_j)p_0(\mathbf{k}_{j+1}-\mathbf{k}_j)=l_s^{-1}l. \tag{1.71}$$

In the absence of absorption, $l_s^{-1}l$ is exactly equal to 1, that is the evidence of photon weight conservation. Notice that it is the close affinity of the expansion parameter $l_s^{-1}l$ to 1, that brings about all difficulties with the analytical solution of the Bethe-Salpeter equation. That is, the series (1.64) does not converge if the finite number of the terms is involved in consideration.

Calculation of the temporal intensity correlation function with MC is similar to the diffuse reflectance simulation. However, after each scattering event, the direction of a photon packet is determined by a more generalized phase function $p(\mathbf{k}_j-\mathbf{k}_{j-1},t)$, which is dependent on the time delay t.

In most applications such as DWS [143, 144, 148], one studies temporal evolution of inhomogeneities within a medium and considers the Brownian mechanism of temporal decay of inhomogeneity fluctuations. Under these conditions, the temporal permittivity correlation function can be represented as a product of the static correlator $G(q,0)$ and exponential function (see eq. 1.63):

$$p(q,t) \approx p_0(q)\exp(-D_s q^2 t), \tag{1.72}$$

where D_s is a self-diffusion coefficient, and $q = |\mathbf{q}|$ is the wave vector transfer $\mathbf{q} = \mathbf{k}_i - \mathbf{k}_s$, $q = 2k\sin\theta_s/2$.

Thus, to proceed from calculation of the intensity to calculation of the temporal field correlation function one has to replace the phase function according to:

$$p_0(\mathbf{k}_{j-1} - \mathbf{k}_j) \to p_0(\mathbf{k}_{j-1} - \mathbf{k}_j)\exp(-D_s|\mathbf{k}_{j-1} - \mathbf{k}_j|^2 t). \tag{1.73}$$

In the diffusion approximation the momentum transfer is changed to its average:

$$\exp\left(-D_s|\mathbf{k}_{j-1} - \mathbf{k}_j|^2 t\right) \to \exp\left(-2(t/\tau)(1-\overline{\cos\theta_s})\right) \to \exp\left(-2(t/\tau)(l/l^*)\right), \tag{1.74}$$

where $\tau = (D_s k^2)^{-1}$ is the characteristic time of scattering particle diffusion at distance comparable to the wavelength, $\overline{\cos\theta_s} = g$ is the mean cosine of the scattering angle θ_s, and $l^* = l_s(1-g)^{-1}$ is the transport length.

Thus, in the MC simulation the temporal field correlation function is given by:

$$g_1(t) = \sum_{i=1}^{N_{ph}} W_{di}\exp\left(-2\frac{t}{\tau}n_i\left[1 - \frac{1}{n_i}\sum_{j=1}^{n_i}\cos\theta_j\right]\right), \tag{1.75}$$

where n_i is the number of scattering events experienced by the i-th photon packet, W_{di} is its statistical weight, and θ_j is the scattering angle at the j-th scattering event.

If the interferential component (1.67) is to be modeled then, one notices that the sole difference from the intensity of the non-coherent component (1.66) is a factor $\exp(i\mathbf{k}_\perp\mathbf{R}_\perp)$, where $\mathbf{k}_\perp = (\mathbf{k}_i + \mathbf{k}_s)_\perp$ and $\mathbf{R}_\perp = (\mathbf{R}_1 - \mathbf{R}_2)_\perp$. Due to the translational invariance of $\mathbf{R}_\perp$ in the xy plane, a factor $\exp(i\mathbf{k}_\perp\mathbf{R}_\perp)$ can be substituted with a factor $\cos(\mathbf{k}_\perp\mathbf{R}_\perp)$. Thus, the MC simulation of the CBS intensity can be realized in the following manner. First, one has to exclude the single scattering from the detected signal, as it does not take part in interference. In the case of normal incidence and a small backscattering angle θ_s, the statistical weight of the i-th photon packet, detected at the outer boundary with the wave vector $\mathbf{k}_s$ at the distance $|(\mathbf{R}_S - \mathbf{R}_D^{(i)})_\perp|$ from the source point $\mathbf{R}_S$, is multiplied by a factor $\cos(\mathbf{q}_\perp(\mathbf{R}_S - \mathbf{R}_D^{(i)})_\perp)$. The expression for the CBS intensity is a sum of contributions from all detected photons:

$$I^{CBS}(\theta_s) = \sum_{i=1}^{N_{ph}} W_{di}\cos(\mathbf{k}_\perp(\mathbf{R}_S - \mathbf{R}_D^{(i)})_\perp)(1 - \delta_{n_i,1}), \tag{1.76}$$

where $(1 - \delta_{n_i,1})$ naturally excludes contribution from the singly scattered photons.

The CBS peak or enhancement factor is defined as

$$h^{CBS} = \frac{2I - I_{single}}{I}, \tag{1.77}$$

where I is the non-coherent intensity (1.66) and I_{single} is the intensity of the singly scattered photons.

1.3.3 Polarization

In the case of electromagnetic field, as opposed to scalar field, additional effort has to be made to trace the direction of the electromagnetic field along the photon path that is given by the polarization vector. According to (1.58) it can be achieved if one calculates the results of n sequential operators applied to the incident field [138]:

$$\prod_{j=1}^{n}\left(\widehat{I}-(\mathbf{R}_{j+1}-\mathbf{R}_j)\otimes(\mathbf{R}_{j+1}-\mathbf{R}_j)|\mathbf{R}_{j+1}-\mathbf{R}_j|^{-2}\right), \tag{1.78}$$

assuming that the photon has experienced n scattering events.

For electromagnetic field, a phase space of a given photon is supplemented with the polarization vector $\mathbf{P}$. In general, $\mathbf{P}$ is a 3-vector and for linear polarization along x axis $\mathbf{P}^{(in)}=(1;0;0)$.

Polarization of the electromagnetic field changes every time after the scattering event. Thus, after each scattering event, when a new direction is determined, a new polarization vector $\mathbf{P}_{j+1}$ is related to $\mathbf{P}_j$ through transformation:

$$\mathbf{P}_{j+1}=\left(\widehat{I}-(\mathbf{R}_{j+1}-\mathbf{R}_j)\otimes(\mathbf{R}_{j+1}-\mathbf{R}_j)|\mathbf{R}_{j+1}-\mathbf{R}_j|^{-2}\right)\mathbf{P}_j. \tag{1.79}$$

Hence, after n scattering events (Fig. 1.13), when a photon packet is detected at a point $\mathbf{R}_D$ the polarization vector is given by:

$$\mathbf{P}^{(out)}=\prod_{j=1}^{n}\left(\widehat{I}-(\mathbf{R}_{j+1}-\mathbf{R}_j)\otimes(\mathbf{R}_{j+1}-\mathbf{R}_j)|\mathbf{R}_{j+1}-\mathbf{R}_j|^{-2}\right)\mathbf{P}^{(in)}. \tag{1.80}$$

If W_{di} is the statistical weight of the detected "scalar" photon, the polarized and depolarized intensities are defined by

$$\begin{aligned} I_{pol}=I_{XX}&=\sum_{i=1}^{N_{ph}}W_{di}P_{ix}^2\Gamma_R^{n_i},\\ I_{depol}=I_{YX}&=\sum_{i=1}^{N_{ph}}W_{di}P_{iy}^2\Gamma_R^{n_i}, \end{aligned} \tag{1.81}$$

where superscript (out) is omitted for brevity. Equations (1.81) describe the non-coherent contribution of ladder diagrams $I_{\beta\alpha}=C^{(L)}_{\beta\beta\alpha\alpha}(0|\mathbf{k}_s,\mathbf{k}_i)$ (eq. 1.66). Notice that for the exact backscattering direction, the Z component is exactly equal to zero.

In the MC simulation the following expressions are used for polarized and depolarized temporal field correlation functions of the electromagnetic field:

$$\begin{aligned} g^{(1)}_{pol}(t)=g^{(1)}_{XX}(t)&=\sum_{i=1}^{N_{ph}}W_{di}P_{ix}^2\Gamma_R^{n_i}\exp(-2\frac{t}{\tau}n_i(1-\frac{1}{n_i}\sum_{j=1}^{n_i}\cos\theta_j)),\\ g^{(1)}_{depol}(t)=g^{(1)}_{YX}(t)&=\sum_{i=1}^{N_{ph}}W_{di}P_{iy}^2\Gamma_R^{n_i}\exp(-2\frac{t}{\tau}n_i(1-\frac{1}{n_i}\sum_{j=1}^{n_i}\cos\theta_j)), \end{aligned} \tag{1.82}$$

where $P_{i\alpha}$ is the polarization vector of the i-th photon with polarization α. $P_{i\alpha}$ is a result of n_i tensor operators (1.78) applied to the initial polarization, and θ_j is the scattering angle at the j-th scattering event (Fig. 1.13).

1.3.4 Simulation of OCT images

The OCT signal in terms of probing depth z can be presented as an interference term of optical signals coming from the sample and reference arms [149, 150]:

$$I(z)=(\langle I_r\rangle\langle I_s\rangle)^{1/2}\mathrm{Re}\{C(z,l_c)\}. \tag{1.83}$$

Here $\langle I_s \rangle$ and $\langle I_r \rangle$ are the mean intensities returning from the sample and reference arms of the interferometer, $C(z, l_c)$ is the normalized coherence function and l_c is the coherence length of probing radiation [151]:

$$l_c = \frac{2\ln 2}{\pi}\frac{\lambda^2}{\Delta\lambda}, \tag{1.84}$$

where $\Delta\lambda$ is the full width at half maximum (FWHM) of the spectrum of source radiation. When performing the MC simulation described above the OCT signal detected at the definite transversal position of the probing beam (A-scan) is calculated for randomly polarized radiation as [152]:

$$I(z) = I_0 \sum_{i=1}^{N_{ph}} \sqrt{W_i} \cos\left(\frac{2\pi}{\lambda}(2z - L_i)\right) \exp\left(-\left(\frac{2z - L_i}{l_c}\right)^2\right), \tag{1.85}$$

where N_{ph} is the number of photons launched, I_0 is a constant defined by instrumental properties of the OCT system, W_i is the weight of i-th detected photon with optical pathlength L_i and $2z$ is the optical pathlength in the reference arm. If one neglects "speckle structure" of the OCT-signal defined by the cosine item, the result can be presented as a superposition of envelopes of partial detected photon contributions [153]:

$$I(z) = I_0 \sum_{i=1}^{N_{ph}} \sqrt{W_i} \exp\left(-\left(\frac{2z - L_i}{l_c}\right)^2\right). \tag{1.86}$$

In order to simulate the 2D OCT image consequent A-scans are simulated with the definite transversal step in probing position. The total number of simulated A-scans and the transversal step between them are predefined regarding the width (FWHM) of the probing beam diameter.

1.3.5 Simulation of polarization dependent OCT signal

Polarization of an electromagnetic wave is typically described in framework of the Stokes-Mueller or Jones formalism [23, 154]. Stokes-Mueller formalism was applied to study polarization in birefringent turbid media for potential application to polarization-sensitive optical imaging [155]. The experimental and numerical studies were carried out to observe the backscattering polarization patterns presented in a form of the Mueller matrices [156, 157]. The residual polarization degree of the backscattered light and its connection to the optical properties of the scattering medium was studied in [158]. To explore the possibility of retrieving the birefringence properties of layered tissue with the depth-resolved polarization-sensitive OCT (PS-OCT) Jones formalism was implemented to reduce long calculation time, typically required in the full Stokes-Mueller approach [159].

Schmitt et al. proposed a method for discriminating short and long path photons that is based on the relationship between the polarization states of incident and forward scattered light [160]. Discussing coherent backscattering and its dependence on the state of polarization of an incident linearly polarized light, Akkermans et al. assumed that for both states of polarization the corresponding intensity can be represented as a product of the intensity of a scalar wave, which does not depend on the polarization state, and a corresponding multiplicative factor (weighting function) describing polarization transfer [138]. These factors are specific for a given polarization state and generally depend on the properties of scattering particles, e.g. size, shape [161, 162]. The expression for the co- and cross-polarized intensities derived from the expression proposed in [162] has been successfully used in [163], whereas the experimental results [164] proved the adequacy of the Akkermans' conjecture of time scales involved in the depolarization process of the backscattered light. Consider a plane electromagnetic wave polarized in the x direction that enters the medium along positive direction of z axis normal to the interface. By a co-polarized wave we understand a linearly polarized scattered wave with the same orientation of polarization as the incident wave, and a cross-polarized wave is perpendicular to the incident wave direction of polarization [154]. Thus, waves scattered in xz and yz planes define co-polarized and cross-polarized components of the scattered electromagnetic wave, respectively.

To account for the depolarization effect in PS-OCT images we adopted the polarization vector formalism where the polarization is described in terms of a polarization vector $\vec{P}$ undergoing a sequence of transformations after each scattering event [154]. The trajectories of the polarized photons are weighted in accordance with their polarization state. Within the far-field or Fraunhofer approximation the polarization vector of the scattered wave $\vec{P}_{i-1}$ is transformed upon the i-th scattering event into $\vec{P}_i$ as [14, 138]:

$$\vec{P}_i = -\vec{e}_i \times [\vec{e}_i \times \vec{P}_{i-1}] = [\hat{I} - \vec{e}_i \otimes \vec{e}_i]\vec{P}_{i-1}, \tag{1.87}$$

where $\vec{e}_i$ is the unit vector along the propagation direction between $(i-1)$-th and i–th scattering events. Note that although the expression is rigorously introduced for the case of pure Rayleigh scattering, it can also be applied as the first approximation in case of Rayleigh-Gans-Debye (RGD) scattering valid for soft scattering particles with the size comparable to or a few times larger than the wavelength [14]. Namely, the size D of the particles should obey the relation $(\varepsilon_r - 1)D/\lambda \gg 1$ where $(\varepsilon_r - 1)$ is the relative fluctuation of dielectric permittivity between the scatterer (e.g., cell component such as nucleus or mitochondria) and the surrounding medium (e.g., cytoplasm). Typically in biotissues the value of $(\varepsilon_r - 1)$ is less than 0.1 [90] therefore RGD approximation is quite reasonable for the particles with the sizes of units of λ which are characterized by non-isotropic scattering phase function. At the same time, implementation for strongly scattering large inclusions may lead to some discrepancy in the final results; however, this approximation can be applied to qualitatively estimate the effects of depolarization in OCT images. Explicitly, the tensor $\mathbf{S}_i = [\hat{I} - \vec{e}_i \otimes \vec{e}_i]$ is presented as

$$S_i = \begin{pmatrix} 1 - e_{iX}^2 & -e_{iX}e_{iY} & -e_{iX}e_{iZ} \\ -e_{iX}e_{iY} & 1 - e_{iY}^2 & -e_{iY}e_{iZ} \\ -e_{iX}e_{iZ} & e_{iX}e_{iZ} & 1 - e_{iZ}^2 \end{pmatrix}. \tag{1.88}$$

It guarantees that the electromagnetic field remains transversal experiencing the i-th scattering event. The chain $\mathbf{T}(n) = S_n S_{n-1} ... S_1$ of projection operators $\mathbf{S}_i$ transforms the initial polarization upon a sequence of n scattering events to the final polarization:

$$\vec{P}_n = S_n S_{n-1} ... S_1 \vec{P}_0. \tag{1.89}$$

Consequently, propagation of co-polarized and cross-polarized components of the electromagnetic field in the medium is described along the same trajectories obtained for the scalar field. The vector nature of electromagnetic field can be taken into account by multiplying the statistical weight of each trajectory by the square of the matrix element of tensor $\mathbf{T}(n)$: $T_{xx}(n)$ for co-polarized component and $T_{yx}(n)$ for cross-polarized one.

In order to link vector and scalar approaches in simulation of PS-OCT images it should be pointed out that in accordance with the optical theorem [165] the scalar approach yields [136, 161]:

$$k_0^4 \int G(k_i - k_s) d\Omega_s = \frac{1}{s}, \tag{1.90}$$

whereas for the electromagnetic field [136, 163]:

$$k_0^4 \int G(k_i - k_s) d\Omega_s = \frac{2}{1 + \cos^2\theta} \frac{1}{s}. \tag{1.91}$$

Therefore, at every scattering event the multiplicative factor should be included:

$$\Gamma = \frac{2}{1+\cos^2\theta} \tag{1.92}$$

Finally, for linearly polarized probing radiation the expression (1.86) can be re-written separately for co- and cross-polarized detected OCT signal:

$$I_{co}(z) = I_0 \sum_{i=1}^{N_{ph}} \sqrt{W_i \Gamma^{n_i} T_{xx}(n_i)^2} \exp\left(-\left(\frac{2z-L_i}{l_c}\right)^2\right) \tag{1.93}$$

for co-polarized component and

$$I_{cross}(z) = I_0 \sum_{i=1}^{N_{ph}} \sqrt{W_i \Gamma^{n_i} T_{yx}(n_i)^2} \exp\left(-\left(\frac{2z-L_i}{l_c}\right)^2\right) \tag{1.94}$$

for cross-polarized one, where n_i is the number of scattering events for i-th detected photon.

1.3.6 Termination

In order to keep the simulation time within reasonable bounds, a test based on prerequisite cut-off criterion is performed after each photon interaction. If the statistical weight W of the packet is less than a minimal value, typically $W_{min} = 0.0001$ or if the total number of scattering events exceeds the maximum value $N_{max\ scat} = 10000$ it is assumed that the packet no longer significantly contributes to the detected signal and can be terminated. After a number of photon packets has been traced in the medium (typically 10^9–10^{11}), the parameters of interest are scored from the accumulated photon histories.

1.4 Online Object Oriented Monte Carlo Computational Tool for the Needs of Biomedical Optics

As one can see, due to a number of practical OD applications the MC model undergoes continuous modifications and changes dedicated to inclusion of diverse properties of incident optical/laser radiation, configuration of the sources and detectors, structure of the medium and the conditions of light detection [99, 104, 108, 135, 137, 152, 153, 165–174]. Past attempts to unify these MC codes are mainly based on the use of structured programming [175]. While structured programming has been known for years, it limits the ability to handle a large code without decreasing its functionality and manageability [176]. In practice, the increasing diversity of the MC applications results in a substantial growth of the model's source code and leads to the development of a set of separate MC codes each dedicated to a particular purpose.

1.4.1 Object oriented concept of Monte Carlo modeling

To generalize, unify and implement MC modeling for a multi-purpose use in various biomedical optics applications we apply the Object Oriented Programming (OOP) concept [177, 178]. The OOP is widely used in mainstream application development and has been found extremely effective in design of complex multi-parametric systems, providing a highly intuitive approach of programming [176, 179]. The key features of OOP allow the MC to be separated into logical components, described by objects.

Thus, each photon packet has been defined as an object interacting with medium or medium components also defined as objects. Splitting the medium into the objects allows developing the tissue model more iteratively and uniformly. The distribution of scattering centers, macro-inhomogeneities, such as blood vessels, tumors, aneurisms, etc. can be formed by combination of 3D elementary volumes (objects) presenting spatial variations in the tissues. Moreover, actual structure of a biological tissue can be imported into the model as an object (image) provided by OCT, Photo-Acoustic Tomography (PAT), ultrasound, MRI, etc.

Utilizing the inheritance feature of OOP the smart hierarchy structure of the code has been created to prevent creation of multiple classes for similar tasks. The hierarchy allows "allied" objects to share variables and members, significantly reducing the amount of source code and paving the way to extend and generalize the MC for various OD applications. In addition, the variations of scattering phase functions, such as Mie, Rayleigh and Henyey-Greenstein [171] have been defined using the polymorphism feature of OOP that allows one to handle the modeling with no changes of the source code.

Thus, the OOP approach significantly increases the efficiency of the model manageability and provides superior opportunities to generalize MC to combine previously developed MC models as a way to imitate a particular OD experiment taking into account various features of optical radiation and light-tissue interaction. Schematically the structure of the generalized MC approach is shown in Figure 1.14.

As one can see, first, by the selection of a certain application the parameters of the Source, Detector and Scattering medium are entered. Depending on the application, the objects are tuned to the appropriate feature of light-tissue interaction and the simulation is performed. By completing, the output data are prepared in the format utilized in the corresponding OD experiment/application. The OOP MC version supports the estimation of sampling volume offered by a reflectance and/or transmittance geometry (e.g. for fiber optic probe with a small mm source-detector spacing); simulation of reflectance or transmittance optical/near-infrared spectra of the multi-layered media like human skin; modeling of skin color depending on volume fraction of melanin and blood, blood oxygen saturation; modeling of OCT images with regards coherence and polarization properties of probing light, imitation of spatial localization of skin tissue fluorescence excitation and simulation of coherent effects of multiple scattering.

1.4.2 Graphics Processing Unit acceleration of the Monte Carlo model

Launching of a large number of photon packets (typically 10^9-10^{11}) and computing their interaction with the medium and with the probe is a highly intensive computational process. Due to the task intensity, processing time is always a significant issue in stochastic modeling, taking a few days to complete at the standard CPU. To achieve supreme performance of simulation a number of programming approaches and optimizations of algorithms have been used in the past, including parallel and cluster computing [180, 181]. The recently developed parallel computing framework, known as Compute Unified Device Architecture (CUDA), introduced by NVIDEA Corporation has been applied. NVIDEA CUDA technology provides an unlimited access to computational resources of the graphic card: processor cores, different types of memory (of various capacity and speed) making the Graphics Processing Unit (GPU) a massive co-processor in parallel computations [180, 181].

We utilize the recent, introduced in 2010, CUDA generation, so-called architecture codename Fermi. Designed for C/C++ development and easily integrated with the Microsoft Visual Studio it makes parallel programming significantly easier, especially in terms of project management and debugging. The latest CUDA generation supports most of the OOP features like creating classes, inheritance, and polymorphism and keeps all dramatic performance gains of the CUDA computing [177]. The OOP MC model has been developed using CUDA 4.1 C/C++ and supports multiple GPUs, providing user's interface and delivering the modeling output. The hardware is presented by two Tesla M2090 / GeForce GTX 480 graphic cards with NVIDIA CUDA computing capability

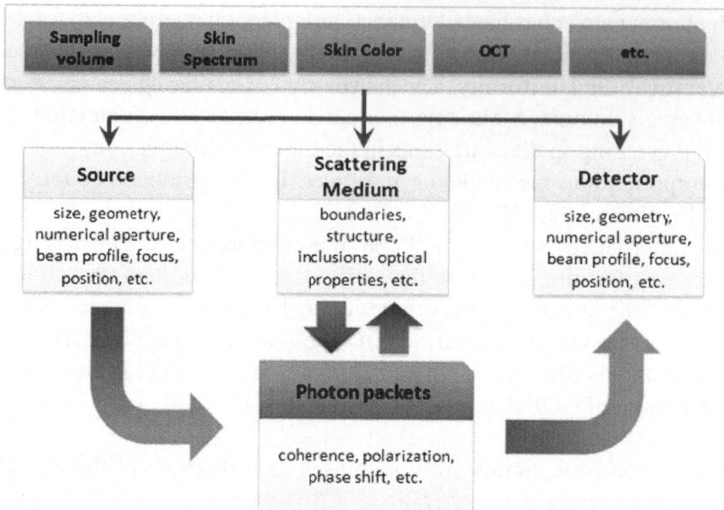

Figure 1.14: Schematic presentation of the generalized object-oriented MC model structure. Data Input and selection of a particular application; Class objects represent exact experimental conditions including source-detector geometry and configuration, medium structure, properties of incident radiation, etc.

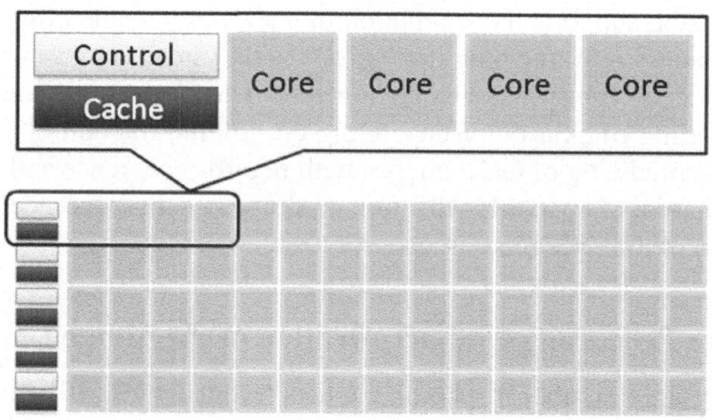

Figure 1.15: Schematic presentation of used GPU logically divided into hundreds of independent cores allowing creation of thousands of lightweight parallel threads.

2.0 having up to 6.0 Tflops of computational power on board (single precision). The graphic chip is logically divided into hundreds of CUDA cores (in our case up to 500 per card), schematically presented in Figure 1.15. Therefore, it executes up to twenty thousand threads simultaneously, without context switch performance losses and very fast (up to 4 Gbit/s) on-chip GDDR memory. The graphic chip's shared memory has been used to store the intermediate results; constant memory is applied for data input, whereas the global memory is used to store parameters of photon objects (e.g. path-length, state of polarization, outlet angles etc.). The tiling and cutoff techniques are used to process large datasets and avoid memory bandwidth limitations [180, 181]. Such a design allows simulating propagation of thousands (15 to 20 depending on application and detector parameters) of photon objects in the medium simultaneously that provides an opportunity for direct imitation of image or wave front transfer in the scattering medium or OCT image modeling.

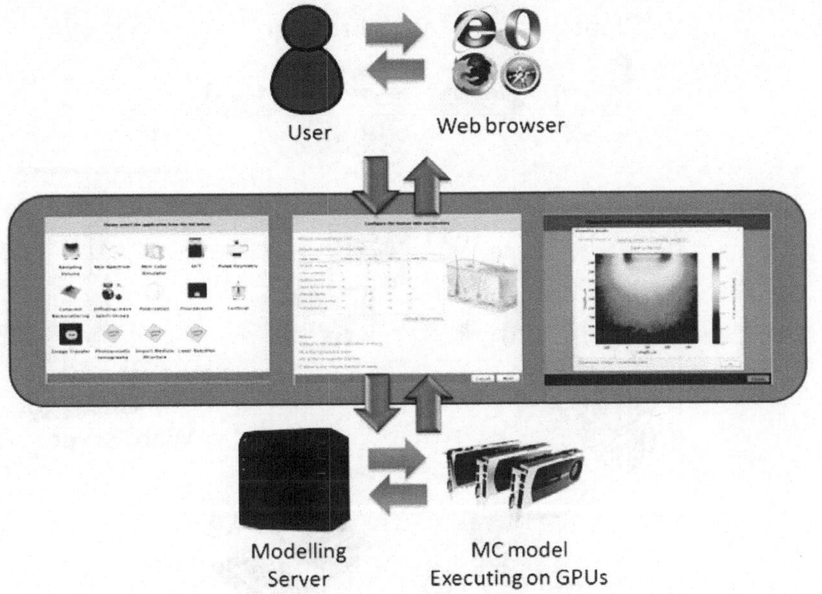

Figure 1.16: Schematic presentation of the key components of the online MC solution. The server hosts a web front end, which accepts user simulation requests and retrieves results. The developed components provide interoperability between the interactive user interface and GPUs.

Specially designed for 3D graphic applications mainly for computer games and professional software designing this cutting edge graphic technology also incorporates a powerful set of instruments applied for optimized simulation of object motion, rotation, reflection, ray-tracing, etc. The NVIDEA CUDA provides GPU-accelerated mathematical libraries, such as CULA, CUBLAS - Linear Algebra, CUFFT - Fast Furrier Transform, CURAND - Random Number Generators [182]. Their incorporation into MC allows speeding up the simulation of each photon packet up to 1000 times.

1.4.3 Online solution and web integration

A flow chart of the online solution is schematically presented on Figure 1.16.

The MC modeling server provides major hardware acceleration by CUDA supporting GPUs. The developed server software consists of the web front end, management part, GPU-web integration and the CUDA-based MC core described above.

The front end of the MC is developed by using Microsoft ASP.NET and Microsoft Silverlight technologies [183–186]. Microsoft Silverlight is used for creation of a cross-platform lightweight interactive interface to access a particular MC application [186], whereas ASP.NET is employed to meet modern design and security requirements [185].

The management part of the MC modeling server consists of the Input / Output (I/O) and Load Balancing systems. The I/O is created to accept and validate user credentials and online input of modeling parameters; to log and store computation enquiries and output data into a server database; to deliver the results of the simulation back to the front end. The I/O works in tandem with the Load Balancing which allows one to manage the server load, monitor running simulations and check the GPU availability. To make the online MC less vulnerable to common network threats and overloads, the management part has been developed utilizing recently added .NET 4.0 features, such as Windows Presentation Foundation (WPF) and Windows Communication Foundation (WCF)

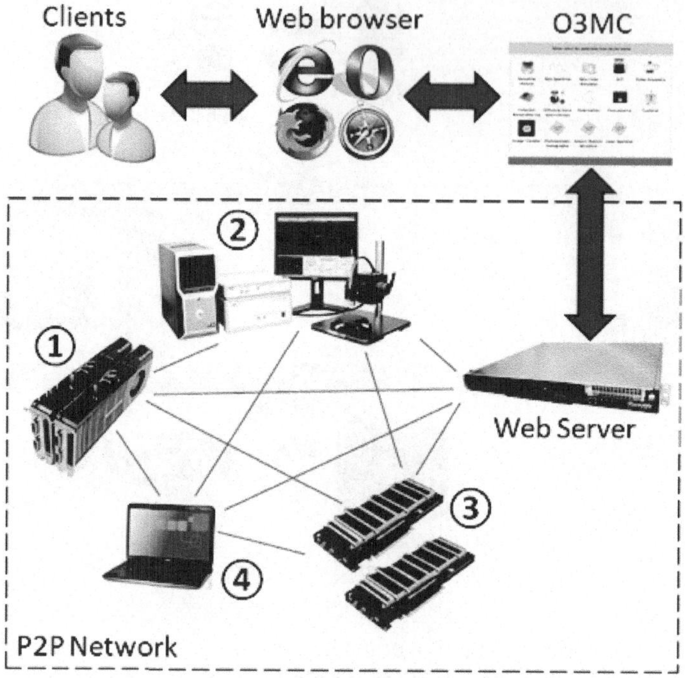

Figure 1.17: Schematic presentation of P2P O3MC implementation. Clients interact with the O3MC web interface via a preferred web browser. The server accepts O3MC simulation requests and keeps track of the participating peers. The P2P network consists of different computers equipped with the CUDA-supporting GPUs: (1) a workstation with two GeForce GTX 480 GPUs each 480 CUDA cores, 1540 Gigaflops of the peak single precision FPP / 85 Gigaflops double precision FPP, 1536 GB of GDDR5 memory; (2) Thorlabs OCT imaging system workstation with Quadro FX580 featuring 32 CUDA cores, 512 MB GDDR3 memory; (3) computational server equipped with two Tesla M2090 GPUs each 512 CUDA cores, 1331 Gigaflops of the peak single precision floating point performance (FPP) / 665 Gigaflops double precision FPP, 6 GB of GDDR5 memory; (4) Dell laptop with GeForce GT555M featuring 144 CUDA cores, 3072 GB GDDR3 memory. Images are adopted from manufacturer websites and/or have a free license.

[187, 188].

It should be pointed out that .NET solutions are executed in the Common Language Runtime (CLR), the core of .NET [184]. Known as a safe managed programming environment the CLR has no direct access to GPUs and other hardware resources. Therefore, to provide the interoperability between the web front end and graphic cards the GPU-web integration component has been developed. The Component Object Model (COM) [189] and .NET interoperability have been used to provide interaction between the binaries produced by C sharp and CUDA compilers. The proposed solution allows multiple users to access GPU computational resources online within a reasonable time (in a range from a few seconds to several minutes). The developed Online Object Oriented MC (O3MC) computational tool is now available at www.biophotonics.ac.nz, and can be used for various applications in biomedical optics as well as in biophotonics and optical engineering [177].

1.4.4 Peer-to-Peer computing infrastructure for the Monte Carlo modeling tool

OOP and GPU implementations enable one to significantly speed up the MC simulation. However, due to the multi-user architecture of the online solution, concurrent simulations by multiple clients could degrade performance of O3MC. For example, if one user accessing the O3MC can get the results in 4.3 seconds on TESLA M2090 GPU, 100 users accessing O3MC at the same time can be stacked in a queue and wait for 10-15 minutes. Therefore, in framework of further development of a tool (available online at: www.biophotonics.ac.nz) to deal with the multi-user access we apply a peer-to-peer (P2P) network. A typical P2P network consists of a set of computers, called nodes or peers, which communicate and share their GPUs (Figure 1.17). The peers in a P2P network are equal among each other, acting both as clients and servers [190]. This approach has gained a lot of popularity in recent years, especially in terms of multimedia content delivery and communication (e.g. BitTorrent, Skype, etc.). With current development we, for the first time to our knowledge, apply a hybrid P2P network (Figure 1.17) utilizing different types of peers for MC simulation.

The web server hosts the online MC tool user interface, accepts O3MC simulation requests from clients and keeps track of the other nodes (Figure 1.17). The nodes are responsible for sharing the information about currently queuing MC simulations, processing them on GPUs, uploading, downloading and hosting the outcomes (presented in a typical journal-paper format) among themselves without the need of the central server. To develop the P2P Network (Figure 1.17) the recently introduced P2P features of .NET 4.0 Windows Communication Foundation (WCF) [191] were applied. This allows integrating the P2P Network with the Load Balancing part of O3MC as both are written in managed code using .NET Framework APIs [177]. Thus, a number of MC simulations can be executed simultaneously on peers without queuing. A specially developed load balancing procedure manages the number of running applications and their distribution on peers/GPUs. Further development of such a network worldwide could be a base for a computational platform for biomedical optics and optical diagnostic community.

1.5 Results of Monte Carlo Simulation

1.5.1 Validation of the technique

To validate the MC model, presented in this chapter, the results of simulations were compared to the predictions of the time-independent diffusion equation for a semi-infinite medium, given by (1.24).

The results of the spatially resolved diffuse reflectance obtained by the MC model directly agree with the results of the steady-state diffusion equation. Figure 1.18 presents a spatially resolved reflectance $R(\rho)$ plotted as a function of the radial distance ρ, where $R(\rho) = \int_0^\infty R(\rho,t)dt$ (see (1.24)). In order to provide better visualization, the simulation was also carried out for the index-matched and index-mismatched medium boundary and the results are presented in terms of natural logarithm of the reflectance multiplied by the square of the radial distance $\ln\left[\rho^2 R(\rho)\right]$ (see Fig. 1.18 b).

Values of R_ϕ, R_j, R_{eff}, C_ϕ, and C_j for typical mismatches of refractive index on the medium boundary are presented in Table 1.4.

Figure 1.19 (a) shows the comparison of time-resolved diffuse reflectance calculated by the diffusion theory, $R(t) = \int_0^\infty R(\rho,t)2\pi\rho d\rho$. Figure 1.19 (b) presents the time dependence of reflectance for a given source-detector separation $\rho = 5$ mm, $R(\rho,t)$, is calculated from the diffusion equation (1.24) and is compared against the results of the MC simulation for a semi-infinite medium with the optical parameters: $\mu_s' = 0.5$ mm^{-1}, $\mu_a = 0.02$ mm^{-1}, $g = 0.92$, $n = 1$.

Good agreement is obtained in all ranges of time. At least 10 scattering events are required

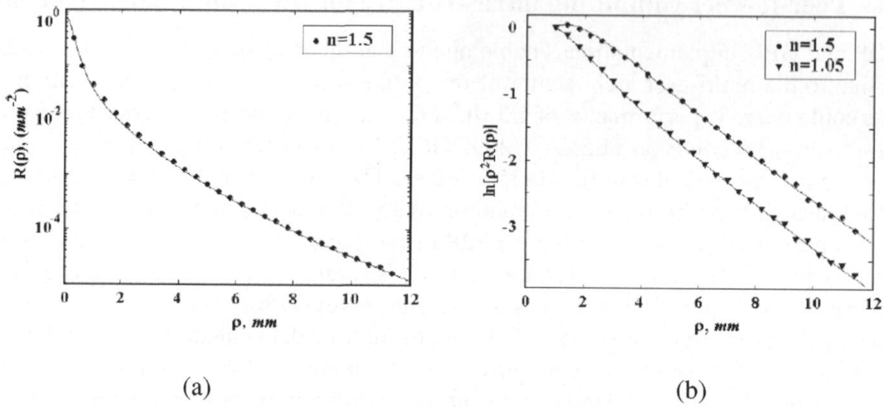

Figure 1.18: Comparison of the results from MC simulation and the diffusion theory for spatially resolved reflectance from index-mismatched interface of semi-infinite medium: (a) spatially resolved diffuse reflectance $R(\rho)$, (b) a natural logarithm of the reflectance multiplied by the square of the radial distance ρ, $\ln\left[\rho^2 R(\rho)\right]$. The symbols show the results of the MC simulation, and the solid lines are the results of the diffusion theory prediction. The optical parameters are: $\mu_s = 30$ mm^{-1}, $\mu_a = 0.01$ mm^{-1}, $g = 0.9$, $n = 1.5$ (•), and $n = 1.05$ (▼).

TABLE 1.4: $R_\phi, R_j, R_{eff}, C_\phi$, and C_j for the refractive index n of a medium, air ($n_{air} = 1$).

n	R_ϕ	R_j	R_{eff}	C_ϕ	C_j
1	0	0	0	0.25	0.5
1.05	0.1056	0.0355	0.0731	0.2236	0.4822
1.37	0.5057	0.3636	0.4679	0.1236	0.3182
1.4	0.529	0.3888	0.4935	0.1178	0.3056
1.45	0.5645	0.4281	0.5326	0.1089	0.2859
1.5	0.5964	0.4644	0.5678	0.1009	0.2678
1.55	0.625	0.4979	0.5996	0.0937	0.251

to occur before a photon can be qualified as a diffuse photon. Indeed, after 75 *ps* a photon has traveled approximately 23 mm, that for a medium of $\mu_s' = 0.5$ mm^{-1} is equivalent to approximately 10 scattering events.

The results of MC modeling are also well agreed with the theoretical predictions for diffuse reflectance and transmittance performed for an isotropic scattering slab [195]. The solution to the diffusion equation for a finite slab was taken from [195], originally derived by [13]. Albedo $a = \frac{\mu_s}{\mu_s+\mu_a}$ was taken 0.9976, and two different optical thicknesses $\tau = 10$, 20, have been considered, where $\tau = (\mu_s + \mu_a)d$ and d is thickness of a slab (Figure 1.20).

Table 1.5 shows the values for transmittance and reflectance obtained by the MC model in comparison with data tabulated by van der Hulst [192], the results of the adding-doubling method [194, 196], and the MC programs developed by van der Zee [193] and Wang et al. [69] for relative refractive index of 1, a set of four values for albedo a, and four values of a slab thickness for each albedo, respectively.

Van der Hulst [192] obtained the values for the diffuse reflectance and transmittance, for a slab illuminated with a collimated light source normally incident on the medium surface, by the doubling method, which is a representative of an adding-doubling methods family. This was done for the case

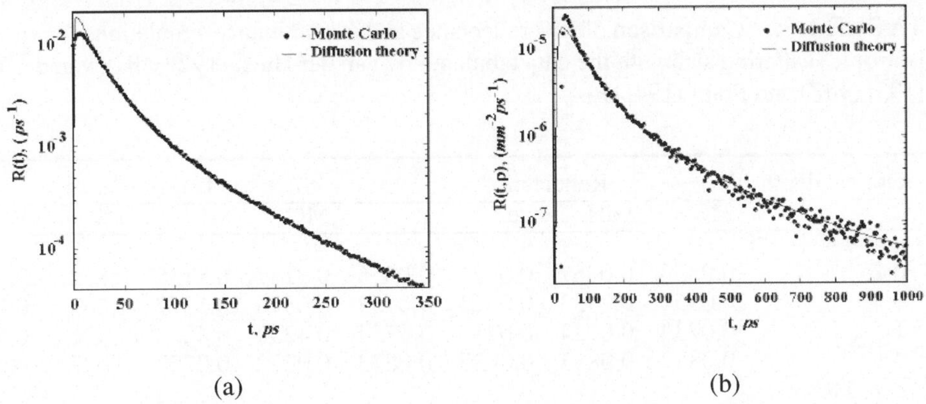

Figure 1.19: Comparison of the time-resolved results of the MC simulation with that of the diffusion equation: (a) time resolved reflectance $R(t)$, (b) time dependence at a source-detector separation $\rho = 5$ mm, $R(\rho, t)$.

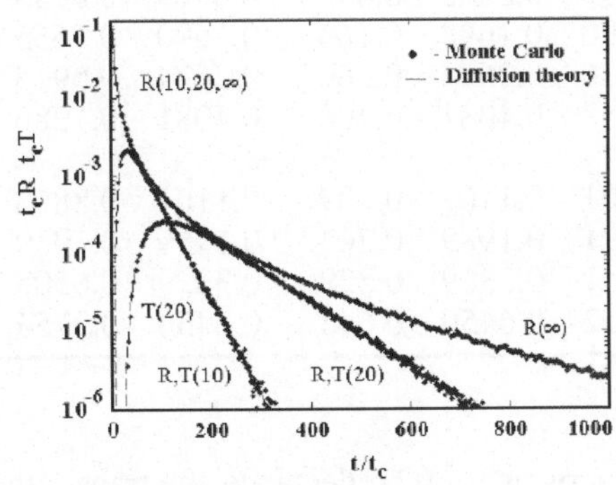

Figure 1.20: Time resolved reflectance and transmittance from an isotropic scattering slab with a plane wave pulse irradiation. Symbols are the MC results, lines are diffusion theory predictions. $R(10,20,\infty)$ and $T(10,20)$ are reflectance and transmittance for $\tau = 10$, 20, and ∞. $t_c = c^{-1}(\mu_s + \mu_a)^{-1}$.

of isotropic and anisotropic scattering, where the HG scattering phase function is used. The values are tabulated as a function of optical depth $\tau = (\mu_s + \mu_a)d$, and albedo $a = \frac{\mu_s}{\mu_s + \mu_a}$ as a parameter, where d is the slab thickness. In all calculations ten MC simulations of 10^6 photon packets each were completed to compute the average and the standard error of the total diffuse reflectance.

In Table 1.6 results are presented for the HG scattering phase function with g values of 0.5, 0.875, and for albedo $a = 0.9, 0.99$. Good agreement can be seen for all these different cases. All digits in the results are meaningful, however, the results of the van der Zee MC code are given with a varying number of accurate digits since no better data have been available to the authors.

The verification of the total diffuse reflectance was carried out for a semi-infinite scattering medium. The average and the standard error of the total diffuse reflectance were computed and compared in the table below with prediction of analytical results of [197], results of the adding-doubling method of [194], and that of the MC code (MCML) developed by [69] versus the developed MC. The medium has the following optical parameters: $\mu_s = 9$ mm^{-1}, $\mu_a = 1$ mm^{-1}, $g = 0.0$ (isotropic scattering), $n = 1.5$. The results are presented in Table 1.7.

TABLE 1.5: Comparison of MC reflectance and transmittance simulations for an isotropic scattering slab with the data tabulated by van der Hulst [192](vdH), van der Zee [193] (vdZ) and Prahl [194] (P).

Optical depth	Reflectance				Transmittance			
τ	MC	vdH	vdZ	P	MC	vdH	vdZ	P
$a = 0.4$								
0.25	0.0356	0.0357	0.037	0.0356	0.8137	0.8136	0.812	0.8136
0.5	0.0554	0.0553	0.0524	0.0553	0.6576	0.6577	0.661	0.6577
1	0.0732	0.0734	0.0716	0.0734	0.4252	0.4250	0.426	0.4251
4	0.0832	0.0833	0.0837	0.0833	0.0272	0.0272	0.0272	0.0272
$a = 0.8$								
0.25	0.0824	0.0824	0.0837	0.0824	0.8594	0.8594	0.858	0.8595
0.5	0.1402	0.1401	0.143	0.1401	0.7377	0.7378	0.734	0.7378
1	0.2108	0.2109	0.209	0.2108	0.5414	0.5414	0.544	0.5414
4	0.2842	0.2840	0.287	0.2840	0.0750	0.0751	0.0754	0.0751
$a = 0.9$								
0.25	0.0965	0.0965	0.0975	0.0965	0.8733	0.8733	0.873	0.8733
0.5	0.1690	0.1690	0.165	0.1690	0.7655	0.7653	0.771	0.7654
1	0.2676	0.2674	0.266	0.2674	0.5915	0.5916	0.594	0.5916
4	0.4082	0.4081	0.408	0.4081	0.1286	0.1285	0.126	0.1285
$a = 0.99$								
0.25	0.1101	0.1101	0.109	0.1101	0.8868	0.8867	0.886	0.8867
0.5	0.1991	0.1989	0.203	0.1989	0.7939	0.7940	0.790	0.7941
1	0.3331	0.3329	0.329	0.3329	0.6508	0.6509	0.655	0.6510
4	0.6452	0.6450	0.645	0.6450	0.2754	0.2755	0.276	0.2755

TABLE 1.6: Comparison of MC reflectance and transmittance simulations for an anisotropic scattering slab, $g = 0.5$ and $g = 0.875$ with the data tabulated by van der Hulst [192] (vdH), van der Zee [193] (vdZ) and Prahl [194] (P).

optical depth	Reflectance				Transmittance			
τ	MC	vdH	vdZ	P	MC	vdH	vdZ	P
$a = 0.9$				$g = 0.5$				
0.5	0.0720	0.0720	0.0739	0.0720	0.8672	0.8672	0.865	0.8672
1	0.1299	0.1298	0.129	0.1298	0.7390	0.7391	0.739	0.7391
4	0.2612	0.2612	0.262	0.2612	0.2505	0.2505	0.249	0.2505
$a = 0.99$				$g = 0.5$				
0.5	0.0879	0.0879	0.0874	0.0878	0.9057	0.9057	0.906	0.9057
1	0.1706	0.1707	0.169	0.1707	0.8147	0.8145	0.816	0.8145
4	0.4700	0.4698	0.467	0.4698	0.4524	0.4527	0.455	0.4527
$a = 0.9$				$g = 0.875$				
0.5	0.0125	0.0125	0.0110	0.0125	0.9354	0.9354	0.935	0.9354
1	0.0238	0.0238	0.0226	0.0238	0.8702	0.8701	0.869	0.8702
4	0.0658	0.0657	0.0650	0.0658	0.5212	0.5212	0.522	0.5212
$a = 0.99$				$g = 0.875$				
0.5	0.0157	0.0157	0.0155	0.0157	0.9789	0.9789	0.979	0.9790
1	0.0327	0.0327	0.0322	0.0327	0.9558	0.9558	0.956	0.9558
4	0.1416	0.1417	0.140	0.1417	0.8003	0.8001	0.802	0.8002

TABLE 1.7: Comparison of the total diffuse reflectance given by analytical results [197], results of the adding-doubling method [194], and MCML [69] versus the developed O3MC [177].

Source	R_d	*error*
Giovanelli [197]	0.2600	–
MCML [69]	0.25907	0.00170
Adding-doubling [194]	0.26079	0.00079
O3MC [177]	0.25957	0.00043

TABLE 1.8: Comparison of the total diffuse reflectance and transmittance given by tabulated data [192], results of the adding-doubling method [194], and MCML [69] versus the developed O3MC [177].

Source	R_d	*error*	T_d	*error*
Van der Hulst [192]	0.09739	–	0.66096	–
MCML [69]	0.09734	0.00035	0.66096	0.00020
Adding-doubling [194]	0.09711	0.00033	0.66159	0.00049
O3MC [177]	0.09741	0.00027	0.66096	0.00017

The columns R_d and *error* are the average and the standard error of the total diffuse reflectance. The average values and error were computed similarly after ten MC simulations of 50000 photon packets each. The medium has the following optical parameters: $\mu_s = 9$ mm^{-1}, $\mu_a = 1$ mm^{-1}, $g = 0.75$ (anisotropic scattering), $n = 1$, and slab thickness $d = 0.2$ mm.

1.5.2 Comparison with the human skin diffuse reflectance spectrum and color measured *in vivo*

Skin diffuse reflectance spectra was simulated by the MC technique assuming a wavelength-independent scattering coefficient for the different skin tissues and using the known wavelength dependence of the absorption coefficients of main skin tissue absorbers, such as oxy- and deoxy-hemoglobin, melanin and water (see Figure 1.8). The results of skin diffuse reflectance spectra, measured *in vivo* by the experimental setup presented in Figure 1.21, have been used to compare with the results of MC. The resulting images have been textured using a human skin surface BRDF mask (see Fig. 1.23 and Fig. 1.24). Converting the spectral power distribution to the CIE XYZ coordinates and then to the actual RGB-gamut color images is done using the standard observer/tristimulus values utilizing D65 illuminant (Figure 1.22).

The absorption properties of skin tissues in the visible and NIR spectral region were estimated by taking into account the anatomical structure of skin as determined from histology, including the spatial distribution of blood vessels, water and melanin content. Reasonable estimates for oxygen saturation (based on likely metabolic demand) and hematocrit are also included, although these parameters are less well defined than the others as they cannot be determined from post-mortem samples. It has been demonstrated that when a computational model of skin is used with reasonable physical and structural parameters, as described above, the results of skin diffuse reflectance spectra MC simulation are reasonably well-fitted with the results of *in vivo* skin spectra measurements [99].

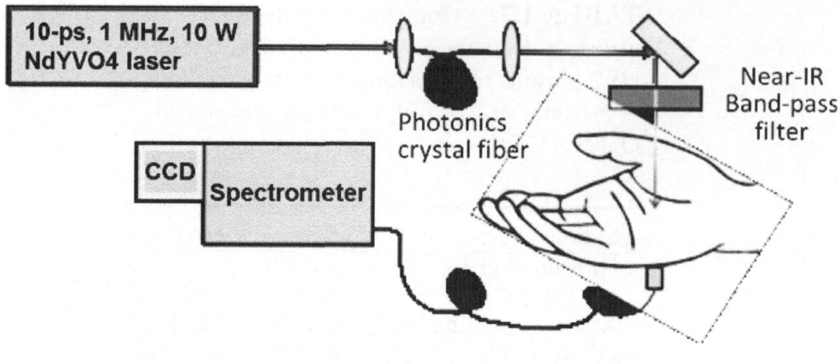

Figure 1.21: Schematic diagram of the experimental set-up. A stable white-light continuum is generated using a large-area photonic crystal fiber and using the near-IR (650-1000 nm) portion of this continuum (roughly, 0.7 W average power) for tissue illumination, while employing a TE-cooled CCD camera (Andor, Inc.) attached to a spectrometer (Horiba, Inc.) for signal detection. An 0.6-mm2-area multimode fiber bundle was used to collect light on the back of the tissue under study. For all the described measurements, the signal was corrected for a background, normalized to the incident light and averaged over 20-s to maximize the signal-to-noise-ratio.

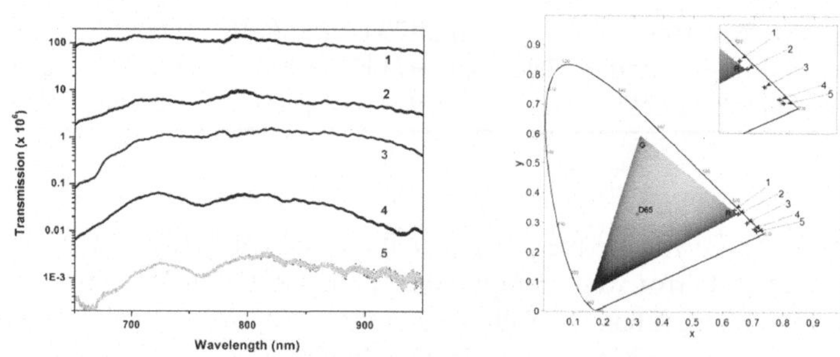

Figure 1.22: The experimental results of transmittance spectra measured for fingernail (1), finger (2), palm (3), wrist (4) and arm (5) *in vivo* (left), and corresponding chromaticity coordinates measured *in vivo* (crosses) and simulated by MC (circles) presented on the CIE 1931 color space (right, represented as gray scale).

The results of the simulation are remarkably similar to the experimentally measured skin spectra in the visible 450-600 nm. The difference in the results of the simulation and the experimental data in the NIR spectral region are explained by the choice of the optical properties of the skin layers, i.e. it was that the scattering properties of all skin layers (i.e. μ_s and g) are wavelength independent.

Thus, based on the transmittance spectra obtained for fingernail, palm, wrist and arm *in vivo*, the chromaticity coordinates are calculated and the regularities of color variation are analyzed by MC simulation. The spectral color composition of biological tissues can be used for express-analysis of their functional physiological condition and identification of the most optimal conditions for diagnostics and treatment.

1.5.3 Sampling volume

Figure 1.25 schematically presents an example of the medium with a fiber optic probe. Due to multiple scattering in the medium, optical radiation is distributed within a certain region G (see

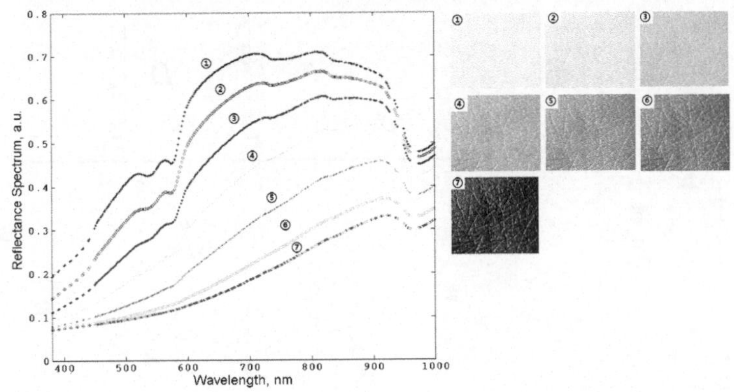

Figure 1.23: The results of MC simulation of human skin spectra (left) and corresponding colors (right, represented as gray scale) while varying the melanin content in Living epidermis.

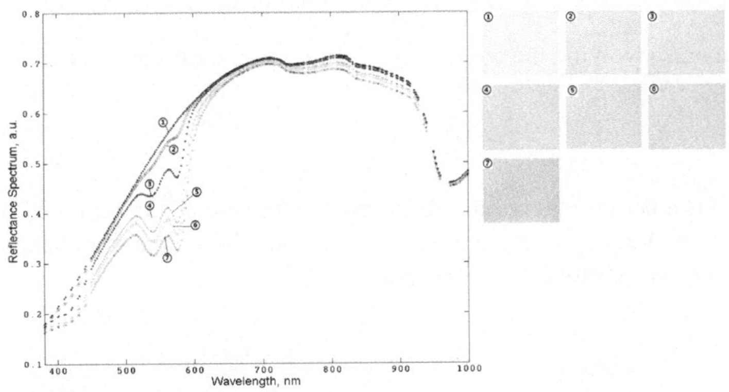

Figure 1.24: The results of MC simulation of human skin spectra (left) and corresponding colors (right, represented as gray scale) while varying the blood concentration in the layers from papillary dermis to subcutaneous tissue.

Fig. 1.25). The region G and the features of the optical radiation distributed within the medium are of predominant interest in dosimetry applications [90].

For OD applications, the spatial distribution of the detected signal (the sampling volume) J is of greater importance. The sampling volume J is formed by the so-called effective optical paths, which are those paths that photons have followed after being emitted at the source and ultimately received by the detector (Fig. 1.25). These photons can traverse many different paths between the source and the detector, some paths being more likely than others. Arridge [198] demonstrated that if represented as a function of a point $\mathbf{r}'$ *in* the medium, the sampling volume $J(\mathbf{r}')$ can be interpreted as the measure (conditional pdf) of the sensitivity of a surface measurement to the interrogated volume of a tissue located at the depth $\mathbf{r}'$. If the region $\delta V(\mathbf{r}')$ attenuates photons at rate α (due to absorption), then the measurement is perturbed, and in the limit $\alpha \to 0$, the rate change of the measurement with the perturbation is given by $J(\mathbf{r_q}, \mathbf{r_m}, \mathbf{r}')$. Note, that only photons that originally passed through $\delta V(\mathbf{r}')$ could have contributed to the change in signal measurement. Hence $J(\mathbf{r_q}, \mathbf{r_m}, \mathbf{r}')$ represents a conditional pdf with the maximum value in the region, which is the most probable origin of the detected signal.

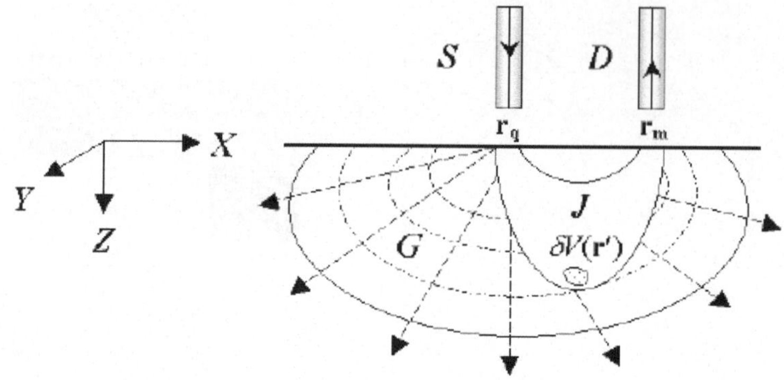

Figure 1.25: Diagram presenting the definition of sampling volume. G is the spatial distribution within semi-infinite scattering medium: J ($J \subset G$) is the spatial distribution of the effective optical paths, passed through a volume $\delta V(\mathbf{r}')$ ($\forall \mathbf{r}' \in J$), source ($S$), detector ($D$).

For experiments involving the backscattered intensity measurements $J(\mathbf{r}')$ is defined as:

$$J(\mathbf{r_q}, \mathbf{r_m}, \mathbf{r}') = \frac{\partial A(\mathbf{r_q}, \mathbf{r_m})}{\partial \mu_a(\mathbf{r}')}, \tag{1.95}$$

where $\partial \mu_a(\mathbf{r}')$ is a perturbation of the absorption coefficient at a point $\mathbf{r}'$. $\partial A(\mathbf{r_q}, \mathbf{r_m})$ is a perturbation of attenuation A at a point $\mathbf{r_m}$ of the detector, while the source of radiation is located at a point $\mathbf{r_q}$ [67, 198, 199]. Attenuation A is defined as

$$A(\mathbf{r_q}, \mathbf{r_m}) = -\ln\left(\frac{I(\mathbf{r_m})}{I_0(\mathbf{r_q})}\right). \tag{1.96}$$

Here, $I_0(\mathbf{r_q})$ is the intensity of incident radiation at a point $\mathbf{r_q}$, $I(\mathbf{r_m})$ is the intensity of the detected backscattered radiation at a point $\mathbf{r_m}$ (see Fig. 1.25). Combining (1.95) and (1.96), $J(\mathbf{r_q}, \mathbf{r_m}, \mathbf{r}')$ takes the form of

$$J(\mathbf{r_q}, \mathbf{r_m}, \mathbf{r}') = -\frac{1}{I(\mathbf{r_m})} \frac{\partial I(\mathbf{r_m})}{\partial \mu_a(\mathbf{r}')}. \tag{1.97}$$

A short form of coordinate dependence of the sampling volume is used further in the text, i.e. $J(\mathbf{r}')$ instead of $J(\mathbf{r_q}, \mathbf{r_m}, \mathbf{r}')$.

Thus, the sampling volume $J(\mathbf{r}')$ is defined as the gradient of the specific radiation flux, which is registered by the detector, with respect to the absorption coefficient $\delta V(\mathbf{r}')$ in the medium at point $\mathbf{r}'$, $\mathbf{r}' \in G$. As a function of $\mathbf{r}'$, $J(\mathbf{r}')$ characterizes the complete spatial distribution of the detected optical radiation in the medium and is determined by the spatial distribution of the effective optical paths. For a heterogeneous medium, which consists of several homogeneous components of different optical properties, e.g. seven optically homogeneous layers of skin, the partial components of the sampling volume $J_k(\mathbf{r}')$ are considered, as:

$$J_k(\mathbf{r}') = -\frac{1}{I(\mathbf{r_m})} \frac{\partial I(\mathbf{r_m})}{\partial \mu_{ak}(\mathbf{r}')}. \tag{1.98}$$

The sampling volume $J_k(\mathbf{r}')$ is equal to $< L(\mathbf{r}') >$, which is the mean "effective path length" of the photons of optical radiation traveling through a small volume $\delta V(\mathbf{r}')$ [67]. This gives a recipe for a practical implementation of numerical calculation of the sampling volume.

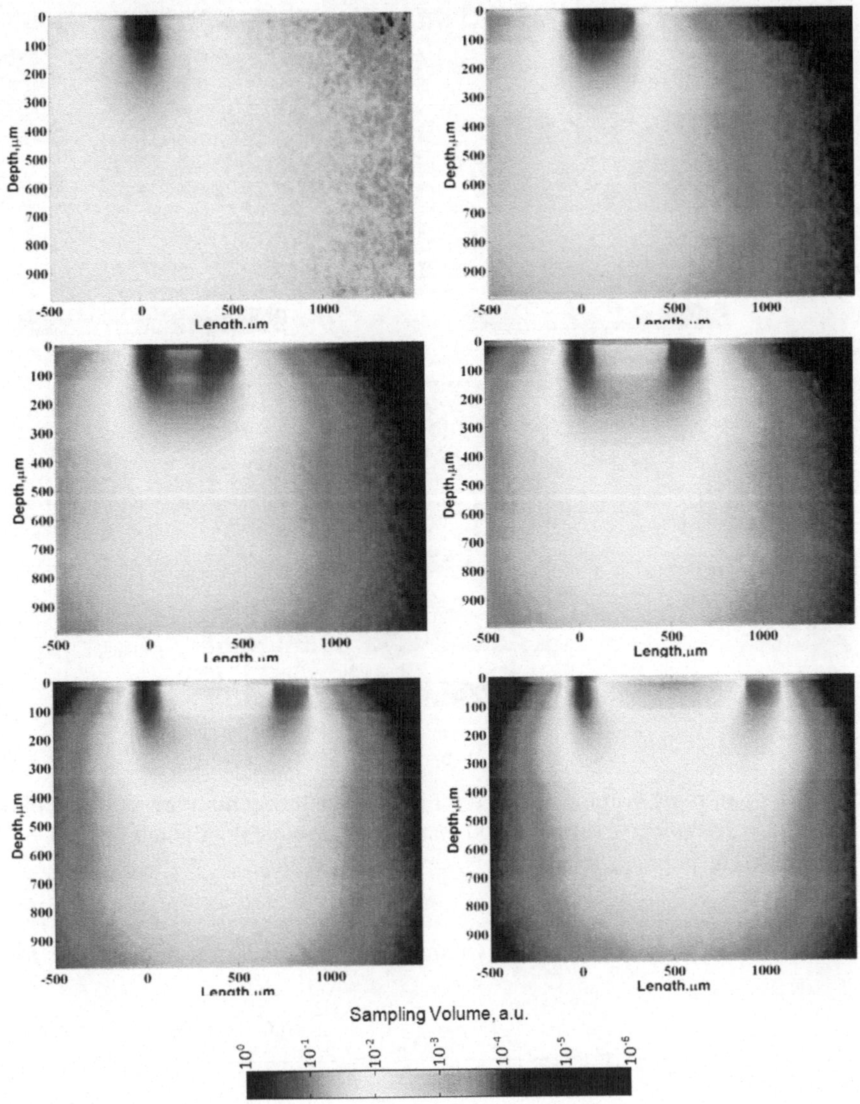

Figure 1.26: (See color insert.) The results of the MC simulation of detector depth sensitivity for a particular optical probe for human skin while varying the separation between source (200 μm) and detector (200 μm): (a) 0.0 μm, (b) 200 μm, (c) 300 μm, (d) 400 μm, (e) 600 μm, (f) 800 μm, (g) 1000 μm, respectively.

MC numerical simulation is the optimal technique for estimation of the pdf of the effective optical paths, i.e. the sampling volume. Once a photon packet is registered by the detector, its trajectory from the source to the detector is weighted by the final statistical weight. Having divided the modeling medium into pixels (e.g. $10\mu m \times 10\mu m \times 10\mu m$) and following the trajectory of each photon

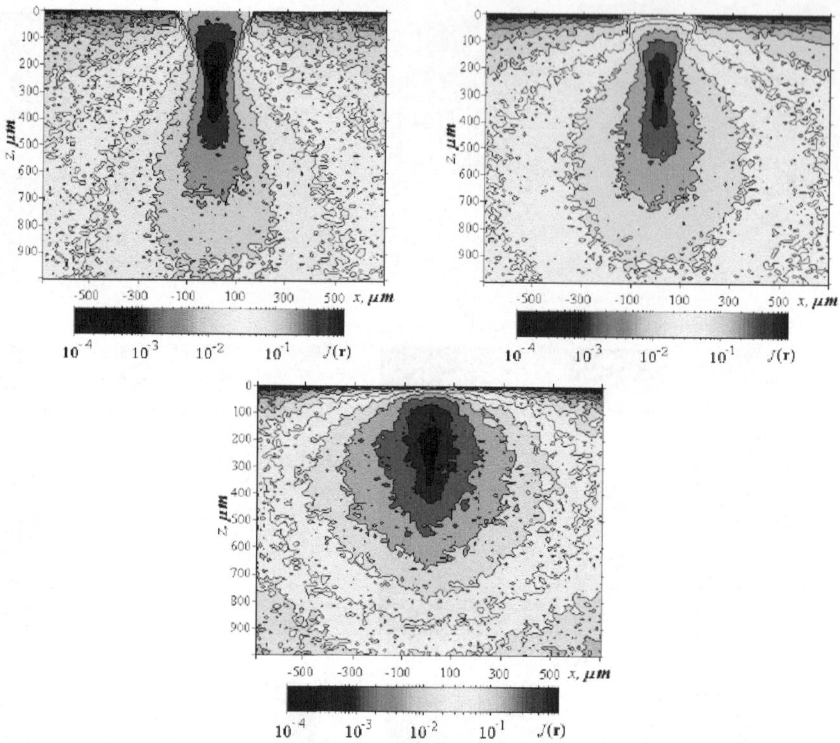

Figure 1.27: Sampling volume $J(x,z)$ for a highly scattering homogeneous medium: (a) $\mu_s = 10$ mm^{-1}; (b) $\mu_s = 26.6\ mm^{-1}$; (c) $\mu_s = 100\ mm^{-1}$. Other optical parameters are $g = 0.9$, $\mu_a = 0.01$ mm^{-1}, $n = 1.4$. The depth of focal plane $z_f = 300\ \mu$m.

packet from pixel to pixel, the sampling volume $J(\mathbf{r}')$ in a pixel is accumulated as follows:

$$J(\mathbf{r}') = -\frac{1}{I(\mathbf{r_m})}\frac{\partial I(\mathbf{r_m})}{\partial \mu_a(\mathbf{r}')} = \frac{\sum\limits_{i=1}^{N_{ph}} l_i(\mathbf{r}')W_{di}(\mathbf{r_m})}{l_0 \sum\limits_{i=1}^{N_{ph}} W_{di}(\mathbf{r_m})}. \tag{1.99}$$

Here W_{di} is the final weight of the i-th detected photon packet given by (1.46), N_{ph} is the total number of the detected photon packets, $l_i(\mathbf{r}')$ is a path length traversed by the i-th photon packet in a pixel with a center at $\mathbf{r}'$, l_0 is the size of the pixel. Finally, the sampling volume is represented by a 2D cross section map $J(x,z)$, where x is the horizontal axis and z is the depth direction. To determine the path length l_i in a pixel, the algorithm based on the Cohen-Sutherland line clipping method is implemented. The results of the sampling volume modeling for an optical probe for human skin (see the parameters in Table 1.2) are shown in Figure 1.26.

The results of numerical simulation of the sampling volume $J(x,z)$ for confocal probe [200, 201] are presented in Fig. 1.27. The parameters were taken close to those of a typical confocal scheme [202]. Optical parameters of the medium were estimated in accordance with experimental data [203] that defines the maximum penetration depth of confocal probe.

As expected, when the depth of focal plane z_f is less than 3-4 mean photon path lengths l ($\mu_s \leq 10$ mm^{-1} or $l \geq 100\ \mu$m), sampling volume $J(x,z)$ reveals a distinct region at the depth of 300 μm, where the majority of the detector photons have been focused. Increasing z_f, the depth of focal plane in the medium, up to about 8-20 mean photon path lengths l (μ_s = 26.6-40 mm^{-1} or l =

25-37.5 μm) does not affect $J(x,z)$ so that the general tendency for photon localization remains unchanged. However, in this case the contrast of the image is expected to reduce because the central focal spot has been enlarged (see Fig. 1.27 b). Increasing the depth of focal plane z_f even further ($\mu_s > 100\ mm^{-1}$ or $l < 1\ \mu$m) will result in a complete refocusing of the incident optical radiation, though it is still well focused.

These results give a perception of how the signal detected during confocal probing localizes in the homogeneous medium. They are also in agreement with the experimental data and the predications of alternative modeling techniques [61, 204, 205].

1.5.4 Fluorescence

Earlier MC schemes of fluorescence modeling consist of the three simulation steps [206, 207, 208, 209]. First, the fluence rate distribution within a tissue volume is calculated by the standard MC scheme [63, 69]. At the second step, spatial fluorescence distribution is obtained by multiplying the fluence rate distribution by the intrinsic fluorescence profile, which is defined as the product of the absorption coefficient of the fluorophore at the excitation wavelength and its quantum yield at the emission wavelength. Finally, the detected fluorescence is calculated as the convolution of the fluorescence source distribution throughout the tissue with the Green's function. In the framework of this model, the intensity of the simulated local fluorescence is proportional to the fraction of the absorbed energy that is determined by the quantum yield of the fluorophore. The fluorescence source distribution within the medium is mainly dependent on the fluence rate distribution. Crille et al. [210] employed the MC fluorescence forward-adjoin model. This MC scheme utilizes the solution of a transport equation both in forward (excitation photon) and in adjoin (fluorescent photon) calculations. The solution of the adjoin transport equation is obtained for those fluorescence photons that contribute to the detected fluorescence signal.

Another scheme of an independent simulation of the fluorescence acts has been proposed [211]. In this approach, the emission of the fluorescence photons occurs at the scattering sites and the quantum yield of a fluorophore γ serves as the fluorescence threshold probability (Figure 1.28 a). The intensity of simulated fluorescence is defined by the fraction of the absorbed radiation $W_{i-1} - W_i$ (see Fig. 1.28 a). In a more plausible model of fluorescence simulation [212, 213], the fluorophore absorption μ_{af} is separated from the total medium/layer absorption by the standard rejection scheme based on the fluorophore absorption threshold $P_a = (1 - \exp(-\mu_{af} l_i))$ (Fig. 1.28 b). Here, the intensity of generated fluorescence is equal to the product of the quantum yield and the intensity of the incident radiation, γW_{i-1}. In this model, each photon packet produces only one fluorescence photon. Both models have assumed that the fluorescence is emitted uniformly from the scattering sites in random directions (see Fig. 1.28 a, b).

A possibility to incorporate in MC spatial distribution of fluorescence has been suggested in [166, 214]. The fluorescence excitation is determined as:

$$W_{em}(\mathbf{r}) = W(\mathbf{r}) P_a P_\rho P_\gamma, \tag{1.100}$$

where $W(\mathbf{r})$ is the photon weight at a point $\mathbf{r}$ and is equal to the probability that the photon packet has reached a point $\mathbf{r} = \mathbf{r}(x,y,z)$ in the medium; P_a is the probability of the photon packet absorption at the i-th step; P_ρ is the probability of absorption by the fluorophore non-uniformly distributed within the medium; P_γ is the probability of the fluorescence excitation determined by the fluorophore quantum yield γ. The probabilities P_a, P_ρ, P_γ are calculated by the standard rejection scheme [72]. In contrast to the models [206–213] (Fig. 1.28 a and b), where fluorescence is emitted between scattering events, following spatial distribution of fluorophores in tissues (Figure 1.29), e.g. collagen distribution for autofluorescence [166, 214].

spatial distribution of the fluorophores is described as $\cos(k\rho)\cos(kz)$, where $k = \pi/d$; d is the collagen fiber diameter; $\rho = \rho(x,y)$ and z are the coordinates of a point in the medium. The non-homogeneous distribution of fluorescence within the dermal layers is clearly illustrated in the ex-

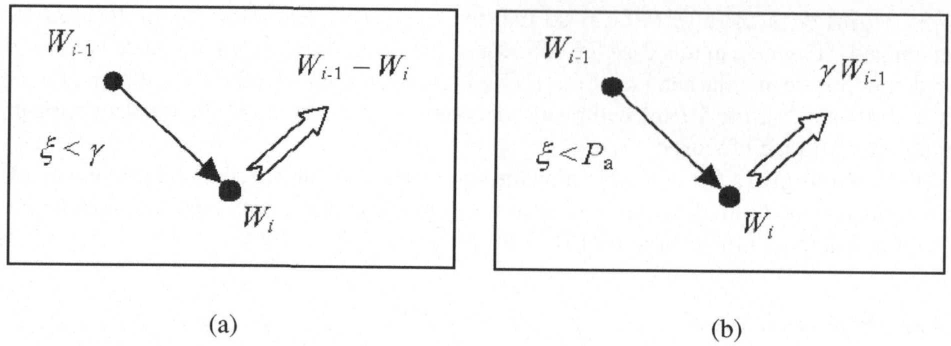

Figure 1.28: Schematic representation of the MC fluorescence simulation: (a) the fluorescence probability is determined by quantum yield γ of a fluorophore [211]; (b) each fluorescence event is determined by the probability of the photon packet absorption $P_a = (1 - \exp(-\mu_{af} l_i))$ [212, 213]. W_{i-1} and W_i are the statistical photon weights at the $(i-1)$-th and i-th steps of the photon packet; μ_{af} is the fluorophore absorption coefficient; l_i is the path length of a photon between the scattering events; $\xi\,(0 \leq \xi \leq 1)$ is the uniformly distributed random number used in the rejection scheme.

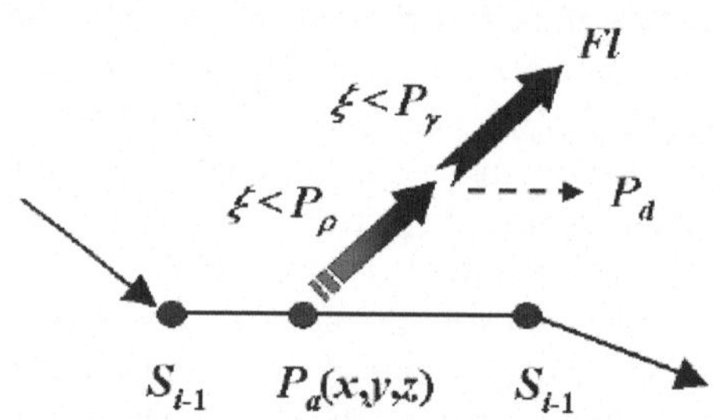

Figure 1.29: Schematic representation of the fluorescence modeling: P_a is probability of the photon packet absorption between two scattering sites S_{i-1} and S_i; P_r is the probability of the absorption by the fluorophore; P_γ is the probability of the fluorophore fluorescence determined by the fluorophore quantum yield γ; $P_d = (1 - P_\gamma)$ is the probability of dissipation determining a fraction of absorbed energy exerted non-radiative relaxation through other mechanisms, e.g. thermal excitation or phosphorescence, etc.; $\rho\,(x, y, z)$ determines spatial fluorophore distribution within the medium.

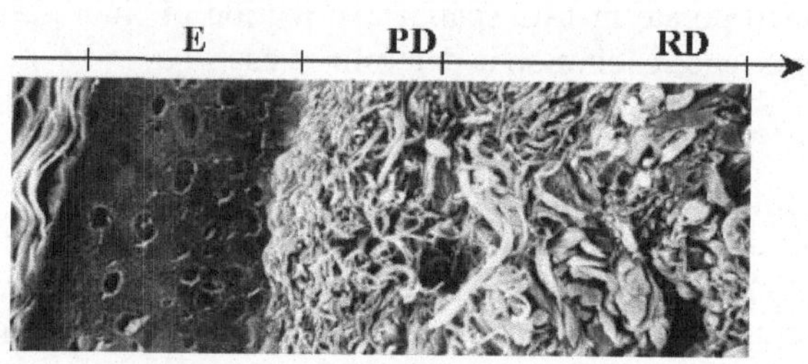

Figure 1.30: The scanning electron micrograph taken from [215] shows the arrangement of collagen fibers in the dermis (with permission). Fiber bundle diameters and density of packing in the papillary dermis (PD) and reticular dermis (RD) are different. Collagen is organized in long, wavy bundles, which vary in diameter from about 1-40 μm. Collagen bundles interweave in a complex and random manner to form a three-dimensional irregular meshwork [107, 216].

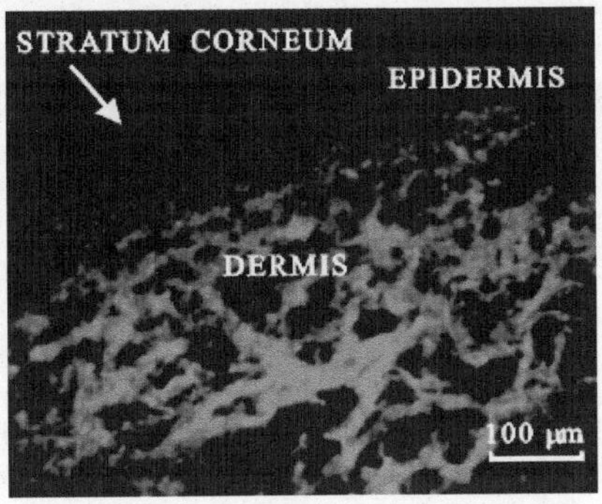

Figure 1.31: Experimental autofluorescence image of skin tissue section under illumination of 442 nm laser radiation. (Courtesy of Dr. H. Zeng, from [208]. With permission).

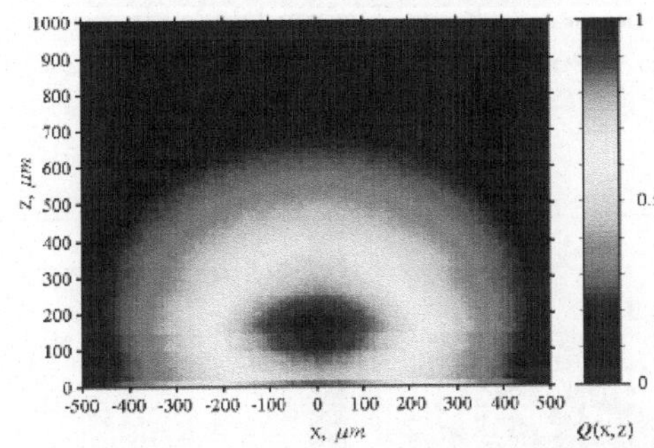

Figure 1.32: Two-dimensional distributions of the spatial depth sensitivity $Q(x,z)$. The optical parameters of skin layers were chosen for 488 nm. The fractions of fluorescence that are sensitive to sensor and topical dermal layers are close. The diameter and numerical aperture of detector are equal to $D = 1000\ \mu$m and $NA = 0.63$; acceptance angle $\theta_d = \sin^{-1}(NA/n_0) = 40^0$.

perimental images of autofluorescence of human skin (Figure 1.31), whereas the distribution of fluorophores in the stratum corneum and the epidermis seems to be homogeneous [208].

The fluorescence photons are emitted isotropically from the source points, which agrees with the assumptions proposed in earlier works [206–213].

The spatial distribution of fluorescence excitation is accumulated as a set of coordinates (x,y,z) and photon weights W_{em}. The fluorescence photons are emitted until the necessary number of photon packets collected by a detector is achieved. The MC method is employed to propagate fluorescence photons, however, new values of the optical parameters corresponding to emission wavelength are used.

To express the sensitivity of a surface measurement (a detection system) to interrogated volume of the tissue the detector depth sensitivity (the sampling volume) is employed. Here, the sampling volume $Q(\mathbf{r})$ is defined as the gradient of fluorescent radiation density with respect to the absorption coefficient of a small region of medium at the point **r**.

The described MC model has been applied to assess spatial distribution of both skin tissue autofluorescence and fluorescence excitation of the smart "tattoo" sensor layer. Optical parameters of skin tissues used in the simulation are shown in [166, 214].

Additional MC simulation was carried out to illustrate how the localization of fluorescence excitation and the sampling volume are affected by excitation at longer wavelength. For this case the

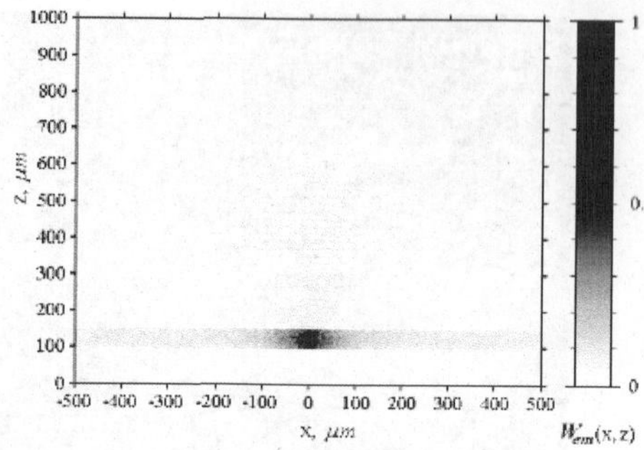

Figure 1.33: Spatial distribution $W_{em}(x,z)$ of the fluorescence excitation of the "tattoo" sensor layer and autofluorescence excitation in human skin in the near infrared spectral region. Excitation of autofluorescence in the dermal layers is highly ($\sim$ 4-5 times) suppressed due to the low fluorescence efficiency of natural fluorophores in the near infrared spectral region. The main fluorescence excitation is localized in the sensor layer. The modeled skin tissue's optical properties were chosen for 700 nm. The diameter of source is equal to 200 μm. The incident beam has a uniform geometry profile.

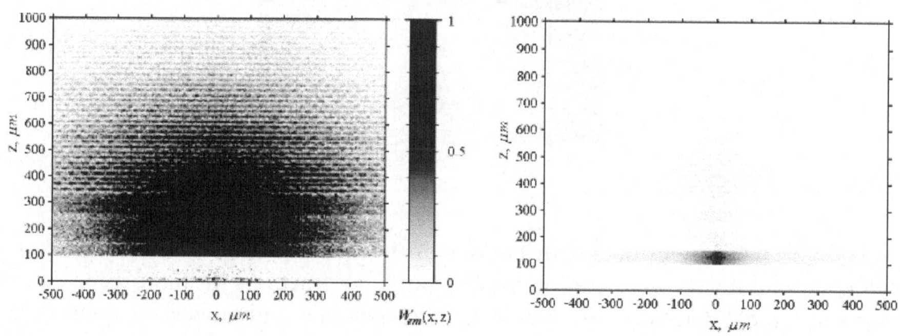

(a) (b)

Figure 1.34: Spatial distribution of the fluorescence excitation for the refractive index matching ($n = 1.5$): (a) - visible spectral region 488 nm; (b) - near infrared spectral region 700 nm.

modeled skin tissue's optical properties were chosen for 700 nm. Due to the monotonically decreasing scattering of skin tissue with wavelength in the range 450-1100 nm [68, 114] the scattering coefficients μ_s are reduced by a factor of 2–3, whereas the absorption coefficients of the skin layers are taken to be a factor of ten less [90]. Scattering of the sensor layer was believed to be close to that of the epidermis, while its absorption coefficient was taken unchanged, that presumed the usage of the near infrared fluorophore [217]. The low fluorescence efficiency of endogenous fluorophores in the near infrared spectral region [218] was simulated by their reduced absorption; quantum yields of biotissues were kept unchanged.

The results of the simulation are presented in Figure 1.33. The results show that excitation of autofluorescence in the dermal layers is highly ($\sim$ 4-5 times) suppressed due to the low fluorescence efficiency of natural fluorophores in the near infrared spectral region [218] and the main fluorescence excitation is localized in the sensor layer. Nevertheless, the periodic structure of fluorescence excitation in the dermal layers is still observed.

The MC technique has been applied for modeling the fluorescence excitation and assessing of the sampling volume within the skin. The simulation results show that the maximum of the fluorescence excitation sources is localized in the topical dermal and in the "smart" sensor ("tattoo") layers. Spatial distribution of the fluorescence excitation within dermal layers demonstrates a good correlation to experimental autofluorescence image of skin tissue. When moving to the near infrared spectral region, the fraction of the autofluorescence excitation is significantly reduced and the sampled area is predominately localized in the "tattoo" sensor layer. Refractive index matching at skin interface produces a remarkable enhancement of the sampling volume localization. The maximum of the detector depth sensitivity is shifted to the "tattoo" sensor layer and moves away from the stratum corneum and the epidermis. The simulations have revealed a general tendency of optical/fluorescence measurements to localism in a small shallow volume in the "tattoo" sensor layer. It is concluded that the results of this study accompanied by recent progress in biophotonics can be beneficial to a number of applications aimed towards medical diagnostics and general physiological studies.

1.5.5 Coherent effects and polarization

The MC method has been extensively used to simulate the coherent effects of multiple scattering including temporal field correlation function, the CBS intensity and the helicity flip of circularly polarized light [135, 137, 168, 169, 219–224]. For a semi-infinite isotropic, scattering, and non-absorbing medium, the intensity of single and double scattered photons can be estimated analytically:

$$\begin{aligned} I_{single} &= l^{-1} \int dz_1 \int d\mathbf{R}_2 \delta(\mathbf{R}_2 - \mathbf{R}_1) \exp(-\frac{2z_1}{l}) = 1/2, \\ I_{double} &= (4\pi)^{-1} l^{-2} \int dz_1 \int d\mathbf{R}_2 \Lambda_0(\mathbf{R}_2 - \mathbf{R}_1) \exp(-\frac{z_1 + z_2}{l}) = \ln\sqrt{2}, \end{aligned} \tag{1.101}$$

where z_1 and z_2 are the distance from the scattering points. For isotropic scattering the phase function $p_0(\mathbf{k}_i - \mathbf{k}_s) = \frac{1}{4\pi}$. Moreover, for isotropic scattering an exact Milne solution is available that, for example, gives the ratio of the diffuse reflectance and intensity of the single scattered photons $I/I_{single} = 8.455$ [20]. Several MC simulations have been carried out to define the cut-off criterion, i.e. the minimal weight, maximum number of scattering events, etc. Accuracy of not less than 4 significant digits has been achieved for $N_{ph} = 10^5$, $N_{max\ scat} = 5000$, and $W_{min} = 10^{-3}$.

The results of calculation of the temporal field correlation functions for scattering media with different anisotropy factors $g = 0, 0.5$ and 0.9 are presented in Figure 1.35. The optical properties of a medium are: $\mu_s = 30$ mm^{-1}, $\mu_a = 0$, $n = 1$. Thus, the transport of mean free path lengths (MFPs) are $l^* = l/(1-g) = 33.3\ \mu m$, 66.6 μm and 333.3 μm for isotropic $g = 0$, intermediate $= 0.5$ and highly anisotropic $g = 0.9$ scattering media. A semi-infinite medium and a slab of thickness $L = l^*$ are considered.

The obtained results (Fig. 1.35) are reasonably well described by the analytical formula derived from the diffusion approximation [133, 148]:

$$g_1(\tau) \propto \frac{\sinh(\alpha[L + \eta_1 - \eta_0])}{\sinh(\alpha[L + 2\eta_1])}, \tag{1.102}$$

where $\alpha = (3t/(\tau l^{*2}))^{1/2}$, $\eta_0 = l^*$ is the depth at which the incident light is completely diffused, $\eta_1 \approx (2/3)l^*$ is the extrapolated boundary length. Since the influence of the factor of anisotropy g decreases as a slab becomes thicker, there is a tendency for a better agreement between the results of the MC simulation and predictions of the diffusion theory (Fig. 1.35). This was ascribed to the diminishing role of lower order scattering events, which cannot be properly accounted for within the diffusion theory. Nevertheless, the general tendency of independence on the anisotropy factor g is as obvious for a semi-infinite medium as for a slab. Deviation from the expected linear decay at

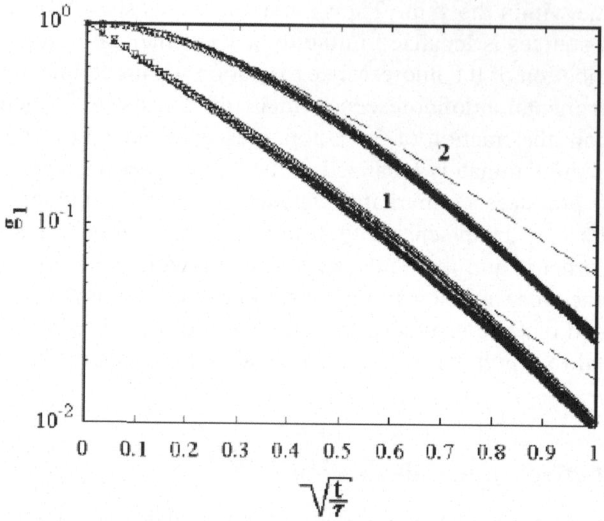

Figure 1.35: The normalized temporal field correlation functions $g_1(t)$ for backscattering radiation versus $(t/\tau)^{1/2}$: semi-infinite medium (1), a slab of thickness $L = l/(1-g)$ (2). Different factors of anisotropy are considered (□) – isotropic $g = 0$, (•) – intermediate $g = 0.5$, and (△) – high anisotropic $g = 0.9$. Dashed lines are approximation (1.102) for a semi-infinite medium and a slab. The optical properties of a medium are: $\mu_s = 30$ mm^{-1}, $\mu_a = 0$, $n = 1$.

some time is attributed to the effect of limited number of longer photon paths, which is a result of finite computation time. In time, the contribution of longer paths diminishes, and the requirement of a large number of long-path photons becomes less strict.

The CBS intensity peak is simulated for the same isotropic, intermediate and high anisotropy semi-infinite scattering media. The results of the MC simulation for isotropic scattering show that h^{CBS} = 1.87, that agrees very well with the results derived from the generalized solution of the Milne problem: h^{CBS} = 1.88 [20]. In limit of $g \to 1$ the theory predicts $h^{CBS} \to 2$, that corresponds with the results of the MC simulation $h^{CBS} = 1.99$ for $g = 0.9$.

Expressed in terms of the dimensionless parameter $\tilde{q} = kl^* \sin\theta_s$, the simulated angular dependence of the CBS exposes typical behavior, indicating that it is practically independent of anisotropy (Fig. 1.36). The results of simulation are compared against the results predicted by the analytical approach [225]:

$$I^{(1)}_{CBS} = \exp(-\gamma kl^* \sin\theta_s) \tag{1.103}$$

or in its linear approximation:

$$I^{(2)}_{CBS} = 1 - \gamma kl^* \sin\theta_s, \tag{1.104}$$

where $\gamma \approx 2$ is the relative slope of the CBS decay (Fig. 1.36). The results of simulation also indicate a universal decreasing trend, whereas the diffusion approximation predicts that the CBS peak falls down with different slope values for different values of the anisotropy factor. Notice that this dependence strongly disagrees with the predictions of the diffusion approximation [138]:

$$I^{(diff)}_{CBS} \propto 1 - 2\frac{(1+z^*)^2}{1+2z^*} kl^* \sin\theta_s, \tag{1.105}$$

which yields the slope $\gamma^{(diff)} \approx 2.3$ for $g = 0$ and $\gamma^{(diff)} \approx 0.71$ for $g \to 1$, where $z^* = 0.71(1-g)^{-1}$ is the Milne extrapolation parameter [226]. To some extent, the results obtained also demonstrate

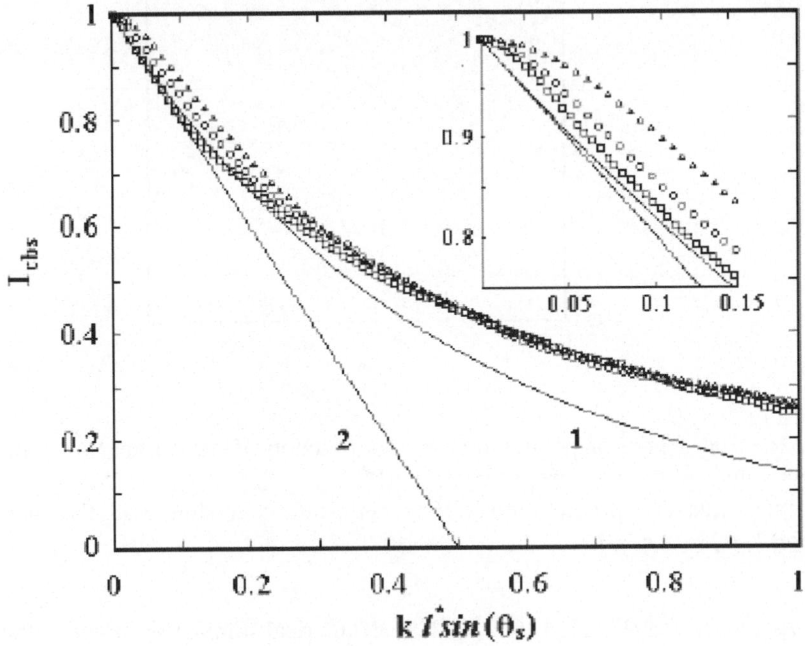

Figure 1.36: The peak of the CBS intensity (I_{CBS}) as a function of $kl^* \sin\theta_s$: (□) – $g = 0$, (○) – $g = 0.5$; (▲) – $g = 0.9$. Solid lines present: (1) – (1.103) and (2) – (1.104) with slope $\gamma = 2$. The optical properties of a medium are: $\mu_s = 30$ mm^{-1}, $\mu_a = 0$, $n = 1$; $\lambda = 0.6$ μm.

the decrease in the CBS slope with the increase in the anisotropy factor g as seen in the inset of Figure 1.36.

[138] have made a conjecture that for both states of polarization the corresponding intensities (1.81) can be represented as a product of the intensity of a scalar field and two multiplicative factors (weighting functions) describing the polarization transfer. These factors (functions) are specific for a given polarization state and generally depend on the properties of scattering particles, e.g. size, shape [138, 161]. Experimental results for the study of time scales involved into depolarization process of the backscattered light have proved the adequacy of the Akkermans' conjecture [164]. For isotropic scattering, after n scattering events the degree of polarization ratio also called residual polarization is given by [138]:

$$P(n) = \frac{I_{pol}(n) - I_{depol}(n)}{I_{pol}(n) + I_{depol}(n)} = \frac{3(0.7)^{n-1}}{2+(0.7)^{n-1}}. \tag{1.106}$$

Figure 1.37 illustrates the degree of polarization P as a function of the number of scattering events n for different values of the anisotropy factor g. The degree of polarization P has indeed an exponential decay as demonstrated in Figure 1.37, however, the decay slope is less than predicated by the diffusion approximation for anisotropic media. Increasing the anisotropy factor leads to increase of the characteristic polarization length [138, 227] since at higher g a photon has to scatter more by a factor $(1-g)^{-1}$ to change its direction. As a consequence (1.79), the polarization vector changes at a slower rate.

To verify the results of simulation, they are compared against the exact solutions for point-like Rayleigh scatters. For Rayleigh scatters, normal incidence and exact backscattering detection, the generalized Milne solution for electromagnetic field gives the ratio of polarized and depolarized

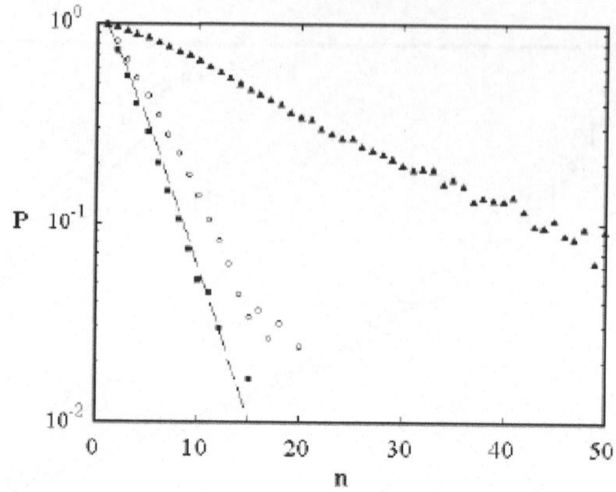

Figure 1.37: The degree of polarization P as a function of the number of scattering events n for different values of the anisotropy factor g: (■) – $g = 0$, (○) – $g = 0.5$; (▲) – $g = 0.9$. Solid line represents diffusion approximation (1.106). Semi-infinite medium with the optical parameters: $\mu_s = 30\ \text{mm}^{-1}$, $\mu_a = 0$, $n = 1$.

intensities $I_{pol}/I_{depol} \approx 1.92$ [19, 136, 228, 229]. Numerical stimulation suggests that $I_{pol}/I_{depol} =$ 1.94 with all significant digits. An alternative to the degree of polarization P is the (full-intensity) depolarization ratio of the backscattered intensities:

$$d = \frac{I_{pol} - I_{depol}}{I_{pol} + I_{depol}}. \tag{1.107}$$

The generalized Milne solution gives $d = 0.31$ [19, 136, 228, 229], while simulation results suggested $d = 0.326$. Notice that numerically close value $d = 0.33$ was obtained by Rojas-Ochoa et al. [227].

Peak maximum of the polarized CBS intensity is defined as

$$h_{pol}^{CBS} = \frac{2I_{pol} - I_{single}}{I_{pol}}. \tag{1.108}$$

Theoretically predicted value for h_{pol}^{CBS} is 1.75 [19, 136, 228, 229]. Iwai et al. [132] have estimated the value of peak maximum of the polarized CBS intensity by numerical MC simulation and have found $h_{pol}^{CBS} = 1.4$. A value $h_{pol}^{CBS} = 1.69$ was found by Lenke and Maret [130]. The developed MC method gave $h_{pol}^{CBS} = 1.746$ that is in excellent agreement with the theory.

Figure 1.38 demonstrates the simulation results of the temporal field correlation functions of polarized and depolarized components for Rayleigh scatters, $g = 0$, and for a strongly anisotropic scattering medium, $g = 0.9$. Clearly, polarization effects modify the path-length distribution and therefore strongly influence the decay of the temporal field correlation function.

As compared to the temporal field correlation function for scalar field (Fig. 1.35), a strong dependence of the correlation function on the anisotropy factor is observed (Fig. 1.38). Similar dependence of the simulation results on g was demonstrated by Rojas-Ochoa et al. [227]. Interestingly, the shape of $g_{pol}^{(1)}(t)$ and $g_{depol}^{(1)}(t)$ is similar to the shape of $g_1(t)$ (Fig. 1.35).

The diffusion nature of optical radiation propagation in multiple scattering media results in a linear decay of the temporal correlation function $g_{(1)}(t)$ in the limit $\sqrt{6t/\tau} \ll 1$, $g_{(1)}(t) \sim 1 - \gamma\sqrt{6t/\tau}$, where γ is the slope ([142, 144]). Notice that according to (1.74) and (1.75), in the case of strong anisotropy, $1 - g \ll 1$, the factor $(t/\tau)(l/l^*)$ is still small enough, even if $t/\tau \sim 1$, when $g_{(1)}(t)$ as a function of $\sqrt{t/\tau}$ does not exhibit linear behavior.

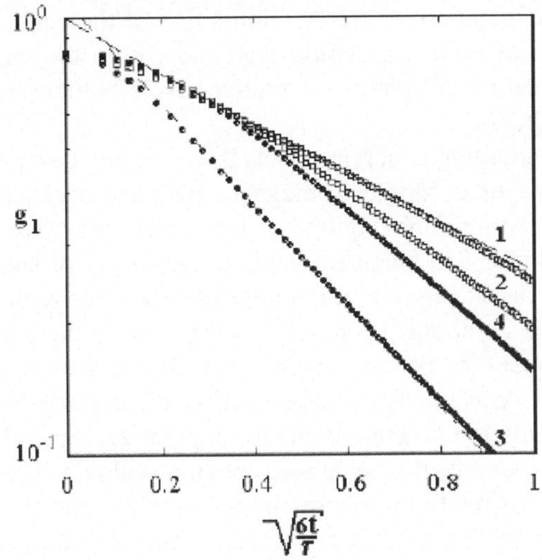

Figure 1.38: Temporal field correlation function of electromagnetic field: isotropic scattering medium, $g = 0$, (□) – $g^{(1)}_{pol}(t)$ (1) and (•) – $g^{(1)}_{depol}(t)$ (3); anisotropic scattering medium, $g = 0.9$, (□) – $g^{(1)}_{pol}(t)$ (2) and (•) – $g^{(1)}_{depol}(t)$ (4). Dashed lines demonstrate the slopes $\gamma_{pol} \approx 1.42$ of $g^{(1)}_{pol}(t)$ and $\gamma_{depol} \approx 2.68$ of $g^{(1)}_{depol}(t)$ for an isotropic scattering medium. Semi-infinite medium with the optical parameters: $\mu_s = 30$ mm^{-1}, $\mu_a = 0$, $n = 1$.

For Rayleigh scatters theoretical predictions of the slope for the polarized temporal correlation function $g^{(1)}_{pol}(t)$ and for the depolarized temporal correlation function $g^{(1)}_{depol}(t)$ are $\gamma_{pol} \approx 1.44$ and $\gamma_{depol} \approx 2.75$, respectively [19, 136]. Diffusion approximation yields $\gamma_{pol} \approx 1.6$ and $\gamma_{depol} \approx 2.7$ [162], which are close to experimental data $\gamma_{pol} \approx 1.6 \pm 0.1$? $\gamma_{depol} \approx 2.8 \pm 0.2$. These experimental results were obtained for suspension of latex particles with diameter of $a = 0.091$ μm, that is far less than the wavelength 488 nm, which implies Rayleigh scattering in the suspension.

Note that similar to the experiment conducted by [144], a deviation from a linear behavior is observed for small value of $\sqrt{t/\tau}$. It is explained by a finite numerical aperture and small statistics of photons with a large number of scattering events. In Figure 1.38, linear parts of $g^{(1)}_{pol}(t)$ and $g^{(1)}_{depol}(t)$ start from $\sqrt{t/\tau} \approx 0.15$, and have slopes $\gamma_{pol} \approx 1.42$ and $\gamma_{depol} \approx 2.68$, respectively. Increasing the anisotropy factor g increases γ_{pol} and decreases γ_{depol}.

Cycle diagrams related to the interferential component of backscattering [136, 230] and diagrams related to the field correlation effects [161] can be represented as ladder diagrams within the theory of coherent effects in multiple scattering [137]. This allows one to employ the Bethe-Salpeter equation to describe coherent effects of electromagnetic or scalar fields. A formal difference from the original ladder diagrams related to the main non-coherent component of the scattered field is an additional factor in the vertexes of ladder diagrams. This factor describes the phase shift of the fields which are part of the propagator of the Bethe-Salpeter equation (1.57).

Using a combination of the stochastic MC technique and the iteration procedure of the solution to the Bethe-Salpeter equation, a numerical method has been developed for stochastic modeling of coherent effects in a multiple scattering medium. It has been shown that additional phase-related factors in the ladder diagrams are equivalent in the stochastic modeling to multiplication of the statistical weights by corresponding factors after each scattering event during the random walk of a photon packet.

The MC technique is generalized for the simulation of the coherent backscattering and temporal correlation function of optical radiation scattered within the randomly inhomogeneous turbid medium. The developed model yields qualitative results which are ready for direct comparison against theoretical predictions.

Multiple scattering including coherent effects is commonly described in terms of scalar field. As a result of the study presented, for electromagnetic field and backscattering geometry a completely different quantitative description is required to account for the wave nature of light as compared to the case of the scalar field. The main reason is the presence of significant contribution of lower-order scattering in the backscattered radiation [138]. The decay of the temporal field correlation function of the polarized component is much less than that of the scalar field. At the same time, for the depolarized component the decay is bigger than that of scalar field. Intensity of the polarized component is almost twice as much as the intensity of the depolarized component.

As compared to attenuation measurements for unpolarized optical radiation which give estimate of the photon transport length, the developed method yields some extra useful information. For example, it is possible to relate the degree of polarization and the number of scattering events. To conclude, the developed method introduces a possibility for a less sophisticated modeling of radiation transfer (coherent and field correlation effects) in such multiple scattering media as liquid crystals, biological tissues, etc.

1.5.6 Modeling of OCT images

MC modeling of the OCT images of skin in non-, co- and cross-polarized modes was performed in [150, 153]. Instrumental parameters used in simulation are taken in accordance with the characteristics of the reference experimental cross-polarization OCT setup. The incidence of radiation at the surface of turbid medium is considered normal. This situation corresponds to the case of collimated probing beam. The case when imaging is performed with the focused Gaussian-shaped probing beam which beam waist is located at some depth inside the medium can be simulated using, for example, the ray-optics approach proposed in [231]. For simulation of an A-scan 50,000 photons were employed; 50 A-scans were obtained to construct each 2D OCT image.

Simulated OCT images of skin in non-polarized mode were implemented without account for speckle effects as presented in Figure 1.39 for four various values of coherence lengths.

Introduction of "speckle effects" into the Monte Carlo simulation process with accordance to expression causes additional noise observed in the obtained OCT images for all considered coherence length values (see Figure 1.40). These results are in qualitative agreement with the images simulated without account of the "speckle noise," which on the one hand confirms the adequacy of the proposed algorithm and on the other hand demonstrates its ability for quantitative study of "speckle effects" in OCT image formation. In experimental setups "speckle effects" are usually reduced by spatial averaging of the signal and additional numerical processing.

Figure 1.41 demonstrates the simulated OCT images obtained in non-, co- and cross- polarization modes correspondingly. These images qualitatively agree with the experimental ones. Note that both experimental and simulated images obtained in cross-polarization mode demonstrate the same features: relatively low signal from the top boundary and bright epidermis layer. However, the simulated cross-polarization mode image exhibits lower absolute intensity compared to the experimental one which possibly originates from the assumption of soft scatterers. In reality the rate of depolarization appears to be higher compared to the value accounted in the simulations.

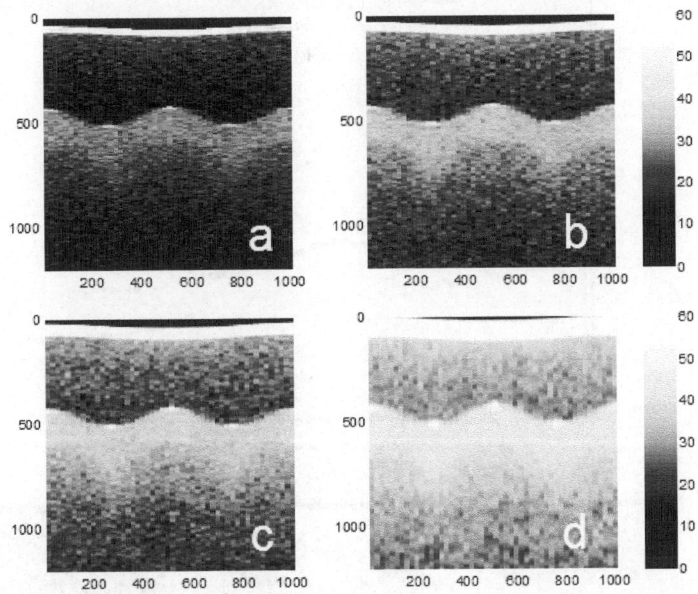

Figure 1.39: Simulated 2D OCT images of skin without account for speckle effects for various coherence lengths of low-coherent light source: 5 μm (a), 10 μm (b), 15 μm (c), 30 μm (d).

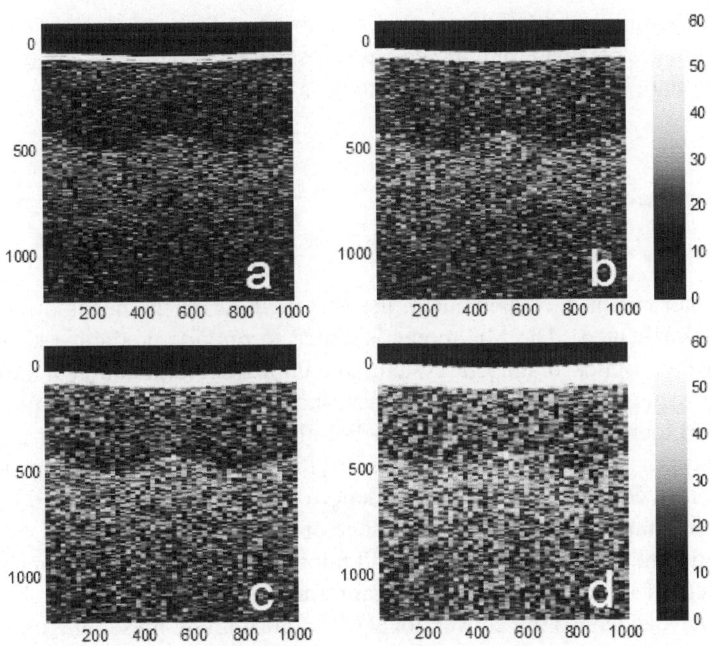

Figure 1.40: Simulated 2D OCT images of skin with account for "speckle effects" for various coherence lengths of low-coherent light source: 5 μm (a), 10 μm (b), 15 μm (c), 30 μm (d).

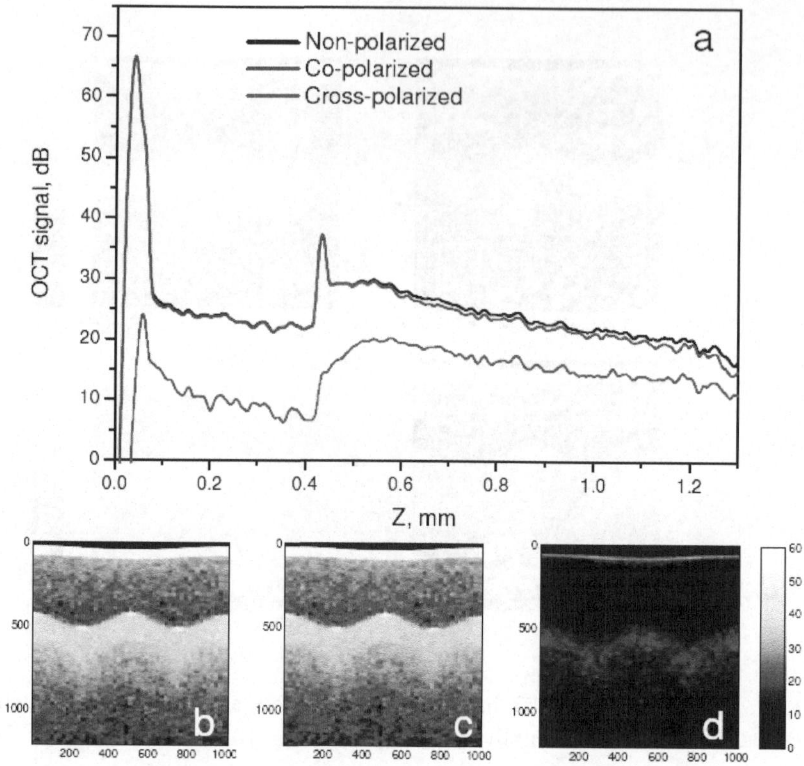

Figure 1.41: A-scan of an OCT image of skin obtained for non-, co- and cross- polarized modes (a); 2D OCT images obtained for non-, co- and cross- polarized modes: (b), (c) and (d) respectively; coherence length of low-coherent light source is 15 μm.

1.6 Summary

In this chapter recent developments in the MC method for the needs of biomedical optics and OD have been presented. The MC model is aimed to provide predictive information to optimize clinical/biomedical optical diagnostic systems and improve interpretation of the experimental results especially for express non-invasive biomedical diagnostics. It should be pointed out that MC is not applied to biomedical applications only but also can be used in other applications including industrial sprays or imitation of image transfer [170, 232–237]. Each part of the MC model has been implemented computationally independent from others so that further development of the MC does not require major changes. Versatile usage of the developed MC model has been exemplified by its application to fiber optics, confocal and fluorescence probes, including also polarization and coherent effects of optical radiation propagating in a scattering medium. In terms of modeling, these studies have extended the conventional MC algorithm by presenting new models of coherent backscattering and field correlation functions constructed by step-by-step comparison against the Bethe-Salpeter equation. Polarization dependence, formation of OCT images has been formulated and introduced into the model of coherent effects. The developed model yields qualitative results which can be readily compared against theoretical predications.

To generalize MC modeling for multipurpose use, we applied the concept of object-oriented programming. This allows the user to describe photon migration and light-tissue interaction as interacting objects. The photon object propagates through the object medium and interacts with its constituents, such as cells, blood vessels, collagen fiber and tumors. Dividing up the medium into objects makes it possible to develop realistic tissue models presenting 3D spatial variations of biological structure. Moreover, defining the actual structure of biological tissue as an object enables it to be imported into the model from any of several imaging modalities, such as electron microscopy, magnetic resonance imaging, and OCT. We used the inheritance feature of object-oriented programming to create a "smart" hierarchical structure of the MC code to avoid having multiple classes for similar tasks. The hierarchy allows "allied" objects to share variables and members, significantly reducing the amount of source code and paving the way to extend and generalize the MC. Depending on the application, objects can be tuned to an appropriate state of light-tissue interaction and to a particular optical diagnostic technique.This approach is a unification of radiative transfer modeling within different OD techniques. It allows theoretical studies and optical engineering concepts to be readily processed by one computational code.

To achieve optical simulation performance, a recently developed parallel computing framework known as CUDA has been employed. Specially designed for professional 3D graphics applications, this technology allows each graphic chip to be logically divided into hundreds of cores, turning the graphics processing unit into a massive co-processor for parallel computations. This capability enables simulation of thousands of objects, i.e. simultaneous propagation of photons in the medium that speeds the process of simulation up to 10^3 times.

Thus, the developed Monte Carlo can be used online to imitate various aspects of optical radiation propagation within complex highly scattering media such as biological tissues. It is felt that the developed model will assists in broadening the range of applications of the coherent and correlation based methods. To conclude, the developed method introduces a possibility for a less sophisticated modeling of radiation transfer (coherent and field correlation effects) in such multiple scattering media as liquid crystals, biological tissues, etc.

References

[1] M. Ohzu and S. Komatsu, *Optical Methods in Biomedical and Environmental Sciences,* Elsevier (1994).

[2] V. Tuchin, Ed., *Handbook of Optical Biomedical Diagnostics,* vol. PM107, SPIE Press, Washington (2002).

[3] A. Yodh and D. Boas, "Functional imaging with diffusing light," in *Biomedical Photonics Handbook, T.* Vo-Dinh, Ed., ch. 21, 1–45, CRC Press (2003).

[4] K. Mudry, R. Plonsey, and J. Bronzino, Eds., *Biomedical Imaging,* CRC Press (2003).

[5] T. Vo-Dinh, Ed., *Biomedical Photonics Handbook,* CRC Press (2003).

[6] R. Verdaasdonk and C. van Swol, "Laser light delivery systems for medical applications," *Physics in Medicine and Biology* **42** (5), 869–894 (1997).

[7] A. Mignani and F. Baldini, "Biomedical sensors using optical fibres," *Reports on Progress in Physics* **59** (1), 1–28 (1996).

[8] R. Waynant, *Lasers in Medicine,* CRC Press (2002).

[9] A. Schuster, "Radiation through a foggy atmosphere," *Astrophysical Journal* **21**, 1–22 (1905).

[10] A. Kim, "Transport theory for light propagation in biological tissue," *Journal of the Optical Society of America A* **21** (5), 820–827 (2004).

[11] V. Kuzmin and V. Romanov, "Coherent phenomena in light scattering from disordered systems," *Physics-Uspekhi* **39** (3), 231–260 (1996).

[12] K. Furutsu and Y. Yamada, "Diffusion approximation for a dissipative random medium and the application," *Physical Review E* **50** (5), 3634–3640 (1994).

[13] S. Ito and K. Furutsu, "Theory of light pulse propagation through thick clouds," *Journal of the Optical Society of America* **70** (4), 366–374 (1980).

[14] A. Ishimaru, *Wave Propagation and Scattering in Random Media,* Academic Press, New York (1978).

[15] S. Chandrasekhar, *Radiative Transfer,* Dover Publications (1978).

[16] R. Fante, "Electromagnetic beam propagation in turbulent media," *Proceedings IEEE* **63**, 1669–1692 (1975).

[17] V. Kourganoff, *Introduction to the General Theory of Particle Transfer,* Gordon & Breach, New York (1969).

[18] A. Ishimaru, "Diffusion of light in turbid material," *Applied Optics* **28** (12), 2210–2215 (1989).

[19] E. Amic, J. Luck, and T. M. Nieuwenhuizen, "Anisotropic multiple scattering in diffusive media," *Journal of Physics A: Mathematical and General* **29** (16), 4915–4955 (1996).

[20] M. Rossum and T. Nieuwenhuizen, "Multiple scattering of classical waves: microscopy, mesoscopy, and diffusion," *Reviews of Modern Physics* **71** (1), 313–370 (1999).

[21] B. van Tiggelen, A. Lagendijk, and A. Tip, "Multiple-scattering effects for the propagation of light in 3D slabs," *Journal of Physics: Condensed Matter* **2** (37), 7653–7677 (1990).

[22] S. Arridge, M. Cope, and D. Delpy, "Theoretical basis for the determination of optical pathlengths in tissue: temporal and frequency analysis," *Physics in Medicine and Biology* **37** (7), 1531–1560 (1992).

[23] C. Bohren and D. Huffman, *Absorption and Scattering of Light by Small Particles,* John Wiley & Sons, New York (1983).

[24] M. Born and E. Wolf, *Principles of Optics: Electromagnetic Theory of Propagation, Interference and Diffraction of Light,* Pergamon Press, London, 6th ed. (1986).

[25] J. Beuthan, O. Minet, J. Helfmann, M. Herrig, and G. Muller, "The spatial variation of the refractive index in biological cells," *Physics in Medicine and Biology* **41** (3), 369–382 (1996).

[26] A. Hielscher, J. Mourant, and I. Bigio, "Influence of particle size and concentration on the diffuse backscattering of polarized light from tissue phantoms and biological cell suspensions," *Applied Optics* **36** (1), 125–135 (1997).

[27] M. Kohl, M. Essenpreis, and M. Cope, "The influence of glucose concentration upon the transport of light in tissue-simulating phantoms," *Physics in Medicine and Biology* **40** (7), 1267–1287 (1995).

[28] M. Hammer, D. Schweitzer, B. Michel, E. Thamm, and A. Kolb, "Single scattering by red blood cells," *Applied Optics* **37** (31), 7410–7418 (1998).

[29] G. Pomraning, *The Equations of Radiation Hydrodynamics,* Pergamon Press, Oxford (1973).

[30] K. Case and P. Zweifel, *Linear Transport Theory,* Addison-Wesley (1967).

[31] R. Fante, "Relationship between radiative-transport theory and Maxwell's equations in dielectric media," *Journal of the Optical Society of America* **71**, 460–468 (1981).

[32] G. Wing, Ed., *An Introduction to Transport Theory,* John Wiley Pub. Co., London (1962).

[33] K. Mitra and S. Kumar, "Development and comparison of models for light-pulse transport through scattering absorbing media," *Applied Optics* **38** (1), 188–196 (1999).

[34] M. Patterson, B. Wilson, and D. Wyman, "The propagation of optical radiation in tissue I. Models of radiation transport and their application," *Lasers in Medical Science* **6**, 155–167 (1991).

[35] P. Kubelka, "New contributions to the optics of intensely light-scattering materials. Part I," *Journal of the Optical Society of America* **38** (5), 448–457 (1948).

[36] P. Kubelka, "New contributions to the optics of intensely light-scattering materials. Part II," *Journal of the Optical Society of America* **44** (4), 330–335 (1954).

[37] A. Klose and A. Hielscher, "Iterative reconstruction scheme for optical tomography based on the equation of radiative transfer," *Medical Physics* **26** (8), 1698–1707 (1999).

[38] A. Welch and M. van Gemert, Eds., *Optical-Thermal Response of Laser Irradiate Tissue,* Plenum Press, New York (1995).

[39] M. Abramowitz and I. Stegun, Eds., *Handbook of Mathematical Functions with Formulas, Graphs, and Mathematical Tables,* Dover, New York (1965).

[40] W. Star, "Diffusion theory of light transport," in *Optical-Thermal Response of Laser Irradiate Tissue,* A. Welch and M. van Gemert, Eds., 131–206, Plenum Press, New York (1995).

[41] T. Durduran, A. Yodh, B. Chance, and D. Boas, "Does the photon-diffusion coefficient depend on absorption," *Journal of the Optical Society of America A* **14** (12), 3358–3365 (1997).

[42] R. Haskell, L. Svaasand, T.-T. Tsay, T.-C. Feng, and M. McAdams, "Boundary conditions for the diffusion equation in the radiative transfer," *Journal of the Optical Society of America A* **11** (10), 2727–2741 (1994).

[43] A. Kienle and M. Patterson, "Improved solutions of the steady-state and the time-resolved diffusion equations for reflectance from semi-infinite turbid medium," *Journal of the Optical Society of America A* **14** (1), 246–254 (1997).

[44] A. Kienle, L. Lilge, M. Patterson, R. H. R. Steiner, and B. Wilson, "Spatially resolved absolute diffuse reflectance measurements for noninvasive determination of the optical scattering and absorption coefficients of biological tissue," *Applied Optics* **35** (13), 2304–2314 (1996).

[45] M. Patterson, B. Chance, and B. Wilson, "Time resolved reflectance and transmittance for the non-invasive measurement of tissue optical properties," *Applied Optics* **28** (12), 2331–2336 (1989).

[46] R. Aronson and N. Corngold, "Photon diffusion coefficient in an absorbing medium," *Journal of the Optical Society of America A* **16** (5), 1066–1071 (1999).

[47] W. Cai, M. Xu, M. Lax, and R. Alfano, "Diffusion coefficient depends on time, not on absorption," *Optics Letters* **27** (9), 731–733 (2002).

[48] K. Yoo, F. Liu, and R. Alfano, "When does the diffusion approximation fail to describe photon transport in random media?," *Physical Review Letters* **64** (22), 2647–2650 (1990).

[49] B. Chen, K. Stamnes, and J. Stamnes, "Validity of the diffusion approximation in bio-optical imaging," *Applied Optics* **40** (34), 6356–6366 (2001).

[50] D. Durian and J. Rudnick, "Photon migration at short times and distances and in cases of strong absorption," *Journal of the Optical Society of America A* **14**, 235–245 (1997).

[51] J. Hebden, S. Arridge, and D. Delpy, "Optical imaging in medicine: II. Modelling and reconstruction," *Physics in Medicine and Biology* **42** (5), 841–853 (1997).

[52] R. Bonner, R. Nossal, S. Havlin, and G. Weiss, "Model for photon migration in turbid biological media," *Journal of the Optical Society of America A* **4** (3), 423–432 (1987).

[53] A. Gandjbakhche and G. Weiss, "Random walk and diffusion-like model of photon migration in turbid media," in *Progress in Optics,* E. Wolf, Ed., **34**, 333–402, Elsevier Science (1995).

[54] L. Dagdug, G. Weiss, and A. Gandjbakhche, "Effects of anisotropic optical properties on photon migration in structured tissues," *Physics in Medicine and Biology* **48** (10), 1361–1370 (2003).

[55] L. Perelman, J. Wu, I. Itzkan, and M. Feld, "Photon migration in turbid media using path integrals," *Physical Review Letters* **72** (9), 1341–1344 (1994).

[56] L. Perelman, J. Wu, Y. Wang, I. Itzkan, R. Dasari, and M. Feld, "Time-dependent photon migration using path-integrals," *Physical Review E* **51** (6), 6134–6141 (1995).

[57] L. Perelman, J. Winn, J. Wu, R. Dasari, and M. Feld, "Photon migration of near-diffusive photons in turbid media: A Lagrangian-based approach," *Journal of the Optical Society of America A* **14** (1), 224–229 (1997).

[58] J. Winn, L. Perelman, K. Chen, J. Wu, R. Dasari, and M. Feld, "Distribution of the paths of early-arriving photons traversing a turbid medium," *Applied Optics* **37** (34), 8085–8091 (1998).

[59] S. Jacques and X. Wang, "Path integral description of light transport versus Monte Carlo and diffusion theory," in *Optical Tomography and Spectroscopy of Tissue: Theory, Instrumentation, Model, and Human Studies II*, **2979**, 488–499 (1997).

[60] M. Wilson and R. Wang, "A path-integral model of light scattered by turbid media," *Journal of Physics B* **34** (8), 1453–1472 (2001).

[61] G. Marchuk, G. Mikhailov, M. Nazaraliev, R. Darbinjan, B. Kagrin, and B. Elepov, *The Monte Carlo Methods in Atmospheric Optics*, Springer-Verlag, Berlin (1980).

[62] S. Feng, Z. Fanan, and B. Chance, "Monte Carlo simulations of photon migration path distributions in multiple scattering media," *SPIE Proceedings* **1888,** 78–89 (1993).

[63] S. Prahl, M. Keijzer, S. Jacques, and A. Welch, "A Monte Carlo model of light propagation in tissue," in *SPIE Proceedings of Dosimetry of Laser Radiation in Medicine and Biology*, G. Muller and D. Sliney, Eds., **IS 5**, 102–111, Plenum Press, New York (1989).

[64] M. Keijzer, S. Jacques, S. Prahl, and A. Welch, "Light distributions in artery tissue: Monte Carlo simulations for finite-diameter laser beams," *Lasers in Surgery and Medicine* **9** (2), 148–154 (1989).

[65] S. Flock, M. Patterson, B. Wilson, and D. Wyman, "Monte Carlo modeling of light propagation in highly scattering tissue-I: Model predictions and comparison with diffusion theory," *IEEE Transactions on Biomedical Engineering* **36** (12), 1162–1168 (1989).

[66] R. Graaff, A. Dassel, M. Koelink, F. de Mul, J. Aarnoudse, and W. Zijlstra, "Condensed Monte Carlo simulations for the description of light transport," *Applied Optics* **32** (4), 426–434 (1993).

[67] M. Hiraoka, M. Firbank, M. Essenpreis, M. Cope, S. Arridge, P. van der Zee, and D. T. Delpy, "A Monte Carlo investigation of optical pathlength in inhomogeneous tissue and its application to near-infrared spectroscopy," *Physics in Medicine and Biology* **38** (12), 1859–1876 (1993).

[68] C. Simpson, M. Kohl, M. Essenpreis, and M. Cope, "Near-infrared optical properties of *ex vivo* human skin and subcutaneous tissues measured using the Monte Carlo inversion technique," *Physics in Medicine and Biology* **43** (9), 2465–2478 (1998).

[69] L. Wang, S. Jacques, and L. Zheng, "MCML - Monte Carlo modelling of light transport in multi-layered tissues," *Computer Methods and Programs in Biomedicine* **47** (2), 131–146 (1995).

[70] I. Lux and L. Koblinger, *Monte Carlo Particle Transport Methods: Neutron and Photon Calculations*, CRC Press (1991).

[71] I. Sobol, *The Monte Carlo Method*, The University of Chicago Press (1974).

[72] K. Stenn, "The skin," in *Cell and Tissue Biology: A Textbook of Histology*, L. Weiss, Ed., 539–572, Urban & Schwarzenberg, Baltimore (1988).

[73] F. A. Duck, *Physical Properties of Tissue: A Comprehensive Reference Book*, Academic Press, London (1990).

[74] B. Beauvoit, S. Evans, T. Jenkins, E. Miller, and B. Chance, "Correlation between the light scattering and the mitochondrial content of normal tissues and transplantable rodent tumors," *Analytical Biochemistry* **226** (1), 167–174 (1995).

[75] T. Kitai, B. Beauvoit, and B. Chance, "Optical determination of fatty change of the graft liver with near-infrared time-resolved spectroscopy," *Transplantation* **62**, 642–677 (1996).

[76] G. Kumar and J. Schmitt, "Micro-optical properties of tissue," in *Advances in Laser and Light Spectroscopy to Diagnose Cancer and Other Diseases III: Optical Biopsy*, **2679**, 106–116 (1996).

[77] S. Jacques, "Origins of tissue optical properties in the UVA, visible and NIR regions," in *Advances in Optical Imaging and Photon Migration,* R. Alfano and J. Fujimoto, Eds., **2**, 364–370, OSA, Washington, DC (1996).

[78] I. Saidi, S. Jacques, and F. Tittel, "Mie and Rayleigh modeling of visible-light scattering in neonatal skin," *Applied Optics* **34** (31), 7410–7418 (1995).

[79] Y. Yarker, R. Aspden, and D. Hukins, "Birefringence of articular cartilage and the distribution on collagen fibril orientations," *Connective Tissue Research* **11** (2-3), 207–213 (1983).

[80] A. Jones, "Light-scattering for particle characterization," *Progress in Energy and Combustion Science* **25** (1), 1–53 (1999).

[81] A. Dunn, C. Smithpeter, A. Welch, and R. Richards-Kortum, "Finite-difference time-domain simulation of light scattering from single cells," *Journal of Biomedical Optics* **2** (3), 262–266 (1997).

[82] P. Sloot, A. Hoekstra, and C. Figdor, "Osmotic response of lymphocytes measured by means of forward light scattering: Theoretical considerations," *Cytometry* **9**, 636–641 (1988).

[83] S. Flock, B. Wilson, and M. Patterson, "Total attenuation coefficients and scattering phase functions of tissues and phantom materials at 633 nm," *Medical Physics* **14** (5), 835–841 (1987).

[84] R. Anderson and J. Parrish, "Optical properties of human skin," in *The Science of Photomedicine,* J. Regan and J. Parrish, Eds., 147–194, Plenum Press, New York (1982).

[85] W. Bruls and J. van der Leun, "Forward scattering properties of human epidermal layers," *Photochemistry and Photobiology* **40** (2), 231–242 (1984).

[86] M. van Gemert, S. Jacques, H. Sterenborg, and W. Star, "Skin optics," *IEEE Transactions on Biomedical Engineering* **36** (12), 1146–1154 (1989).

[87] L. Henyey and J. Greenstein, "Diffuse radiation in the galaxy," *Astrophysical Journal* **93**, 70–83 (1941).

[88] G. Tearney, M. Brezinski, J. Southern, B. Bouma, M. Hee, and J. Fujimoto, "Determination of the refractive index of highly scattering tissue by optical coherence tomography," *Optics Letters* **20** (21), 2258–2261 (1995).

[89] S. Gonzalez, M. Rajadhyaksha, and R. Anderson, "Non-invasive (real-time) imaging of histologic margin of a proliferative skin lesion *in vivo*," *Journal of Investigative Dermatology* **111** (3), 538–539 (1998).

[90] V. Tuchin, *Tissue Optics: Light Scattering Methods and Instruments for Medical Diagnosis, Second Edition,* SPIE Press, Washington (2007).

[91] Z. Song, K. Dong, X. Hu, and J. Lu, "Monte Carlo simulation of converging laser beams propagating in biological materials," *Applied Optics* **38** (13), 2944–2949 (1999).

[92] E. Cashwell and C. Everett, Eds., *A Practical Manual on the Monte Carlo Method for Random Walk Problems,* Pergamon Press, New York (1959).

[93] J. Foley and A. van Dam, Eds., *Computer Graphics: Principles and Practice,* Addison Wesley, Reading, MA (1990).

[94] R. Plastock and G. Kalley, Eds., *Theory and Problems of Computer Graphics,* McGraw-Hill, New York (1986).

[95] D. Toublanc, "Henyey Greenstein and the Mie phase function in Monte Carlo radiative transfer computations," *Applied Optics* **35** (18), 3271–3274 (1996).

[96] J. Zijp and J. ten Bosch, "Use of tabulated cumulative density functions to generate presudo-random numbers obeying specific distributions for Monte Carlo simulations," *Applied Optics* **33** (3), 533–534 (1994).

[97] S. Jacques, "The role of skin optics in diagnostic and therapeutic use of lasers," in *Lasers in Dermatology,* R. W. Steiner, R. Kaufmann, M. Landthaler, and O. Braun-Falco, Eds., 1–21, Springer-Verlag, Berlin (1991).

[98] S. Matcher, M. Cope, and D. Delpy, "*In vivo* measurements of the wavelength dependence of tissue-scattering coefficients between 760 and 900 *nm* measured with time-resolved spectroscopy," *Applied Optics* **36** (1), 386–396 (1997).

[99] I. Meglinski and S. Matcher, "Quantitative assessment of skin layers absorption and skin reflectance spectra simulation in visible and near-infrared spectral region," *Physiological Measurements* **23** (4), 741–753 (2002).

[100] B. Wilson and G. Adam, "A Monte Carlo model for the absorption and flux distributions of light in tissue," *Medical Physics* **10** (6), 824–830 (1983).

[101] R. Meier, J. Lee, and D. Anderson, "Atmospheric scattering of middle UV radiation from an internal source," *Applied Optics* **17** (20), 3216–3225 (1978).

[102] R. Groenhuis, H. Ferwerda, and J. T. Bosch, "Scattering and absorption of turbid materials determined from reflection measurements. I: Theory," *Applied Optics* **22** (16), 2456–2462 (1983).

[103] E. Okada, M. Firbank, M. Schweiger, S. Arridge, M. Cope, and D. Deply, "Theoretical and experimental investigation of near-infrared propagation in a model of the adult head," *Applied Optics* **36** (1), 21–31 (1997).

[104] I. Meglinsky and S. Matcher, "Modelling the sampling volume for skin blood oxygenation measurements," *Medical and Biological Engineering and Computing* **39** (1), 44–50 (2001).

[105] H. Hasegawa, Y. Yamada, M. Tamura, and Y. Nomura, "Monte Carlo simulation of light transmission through living tissues," *Applied Optics* **30** (31), 4515–4520 (1991).

[106] J. Whitton and J. Everall, "The thickness of the epidermis," *British Journal of Dermatology* **89** (5), 467–476 (1973).

[107] G. Odland, "Structure of the skin," in *Physiology, Biochemistry, and Molecular Biology of the Skin,* L. Goldsmith, Ed., 1, ch. 1, 3–62, SPIE Press (1991).

[108] I. Meglinski and S. Matcher, "Computer simulation of the skin reflectance spectra," *Computer Methods and Programs in Biomedicine* **70** (2), 179–186 (2003).

[109] R. Anderson, J. Hu, and J. Parrish, "Optical radiation transfer in the human skin and applications in *in vivo* remittance spectroscopy," in *Bioengineering and the Skin,* R. Marks and P. Payne, Eds., 253–265, MTP Press, Lancaster (1981).

[110] J. Feather, J. Dawson, and D. B. J. Cotterill, "Theoretical and experimental study of the optical properties of *in vivo* skin," in *Bioengineering and the Skin,* R. Marks and P. Payne, Eds., 275–281, MTP Press, Lancaster (1981).

[111] R. Graaff, M. Koelink, F. de Mul, W. Zijlstra, A. Dassel, and J. Aarnoudse, "Optical properties of human dermis *in vitro* and *in vivo*," *Applied Optics* **32** (4), 435–447 (1993).

[112] M. Rajadhyaksha and J. Zavislan, "Confocal reflectance microscopy of unstained tissue *in vivo*," *Retinoids and Lipid-Soluble Vitamins in Clinical Practice* **14** (1), 26–30 (1998).

[113] J. Schmitt and G. Kumar, "Optical scattering properties of soft tissue: A discrete particle model," *Applied Optics* **37** (13), 2788–2797 (1998).

[114] R. Doornbos, R. Lang, M. Aalders, F. Cross, and H. J. Sterenborg, "The determination of *in vivo* human tissue optical properties and absolute chromophore concentrations using spatially resolved steady-state diffuse reflectance spectroscopy," *Physics in Medicine and Biology* **44** (4), 967–981 (1999).

[115] W. Cheong, S. Prahl, and A. Welch, "A review of the optical properties of biological tissues," *IEEE Journal of Quantum Electronics* **26** (12), 2166–2185 (1990).

[116] L. Douven and G. Lucassen, "Retrieval of optical properties of skin from measurement and modeling the diffuse reflectance," in *Laser-Tissue Interaction XI: Photochemical, Photothermal, and Photomechanical,* **3914**, 312–323 (2000).

[117] G. Chapman, *The Body Fluids and Their Functions,* Edward Arnold, Oxford *(1980).*

[118] T. Ryan, "Cutaneous circulation," in *Physiology, Biochemistry, and Molecular Biology of the Skin,* L. Goldsmith, Ed., **2**, 1019–1084, SPIE Press (1991).

[119] M. Shimada, Y. Yamada, M. Itoh, and T. Yatagai, "Melanin and blood concentration in human skin studied by multiple regression analysis: Experiments," *Physics in Medicine and Biology* **46** (9), 2385–2395 (2001).

[120] M. Shimada, Y. Yamada, M. Itoh, and T. Yatagai, "Melanin and blood concentration in a human skin model studied by multiple regression analysis: Assessment by Monte Carlo simulation," *Physics in Medicine and Biology* **46** (9), 2397–2406 (2001).

[121] R. Potts, "Stratum corneum hydration: Experimental techniques and interpretations of results," *Journal of the Society of Cosmetic Chemists* **37**, 9–33 (1985).

[122] F. Bolin, L. Preuss, R. Taylor, and R. Ference, "Refractive index of some mammalian tissues using a fiber optic cladding method," *Applied Optics* **28** (12), 2297–2303 (1989).

[123] D. Churmakov, I. Meglinski, and D. Greenhalgh, "Influence of refractive index matching on the photon diffuse reflectance," *Physics in Medicine and Biology* **47** (33), 4271–4285 (2002).

[124] B. van Tiggelen and S. Skipetrov, Eds., *Wave Scattering in Complex Media: From Theory to Applications,* Kluwer Academic Publisher, Dodrecht (2003).

[125] P. Wolf and G. Maret, "Weak localization and coherent backscattering of photons in disordered media," *Physical Review Letters* **55**, 2696–2699 (1985).

[126] M. van Albada and A. Lagendijk, "Observation of weak localization of light in a random medium," *Physical Review Letters* **55**, 2692–2695 (1985).

[127] M. Ospeck and S. Fraden, "Influence of reflecting boundaries and finite interfacial thickness on the coherent back-scattering cone," *Physical Review E* **49** (5), 4578–4589 (1994).

[128] D. Boas, I. Meglinsky, L. Zemany, L. Campbell, B. Chance, and A. Yodh, "Diffusion of temporal field correlation with selected applications," in *Proceedings SPIE: CIS Selected Papers: Coherence-Domain Methods in Biomedical Optics*, V. Tuchin, Ed., **2732**, 34–46, SPIE Press, Bellingham (1996).

[129] R. Lenke and G. Maret, "Multiple scattering of light: Coherent backscattering and transmission," in *Scattering in Polymeric and Colloidal Systems, W.* Brown and K. Mortensen, Eds., ch. 1, 1–73, Gordon and Breach Science Publishers (2000).

[130] R. Lenke and G. Maret, "Magnetic field effects on coherent backscattering of light," *The European Physical Journal B* **17** (1), 171–185 (2000).

[131] K. Ishii, T. Iwai, and T. Asakura, "Angular polarization properties of dynamic light scattering under influence of enhanced backscattering," *Optics Communication* **140**, 99–109 (1997).

[132] T. Iwai, H. Furukawa, and T. Asakura, "Numerical analysis on enhanced backscatterings of light based on Rayleigh-Debye scattering theory," *Optical Review* **2** (6), 413–419 (1995).

[133] S. Skipetrov and S. Chesnokov, "Analysis, by the Monte Carlo method, of the validity of the diffusion approximation in a study of dynamic multiple scattering of light in randomly inhomogeneous media," *Quantum Electronics* **25** (8), 753–757 (1998).

[134] D. Zimnyakov, J.-T. Oh, Y. Sinichkin, V. Trifonov, and E. Gurianov, "Polarization-sensitive speckle spectroscopy of scattering media beyond the diffusion limit," *Journal of the Optical Society of America A* **21** (1), 59–70 (2004).

[135] V. Kuzmin and I. Meglinski, "Coherent multiple scattering effects and Monte Carlo method," *JETP Letters* **79** (3), 109–113 (2004).

[136] V. Kuzmin and E. Aksenova, "A generalized Milne solution for the correlation effects of multiple light scattering with polarization," *Journal of Experimental and Theoretical Physics* **96** (5), 816–831 (2003).

[137] I. Meglinski, V. Kuzmin, D. Churmakov, and D. Greenhalgh, "Monte Carlo simulation of coherent effects in multiple scattering," *Proceeding of Royal Society A* **461** (2053), 43–53 (2005).

[138] E. Akkermans, P. W. R. Maynard, and G. Maret, "Theoretical study of the coherent backscattering of light by disordered media," *Journal of Physics France* **49**, 77–98 (1988).

[139] Y. Barabanenkov and V. Ozrin *Sov. Phys. JETP* **67**, 1117 (1988).

[140] B. Berne and R. Pecora, Eds., *Dynamic Light Scattering,* Dover Publications (2000).

[141] R. Pecora, Ed., *Dynamic Light Scattering and Velocimetry,* Plenum Press, New York (1985).

[142] W. Brown, *Dynamic Light Scattering: The Method and Some Applications,* Clarendon Press, Oxford (1993).

[143] G. Maret and P. Wolf, "Multiple light scattering from disordered media. The effect of Brownian motion of scatterers," *Zeitschriftfur Physik B - Condensed Matter* **65** (4), 409–413 (1987).

[144] D. Pine, D. Weitz, P. Chaikin, and E. Herbolzheimer, "Diffusing wave spectroscopy," *Physical Review Letters* **60** (12), 1134–1137 (1988).

[145] H. Cummins and E. Pike, *Photon Correlation and Light Beating Spectroscopy,* Plenum Press, New York (1974).

[146] D. Boas and A. Yodh, "Spatially varying dynamical properties of turbid media probed with diffusing temporal light correlation," *Journal of the Optical Society of America A* **14** (1), 192–215 (1997).

[147] B. van Tiggelen and R. Maynard, "Reciprocity and coherent backscattering of light," in *Wave Propagation in Complex Media (IMA Volumes in Mathematics and its Applications),* G. Papanicolaou, Ed., **96**, 247–271, Springer, New York (1997).

[148] D. J. Pine, D. Weitz, J. Zhu, and E. Herbolzheimer, "Diffusing-wave spectroscopy: Dynamic light scattering in the multiple scattering limit," *Journal of Physics of France* **51**, 2101–2127 (1990).

[149] B. Bouma and G. Tearney, *Handbook of Optical Coherence Tomography,* Marcel Dekker, New York *(2001).*

[150] I. Meglinski, M. Kirillin, V.L. Kuzmin, R. Myllyla, "Simulation of polarization-sensitive optical coherence tomography images by a Monte Carlo method," *Optics Letters* **33** (2), 1581–1583 (2008).

[151] J.W. Goodman, Ed., *Statistical Optics,* Wiley-Interscience (1985).

[152] M.Y. Kirillin, I.V. Meglinski, A.V. Priezzhev, "Effect of photons of different scattering orders on the formation of a signal in optical low-coherence tomography of highly scattering media," *Quantum Electronics* **36** (3), 247–252 (2006).

[153] M. Kirillin, I. Meglinski, E. Sergeeva, V.L. Kuzmin, R. Myllyla, "Simulation of optical coherence tomography images by Monte Carlo modeling based on polarization vector approach," *Optics Express* **18** (2), 21714–21724 (2010).

[154] C. Brosseau, *Fundamentals of Polarized Light: A Statistical Optics Approach,* John Wiley & Sons, New York (1998).

[155] X. Wang and L. Wang, "Propagation of polarized light in birefringent turbid media: A Monte Carlo study," *Journal of Biomedical Optics* **7** (3), 279–290 (2002).

[156] M. Rakovic, G. Kattawar, M. Mehrubeoglu, B. Cameron, L. Wang, S. Rastegar, and G. Cote, "Light backscattering polarization patterns from turbid media: Theory and experiment," *Applied Optics* **38** (15), 3399–3408 (1999).

[157] S. Bartel and A. Hielscher, "Monte Carlo simulations of the diffuse backscattering Mueller matrix for highly scattering media," *Applied Optics* **39** (10), 1580–1588 (2000).

[158] D. Zimnyakov, Y. Sinichkin, P. Zakharov, and D. Agafonov, "Residual polarization of non-coherently backscattered linearly polarized light: The influence of the anisotropy parameter of the scattering medium," *Waves in Random Media* **11** (4), 395–412 (2001).

[159] S. Gangnus, S. Matcher, and I. Meglinski, "Monte Carlo modeling of polarized light propagation in biological tissues," *Laser Physics* **14** (6), 1–6 (2004).

[160] J. Schmitt, A. Gandjbakhche, and R. Bonner, "Use of polarized light to discriminate short-path photons in a multiply scattering medium," *Applied Optics* **31** (30), 6535–6546 (1992).

[161] M. Stephen and G. Cwilich, "Rayleigh scattering and weak localization: Effects of polarization," *Physical Review B* **34** (11), 7564–7572 (1986).

[162] F. MacKintosh and S. John, "Diffusing-wave spectroscopy and multiple scattering of light in correlated random media," *Physical Review B* **40** (4), 2383–2406 (1989).

[163] D. Zimnyakov and Y. Sinichkin, "A study of polarization decay as applied to improved imaging in scattering media," *Journal of Optics A: Pure and Applied Optics* **2** (3), 200–208 (2000).

[164] A. Dogariu, C. Kutsche, P. Likamwa, G. Boreman, and B. Moudgil, "Time-domain depolarization of waves retroreflected from dense colloidal media," *Optics Letters* **22** (9), 585–587 (1997).

[165] V. Kuzmin and I. Meglinski, "Helicity flip of backscattered circularly polarized light," *SPIE Proceedings* **7573**, 75730 (2010).

[166] D. Churmakov, I. Meglinski, and D. Greenhalgh, "Amending of fluorescence localization by the refractive index matching," *Journal of Biomedical Optics* **9** (2), 339–346 (2004).

[167] V. Kuzmin and I. Meglinski, "Anomalous polarization phenomena of light scattered in random media," *Journal of Experimental and Theoretical Physics* **137** (2), 742–753 (2010).

[168] V. Kuzmin and I. Meglinski, "Coherent effects of multiple scattering for scalar and electromagnetic fields: Monte-Carlo simulation and Milne-like solutions," *Optics Communications* **273**, 307–310 (2007).

[169] V.L. Kuzmin, I. Meglinski, and D.Y. Churmakov, "Stochastic modeling of coherent phenomena in strongly inhomogeneous media," *Journal of Experimental and Theoretical Physics* **101**, 22–32 (2005).

[170] E. Berrocal, I. Meglinski, D.A. Greenhalgh, and M.A. Linne, "Image transfer through the complex scattering turbid media," *Laser Physics Letters* **3**, 464–468 (2006).

[171] E. Berrocal, D. Sedarsky, M. Paciaroni, I. Meglinski, and M.A. Linne, "Imaging through the turbid scattering media: Part I: Experimental and simulated results for the spatial intensity distribution," *Optics Express* **15**, 10649–10665 (2007).

[172] D. Boas, J. Culver, J. Stott, and A. Dunn, "Three dimensional Monte Carlo code for photon migration through complex heterogeneous media including the adult human head," *Optics Express* **10**, 159–170 (2002).

[173] S. P. J. Ramella-Roman and S. Jacques, "Three Monte Carlo programs of polarized light transport into scattering media: Part I," *Optics Express* **13**, 4420–4438 (2005).

[174] H. Shen and G. Wang, "A study on tetrahedron-based inhomogeneous Monte Carlo optical simulation," *Biomedical Optics Express* **2**, 44–57 (2011).

[175] I. Meglinski, M. Kirillin, and V.L. Kuzmin, "The concept of a unified modelling of optical radiation propagation in complex turbid media," *SPIE Proceedings* **7142**, 714204 (2008).

[176] S. Schach, *Object-Oriented and Classical Software Engineering, Seventh Ed.*, McGraw-Hill (2006).

[177] A. Doronin and I. Meglinski, "Online object oriented Monte Carlo computational tool for the needs of biomedical optics," *Biomedical Optics Express* **2**, 2461–2469 (2011).

[178] A. Doronin and I. Meglinski, "Monte Carlo simulation of photon migration in turbid random media based on the object-oriented programming paradigm," *SPIE Proceedings* **7907**, 790709 (2011).

[179] S. McConnell, *Code Complete, Second ed.*, Microsoft Press (2004).

[180] D. B. Kirk and W. Hwu, *Programming Massively Parallel Processors: A Hands-On Approach,* MK Publishers (2010).

[181] J. Sanders and E. Kandrot, *CUDA by Example: An Introduction to General-Purpose GPU Programming,* Addison-Wesley (2010).

[182] NVIDIA, *CUDA C Programming Guide, CUBLAS Library, CUFFT Library, CURAND Library,* NVIDIA Corporation (2012).

[183] L. Shklar and R. Rosen, *Web Application Architecture: Principles, Protocols and Practices,* John Wiley and Sons Ltd. (2009).

[184] A. Troelsen, *Pro C 2010 and the .NET 4 Platform,* APRESS (2010).

[185] A. F. M. MacDonald and M. Szpuszta, *Pro* ASP.NET *4 in C 2010, Fourth ed.,* APRESS (2010).

[186] L. Moroney, *Microsoft Silverlight 4 Step by Step,* Microsoft Press (2010).

[187] N. Pathak, *Pro WCF 4: Practical Microsoft SOA Implementation,* APRESS (2011).

[188] N. Pathak, *Pro WPF in C 2010: Windows Presentation Foundation in .NET 4,* APRESS (2010).

[189] A. Troelsen, *Developer's Workshop to COM and ATL 3.0,* Wordware Publishing (2000).

[190] T. H. K. Ragab and A. Hassanien, Eds., *Developing Advanced Web Services through P2P Computing and Autonomous Agents: Trends and Innovations,* Information Science Reference (2010).

[191] M. Neely, "Peer fun: A peer-to-peer work processing app with wcf," *MSDN Magazine* 6 (2009).

[192] H. van de Hulst, *Light Scattering by Small Particles,* Dover, New York (1957).

[193] P. van der Zee, *Measurements and modelling of the optical properties of human tissue in the near-infrared.* PhD thesis, University of London (1992).

[194] S. Prahl, "The adding-doubling method," in *Optical-Thermal Response of Laser Irradiate Tissue,* A. Welch and M. van Gemert, Eds., ch. 5, 101–125, Plenum Press, New York (1995).

[195] M. Brewster and Y. Yamada, "Optical properties of thick, turbid media from picosecond time-resolved light scattering measurements," *International Journal of Heat and Mass Transfer* **38** (14), 2569–2581 (1995).

[196] S. Prahl, *Light transport in tissue.* PhD thesis, University of Texas at Austin (1988).

[197] R. Giovanelli, "Reflection by semi-infinite diffusers," *Optica Acta* **2**, 153–162 (1995).

[198] S. Arridge, "Photon-measurement density functions. Part I: Analytical forms," *Applied Optics* **34** (31), 7395–7409 (1995).

[199] M. Firbank, E. Okada, and D. Delpy, "A theoretical study of the signal contribution of regions of the adult head to near-infrared spectroscopy studies of visual evoked responses," *Neuroimage* **8** (1), 69–78 (1998).

[200] I. Meglinski, A. Bashkatov, E. Genina, D. Churmakov, and V. Tuchin, "Study of the possibility of increasing the probing depth by the method of reflection confocal microscopy upon immersion clearing of near-surface human skin layers," *Quantum Electronics* **32** (10), 875–882 (2002).

[201] I. Meglinski, A. Bashkatov, E. Genina, D. Churmakov, and V. V. Tuchin, "The enhancement of confocal images of tissues at bulk optical immersion," *Laser Physics* **13** (1), 65–69 (2003).

[202] J. Pawley, *Handbook of Biological Confocal Microscopy,* Plenum Press, New York (1995).

[203] J. Schmitt, A. Knuttel, and M. Yadlowski, "Confocal microscopy in turbid media," *Journal of the Optical Society of America A* **11** (8), 2226–2235 (1994).

[204] J. Schmitt and K. Ben-Letaief, "Efficient Monte Carlo simulation of confocal microscopy in biological tissue," *Journal of the Optical Society of America A* **13** (5), 952–961 (1996).

[205] A. Dunn, C. Smithpeter, A. Welch, and R. Richards-Kortum, "Sources of contrast in confocal reflectance imaging," *Applied Optics* **35** (19), 3441–3446 (1996).

[206] R. Richards-Kortum, "Fluorescence spectroscopy of turbid media," in *Optical-Thermal Response of Laser Irradiate Tissue*, A. Welch and M. van Gemert, Eds., ch. 20, 667–707, Plenum Press, New York (1995).

[207] J. Qu, C. MacAulay, S. Lam, and B. Palcic, "Laser-induced fluorescence spectroscopy at endoscopy: Tissue optics, Monte Carlo modelling, and *in vivo* measurements," *Optical Engineering* **34** (11), 3334–3343 (1995).

[208] H. Zeng, C. MacAulay, D. McLean, and B. Palcic, "Reconstruction of *in vivo* skin autofluorescence spectrum from microscopic properties by Monte Carlo simulation," *Journal of Photochemistry and Photobiology B* **38** (3), 234–240 (1997).

[209] A. Welch, C. Gardner, R. Richards-Kortum, E. Chan, G. Criswell, J. Pfefer, and S. Warren, "Propagation of fluorescent light," *Lasers in Surgery and Medicine* **21** (2), 166–178 (1997).

[210] R. Crilly, W. Cheong, B. Wilson, and J. Spears, "Forward-adjoin fluorescence model: Monte Carlo integration and experimental validation," *Applied Optics* **36** (25), 6513–6519 (1997).

[211] M. McShane, S. Rastegar, M. Pishko, and G. Cote, "Monte Carlo modeling of implantable fluorescent analyte sensors," *IEEE Transactions on Biomedical Engineering* **47** (5), 624–632 (2000).

[212] B. Pogue and G. Burke, "Fiber-optic bundle design for quantitative fluorescence measurement from tissue," *Applied Optics* **37** (31), 7429–7436 (1998).

[213] K. Vishwanath, B. Pogue, and M. Mycek, "Quantitative fluorescence spectroscopy in turbid media: Comparison of theoretical, experimental and computational methods," *Physics in Medicine and Biology* **47** (18), 3387–3405 (2002).

[214] D. Churmakov, I. Meglinski, S. Piletsky, and D. Greenhalgh, "Analysis of skin tissues spatial fluorescence distribution by the MC simulation," *Journal of Physics D: Applied Physics* **36** (14), 1722–1728 (2003).

[215] L. Smith, K. Holbrook, and P. Byers, "Structure of dermal matrix during development and in the adult," *Journal of Investigative Dermatology* **79**, 930–1040 (1982).

[216] W. Montagna, A. Kligman, and K. Carlisle, *Atlas of Normal Human Skin,* Springer-Verlag, Berlin (1992).

[217] G. Casay, D. Shealy, and G. Patonay, "Near-infrared fluorescence probes," in *Topics in Fluorescence Spectroscopy,* J. Lakowicz, Ed., 4, ch. 7, 183–222, Plenum Press, New York (1994).

[218] J. Lakowicz, *Principles of Fluorescence Spectroscopy,* Kluwer Academic, New York (1999).

[219] V. Kuzmin and I. Meglinski, "Numerical simulation of coherent effects under the multiple scattering conditions," *Optics and Spectroscopy* **97** (1), 101–106 (2004).

[220] V. Kuzmin and I. Meglinski, "Numerical simulation of coherent back-scattering and temporal intensity correlations in random media (overview)," *Quantum Electronics* **36** (11), 990–1002 (2006).

[221] V. Kuzmin and I. Meglinski, "Backscattering of linearly and circularly polarized light in randomly inhomogeneous media," *Optics and Spectroscopy* **106** (2), 257–267 (2009).

[222] V. Kuzmin and I. Meglinski, "Helicity flip of backscattered circularly polarized light," *SPIE Proceedings* **7573**, 75730 (2010).

[223] V. Kuzmin and I. Meglinski, "Anomalous polarization phenomena of light scattered in random media," *JETP* **137** (5), 742–753 (2010).

[224] V. Kuzmin and I. Meglinski, "Dependence of the circular polarization of backscattered light in random media on anisotropy of scatterers," *Optics and Spectroscopy* **108** (1), 99–106 (2010).

[225] F. MacKintosh, J. Zhu, and D. Pine, "Polarization memory of multiply scattered light," *Physical Review B* **40** (13), 9342–9345 (1989).

[226] M. Mishchenko, "Diffuse and coherent backscattering by discrete random media. I. Radar reflectivity, polarization ratios, and enhancement factors for a half-space of polydisperse, non-absorbing and absorbing spherical particles," *Journal of Quantitative Spectroscopy and Radiative Transfer* **56** (5), 673–702 (1996).

[227] L. Rojas-Ochoa, D. Lacoste, R. Lenke, P. Schurtenberger, and F. Schefford, "Depolarization of backscattered linearly polarized light," *Journal of the Optical Society of America A* **21** (9), 1799–1804 (2004).

[228] V. Kuzmin, "The Milne problem solution for the temporal correlation function of an electromagnetic field," *Optics and Spectroscopy* **93** (3), 439–448 (2002).

[229] T. Nieuwenhuizen and J. Luck, "Skin layer of diffusive media," *Physical Review E* **48** (1), 569–588 (1993).

[230] A. Golubentzev, "Reflection by semi-infinite diffusers," *Zh. Eksp. Teor. Fiz.* **86**, 47 (1984).

[231] V. Kuzmin, V. Romanov, and L. Zubkov, "Propagation and scattering of light in fluctuating media," *Physics Reports* **248**, 71–368 (1994).

[232] M. Jermy and A. Allen, "Simulating the effects of *multiple scattering* on images of dense sprays and particle fields," *Applied Optics* **41** (20), 4188–4196 (2002).

[233] E. Berrocal, D.Y. Churmakov, V.P. Romanov, M.C. Jermy, and I. Meglinski, "Crossed source detector geometry for novel spray diagnostic: Monte Carlo simulation and analytical results," *Applied Optics* **44** (13), 2519–2529 (2005).

[234] I. Meglinski, V. Romanov, D. Churmakov, E. Berrocal, M. Jermy, and D. Greenhalgh, "Low and high orders light scattering in the dispersible media," *Laser Physics Letters* **1** (8), 387–390 (2004).

[235] E. Berrocal, M.C. Jermy, and I. Meglinski, "New model of light propagation within highly inhomogeneous polydisperse turbid medium: Application for dense sprays diagnostics," *Optics Express* **13** (23), 9181–9195 (2005).

[236] E. Berrocal, D. Sedarsky, M. Paciaroni, I. Meglinski and M. Linne, "Laser light scattering in turbid media Part I: Experimental and simulated results for the spatial intensity distribution," *Optics Express* **15** (17), 10649–10665 (2007).

[237] I. Meglinski, E. Berrocal, D.A. Greenhalgh, and M.A. Linne, "Image transfer through the complex scattering turbid media," *SPIE Proceedings* **6535**, 65350 (2007).

2

Quantitative Polarimetry for Tissue Characterization and Diagnosis

David Layden

Department of Physics and Astronomy, University of Waterloo, 200 University Avenue West, Waterloo, Ontario, Canada

Nirmalya Ghosh

Department of Physical Sciences, Indian Institute of Science Education and Research (IISER), Kolkata, Mohanpur, West Bengal, India

Alex Vitkin

Division of Biophysics and Bioimaging, Ontario Cancer Institute; Department of Medical Biophysics and Radiation Oncology, University of Toronto, 610 University Avenue, Toronto, Ontario M5G 2M9, Canada

Studies of polarization properties of scattered light from turbid materials such as biological tissues have received considerable recent attention, because of the potential of polarimetric approaches for tissue imaging, characterization, and diagnosis. Polarization can be used as an effective tool to discriminate against multiply scattered light (acting as a gating / contrast mechanism) and thus may facilitate enhancement of contrast and resolution in tissue imaging. Moreover, the intrinsic tissue polarimetry characteristics contain a wealth of morphological and functional information, which can be exploited for quantitative tissue characterization and assessment. However, in a complex random medium like tissue, numerous complexities due to multiple scattering and spatially inhomogeneous birefringence, as well as simultaneous occurrences of several polarization events, present formidable challenges for biomedical tissue polarimetry. In this chapter, we discuss advances in polarized light methodologies to overcome some of these challenges, and present illustrative examples of biomedical applications. Specifically, we review the basic polarimetry formalisms, outline the specific issues in tissue polarimetry, discuss the Stokes and Mueller experimental systems, and describe forward modeling of polarized light propagation in tissue. We then focus on inverse analysis for polarimetric results quantification and applications to quantitative tissue assessment. The other classes of polarization applications in biomedicine, that of tissue imaging and polarization microscopy, are also mentioned in passing, with sufficient references to corresponding recent reviews of these topics.

Key words: polarization, multiple scattering, retardance and birefringence, turbid polarimetry, Monte Carlo simulations, Stokes vector, Mueller matrix, polar decomposition, tissue anisotropy, biological and medical applications

2.1 Introduction

Polarization of light has not been exploited to its full extent in biomedicine, partly because of the highly depolarizing nature of most biological tissues. This is unfortunate, because polarization offers an interesting contrast mechanism for tissue imaging and a rich abundance of important biophysical information of potential relevance to tissue diagnosis and characterization. Its partial neglect in biomedicine is slowly being redressed, however, as better experimental techniques of partial polarization detection and quantification, improved models of polarized light-tissue interactions, and refined interpretation of tissue polarization data are emerging. As such, several attractive applications of this improved polarimetric methodology become feasible. In this chapter, we review polarized light fundamentals and mathematical formulations of polarized light propagation in biological tissues, describe forward and inverse problems in polarimetry of turbid media, discuss advances in various emerging polarimetric measurement systems, and focus on applications related to tissue diagnosis and assessment.

2.2 Fundamentals of Polarization

The definitions and properties of polarized light have been discussed at length in literature [1, 2, 3, 4], and so only a brief overview is provided here. In its classical description, polarization is a consequence of electromagnetic (EM) wave nature of light, in which the transverse oscillations of the electric and magnetic field vectors ($\vec{E}$ and $\vec{B}$) trace out stationary curves. If these vectors instead follow random paths in their temporal evolution, the resulting light is said to be unpolarized. The shape of the function traced out by the vectors defines the polarization state of the beam in question.

2.2.1 Polarization states

When the electric field vector $\vec{E}$ of an EM wave is confined to a plane, the resulting light is said to be linearly polarized, and when temporal evolution of the $\vec{E}$ vector traces out circles normal to the direction of the wave's propagation, the resulting beam is called circularly polarized. Linear and circular polarization are special cases of the more general elliptical polarization, in which $\vec{E}$ follows an ellipse as the wave propagates.

In the quantized description of polarization, each individual photon is polarized, and its associated state vector corresponds to one of the classical polarized states [5, 6]. When a large number of photons are considered, their collective behavior is consistent with the classical limit (the wave solution to Maxwell's equations), and in the case when all of the photons in a beam of light exhibit the same polarization, the light is said to be fully polarized. On the other hand, when there are photons of different polarizations, but with a distribution favoring one particular state, the light is called partially polarized. Finally, when the photons are uniformly distributed over all possible polarization states the light is said to be unpolarized. A useful quantification of this distribution is the degree of polarization, which measures the uniformity, or lack thereof, the photon polarizations in a beam: the degree of polarization of fully polarized light is 1, and that of unpolarized light is 0. Depending on the magnitude of the relative surplus of a particular polarization state, a partially polarized beam of light can fall somewhere between these two extremes.

There are two mathematical formalisms commonly used to describe polarization: the Jones calculus [3, 5, 6], a field-based model which assumes coherent addition of the phase and amplitude of EM waves, and the Stokes-Mueller calculus [3, 5, 6, 8, 9, 10], an intensity-based model which instead utilized incoherent addition of intensities. While theoretically interesting, the Jones formalism is limited in that it can describe pure polarization states, and it is thus ill suited for applications in which it is necessary to consider partial polarization. In general, biological tissues tend to be depolarizing, and so Jones calculus is rarely used in tissue polarimetry. Fortunately, the Stokes-Mueller formalism is capable of fully describing polarized light and its interaction with arbitrary materials, and so it is the mathematical system of choice in biomedical polarimetry.

2.2.2 Stokes-Mueller formalism

In this experimentally oriented formalism, polarization states are described by four measurable quantities, known as the Stokes parameters (introduced by G. G. Stokes in 1852). The four parameters, denoted I, Q, U, and V, are defined relative to six different intensity measurements, each corresponding to the intensity of a beam in question after it has passed through various ideal polarizers: I_H is the intensity through a horizontal linear polarizer, I_V through a vertical linear polarizer, I_P and I_M through linear polarizers at 45° and 135° (or −45°) respectively, and finally I_R and I_L through right and left circular polarizers, respectively. The Stokes parameters are often combined into a four-dimensional vector, called a Stokes vector, in which the parameters can be written as

$$S = \begin{bmatrix} I \\ Q \\ U \\ V \end{bmatrix} = \begin{bmatrix} I_H + I_V \\ I_H - I_V \\ I_P - I_M \\ I_R - I_L \end{bmatrix}. \tag{2.1}$$

Thus, I represents the total intensity of the light, Q and U represent the degree and orientation of linear polarization, and V represents the degree and direction of circular polarization. Note that I is given above as a sum of horizontal and vertical polarized intensities, even though a sum of any two orthogonal polarization states would do; also note that S is not a vector in the classical sense (not a directional quality), but in the column-matrix sense of the word. The Stokes parameters are related by

$$I^2 \geq Q^2 + U^2 + V^2, \tag{2.2}$$

where the equality holds in the case of full polarization, and the inequality for partial polarization. Thus, the degree of polarization is defined as a function of the Stokes parameters by

$$DOP = \frac{\sqrt{Q^2 + U^2 + V^2}}{I}, \tag{2.3}$$

so when a beam is unpolarized ($DOP = 0$), we have that $Q = U = V = 0$. Further, the degree of linear polarization is defined by

$$DOLP = \frac{\sqrt{Q^2 + U^2}}{I}, \tag{2.4}$$

and the degree of circular polarization by

$$DOCP = \frac{V}{I}. \tag{2.5}$$

When light described by the Stokes vector S_{in} interacts with a material, its polarization state is usually modified, and the resulting light can be described by the Stokes vector S_{out}. The transfer function between the input and output states can be written as a linear equation

$$S_{out} = \mathbf{M}S_{in}, \tag{2.6}$$

where $\mathbf{M}$ is a 4×4 matrix known as a Mueller matrix (named after its inventor Hans Mueller, who introduced it in the 1940s). Expanding Eq. (2.6) into its components gives

$$\begin{bmatrix} I_{out} \\ Q_{out} \\ U_{out} \\ V_{out} \end{bmatrix} = \begin{bmatrix} M_{1,1} & M_{1,2} & M_{1,3} & M_{1,4} \\ M_{2,1} & M_{2,2} & M_{2,3} & M_{2,4} \\ M_{3,1} & M_{3,2} & M_{3,3} & M_{3,4} \\ M_{4,1} & M_{4,2} & M_{4,3} & M_{4,4} \end{bmatrix} \begin{bmatrix} I_{in} \\ Q_{in} \\ U_{in} \\ V_{in} \end{bmatrix}. \tag{2.7}$$

The effects of a material on polarized light are completely described by its corresponding Mueller matrix [3, 6, 10], and so the matrix's 16 elements (15 if the change in absolute intensity is excluded) serve as the sample's "polarization fingerprint," from which it is possible to infer information about its physical nature.

It is important to note that not every real 4×4 matrix is a physically realizable Mueller matrix. The fundamental requirement for these matrices is that they map to a physically significant Stokes vector (i.e., one satisfying Eq. (2.2)) for every possible incident polarization state [9, 10].

While both the Jones and the Stokes-Mueller formalisms describe polarization change using matrix/vector equations, the latter provides a framework with which depolarizing materials (e.g., biological samples) can be described. So while the 2×2 transfer matrices of Jones calculus can potentially be a useful theoretical tool, their practical applications have been limited to describing specular reflections, clear media, and thin films where depolarization is not an issue. Mueller matrices, on the other hand, not only provide a complete description of a much wider range of physical materials, but their elements are associated with various intensities (rather than amplitudes), and so they can be experimentally determined with relative ease using intensity-measuring conventional (square-law detector) instruments, such as polarimeters, spectrometers and radiometers. Thus, for the purposes of this chapter, we will employ the Stokes-Mueller formalism exclusively for describing biomedical polarimetry.

2.2.3 Fundamental polarimetric characteristics

There are three principle characteristics of interest that a Mueller matrix can encode: depolarization, diattenuation and retardance, all of which will be examined in further detail.

2.2.3.1 Depolarization

If the degree of polarization of a beam incident on a sample is equal to m (where m is between 0 and 1), and the light resulting from the interaction has a degree of polarization n, where $m > n$, then the sample is said to be depolarizing. For the incident beam

$$m = \frac{\sqrt{Q_{in}^2 + U_{in}^2 + V_{in}^2}}{I}, \tag{2.8}$$

and so in the case that the intensity is unchanged, the degree of polarization of the resulting light can be written as

$$n = \frac{\sqrt{Q_{out}^2 + U_{out}^2 + V_{out}^2}}{I} = \frac{\sqrt{(aQ_{in})^2 + (bU_{in})^2 + (cQ_{in})^2}}{I}, \tag{2.9}$$

where $|a|, |b|, |c| \leq 1$. This relation can be cast in matrix form (like that of Eq. (2.6)) by taking the Mueller matrix of the sample to be [9, 11]

$$\mathbf{M}_\Delta = \begin{bmatrix} 1 & 0 & 0 & 0 \\ 0 & a & 0 & 0 \\ 0 & 0 & b & 0 \\ 0 & 0 & 0 & c \end{bmatrix} \quad |a|, |b|, |c| \leq 1 \tag{2.10}$$

Thus, $1-|a|$ and $1-|b|$ are the linear depolarization factors (for horizontal/vertical and ±45° respectively), and $1-|c|$ is the circular depolarization factor. The net depolarization, denoted Δ, is usually defined as

$$\Delta = 1 - \frac{|a|+|b|+|c|}{3} = 1 - \frac{|Tr(\mathbf{M}_\Delta) - 1|}{3}, \tag{2.11}$$

so Δ remains between 0 and 1.

Note that this *depolarization factor of the medium* is not the same as the various Stokes degrees of polarization in Eqs. (2.3)–(2.5). The latter quantify the amount of *polarization of the light beam*, whereas the former describes the tendency of a material to depolarize light, in a manner that is somewhat independent of the polarization state of the incident light. In general, the two quantities can be approximately related as $DOP_{light} \sim 1 - \Delta_{medium}$, although this relation only holds as an equality in special cases. In biomedical polarimetry, the dominant processes causing depolarization are multiple scattering and spatially heterogeneous arrangements of uniaxially birefringent domains. A material with a large value of Δ is significantly depolarizing, and so in general, the degree of polarization of light after interaction with such a medium will tend to be low.

2.2.3.2 Diattenuation

The following two polarization effects, namely diattenuation and retardance, are both the result of differences in the refractive indices for different polarization states, and are often described in terms of ordinary and extraordinary axis and indices. Differences in the real parts of said indices result in linear and circular birefringence (retardance), whereas differences in the imaginary parts can cause linear and circular dichroism (which manifests itself as diattenuation). Diattenuation is analogous to dichroism, which is the differential absorption of two orthogonal polarization states (linear or circular); however, diattenuation is more general, since the differential attenuation need not be caused by absorption, but rather, it can be the result of various other effects (e.g, scattering).

The diattenuation (d) of an optical element is a measure of the differential attenuation of orthogonal polarization states, for both linear and circular polarization. Thus, linear diattenuation is defined as the differential attenuation of two orthogonal linear polarization states (e.g., ±45°), and circular diattenuation is defined as the differential attenuation of right and left circular polarization states. The Mueller matrix of an ideal diattenuator can be defined using three parameters: q and r, the intensity transmittance (or reflectance) of the two incident orthogonal polarization states in question (be they linear or circular), and θ, the angle (with respect to the horizontal) at which the principle axis is oriented. For a linear diattenuation, the Mueller matrix is defined as [9, 11]

$$\begin{bmatrix} q+r & (q-r)\cos(2\theta) & (q-r)\sin(2\theta) & 0 \\ (q-r)\cos(2\theta) & (q+r)\cos^2(2\theta)+2\sqrt{qr}\sin^2(2\theta) & (q+r-2\sqrt{qr}\sin(2\theta)\cos(2\theta) & 0 \\ (q-r)\sin(2\theta) & (q+r-2\sqrt{qr}\sin(2\theta)\cos(2\theta) & (q+r)\cos^2(2\theta)+2\sqrt{qr}\sin^2(2\theta) & 0 \\ 0 & 0 & 0 & 2\sqrt{qr} \end{bmatrix}. \tag{2.12}$$

In the circular case, the dependence on θ disappears due to rotational symmetry, and so the general

Mueller matrix for a circular diattenuator is [9, 11]

$$\mathbf{M}_\mathrm{D} = \begin{bmatrix} q+r & 0 & 0 & q-r \\ 0 & 2\sqrt{qr} & 0 & 0 \\ 0 & 0 & \sqrt{qr} & 0 \\ q-r & 0 & 0 & q+r \end{bmatrix}. \tag{2.13}$$

A common example of a diattenuator is an ideal polarizer, which can transform an unpolarized incident beam to fully polarized light ($d = 1$ in this case), albeit often with a significant decrease in the intensity I.

2.2.3.3 Retardance (birefringence)

Retardance, closely related to birefringence, is the property in which a material introduces a phase shift between two orthogonal polarization states when it interacts with incident light. Mathematically, the two are related simply via $\delta = kL\Delta n$, where δ is the retardance, k is the wave vector of the light, L is the pathlength in the medium, and Δn is the difference in the real parts of the refractive index known as birefringence. Linear retardance (or linear birefringence), denoted δ, takes place between linear polarization components separated by a geometric angle of 90° (e.g., horizontal and vertical linear polarization components). Note that linear birefringence (retardance) is a vector quantity, possessing both a magnitude and a direction (orientation). The general Mueller matrix of a pure linear retarder with retardance δ and a fast axis oriented at an angle θ is [9, 11]

$$\begin{bmatrix} 1 & 0 & 0 & 0 \\ 0 & \cos^2(2\theta)+\sin^2(2\theta)\cos(\delta) & \sin(2\theta)\cos(2\theta)\,[1-\cos(\delta)\,] & -\sin(2\theta)\sin(\delta) \\ 0 & \sin(2\theta)\cos(2\theta)\,[1-\cos(\delta)\,] & \sin^2(2\theta)+\cos^2(2\theta)\cos(\delta) & \cos(2\theta)\sin(\delta) \\ 0 & \sin(2\theta)\sin(\delta) & -\cos(2\theta)\sin(\delta) & \cos(\delta) \end{bmatrix} \tag{2.14}$$

Circular retardance (optical rotation), denoted ψ, arises from phase differences between right circularly polarized (RCP) and left circularly polarized (LCP) states. The Mueller matrix of a circular retarder with an optical rotation of ψ is [9, 11]

$$\begin{bmatrix} 1 & 0 & 0 & 0 \\ 0 & \cos(2\psi) & -\sin(2\psi) & 0 \\ 0 & \sin(2\psi) & \cos(2\psi) & 0 \\ 0 & 0 & 0 & 1 \end{bmatrix} \tag{2.15}$$

2.3 Experimental Polarimetry

There are two principle applications in biomedical polarimetry research: tissue imaging and tissue characterization. Both of these require highly accurate measurements of the polarization retaining signals, as biological tissues tend to be strongly depolarizing due to multiple scattering and/or birefringence domains of varying magnitude and orientation, thus creating a large depolarized source of noise which can inhibit the detection of the weak remaining information-carrying polarization signal. Thus, many traditional polarimetry systems (e.g., crossed linear polarizers used in microscopy for examining thin fixed *ex-vivo* tissue slices) are poorly suited for these applications.

Polarimetric approaches offer an additional contrast mechanism that confers two main advantages over intensity-only polarization-insensitive methods: they allow for some discrimination against multiply scattered light, which can enable higher resolution imaging of tissues and their underlying structures [12], and they provide a method for non-invasive and quantitative tissue diagnosis, since the polarimetric characteristics of tissues can encode a large amount of biochemical, morphological, and functional information [13, 14, 15]. A variety of experimental tools for exploiting these advantages have been developed, which are capable of performing reliable measurements of polarimetric tissue data, despite the aforementioned technical and biophysical challenges. Such instruments can be used to measure the Stokes vector of a beam upon interacting with the sample in question, and/or the Mueller matrix of the sample itself.

2.3.1 Stokes polarimeters

As discussed in Section 2.2.2, the Stokes parameters corresponding to a beam of light can be determined by performing six intensity measurements through linear and circular polarizers (I_H, I_V, I_P, I_M, I_R, I_L) [10]. By exploiting the property that $I_H + I_V = I_P + I_M = I_L + I_R$, it is possible to determine the Stokes parameters of a beam with only four measurements, using a linear polarizer, with transmission axis aligned at $+45°$ above the horizontal axis, followed by a quarter wave plate, with its fast axis oriented horizontally. Combined, these two elements form a circular polarizer. Three sets of intensity measurements (denoted $I_{cir}(\alpha)$, where α is the angle of the combined polarizer's fast axis above the horizontal) are performed by varying the angle (α) of the circular polarizer with respect to the horizontal axis. The first three measurements are at $\alpha = 0°$, $45°$, and $90°$, and the final measurement, denoted $I_{lin}(\alpha)$, is performed by turning the combined polarizer around and setting α to $0°$. The Stokes parameters can be inferred from these intensity measurements by

$$\begin{bmatrix} I \\ Q \\ U \\ V \end{bmatrix} = \begin{bmatrix} I_{cir}(0°) + I_{cir}(90°) \\ I - 2I_{cir}(45°) \\ I_{cir}(0°) - I_{cir}(90°) \\ -I + 2I_{lin}(0°) \end{bmatrix}. \tag{2.16}$$

This measurement scheme, first proposed by Collett [16], has been used to measure the Stokes parameters of transmitted (or backscattered) light from tissue and tissue-like turbid media [17, 18, 19, 20, 21]. However, in order to accurately quantify tissue polarimetric characteristics, it is generally desirable to use a more sensitive detection method.

One method that shows promise in performing measurements in the challenging biomedical environment is the use of polarization modulation with synchronous detection. Various sensitive detection schemes are possible with this approach; some perform polarization modulation on the beam that is incident on the sample, whereas others modulate the sample-emerging light by placing the polarization modulator between the sample and the detector. The resulting periodic signal can be synchronously monitored with a phase-sensitive (lock-in amplifier based) detection method, and then analyzed to extract the polarization properties of the beam (Stokes polarimetry) or of the sample (Mueller polarimetry) that are linked to the physical quantities of interest.

A schematic diagram of one particular polarimeter employing polarization modulation and synchronous lock-in amplification is shown in Fig. 2.1 [22]. The system is seeded with unpolarized light from the laser, which then passes through a mechanical chopper operating at a low frequency f_c (typically in the tens-hundreds of Hz range, exact value unimportant). The chopper is used in conjunction with lock-in detection to accurately establish the overall signal intensity (I), while eliminating the contributions of the output or background fluctuations and any dark current. The input optics, comprised of a linear polarizer (P_1) and an orientation-adjustable quarter wave plate (QWP_1) enable the generation of any input polarization state (with $DOP = 1$). Following the light-tissue interactions, the beam enters the detection optics, which consist of a removable quarter wave plate (QWP_2), with its fast axis oriented at $-45°$, followed by a photoelastic modulator (PEM), a linearly birefringent resonant device operating in the kilohertz range (e.g., $f_p \sim 50$ kHz), whose fast axis is horizontal (0°) and whose retardation (δ_{PEM}) is modulated sinusoidally according to the function $\delta_{PEM}(t) = \delta_o \sin(\omega t)$, where $\omega = 2\pi f_p$ and δ_o is the PEM's user-specific amplitude of maximum

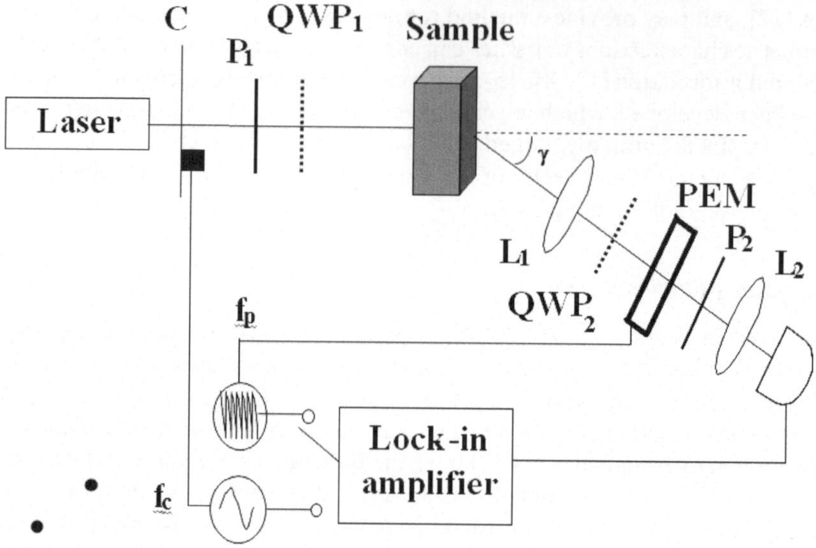

Figure 2.1: A polarimeter employing polarization modulation and synchronous detection to measure Stokes parameters. C_1 is a mechanical chopper, P_1 and P_2 are linear polarizers, QWP_1 and QWP_2 are removable quarter wave plates, L_1 and L_2 are lenses, PEM is a photoelastic modulator, and APD a photodetector. The chopper and the PEM modulate the signal with frequencies f_c and f_p respectively. The detection optics can be rotated by an angle γ around the sample (Adapted from [14]).

retardation. When measuring the Stokes parameters Q and U, the fast axis of QWP_2 is oriented at $-45°$, and when measuring V, said retarder is removed altogether. The PEM is followed by a linear polarizer (referred to as an analyzer) oriented at 45°, which converts the polarization modulation from the PEM into intensity modulation suitable for photodetection. The resulting light is collected using a pair of lenses, and focused onto a photodetector (e.g., an avalanche photodiode), the signal from which is sent to a lock-in amplifier. In order to extract the Stokes parameters from the alternating photocurrent, the reference input of the lock-in amplifier is toggled between the chopper frequency (f_c) and the PEM modulation frequency (f_p) and its harmonics.

In this experimental arrangement, the Stokes vector of the beam entering the detector, denoted $S_f = \left[I_f\ Q_f\ U_f\ V_f\right]^T$, can be related to that of the sample-emerging light, denoted $S = \left[I\ Q\ U\ V\right]^T$, by multiplying the vector representing the input state by the Mueller matrices of the optical elements [22]. When the QWP_2 is in place, the relation is

$$\begin{bmatrix} I_f \\ Q_f \\ U_f \\ V_f \end{bmatrix} = \frac{1}{2}\begin{bmatrix} 1&0&1&0 \\ 0&0&0&0 \\ 1&0&1&0 \\ 0&0&0&0 \end{bmatrix}\begin{bmatrix} 1&0&0&0 \\ 0&1&0&0 \\ 0&0&\cos(\delta)&\sin(\delta) \\ 0&0&-\sin(\delta)&\cos(\delta) \end{bmatrix}\begin{bmatrix} 1&0&0&0 \\ 0&0&0&1 \\ 0&0&1&0 \\ 0&-1&0&0 \end{bmatrix}\begin{bmatrix} I \\ Q \\ U \\ V \end{bmatrix}, \tag{2.17}$$

and when QWP_2 is removed it is

$$\begin{bmatrix} I_{fr} \\ Q_{fr} \\ U_{fr} \\ V_{fr} \end{bmatrix} = \frac{1}{2}\begin{bmatrix} 1&0&1&0 \\ 0&0&0&0 \\ 1&0&1&0 \\ 0&0&0&0 \end{bmatrix}\begin{bmatrix} 1&0&0&0 \\ 0&1&0&0 \\ 0&0&\cos(\delta)&\sin(\delta) \\ 0&0&-\sin(\delta)&\cos(\delta) \end{bmatrix}\begin{bmatrix} I \\ Q \\ U \\ V \end{bmatrix}. \tag{2.18}$$

Thus, the intensity measured by the photodetector is

$$I_f = \frac{I}{2}[1 - q\sin\delta_{PEM} + u\cos\delta_{PEM}], \tag{2.19}$$

with QWP_2 in place, and

$$I_{fr} = \frac{I}{2}[1 - v\sin\delta_{PEM} + u\cos\delta_{PEM}], \tag{2.20}$$

when it is removed. Here q, u, and v are the normalized polarization parameters, defined as $q = Q/I$, $u = U/I$, and $v = V/I$. These parameters can be recovered from I_f and I_{fr} by expressing Eqs. (2.19) and (2.20) as Fourier series whose coefficients are given by Bessel functions (this follows since a periodic function whose argument is itself periodic is represented as a series of harmonics with Bessel coefficients [23]). By setting the peak modulation retardance to $\delta_o = 2.405$ radians (corresponding to the first root of the zeroth-order Bessel function), the normalized polarization parameters can be expressed as functions of the synchronously-detected signals at the chopper frequency V_{f_c}, as well as the first and second harmonics of the photoelastic modulation frequency, $V_{f_{PEM}}$ and $V_{2f_{PEM}}$ respectively. When the detection wave plate is in place, we have [22]

$$q = \frac{V_{f_{PEM}}}{V_{f_c}\sqrt{2}\,J_1(\delta_o)}, \tag{2.21}$$

$$u = \frac{V_{2f_{PEM}}}{V_{f_c}\sqrt{2}\,J_2(\delta_o)}, \tag{2.22}$$

and with QWP_2 removed:

$$v = \frac{V_{f_{PEM}}}{V_{f_c}\sqrt{2}\,J_1(\delta_o)}. \tag{2.23}$$

Thus, the synchronous lock-in detected signals recovered at the first and second harmonics of the polarization modulation frequency, along with that at the chopper frequency, can be used to determine the Stokes parameters of a beam with high SNR for any given state of polarization [22].

While this single PEM scheme is faster and more accurate than sequential DC measurements, it does not allow one to measure all four Stokes parameters simultaneously, as the measurement of circular polarization requires the manual addition of a wave plate in the beam path, making it difficult to automate measurements, and rendering the method inaccurate for time-varying Stokes vectors. Fortunately, the system described above has been generalized to include a second photoelastic modulator (placed directly after the first), which allows for the quasi-simultaneous automated measurement of the complete Stokes vectors with a high SNR [24]. The second PEM removes the need for a quarter wave plate, as the bi-periodic intensity oscillations produced by the dual PEMs along with the linear polarizer contain sufficient information to fully describe the polarization state of the beam in question. Such a system has proven to be useful as it allows for rapid and flexible measurement of Stokes vectors, which is useful in itself, and/or can be processed further to enable Mueller polarimetry.

2.3.2 Mueller polarimeters

While knowing the Stokes vector of a beam after it has interacted with a sample can be very informative, this information is dependent on sample properties *and* on the input light beam (as evident from Eq. (2.6)). Thus, it is often desirable to determine the sample's Mueller matrix itself, which provides a comprehensive description of its polarimetric properties independent of incident light polarization (its true polarization transfer function). Devices capable of performing such measurements, known as Mueller matrix polarimeters, have successfully used both DC (using sequential static measurements) and AC polarization modulation techniques.

The central difference between Stokes and Mueller experimental polarimetry is that the latter requires knowledge of the polarimetric state of a beam both before and after its interaction with the sample. In general, it is necessary to know at least 16 independent polarization parameters for both the input and the output states [1, 3, 9]. That is, if one knows the Stokes vectors of at least four (suitably selected) input beams before they interact with the sample and then after they do so, then it is possible to determine the transfer function (the Mueller matrix) of the material in question. In general, if S^i_{in} is the Stokes vector corresponding to the i-th input beam and S^i_{out} is that of the corresponding output state, then the two vectors can be related as

$$S^i_{out} = \mathbf{M}S^i_{in} \tag{2.24}$$

If the input and output vectors are known for n beams (i.e., $1 \leq i \leq n$), then each input/output pair can be related using Eq. (2.24). The resulting n linear equations can be combined in matrix form as

$$\left[S^1_{out} \cdots S^n_{out}\right] = \left[\mathbf{M}S^1_{in} \cdots \mathbf{M}S^n_{in}\right] = \mathbf{M}\left[S^1_{in} \cdots S^n_{in}\right], \tag{2.25}$$

and so the sample Mueller matrix is given by

$$\mathbf{M} = \left[S^1_{out} \cdots S^n_{out}\right] \left[S^1_{in} \cdots S^n_{in}\right]^{-1}, \tag{2.26}$$

provided $\left[S^1_{in} \cdots S^n_{in}\right]$ is invertible (so n must equal 4). In practice, the invertability of a matrix is not binary (i.e., either invertible or not), but rather presents a continuum in which some matrices are more invertible than others. Given the imperfect nature of experimental measurements, a matrix ill-suited for inversion (known as poorly-conditioned) will tend to amplify Stokes measurement errors into the determined Mueller matrix, whereas a well-conditioned matrix will minimize their impact. Several authors have addressed the issue of robust Mueller polarimetry based on optimum selection of input Stokes states [25, 26, 27]; some results from a recent study by Layden et al. [28] are summarized here. In Mueller polarimetry, a globally well-conditioned matrix $\left[S^1_{in} \cdots S^n_{in}\right]$ is one whose Stokes vectors (columns) are evenly distributed over the Poincaré sphere [29]. It is possible, and sometimes advantageous, to generalize Eq. (2.26) to the case of $n \geq 4$ by replacing the traditional inverse with the Moore-Penrose pseudoinverse defined as

$$\mathbf{A}^{+} = \mathbf{A}^T\left(\mathbf{A}\mathbf{A}^T\right)^{-1}, \tag{2.27}$$

where $\mathbf{A}^{+}$ is said to be the pseudoinverse of the matrix $\mathbf{A}$. In order to quantify the robustness of a Mueller matrix determined from a given set of input Stokes vectors (and their corresponding output vectors), one can perturb the elements in Eq. (2.26) by incorporating measurement errors. Thus, each Stokes vector S^i becomes $S^i + \delta S^i$, where δS^i represents the measurement error associated with the given polarization state. Naturally, the measurement errors in these vectors propagate into the inferred Mueller matrix, which takes the form

$$\mathbf{M}+\delta\mathbf{M} = \left[S^1_{out} + \delta S^1_{out} \cdots S^n_{out} + \delta S^n_{out}\right] \left[S^1_{in} + \delta S^1_{in} \cdots S^n_{in} + \delta S^n_{in}\right]^{+}, \tag{2.28}$$

where $\delta\mathbf{M}$ is the 4×4 matrix representing the deviation from the sample's true transfer function. To maximize the robustness of such a polarimeter, the root mean square of the error $\delta\mathbf{M}$ can be minimized by choosing input Stokes vectors which form the vertices of Platonic solids on the Poincaré sphere [28].

The polarization modulation experimental setups described in Section 2.3.1 can be used to measure the Mueller matrix of a sample by first selecting at least 4 different polarization state generator configurations and measuring their resulting Stokes vectors, and then by sequentially shining those same beams onto a sample, and measuring the corresponding Stokes vectors of the resulting light. This approach has been used in complex tissue-like turbid media and in actual tissues [30, 31] and some of the representative results are presented in Section 2.6. Different Mueller polarimeters employing photoelastic modulators have been explored, some of which modulate not only the light emerging from the sample, but also the original beam, before it is incident on the material of interest. Thus, by putting the sample between two or more PEMs, it can be possible to monitor the various modulation frequencies (and their harmonics) to directly recover the elements of the sample Mueller matrix, while bypassing Stokes vector measurements altogether.

Another type of modulation-based Mueller polarimeter involves the use of dual rotating retarders. In this approach, which has been widely used in tissue polarimetry [32, 33, 34], the polarization of the sample-incident light is modulated by passing a beam through a fixed linear polarizer, followed by a wave plate (with retardation δ_1) rotating at an angular velocity of ω_1. This beam is then incident on the sample, and the resulting light is directed through the analyzing optics, which consist of another rotating wave plate (with retardation δ_2, rotating at angular velocity ω_2) and a linear polarizer, which is held fixed. The rotation of the two wave plates results in a periodic variation in the measured intensity, which can be analyzed by multiplying the Mueller matrices corresponding to the elements in the optical path (i.e., the polarizers, wave plates, and the sample). In the most common configurations, the axes of the polarizers are set parallel, the wave plates are both chosen to have a quarter wave retardance ($\delta_1 = \delta_2 = \frac{\pi}{2}$) and their angular velocities are set at a 5:1 ratio ($5\omega_1 = \omega_2$) [32, 34]. It has been shown that this ratio of angular velocities allows for the recovery of all sixteen Mueller matrix elements from the amplitudes and phases of the twelve frequencies in the intensity signal. In order to compute these elements, the detected signal is Fourier analyzed, and the elements of the Mueller matrix can be inferred from the resulting coefficients. A more generalized version of this measurement scheme could use arbitrary values of retardation and polarizer orientations, as well as a different ratio of angular velocities, in order to determine prioritized Mueller matrix elements with greater precision and/or higher SNR [32, 34].

Another noteworthy polarimetric measurement scheme that employs polarization modulation is the snapshot Mueller matrix polarimeter [35]. This measurement method encodes polarimetric information in different wavelengths of a beam, allowing for highly sensitive and instantaneous measurement of all sixteen Mueller matrix elements simultaneously. To do so, a broadband spectrum source is used in conjunction with two birefringent retarders and a linear polarizer to produce the incident beam, and the light emerging from the sample is analyzed using a similar combination of birefringent retarders and a linear polarizer. The thickness of the retarders on either side of the sample are optimized to recover and analyze sufficiently many polarization states, and the resulting spectral signals (over a narrow range of $\Delta\lambda \sim 10$nm), which are recorded using a spectrometer, are Fourier analyzed to produce all sixteen Mueller matrix elements.

While modulation based Mueller polarimeters show great promise in point measurements, they usually involve synchronous detection, which can make them poorly suited for imaging larger areas. Instead, such measurements are usually performed with DC-based polarimeters, by sequentially measuring the intensities with at least sixteen different configurations of source polarizers and detection analyzers [36]. Unfortunately, such an approach results in fairly low sensitivity measurements, and alternative methods have been investigated. One such method involves liquid crystal variable retarders, which enables the measurement of Mueller matrices with higher sensitivity and precision [37, 38, 39]. Such a polarimeter is comprised of a polarization state generator (PSG) unit, a polarization state analyzer (PSA) unit and an imaging camera, for spatially resolved signal detection. The PSG, which polarizes the light incident on the sample, is composed of a linear polarizer (P_1) and two liquid crystal variable retarders (LC_1 and LC_2), with adjustable retardances of δ_1 and δ_2 respectively, whose birefringent axes are aligned at angles θ_1 and θ_2 with the axis of the polarizer [38]. A schematic of such a measurement scheme is shown in Fig. 2.2.

One widely used configuration involves setting $\theta_1 = 45°$ and $\theta_2 = 0°$, in which case the Stokes vector, S_{in}, of the light incident on the sample can be expressed as a simple function of the retar-

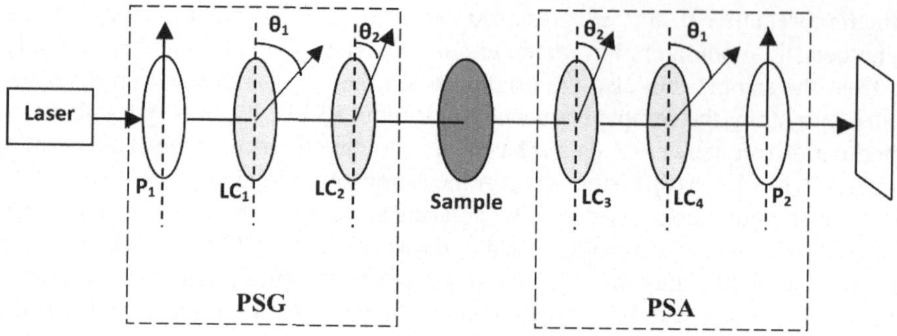

Figure 2.2: A liquid crystal variable retarder polarimeter, where P_1 and P_2 are linear polarizers, and LC_1–LC_4 are liquid crystal variable retarders. Together, P_1, LC_1 (having retardance of δ_1 and orientation angle θ_1), and LC_2 (having retardance of δ_2 and orientation angle θ_2) comprise the polarization state generator (PSG). Likewise, LC_3 (having retardance of δ_2 and orientation angle θ_2), LC_4 (having retardance of δ_1 and orientation angle θ_1), and P_2 collectively form the polarization state analyzer (PSA). While the above schematic depicts transmission measurements, other detection geometries are possible using this measurement scheme.

dances [39]

$$S_{in} = \begin{bmatrix} 1 & 0 & 0 & 0 \\ 0 & 1 & 0 & 0 \\ 0 & 0 & \cos\,\delta_2 & \sin\,\delta_2 \\ 0 & 0 & -\sin\,\delta_2 & \cos\,\delta_2 \end{bmatrix} \begin{bmatrix} 1 & 0 & 0 & 0 \\ 0 & \cos\,\delta_1 & 0 & -\sin\,\delta_1 \\ 0 & 0 & 1 & 0 \\ 0 & \sin\,\delta_1 & 0 & \cos\,\delta_1 \end{bmatrix} \begin{bmatrix} 1 \\ 1 \\ 0 \\ 0 \end{bmatrix} = \begin{bmatrix} 1 \\ \cos\,\delta_1 \\ \sin\,\delta_1 \sin\delta_2 \\ \sin\,\delta_1 \cos\delta_2 \end{bmatrix} \tag{2.29}$$

It is apparent from Eq. (2.29) that any possible polarization state on the Poincaré sphere can be generated with the proper choice of δ_1 and δ_2. The system's PSA consists of a similar arrangement of liquid crystal variable retarders (LC_3 and LC_4) and a linear polarizer, but positioned in the reverse order with respect to the incoming light. It is followed by a detector, which, for imaging applications, is a CCD camera.

The PSG unit can be used to produce four unique Stokes vectors, which can be grouped into a 4×4 generator matrix $\mathbf{W}$, where the i-th column of $\mathbf{W}$ corresponds to the i-th polarization state. Similarly, after sample interactions, the PSA results can be described by a 4×4 analyzer matrix $\mathbf{A}$. The Stokes vectors of the light to be analyzed are projected onto four basis states, given by the rows of $\mathbf{A}$. The sixteen intensity measurements required for the construction of a full Mueller matrix are grouped into the measurement matrix $\mathbf{M}_i$, which can be related to PSA/PSG matrices $\mathbf{W}$ and $\mathbf{A}$, as well as the sample Mueller matrix $\mathbf{M}$ by [9, 40]

$$\mathbf{M}_i = \mathbf{A}\,\mathbf{M}\,\mathbf{W}. \tag{2.30}$$

The sample Mueller matrix can be represented as a 16 element column vector M^{vec}, which can be related to the corresponding 16×1 intensity measurement vector M_i^{vec} as

$$M_i^{vec} = \mathbf{Q} M^{vec}, \tag{2.31}$$

where $\mathbf{Q}$ is the 16×16 matrix given by the Kronecker product of $\mathbf{A}$ with the transpose of $\mathbf{W}$:

$$\mathbf{Q} = \mathbf{A} \otimes \mathbf{W}^T \tag{2.32}$$

Once the exact forms of the system A and W matrices are known, all the sixteen elements of the sample Mueller matrix (M^{vec}, written in column vector form) can be determined from the sixteen measurements (M_i^{vec}). The 4×4 sample Mueller matrix is obtained by rearranging the elements of M^{vec}. One important advantage of this approach is that, it allows for calibration and determination of the exact forms of the system PSG and PSA matrices [38]. This can be accomplished by the so-called "eigenvalue calibration method," wherein the exact forms of the system PSG (**W**) and PSA (**A**) matrices are determined from measurements on calibrating samples having known forms of Mueller matrices (e.g., a set of quarter wave plates and polarizers) [37, 38, 40]. As is apparent, several specific measurement schemes are possible under this general approach, depending on the selected values of δ_1 and δ_2, as well as θ_1 and θ_2. Several such configurations have therefore been examined, and some authors have determined the values of the system parameters (elements of **A** and **W** matrices), which optimize the polarimeter and minimize the noise in the resulting Mueller matrix, resulting in more accurate tissue measurements [37].

Recently, a modulation-based polarimetric imaging scheme employing stroboscopic illumination has been explored for large surface area measurements [41]. In this novel approach, the sample is illuminated by a laser, whose pulses are precisely controlled by a programmable pulse generator. The temporal reference is triggered by the controller of a photoelastic modulator (PEM) operating at 50 kHz, and the resulting synchronization facilitates "freezing" the intensity variation of the modulated signal at desirable temporal phases. The intensity is measured (with a CCD camera) at four specific temporal phases, which are made effectively static via stroboscopic illumination, and the resulting data is used to infer two-dimensional images of ellipsometric parameters [41, 42]. While this approach may hold promise, it has not yet been employed for complete (sixteen element) Mueller matrix imaging.

2.4 Forward Modeling of Polarization Transfer in Complex Random Media

Accurate modeling of interaction of polarized light with tissue micro-structures and its propagation through turbid tissue is extremely useful for the applications of polarized light methods for tissue imaging, characterization and diagnosis. The insight gained from such *forward models* helps in designing and optimizing experiments, and analyzing/interpreting measured data, for specific applications.

A rigorous, electromagnetic theory based approach for analyzing light propagation in tissue will need to identify and incorporate the spatio-temporal distribution of complex tissue dielectric structures (different cells and subcellular structures, connective stromal tissues / extra-cellular matrix, blood and lymphatic networks, interstitial fluids, etc.) and their absorption and scattering properties. Clearly this is a formidable task. Due to the ensuing complexity, heuristic approaches with different levels of approximations have been developed to model light transport in tissues. Radiative transport theory and its simplified variant, the diffusion equation, are often used to model light propagation in tissue [43, 44, 45]. However, both of these are intensity based (scalar) techniques, and typically neglect the vector nature of light (polarization). Some attempts have been made to use the vector radiative transfer equation (VRTE) in this framework to incorporate polarization information by describing transport of the Stokes vectors of light (photon packets) through a random medium [43, 45]. However, solving the VRTE in real systems is rather complex, and the solutions are often too slow and insufficiently flexible to handle the necessary boundary conditions for arbitrary geometries and arbitrary optical properties as desirable in case of tissue [43]. Alternative analytical approaches based on photon diffusion formalisms, random walk models, and maximum entropy principles have been explored for modeling polarized light transport in random media such as tissues [43, 46, 47, 48, 49]. In these analytical/heuristic approaches, tissue is typically modeled as a turbid medium having bulk-average scattering and absorption properties, where propagation leads to depolarization as a result of strong multiple scattering events (birefringence effects are often ignored). These approaches have derived simplified analytical relationships between various quantities of practical interests such as the degree of polarization (either linear or circular) of forward-scattered or back-scattered light from a turbid medium, average path lengths, the optical transport parameters of the medium, and so forth [46, 48, 49]. The main aim of these approximate analytical approaches has been to understand the overall depolarization trends, its dependence on the scattering properties of the media, and on the incident state of polarization, and to design / optimize general polarization schemes to discriminate against multiply scattered photons for tissue imaging in 'simple' geometries. These approaches, while useful, are approximate by their very nature and typically neglect other simultaneously occurring complex tissue polarimetry events (such as linear birefringence, optical activity, etc.). The applications of these models have thus been restricted to the 'tissue imaging' domain (employing polarization gating methods and various other co/cross polarization detection schemes). Interested readers are referred to references [43, 46, 47, 48, 49, 50] for the details of these models.

A more encompassing, accurate method is clearly needed for polarimetry applications involving quantitative assessment of tissue composition and micro-architecture. This can be accomplished by the polarization-sensitive Monte Carlo (PSMC) techniques. Monte Carlo (MC) technique is a general and robust approach for modeling light transport in a random medium [44, 51], with its advantage of applicability to arbitrary geometries and arbitrary optical properties. In this statistical approach to radiative transfer, the multiple scattering trajectories of individual photons are determined using random numbers to predict the probability of each scattering event. It is also assumed that scattering events occur independently and exhibit no coherence effects. The superposition of many photon paths approaches the actual photon distribution in time and space. The initial Monte Carlo biophotonic models were developed for intensity calculations only and neglected polarization information [51], which has recently been incorporated in a number of implementations by keeping track of the Stokes vectors of propagating photon packets [50, 52, 53, 54, 55, 56]. A typical flowchart for a PSMC model is shown in Fig. 2.3. Briefly in this model, position, propagation direction, and polarization of each photon are initialized and modified as the photon propagates through the medium. The photon's polarization, with respect to a set of arbitrary orthonormal axes defining its reference frame, is represented as a Stokes vector **S** and polarization effects are applied using medium Mueller matrices **M** [13]. The photon propagates in the sample between scattering events a distance sampled from the probability distribution $\exp(-\mu_t d)$, where the extinction coefficient μ_t is the sum of the absorption μ_a and scattering μ_s coefficients and d is the distance traveled by the photon between scattering events [50, 51]. Upon encountering a scattering event, a scattering plane and angle are statistically sampled based on the polarization state of the photon and the Mueller matrix of the scatterer. The photon's reference frame is first expressed in the scattering plane and then transformed to the laboratory (experimentally observable) frame through multiplication of appropriate rotation matrices (reference frame manipulation) and by the Mueller matrix corresponding to the scattering event. Usually, the scattering Mueller matrix **M** is computed using Mie theory [4], which assumes the scattering medium to be comprised of discrete spherical scatterers. In principle, incorporation of scattering Mueller matrices for other non-spherical scatterers or the scattering matrices for other continuously fluctuating medium is also possible [50, 52]. Nevertheless, the evolution of polarization state of each photon packet is tracked (via the Stokes vectors) following successive scattering events. The absorption effects are incorporated after successive scattering events by reducing the photon weight by a factor $W = \frac{\mu_a}{\mu_a+\mu_s}$, as conventionally done in intensity-based MC models also [44, 51]. Upon encountering an interface (either an internal one, representing tissue layers of different optical properties, or an external one, representing external boundary), the probability of either reflection or transmission is calculated using Fresnel coefficients. Assuming no interference effects, the final Stokes vectors for light exiting the sample in a particular direction are computed as the sum of all the appropriate sub-populations of photons. The sample Mueller matrix can then be calculated by sequentially changing the input polarization, recording the corresponding output

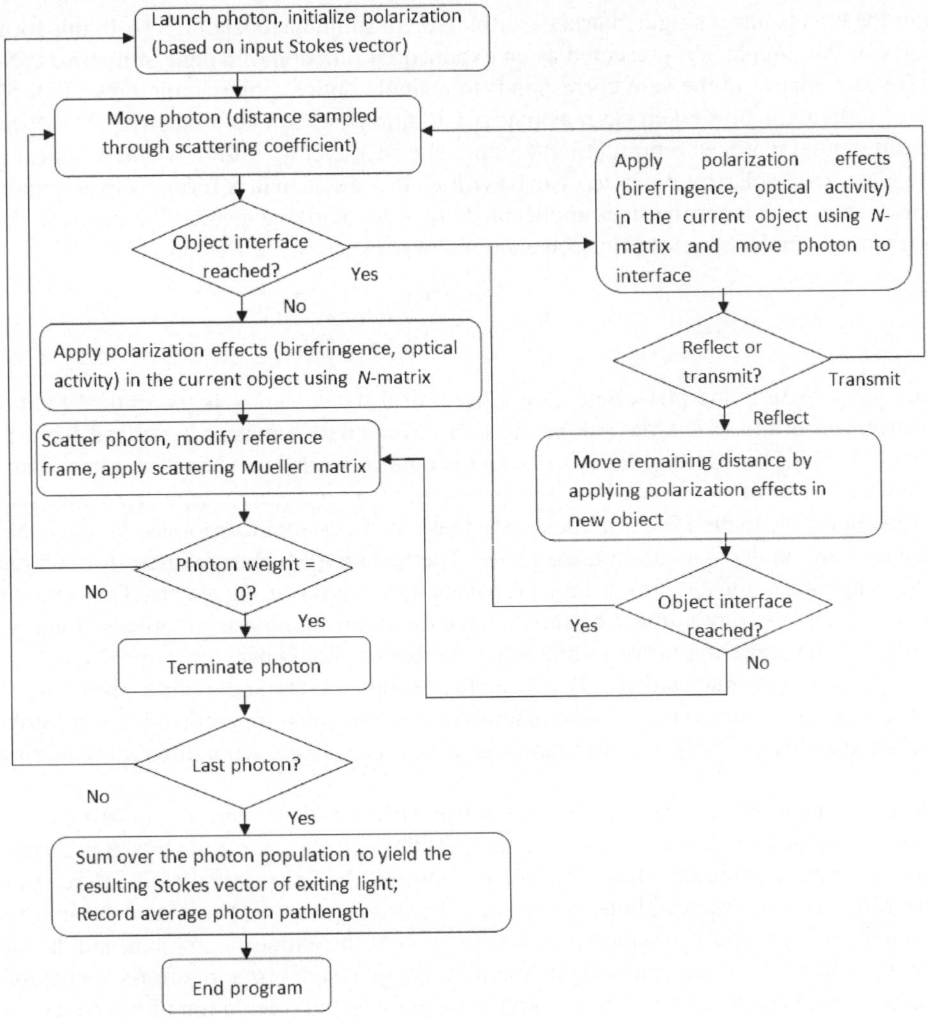

Figure 2.3: A flowchart representing the polarization-sensitive Monte Carlo model. (Adapted from [13].)

Stokes vectors for each respective input state, and performing algebraic manipulations as described previously [53].

While the effects of scattering on the polarization evolution after successive scattering events can be modeled by the scattering Mueller matrix **M**, the effects of other medium polarimetry effects such as linear birefringence and optical activity can also be incorporated by including their corresponding Mueller matrices. However, this is not an obvious modeling step. Specifically, problems arise in modeling simultaneous polarization events in the presence of multiple scattering. Matrix multiplication of the Mueller matrices for individual polarization effects is not commutative ($\mathbf{M_A}\,\mathbf{M_B} \neq \mathbf{M_B}\mathbf{M_A}$), thus, different orders in which these effects are applied will have different effects on the output polarization. Yet in biological tissue, effects such as optical activity due to chiral molecules (e.g., glucose and proteins) and linear birefringence due to anisotropic tissue structures (e.g., collagen, elastin, and muscle fibers) must be incorporated into the model in the presence of scattering. This problem is tackled through the use of so-called N-matrix formalism, which combines the effects into a single matrix describing them simultaneously [1, 57]. In this formalism, the matrix of the sample is represented as an exponential function of a sum of matrices (N-matrices), where each matrix in the sum corresponds to a single optical polarization effect [53, 57]. The issue of ordering is thus taken care, as matrix addition is always commutative. The N-matrices are the differential matrices representing the optical effect over an infinitely small optical pathlength, wherein several polarization effects can be written in a single matrix form. Conventionally, these N-matrices are 2×2 Jones matrices applicable to non-depolarizing media. For example, the N-matrix representing combined linear birefringence and optical activity is written as [1, 57]

$$N_{OA+LB} = \frac{1}{2}\begin{bmatrix} ig_0 & \chi \\ -\chi & -ig_0 \end{bmatrix} \tag{2.33}$$

Here, $g_0 = \frac{2\pi}{\lambda}\Delta n$ is the phase retardation per unit distance and χ is the optical rotation per unit distance. From this N-matrix, the parent non-differential M matrix is derived for the combined effect [53, 57]. The resulting Jones M-matrix is then converted to a Mueller matrix. Note that such a conversion from Jones to Mueller matrix is possible only for non-depolarizing matrices. This is indeed applicable to the PSMC model, since these matrices are incorporated *between* the scattering events, where no depolarization takes place. The resulting Mueller matrices for combined effects are thus applied to the photons as they propagate between scattering events. This approach enabled the combination of any number of simultaneously occurring polarizing effects. Finally, as shown in Fig. 2.3, the scattering histories of a large number of photon packets (typically 10^7–10^9 photons are required to generate statistically acceptable results) are tracked as they propagate through the medium and are summed to yield the macroscopic parameters of practical interest (Stokes vectors, Mueller matrices, pathlength distributions, polarization statistics from different scattering histories, etc.).

In the simulation, circular and linear birefringence (these are the two most tissue polarimetry effects in addition to depolarization) are modeled through the optical activity χ in degrees per centimeter, and through the anisotropy in refractive indices (Δn), respectively [53]. Here, $\Delta n = (n_e - n_o)$ is the difference in refractive index along the extraordinary axis (n_e) and the ordinary axis (n_o). For simplicity, it is generally assumed that the direction of the extraordinary axis and the value for Δn is constant throughout the scattering medium (although recent research efforts are exploring the effects of multiple uniaxial domains of varying magnitude and orientation of birefringence). In each simulation, n_e and n_o are taken as input parameters and a specific direction of the extraordinary axis is chosen. As photons propagate between scattering events, the difference in refractive indices seen by the photons depends on the propagation direction with respect to the extraordinary axis. The effect is usually modeled using standard formulae describing the angular variation of refractive index in uni-axial medium [50, 53]. Similar to the conventional MC model, the scattering and absorption properties are modeled using the optical transport parameters, scattering coefficient (μ_s) and absorption coefficient (μ_a).

The validity of the above PSMC model has been tested on experimental tissue simulating phantoms exhibiting simultaneous scattering and polarization properties, which are known and user-controlled *a priori* [13, 14, 30, 53]. These solid optical phantoms were developed using polyacrylamide as a base medium, with sucrose-induced optical activity, polystyrene microspheres-induced scattering and mechanical stretching to cause linear birefringence [53]. These phantom systems mimic the complexity of biological tissues, in that they exhibit simultaneous effects of linear birefringence, optical activity and depolarization due to multiple scattering. The experimental results of Mueller matrix measurements from these tissue phantoms and corresponding MC simulation results of analogous turbid media are presented and discussed subsequently.

2.5 Interpretation and Decomposition of Mueller Matrices

Polarimetric quantities, such as depolarization, optical activity, and linear birefringence can potentially serve as valuable metrics in biomedical applications. For example, changes in tissue mechanical anisotropy (resulting from disease progression or treatment response) can be probed with birefringence measurements [13, 58], and blood sugar levels can potentially be determined by measuring the optical rotation induced by the chiral glucose molecules [14, 15]. Despite the wealth of important properties which can be determined via tissue polarimetry, numerous complexities inhibit their straightforward extraction and interpretation.

Multiple scattering, a common phenomenon in biomedical polarimetry, not only causes extensive depolarization, but alters the state of the remaining polarized signal in a complex manner, for example, by scattering-induced diattenuation and by scattering-induced changes in the orientation of the polarization vector [22, 59]. Not only are polarimetric quantities difficult to measure reliably, but their co-occurrence in biomedical samples greatly complicates their unique interpretation. This problem manifests itself most clearly in trying to interpret the Mueller matrices of such samples: while the materials' transfer functions may qualitatively resemble those of one (or many) of the fundamental characteristics discussed in Section 2.2.3, their measured Mueller matrices generally look nothing like that of the idealized versions. Instead, they contain a convolved mix of otherwise individually recognizable properties, with much 'inter-element cross talk' obscuring potentially interesting polarization biometrics and hindering their interpretation. Thus, methods accounting for multiple scattering-induced effects, and capable of decoupling the individual contributions of simultaneously occurring basic polarimetric characteristics are required.

2.5.1 Decomposition into basic polarimetric components

Previous attempts at tissue polarimetry analysis have mostly utilized semi-empirical approaches by selectively measuring particular Stokes vectors or Mueller matrix elements of interest, based on the purported polarimetric signatures associated with various tissue anatomical or compositional characteristics [60]. However, recent studies have employed more general models to extract, quantify and interpret intrinsic tissue polarimetry characteristics by decomposing their measured Mueller matrices into more easily interpretable "basis" matrices [30, 31].

One particularly noteworthy method of Mueller matrix decomposition is known as the product, or Lu-Chipman, decomposition, after its inventors, who first demonstrated its validity in optically clear media [11]. This method consists of representing a sample Mueller matrix $\mathbf{M}$ as a product of three basis matrices

$$\mathbf{M} = \mathbf{M}_{\Delta}\mathbf{M}_{R}\mathbf{M}_{D}, \tag{2.34}$$

where the depolarizer matrix $\mathbf{M}_{\Delta}$ encodes the depolarizing effects of the medium, the retarder matrix $\mathbf{M}_{\mathrm{R}}$ describes its linear birefringence and optical activity, and the diattenuator matrix $\mathbf{M}_{\mathrm{D}}$ accounts for the effects of linear and circular diattenuation.

The diattenuation matrix $\mathbf{M}_{\mathrm{D}}$ is defined as

$$\mathbf{M}_{D}= \begin{bmatrix} 1 & \vec{d}^{T} \\ \vec{d} & \mathbf{m}_{\mathrm{D}} \end{bmatrix}, \tag{2.35}$$

where $\mathbf{m}_{D}$ is the 3×3 matrix usually expressed as

$$\mathbf{m}_{D}=\sqrt{1-d^{2}}\,\mathbf{I}+\left(1-\sqrt{1-d^{2}}\right)\hat{d}\hat{d}^{T} \tag{2.36}$$

Here **I** is the 3×3 identity matrix, and $\vec{d}$ is the diattenuation vector defined as

$$\vec{d} = \frac{1}{m_{1,1}} \left[m_{1,2} \; m_{1,3} \; m_{1,4} \right]^T, \tag{2.37}$$

where $\hat{d}$ is its corresponding unit vector, determined by dividing the diattenuation vector by its magnitude d, given by

$$d = \frac{1}{m_{1,1}} \sqrt{m_{1,2}^2 + m_{1,3}^2 + m_{1,4}^2} \tag{2.38}$$

(The scalar m_{ij} is the element of the sample Mueller matrix in the i-th row and the j-th column.) The elements $m_{1,2}$ and $m_{1,3}$ represent the linear diattenuation for horizontal/vertical and $\pm 45°$ linear polarization respectively, and $m_{1,4}$ represents the circular diattenuation.

The product of the two remaining matrices in the decomposition can be expressed by right-multiplying the sample Mueller matrix by the inverse of $\mathbf{M}_D$, which motivates the following definition:

$$\mathbf{M}' = \mathbf{M}_\Delta \mathbf{M}_R = \mathbf{M}\mathbf{M}_D^{-1}. \tag{2.39}$$

The matrices $\mathbf{M}_\Delta$, $\mathbf{M}_\mathrm{R}$ and $\mathbf{M}'$ take the following form:

$$\mathbf{M}_\Delta = \begin{bmatrix} 1 & \vec{0}^T \\ P_\Delta & \mathbf{m}_\Delta \end{bmatrix}; \;\; \mathbf{M}_\mathrm{R} = \begin{bmatrix} 1 & \vec{0}^T \\ \vec{0} & \mathbf{m}_\mathrm{R} \end{bmatrix}; \;\; \text{and } \mathbf{M}' = \begin{bmatrix} 1 & \vec{0}^T \\ P_\Delta & \mathbf{m}' \end{bmatrix}, \tag{2.40}$$

where $P_\Delta = \frac{\vec{P} - m\vec{d}}{1-d^2}$, and the polarizance vector $\vec{P}$ is given by

$$\vec{P} = \frac{1}{m_{1,1}} \left[m_{2,1} \; m_{3,1} \; m_{4,1} \right]^T \tag{2.41}$$

The blocks in Eq. (2.40) are naturally related as $\mathbf{m}' = \mathbf{m}_\Delta \mathbf{m}_R$. The matrix $\mathbf{m}_\Delta$ can be formed using the eigenvalues of $\mathbf{m}'\mathbf{m}'^T$ [11]; then, $\mathbf{M}_\Delta$ can be constructed and used to extract the net depolarization coefficient Δ, another potentially useful biometric, using Eq. (2.11).

The remaining matrix $\mathbf{M}_\mathrm{R}$, which encodes the retardance, can be computed from Eq. (2.39), and the scalar value of the total retardance R (representing the combined effect of linear and circular birefringence) is calculated as

$$R = \arccos\left(\frac{\mathrm{Tr}(\mathbf{M}_\mathrm{R})}{2} - 1 \right) \tag{2.42}$$

The matrix $\mathbf{M}_\mathrm{R}$ can be further analyzed to extract the corresponding linear retardance δ, as well as the optical rotation ψ, by separating it into the standard Mueller matrices corresponding to said parameters (Eqs. (2.14) and (2.15)). The values of these numbers can then be expressed directly in terms of the elements of $\mathbf{M}_\mathrm{R}$ as [30]

$$\delta = \arccos(\sqrt{(m_{\mathrm{R}2,2} + m_{\mathrm{R}3,3})^2 + (m_{\mathrm{R}3,2} - m_{\mathrm{R}2,3})^2} - 1) \tag{2.43}$$

and

$$\psi = \arctan\left(\frac{m_{\mathrm{R}3,2} - m_{\mathrm{R}2,3}}{m_{\mathrm{R}2,2} + m_{\mathrm{R}3,3}} \right). \tag{2.44}$$

In summary, the above decomposition (Eqs. (2.34)–(2.44)) operates on a sample Mueller matrix, and extracts several medium-specific polarimetry metrics of promising biomedical value, namely diattenuation (d), linear, circular and total depolarization (Δ), linear retardance and its orientation (δ and θ), and optical rotation (ψ).

Due to the non-commutative nature of matrix multiplication (i.e., $\mathbf{AB} \neq \mathbf{BA}$ in general), the order of the basis matrices in Eq. (2.34) is only one of six possible (distinct) permutations. The arrangements are classified into two families: those where the diattenuator matrix is placed before the depolarizer (this includes Eq. (2.34)), and those where it is placed after [61]. The two groups are shown below:

$$\Delta D\ Family = \begin{cases} \mathbf{M}_\Delta \mathbf{M}_R \mathbf{M}_D \\ \mathbf{M}_\Delta \mathbf{M}_D \mathbf{M}_R \\ \mathbf{M}_R \mathbf{M}_\Delta \mathbf{M}_D \end{cases} \quad D\Delta\ Family = \begin{cases} \mathbf{M}_D \mathbf{M}_R \mathbf{M}_\Delta \\ \mathbf{M}_R \mathbf{M}_D \mathbf{M}_\Delta \\ \mathbf{M}_D \mathbf{M}_\Delta \mathbf{M}_R \end{cases} \tag{2.45}$$

It has been shown that of the six possible multiplicative orders, the Lu-Chipman decomposition and its reversal ($\mathbf{M}_D\mathbf{M}_R\mathbf{M}_\Delta$), known as the reverse decomposition, always produce physically realizable Mueller matrices [61]. The other four decompositions can be obtained from the aforementioned two by employing similarity transformations. It has been found that in tissue polarimetry (in the absence of large d-values), the Lu-Chipman and reverse decompositions yield the correct description of the medium in question, based on the metrics presented above. The only differences between the forward and reverse orders were occasional sign changes in the derived values, indicating that both approaches extract the magnitudes of the polarization metrics in a self-consistent manner.

In an effort to eliminate any remaining ambiguity associated with the multiplicative order of the basis matrices, a more general kind of decomposition, known as the symmetric decomposition, has been developed, which factors an arbitrary depolarizing Mueller matrix into 5 matrices: a diagonal depolarizer $\mathbf{M}_\Delta$ multiplied to either side by an equivalent optical sequence containing diattenuators and retarders [62]. This decomposition can be expressed as

$$\mathbf{M} = \mathbf{M}_{D2}\mathbf{M}_{R2}\mathbf{M}_\Delta\mathbf{M}_{R1}^T\mathbf{M}_{D1} \tag{2.46}$$

As is apparent from the six different decompositions given in Eq. (2.45), the ambiguity in the derived polarization parameter mainly arises depending upon whether the diattenuator matrix is placed before or after the depolarizer. The symmetric decomposition helps in interpretation and analysis of any experimental Mueller matrix in that it does not impose any restriction on the preferred sequential occurrence of the diattenuation effect. Thus, it allows for extraction of the constituent polarization parameters of any complex system with less ambiguity. However, it should be mentioned, this approach also does not really address the issue of *simultaneously* occurring polarization effects, which is typically encountered in tissue. In order to address this issue, a more general kind of decomposition based on differential matrix formalism of the Mueller calculus, has recently been developed [63]. This formalism was originally proposed by Azzam for non-depolarizing optical media [64]; it has been extended and generalized to incorporate depolarization effects [63]. Within the differential matrix formalism, all elementary polarization and depolarization properties of the medium are contained in a single differential matrix representing them simultaneously. Thus, this approach is expected to be more suitable for Mueller matrix polarimetry analysis of tissues, exhibiting *simultaneous* polarization effects. An interested reader is referred to the literature [63, 64] for the details of the differential Mueller matrix formalism.

There exists another type of product decomposition, known as the Cloude decomposition, which expresses an arbitrary depolarizing Mueller matrix $\mathbf{M}$ as a *sum* of a non-depolarizing Mueller matrix $\mathbf{M}_{n\Delta}$(which can be further decomposed using the above-mentioned process) and an ideal polarizer $\mathbf{M}_\Delta$ [65]. While theoretically interesting and practically attractive (matrix addition is commutative, so there is no order ambiguity as in product-based decompositions), Cloude decomposition has not been used in tissue polarimetry.

The decompositions presented here hold great promise for their ability to extract useful biological metrics from the Mueller matrices of complex samples, but they require comprehensive validation; more specifically, the effects of various decomposition processes, permutations of basis matrices, the detection geometry and the propagation path of multiply scattered photons on the extracted metrics must be thoroughly examined, and above all, the derived parameters must be shown to accurately represent the true polarimetric properties of the medium in question. Several studies have

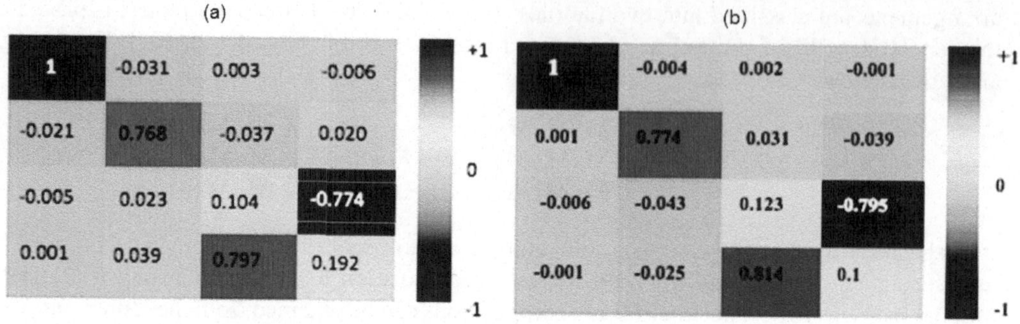

Figure 2.4: The Mueller matrices (a) experimentally recorded in the forward (transmission) detection geometry from birefringent (extension = 4 mm, corresponding to a value of linear retardance δ = 1.345 rad for a clear phantom), chiral concentration of sucrose = 1 M, $\chi = 1.96$ degree cm^{-1} turbid ($\mu_s = 30$ cm^{-1}, $g = 0.95$) phantom of thickness of 1 cm; (b) generated through the PSMC model, using the same controlled input scattering and polarization parameters (linear birefringence $\Delta n = 1.36 \times 10^{-5}$, corresponding to $\delta = 1.345$ rad, $\chi = 1.96$ degree cm^{-1}, $\mu_s = 30$ cm^{-1}, $g = 0.95$) as that of the experimental phantom. The excellent agreement between the experimental and the simulated Mueller matrices emphasizes the capability of the PSMC model in simulating complex tissue polarimetry effects, including simultaneous optical activity and birefringence in the presence of multiple scattering. The results of the decomposition of the experimental Mueller matrix in (a) are presented in Table 2.1.

begun investigating these issues [13, 30, 66] and some of the results are presented in the following section.

2.5.2 Experimental verification of decomposition

Figure 2.4(a) provides an example of an experimentally derived Mueller matrix of a control sample, composed of solid polyacrylomide, and exhibiting simultaneous polarization, linear birefringence, and optical activity. Its Mueller matrix was measured in the forward detection geometry. Figure 2.4(b) shows the corresponding theoretical prediction obtained with the PSMC model, demonstrating excellent agreement of the forward model with the control experimental data. While the sample measured matrix has a rather complex form, with essentially all sixteen elements being non-zero, the resulting basis matrices derived from the Lu-Chipman decomposition (Table 2.1) exhibit simpler features, namely high levels of symmetry and many zero off-diagonal elements. The scalar parameters (Δ, d, δ, and ψ) are also presented in the table, showing excellent agreement of the decomposition-derived parameters with the controlled inputs

The values for parameters δ and ψ determined from the decomposition of Mueller matrices corresponding both to non-scattering (no-microspheres) and turbid ($\mu_s = 30$ cm^{-1}, $g = 0.95$) optically active ($\chi = 1.96$ °cm^{-1}) phantoms with increasing birefringence (sample extension of 0–4 mm, $\delta = 0$–1.34 rad) are displayed in Fig. 2.5 [30]. The values are in close agreement with the controlled experimental inputs ($\psi \approx 1.96°$ and $\delta = 1.34$ rad at 4 mm of extension), for both clear and scattering samples. This result suggests that the depolarizing effects of multiple scattering have been properly isolated and accounted for in the decomposition.

Figure 2.6 shows the derived linear retardance (δ) and optical rotation (ψ) for Monte Carlo generated Mueller matrices, using chiral molecule concentration as the independent variable [31]. As in the experimental case, the values are in excellent agreement with the input parameters (δ = 1.4 rad and $\chi = 1.96°$ cm^{-1} at 1 M sucrose) for both non-scattering and turbid media, showing self-

TABLE 2.1: The upper panel shows the experimentally determined Mueller matrix of Fig. 2.4(a), and its decomposition into three basis matrices. The lower panel presents the polarization parameters extracted from these matrices in the second column, and the corresponding expected values in the third. The input control values for linear retardance δ and optical rotation ψ were obtained from measurement on a clear ($\mu_s = 0$ cm^{-1}) phantom having the same extension (4 mm) and similar concentration of sucrose (1 M) as that of the turbid phantom, and corrected for the increased pathlength due to multiple scattering (determined from Monte Carlo modeling). The expected value for the net depolarization coefficient Δ was determined from the Monte Carlo simulation of the experiment as per Figure 2.4(b). (Adapted from reference [30]).

M (measured)

$$\begin{bmatrix} 1.0000 & -0.0312 & 0.0029 & -0.0066 \\ -0.0214 & 0.7678 & -0.0370 & 0.0204 \\ -0.0055 & 0.0230 & 0.1043 & -0.7735 \\ 0.0014 & 0.0390 & 0.7972 & 0.1920 \end{bmatrix}$$

Polar decomposition process

$\mathbf{M}_\Delta$ $\mathbf{M}_R$ $\mathbf{M}_D$

$$\begin{bmatrix} 1.0000 & 0 & 0 & 0 \\ 0.0028 & 0.7552 & 0 & 0 \\ -0.0102 & 0 & 0.7689 & 0 \\ 0.0016 & 0 & 0 & 0.8454 \end{bmatrix} \begin{bmatrix} 1.0000 & 0 & 0 & 0 \\ 0 & 0.9984 & -0.0513 & 0.0242 \\ 0 & 0.0333 & 0.1844 & -0.9823 \\ 0 & 0.0460 & 0.9815 & 0.1858 \end{bmatrix} \begin{bmatrix} 1.0000 & -0.0312 & 0.0029 & -0.0066 \\ 0.0312 & 1.0000 & -0.0000 & 0.0001 \\ 0.0029 & -0.0000 & 0.9995 & -0.0000 \\ 0.0066 & 0.0001 & -0.0000 & 0.9995 \end{bmatrix}$$

Parameters	Derived parameters	Expected value
d	0.032	0
δ	1.384 rad	1.345 rad
ψ	2.04°	2.07°
Δ	0.21	0.19

consistency in inverse decomposition analysis and successful decoupling. The small increases in optical rotation observed in turbid media (in both the experimental phantoms or the corresponding Monte Carlo simulated scattering media) likely arise from the increased optical pathlength caused by multiple scattering, thus resulting in accumulations of ψ values [30].

The illustrative results discussed above are based on Mueller matrices recorded in the forward detection geometry, but the extension of this approach to backward detection geometry (which is well-suited for *in-situ* measurements) is warranted, and has also been validated [66]. While the later geometry is important for conceptual and practical reasons, it offers additional technical hurdles; notably, the polarization parameters associated with the intrinsic polarimetric properties of the sample in question can be difficult to infer since they are more strongly coupled with scattering-induced effects. At detection positions sufficiently close to the exact backscattering direction, the contribution of the backscattered (singly or weakly scattered) photons can cause large apparent scattering-induced diattenuation and linear retardance effects, even from isotropic ($\Delta n = 0$) scattering samples. This additional contribution masks the intrinsic polarimetric parameters of interest and hinders their accurate determination. However, it has been shown that as one moves away from the exact backscattering geometry, the magnitude of scattering-induced diattenuation and retardance gradually diminish and eventually become weak (magnitudes $d \leq 0.05$, $\delta \leq 0.1$) for detection positions located at distances larger than a transport length away from the point of illumination ($r > l_{tr}$,

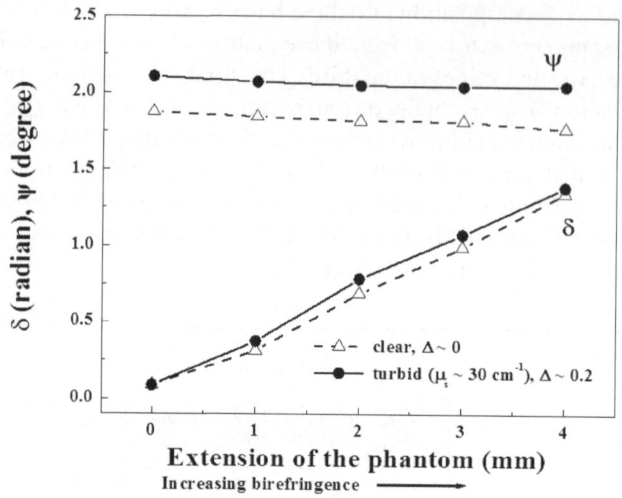

Figure 2.5: Linear retardance δ and optical rotation ψ derived from the decomposition of experimentally determined Mueller matrices of solid chiral (χ = 1.96° cm^{-1}, corresponding to 1 M concentration of sucrose) phantoms with varying degrees of strain-induced birefringence (extension of 0–4 mm, δ = 0–1.345 radian). Results are shown from both clear ($\mu_s = 0$ cm^{-1}) and turbid (μ_s = 30 cm^{-1}, $g = 0.95$) phantoms, and the values for the decomposition-derived depolarization coefficient Δ are also noted. The measurements were performed in the forward detection geometry ($\gamma = 0°$) through a 1 cm×1 cm ×4 cm phantom. The symbols correspond to experimental data and the lines serve to guide the eye. (Adapted from references [13, 31].)

where $l_{tr} = 1/\mu_s(1-g)$ is the transport scaling length). Thus one possible method to accurately measure polarization parameters from a turbid medium using backward detection geometry is to perform measurements at a distance larger than a transport length away from the point of illumination [66].

Ongoing examination of Mueller matrix decomposition for tissue-like complex turbid media (whose constituents properties are controlled and known *a priori*), with both experimental and Monte Carlo-simulated matrices, have shown that in turbid media with weak diattenuation (magnitude $d \leq 0.1$), the decomposition-inferred parameters are essentially independent of the multiplicative order of the basis matrices, and that they accurately reflect the known sample properties. This is an important result, as it suggests that the measurement and decomposition techniques discussed above may be directly applicable to tissues, in which biological molecules (such as nucleic acids, amino acids and proteins) exhibit weak dichroism or diattenuation, which would otherwise be masked by more pronounced polarimetric effects.

By extrapolating the results from Section 2.5.1, one might suspect that the parameters derived from actual tissue should be independent of multiplication order in the decomposition. This conjecture is verified in Table 2.2, which provides an example of a decomposition analysis performed on the Mueller matrix recorded from dermal tissue of an athymic nude mouse [67]. The basis matrices corresponding to Lu-Chipman and reverse decompositions are shown in this table, as well as the corresponding values of the extracted polarization parameters. (The other four permutations in Eq. (2.45) were ruled out in light of physical or mathematical considerations [61, 68].) The similarity between the elements of the basis matrices corresponding to both decompositions suggests that the polarimetric interactions of photons passing through tissue occur simultaneously, rather

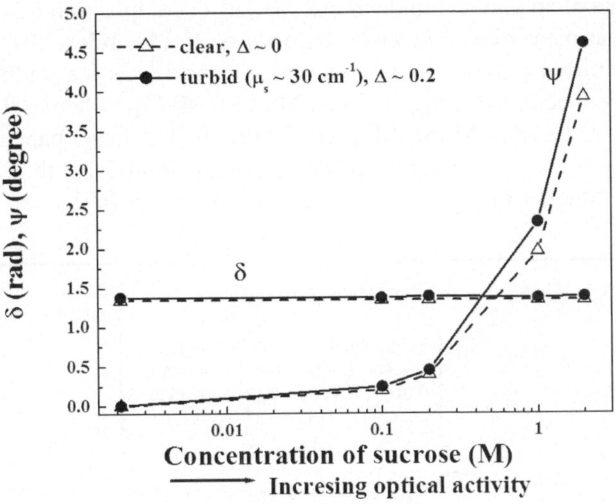

Figure 2.6: The values of δ and ψ extracted from the decomposition of Monte Carlo-generated Mueller matrices from birefringent media (linear birefringence $\Delta n = 1.36 \times 10^{-5}$, corresponding to δ = 1.345 rad for a path length of 1 cm; the axis of linear birefringence was kept along the vertical direction, orientation angle = 90°) with varying levels of chirality (χ = 0, 0.196, 0.392, 1.96, and 3.92° cm^{-1}, corresponding to concentration of sucrose of 0, 0.1, 0.2, 1, and 2 M, respectively). Results are presented for both clear (μ_s = 0 cm^{-1}) and turbid (μ_s = 30 cm^{-1}, $g = 0.95$) media. The symbols represent data points and the lines serve to guide the eye. (Adapted from references [13, 31].)

than in a preferred sequence, as expected. Most importantly, the excellent agreement between the parameters extracted from two decompositions and their true values underscores the validity of the decomposition formalism and its self-consistency with respect to the ambiguity of ordering.

Decoupling and quantification of the individual intrinsic tissue polarimetry characteristics is thus enabled by the polar decomposition analysis, despite their simultaneous occurrence, even in the presence of the numerous complexities due to multiple scattering. The ability to isolate individual polarization properties provides a potentially valuable non-invasive tool for biological tissue examinations. The following section examines the ongoing and prospective biomedical applications of the intrinsic tissue polarimetry characteristics.

2.6 Biomedical Applications of Polarimetric Measurements

A widely-pursued application of polarized light methods is for tissue imaging, which we only mention in passing (with sufficient citations to refer an interested reader). These imaging approaches encompass polarization-gating and various parallel/cross linear polarization arrangements for enhancing skin examinations in dermatology and tumor margins imaging, specifically intraoperatively / following surgical resections. An interested reader is referred to a recent review on polarized light imaging of biological tissues by Jacques [69]. Another imaging-related biomedical application of

TABLE 2.2: The upper panel shows an experimentally determined Mueller matrix measured from dermal tissue of an athymic nude mouse, and its decomposition into three basis matrices. The original matrix was measured *in vivo* from a dorsal skinfold window chamber mouse model, using a high sensitivity turbid-polarimetry system [66]. The basis matrices in the uppermost decomposition were obtained using the order $\mathbf{M} = \mathbf{M}_\Delta \mathbf{M}_R \mathbf{M}_D$, whereas those in the lower set correspond to the order $\mathbf{M} = \mathbf{M}_D \mathbf{M}_R \mathbf{M}_\Delta$, see Eq. (2.46). The lower panel shows the derived polarimetric parameters corresponding to each decomposition. Note that this is the first demonstration of Mueller matrix decomposition in live tissues [67].

M (measured)

$$\begin{bmatrix} 1 & 0.0707 & 0.0348 & -0.0060 \\ 0.0480 & 0.4099 & 0.0077 & 0.0650 \\ 0.0162 & -0.0184 & 0.2243 & -0.3580 \\ 0.0021 & -0.0465 & 0.3571 & 0.1783 \end{bmatrix}$$

M_Δ $\quad$ M_R $\quad$ M_D

$$\begin{bmatrix} 1 & 0 & 0 & 0 \\ 0.0193 & 0.4006 & 0 & 0 \\ 0.0076 & 0 & 0.4596 & 0 \\ -0.0060 & 0 & 0 & 0.3768 \end{bmatrix} \begin{bmatrix} 1 & 0 & 0 & 0 \\ 0 & 0.9935 & 0.0697 & 0.0897 \\ 0 & 0.0435 & 0.4960 & -0.8673 \\ 0 & -0.1049 & 0.8655 & 0.4897 \end{bmatrix} \begin{bmatrix} 1 & 0.0707 & 0.0348 & -0.0060 \\ 0.0707 & 0.9994 & 0.0012 & 0 \\ 0.0348 & 0.0012 & 0.9975 & 0 \\ -0.0060 & 0 & 0 & 0.9969 \end{bmatrix}$$

$$\begin{bmatrix} 1 & 0.0516 & 0.0301 & -0.0037 \\ 0 & 0.3994 & 0 & 0 \\ 0 & 0 & 0.4588 & 0 \\ 0 & 0 & 0 & 0.3758 \end{bmatrix} \begin{bmatrix} 1 & 0 & 0 & 0 \\ 0 & 0.9935 & 0.0701 & 0.0898 \\ 0 & 0.0436 & 0.4960 & -0.8672 \\ 0 & -0.1047 & 0.8655 & 0.4898 \end{bmatrix} \begin{bmatrix} 1 & 0.0480 & 0.0162 & 0.0021 \\ 0.0480 & 0.9999 & 0.0004 & 0 \\ 0.0162 & 0.0004 & 0.9988 & 0 \\ 0.0021 & 0 & 0 & 0.9987 \end{bmatrix}$$

Parameters	Derived parameters using the order $\mathbf{M}_\Delta \mathbf{M}_R \mathbf{M}_D$	Derived parameters using the order $\mathbf{M}_D \mathbf{M}_R \mathbf{M}_\Delta$
d	0.079	0.051
δ	1.06 rad	1.058 rad
ψ	0.51°	0.50°
Δ	0.58	0.59

polarimetry is its use in microscopy, especially nonlinear microscopy. Again, the reader is referred to an excellent and comprehensive review of recent developments in this exciting field [71]. Outside the tissue imaging domain, quantitative assessment of tissue composition and micro-architecture are two particularly attractive and promising applications of polarized light methods in medicine, and these tissue characterization approaches will be reviewed below.

2.6.1 Quantitative glucose sensing with Stokes-Mueller polarimetry

Glucose is an optically active (chiral) molecule, and its structural asymmetry imposes a unique "fingerprint" on polarized light that interacts with it. For example, the plane of polarization of linearly polarized light is rotated upon passage through a glucose solution, by an amount proportional to the light interaction length, its concentration, and its wavelength-dependent rotatory power (a known quantity). As such, the glucose concentration in clear media can be easily determined by polarimetric measurements of optical rotation (this is routinely done, for example in biochemical laboratories and in the food industry [1, 72]). Can a similar polarized light approach be used in biomedicine, for example to noninvasively determine blood glucose levels in diabetic patients? If yes, this would represent a tremendous advance, as noninvasive glucose sensing remains arguably

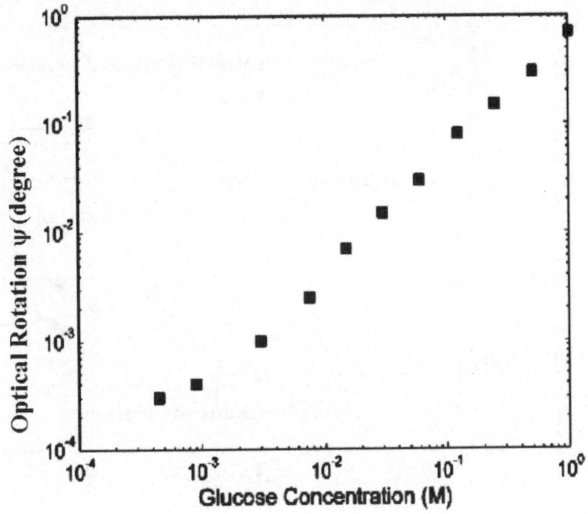

Figure 2.7: Logarithmic plot of experimentally determined optical rotation as a function of glucose concentration in scattering media (1.4 μm diameter polystyrene microspheres in water, $\mu_s \sim 28$ cm^{-1}) down to physiological glucose levels. Measurements were performed using forward detection geometry ($\gamma = 0°$) through 1 cm of turbid media in a quartz cuvette. (Adapted from [14, 73].)

one of the most pressing unsolved problems in clinical medicine. Numerous approaches have been, and are being actively explored to address this difficult challenge [15].

Unfortunately, the polarimetric approach for biomedical glucometry is also fraught with difficulties. Unlike its "easy" transparent media counterpart, light propagating in tissue does not have a unique interaction length which is needed to convert measured optical rotation to glucose concentration; other dominant and complex tissue effects such as multiple scattering and inhomogeneous birefringence depolarize the light and alter its polarization properties (including causing chirality-unrelated apparent rotation of its linear polarized fraction), the glucose chirality effects are rather weak (owing to the low physiologic levels of blood glucose, in the range of 3–30 mM, or ~0.5–5 gm/L of blood, yielding optical rotations in the milli-degree range), and other chiral molecules present in tissue mask the already-weak glucose signal. Nevertheless, we and others have performed careful fundamental feasibility studies towards polarimetric tissue glucometry, as briefly summarized below.

Figure 2.7 shows milli-degree-level optical rotations ψ induced by physiological (millimolar) glucose concentrations in a 1-cm-thick polystyrene microsphere scattering phantom ($\mu_s \sim 30$ cm^{-1}) [73]. This study was performed with a sensitive polarimetric system that utilized polarization modulation and synchronous detection with a dual balanced photodetector approach, optimized to measure weak polarization signals in largely depolarized background. The results shown are for the forward-direction transmission geometry, with the rotations calculated from the determined Stokes vectors via $\psi = 0.5 \tan^{-1}(u/q)$. The forward transmission direction was selected to enable direct results interpretation (pathlength $\geq$ cuvette thickness, rotation directly proportional to glucose concentration) and to minimize rotation artefacts unrelated to chirality. The drawback of transmission geometry is severe depolarization, limiting polarimetric measurements to 2–3 mm thicknesses of tissue [19, 22, 67]; this is why the scattering coefficient for this study in 1-cm-thick cuvette was lowered to $\sim 30\%$ of typical tissue levels. Nevertheless, this preliminary study shows the polarimetric potential for measuring physiological glucose levels in tissue-like scattering media.

Backwards detection geometry in reflection mode is more convenient for practical tissue applica-

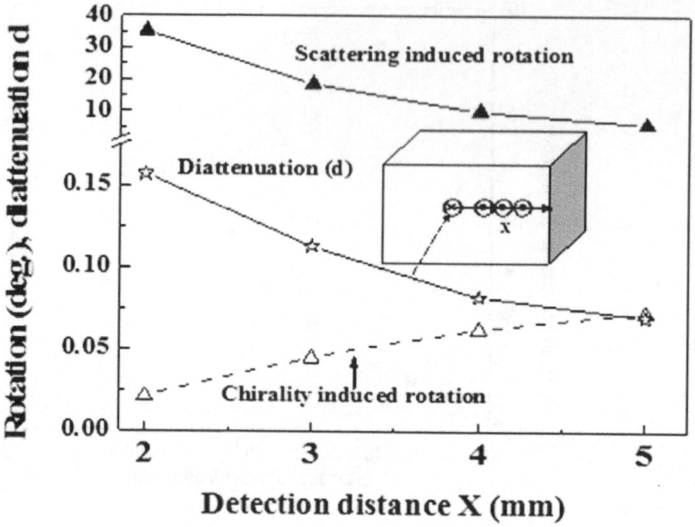

Figure 2.8: Optical rotation (ψ), derived from the decomposition of Monte Carlo generated Mueller matrices (open triangles), of backscattered light as a function of distance from the center of the incident beam of a chiral ($\chi = 0.082$ degree cm^{-1}, corresponding to 100 mM concentration of glucose) isotropic turbid medium ($\mu_s = 30$ cm^{-1}, $g = 0.95$, thickness $t = 1$ cm). The solid triangles represent the corresponding scattering induced rotation of the polarization vector, derived from the Stokes parameters of the scattered light (for incident polarization state $S = [1,0,1,0]^T$). The inset shows the backwards detection geometry. *Decomposition analysis revealed that the large scattering-induced (chirality-unrelated) apparent rotation is due to linear diattenuation (shown by open asterisk), and can be decoupled from the chirality-induced rotation.* The chirality-induced rotation approaches zero as the detection angle approaches the exact backscattering detection. The symbols represent PSMC-generated points and the lines serve to guide the eye. (Adapted from [29, 31, 65].)

tions, yet the chirality-unrelated optical rotation artefacts can be severe [56]. A method to suppress these artefacts is thus essential, and the Mueller matrix polar decomposition methodology can be used to advantage here. Figure 2.8 shows the variations in the scattering induced apparent rotation and in the chirality-induced true optical rotation as a function of offset distance from the point of illumination, in the backscattering direction [13, 31]. As seen, the scattering rotation artefact can be nearly an order of magnitude larger than the small chirality effect, completely dominating and masking the presence of glucose. Yet polar decomposition can effectively separate out these two differently sized contributions, revealing the glucose signal in this important yet artefact-prone detection geometry. Despite the highly preliminary nature of this study – the complicating effects of other chiral confounders, experimental validation of these Monte Carlo simulations results, signal changes due to varying optical absorption, and other complexities yet to be evaluated – this does suggest a method to tease out small glucose specific signals in highly scattering tissues. In combination with Monte Carlo-determined pathlength distributions, we are currently investigating spectroscopic polarimetry coupled with chemometric regression analysis to isolate glucose rotations from contributions of other chiral confounders [74]. Further, given the extremely challenging nature of the noninvasive glucometry problem, it is worthwhile to consider hybrid approaches; that is, combining spectral turbid polarimetry with another diagnostic modality (e.g., photoacoustics) by carefully drawing on each technique's complementary strengths in isolating small tissue glucose levels.

2.6.2 Mueller matrix quantification of structural anisotropy in tissue

Tissue structural asymmetries can stem from aligned orientations of tissue fibrillar components, such as connective tissues composed of collagen, elastin or cartilage, and from elongated asymmetric cells such as smooth muscle or neurons. These structural alignments often result in tissue birefringence, which can be probed with polarized light. Since the structural and functional properties of these tissues change with disease initiation and progression or in response to therapies, birefringence measurements may represent a sensitive metric for assessing tissue status. The polar decomposition platform is the preferred methodology in this context for two reasons: (1) it is essential to separate out the birefringence signature from other complex and simultaneously-occurring compounding effects, and (2) other tissue metrics that are derived "for free" using this methodology (e.g., diattenuation, depolarization, and potentially other metrics not discussed above, such as retardance ellipticity [11, 77]) may offer additional complementary biophysical information that can help generate a more complete picture of the complex nature of the interrogated biological tissue. Below we present a cardiologic and a urological study to demonstrate the utility of polarimetric monitoring of tissue anisotropy.

2.6.2.1 Cardiologic studies in the heart

Myocardial muscle is highly structured and anisotropic, due in part to the aligned arrangement of cardiomyocytes and collagen fibers. It thus exhibits high levels of linear birefringence in its natural healthy state. Following a heart attack, there is significant structural remodelling, with cardiomyocyte atrophy and an increase in fibrotic collagen content (scar tissue), often arranged in chaotic and random fashion. One thus expects a lowering of structural anisotropy, manifest as a decrease in polarimetrically-derived linear birefringence levels. Further, various post-infarct therapies (e.g., stem cell tissue regeneration) aim to restore heart muscle towards its normal structure, and more importantly restore some of its functional status [78]. It is thus interesting to apply the polarimetric polar-decomposition methodology to quantify cardiac linear birefringence, and test its utility to monitor the severity of heart infarct and to gauge the success of subsequent regenerative treatments.

Figure 2.9 summarizes the pertinent results from such a study, performed in transmission through 1-mm thick *ex-vivo* slabs of Lewis rat hearts after myocardial infarction, both with and without stem cell treatments [31]. Point polarimetry measurements (obtained with PEM-based polarization modulation and synchronous detection system) and imaging results (with static polarization components and a camera system) are shown, with both sets analyzed via the Mueller matrix polar decomposition approach. The reader is referred to the original literature for the many details of biological model and measurement specifics [31, 79]. Several interesting trends are evident from Fig. 2.9. These include the high levels of native linear birefringence, a dramatic decrease in the affected areas following the infarct, and partial recovery of these up towards pre-infarct birefringence levels following stem cell regenerative treatments. This birefringence increase suggests myocardial microstructural remodelling caused by therapeutic stem cell injection, and was subsequently confirmed by histology [79, 80]. Monitoring the micro-organizational state of cardiac tissue via tissue polarimetry thus appears possible, with the important added advantage (not feasible with many other techniques) of being able to assess and quantify regenerative treatments of infarcted myocardium.

Additional metrics that emerge from the polar decomposition analysis essentially for "free," for example diattenuation and depolarization (and circular birefringence/optical rotation, if any), contain useful biological microstructural and compositional information that can supplement the linear birefringence results [67]. We are currently examining optimal means of combining these various polarimetric tissue characterization metrics; suffice it to say for now that the measurement and quantification of tissue linear birefringence offers a promising means of assessing the health, and pathology, of aligned biological tissues such as found in the heart. Similar trends are emerging in oncology, with several recent reports detailing polarimetric contrast between normal and cancerous tissues in the oral and cervical cavities [81, 82], with potential application for early diag-

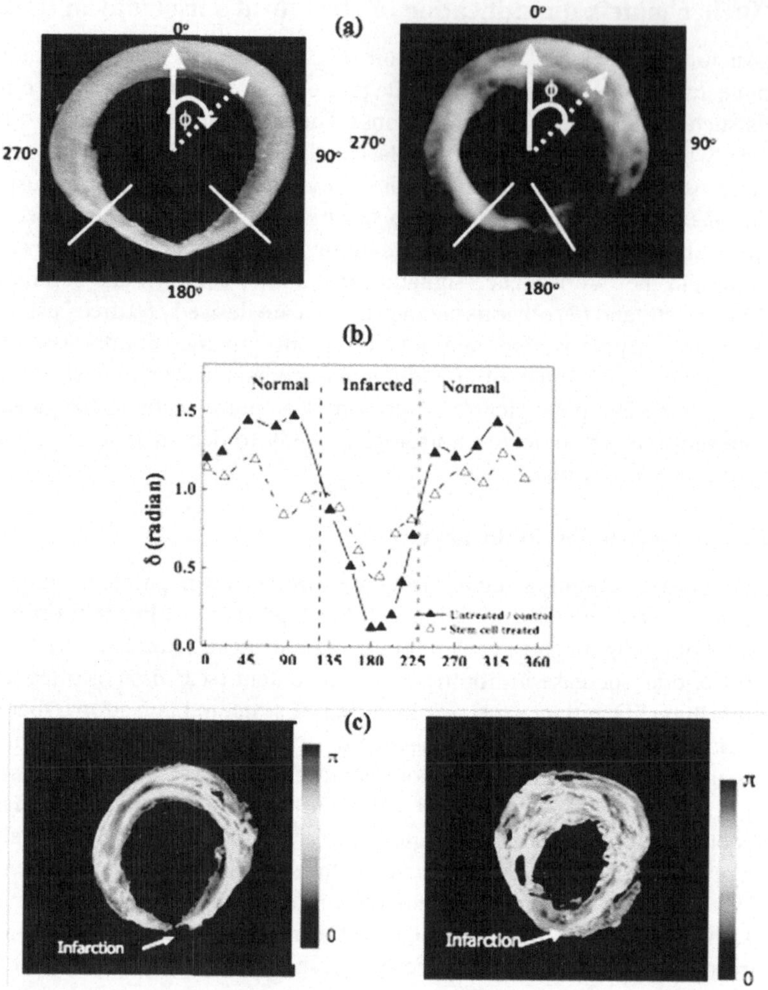

Figure 2.9: (See color insert.) Linear retardance δ extracted from experimentally determined Mueller matrices corresponding to 1 mm-thick tissue sections from Lewis rat hearts following myocardial infarction. (a) White-light photographs of untreated (left panel) and stem cell treated (right panel) tissue. (b) Mueller matrix-derived linear retardance (δ) values at different angular positions from the untreated (solid triangles) and treated (open triangles) samples. (c) The corresponding linear retardance (δ) images for the same tissue, derived from imaging polarimetry measurements. (Adapted from [31, 74].)

nosis/detection and for intraoperative surgical margins assessment [82]. However, many technical and conceptual challenges in quantifying biological anisotropy via the linear birefringence approach remain; for example, additional studies dealing with nonlinear microscopy validation, unique determination of true birefringence magnitude and orientation, comparisons with diffusion-tensor MR, and effects of spatially heterogeneous birefringence, have recently been undertaken [83, 84, 85].

2.6.2.2 Urologic studies in the bladder

The bladder is another internal organ whose structure and function engenders anisotropic tissue structure. Its purpose is to store and then expel urine, and its wall layers extend and then contract to allow this to happen. Microstructural remodelling in its epithelial layers is known to occur under mechanical distension and during various disease processes (e.g., bladder outlet obstruction) [86, 87, 88, 89, 90]. As a step towards developing a turbid polarimetry platform for human bladder pathology studies, we have recently obtained birefringence maps in normal *ex vivo* distended rat bladders that demonstrate the differential response of different bladder regions (dome, ventral and dorsal locations) to changes in filling pressure [91]. The results of Fig. 2.10 were obtained under pressures that represent typical physiological ranges in normal rodent (and human) bladders; as we progress to examine pathological cases, the upper end of the pressure range will likely have to increase. As seen, the dome region of the bladder shows maximum birefringence when the bladder is distended to high pressures, whereas the ventral tissues remains roughly isotropic during distension. In addition, the average anisotropy direction is longitudinal, along the urethra to dome. Using the analysis in Section 2.2.3.3, we converted the retardance values (derived from polar decomposition) to birefringence by measuring the bladder wall thickness with OCT, and by estimating the average photon pathlength in this reflection geometry via our polarization-sensitive Monte Carlo model (Section 2.4). The derived wall anisotropy trends thus represent an intrinsic tissue property of its anisotropy/organization independent of thickness, to better aid in understanding the structure-functions relation in healthy bladders. These new insights into the wall microstructure anisotropy of *ex vivo* distending bladders may also help improve the functionality of the artificially engineered bladder tissues [92, 93].

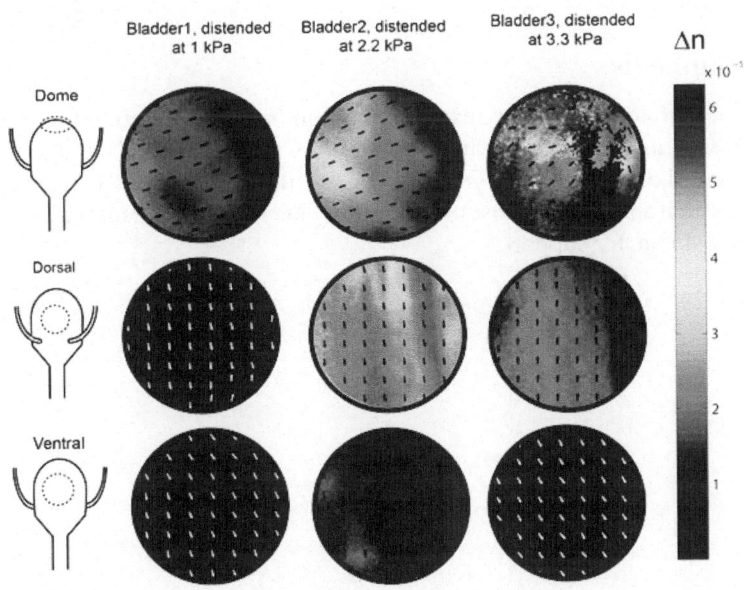

Figure 2.10: (See color insert.) Regional anisotropy (birefringence) images of healthy *ex vivo* intact rat bladders distended to 1.0, 2.2, and 3.3 kPa. The polarization measurements were performed in reflection geometry (25° off the exact backscattering direction). Retardance maps were derived by polar decomposition analysis, and converted to birefringence using OCT-measured bladder wall thickness and Monte Carlo-derived average pathlength. The rows show the birefringence images from the anatomical region indicated by the dotted contour on the *ex vivo* bladder cartoon in the left column. The color represents the value of Δn (color bar on right), and the arrows indicate the anisotropy direction. The field of view is 2 mm in diameter. Note the maximum birefringence in the dome region upon maximum distension, and the overall longitudinal anisotropy orientation (along urethra-dome axis). (Adapted from [91].)

2.7 Conclusion

Biological tissues are not easily amenable to polarimetric investigation, owing to extensive polarization loss caused by multiple scattering and by spatially-varying birefringence. Nevertheless, it is possible in many circumstances to reliably detect some surviving polarization states after fully polarized (linear, circular, elliptical) light is shone on tissue. Several issues then emerge, including (1) how to reliably measure and characterize this surviving fraction, (2) how to interpret these measured polarization signals and relate them to tissue properties of interest, and (3) how to apply this emerging methodology to biomedical problems of interest. We have addressed various aspects of (1)–(3) in this chapter, concentrating on applications pertaining to polarimetric detection of optical activity (for glucose sensing) and birefringence imaging (for tissue anisotropy assessment). The general trend towards polarization quantification, exemplified by Mueller matrix decomposition, has been noted, as is essential for further advances in this challenging field. Coupled with improvements in experimental methods and theoretical models, recent resurgence of interest and research activity, and expanding range of exciting biomedical applications, the near- and long-term future of tissue polarimetry appears promising.

Acknowledgments

The Toronto turbid polarimetry research program has been supported by funds from the Natural Sciences and Engineering Research Council of Canada (NSERC) and the Premier's Research Excellence Award (Government of Ontario). NG would like to acknowledge IISER Kolkata, an autonomous research and teaching institute funded by the Ministry of Human Resource Development, Government of India, for support.

References

[1] D.S. Kliger, J.W. Lewis, and C.E. Randall, *Polarized Light in Optics and Spectroscopy*, Academic Press–Harcourt Brace Jovanovich, New York (1990).

[2] C. Brouseau, *Fundamentals of Polarized Light, a Statistical Optics Approach*, Wiley, New York (1998).

[3] E. Collett, *Polarized Light: Fundamentals and Applications*, Marcel Dekker Inc., New York (1990).

[4] C.F. Bohren and D.R. Huffman, *Absorption and Scattering of Light by Small Particles*, Wiley, New York (1983).

[5] V. Ronchi, *The Nature of Light*, Harvard University Press, Cambridge, Massachusetts (1970).

[6] E. Hecht, *Optics*, 4th edition, Addison-Wesley, San Francisco (2002).

[7] E.W. Thulstrup and J. Michl, *Elementary Polarization Spectroscopy*, 2nd edition, Wiley, New York (1997).

[8] R.A. Chipman, "Polarimetry," Chap. 22 in *Handbook of Optics*, 2nd ed., M. Bass, Ed., Vol. 2, pp. 22.1–22.37, McGraw-Hill, New York (1994).

[9] W.S. Bickel and W.M. Bailey, "Stokes vectors, Mueller matrices, and polarization of scattered light," *Am. J. Phys.* **53**, 468–478 (1985).

[10] S. Yau Lu and R.A. Chipman, "Interpretation of Mueller matrices based on polar decomposition," *J. Opt. Soc. Am. A* **13**, 1106–1113 (1996).

[11] S.L. Jacques, J.C. Ramella-Roman, and K. Lee, "Imaging skin pathology with polarized light," *J. Biomed. Opt.* **7**, 329–340 (2002).

[12] N. Ghosh, M.F.G. Wood, and I.A. Vitkin, "Polarized light assessment of complex turbid media such as biological tissues using Mueller matrix decomposition"; Chapter 9, *Handbook of Photonics for Biomedical Science*, Ed. by Valery V. Tuchin, CRC Press, Taylor & Francis Group, London, pp.253–282 (2010).

[13] M.F.G. Wood, N. Ghosh, X. Guo, and I.A. Vitkin, "Towards noninvasive glucose sensing using polarization analysis of multiply scattered light"; Chapter 17, *Handbook of Optical Sensing of Glucose in Biological Fluids and Tissues*, Ed. by Valery V. Tuchin, Series in Medical Physics and Biomedical Engineering Volume: 12, CRC Press, Taylor & Francis Group, London (2008), pp. 527–558.

[14] R.J. McNichols and G.L. Côté, "Optical glucose sensing in biological fluids: an overview," *J. Biomed. Opt.* **5**, 5–16 (2000).

[15] E. Collett, "Measurement of the four Stokes polarization parameters with a single circular polarizer," *Opt. Commun.* **52**, 77–80 (1984).

[16] V. Sankaran, K. Schonenberger, J.T. Walsh Jr., and D.J. Maitland, "Polarization discrimination of coherently propagating light in turbid media," *Appl. Opt.* **38**, 4252–4261 (1999).

[17] V. Sankaran, J.T. Walsh, Jr., and D.J. Maitland, "Comparative study of polarized light propagation in biological tissues," *J. Biomed. Opt.* **7**, 300–306 (2002).

[18] N. Ghosh, A. Pradhan, P.K. Gupta, S. Gupta, V. Jaiswal, and R.P. Singh, "Depolarization of light in a multiply scattering medium: effect of refractive index of scatterer," *Phys. Rev. E*, **70**, 066607 (2004).

[19] N. Ghosh, P.K. Gupta, A. Pradhan, and S.K. Majumder, "Anomalous behavior of depolarization of light in a turbid medium," *Phys. Lett. A* **354**, 236–242 (2006).

[20] N. Ghosh, H.S. Patel, and P.K. Gupta, "Depolarization of light in tissue phantoms – effect of a distribution in the size of scatterers," *Opt. Exp.* **11**, 2198–2205 (2003).

[21] X. Guo, M. F. G. Wood, and I. A. Vitkin, "Angular measurement of light scattered by turbid chiral media using linear Stokes polarimetry," *J. Biomed. Opt.* **11**, 041105 (2006).

[22] M. Abramowitz and I. Stegun, *Handbook of Mathematical Functions with Formulas, Graphs, and Mathematical Tables*, National Institute of Standards and Technology, Washington, D.C., 1964.

[23] W. Guan, G.A. Jones, Y. Liu, and T.H. Shen, "The measurement of the Stokes parameters: a generalized methodology using a dual photoelastic modulator system," *J. Appl. Phys.* **103**, 043104 (2008).

[24] A. Ambirajan and D.C. Look, Jr., "Optimum angles for a polarimeter: part I," *Opt. Eng.*, **34**, 1651–1655 (1995).

[25] D.S. Sabatke, M.R. Descour, E.L. Dereniak, W.C. Sweatt, S.A. Kemme, and G.S. Phipps, "Optimization of retardance for a complete Stokes polarimeter," Opt. Lett. **25**, 802–804 (2000).

[26] S.N. Savenkov, "Optimization and structuring of the instrument matrix for polarimetric measurements," *Opt. Eng.*, **41**, 965–972 (2002).

[27] D. Layden, M.F.G. Wood, and I.A. Vitkin, "Optimum selection of input polarization states in determining the sample Mueller matrix: a dual photoelastic polarimeter approach," *Opt. Exp.* (2012, in press).

[28] E. Collett, *Field Guide to Polarization*, SPIE Press: Bellingham, WA (2005).

[29] N. Ghosh, M.F.G. Wood, and I.A. Vitkin, "Mueller matrix decomposition for extraction of individual polarization parameters from complex turbid media exhibiting multiple scattering, optical activity and linear birefringence," *J. Biomed. Opt.* **13**, 044036 (2008).

[30] N. Ghosh, M.F.G. Wood, S.-H. Li, R.D. Weisel, B.C. Wilson, Ren-Ke Li, and I.A. Vitkin, "Mueller matrix decomposition for polarized light assessment of biological tissues," *J. Biophotonics,* **2**, 145–156 (2009).

[31] R.M.A. Azzam, "Photopolarimetric measurement of the Mueller matrix by Fourier analysis of a single detected signal," *Opt. Lett.* **2**, 148–150 (1978).

[32] D.H. Goldstein, "Mueller matrix dual-rotating retarder polarimeter," *Appl. Opt.* **31**, 6676–6683 (1990).

[33] M.H. Smith, "Optimization of a dual-rotating-retarder Mueller matrix polarimeter," *Appl. Opt.* **41**, 2488–2493 (2002).

[34] M. Dubreuil, S. Rivet, B. Le Jeune, and J. Cariou, "Snapshot Mueller matrix polarimeter by wavelength polarization coding," *Opt. Express*, **15,** 13660 (2007).

[35] J.S. Baba, J.R. Chung, A.H. DeLaughter, B.D. Cameron, and G.L. Côté, "Development and calibration of an automated Mueller matrix polarization imaging system," *J. Biomed. Opt.* **7**, 341–348 (2002).

[36] A. De Martino, E. Garcia-Caurel, B. Laude, and B. Drévillon, "General methods for optimized design and calibration of Mueller polarimeters," *Thin Solid Films* **455**, 112–119 (2004).

[37] B. Laude-Boulesteix, A. de Martino, B. Drévillon, and L. Schwartz, "Mueller polarimetric imaging system with liquid crystals," *Appl. Opt.* **43**, 2824–2832 (2004).

[38] M. Mujat and A. Dogariu, "Real-time measurement of the polarization transfer function," *Appl. Opt.* **40**, 34–44 (2001).

[39] E. Compain, S. Poirier, and B. Drevillon, "General and self-consistent method for the calibration of polarization modulators, polarimeters, and Mueller-matrix ellipsometers," *Appl. Opt.* **38**, 3490–3502 (1999).

[40] C.-Y. Han and Y.-F. Chao, "Photoelastic modulated imaging ellipsometry by stroboscopic illumination technique," *Rev. Sci. Instrum.* **77**, 023107 (2006).

[41] R.M. Azzam and N.M. Bashara, *Ellipsometry and Polarized Light*, North Holland, Amsterdam (1979).

[42] V.V. Tuchin, L. Wang, and D.A. Zimnyakov, *Optical Polarization in Biomedical Applications*, Springer-Verlag, New York (2006).

[43] A.J. Welch, M.J.C Van Germert, W.M. Star and B.C. Wilson, "Overview of tissue optical properties," in *Optical Thermal Response of Laser Irradiated Tissue*, A.J. Welch and M.J.C. Van Germert, Eds., Plenum, New York (1995).

[44] A. Ishimaru, *Wave Propagation and Scattering in Random Media*, Academic Press, New York (1978).

[45] D. Bicout, C. Brosseau, A.S. Martinez, and J.M. Schmitt, "Depolarization of multiply scattered waves by spherical diffusers: Influence of size parameter," *Phys. Rev. E* **49**, 1767–1770 (1994).

[46] E.E. Gorodnichev, A.I. Kuzolov, and D.B. Rozozkin, "Diffusion of circularly polarized light in a disordered medium with large scale inhomogeneities," *JETP Letters* **68**, 22–28 (1998).

[47] A.D. Kim and M. Moscoso, "Influence of the refractive index on the depolarization of multiply scattered wave," *Phys. Rev. E* **64**, 026612 (2001).

[48] M. Xu and R. R. Alfano, "Random walk of polarized light in turbid media," *Phys. Rev. Lett.* **95**, 213901 (2005).

[49] N. Ghosh and I.A. Vitkin, "Tissue polarimetry: concepts, challenges, applications and outlook," *J. Biomed. Opt.* **16**, 110801 (2011).

[50] L. Wang, S.L. Jacques, and L. Zheng, "MCML—Monte Carlo modeling of light transport in multi-layered tissues," *Comput. Methods Programs Biomed.* **47**, 131–146 (1995).

[51] M. Moscoso, J.B. Keller, and G. Papanicolaou, "Depolarization and blurring of optical images by biological tissue," *J. Opt. Soc. Am. A* **18**, 948–960 (2001).

[52] M.F.G. Wood, X. Guo, and I.A. Vitkin, "Polarized light propagation in multiply scattering media exhibiting both linear birefringence and optical activity: Monte Carlo model and experimental methodology," *J. Biomed. Opt.* **12**, 014029 (2007).

[53] M. Xu, "Electric field Monte Carlo for polarized light propagation in turbid media," *Opt. Exp.* **12**, 6530–6539 (2004).

[54] J.C. Ramella-Roman, S.A. Prahl, and S.L. Jacques, ''Three Monte Carlo programs of polarized light transport into scattering media: part I," *Opt. Exp.* **13**, 4420–4438 (2005).

[55] D. Côté and I.A. Vitkin, "Robust concentration determination of optically active molecules in turbid media with validated three-dimensional polarization sensitive Monte Carlo calculations," *Opt. Express* **13**, 148-163 (2005).

[56] R. Clark Jones, "New calculus for the treatment of optical systems. VII. Properties of the N-matrices," *J. Opt. Soc. Am.* **38**, 671–685 (1948).

[57] L.V. Wang, G.L Côté, and S. L. Jacques, "Special section guest editorial: tissue polarimetry," *J. Biomed. Opt.* **7**, 278 (2002).

[58] S. Manhas, M.K. Swami, P. Buddhiwant, N. Ghosh, P.K. Gupta, and K. Singh, "Mueller matrix approach for determination of optical rotation in chiral turbid media in backscattering geometry," *Opt. Exp.* **14**, 190–202 (2006).

[59] P.J. Wu and J.T. Walsh Jr.,"Stokes polarimetry imaging of rat tail tissue in a turbid medium: degree of linear polarization image maps using incident linearly polarized light," *J. Biomed. Opt.* **11**, 014031 (2006).

[60] R. Ossikovski, A. De Martino, and S. Guyot, "Forward and reverse product decompositions of depolarizing Mueller matrices," *Opt. Lett.* **32**, 689–691 (2007).

[61] R. Ossikovski, "Analysis of depolarizing Mueller matrices through a symmetric decomposition," *J. Opt. Soc. Am. A* **26**, 1109–1118 (2009).

[62] R. Ossikovski, "Differential matrix formalism for depolarizing anisotropic media," *Opt. Lett.* **36**, 2330–2332 (2011).

[63] R.M.A. Azzam, "Propagation of partially polarized light through anisotropic media with or without depolarization: A differential 4×4 matrix calculus," *J. Opt. Soc. Am.* **68**, 1756–1767 (1978).

[64] R. Ossikovski et al., "Depolarizing Mueller matrices: how to decompose them?," *Phys. Stat. Sol.* (a) **205**, 720–727 (2008).

[65] N. Ghosh, M.F.G. Wood, and I.A. Vitkin, "Polarimetry in turbid, birefringent, optically active media: a Monte Carlo study of Mueller matrix decomposition in the backscattering geometry," *J. Appl. Phys.* **105**, 102023 (2009).

[66] M.F.G. Wood, N. Ghosh, E.H. Moriyama, B.C. Wilson, and I.A. Vitkin, "Proof-of-principle demonstration of a Mueller matrix decomposition method for polarized light tissue characterization *in vivo*," *J. Biomed. Opt.* **14**, 014029 (2009).

[67] N. Ghosh, M.F.G. Wood, and I.A. Vitkin, "Influence of the order of the constituent basis matrices on the Mueller matrix decomposition-derived polarization parameters in complex turbid media such as biological tissues," *Opt. Commun.* **283**, 1200–1208 (2010).

[68] S.L. Jacques, "Polarized light imaging of biological tissues," in *Handbook of Biomedical Optics*, chapter 30, edited by D. Boas, C. Pitris and N. Ramanujam, CRC Press, Boca Raton, Florida (2011).

[69] S. Brasselet , "Polarization-resolved nonlinear microscopy: application to structural molecular and biological imaging," *Advances in Optics and Photonics* **3**, 205–271 (2011).

[70] C.A. Browne and F.W. Zerban, *Physical and Chemical Methods of Sugar Analysis*, Wiley, New York (1941).

[71] D. Côté and I.A. Vitkin, "Balanced detection for low-noise precision polarimetric measurements of optically active, multiply scattering tissue phantoms," *J. Biomed. Opt.* **9**, 213–220 (2004).

[72] M.F.G. Wood, D. Côté, and I.A. Vitkin, "Combined optical intensity and polarization methodology for analyte concentration determination in simulated optically clear and turbid biological media," *J. Biomed. Opt.* **13**, 044037 (2008).

[73] D. Goldstein, *Polarized Light*, 2nd edition, Marcel Dekker, New York (2003).

[74] D. Orlic et al., "Bone marrow cells regenerate infarcted myocardium," *Nature* **410**, 701–705 (2001).

[75] M.F.G. Wood, N. Ghosh, M.A. Wallenburg, S.-H. Li, R.D. Weisel, B.C. Wilson, R.-K. Li, and I.A. Vitkin, "Polarization birefringence measurements for characterizing the myocardium, including healthy, infracted, and stem cell treated regenerating cardiac tissues," *J. Biomed. Opt.* **15**, 047009 (2010).

[76] S.-H. Li, Z. Sun, L. Guo, M. Han, M.F.G. Wood, N. Ghosh, I.A. Vitkin, R.D. Weisel, and R.-K. Li, "Elastin gene over-expression during cell therapy prevents scar expansion and ventricular dysfunction after myocardial infarction," *J. Molec. Cell Cardiol.* 2012 (in press).

[77] J. Chung et al., "Use of polar decomposition for the diagnosis of oral precancer," *Appl. Opt.* **46**, 3038–3044 (2007).

[78] P. Shukla and A. Pradhan, "Mueller decomposition images for cervical tissue: Potential for discriminating normal and dysplastic states," *Opt. Exp.* **17**, 1600–1609 (2009).

[79] S. Manhas, M.K. Swami, H.S. Patel, A. Uppal, N. Ghosh, and P.K. Gupta, "Polarized diffuse reflectance measurements on cancerous and noncancerous tissues," *J. Biophotonics* **2**, 581–587 (2009).

[80] M.A. Wallenburg, M.F.G. Wood, N. Ghosh, and I.A. Vitkin, "Polarimetry-based method to extract geometry-independent metrics of tissue anisotropy," *Opt. Lett.*, **35**, 2570–2572 (2010).

[81] M.A. Wallenburg, M. Pop, M.F.G. Wood, N. Ghosh, G.A. Wright, and I.A. Vitkin, "Comparison of optical polarimetry and diffusion tensor MR imaging for assessing myocardial anisotropy," *J. Innov. Opt. Health Sci.* **3,** 109–121 (2010).

[82] M.A. Wallenburg, S.-H. Li, R.-K. Li, and I. A. Vitkin, "Two photon microscopy of healthy, infarcted, and regenerating myocardium," *J. Biophoton.* **4**, 297–304, (2011).

[83] K.J. Aitken and D.J. Bagli, "The bladder extracellular matrix. Part I: architecture, development and disease," *Nat. Rev. Urol.* **6**, 596–611 (2009).

[84] K.J. Aitken and D.J. Bagli, "The bladder extracellular matrix. Part II: regenerative applications," *Nat. Rev. Urol.* **6**, 612–21 (2009).

[85] T. Berrocal, P. Lopez-Pereira, A. Arjonilla, and J. Gutierrez, "Anomalies of the distal ureter, bladder, and urethra in children: embryologic, radiologic, and pathologic features," *Radiographics* **22**, 1139–1164 (2002).

[86] A. Tubaro, C. De Nunzio, A. Trucchi, G. Palleschi, and L. Miano, "The effect of bladder outlet obstruction treatment on ultrasound-determined bladder wall thickness," *Rev. Urol.* **7**, S35-42 (2005).

[87] C.C. Wang, J. Nagatomi, K.K. Toosi, N. Yoshimura, J.H. Hsieh, M.B. Chancellor, and M. Sacks, "Diabetes-induced alternations in biomechanical properties of urinary bladder wall in rats," *Urology* **73**, 911-915 (2009).

[88] S. Alali, K. Aitken, D. Bagli, and I.A. Vitkin, "Optical assessment of anisotropy in ex-vivo distended rat bladders," *J. Biomed. Opt.* (2012, in press).

[89] G.S. Jack, R. Zhang, M. Lee, Y. Xu, B.M. Wu, and L.V. Rodrigues, "Urinary bladder smooth muscle engineered from adipose stem cells and a three dimensional synthetic composite," *Biomaterials* **30**, 3259-70 (2009).

[90] R.L. Heise, J. Ivanova, A. Parek, and M.A. Sacks, "Generating elastin-rich small intestinal submucosa-based smooth muscle constructs utilizing exogenous growth factors and cyclic mechanical stimulation," *Tissue Eng. Part A* **15,** 3951-60 (2009).

3

Spatial and Temporal Frequency Domain Tissue Optical Imaging

Amaan Mazhar
Beckman Laser Institute and Medical Clinic, University of California, Irvine

David J. Cuccia
Modulated Imaging Inc., Irvine, CA

Anthony J. Durkin, Bruce J. Tromberg
Beckman Laser Institute and Medical Clinic, University of California, Irvine

The medical field has been revolutionized by technologies that visualize tissue for diagnostic purposes. However, quantitative characterization of tissue structure and function remains a challenge due to structural heterogeneity and functional diversity across spatial scales. Optical technologies have proven to be an inexpensive and safe method to visualize tissue at a multitude of spatial scales. The focus of this chapter is on meso- to macroscopic ($\sim$0.1–5 cm) imaging of tissue. Over these length scales, light is multiply scattered, thus rendering the resulting images blurry and more difficult to interpret. The loss of structural information is balanced, in part, by the exquisite sensitivity of multiply scattered "diffuse" light to small changes in tissue functional properties. Thus, quantitative characterization of tissue optical scattering and absorption can provide the key to understanding tissue structure and function, respectively. There has been extensive work on a number of measurement methods to characterize light transport in tissue. In this chapter, we will review some general approaches used to characterize thick tissue and will focus in detail on frequency domain spatial and temporal techniques for quantitative tissue analysis.

Key words: spatial frequency domain imaging, diffuse optical imaging, frequency domain photon migration

3.1 Background

The use of light for medical diagnostic imaging has grown substantially over the past 2 decades driven, in part, by the development of new methods for characterizing tissue structure and function beneath the surface [1, 2, 3]. For thick tissue imaging (>1 mm depth), near-infrared (NIR) light (~650 nm–1000 nm) is often used because tissue has relatively low absorption in this regime and NIR light is able to propagate more deeply compared to ultraviolet (UV) and visible (VIS) light.

Absorption in turbid systems is characterized by the absorption coefficient (μ_a). This value represents the probability per unit length that an absorption event will occur and is often given in units of mm^{-1} or cm^{-1}. The measured absorption spectra are linear combinations of the component chromophore spectra. Multispectral measurement of absorption coefficients combined with knowledge of the wavelength-dependent molar extinction (ε) values of tissue chromophores enables the calculation of tissue chromophore concentration (*C*) using equation (3.1)

$$\vec{\mu}_a(\lambda) = 2.303[\varepsilon(\lambda)]\vec{C}, \tag{3.1}$$

where the brackets [ ] represent a matrix, the upper arrows indicate a vector, and λ is the wavelength. This equation can be solved by adjusting μ_a and C into the appropriate vectors, ε into a matrix, and solving the linear algebra equation. If the absorption coefficient and chromophores are homogenously distributed in tissue volume, no *a priori* knowledge about chromophore concentration needs to be assumed. The primary NIR tissue chromophores are oxyhemoglobin (ctO_2Hb), deoxyhemoglobin (ctHHb), water (ctH_2O), melanin (fmel), and bulk lipid (fLipid). Useful indices such as total hemoglobin (ctTHb= ctO_2Hb + ctHHb), and % oxygen saturation ($stO_2=100\times ctO_2Hb/ctTHb$) can also be determined.

Concentrations (or tissue % fraction) of these chromophores can be calculated using published values of basis spectra. As an example, hemoglobin concentration is often calculated using published hemoglobin extinction coefficients [4]. Water content and bulk lipid (fLipid) are determined from tissue absorption spectra using pure water and lipid spectra [5, 6, 7]. Lipid extinction coefficient values can also be obtained from mammalian fat spectra [8]. Melanin absorption has been shown to have an exponential dependence on wavelength [9]. Typical absorption spectra for each constituent in the NIR and a composite tissue absorption spectrum are shown in Fig. 3.1.

Accurate measurements of absorption in tissue are complicated by distortions from multiple light scattering. Scattering arises from variations in refractive index that occur due to the heterogeneous distribution, size, and composition of cellular and extracellular components. The scattering coefficient μ_s is the product of the number of scattering particles in a medium and the cross sectional area. Scattering interactions also are directional which is described by the value of anisotropy, *g*. The value *g* varies from -1 to 1, where 1 is completely forward scattering, 0 is isotropic, and -1 is back scattering. In biomedical optics, the amount of scattering is often described by the reduced scattering coefficient μ_s' which is equal to $\mu_s(1-g)$. In tissue, scattering is mostly forward scattering ($g \sim 0.9$) and is dependent on cellular structure, size, and distribution [10]. In the NIR, scattering lengths in tissue are three to five orders of magnitude shorter than absorption lengths.

The presence of multiple scattering results in a number of measurement related implications. First, light can be detected in both an epi- or trans-illumination geometry. Second, there is degradation in spatial resolution due to multiple scattering. Lastly, the attenuation of reflected or transmitted light intensity is due to a combination of absorption and scattering. In an epi-illumination (reflection) geometry, the reflectance is the fraction of incident light that is remitted back through the surface. The overall light attenuation is due to a combination of absorption and scattering and is often described by the effective attenuation coefficient:

$$\mu_{eff}^2 = 3\mu_a(\mu_a + \mu_s') \tag{3.2}$$

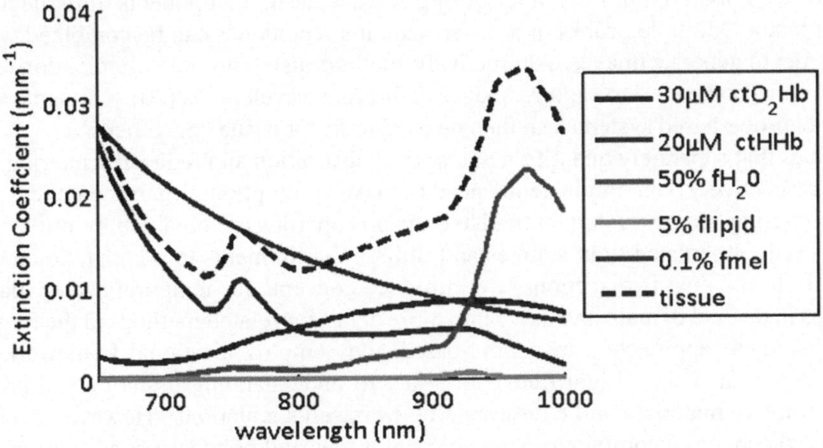

Figure 3.1: An example of typical individual tissue chromophore absorption coefficients.

Absorption and scattering cannot be separated with a single reflectance measurement at a single wavelength. However, the measurement of light absorption contains unique information regarding tissue functional content. Consequently, there are many approaches for obtaining tissue absorption spectra. For example, assumptions can be made about scattering so that all changes in reflectance are attributed solely to changes in absorption. These absorption changes are then correlated to relevant tissue chromophores. This method relies on *a priori* knowledge of scattering and is susceptible to errors due to the natural variation in reduced scattering values within a given tissue and between subjects.

A popular strategy in clinical settings is to measure reflected or transmitted light compared to a baseline value. Changes in reflectance at single wavelengths are then assumed to be primarily due to absorption. Changes in the concentration of multiple chromophores must then be calculated by taking measurements at several wavelengths. This method suffers from a lack of exact knowledge of the spectrally dependent optical path length. A great deal of research has been done to quantify the correct set of wavelengths that minimize error [11, 12]. This method is valuable for dynamic trending measurements but has limited utility for a single 'snapshot' measurement and for comparing absolute values between subjects.

Another approach to recover tissue chromophores is to use spectral constraints. In this method, reduced scattering is assumed to follow a power-law dependence:

$$\mu_s'(\lambda) = A\lambda^{-b} \tag{3.3}$$

where A is a representative of the number density of scatterers and b represents the average size of the scattering particles. The power law dependence of scattering in tissue has been found to be applicable for large wavelength ranges [13, 14, 15]. Another assumption for this type of measurement is *a priori* knowledge of constituent tissue chromophores. The main absorbers in tissue are fit for directly using component spectra instead of determining absorption and scattering values at specific wavelengths. This concept has also been extended to direct three-dimensional reconstruction of chromophore values in turbid media [16]. The choice of wavelengths is critical for accurate reconstruction and has been investigated thoroughly by looking at the relevant extinction coefficients of absorbing chromophores [17, 18]. Additional wavelengths are required to fit for the scattering power law and the relatively coupled space for scattering parameters (A, b) can make inversion a challenge. Modified scattering terms have also been presented in order to make this space more linear [19]. A key advantage remains that measurements are only required for one source and detector pair. However, assumptions about absorbing and scattering components of tissue are potentially a limiting factor. Multiple probes or a raster scanning techniques can be combined with these methods in order to generate images. Alternatively, methods using discrete illumination or multi-spectral cameras can also be used to capture images at discrete wavelengths [20]. The same algorithms used in contact probe-based systems can then be used to fit for tissue constituents.

Methods that separately quantify tissue optical absorption and reduced scattering parameters (μ_a and μ_s', respectively) can eliminate the need to make assumptions regarding optical path length and tissue scattering. In general, quantitative optical properties are obtained by utilizing spatially and or temporally modulated light sources and fitting measurements to computational models of light transport. In the next two sections, we introduce concepts for temporal and spatial measurement strategies in the real domain and delve into more detail for related methods in the frequency domain.

Because these approaches are model-based, they employ a rational framework for describing light transport in tissue. Light transport is key to understanding tissue optical properties. Light transport in any material can be described by Maxwell's equations. However, dense scattering in turbid media creates a complex superposition of waves and boundary conditions that cannot easily be solved analytically or numerically. The radiative transfer equation (RTE, or Boltzmann equation) is an approximation to Maxwell's equations, based upon conservation of energy, describing the propagation of photons and energy through space and time. While it is also difficult to solve the full expression analytically and numerically [21], assumptions can be made to the RTE that are applicable to photon transport in tissue and result in simpler analytical solutions. The most commonly used is the P_1 approximation, which keeps the first-order term of a spherical expansion of the RTE (called the P_n approximation) and reviewed in detail [22, 23]. Stochastic approaches such as Monte Carlo simulations can also be used to simulate light transport.

3.2 Temporal Methods for Optical Property Determination

Time-domain (TD) measurements methods (Fig. 3.2) measure the time of flight of photons as they traverse through tissue [24]. In this configuration, an NIR source and detector are placed at fixed positions. A short pulse ($\sim$ 1 ps) of light is sent into the tissue and the remitted signal, the temporal spread function (t-PSF) is measured as a function of time by a detector. Because NIR scattering lengths in tissue are short, i.e., $\sim$20–40 μm, the early portion of the t-PSF is primarily affected by tissue scattering and the tissue scattering coefficient is related to the time taken to achieve the reflectance maximum. NIR absorption lengths in tissue are much longer, $\sim$10 cm, and therefore the tissue absorption coefficient is proportional to the logarithmic slope of the pulse decay. This method was first used in the late 1980s to determine tissue hemoglobin concentration *in vivo* by evaluating the logarithmic slope of the pulse decay [25].

TD measurements were also used to obtain a differential path length factor (DPF) that describes the actual path length of light propagation which is much greater than the linear distance between source and detector [26]. When used in conjunction with Beer's Law, the DPF facilitates determination of tissue chromophores [27]. Subsequent advances in "photon migration" models for light transport have led to model-based time domain methods. Time domain photon migration (TDPM) measurements rely on the conceptual framework that the temporal dispersion of the pulse is unique to a set of tissue optical properties. The entire temporal point spread function is fit to a model in order to calculate tissue absorption and scattering properties. This approach has been shown to be accurate in phantoms [28] and tissues [29, 26]. It has been applied to measure multiple tissue types such as the prostate [30, 31] and breast [30]. Depth information is intrinsically stored in temporal data. Photons that travel deeper into tissue have longer flight times and can be analyzed separately

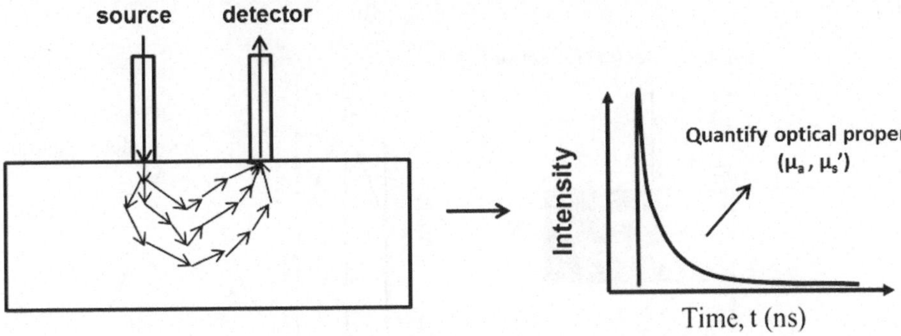

Figure 3.2: Measurement of Optical Properties with time-resolved measurements. The peak amplitude and slope of decay for the detected signal are used to fit for optical properties of the sample.

to assess deeper tissue [32]. This concept has been applied to layered systems [33]. In general, time-resolved measurements are used in a point-based geometry and employ multiple detectors or scanning in order to generate images.

Frequency domain (FD) methods are also used to measure the temporal dispersion of light propagation in tissue. FD techniques employ intensity modulated (MHz-GHz) sources, phase-sensitive detection, and photon migration models. Frequency domain photon migration (FDPM) is based on the conceptual framework of scalar diffuse photon density waves (PDW) that propagate in turbid materials with a coherent front. PDW modulation wavelength and phase velocity are defined by the tissue optical properties and source modulation frequency. They display properties of interference [34], refraction [35], scattering [36], diffraction [37], and dispersion [38, 39].

In FDPM measurements, an intensity modulated is introduced into the tissue. The resulting PDWs will be diminished in amplitude and delayed in phase at the detector (Fig. 3.4), but at the same modulation frequency. The changes in amplitude and phase can be measured at multiple frequencies (MHz-GHz) and fit to photon migration models to determine optical properties [40, 41, 42]. The frequency domain measurement is related to the time domain via a Fourier transform. FDPM models have been developed to separate absorption from scattering in turbid media analogous to steady-state solutions [43] and then applied to living tissue [44]. Two-dimensional images can be generated by scanning sources and detectors over a field of view, using multiple sources and detectors, or using an imaging detector with temporally modulated gain [45].

A major advantage of FDPM is the ability to extract optical properties independent of spectral constraints. However, measurements at multiple wavelengths are still needed to calculate chromophore concentrations. In order to improve spectral density, an approach that combines FDPM with time-independent reflectance spectroscopy (CW-NIRS) has been developed [42]. The FDPM component of the system measures $\mu_a(\lambda)$ and $\mu_s'(\lambda)$ at specific laser diode wavelengths (typically 5–6 wavelengths). The scattering coefficients measured at specific laser diode wavelengths are then fit to a standard power law (Eq. (3.3)) to determine the full $\mu_s'(\lambda)$ spectrum. The power law dependence of scattering in tissue has been found to be applicable for large wavelength ranges [13, 14, 15]. In general, the A parameter is correlated to scatter density and the b parameter is correlated to average scatter size. The $\mu_s'(\lambda)$ spectrum is combined with time-independent (CW) reflectance data in order to calculate broadband absorption spectra. Using this method, $\mu_a(\lambda)$ and $\mu_s'(\lambda)$ are measured over the entire NIR, typically 650–1000 nm, with potentially very high spectral resolution. This method is often referred to as broadband Diffuse Optical Spectroscopy (DOS).

FDPM technologies have been widely used in tissue characterization due to the fact that it can provide non-invasive measurements of hemodynamics. FDPM measures the microvascular status

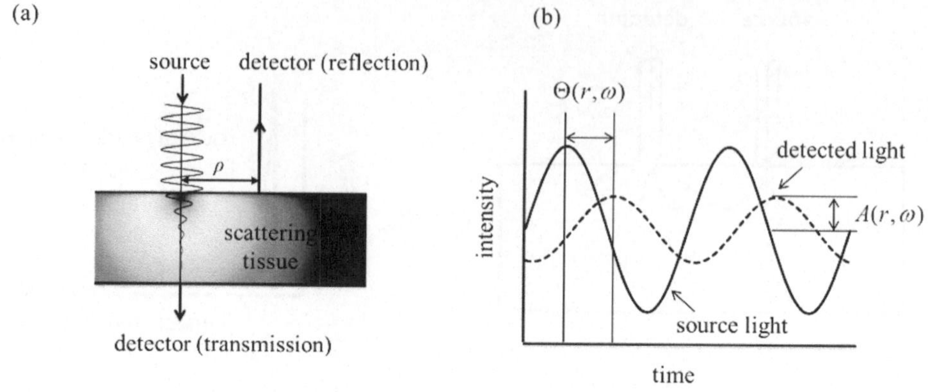

Figure 3.3: Measurement of optical properties with Frequency Domain Photon Migration (FDPM); a) A temporally-modulated light source creates photon density wave (PDWs) which are attenuated in the tissue. The attenuated light can be detected in either reflection or transmission geometries. b) The detected signal is diminished in amplitude and delayed in phase $A(r, \omega)$ with respect to the source. These amplitude and phase shifts are used to fit for optical properties. This figure is from publication [46].

of tissue and is a direct measure of tissue perfusion and metabolism [47, 48, 49]. The changes in tumor hemoglobin content have been measured for chemotherapy agents that are known to possess anti-angiogenic capabilities [7]. Hemoglobin changes can be detected as early as one-day after beginning treatment and the rate of change can be used to predict pathological response [50].

Tissue concentrations of water and lipids have also been found to be substantially different in breast cancer vs. normal tissue [51, 52]. Broadband FDPM methods, also known as broadband Diffuse Optical Spectroscopy (DOS), can reveal absorption spectral signatures that are unique to cancerous breast tissue [53]. The changes in breast tissue water and lipids have been associated with long-term alterations during neoadjuvant chemotherapy as seen with both DOS [54] and MRI [55]. Tumor water concentration and water binding state as measured by DOS scales with the Nottingham Bloom-Richardson histopathology score and may be a correlate to tissue cellularity and extracellular matrix composition [52, 56, 57]. Finally, the extent of water macromolecular binding determined from DOS spectral content has been found to be similar to MRI measures of water Apparent Diffusion Coefficient (ADC). These water spectral variations can be used to measure deep tissue temperature [58, 57]. This list of applications is certainly not exhaustive as FDPM has been extended to many problems including understanding muscle function [59], functional studies of the brain [60, 61], diabetic foot ulcers [62, 63], and others. The use of FDPM technology in Diffuse Optical Tomography (DOT) is also an active area of investigation and has been extensively reviewed [64, 65].

3.3 Spatially-Resolved Methods for Optical Property Determination

The concept of spatially-resolved diffuse reflectance (SRDR) to measure optical properties is well established [66, 67, 14, 68]. In this framework, reflectance is measured at multiple distances ρ from a well-defined source location (Fig. 3.4). Detection can be performed using several source-detector pairs/positions [14, 69] or by binning pixels from a camera-based image [67]. The slope

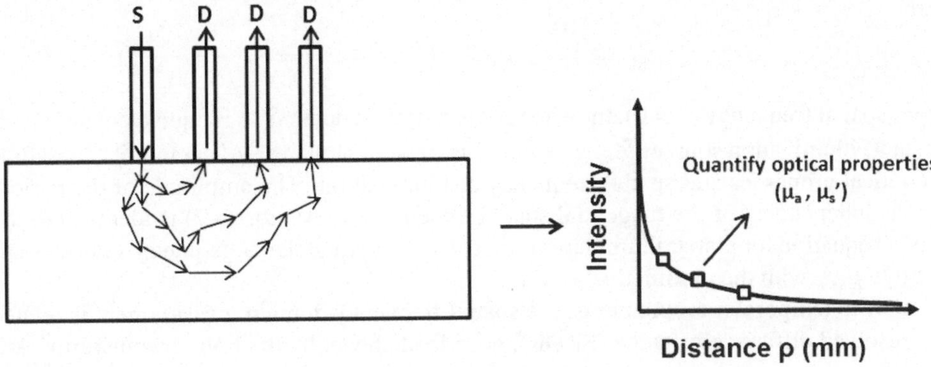

Figure 3.4: Schematic of SRDR Measurement. The spatial point spread function (s-PSF) is measured for multiple distances ρ. This distance-dependent decay is unique to a set of tissue optical properties.

of the reflectance decay, as a function of distance ρ from the source is unique to a set of absorption and scattering properties. Monte Carlo models, diffusion models, and neural network models can be used to predict slope and recover optical properties. SRDR also has some inherent depth sensitivity. A single source-detector pair interrogates a volume of tissue that is often represented by a "photon banana." The source-detector pairs that are further apart detect photons that have travelled further and have probed deeper volumes. In order to generate images, multiple sources and detectors must be combined or raster scanned over a tissue surface. Technologies such as Laminar Optical Tomography (LOT) have utilized this scanning principle to perform depth-resolved imaging and tomography of tissue volumes [70, 71].

As described above, the temporally modulated scalar photon density wave is a well-established frequency-domain concept. Time-independent spatially modulated photon density waves can be presented in a similar conceptual framework to recover optical properties.

In the diffusion regime, the time-independent form of the diffusion equation for a homogeneous medium is given by

$$\nabla^2 \varphi - \mu_{eff}^2 \varphi = -3\mu_{tr} q, \tag{3.4}$$

where φ is the fluence rate, q is the source, $\mu_{tr} = \mu_a + \mu_s'$ is the transport coefficient, $\mu_{eff} = [3\mu_a \mu_{tr}]^{1/2}$, μ_a is the absorption coefficient, $\mu_s' = \mu_s(1-g)$ is the reduced scattering coefficient, and g is the cosine of the average scattering angle. Imposing a semi-infinite geometry, a normally-incident, periodically-varying plane wave source can be introduced and described as:

$$q = q_0(z)\cos(kx + \alpha) \tag{3.5}$$

with spatial frequency $f_x = k/2\pi$ and spatial phase α, extending infinitely in the tangential spatial dimension, x, with some arbitrary dependence on depth, z. A sinusoidal source will give rise to a diffuse fluence rate with the same frequency:

$$\varphi = \varphi_0(z)\cos(kx + \alpha) \tag{3.6}$$

Insertion of Eqs. (3.5) and (3.6) into Eq. (3.4) yields a 1D second-order Helmholtz equation for the fluence rate as a function of depth, z:

$$\frac{d^2}{dz^2}\varphi_0(z) - \mu'^2_{eff}\varphi_0(z) = -3\mu_{tr} q_0(z), \tag{3.7}$$

where

$$\mu'_{eff} = \left(\mu^2_{eff} + k^2\right)^{1/2} \equiv \frac{1}{\delta_{eff}'}. \tag{3.8}$$

At zero spatial frequency ($k = 0$), the effective penetration depth δ'_{eff} is equivalent to that of a planar (constant) illumination source, $\delta_{eff} = 1/\mu_{eff}$. In general, however, μ'_{eff} (and δ'_{eff}) are functions of both optical properties and spatial frequency of illumination. The amplitude of the periodic wave, $\varphi_0(z)$, is independent of the tangential spatial dimension x. As Eq. (3.7) is identical to the photon diffusion equation for planar illumination, we can use existing planar geometry solutions and simply substitute μ_{eff} with the modified μ'_{eff} term.

Similar to temporal measurements, the spatial frequency domain measurement is related to spatially resolved diffuse reflectance (SRDR), described above, by the Fourier transform. Analysis of spatial frequency patterns to recover spatially-averaged tissue optical properties was first demonstrated by Dognitz and Wagnieres [72]. A slide projector was used to project circular patterns of light with fixed spacing (frequency) onto the tissue. The average reflected intensity was recorded on a camera and used to measure the optical properties of a bulk sample. A similar device has recently been described using a single pixel detector and spectrometer. This method, Spatially Modulated Quantitative Spectroscopy (SMoQS), has combined broadband spectroscopy with spatial frequency modulation to recover optical properties of bulk tissue at a single point with high spectral content [73].

3.3.1 Spatial Frequency Domain Imaging (SFDI)

The major benefit of measurements in the spatial frequency domain is that it is amenable to a wide-field, non-contact imaging geometry with a scalable field of view. Spatial Frequency Domain Imaging (SFDI) technology consists of three basic components: a light source, spatial light modulator (SLM), and a charge-coupled device (CCD) camera. In one version of this method, spatially-modulated structured illumination patterns are projected onto tissue at a number of frequencies and phases in the form:

$$S = \frac{S_o}{2}[1 + M_0 \cos(2\pi f_x + \alpha)] \tag{3.9}$$

where S_0, M_0, f_x, and α are the illumination source intensity, modulation depth, spatial frequency, and spatial phase, respectively. The remitted light, or diffuse reflectance, from the sample is then captured by a CCD camera. This reflected light, I, is composed of AC and DC components:

$$I = I_{AC} + I_{DC} \tag{3.10}$$

The measured AC component of the reflected intensity, I_{AC}, can be characterized as:

$$I_{AC} = M_{AC}(x, f_x) * \cos(2\pi f_x + \alpha) \tag{3.11}$$

where $M_{AC}(x, f_x)$ represents the Modulation Transfer Function (MTF) of the diffusively reflected photon density waves (PDW). The MTF depends on the optical properties of the tissue.

As an example, linear sinusoidal patterns of light can be projected onto tissue and then used to generate images of spatially varying tissue optical properties. The tissue is illuminated with a sinusoidal patterns at different spatial frequencies with three phase offsets $\alpha = 0$, $2\pi/3$, and $4\pi/3$ radians. $M_{AC}(x, f_x)$ across an entire image is then calculated using a common demodulation expression [74]

$$M_{AC}(x, f_x) = \frac{\sqrt{2}}{3}[(I_1 - I_2)^2 + (I_2 - I_3)^2 + (I_3 - I_2)^2]^{1/2} \tag{3.12}$$

In practice, a spatial light modulator is used to generate the structured light patterns. Developer kits that use Digital Micromirror Devices (DMD) and LCoS (Liquid Crystal on Silicon) technologies are

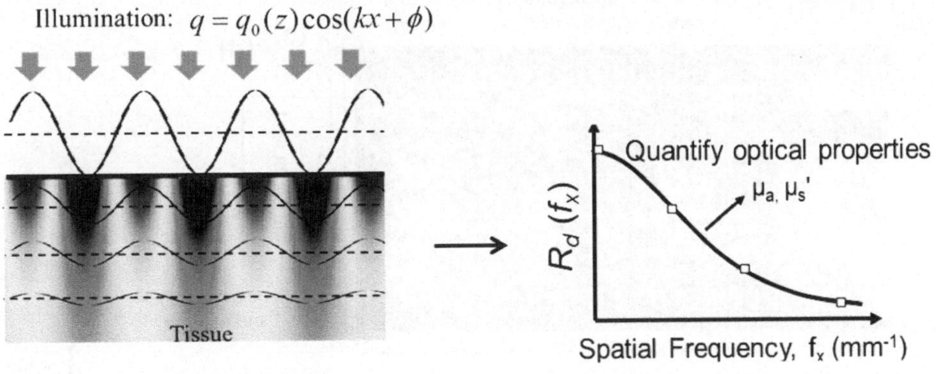

Figure 3.5: Schematic of SFDI Measurement. In this embodiment, spatially modulated waves with multiple frequencies (f_x) are impinged on tissue (only 1 f_x shown) at multiple frequencies. The amplitude decay of the remitted light as a function of frequency is characteristic of a set of tissue optical properties.

pervasive in the market and both are excellent tools for generating any pattern desired by the user. Film slides and patterned masks can also be used to generate projection patterns but are limiting as they are less flexible.

In order to recover tissue optical properties across an image, $M_{AC}(x, f_x)$ is measured at multiple spatial frequencies, f_x, at each pixel of the camera. After a calibration to a known standard, the resulting curve is fit using a least-squares approximation to a given forward light transport model. In principal, low spatial frequencies have high sensitivity to absorption and scattering in homogenous turbid media. At high frequencies, this contrast is limited to scattering – providing the main premise for extracting optical properties (Fig. 3.5). Look-up table (LUT) approaches using models at two spatial frequencies can be used to accurately invert for optical properties [75, 76]. In the case of a homogenous medium, this method has shown substantial equivalence to a least squares fitting method [75]. A flowchart of the SFDI Imaging method is shown in Fig. 3.6.

SFDI is an intensity-based technique and requires a stabilized light source. Incoherent sources are preferred as speckle from coherent sources can provide intensity fluctuations on the field of view. Although this is not ideal, the fluctuations can be addressed with some post-processing and smoothing which is described later. Typically, a cross-polarized illumination and detection scheme is implemented to eliminate specular reflections and isolate photons that traverse through the tissue. The SFDI imaging method is meant to measure optical properties at a single wavelength. Thus, the choice of illumination wavelength ultimately depends on spectroscopic needs. Multi-spectral illumination can be achieved with 2 strategies: 1) a broadband light source coupled with filtered detection or 2) monochromatic light source.

As described above, detection is typically carried out using a CCD camera. Each pixel is treated as an individual detector and reflects a unique inverse problem. In general, CCD requirements are not stringent and really depend on applications. Most studies have used uncooled 12-bit dynamic range cameras with success. For clinical imaging, the relative NIR sensitivity of the CCD may be important to minimize acquisition times. Higher dynamic range cameras may be necessary for low light level applications such as fluorescence imaging. Faster read-out cameras or frame-transfer cameras may be needed to measure dynamic events on short time scales.

Most *in vivo* SFDI research has been performed using NIR light. As described above, the primary endogenous sources of NIR contrast in tissue are oxyhemoglobin (ctO_2Hb), deoxyhemoglobin (ctHHb), water (ctH_2O), melanin and lipids. The absorption at a single wavelength is due to the sum

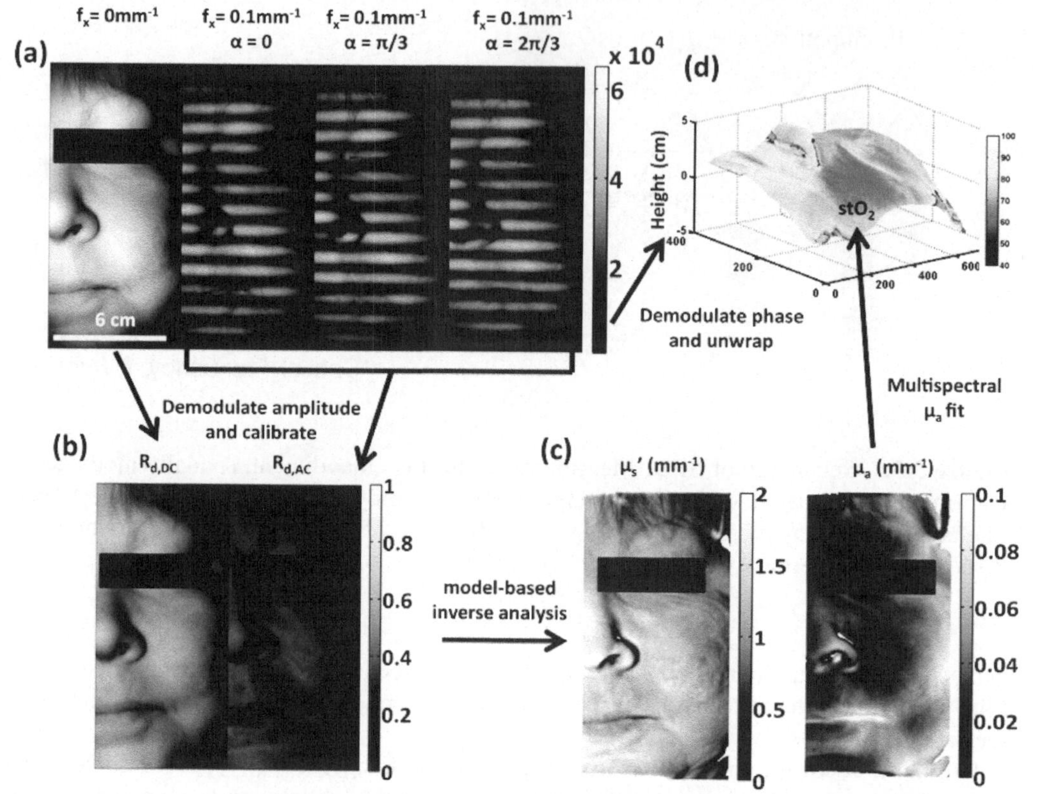

Figure 3.6: Flowchart of SFDI data processing and typical SFDI data products a) modulated intensity patterns are projected onto the surface at each frequency (three phase images per frequency) are b) amplitude demodulated and calibrated, and c) fit to a multi-frequency model to determine optical properties. Separately, d) phase demodulation provides information on tissue height, which can be used for both curvature calibration and visualization. Data are processed separately for each pixel, generating spatial maps of optical properties. This figure is from publication [77].

of the absorption of these intrinsic chromophores. Thus, system performance in extracting these chromophores is highly dependent on wavelength optimization. Optimal wavelengths can be determined based on singular value decomposition of a matrix consisting of the basis tissue chromophore extinction coefficients. This approach was first described by Corlu et al. for spectrally-constrained CW measurements [17, 19]. Corlu et al. also described a calculation of a residual term to account for fitting the scattering term which in general meant more wavelengths were required to fit the inverse problem. Scattering can be recovered independently using SFDI; thus no residual is calculated in this framework and the number of wavelengths required is reduced compared to CW measurements. Ideal wavelength pairs for hemodynamic measurements have been shown for hemoglobin recovery for certain hemoglobin measurements in tissue [78].

Based on this analysis, a fast ($\sim$1 s acquisition) SFDI hemodynamic system can be built using two wavelengths optimized for fitting hemoglobin assuming fixed amounts of water, melanin and lipid. In one case, the combinations of 670 nm/850 nm and 730 nm/850 nm were shown equivalent to using a spectrally dense 34 wavelength data set for the recovery of blood volume and saturation *in vivo* [78]. The design requirement for additional wavelengths ultimately depends on the application and the sources of endogenous contrast such as hemoglobin, water, lipid, or melanin to be measured.

A framework using singular value decomposition of basis spectra as described above can be adopted to optimize these wavelengths.

These improvements are critical as rapid SFDI measurements can greatly benefit clinical applications. Subject motion poses a challenge in clinical imaging and can cause errors in recovered optical property images. Several strategies have been proposed to correct for motion artifact. Fiducial markers have been placed in the field of view and used to correct for movement artifacts in SFDI [79]. Motion-gated methods have also been proposed to reduce motion artifacts in optical imaging [80]. Ultimately, a short imaging time is still preferred to minimize errors due to motion artifacts.

As described above, there are two general strategies for multi spectral imaging measurements: 1) a broadband source can used to illuminate the sample coupled with filtered detection or 2) discrete wavelength light sources can be used to illuminate the sample sequentially. Both approaches are viable and have been used in SFDI measurements. Discrete light sources such as light emitting diodes (LED's) and laser diodes are attractive as they generally have higher powers and can reduce imaging times for large fields of view. Systems with both discrete LED's and laser sources have been described in the literature [81, 77, 82]. Broadband sources retain much greater spectral flexibility but are usually less powerful when filtered at specific wavelengths which, in turn, can increase imaging time. Broadband sources have also been paired with scan-free hyperspectral imaging cameras such as the computed tomographic imaging spectrometer (CTIS) and the Image Mapping Spectrometer (IMS) to generate high spectral and spatial resolution SFD images [83, 84]. However, in this case there is still a need to balance the source spectral output with the sensitivity and dynamic range of the detector in order to optimize overall system performance. In this configuration, cost can become a consideration as the detection hardware is much more advanced and specialized.

In some cases, measuring dynamic changes in tissue over relatively short time scales (<5 s) are of interest. Short imaging times improve the ability to capture fast-occurring hemodynamic changes. In the case of skin flap monitoring, SFDI was able to detect and identify vascular occlusion *in vivo* within minutes of an occlusion in a preclinical model [85]. SFDI was also used to assess tissue health quantitatively after a certain period of vascular ischemia followed by saline treatment [86]. In this study, SFDI hemodynamic measurements were also validated in pre-clinical settings with an FDA-cleared (US approval) device (Fig. 3.7). This was then applied intra-operatively to a human Transverse Rectus Abdominis Myocutaneous (TRAM) flap procedure [87]. Pre-clinical imaging of endogenous contrast has also been demonstrated while measuring functional brain activation in mice [88]. In this study, it was shown that there are scattering and absorption changes that happen in the brain during an ischemic event. In an Alzheimer's study, functional activation can also be used to differentiate between healthy and diseased brains in mice [89]. Finally, the ability of SFDI to measure scattering, and particularly the spatial orientation of scattering structures, has shown potential moving forward [90].

In large field of view clinical applications, height correction is also a key element for non-contact imaging systems such as SFDI [87]. A handful of methods have been advanced to deal with this problem. Surface profilometry using angled illumination and detection of phase shifts of structured illumination is a good match with SFDI and has been used to correct for height-dependent, angle dependent, and illumination frequency dependent intensity changes [91]. Broad shapes of intensity changes have also been used to measure topology and correct for height artifacts in planar multi-spectral imaging. This method assumes that changes in the light field and spatially variant optical properties are on a smaller scale than the height dependent broad intensity changes [92].

3.3.2 Depth resolved SFDI

SFDI imaging methods have been shown to perform depth sensitive imaging of optical property contrast [93]. Tissue behaves as a low pass filter meaning high illumination frequencies (f_x) are essentially gated by the tissue (Fig. 3.8). Based on this concept, multi-frequency illumination allows differentiation between photons that have traveled longer path lengths (f_x is low) and shorter

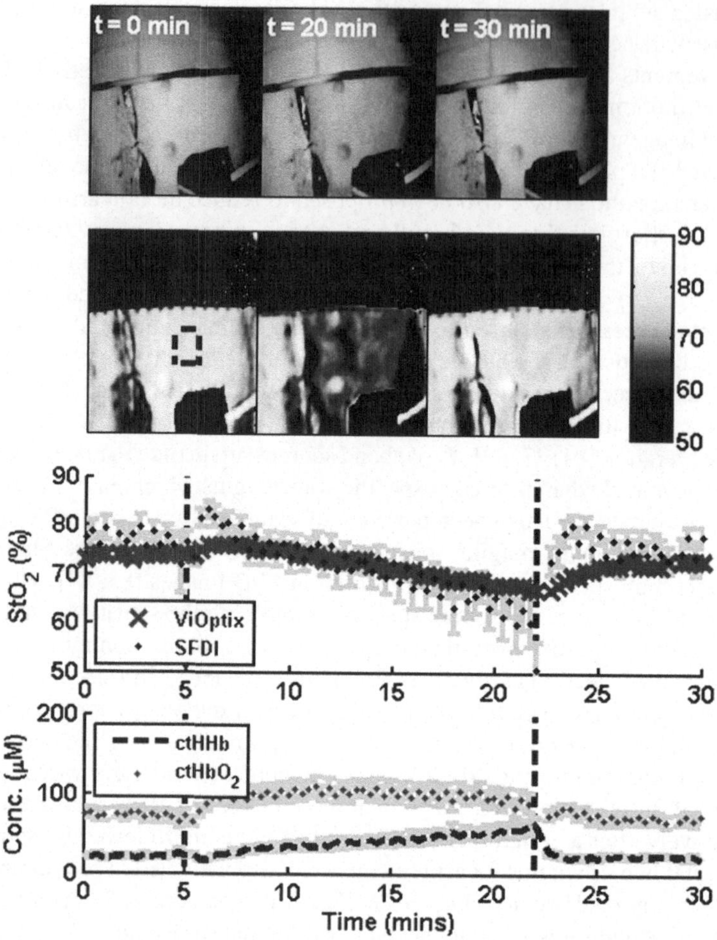

Figure 3.7: (See color insert.) Example of a venous occlusion in a pre-clinical tissue flap model. Recovered stO_2 values in a region of interest (ROI) are validated with FDA probe and recovered blood volume changes are consistent with venous congestion [87].

path lengths (f_x is high).

This has two main consequences. As described in examples above, we have used this relationship to extract optical properties of a homogenous medium in a wide-field manner for NIR wavelengths. This is because absorption path lengths are much greater than scattering path lengths in the NIR. Thus, contrast related to shorter average path lengths (i.e., scattering) can be isolated using high frequency illumination allowing recovery of depth averaged optical properties. Due to shorter mean photon path lengths, high frequency illumination can be used to interrogate superficial volumes of tissue enabling depth sensitive imaging. Although homogenous models for SFDI have proven to be useful in presented work so far, the possibility of advanced models with depth discrimination show promise as a way to improve further quantitation. Layered models are particularly interesting as they mimic the geometry commonly found in skin.

For example, a simple model of skin can assume two distinct layers 1) a top layer representing the epidermis that primarily consists of melanin and 2) a bottom layer representing the dermis which constitutes the bulk of the microvasculature. The validity of two-layer forward models in the diffusion regime has been demonstrated in a set of phantom studies for SFDI [94]. Inverse models

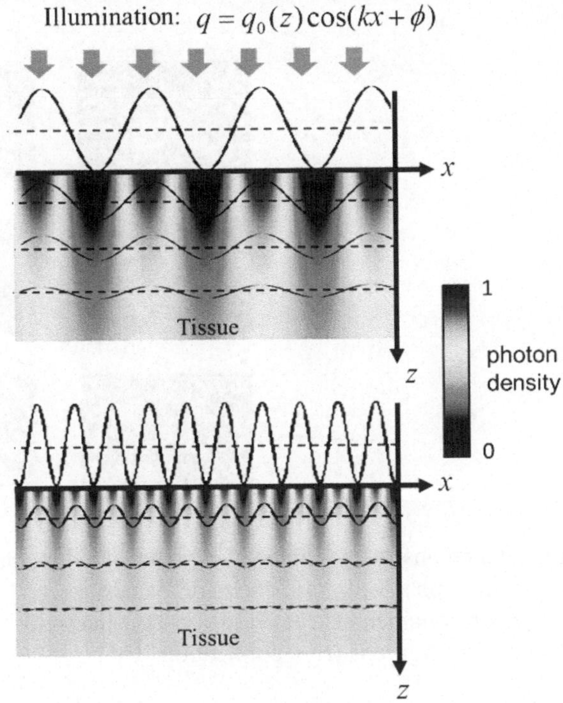

Figure 3.8: Illustration of how tissue acts like a low pass filter to spatially modulated illumination. Patterns with lower spatial frequencies propagate deeper into tissue [46].

showed that optical properties for two layers could be recovered accurately with some *a priori* estimates of top layer thickness. This model was also applied in a pilot study for a volar forearm measurement. A neural network model based on Monte Carlo simulations has also been proposed and applied for two-layer structures in the spatial frequency domain [95]. *In vivo* applications of this model showed improved recovery of tissue hemoglobin and melanin content for a multitude of skin types [96]. Hybrid diffusion and two-flux approximations to multi-layered geometries have also been developed [97].

Beyond layers, spatial frequency domain tomographic approaches have also been developed for quantitative reconstruction of absorption perturbations. Traditionally, the field of diffuse optical tomography (DOT) has adopted methods that include the use of multiple fibers and detectors to generate many unique "views" of the turbid sample [98]. This is applicable to all the methods described thus far: time-domain, steady-state, and frequency domain measurements. Spatial frequency domain imaging provides an alternative method to compress this data. The concept of propagating plane waves in the spatial Fourier domain has been well described [99, 100, 101]. These algorithms were first applied using raster scanned sources and Fourier transforms to generate data [102, 103]. More recently, the concept of a structured illumination source was proposed for direct three dimensional reconstruction of objects [104]. These types of algorithms using structured light were then applied to measure phantoms in reflectance mode and shown to reconstruct buried absorbing tubes with enhanced resolution and more accurate quantitation compared to traditional homogenous models (Fig. 3.9) [105]. The algorithm has been advanced to reconstruct arbitrarily oriented buried structures [106] and has also been used to image mice in transmittance mode [107, 108].

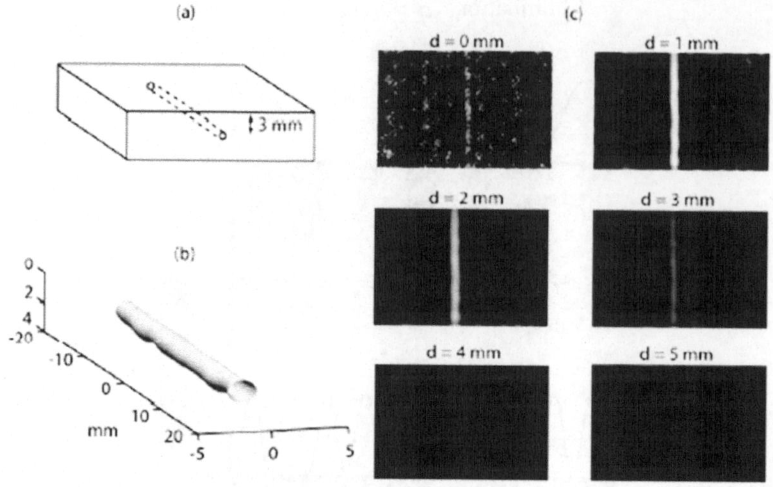

Figure 3.9: Example of a reconstructed image of a single absorbing tube located 3 mm below the surface of a tissue simulating phantom. (a) schematic of tissue simulating phantom. (b) volume rendering of the three dimensional reconstructed image. (c) slices through the reconstructed image at depths of $d = 1$–5 mm. This figure is from publication [105].

3.3.3 Fluorescence SFDI

The growth of NIR fluorescent probes has stimulated considerable activity in the development of *in vivo* fluorescence imaging and tomography technologies for clinical and pre-clinical research [109, 110]. As mentioned above, photon penetration is maximized in the NIR due to low absorption and relatively high scattering. Thus, accurate mapping of sub-surface (i.e., mm to cm) fluorescence with high spatial resolution remains a critical challenge; particularly in the near infrared. This is due to the fact that lateral and axial localization of fluorescence is "blurred" by multiple light scattering. In order to address this limitation, imaging systems that utilize multiple detectors, source scanning, and time/frequency domain techniques have been successfully implemented based on diffuse optical tomography principles [111, 112, 113].

SFDI offers a simple non-scanning alternative method to improve axial and transverse resolution of buried fluorescent inhomogeneities. This approach utilizes similar principles to technologies employing structured illumination developed for the diffraction regime [114, 115]. However, in this case lateral and axial resolution improvements are obtained from thick, turbid materials using principles of scalar photon density waves propagating in the diffusion regime [93, 116, 75]. As described above, tissue behaves as a low pass filter. Thus, structured illumination can be used to specifically impact the depth dependent excitation fluence rate. As an example, a forward fluence model for spatially modulated light – specifically sinusoidal waves - can be adapted from a 1D second-order Helmholtz equation in order to calculate fluence rate (ϕ) as a function of depth, z [75]. An example of relative fluence decay for two spatial frequencies is shown for a given set of optical properties (Fig. 3.8). As the illumination spatial frequency increases, the normalized fluence rate of excitation decays more rapidly with depth. Since tissue acts as a low pass spatial filter, the excitation intensity delivered to deeper structures can be tuned by the illumination frequency, allowing depth-sensitive excitation of fluorophores. Qualitatively, application of this concept has shown to improve spatial resolution and contrast of buried fluorescence objects in phantoms by reducing the effects background scattering and fluorescence (Fig. 3.10) [117].

A number of quantitative tomographic algorithms using structured illumination have recently

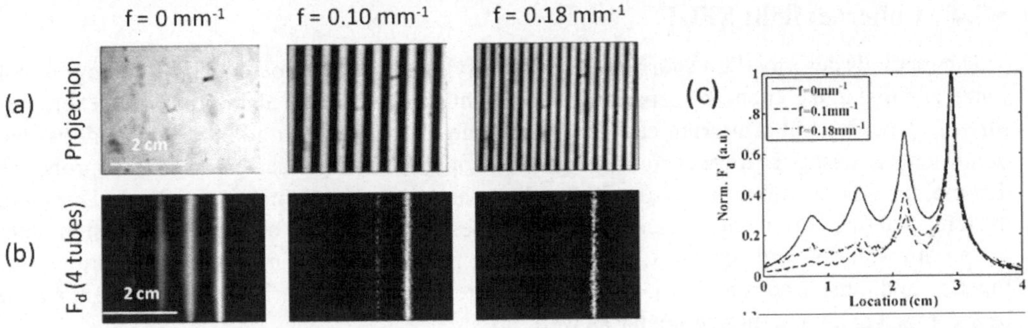

Figure 3.10: Demodulated and calibrated fluorescence maps of phantoms at multiple spatial frequencies. (a) Illumination at three frequencies phase result in depth sensitive imaging along with improved transverse resolution. (b) Images and (c) horizontal line profiles of the four tube phantom demonstrate reduced sensitivity to deep structures [117].

been proposed and implemented. Patterns such as bars [118], scanning Gaussians [119], checkerboards [108], sine waves [107, 105], and wavelet bases [120] have all been proposed as alternatives to raster-scanned sources. Advances in choosing the right type and number of patterns have tremendously reduced acquisition times while maintaining the same information content as a raster-scanned source [121]. Illumination patterns have also been coupled with advanced image compression to further improve imaging and reconstruction times [108].

Fluorescence imaging using a simple planar reflectance geometry has grown in popularity as an approach for surgical guidance *in vivo*. NIR fluorescence imaging using NIR light has been translated successfully for small animal imaging [122], intra-operative sentinel lymph node mapping [123, 124, 125], and imaging of lymphatic flow [126, 127]. As a result, planar fluorescence imaging technologies are fairly pervasive in the commercial market. Although much more challenging, quantitative recovery of fluorescence in tissue is highly desirable as it can provide information on tissue function and correct for light delivery to the fluorophore at the excitation wavelength, the concentration of fluorophore, the quantum efficiency of fluorophore, and the light transport of the emitted photons to the detector. In principle, planar steady-state wide-field fluorescence imaging methods cannot decouple these parameters rendering these imaging modalities essentially qualitative. Some planar reflectance imaging methods have used maps of reflectance at absorption wavelengths to normalize data. Researchers have shown that a priori knowledge of optical properties can enable improved quantitation of buried fluorescence objects [128, 129].

In the field of neurosurgery, 5-aminolevulinic acid (ALA)-induced protoporphyrin IX (PpIX) is gaining popularity as a surgical adjunct to improve the extent of tumor resection. Probe-based optical property corrected measurements of fluorescence have proven to be quantitative and shown much higher accuracy at detecting high grade gliomas compared to qualitative methods [130]. The need to detect buried gliomas at depth will significantly enhance intra-operative guidance of tumor removal. Widefield methods that use multi-spectral modeling of light propagation improve depth discrimination of buried gliomas [131, 132]. SFDI has also been applied to this problem as it provides both depth discrimination and optical property characterization in a wide-field manner. SFDI tomography for detection of orthotopic tumors has been shown in a pre-clinical glioma model [133]. Similarly, SFDI derived optical property maps have also been used to correct for wide-field images of PpIX fluorescence concentrations for topical skin cancer applications [134].

3.3.4 Coherent light SFDI

The methods described thus far focus on quantifying tissue composition, e.g., hemoglobin, lipid, water, and melanin content, by separating static light scattering from absorption. However, the measure of dynamic light scattering can provide unique insight regarding blood flow and the delivery of nutrients to tissue. Diffuse correlation spectroscopy (DCS) is a fiber-based contact probe method that measures both amount of tissue chromophore and the rate at which it is delivered by modeling the temporal fluctuations of an incident light source. DCS measures changes in perfusion with high temporal resolution and low (~5–10 mm) spatial resolution with important applications in brain function and muscle activity [135, 136, 137]. The temporal characteristics of a coherent source can be leveraged in an imaging geometry as well.

When a coherent light source interacts with a scattering sample, a speckle pattern is produced due to the constructive and destructive interference of light waves propagating along different paths. Fercher and Briers introduced the concept of Laser Speckle Imaging (LSI) using spatial statistics to characterize the fluctuations at the surface [138]. The hardware for a traditional LSI system is very similar to a typical SFDI system. A CCD camera is used to image the interference (i.e., speckle) patterns produced by the coherent addition of scattered laser light propagating with varying path lengths. The motion of scattering particles causes intensity fluctuations in the speckle pattern that can be analyzed with temporal, spatial, or combined spatiotemporal algorithms [139]. The LSI technique has been used to track relative changes in blood flow in tissues such as skin and brain over a specified time [140, 141].

LSI enables imaging of two-dimensional structure and flow. A single snapshot, taken at an exposure time on the order of the speckle correlation time, is analyzed using spatial statistics. The local speckle contrast, K, is calculated from a reflectance image as:

$$K = \frac{\sigma_s}{\langle I \rangle} \tag{3.13}$$

where σ_s and $\langle I \rangle$ represent the spatial standard deviation and mean pixel intensity in a region of interest. In practice, a speckle contrast image is calculated with the use of a sliding window operator moved across the entire image. In principle, regions with increased flow result in more rapid intensity fluctuations. During a single camera exposure (typically on the order of 1–20 ms), these fluctuations will reduce speckle visibility as compared with regions with relatively less motion. Thus, speckle contrast is inversely proportional to motion in a sample.

Several methods have been suggested to convert speckle contrast to a measure of flow in tissue [142]. Assumptions must be made to describe the nature of the motion. Methods using Gaussian, Lorentzian, hybrid, random, and calibration models of perfusion have been described but absolute flow quantification remains difficult [143, 142]. In general, the speckle contrast value is inversely proportional to blood flow and a metric such as the Speckle Flow Index (SFI) can be defined to assess relative flow in an image [144]. Regardless of the model used, the calculation of an accurate speckle contrast remains a major obstacle.

Measurement and model considerations for quantifying speckle contrast depend on many factors. These include the ratio of speckle size to pixel size [145], speckle window size, choice of dynamic model, noise [146], and effects of static scattering [147, 148, 149]. Comprehensive reviews of image processing algorithms and applications have covered many of these studies [150, 151].

Recent work on Laser Doppler Flowmetry (LDF) has shown that optical path length is an important consideration during measurements [152, 153]. LDF is another optical fiber-based correlate to LSI. In practice, LSI is similar to LDF and is used to measure many types of tissue such as brain and skin. These tissue types span a large range of optical properties and different optical path lengths. Dynamic physiological measurements can also result in changes in optical path lengths. Coherent Spatial Frequency Domain Imaging (cSFDI) has shown potential as a method to help quantify optical path lengths in the context of measuring speckle contrast. The introduction of spatially modulated coherent light results in two major implications. First, similar to depth-sensitive absorption contrast, the introduction of spatial frequencies is able to perform qualitative crude sectioning of speckle contrast. This has been demonstrated in phantom measurements [154]. Additionally, static optical properties can be fit using diffusion and Monte Carlo models to help further quantify speckle contrast independent of baseline optical properties.

In the diffusion regime, the speckle contrast term can be derived in terms of optical properties using knowledge of the electric field temporal autocorrelation function, $G_1(\tau)$, and camera exposure time, T, as derived in previous literature [139, 147, 143]: $G_1(\tau)$ is related to the intensity autocorrelation function, $G_2(\tau)$, via the Siegert relationship and has been shown to obey the correlation diffusion equation in a turbid media [155]:

$$\nabla^2 G_1(\tau) - \mu_{eff} G_1(\tau) = q \tag{3.14}$$

In these equations, q is the source, $\mu_{tr} = \mu_a + \mu_s'$ the transport or total attenuation coefficient, μ_a the absorption coefficient, μ'_s, the reduced scattering coefficient, $\mu_{a,dyn}$ is the dynamic absorption term, and $\mu_{eff} = [3\mu_{a,dyn}\mu_{tr}]^{1/2}$. The $mu_{a,dyn}$ term is unique to this framework as it incorporates the motion in the turbid system:

$$\mu_{a,dyn} \rightarrow \mu_a + \frac{1}{3}\mu_s' k_o^2 \left\langle \Delta r^2(\tau) \right\rangle \tag{3.15}$$

Here $k_o = \frac{2\pi n}{\lambda}$ is the wave number of the propagating photons, and $\left\langle \Delta r^2(\tau) \right\rangle$ is the mean square displacement of the dynamic scattering particles. Note that for Brownian motion $\left\langle \Delta r^2(\tau) \right\rangle = 6D_B\tau$, where D_B is the Brownian diffusion coefficient. The solution for Eq. (3.14) is in the same form as typical photon fluence equation in the diffuse regime (Eq. (3.3)), except that the absorption term is modified [155]. Thus, the solution derived in the SFD can be applied to this equation.

However, just as in photon diffusion models, if the dynamic absorption term is too high (i.e., high absorption, high flow, or longer exposure times) Monte Carlo modeling of these phenomena is more appropriate. This can be done by tracking the momentum transfer of a photon-scatterer collision directly which has been shown to accurately predict speckle contrast in liquid phantoms in the spatial frequency domain [156]. Additionally, these models have also demonstrated the impact of illumination inhomogeneity on measured speckle contrast [157]. In principle, cSFDI is a single platform that is able to image both optical properties (absorption and reduced scattering) and speckle contrast. In future work, we expect that this method will be able to image both changes in tissue oxygenation and flow to unlock more information about metabolism as is done with DCS (Fig. 3.11). Because of its fiber-based geometry, DCS in the NIR is typically more sensitive to flow in deep tissue such as brain and muscle. In contrast, cSFDI is performed in a planar illumination geometry and has more superficial sensitivity with applications in cutaneous wounds, port-wine stains, skin flaps and exposed tissue in intraoperative settings.

3.4 Summary and Future Perspectives

In this chapter, we have described a general set of methods for quantitatively measuring optical parameters of tissue based on spatial and temporal modulation of light. The utility of each method depends on how well the technology matches a given application. For example, contact probe based time domain techniques such as FDPM are well-suited for functional interrogation of deeper tissue structures such as brain, breast, and muscle. Widefield imaging methods such as SFDI and speckle are most effective for characterizing spatially heterogenous tissue over large and scalable fields of view. Skin imaging, particularly of wounds, and image-guided surgery are examples of

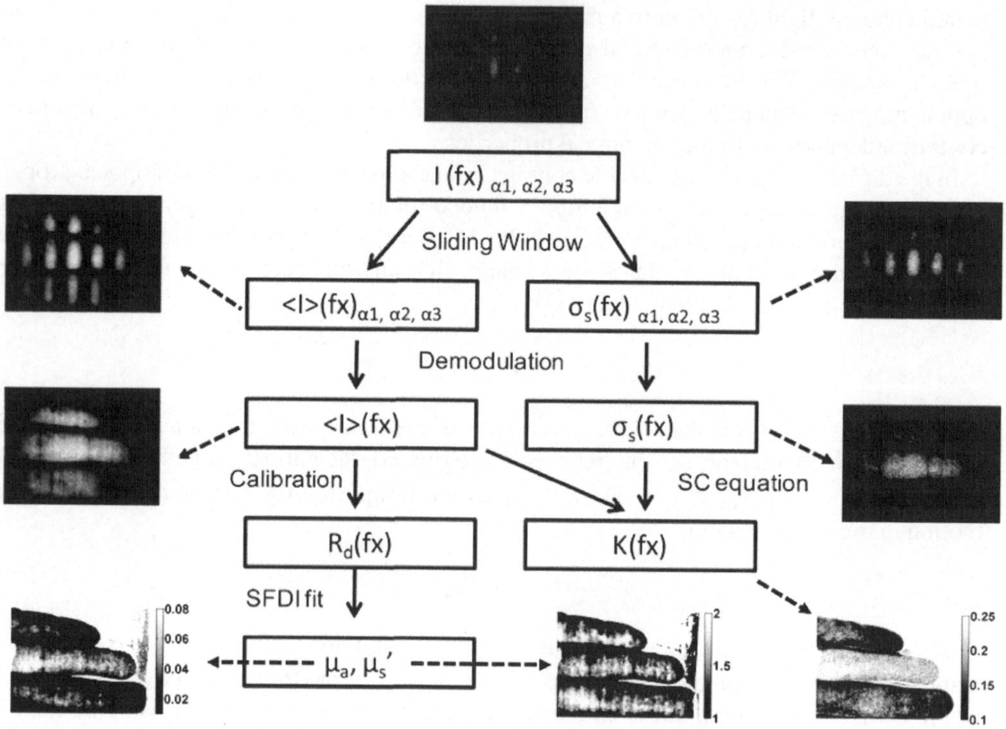

Figure 3.11: Analysis steps for cSFDI data. In this framework, both optical properties and flow can be measured using the same imaging modality. This figure is from publication [154].

clinical applications that are an excellent match for this type of non-contact technology. Pre-clinical imaging of small animals is also an important application for wide-field imaging technologies.

Continued improvements in hardware will help further advance these technologies into the clinic as they are miniaturized and become point of care devices. However, advances in modeling and computation may have the greatest impact on these model-based technologies that rely on multiply-scattered light. This is due to the fact that current methods primarily employ relatively simple diffusion-based approaches. As modeling accuracy improves, we anticipate better measurement performance for resolving subsurface structures and acquiring greater functional information content. This may lead to new contrast elements that describe previously unseen features such as the orientation and connectivity of subsurface scatterers, depth-resolved localization of blood flow, and improved accuracy and sensitivity to cellular function and organization. These advances will allow us to gain a deeper understanding of the various sources of static and dynamic optical contrast in tissue while bringing us closer to our long-term goal of extracting spatially-localized cellular and molecular information content using deeply-penetrating, multiply-scattered light.

Acknowledgments

The authors wish to thank our colleagues and collaborators who have contributed so much to our field. We would particularly like to thank our colleagues Albert Cerussi, Bernard Choi, John

Frangioni, Sylvain Gioux, Soren Konecky, Tom O'Sullivan, Rolf Saager, and Tyler Rice. This work was supported by National Institutes of Health Grants P41RR01192 and P41EB015890 (Laser Microbeam and Medical Program), R01-CA142989, R21 EB014440, R21-CA129758, R43RR025985, 2R42GM077713, and Air Force Research Laboratory Agreement Number FA9550-04-1-0101. Beckman Laser Institute programmatic support from the Arnold and Mabel Beckman Foundation is gratefully acknowledged.

Conflict of Interest Statement

B.T., A.D., and D.C. report patents, which are owned by the University of California, that are related to the technology and analysis methods described in this tutorial. The diffuse optical imaging instrumentation described was constructed in a university laboratory using federal grant support. The University of California has licensed SFDI technologies and analysis methods to Modulated Imaging, Inc. B.T., A.D., and D.C. are co-founders of Modulated Imaging.

References

[1] A. Gibson and H. Dehghani, "Diffuse optical imaging," *Philos. Transact. A Math. Phys. Eng. Sci.* **367** (1900), 3055–3072 (2009).

[2] D.A. Boas, C. Pitris, et al., "Handbook of Biomedical Optics," *J. Biomed. Opt.* **16** (12), 129901 (2011).

[3] C.E. Elwell and C.E. Cooper, "Making light work: illuminating the future of biomedical optics," *Philos. Transact. A Math. Phys. Eng. Sci.* **369**, 4358–4379 (2011).

[4] W.G. Zijlistra, A. Buursma, et al. *Visible and Near Infrared Absorption Spectra of Human and Animal Haemoglobin: Determination and Application*, VSP (2000).

[5] R. Cubeddu, C. D'Andrea, et al., "Effects of the menstrual cycle on the red and near-infrared optical properties of the human breast," *Photochemistry and Photobiology* **72** (3), 383–391 (2000).

[6] A.E. Cerussi, D. Jakubowski, et al., "Spectroscopy enhances the information content of optical mammography," *J. Biomed. Opt.* **7** (1), 60–71 (2002).

[7] A. Cerussi, D. Hsiang, et al., "Predicting response to breast cancer neoadjuvant chemotherapy using diffuse optical spectroscopy," *Proc. Natl. Acad. Sci. U.S.A.* **104** (10), 4014–4019 (2007).

[8] R.L. van Veen, H.J. Sterenborg, et al., "Determination of visible near-IR absorption coefficients of mammalian fat using time- and spatially resolved diffuse reflectance and transmission spectroscopy," *J. Biomed. Opt.* **10** (5), 054004 (2005).

[9] G. Zonios, A. Dimou, et al., "Melanin absorption spectroscopy: new method for noninvasive skin investigation and melanoma detection," *J. Biomed. Opt.* **13** (1), 014017 (2008).

[10] R. Drezek, A. Dunn, et al., "Light scattering from cells: finite-difference time-domain simulations and goniometric measurements," *Appl. Opt.* **38** (16), 3651–3661 (1999).

[11] D.A. Boas, A.M. Dale, et al., "Diffuse optical imaging of brain activation: approaches to optimizing image sensitivity, resolution, and accuracy," *Neuroimage* **23** Suppl 1, S275–S288 (2004).

[12] K. Uludag, J. Steinbrink, et al.,"Separability and cross talk: optimizing dual wavelength combinations for near-infrared spectroscopy of the adult head," *Neuroimage* **22** (2), 583–589 (2004).

[13] J.R. Mourant, T. Fuselier, et al., "Predictions and measurements of scattering and absorption over broad wavelength ranges in tissue phantoms," *Appl. Opt.* **36** (4), 949–957 (1997).

[14] R.M. Doornbos, R. Lang, et al., "The determination of in vivo human tissue optical properties and absolute chromophore concentrations using spatially resolved steady-state diffuse reflectance spectroscopy," *Phys. Med. Biol.* **44** (4), 967–981 (1999).

[15] R. Reif, O. A'Amar, et al., "Analytical model of light reflectance for extraction of the optical properties in small volumes of turbid media," *Appl. Opt.* **46** (29) 7317–7328 (2007).

[16] A. Li, Q. Zhang, et al., "Reconstructing chromosphere concentration images directly by continuous-wave diffuse optical tomography," *Opt. Lett.* **29** (3), 256–258 (2004).

[17] A. Corlu, T. Durduran, et al., "Uniqueness and wavelength optimization in continuous-wave multispectral diffuse optical tomography," *Opt. Lett.* **28** (23), 2339–2341 (2003).

[18] M.E. Eames, J. Wang, et al., "Wavelength band optimization in spectral near-infrared optical tomography improves accuracy while reducing data acquisition and computational burden," *J. Biomed. Opt.* **13** (5), 054037 (2008).

[19] A. Corlu, R. Choe, et al., "Diffuse optical tomography with spectral constraints and wavelength optimization," *Appl. Opt.* **44** (11), 2082–2093 (2005).

[20] A. Vogel, V.V. Chernomordik, et al., "Using noninvasive multispectral imaging to quantitatively assess tissue vasculature," *J. Biomed. Opt.*12 (5), 051604 (2007).

[21] A.D. Kim, "Transport theory for light propagation in biological tissue," *J. Opt. Soc. Am. A* **21** (5), 820–827 (2004).

[22] A. Yodh and B. Chance, "Spectroscopy and imaging with diffusing light," *Physics Today* **48** (3), 34–40 (1996).

[23] L.V. Wang and H.-I. Wu *Biomedical Optics: Principles and Imaging*, Hoboken, NJ, John Wiley & Sons Inc. (2007).

[24] M.S. Patterson, B. Chance, et al., "Time resolved reflectance and transmittance for the non-invasive measurement of tissue optical properties," *Appl. Opt.* **28** (12), 2331–2336 (1989).

[25] B. Chance, J.S. Leigh, et al., "Comparison of time-resolved and -unresolved measurements of deoxyhemoglobin in brain," *Proc. Natl. Acad. Sci. U.S.A.* **85** (14), 4971–4975 (1988).

[26] D.T. Delpy, M. Cope, et al., "Estimation of optical pathlength through tissue from direct time of flight measurement," *Phys. Med. Biol.* **33** (12,)1433–1442 (1988).

[27] A. Duncan, J.H. Meek, et al., "Optical pathlength measurements on adult head, calf and forearm and the head of the newborn infant using phase resolved optical spectroscopy," *Phys. Med. Biol.* **40** (2), 295–304 (1995).

[28] S.J. Madsen, B.C. Wilson, et al., "Experimental tests of a simple diffusion model for the estimation of scattering and absorption coefficients of turbid media from time-resolved diffuse reflectance measurements," *Appl. Opt.* **31** (18), 3509–3517 (1992).

[29] B. Chance, S. Nioka, et al., "Time-resolved spectroscopy of hemoglobin and myoglobin in resting and ischemic muscle," *Anal. Biochem.* **174** (2), 698–707 (1988).

[30] T. Svensson, J. Swartling, et al., "Characterization of normal breast tissue heterogeneity using time-resolved near-infrared spectroscopy," *Phys. Med. Biol.* **50** (11), 2559–2571 (2005).

[31] T. Svensson, S. Andersson-Engels, et al., "In vivo optical characterization of human prostate tissue using near-infrared time-resolved spectroscopy," *J. Biomed. Opt.* **12** (1), 014022 (2007).

[32] E.M. Hillman, J. C. Hebden, et al., "Time resolved optical tomography of the human forearm," *Phys. Med. Biol.* **46**(4), 1117–1130 (2001).

[33] F. Martelli, S. Del Bianco, et al., "Phantom validation and in vivo application of an inversion procedure for retrieving the optical properties of diffusive layered media from time-resolved reflectance measurements," *Opt. Lett.* **29** (17), 2037–2039 (2004).

[34] J.M. Schmitt, A. Knüttel, et al., "Interference of diffusive light waves," *J. Opt. Soc. Am. A* **9** (10), 1832–1843 (1992).

[35] M.A. O'Leary, D.A. Boas, et al., "Refraction of diffuse photon density waves," *Phys. Rev. Lett.* **69** (18), 2658–2661 (1992).

[36] D.A.Boas, M.A. O'Leary, et al., "Scattering and wavelength transduction of diffuse photon density waves," *Phys. Rev. E* **47** (5), R2999–R3002 (1993).

[37] J.B. Fishkin and E. Gratton, "Propagation of photon-density waves in strongly scattering media containing an absorbing semi-infinite plane bounded by a straight edge," *Journal of the Optical Society of America A (Optics and Image Science)* **10** (1), 127–140 (1993).

[38] L.O. Svaasand and B.J. Tromberg, "On the properties of optical waves in turbid media," *Proc. SPIE* **1525**, 41–51 (1991).

[39] B.J. Tromberg, L.O. Svaasand, et al., "Properties of photon density waves in multiple-scattering media," *Appl. Opt.* **32** (4) 607–616 (1993).

[40] B.W. Pogue and M.S. Patterson, "Frequency-domain optical absorption spectroscopy of finite tissue volumes using diffusion theory," *Phys. Med. Biol.* **39** (7), 1157–1180 (1994).

[41] J.B. Fishkin, O. Coquoz, et al., "Frequency-domain photon migration measurements of normal and malignant tissue optical properties in a human subject," *Appl. Opt.* **36** (1), 10–20 (1997).

[42] H.P. Tuan, C. Olivier, et al., "Broad bandwidth frequency domain instrument for quantitative tissue optical spectroscopy," *Review of Scientific Instruments* **71** (6), 2500–2513 (2000).

[43] M.S. Patterson, J.D. Moulton, et al., "Frequency-domain reflectance for the determination of the scattering and absorption properties of tissue," *Appl. Opt.* **30** (31), 4474–4476 (1991).

[44] E.M. Sevick, B. Chance, et al., "Quantitation of time- and frequency-resolved optical spectra for the determination of tissue oxygenation," *Analytical Biochemistry* **195** (2), 330–351 (1991).

[45] J. Selb, D.K. Joseph, et al., "Time-gated optical system for depth-resolved functional brain imaging," *J. Biomed. Opt.* **11** (4), 044008 (2006).

[46] T.D. O'Sullivan, A.E. Cerussi, et al., "Diffuse optical imaging using spatially and temporally modulated light," *J. Biomed. Opt.* **17** (7), 071311 (2012).

[47] B.J. Tromberg, N. Shah, et al., "Non-invasive in vivo characterization of breast tumors using photon migration spectroscopy," *Neoplasia* **2** (1-2), 26–40 (2000).

[48] B.W. Pogue, S.P. Poplack, et al., "Quantitative hemoglobin tomography with diffuse near-infrared spectroscopy: pilot results in the breast," *Radiology* **218** (1), 261–266 (2001).

[49] Q. Zhu, S.H. Kurtzma, et al., "Utilizing optical tomography with ultrasound localization to image heterogeneous hemoglobin distribution in large breast cancers," *Neoplasia* **7** (3), 263–270 (2005).

[50] D. Roblyer, S. Ueda, et al., "Optical imaging of breast cancer oxyhemoglobin flare correlates with neoadjuvant chemotherapy response one day after starting treatment," *Proceedings of the National Academy of Sciences* **108** (35), 14626–14631 (2011).

[51] P. Taroni, G. Danesini, et al., "Clinical trial of time-resolved scanning optical mammography at 4 wavelengths between 683 and 975 nm," *J. Biomed. Opt.* **9** (3), 464–473 (2004).

[52] A. Cerussi, N. Shah, et al., "In vivo absorption, scattering, and physiologic properties of 58 malignant breast tumors determined by broadband diffuse optical spectroscopy," *J. Biomed. Opt.* **11** (4), 044005 (2006).

[53] S. Kukreti, A. Cerussi, et al., "Intrinsic tumor biomarkers revealed by novel double-differential spectroscopic analysis of near-infrared spectra," *J. Biomed. Opt.* **12** (2), 020509 (2007).

[54] D.B. Jakubowski, A E. Cerussi, et al., "Monitoring neoadjuvant chemotherapy in breast cancer using quantitative diffuse optical spectroscopy: a case study," *J. Biomed. Opt.* **9** (1), 230–238 (2004).

[55] N.R. Jagannathan, M. Singh, et al., "Volume localized in vivo proton MR spectroscopy of breast carcinoma: variation of water-fat ratio in patients receiving chemotherapy," *NMR Biomed.* **11** (8), 414–422 (1998).

[56] S.H. Chung, A.E. Cerussi, et al., "Tissue bound water studies on breast tumor using diffuse optical spectroscopy," *Proc. SPIE* **6434**, 64341F (2007).

[57] S.H.Chung, A.E. Cerussi, et al., "Non-invasive detection and monitoring of tumor pathological grade during neoadjuvant chemotherapy by measuring tissue water state using diffuse optical spectroscopic imaging," *Cancer Res.* **69** (2), 101S (2009).

[58] S.H. Chung, A.E. Cerussi, et al., "In vivo water state measurements in breast cancer using broadband diffuse optical spectroscopy," *Physics in Medicine and Biology* **53** (23), 6713–6727 (2008).

[59] R.A. De Blasi, S. Fantini, et al., "Cerebral and muscle oxygen saturation measurement by frequency-domain near-infra-red spectrometer," *Med. Biol. Eng. Comput.* **33** (2), 228–230 (1995).

[60] J.P. Culver, T. Durduran, et al.. "Diffuse optical tomography of cerebral blood flow, oxygenation, and metabolism in rat during focal ischemia," *J. Cereb. Blood. Flow. Metab.* **23** (8), 911–924 (2003).

[61] M. Wolf, M. Ferrari, et al., "Progress of near-infrared spectroscopy and topography for brain and muscle clinical applications," *J. Biomed. Opt.* **12** (6), 062104 (2007).

[62] E.S. Papazoglou, M. Neidrauer, et al., "Noninvasive assessment of diabetic foot ulcers with diffuse photon density wave methodology: pilot human study," *J. Biomed. Opt.* **14** (6), 064032 (2009).

[63] M. Neidrauer, L. Zubkov, et al., "Near infrared wound monitor helps clinical assessment of diabetic foot ulcers," *J. Diabetes. Sci. Technol.* **4** (4), 792–798 (2010).

[64] H. Dehghani, S. Srinivasan, et al., "Numerical modelling and image reconstruction in diffuse optical tomography," *Philos. Transact. A Math. Phys. Eng. Sci.* **367** (1900), 3073–3093 (2009).

[65] G. Xu,, D. Piao, et al., "Direct-current-based image reconstruction versus direct-current included or excluded frequency-domain reconstruction in diffuse optical tomography," *Appl. Opt.* **49** (16), 3059–3070 (2010).

[66] T.J. Farrell, M.S. Patterson, et al., "A diffusion theory model of spatially resolved, steady-state diffuse reflectance for the noninvasive determination of tissue optical properties in vivo," *Med. Phys.* **19** (4), 879–888 (1992).

[67] A. Kienle, L. Lilge, et al., "Spatially resolved absolute diffuse reflectance measurements for noninvasive determination of the optical scattering and absorption coefficients of biological tissue," *Appl. Opt.* **35** (13), 2304–2314 (1996).

[68] D.E. Hyde, T.J. Farrell, et al., "A diffusion theory model of spatially resolved fluorescence from depth-dependent fluorophore concentrations," *Phys. Med. Biol.* **46** (2), 369–383 (2001).

[69] T.J. Pfefer, L.S. Matchette, et al., "Reflectance-based determination of optical properties in highly attenuating tissue," *J. Biomed. Opt.* **8** (2), 206–215 (2003).

[70] E.M. Hillman, D.A. Boas, et al., "Laminar optical tomography: demonstration of millimeter-scale depth-resolved imaging in turbid media," *Opt. Lett* **29** (14), 1650–1652 (2004).

[71] E.M. Hillman, A. Devor, et al., "Depth-resolved optical imaging and microscopy of vascular compartment dynamics during somatosensory stimulation," *Neuroimage* **35** (1), 89–104 (2007).

[72] N. Dognitz and G. Wagnieres, "Determination of tissue optical properties by steady-state spatial frequency-domain reflectometry," *Lasers in Medical Science* **13** (1), 55–65 (1998).

[73] R.B. Saager, D.J. Cuccia, et al., "Determination of optical properties of turbid media spanning visible and near-infrared regimes via spatially modulated quantitative spectroscopy," *J. Biomed. Opt.* **15** (1), 017012 (2010).

[74] M.A. Neil, R. Juskaitis, et al., "Method of obtaining optical sectioning by using structured light in a conventional microscope," *Opt. Lett.* **22** (24), 1905–1907 (1997).

[75] D.J. Cuccia, F. Bevilacqua, et al., "Quantitation and mapping of tissue optical properties using modulated imaging," *J. Biomed. Opt.* **14** (2), 024012 (2009).

[76] T.A. Erickson, A. Mazhar, et al., "Lookup-table method for imaging optical properties with structured illumination beyond the diffusion theory regime," *J. Biomed. Opt.* **15** (3), 036013 (2010).

[77] A. Mazhar, S.A. Sharif, et al., "Spatial frequency domain imaging of port wine stain biochemical composition in response to laser therapy: a pilot study," *Lasers Surg. Med.* **44** (8), 611–621 (2012).

[78] A. Mazhar, S. Dell, et al., "Wavelength optimization for rapid chromophore mapping using spatial frequency domain imaging," *J. Biomed. Opt.* **15** (6), 061716 (2010).

[79] J.Q. Nguyen, R.B. Saager, et al., "Effects of motion on optical properties in the spatial frequency domain," *J. Biomed. Opt.* **16** (12), 126009 (2011).

[80] S. Gioux, Y. Ashitate, et al., "Motion-gated acquisition for in vivo optical imaging," *J. Biomed. Opt.* **14** (6), 064038 (2009).

[81] D.J. Cuccia, "Spatial Frequency Domain Imaging (SFDI): a technology overview and validation of an LED-based clinic-friendly device," *Proc. SPIE* **8254**, 825405 (2012).

[82] A. Mazhar, S.A. Sharif, et al., "Implementation of an LED-based clinical spatial frequency domain imaging system," *Proc. SPIE* **8254**, 82540A (2012).

[83] N. Hagen, N. Bedard, et al., "Spectrally-resolved imaging of dynamic turbid media," *Proc. SPIE* **7892**, 789206 (2011).

[84] J.R. Weber, D.J. Cuccia, et al., "Multispectral imaging of tissue absorption and scattering using spatial frequency domain imaging and a computed-tomography imaging spectrometer," *J. Biomed. Opt.* **16** (1), 011015 (2011).

[85] M.R. Pharaon, T. Scholz, et al., "Early detection of complete vascular occlusion in a pedicle flap model using quantitative [corrected] spectral imaging," *Plast. Reconstr. Surg.* **126** (6), 1924–1935 (2010).

[86] A. Yafi, T.S. Vetter, et al., "Postoperative quantitative assessment of reconstructive tissue status in a cutaneous flap model using spatial frequency domain imaging," *Plast. Reconstr. Surg.* **127** (1), 117–130 (2011).

[87] S. Gioux, A. Mazhar, et al., "First-in-human pilot study of a spatial frequency domain oxygenation imaging system," *J. Biomed. Opt.* **16** (8), 086015 (2011).

[88] D. Abookasis, C.C. Lay, et al., "Imaging cortical absorption, scattering, and hemodynamic response during ischemic stroke using spatially modulated near-infrared illumination," *J. Biomed. Opt.* **14** (2), 024033 (2009).

[89] A.J. Lin, M.A. Koike, et al., "Spatial frequency domain imaging of intrinsic optical property contrast in a mouse model of Alzheimer's disease," *Ann. Biomed. Eng.* **39** (4), 1349–1357 (2011).

[90] S.D. Konecky, T. Rice, et al., "Imaging scattering orientation with spatial frequency domain imaging," *J. Biomed. Opt.* **16** (12), 126001 (2011).

[91] S. Gioux, A. Mazhar, et al., "Three-dimensional surface profile intensity correction for spatially modulated imaging," *J. Biomed. Opt.* **14** (3), 034045 (2009).

[92] J. M. Kainerstorfer, F. Amyot, et al., "Direct curvature correction for noncontact imaging modalities applied to multispectral imaging," *J. Biomed. Opt.* **15** (4), 046013 (2010).

[93] D.J. Cuccia, F. Bevilacqua, et al., "Modulated imaging: quantitative analysis and tomography of turbid media in the spatial-frequency domain," *Opt. Lett.* **30** (11), 1354–1356 (2005).

[94] J.R. Weber, D.J. Cuccia, et al., "Noncontact imaging of absorption and scattering in layered tissue using spatially modulated structured light," *Journal of Applied Physics* **105** (10), (2009).

[95] D. Yudovsky and A.J. Durkin, "Spatial frequency domain spectroscopy of two layer media," *J. Biomed. Opt.* **16** (10), 107005 (2011).

[96] D. Yudovsky, J.Q. Nguyen, et al., "In vivo spatial frequency domain spectroscopy of two layer media," *J. Biomed. Opt.* **17** (10), 107006 (2012).

[97] D. Yudovsky, and A.J. Durkin, "Hybrid diffusion and two-flux approximation for multilayered tissue light propagation modeling," *Appl. Opt.* **50** (21), 4237–4245 (2011).

[98] A.H. Hielscher, A.Y. Bluestone, et al., "Near-infrared diffuse optical tomography," *Dis Markers* **18** (5-6), 313–337 (2002).

[99] X. Cheng and D. Boas, "Diffuse optical reflection tomography using continuous wave illumination," *Opt. Express* **3** (3), 118–123 (1998).

[100] J.C. Schotland and V.A. Markel, "Inverse scattering with diffusing waves," *J. Opt. Soc. Am. A, Opt. Image Sci. Vis.* **18** (11), 2767–2777 (2001).

[101] V.A. Markel and J.C. Schotland, "Symmetries, inversion formulas, and image reconstruction for optical tomography," *Phys. Rev. E Stat. Nonlin. Soft Matter Phys.* **70** (5 Pt 2), 056616 (2004).

[102] Z.M. Wang, G.Y. Panasyuk, et al., "Experimental demonstration of an analytic method for image reconstruction in optical diffusion tomography with large data sets," *Opt. Lett.* **30** (24), 3338–3340 (2005).

[103] S.D. Konecky, G.Y. Panasyuk, et al., "Imaging complex structures with diffuse light," *Opt. Express* **16** (7), 5048–5060 (2008).

[104] V. Lukic, V.A. Markel, et al., "Optical tomography with structured illumination," *Opt. Lett.* **34** (7), 983–985 (2009).

[105] S.D. Konecky, A. Mazhar, et al., "Quantitative optical tomography of sub-surface heterogeneities using spatially modulated structured light," *Opt. Express* **17** (17), 14780–14790 (2009).

[106] C. D'Andrea, N. Ducros, et al., "Fast 3D optical reconstruction in turbid media using spatially modulated light," *Biomed. Opt. Express* **1** (2), 471–481 (2010).

[107] A. Bassi, C. D'Andrea, et al., "Detection of inhomogeneities in diffusive media using spatially modulated light," *Opt. Lett.* **34** (14), 2156–2158 (2009).

[108] S. Belanger, M. Abran, et al., "Real-time diffuse optical tomography based on structured illumination," *J. Biomed. Opt.* **15** (1), 016006 (2010).

[109] J.V. Frangioni, "In vivo near-infrared fluorescence imaging," *Curr. Opin. Chem. Biol.* **7**, 626–634 (2003).

[110] V. Ntziachristos, C. Bremer, et al., "Fluorescence imaging with near-infrared light: new technological advances that enable in vivo molecular imaging," *Eur. Radiol.* **13** (1), 195–208 (2003).

[111] E.E. Graves, J. Ripoll, et al., "A submillimeter resolution fluorescence molecular imaging system for small animal imaging," *Med. Phys.* **30** (5), 901–911 (2003).

[112] A.J. Chaudhari, F. Darvas, et al., "Hyperspectral and multispectral bioluminescence optical tomography for small animal imaging," *Phys. Med. Biol.* **50** (23), 5421–5441 (2005).

[113] V. Ntziachristos, J. Ripoll, et al., "Looking and listening to light: the evolution of whole-body photonic imaging," *Nat. Biotechnol.* **23** (3), 313–320 (2005).

[114] M.G. Gustafsson, "Nonlinear structured-illumination microscopy: wide-field fluorescence imaging with theoretically unlimited resolution," *Proc. Natl. Acad. Sci. U.S.A.* **102** (37), 13081–13086 (2005).

[115] S. Delica and C.M. Blanca, "Wide-field depth-sectioning fluorescence microscopy using projector-generated patterned illumination," *Appl. Opt.* **46** (29), 7237–7243 (2007).

[116] A. Bassi, C. D'Andrea, et al., "Temporal propagation of spatial information in turbid media," *Opt. Lett.* **33** (23), 2836–2838 (2008).

[117] A. Mazhar, D.J. Cuccia, et al., "Structured illumination enhances resolution and contrast in thick tissue fluorescence imaging." *J. Biomed. Opt.* **15** (1), 010506 (2010).

[118] A. Joshi, W. Bangerth, et al., "Non-contact fluorescence optical tomography with scanning patterned illumination," *Opt. Express* **14** (14), 6516–6534 (2006).

[119] A. Joshi, W. Bangerth, et al., "Plane-wave fluorescence tomography with adaptive finite elements," *Opt. Lett.* **31** (2), 193–195 (2006).

[120] N. Ducros, C. D'Andrea, et al., "Full-wavelet approach for fluorescence diffuse optical tomography with structured illumination," *Opt. Lett.* **35** (21), 3676–3678 (2010).

[121] J. Dutta, S. Ahn, et al., "Illumination pattern optimization for fluorescence tomography: theory and simulation studies," *Phys. Med. Biol.* **55** (10), 2961–2982 (2010).

[122] R. Weissleder, C.H. Tung, et al., "In vivo imaging of tumors with protease-activated near-infrared fluorescent probes," *Nat. Biotechnol.* **17** (4), 375–378 (1999).

[123] S.L. Troyan, V. Kianzad, et al., "The FLARE intraoperative near-infrared fluorescence imaging system: a first-in-human clinical trial in breast cancer sentinel lymph node mapping," *Ann. Surg. Oncol.* **16** (10), 2943–2952 (2009).

[124] S. Gioux, H.S. Choi, et al., "Image-guided surgery using invisible near-infrared light: fundamentals of clinical translation," *Mol. Imaging.* **9** (5), 237–255 (2010).

[125] B.T. Lee, M. Hutteman, et al., "The FLARE intraoperative near-infrared fluorescence imaging system: a first-in-human clinical trial in perforator flap breast reconstruction," *Plast. Reconstr. Surg.* **126** (5), 1472–1481 (2010).

[126] S. Kwon and E.M. Sevick-Muraca, "Noninvasive quantitative imaging of lymph function in mice," *Lymphat. Res. Biol.* **5** (4), 219–231 (2007).

[127] R. Sharma, W. Wang, et al., "Quantitative imaging of lymph function," *Am. J. Physiol. Heart. Circ. Physiol.* **292** (6), H3109–3118 (2007).

[128] J. Wu, M.S. Feld, et al. "Analytical model for extracting intrinsic fluorescence in turbid media," *Appl. Opt.* **32** (19), 3585–3595 (1993).

[129] A. Kim, M. Khurana, et al., "Quantification of in vivo fluorescence decoupled from the effects of tissue optical properties using fiber-optic spectroscopy measurements," *J. Biomed. Opt.* **15** (6), 067006 (2010).

[130] P.A. Valdes, F. Leblond, et al., "Quantitative fluorescence in intracranial tumor: implications for ALA-induced PpIX as an intraoperative biomarker," *J. Neurosurg.* **115** (1), 11–17 (2011).

[131] A. Kim, M. Roy, et al., "Topographic mapping of subsurface fluorescent structures in tissue using multiwavelength excitation," *J. Biomed. Opt.* **15** (6), 066026 (2010).

[132] F. Leblond, Z. Ovanesyan, et al., "Analytic expression of fluorescence ratio detection correlates with depth in multi-spectral sub-surface imaging," *Phys. Med. Biol.* **56** (21), 6823–6837 (2011).

[133] S.D. Konecky, C.M. Owen, et al., "Spatial frequency domain tomography of protoporphyrin IX fluorescence in preclinical glioma models," *J. Biomed. Opt.* **17** (5), 056008 (2012).

[134] R.B. Saager, D.J. Cuccia, et al., "Quantitative fluorescence imaging of protoporphyrin IX through determination of tissue optical properties in the spatial frequency domain," *J. Biomed. Opt.* **16** (12), 126013 (2011).

[135] C. Zhou, G. Yu, et al., "Diffuse optical correlation tomography of cerebral blood flow during cortical spreading depression in rat brain," *Opt. Express.* **14** (3), 1125–1144 (2006).

[136] G. Yu, T. F. Floyd, et al., "Validation of diffuse correlation spectroscopy for muscle blood flow with concurrent arterial spin labeled perfusion MRI," *Opt. Express.* **15** (3), 1064–1075 (2007).

[137] M.N. Kim, T. Durduran, et al., "Noninvasive measurement of cerebral blood flow and blood oxygenation using near-infrared and diffuse correlation spectroscopies in critically brain-injured adults," *Neurocrit. Care* **12** (2), 173–180 (2010).

[138] J.D. Briers, "Laser Doppler, speckle and related techniques for blood perfusion mapping and imaging," *Physiol. Meas.* **22** (4), R35–66 (2001).

[139] R. Bandyopadhyay, A.S. Gittings, et al., "Speckle-visibility spectroscopy: A tool to study time-varying dynamics," *Review of Scientific Instruments* **76** (9), 093110–093111 (2005).

[140] A.K. Dunn, H. Bolay, et al., "Dynamic imaging of cerebral blood flow using laser speckle," *J. Cereb. Blood. Flow Metab.* **21** (3), 195–201 (2001).

[141] Y.-C. Huang, T.L. Ringold, et al., "Noninvasive blood flow imaging for real-time feedback during laser therapy of port wine stain birthmarks," *Lasers in Surgery and Medicine* **40** (3), 167–173 (2008).

[142] D.D. Duncan, S.J. Kirkpatrick, et al., "Laser speckle contrast imaging for the quantitative assessment of flow," *Proceedings of SPIE* **7176** (1) 717603–717608 (2009).

[143] D.D. Duncan and S.J. Kirkpatrick, "Can laser speckle flowmetry be made a quantitative tool?" *Journal of the Optical Society of America. A, Optics, Image Science, and Vision* **25** (8), 2088–2094 (2008).

[144] B. Choi, J. C. Ramirez-San-Juan, et al., "Linear response range characterization and in vivo application of laser speckle imaging of blood flow dynamics," *J. Biomed. Opt.* **11** (4), 041129 (2006).

[145] S.J. Kirkpatrick, D.D. Duncan, et al., "Detrimental effects of speckle-pixel size matching in laser speckle contrast imaging," *Opt. Lett.* **33** (24), 2886–2888 (2008).

[146] S. Yuan, Y. Chen, et al., "Noise analysis in laser speckle contrast imaging, " *Animals* **7563**, 75630J–75635 (2010).

[147] P. Zakharov, A. Volker, et al., "Quantitative modeling of laser speckle imaging," *Opt. Lett.* **31** (23), 3465–3467 (2006).

[148] D.D. Duncan, S.J. Kirkpatrick, et al., "Statistics of local speckle contrast," *J. Opt. Soc. Am. A Opt. Image Sci. Vis.* **25** (1), 9–15 (2008).

[149] A.B. Parthasarathy, W.J. Tom, et al., "Robust flow measurement with multi-exposure speckle imaging," *Opt. Express* **16** (3), 1975–1989 (2008).

[150] M. Draijer, E. Hondebrink, et al., "Review of laser speckle contrast techniques for visualizing tissue perfusion," *Lasers in Medical Science* **24** (4), 639–651 (2009).

[151] D.A. Boas and A.K. Dunn, "Laser speckle contrast imaging in biomedical optics," *J. Biomed. Opt.* **15** (1), 011109 (2010).

[152] V. Rajan, B. Varghese, et al., "Influence of tissue optical properties on laser Doppler perfusion imaging, accounting for photon penetration depth and the laser speckle phenomenon," *Journal of Biomedical Optics* **13** (2), 024001–024001 (2008).

[153] B. Varghese, V. Rajan, et al., "Measurement of particle flux in a static matrix with suppressed influence of optical properties, using low coherence interferometry," *Optics Express* **18** (3), 2849–2857 (2010).

[154] A. Mazhar, D.J. Cuccia, et al., "Laser speckle imaging in the spatial frequency domain," *Biomed. Opt. Express* **2** (6), 1553–1563 (2011).

[155] D.A. Boas and A.G. Yodh, "Spatially varying dynamical properties of turbid media probed with diffusing temporal light correlation," *J. Opt. Soc. Am. A* **14** (1), 192–215 (1997).

[156] T.B. Rice, S.D. Konecky, et al., "Quantitative determination of dynamical properties using coherent spatial frequency domain imaging," *J. Opt. Soc. Am. A Opt. Image Sci. Vis.* **28** (10) 2108–2114 (2011).

[157] T.B. Rice, S.D. Konecky, et al., "Determination of the effect of source intensity profile on speckle contrast using coherent spatial frequency domain imaging," *Biomed. Opt. Express.* **3** (6) 1340–1349 (2012).

4

Multiphoton Microscopy and SHG

Riccardo Cicchi, Leonardo Sacconi
National Institute of Optics - National Research Council (INO-CNR), Largo E. Fermi 6, Florence, Italy; European Laboratory for Nonlinear Spectroscopy (LENS), University of Florence, Via N. Carrara 1, Sesto Fiorentino, Italy

Francesco S. Pavone
European Laboratory for Nonlinear Spectroscopy (LENS), University of Florence, Via N. Carrara 1, 50019 Sesto Fiorentino, Italy; Department of Physics, University of Florence, Via G. Sansone 1, 50019 Sesto Fiorentino, Italy

Nonlinear microscopy has undergone impressive growth in the last 20 years, making it one of the most used optical tools in biological and biomedical imaging of cells and tissues. The main features offered by this microscopy technique consist in providing an intrinsic optical sectioning, an increased penetration depth in optically turbid samples, and a higher spatial resolution with respect to other laser scanning imaging modalities. The two most used imaging techniques based on nonlinear optical effects are two-photon fluorescence (TPF) and second-harmonic generation (SHG) microscopy. Both TPF and SHG can be used in biological and biomedical imaging by means of signal enhancers such as exogenous fluorophores and harmonophores or by taking advantage of the endogenous tissue components able to emit fluorescence or to generate second-harmonic light.

Key words: nonlinear microscopy, second harmonic generation, biomedical imaging, two-photon fluorescence

4.1 Introduction to Nonlinear Optical Microscopy

Nonlinear optical (NLO) microscopy includes several laser scanning imaging techniques that are based on a nonlinear interaction between light and a biological sample. NLO microscopy is based on a nonlinear effect in which a molecule interacts with two or more photons in the same quantum event, whereas in linear optics the interaction is limited to a single photon. NLO microscopy intrinsically offers several advantages with respect to other laser scanning imaging techniques based on linear optical interaction. First, the signal of interest depends nonlinearly on the intensity of the excitation field with the direct consequence of an excitation volume spatially confined in a small region around the focal point. This feature provides a higher spatial resolution with respect to other conventional microscopy techniques employing similar excitation wavelengths as well as intrinsic optical sectioning capability. In fact, the axial confinement of the excitation volume prevents the interaction of light with molecules located out-of-focus. Hence in NLO microscopy a spatial filter rejecting "out-of-focus" photons as in confocal laser scanning microscopy is not required. This allows one to drastically limit the exposure when performing a 3D scanning of the specimen reducing photo-damage and photo-toxicity effects. Another advantage offered by NLO microscopy is the use of NIR laser wavelengths for exciting electronic transitions with resonances located in the visible range. This allows one to image deeper in highly scattering media such as biological tissues because NIR wavelengths are much less scattered with respect to visible wavelengths. For this reason NLO microscopy offers high penetration depth in biological tissues enabling deep optical sectioning of biological tissues [1, 2]. In addition, scattered photons are unable to reach the focal volume so that they do not contribute to the excitation and the spatial resolution of NLO microscopy remains almost unchanged when imaging deep into an optically dense specimen [3]. For these reasons NLO microscopy allows optical sectioning with micron-scale resolution in deep tissue.

The two most used imaging techniques based on NLO effects are two-photon excited fluorescence (TPF) and second-harmonic generation (SHG) microscopy. TPF microscopy is a good example of modern physics in which the theoretical prediction of the process anticipates its experimental discovery by several years. In fact, the possibility of exciting an electronic transition by simultaneous absorption of two photons, each having one half the resonance energy, was theoretically demonstrated in 1931 by Maria Göppert-Mayer [4]. 30 years passed before the first experimental observation of a two-photon excited transition by Kaiser and Garrett [5]. Another 3 decades passed before Denk, Strickler and Webb took advantage of this process to develop a new microscopic imaging technique [6]. Since its invention in 1990, the use of TPF microscopy has undergone an impressive growth in both biological and biomedical fields [1, 7, 8]. During the last two decades, TPF has been used as a powerful imaging technique in a large set of applications in life science [9, 10, 11, 12, 13]. TPF microscopy is particularly powerful for unstained tissue imaging. Since both cells and extracellular matrix contain several intrinsically fluorescent molecules (NADH, tryptophan, keratins, melanin, elastin, cholecalciferol), biological tissues can be imaged by TPF microscopy without any exogenously added probe [14, 15]. In the years beginning the new century, TPF microscopy started to be used also for *in vivo* imaging. Up to now, the most popular *in vivo* imaging applications are related to skin imaging on living human subjects [16, 17, 18, 19] and to brain imaging of small animals [20, 21]. Recently, several technological developments have been aimed at realizing a TPF endoscopic [22] microscope to be used in clinical diagnostic imaging.

Another powerful NLO imaging technique is represented by second-harmonic generation (SHG) microscopy [23, 24]. SHG microscopy is able to provide background free images of anisotropic biological structures with large hyperpolarizability [25, 26], such as collagen [27, 28, 29], muscle [30, 31, 32, 34, 35], or microtubules [36]. SHG is a nonlinear second-order scattering process occurring in systems that satisfy certain requirements in terms of symmetry. The required conditions for having a detectable SHG signal can be summarized as follows: the single emitter has a large hyperpolarizability at the molecular level and the emitters are organized in an anisotropic structure at the scale of the focal volume. These conditions are satisfied in anisotropic biological molecules such as collagen, muscles or microtubules, making SHG microscopy an ideal tool for investigating the organization of these particular biological systems. SHG has been largely used for imaging non-centrosymmetric molecules inside cells [37, 38, 39], cellular membranes [40, 41, 42, 43, 44], brain [36] and biological tissues [15, 45, 46]. SHG microscopy has been demonstrated extremely powerful to image collagen rich tissues [47] such as cornea [48, 49], tendon [50, 51], and arteries [52]. In fact, because of its fibrillar structure [53], collagen intrinsically has a high hyperpolarizability, providing a strong second-harmonic signal [54] and it can be imaged inside connective tissues using SHG microscopy [15, 55]. Recently, SHG microscopy was also used for studying muscular [56], skeletal

[57, 58], and connective tissues [59, 60] in altered physiological conditions. SHG microscopy can be easily combined with TPF microscopy to make a fantastic imaging tool for connective tissues. In fact, the main components of a connective tissue (elastin and collagen) can be respectively imaged using TPF and SHG microscopy simultaneously.

In this chapter we first provide a brief description of the theoretical background underlying the basis of TPF and SHG microscopy (Section 4.2), including a part (Section 4.3) dedicated to the calculation of the TPF/SHG excitation volume. Then we summarize some peculiar technical features to be taken into account when developing a custom-made TPF/SHG microscope (Section 4.4). In the last part of the chapter (Section 4.5) we describe some biological applications employing both TPF and SHG microscopy. In particular we focus our attention on four specific applications: NLO microscopy of human skin; TPF microscopy of bladder tissue; functional imaging by random access microscopy; probing myosin conformation by SHG.

4.2 Theoretical Background of TPF and SHG

4.2.1 Two-photon absorption

In this section we provide a theoretical description of the two-photon absorption process at the basis of TPF microscopy as treated by Nakamura [61]. We use perturbation theory to describe the two-photon electronic transition induced by an electromagnetic field in fluorescent molecules. The wave function of an electron satisfies the following Schrödinger equation:

$$i\hbar\partial\psi/\partial t = (H_0 + H')\psi, \tag{4.1}$$

where H_0 and H' represent the Hamiltonian for the unperturbed molecular system and for the electromagnetic perturbation, respectively. The Schrödinger equation for a steady state in the unperturbed molecular system is described by:

$$H_0 u_n = \varepsilon_n u_n, \tag{4.2}$$

where ε_n and u_n are eigenvalues and eigenfunctions for the unperturbed system. The generic eigenfunction of the unperturbed system varies in time as follows:

$$\phi = u_n \exp(-i\varepsilon_n t/\hbar). \tag{4.3}$$

Using ϕ, we can write the wave function of a perturbed system as:

$$\psi = \sum a_n(t) u_n \exp(-i\varepsilon_n t/\hbar), \tag{4.4}$$

where $a_n(t)$ can be expanded in series as follows:

$$a_n(t) = a_n^{(0)}(t) + \lambda a_n^{(1)}(t) + \lambda^2 a_n^{(2)}(t) + \ldots. \tag{4.5}$$

Substituting equations (4.4) and (4.5) into equation (4.1), and setting:

$$H'_{kn} = \int u_k^* H' u_n dV; \tag{4.6}$$

$$\omega_{kn} = (\varepsilon_k - \varepsilon_n)/\hbar, \tag{4.7}$$

we find:

$$\partial a_k^{(0)}(t)/\partial t = 0; \tag{4.8}$$

$$\partial a_k^{(l+1)}(t)/\partial t = 1/(i\hbar)\sum H'_{kn}(t)a_n^{(l)}(t)\exp(i\omega_{kn}t). \tag{4.9}$$

Let's suppose that the system occupies the state u_0, which is one of the eigenstates of H_0 at $t=0$, then the coefficient is described by:

$$a_k^{(0)}(t=0) = \delta_{k0}. \tag{4.10}$$

Setting $l=0$ in Eq. (4.9), we obtain:

$$a_k^{(1)}(t) = 1/(i\hbar)\int_0^t H'_{k0}(t')\exp(i\omega_{k0}t')dt'. \tag{4.11}$$

The probability for the electron to occupy the level k at time t is given by:

$$\left|a_k^{(1)}(t)\right|^2 = \left|1/(i\hbar)\int_0^t H'_{k0}(t')\exp(i\omega_{k0}t')dt'\right|^2. \tag{4.12}$$

The corresponding transition probability is:

$$\left|a_k^{(1)}(t)\right|^2/t = 1/t\left|1/(i\hbar)\int_0^t H'_{k0}(t')\exp(i\omega_{k0}t')dt'\right|^2. \tag{4.13}$$

This transition probability is related to a single-photon absorption process. The same approach can be used for two-photon absorption using the second-order perturbation theory. Let's suppose that for an intermediate virtual state m:

$$H'_{m0} \neq 0 \quad \text{and} \quad H'_{km} \neq 0, \tag{4.14}$$

where m is not 0 or k. We obtain:

$$a_m^{(1)}(t) = 1/(i\hbar)\int_0^t H'_{m0}(t'')\exp(i\omega_{m0}t'')dt''. \tag{4.15}$$

Substituting $l=1$ into Eq. (4.9), we obtain the equation:

$$\partial a_k^{(2)}(t)/\partial t = 1/(i\hbar)\sum H'_{kn}(t)a_n^{(1)}(t)\exp(i\omega_{kn}t). \tag{4.16}$$

Substituting Eq. (4.15) for Eq. (4.16) we get:

$$a_k^{(2)}(t) = 1/(i\hbar)^2\sum_m\int_0^t H'_{km}(t')\exp(i\omega_{km}t')dt'\int_0^{t'} H'_{m0}(t'')\exp(i\omega_{m0}t'')dt''. \tag{4.17}$$

Then we can express the transition probability as:

$$\left|a_k^{(2)}(t)\right|^2/t = 1/t\cdot\left|1/(i\hbar)^2\sum_m\int_0^t H'_{km}(t')\exp(i\omega_{km}t')dt'\int_0^{t'} H'_{mo}(t'')\exp(i\omega_{m0}t'')dt''\right|^2. \tag{4.18}$$

For simplicity, we assume the perturbing electromagnetic wave linearly polarized along the z-axis and the molecular dipole moment oriented along this. If the amplitude of the perturbation is E, the perturbation term H' can be expressed as:

$$H' = ezE\sin(\omega t). \tag{4.19}$$

Let's substitute Eq. (4.19) into Eq. (4.18) to obtain the two-photon transition probability as:

$$\begin{aligned}&\left|a_k^{(2)}(t)\right|^2/t = (eE)^4/(\hbar^4 t)\cdot\\&\left|z_{km}\textstyle\int_0^t\sin(\omega t')\exp(i\omega_{km}t')dt' z_{mo}\int_0^{t'}\sin(\omega t'')\exp(i\omega_{m0}t'')dt''\right|^2,\end{aligned} \tag{4.20}$$

where

$$z_{km} = \int u_k^* z u_m dV \text{ and } z_{m0} = \int u_m^* z u_0 dV. \tag{4.21}$$

From this result we can show that the transition probability of the second order perturbation (which corresponds to two-photon absorption through an intermediate virtual state) is proportional to the square of the intensity of the optical field. This result highlights the nonlinearity of TPF microscopy.

4.2.2 Second-harmonic generation

We begin with an overview of the physical background of SHG. In general, molecular harmonic up-conversion originates from the nonlinear dependence of the induced molecular dipole moment μ on a driving optical electric field E. In detail, we can write:

$$\mu = \mu_0 + \alpha E + \tfrac{1}{2}\beta E^2 + \ldots, \tag{4.22}$$

where α is the linear molecular polarizability that describes normal absorption and reflection of light; β is the nonlinear first hyperpolarizability describing SHG, sum and difference frequency generation.

4.2.2.1 Single molecule cross section

We begin by defining the SHG cross section of a single molecule. In particular, a molecule is considered as an elemental dipole emitter driven by the excitation light according to its first hyperpolarizability (β). As before, for simplicity we assume that the excitation field is linearly polarized in the z direction and begin by examining only the β_{zzz} component of β. If the excitation light has frequency ω, the induced dipole moment at the frequency 2ω will be given by:

$$\vec{\mu}_{2\omega} = {}^1\!/\!_2 \beta_{zzz} E_\omega^2 \hat{z}, \tag{4.23}$$

where E_ω is the excitation field amplitude. As derived by Moreaux and co-workers [43], the radiated second-harmonic far field at an inclination θ from the propagation axis x is:

$$\vec{E}_{2\omega}^{(0)}(\theta) = -\frac{\mu_{2\omega}\omega^2}{\pi\varepsilon_0 c^2 r}\sin(\theta)\exp(-i2\omega t), \tag{4.24}$$

where ε_0 is the free-space permittivity, c is the speed of light, r is the distance from the dipole, and t is the corresponding delay time. The resultant power per differential solid angle at an inclination θ, can be expressed as:

$$P_{2\omega}(\theta) = \frac{3}{16\pi}\sigma_{SHG}\sin^2(\theta) I_\omega^2, \tag{4.25}$$

where I_ω is the excitation intensity and

$$\sigma_{SHG} = \frac{4 n_{2\omega}\hbar\omega^5}{3\pi n_\omega^2 \varepsilon_0^3 c^5}\left|\beta_{zzz}\right|^2, \tag{4.26}$$

where n_ω and $n_{2\omega}$ are the refractive indices at ω and 2ω respectively. Equation (4.26) defines the SHG cross section (σ_{SHG}) such that the total SHG power, obtained by integration of Eq. (4.25) over all solid angles, reduces to the simple expression:

$$P_{SHG} = \frac{1}{2}\sigma_{SHG} I_\omega^2. \tag{4.27}$$

It is worth noting that, as in TPF, the emitted power is proportional to the square of the excitation light intensity. Let's consider now the more general case of a collection of identical molecular emitters driven by a field E_ω.

4.2.2.2 Coherent summation

We start with a simple two-dimensional distribution of emitters. In this case we limit the calculation to the geometry in which the dipoles are assumed to be uniformly distributed in a two-dimensional $x-y$ plane and illuminated by a tightly focused excitation beam propagating in x direction and polarized in the $z-y$ plane. In this case we define a local induced dipole moment per unit molecular surface density [43]:

$$\mu_{2\omega,i}(x,y) = \frac{1}{2}E_{\omega}^{2}(x,y)\sum_{j,k}\langle\beta_{ijk}\rangle\,\hat{\varepsilon}_j\hat{\varepsilon}_k, \tag{4.28}$$

where $E_{\omega}(x,y)$ is the complex amplitude of the driving field on the membrane, and $\hat{\varepsilon}_j, \hat{\varepsilon}_k$ are the unit vectors for y and z directions. It has to be noted that the equation (4.28) is very similar to the equation (4.23) for a single emitter, with the only difference that the hyperpolarizability has to be ensemble averaged. We can analyze the simple case in which the molecules in the membrane are perfectly oriented in the z axis. Let's also consider the case in which the field is polarized in the z direction. Under these hypotheses we can write the SHG total power as:

$$P_{SHG} = \frac{1}{2}\Theta_z N^2 \sigma_{SHG} I_{\omega}^{2} \tag{4.29}$$

It has to be noted that the SHG power scales with N^2 and not with N; this is a strong peculiarity of the SHG coherent process. Moreover, from Eq. (4.29) we can observe that the angular pattern of the radiated SHG light is governed mainly by the function [41]:

$$\Theta_z = \frac{3}{8\pi}\int A^2(\vartheta,\varphi)[1-\sin^2\vartheta\cos^2\varphi]\sin\vartheta\, d\vartheta\, d\varphi \tag{4.30}$$

with:

$$A(\vartheta,\varphi) = \exp\left\{-\frac{k_{2\omega}^2}{8}\left[\omega_x^2(\cos\vartheta-\xi')^2+\omega_y^2(\sin\vartheta\sin\varphi)^2\right]\right\}. \tag{4.31}$$

This function governs the angular emission pattern for SHG radiated by a two-dimensional distribution of molecular emitters.

4.3 Spatial Resolution and Image Formation

A molecule excited by a nonlinear transition emits fluorescence light with an intensity proportional to the transition probability, which is in turn proportional to a power of the intensity equal to the number of photons involved in the excitation process (i.e. to the square of the light intensity for TPF and SHG). One of the advantages of a nonlinear excitation, with respect to the corresponding single photon process, is a smaller excitation volume with respect to the beam waist size in the focal volume, resulting in a higher spatial resolution. In fact, the excitation volume is basically determined by the n-th power of the intensity distribution (with n equal to the number of photons involved in the interaction) in the focal volume more than by the intensity distribution itself. A fundamental consequence is that only the molecules enclosed in a small excitation volume (typically of the order of the fl) around the focus are excited, whereas molecules located out of this volume are not. This feature allows intrinsic optical sectioning capability as well as reduced photo-damage or phototoxic effects when scanning large volumes.

In this section we calculate the excitation volume size along the radial and axial directions for a Gaussian beam focused by an aberration-free objective lens considering a second-order nonlinear optical interaction. The problem consists in calculating the intensity distribution $I(x,y,z)$ near the focus for a TEM_{00} laser beam focused by a high numerical aperture objective lens with circular pupil.

If we consider a set of cylindrical coordinates having origin in the focus, we can neglect the angular variable ϕ because the problem is invariant for rotation around this angle and limit our calculation to the radial $I(\rho)$ and axial $I(z)$ dependence of the light intensity near the focus. For simplifying the calculation we can perform a transformation of coordinates from the couple (ρ,z) to the couple of adimensional optical coordinates (v,u), defined by the following relations:

$$v = \frac{2\pi(\mathrm{NA})\rho}{\lambda}; \tag{4.32}$$

$$u = \frac{2\pi(\mathrm{NA})^2 z}{n\lambda}, \tag{4.33}$$

where NA is the numerical aperture of the objective lens, λ is the laser wavelength and n is the refractive index of the surrounding medium. In terms of the new coordinates (v,u) the adimensional profile of the electric field amplitude near the focus of an aberration-free objective lens with circular pupil can be expressed as the following integral [61, 62]:

$$\varepsilon(v,u) = 2\int_0^1 J_0(v\rho)\exp\left(-i\frac{u\rho^2}{2}\right)\rho d\rho, \tag{4.34}$$

where J_0 is the first-type zero-order Bessel function. We can now write the intensity distribution near the focal point as:

$$I(\rho,z) = I(v,u) = I_0\left|\varepsilon(v,u)\right|^2, \tag{4.35}$$

where I_0 is the intensity of the electric field at the focal point $\rho = z = 0$ or $v = u = 0$. In order to calculate the intensity distribution along the radial and axial direction separately, we can solve the integral in Eq. (4.34) substituting $v = 0$ or $u = 0$ alternatively. In this way the radial and axial intensity distributions are expressed as

$$|\varepsilon(v,0)|^2 = \left|2\int_0^1 J_0(v\rho)\rho d\rho\right|^2; \tag{4.36}$$

$$|\varepsilon(0,u)|^2 = \left|2\int_0^1 \exp\left(-i\frac{u\rho^2}{2}\right)\rho d\rho\right|^2. \tag{4.37}$$

Solving the two integrals, we find the following expressions for radial and axial intensity distribution, respectively:

$$|\varepsilon(v,0)|^2 = \left|\frac{2J_1(v)}{v}\right|^2; \tag{4.38}$$

$$|\varepsilon(0,u)|^2 = \left|\frac{\sin(u/4)}{(u/4)}\right|^2. \tag{4.39}$$

Once found the radial and axial intensity distribution in the focal volume, the corresponding excitation volume size for a nonlinear n-order optical interaction can be obtained by considering the n-th power of the intensity distribution. For TPF and SHG microscopy the order to be considered is 2, hence the square of the previous expressions are therefore equal to:

$$PSF_{radial} = \left|\frac{2J_1(v)}{v}\right|^4 \tag{4.40}$$

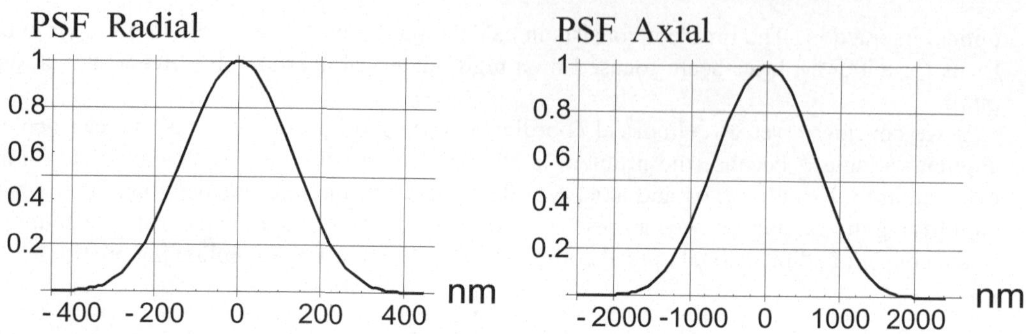

Figure 4.1: Radial (on the left) and axial (on the right) theoretical PSF for two-photon excitation. The two functions were calculated using an excitation wavelength $\lambda = 740$ nm focused by an aberration free lens of NA=0.9 in water ($n = 1.33$).

$$PSF_{axial} = \left| \frac{\sin(u/4)}{(u/4)} \right|^4 \tag{4.41}$$

These two relations express the radial (PSF_{radial}) and axial (PSF_{axial}) point spread functions for TPF or SHG. The behavior of the two point spread functions is plotted in Fig. 4.1 for a Gaussian laser beam with wavelength $\lambda = 740$ nm, focused inside water ($n = 1.33$) by an objective lens of $NA = 0.9$. The radial and axial resolution of the microscope can be taken as the full width at half the maximum (FWHM) of the radial and axial point spread functions, respectively.

4.4 Technical Features of a Nonlinear Microscope

This section describes some peculiar technical features of a NLO microscope. The section is divided in three main parts. After giving a short summary on the laser sources commonly used in a NLO microscope, we then focus our attention on the most critical parts of the microscope: the scanning and the detection systems.

4.4.1 Laser sources

NLO microscopy is based on high-order optical processes so that the probability of exciting a transition is low compared to the equivalent single photon interaction. In order to efficiently excite a NLO process and have a detectable signal level, it is necessary to illuminate the sample with a high spatial and temporal density of photons. While the high spatial photon density is realized by means of a high-NA objective lens, the high temporal photon density requires pulsed ultrafast laser sources, such as femtosecond-pulsed lasers.

The most popular laser source in NLO microscopy is the Ti:Sapphire oscillator. The specifications of this type of laser source depend on the brand and on the model but in general it can provide pulses with a duration in the range of 80–200 fs at a repetition rate of several tens of MHz (in general between 50 MHz and 100 MHz). The Ti:Sapphire laser typically provides an emission power in the range 1–5 W with a broad tuning range (typically in the 700–1000 nm spectral range). This spectral range corresponds to the most suitable range for exciting both TPF and SHG from biological molecules. Because of these features the Ti:Sapphire is probably the best laser source to be used in a NLO microscope. The main drawback is represented by the high cost (typically more than

$100,000).

A possible alternative to the Ti:Sapphire laser is represented by the Cr:Forsterite laser, which is providing femtosecond pulses in a typical wavelength range between 1150 nm and 1300 nm. The Cr:Forsterite emission is comparable to that of the Ti:Sapphire in terms of pulse width and repetition rate, but with a reduced power (typically between hundreds of mW and a 1–2 W). Although longer wavelengths are not the optimal solution for TPF imaging because of a reduced cross-section of biological molecules in this spectral range, their use provides deeper penetration within tissues. Further, the Cr:Forsterite has the advantage of providing an ideal source for third-harmonic generation microscopy [63, 64, 65] at a reduced cost with respect to the Ti:Sapphire oscillator.

A cheaper solution for the laser source is represented by femtosecond-pulsed fiber lasers. These are compact and robust turn-key lasers able to provide train of pulses with a typical width between 100 fs and few ps, a repetition rate in the order of tens of MHz and a maximum power in the order of W. Their cost is about one order of magnitude less with respect to the Ti:Sapphire. The main drawback is that they cannot be tuned, so that their use is limited to applications in which tunability is not required.

Up to now we have considered only laser systems providing a high repetition rate (50–100 MHz) since these are the most commonly used sources in NLO microscopy. However, amplified systems providing pulse width in the range of tens of fs and a repetition rate in the range of few kHz can be used as well [66, 67]. An advantage provided by these systems is the wide spectral range of short pulses offering the possibility to simultaneously excite multiple fluorophores. On the other hand, they can cause stronger unwanted side-effects with respect to the sources described above. In fact, the extremely high peak power increases the probability to induce photo-toxic effects that depend on the 4-th – 5-th or higher power of the excitation intensity.

4.4.2 Scanning system

In this section we are going to describe one of the most important parts of a NLO microscope: the laser scanning system. Starting from basic principles, we then focus our attention on the different elements constituting the scanning head.

4.4.2.1 Basic concepts

In a laser scanning microscope the illumination of the specimen is accomplished by scanning a focused laser beam point-by-point across the sample with a synchronous acquisition of the signal on a single-point detector. The beam scanning is obtained by tilting a collimated laser beam maintaining it centered with respect to the objective back aperture. Using basic principles of optics (as shown in Fig. 4.2A), when a collimated laser beam propagating along the optical axis enters into the objective lens, it is focused in a point corresponding to the intersection of the optical axis with the focal plane. On the other hand, if the collimated beam is tilted with respect to the optical axis, the focal point is located in the focal plane but it is displaced with respect to the optical axis, according to the following relationship:

$$\Delta x = f \tan\theta, \tag{4.42}$$

where Δx is the distance of the focal point from the optical axis, f is the focal length of the objective lens, and θ is the tilting angle of the collimated beam with respect to the optical axis. For small angles, Eq. (4.42) can be approximated to a simpler relationship:

$$\Delta x = f\theta. \tag{4.43}$$

From these equations we can understand that the focal point can be scanned across a specimen located in the focal plane by simply tilting the laser beam with respect to the optical axis. This is in general obtained by means of a scanning system, as described in the following section on scanners.

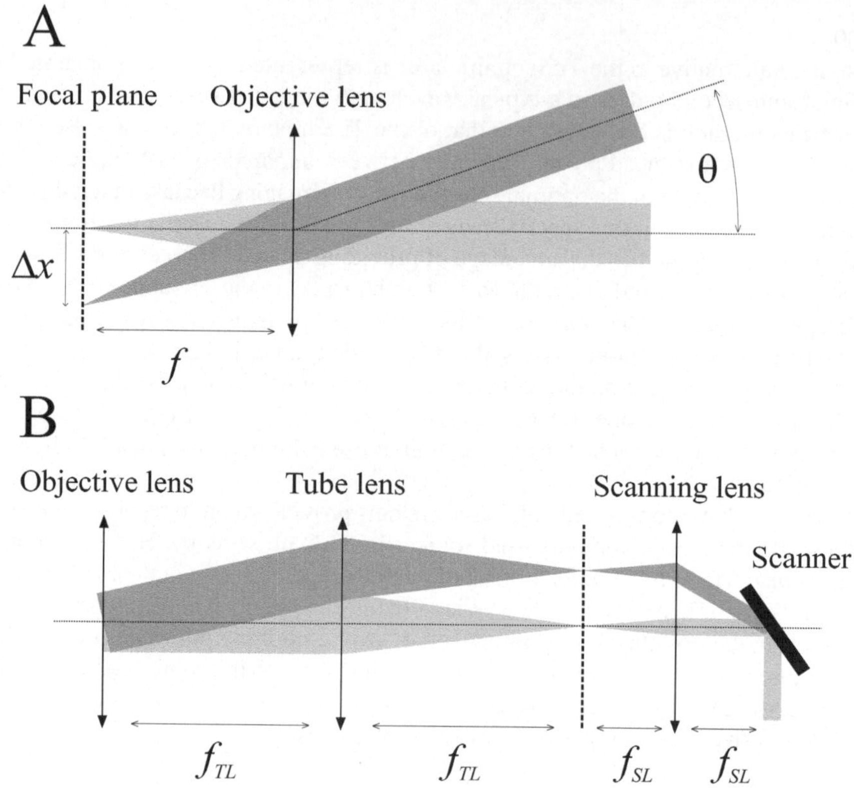

Figure 4.2: (A) Basic optical principle of a laser scanning system. (B) Optical telescope made by the couple (Tube lens - Scanning lens) inserted between the scanning head and the objective lens.

In an experimental setup it is common to insert a 4f telescope between the scanners and the objective lens, as depicted in Fig. 4.2B. Such a telescope provides the following advantages:

1. It allows placing the scanner in a conjugated point with respect to the objective back aperture. In this way the beam is maintained centered with respect to the objective back aperture during scanning, preventing unwanted beam targeting effects.

2. It magnifies the beam size in order to completely fill the objective back aperture. This allows a small beam size on the scanners and to focus the beam to a smaller waist by taking full advantage of the NA offered by the objective lens.

4.4.2.2 Scanners

The scanning head is the part of the microscope allowing the movement of the beam waist across the sample in a controlled manner. The scanning speed is set by the bandwidth of the scanners which is affecting the maximum imaging speed achievable and hence the minimum detectable timescale for the dynamics of interest. Various approaches can be adopted for the scanning system of a custom NLO microscope. The most popular scanners in NLO microscopy are galvanometric mirrors (galvo-mirrors), acousto-optic deflectors (AODs) or polygonal rotating mirrors. In this section we provide a detailed description of the scanners that can be adopted in a custom setup, highlighting advantages and drawbacks of various configurations.

Non-resonant galvanometer-based scanners. The most used scanning system in laser scanning microscopy is made by two orthogonal small mirrors, each of them connected to a galvanometer-based scanner. The galvanometric scanner consists of a current-driven coil mounted around a magnet that allows tilting the position of the small mirror of an angle proportional to the driving current. Most of them include a position sensor for monitoring the angular position of the mirror and a closed-loop servo for enhanced precision. The beam scanning across the specimen can be obtained using various waveforms. The most common is a raster in which one scanner is driven with a saw tooth (or triangular) waveform and the other with a linear ramp. The imaging speed is set by the bandwidth of the faster scanner, which is typically in the range of a few to tens microseconds per pixel. If higher imaging speed is required, a possible alternative to this configuration is represented by resonant scanning, as described below.

Resonant galvanometer-based scanners. In the configuration described above the faster scanner is driven with a saw tooth or with a triangular waveform. Both of them cause the scanner to undergo extreme acceleration or deceleration when the direction of motion is abruptly inverted (at the image edge). This phenomenon drastically limits the maximum scanning speed achievable. A possible solution for increasing imaging speed is represented by resonant scanning which allows always maintaining the scanner acceleration within an upper limit. In resonant scanning the saw tooth (triangular) waveform is substituted with a sine wave with the advantage of higher achievable scan rates without extreme acceleration at the edges of the image. With this configuration the scanner speed is varying according to the sine profile (faster in image center and slower at the edges) with the consequence of a non-uniform scan rate across the image. This effect can be compensated by either limiting the acquisition range to the portion of the sine wave where the profile is almost linear or by synchronizing all the components to the position signal of the resonant scanner.

Acousto-optic deflectors (AODs) scanners. An alternative scanner technology to the galvanometers that allows image speed at video rates consists in tilting the laser beam by means of acousto-optic deflectors (AODs). These devices take advantage of the acousto-optical effect that occurs when a laser beam passes through a crystal in which an ultrasonic wave is traveling. The acoustic wave creates periodic pressure zones in the crystal that locally vary its refractive index causing diffraction of the laser beam. The deflection angle of the first order diffracted beam depends on the periodicity of the refractive index variation so that it can be varied in a controlled manner by changing the frequency of the acoustic wave. The main advantage with respect to galvanometer is that AODs have negligible inertia allowing to reach much higher scanning speed. Further, AODs scanners can produce user-defined deflections to generate customizable scanned regions of interest. The disadvantage is represented by the dispersive properties of the crystals so that AODs are suitable only for monochromatic light. Although these problems have been solved in several experimental instrument designs [68, 69, 71], the concept of using AOD scanners did not become popular among the microscope manufacturers.

Polygonal mirror scanners. A possible scanning solution offering fast imaging speed as AODs without the drawback of dispersion consists in using a polygonal mirror scanner as a fast scanner and a galvanometer as a slow scanner. The polygonal scanning mirror is made by a prism of polygonal basis with mirrors placed onto the external faces. A rotating polygonal mirror causes a laser beam hitting on the external face to be deflected in a similar manner with respect to a galvanometer mirror driven with a saw tooth profile. The advantage is the higher scanning speed achievable with this device in comparison with the galvanometer approach. This approach has the advantage of using an optically simple technology able to reach video-rate speed. The drawback is represented by the complexity of both optical and electronic design for the implementation in an experimental setup.

4.4.3 Detection system

This section focuses on the detectors that can be used in a NLO microscope and on the features to be considered when installing a detector in a custom-made experimental setup.

Photomultiplier Tubes (PMTs). The photomultiplier tube (PMT) is without doubt the most used detector technology in NLO microscopy. In general a PMT is a device maintained under vacuum in which various electrodes find place: a photocathode, constituting the sensitive element of the detector; a number of dynodes for amplifying the signal in a cascade; an anode for the delivering of the output signal. The device needs to be supplied with a high voltage in order to generate an electrical field between the cathode, the dynodes and the anode high enough to generate a signal cascade. A single photo-electron generated by the cathode is accelerated by the electric field and hit on the subsequent dynode inducing the emission of several electrons that are in turn accelerated towards the next dynode. The number of electrons is amplified in each dynode stage in order to achieve a total gain in the order of 10^6–10^8. There are several types of photocathode and dynode geometries available. The features of these elements affect the specifications of the detector. In particular, the sensitivity of the PMT as well as its spectral response depends on the photocathode material, while the dynode geometry affects the overall gain and the temporal response of the detector.

Avalanche photodiodes (APDs). An avalanche photodiode (APD) simply consists in a photodiode driven with a voltage close to or slightly above the breakdown voltage. This allows one to detect very small signal levels as those generated in TPF or SHG. In fact, when a photon hits on the sensitive area of the photodiode an electron-hole pair is generated. The strong electric field generated by the applied voltage accelerates the first pair created so that an avalanche discharge is induced in the device. This amplification system allows one to detect very small signals, down to a single photon. APDs offer a much higher quantum efficiency with respect to the PMTs, especially in the green range of the spectrum (up to 0.7). On the other hand, they have a very small sensitive area.

Micro-channel plates (MCPs). A micro-channel plate (MCP) is a particular family of PMT detectors. The working principle is similar to that of PMTs with a photocathode and an anode but the dynode stage is substituted by a channel with the inner surface coated with a conductive material. The amplification is then generated inside this channel. MCPs offer the advantage of being much faster with respect to traditional PMTs but their cost is normally higher. Further, multiple elements can be assembled in an array fashion in order to make image intensifiers or position-sensitive detectors. The sensitivity is comparable to traditional PMTs.

4.5 Biological Applications

4.5.1 Nonlinear imaging of skin

In the two decades overlapping the beginning of the new millennium, NLO microscopy was successfully used as a powerful technique in skin imaging and optical biopsy by means of a morphological characterization [17, 18, 72, 73] of the tissue under investigation. At the beginning limited to *ex vivo* tissue and to fresh biopsies, NLO imaging has been recently tested and used *in vivo* on human subjects [19]. TPF is particularly useful to image cellular epidermis because cellular NADH can be excited by two-photon absorption in the Ti:Sapphire emission spectral range [9]. When imaging deeper in the papillary dermis, additional morphological information can be provided by SHG, which can be combined with TPF microscopy using the same laser source. SHG was already largely used for imaging anisotropic molecules inside cells [40, 42] and tissues [45, 55]. Collagen fibers produce a high SHG signal [54] with which they can be imaged inside skin dermis. Recently, SHG was also used for investigating collagen fibers orientation and their structural changes in healthy tissues such as human dermis [74, 75, 76, 77] or cornea [48, 78] and in the tumor microenvironment [79, 80, 81, 82, 82, 83, 84, 85]. Combined TPF-SHG microscopy has been applied to skin physiology and pathology, and specifically to the study of normal skin [17, 18, 19, 72, 73], cutaneous photoageing [86, 87, 88, 89], diseased skin [90, 93], and selected skin tumors, including basal cell carcinoma (BCC) [94, 95, 96], and malignant melanoma (MM) [97]. Recently, the *in-vivo*

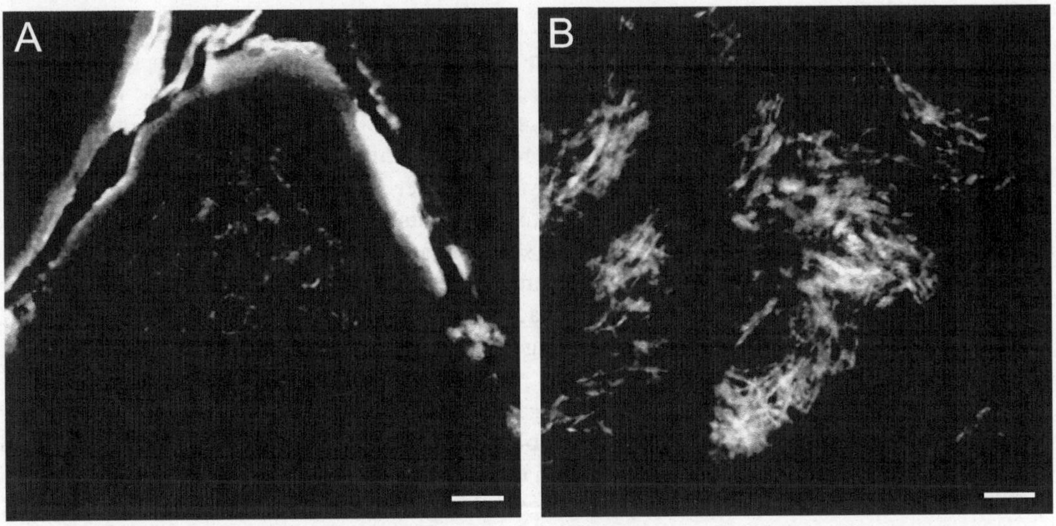

Figure 4.3: (A) TPF image of NADH fluorescence in epidermis acquired at 25 μm depths from skin surface, approximately corresponding to granular layer. Excitation wavelength: 740 nm. Scale bar: 20 μm. (B) SHG image of collagen in papillary dermis acquired at 130 μm depth from skin surface. Excitation wavelength: 900 nm. Scale bar: 40 μm. Figure modified from [131].

use of higher-order harmonic microscopy, together with TPF-SHG, has also been demonstrated to be useful in deep skin imaging [98]. *In vivo* imaging with sub-cellular spatial resolution can be performed by using NLO microscopy up to approximately 200 μm depth from the skin surface. Below we show the capability of NLO microscopy for imaging skin at both epidermal and dermal level by using TPF and SHG microscopy, respectively. The approach described here could become a powerful tool to be used in a dermatological clinic for both early diagnosis and therapy follow-up purposes. Further, new emerging technologies for ultrafast pulsed laser sources, potentially cheaper than the usual solid state Ti:Sapphire oscillator, can help NLO microscopy to find a stable place in the clinical setting.

TPF imaging of epidermis. A representative image of the epidermis, acquired using a water immersion objective lens (NA= 1.2) and an excitation wavelength of 740 nm, is shown in Fig. 4.3A. Signal was collected in the whole spectral range without any filtering in order to have a signal-to-noise ratio as high as possible. Cells are clearly distinguishable and they appear with a fluorescent cytoplasm and a dark nucleus. A morphological analysis enables one to discriminate the epidermal layers. In particular, it is interesting from the physiological point of view to focus the attention on the epidermal layers containing living cells. As expected, the granular layer (Fig. 4.3A) shows cells large in dimension, with a characteristic content of highly fluorescent granuli, and emitting a lower average fluorescence with respect to other epidermal layers. Even if the probability of generating reactive oxygen species by prolonged multi-photon excitation inside skin has already been demonstrated to be not higher than normal sun exposure [99], at the epidermal level it is preferable to limit the acquisition only to a few images because epidermis (especially basal layer) is the most absorbing region inside skin. In addition, in order to reduce the unwanted higher-order NLO effects, TPF images of epidermis should be preferably taken with a reduced power and an increased integration time with respect to the experimental conditions used for fresh *ex vivo* tissue. Further, in order to limit the absorbed power to a minimum dose, a good rule to be adopted for *in vivo* imaging is to reduce power when imaging regions of the body with a high level of pigmentation.

SHG imaging of dermis. A representative image of dermis, acquired using a water immersion objective lens (NA=0.9) and an excitation wavelength of 900 nm, is shown in Fig. 4.3B. Even if 900 nm is not the best wavelength to excite SHG from collagen, this is the optimal wavelength for deep imaging inside dermis because longer wavelengths can penetrate deeper. Further, a slight underfill of the back-aperture of the objective lens has been used in order to increase penetration depth inside tissue. The resolution, even if reduced by this effect, is enough to resolve collagen fibers within dermis. In particular, it is possible to discriminate collagen fibers inside dermis, as well as the contribution of the other filling components. In fact dermis is mainly composed by collagen fibers, arranged to form a sort of skeleton of the tissue, immersed in a matrix mainly composed by water, hyaluronic acid, glicosaminoglicanes and other proteins. Scattering is strongly affected by this matrix and the resulting images are less or more blurry and more or less fibrotic depending on the relative abundance of collagen and other filling components. The signal shown in the images is containing both SHG and TPF, even if the highest contribution is given by SHG. It is clearly distinguishable from the collagen organization in the dermal layer imaged. The particular conformation with holes appearing in the collagen network is probably due to the protrusion of epidermal crests inside dermis. At this depth the skin texture is still visible as demonstrated by the black lines that can be observed in the images. Increasing the acquisition depth, collagen fibers increase more in size and the holes visible in the upper layers are filled by collagen. When imaging deeper the images start becoming blurred and it is difficult to distinguish the collagen network. The maximum imaging depth with these experimental conditions is approximately in the 210–220 μm range, hence enough to image papillary dermis.

4.5.2 Multi-photon imaging of bladder tissue

Bladder cancer is one of the most common cancers in the U.S. [100]. The usual diagnostic method in the clinical routine is based on visual observation of the bladder urothelium through white light cystoscopy, which is the most diffused endoscopic technique for bladder tissue diagnostics. However, cystoscopy is only able to visualize superficial urothelium without the capability to provide a deep optical sectioning of the tissue. New emerging technologies for building miniaturized scanning systems and high-NA optics as well as new designs for delivering pulses through non-dispersive optical fibers have created new insights for NLO endoscopic imaging [101]. Considering the capabilities that NLO microscopy has already demonstrated in providing an "optical biopsy" of a tissue [17, 19, 72, 73], in the future NLO endoscopy has potential for being successfully used in both early diagnosis and therapy follow-up of bladder cancer. Recently, conventional NLO microscopy has been used for the imaging of bladder cell cultures [102] and for bladder tissue samples excised from animals [103, 104].

In this section we present a multimodal analysis for human bladder tissue characterization performed by combining multiple NLO microscopy techniques able to provide optical sectioning. In particular, a morphological analysis of human bladder urothelium is performed by employing TPF and SHG microscopy on fresh biopsies of healthy mucosa (HM) and carcinoma *in situ* (CIS). This multimodal approach allows highlighting differences in morphology, measured in terms of cellular-to-nuclear ratio, between the two tissues. A more detailed analysis helping the discrimination between HM and CIS from the metabolic point of view can be obtained by spectral-resolved detection of endogenous NADH and FAD fluorescence. Multispectral two-photon fluorescence (MTPF) imaging can be performed by detecting tissue endogenous fluorescence on a multichannel spectral-resolved detector. The spectroscopic data offer functional information related to the abundance of fluorescent molecules within the investigated tissue, that are in relation with physiological or pathological states [105]. This multimodal analysis, employing multiple NLO microscopy techniques, may represent a powerful tool, if combined with multi-photon endoscopy, with confocal endoscopy or with fluorescence fiber-based spectroscopy, for the early diagnosis of bladder cancer.

TPF-SHG morphological imaging. The morphological features of the cells can be highlighted in fresh biopsies of bladder urothelium by taking advantage of the endogenous fluorescence pro-

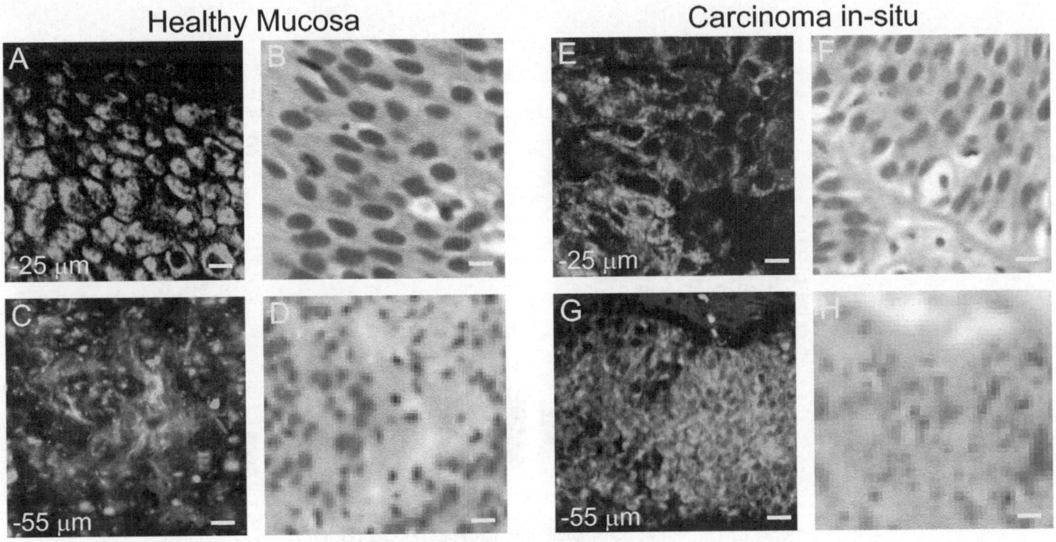

Figure 4.4: (See color insert.) Combined TPF (green-coded) and SHG (blue-coded) images taken from human *ex vivo* fresh biopsies of bladder and the corresponding histological images taken after H&E staining of the same samples. On the left: an optical section of healthy mucosa (A,B) and connective tissue border (C,D) acquired at 25 μm and 55 μm depth from tissue surface, respectively. On the right: an optical section of CIS (E,F) and connective tissue border (G,H) acquired at the same depth as above. Scale bars: 10 μm. Figure modified from [106].

duced by NADH, which can be found inside a fresh tissue biopsy up to 4–5 hours after excision [15, 105]. Both HM and CIS cells give a high fluorescent signal if imaged within 2–3 hours from excision. The images shown in Fig. 4.4 have been acquired using an excitation wavelength of 740 nm and 840 nm for TPF and SHG, respectively. Both TPF and SHG microscopy are able to optically section a thick tissue specimen with micrometric spatial resolution, hence enabling the imaging of bladder urothelium at the sub-cellular level in a very good agreement with common routine histology. The images acquired with combined TPF-SHG microscopy (TPF in green, SHG in blue in Fig. 4.4) are shown together with corresponding H&E images taken after histological examination of the same samples. A particular morphological feature that can be noted is in average a higher SHG signal coming from HM with respect to CIS.

NADH cellular fluorescence imaging shows cells with highly fluorescent cytoplasm and dark nucleus. This allows performing a quantitative analysis of the cellular morphology and in particular to measure the nuclear size against the cellular size. From the acquired images, a larger nuclear size of CIS cells is clearly distinguishable. This morphological signature of tumor cells has already been measured by TPF microscopy in other tissues, such as skin [94], and it could be taken as a typical signature of malignancy. A quantitative measurement of this feature can be obtained by measuring the cellular-to-nuclear dimension ratio. The obtained results are plotted in a bar histogram in Fig. 4.5, showing a smaller ratio for CIS with respect to HM. This interesting result arisen from the morphological analysis is in agreement with the typical signature of malignancy.

MTPF functional imaging. The morphological analysis of a tissue can be extended to functional analysis by means of MTPF detection with two particular excitation wavelengths for selectively exciting NADH and FAD endogenous fluorescence. The selective excitation of NADH and FAD fluorescence can provide functional information on cellular metabolism in a living tissue. In fact NADH and FAD are the main electron donor and acceptor in the oxidative phosphorylation, which is the most efficient metabolic pathway used by biological tissues to produce energy. Oxidative phos-

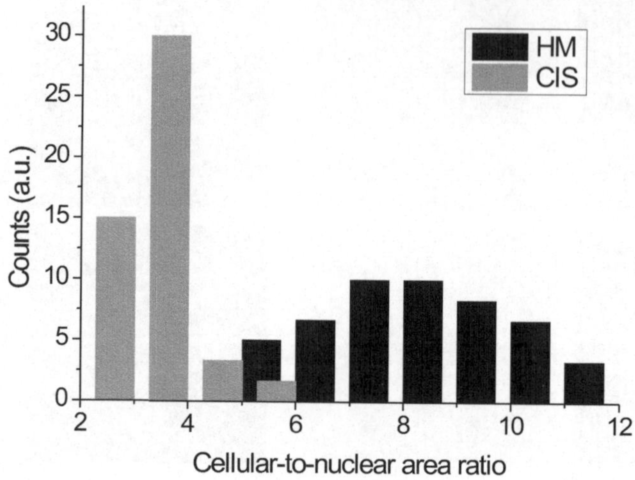

Figure 4.5: Histogram distribution of the cellular-to-nuclear area ratio for CIS (in grey) and for HM (in black), calculated by summing over images acquired in a 20–30 μm range of depth from tissue surface, on 5 samples of CIS and 5 samples of HM and over 10 cells per sample. Figure modified from [106].

phorylation requires oxygen to occur and it involves both NADH and FAD nucleotides as electron carriers. Another less efficient metabolic pathway that can be used by biological tissues for energy production is glycolysis, which does not require oxygen and it involves only NADH as electron carrier. The optical measurement of the relative abundance of NADH and FAD in a biological tissue can be used as an indicator of the metabolic balance between glycolysis and oxidative phosphorylation. An unbalance with respect to a normal condition can be related to diseased conditions, such as cancerous or pre-cancerous. In fact, it is well known that neoplastic tissues have a higher cellular division rate with respect to healthy tissues and correspondingly a higher energy demand. Since the oxygen supply is not enough to produce the required excess of energy through oxidative phosphorylation, neoplastic tissues preferably use glycolysis to satisfy their increased energy demand. As a consequence, the metabolism of a neoplastic tissue has different results from healthy tissues and is unbalanced towards glycolysis. This effect, known as the Warburg effect [107], causes an imbalance in the relative abundance of NADH and FAD that can be optically monitored by means of their fluorescence. The optimal wavelengths for exciting NADH and FAD fluorescence using two-photon excitation are 740 nm and 890 nm, respectively. The fluorescence emission peaks are located in the 460 nm range for NADH and in the 515 nm range for FAD. By selectively exciting and detecting NADH and FAD in two separated spectral channels, it is possible to extract an indicator of the tissue metabolism. In this section NADH-images are intended as the images acquired on a single spectral channel (459–472 nm) of a multispectral PMT detector at 740 nm excitation wavelength, whereas FAD-images are intended as the images acquired on a single spectral channel (508–521 nm) using 890 nm as excitation wavelength. By correcting the numbers of detected photons in the images for the detector spectral response and for the square of the laser power (nonlinear excitation) it is possible to calculate an image representing a map of a normalized index by using the following relationship:

$$ROx = \frac{FAD - NADH}{FAD + NADH}. \tag{4.44}$$

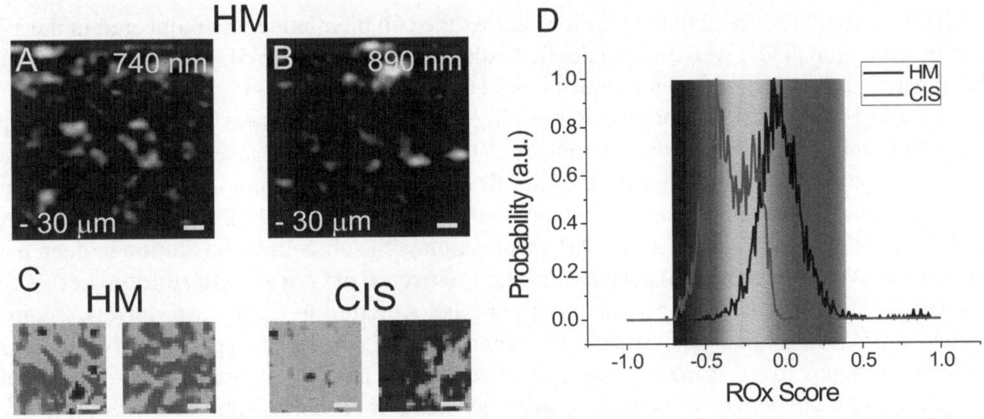

Figure 4.6: (See color insert.) (A) MTPF images of HM acquired at 740 nm excitation wavelength and detected in the 459–472 nm spectral range (NADH-image). (B) MTPF images of HM acquired at 890 nm excitation wavelength and detected in the 511–524 nm spectral range (FAD-image). Scale bars: 2 μm. (C) Two examples of ROx maps, calculated using equation (4.44) for both CIS and HM presented in a color-coded scale. Scale bars: 5 μm. (D) Red-Ox ratio distribution for CIS (red) and for HM (black) with the color-coded scale used in ROx mapping superimposed. Figure modified from [106].

An example of such image processing is shown for bladder tissue in Fig. 4.6. The NADH- and FAD-images are processed using the relationship defined in equation (4.44), and the calculated ROx index is presented as a map in a color-coded scale (Fig. 4.6C for both HS and CIS). The mean distribution of the ROx index, obtained by averaging on 5 samples of HM and 5 samples of CIS is plotted in a histogram in Fig. 4.6D. It is possible to see that the distribution for HM is centered on higher values in comparison to the distribution for CIS. The lower mean value of the index found in CIS confirms a higher relative abundance of NADH in cancer with respect to healthy tissue, corresponding to a higher oxidative stress.

This higher NADH contribution is probably due to a metabolic imbalance towards glycolysis for the cancer, which is in agreement with the Warburg effect. Such a method can be extended to other tissues as well as to other inflammatory and dysplastic tissue conditions. In particular, it has to be noted that this optical non-invasive assessment of the metabolic condition of tissues can provide the possibility to detect cancer in a very early stage.

4.5.3 Functional imaging by random access microscopy

The generation and propagation of an electric impulse, better known as action potential (AP), along the membrane are the main features of an excitable cell. The inter-cellular transmission of action potentials is a fundamental aspect in biology. For example the electrical communication between neurons represents the core of the brain function while the transmission of AP between cardiac cells is crucial for the synchronization of heart contraction.

The most popular method to record electrical activity in neurons is the patch-clamp, introduced by Neher and Sakmann in 1976 [108]. Although this technique allows precise voltage measurements in single cells, it can hardly be applied to many cells at once, given the steric hindrance of the electrodes. Parallel large-area electric measurements are possible using micro electrode arrays [109, 110], which however measure an average electric field rather than the membrane potential of single neurons. Further, the position of the electrodes is imposed by the geometry of the array itself. Current optical techniques for recording membrane potential can overcome these limitations. The use of light to detect electrical field variations across the cell membrane was pioneered in the 1970s by Lawrence Cohen [111], who devised the first voltage sensitive dye (VSD). The VSD is an optical probe in which a change in the membrane potential alters some optically observable parameter (e.g., fluorescence) [112]. VSDs are commonly used in combination with linear microscopy techniques, limiting their application to *in vitro* samples or to the most superficial layers of biological tissues. In fact, the light scattering that occurs into the tissue dramatically degrades the resolution and/or S/N of the acquired images. In the next section we describe how NLO microscopy can be used to optically record inter- and intra-cellular AP propagation with sub-cellular resolution in deep tissue.

Optical recording of electrical activity in intact neuronal networks with random access SHG microscopy. The brain is probably the most complex structure in the known universe, complex enough to coordinate movements, gather and organize lots of sensory data, perform abstract reasoning and develop new ideas. Understanding the mechanisms underlying brain function is therefore one of the biggest challenges of contemporary science. Our current picture of the brain is that of an extremely complex circuit in which elementary computational units (neurons) exchange information between other units in the network through unidirectional links (synapses). The circuit is capable of processing a tremendous amount of information, which is encoded in terms of spikes and transmitted between neurons at synapses. The central question in neuroscience is how simple processes in neurons can generate cognitive functions and form complex memories like those experienced by humans and animals. In principle, if one were able to record from all the neurons in a network involved in a given behavior, it would be possible to reconstruct the related computations.

The main NLO techniques used in combination with VSDs are TPF and SHG. As described before, the former is an incoherent process in which two photons are absorbed almost simultaneously by the molecule to reach an excited state, and a single photon is spontaneously emitted after a variable amount of time (of the order of ns). On the other hand, SHG is a coherent phenomenon where two low-energy photons are transformed in a single high-energy one, without absorption. Due to the coherence properties, SHG signal is much stronger when molecular emitters (molecules operating the frequency doubling) are positioned in an ordered rather than random fashion. SHG thus gives a more contrasted image of cell membranes than TPF [113, 114]. For this reason, SHG imaging of VSDs has been recently exploited to optically detect APs in model membranes [115], in cultured neurons of *Aplysia* [116, 117] and in mammalian intact neuronal systems [118, 119]. In these examples, the optical recording of neuronal APs was performed only in a single position of the neuron using a line scanning procedure. In principle, APs in several neurons can be recorded at a sampling

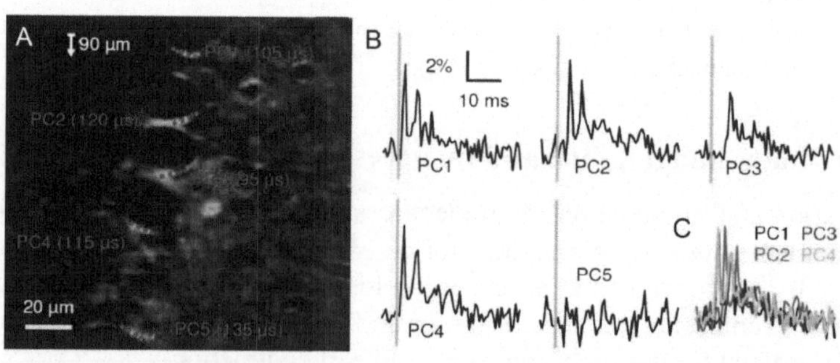

Figure 4.7: (See color insert.) Optical recording of electrical activity in multiple neurons. (A) SHG image of a cerebellar slice taken at a depth of 90 μm. SHG recording was carried out from the lines drawn (dotted) on the 5 neurons, with the integration time per membrane pass indicated. (B) Multiplexed recording of APs from the 5 neurons following electrical stimulation (vertical lines). Each trace represents the average of 20 trials for each neuron. (C) Superposition of SHG traces. Figure modified from [121].

frequency of more than 1 kHz by scanning the beam waist in multiple selected lines. This cannot be achieved with a standard galvanometric mirror since the time required to reach and stabilize a new position is about 1 ms. Scanning a set of points within a plane at high speed is possible using acousto-optic deflectors (AODs). As described above, in an AOD, a propagating ultrasonic wave establishes a grating that diffracts a laser beam at a precise angle which can be changed within a few microseconds. The first implementation of a high-speed, random-access, laser-scanning fluorescence microscope configured to record fast physiological signals from small neuronal structures with high spatiotemporal resolution has been presented by Bullen et al. [120]. Recently, the advantages of SHG were combined with a random access excitation scheme [121] to develop a new microscope (RASH) capable of recording neuronal electrical activity in living tissue, in several cells simultaneously, with a high spatial (sub-cellular) and temporal (sub-millisecond) resolution. The RASH microscope, in combination with a SHG VSD (FM4-64), was used to simultaneously record evoked electrical activity from clusters of Purkinje cells in acute cerebellar slices. The AODs rapidly scanned between lines drawn in the membranes of neurons to perform multiplex measurements of the emitted signal. As shown in Fig. 4.7, both synchronous and asynchronous APs were optically recorded across a given population of neurons averaging 20 trials.

This result shows the strength of this technique in probing the temporal dynamics of neuronal assemblies opening promising prospects in understanding the computations of neuronal networks. The random access modality can be used not only to explore the electrical coupling between neurons but also to study intra-cellular propagation of AP in cardiac cells.

Probing the intra-cellular AP propagation in cardiac cells by random access TPF. Differently from neurons, in cardiac cells APs have a direct consequence: the contraction of the cell itself. The chain reaction that makes possible this event is called excitation-contraction (EC) coupling. This process is fundamental to muscle physiology, whereby the electrical stimulus is usually an AP and the mechanical response is contraction. The general scheme is that an AP arrives to depolarize the cell membrane. This depolarization results in an increase in cytosolic calcium ions (calcium transient). This increase in calcium activates calcium-sensitive contractile proteins to cause cell shortening (contraction). In cardiac muscle, the contraction depends on a phenomenon called calcium-induced calcium release, which involves the conduction of calcium ions into the cell triggering further release of ions into the cytoplasm (about 75% of calcium present in the cytoplasm during contraction is released from the sarcoplasmic reticulum). In this way the simultaneous contraction of all the areas within each cell occurs. Nevertheless, until now it was not yet clear how the simultaneous contraction of the subcellular areas of the cardiac cell was performed itself.

In fact, cardiac cells present deep invagination of the plasma membrane, known as T-tubules, creating an elaborated tridimensional network inside the cell. Several studies in skeletal and cardiac muscle cells highlighted a heterogeneous distribution of the AP-relevant channels between membrane surface and T-tubules. These findings in combination with the limited T-tubular extracellular space point out a possible alteration of the AP features in the excitation-contraction coupling network. Simultaneous recording of membrane potential in these two membrane domains can reveal potential peculiarities of T-tubules electrophysiology. Although current optical techniques for probing membrane potential allow intracellular recording, most approaches lack the spatiotemporal resolution and signal to noise ratio needed for regional assessment of action potential (AP) profile. An ultrafast random access multi-photon (RAMP) microscope was recently used to optically record fast membrane potential transients in multiple positions of the cell membrane with μm spatial resolution [122]. The RAMP microscopy, in combination with a novel VSD, was used to simultaneously record APs in membrane surface and T-tubules in intact cardiac tissue with sub-millisecond time resolution (see Fig. 4.8).

The authors found that APs in the T-tubules have identical amplitude and kinetics as in the membrane surface, indicating that the tight electrical coupling between the two membrane domains prevails over the inhomogeneous distribution of ion channels.

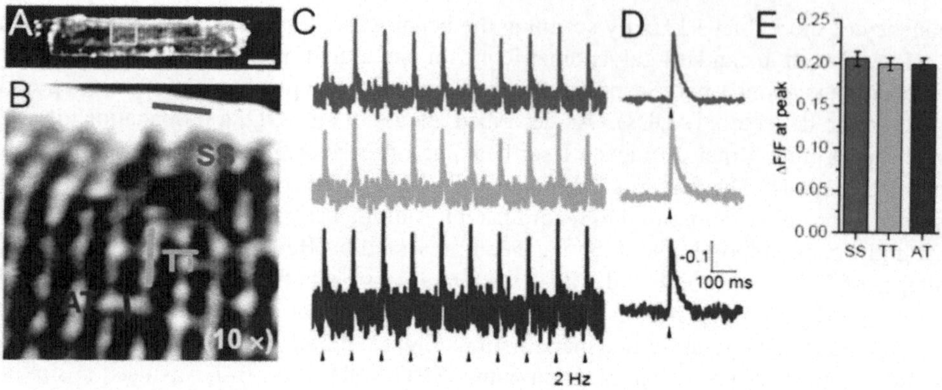

Figure 4.8: (See color insert.) Electrical properties of cardiac cell. (A) TPF image of a stained cardiac cell. (Scale bar: 10 μm.) (B) The region in the yellow box of A is shown magnified 10×. The lines mark the probed sarcolemma regions: superficial membrane (SS) in red, transversal tubule (TT) in green, and axial tubule (AT) in blue. (C) Normalized fluorescence traces from the scanned line indicated in B. APs were electrically stimulated at 2 Hz, corresponding to the black arrowheads. (D) Average of 10 sequential APs shown in C. (E) Relative fluorescence change ($\Delta F/F$) at the peak of APs from the three different membrane regions. Each bar represents the mean ± SE. Figure modified from [122].

4.5.4 Probing the myosin conformation by SHG microscopy

Understanding of complex biological processes requires knowledge of molecular structures and measurement of their dynamics *in vivo*. Generally, several techniques must be used to encompass the spatial and temporal scales involved in such processes. In fact, protein crystallography provides static structures with atomic resolution, while complementary techniques are needed to follow structural dynamics in the cellular context.

Recently, Nucciotti et al. probed structural dynamics *in vivo* using a label-free imaging method [33]. They employed the order-based contrast enhancement by SHG for the functional imaging of muscle cells in different physiological states. In fact, strong SHG signal has been detected from the myosin-based A-band of unstained muscle cells and myofibrils [123, 124]. The possibility of using SHG for the measurement of myosin structural conformation relies on the location of the SHG emitters within the myosin molecule. In fact, this protein is constituted by a passive portion and a catalytically active actin-binding site. Information on the spatial distribution of the emitters can be obtained from SHG polarization anisotropy (SPA) measurements [125]. In a cylindrically symmetric system (such as a muscle fiber), SPA yields a geometrical factor γ related to the average angle of emitters with respect to the fiber axis. In fact, by combining muscle symmetry invariance under rotation around the y-axis (fiber axis, in a system of coordinate with the z-axis along the laser propagation direction), the second order susceptibility tensor can be expressed as [114]:

$$\chi^{(2)} = \begin{pmatrix} 0 & 0 & 0 & 0 & 0 & \chi^{(2)}_{yxx} \\ \chi^{(2)}_{yxx} & \chi^{(2)}_{yyy} & \chi^{(2)}_{yxx} & 0 & 0 & 0 \\ 0 & 0 & 0 & \chi^{(2)}_{yxx} & 0 & 0 \end{pmatrix}. \tag{4.45}$$

The total SHG intensity (I_{SHG}, proportional to the square of the second order induced polarization), can be expressed as a function of the angle φ between the fiber axis and the laser polarization:

$$I_{SHG}(\varphi) \propto \left(\sin^2(\varphi) + \gamma\cos^2(\varphi)\right)^2 + \sin^2(2\varphi) \tag{4.46}$$

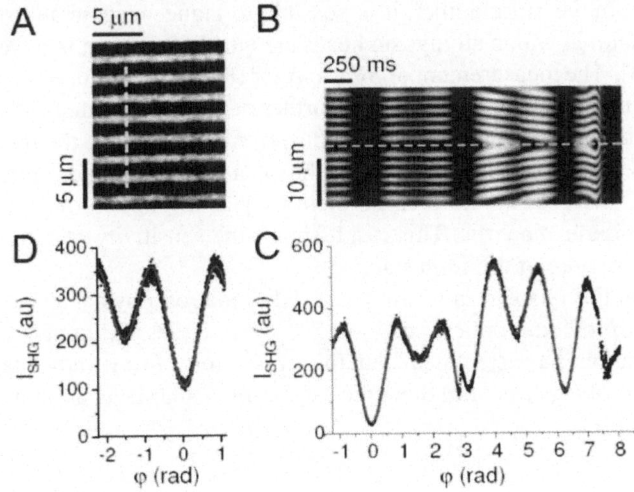

Figure 4.9: Experimental SPA recordings. (A) SHG image of a portion of unstained muscle fiber. (B) Line scan (vertical dashed line in panel A) measurement of SHG intensity at rest and during contraction. The horizontal dashed line shows the point of inversion of scanning direction. (C) SPA measurement: SHG intensity was measured from integration over each line of the scan. The solid line shows the best fit of Eq. (4.46) to a portion of data covering a φ range of π for the resting and the active state. (D) SPA measurement in rigor. Figure modified from [33].

with $\gamma \equiv \chi^{(2)}_{yyy}/\chi^{(2)}_{yxx}$. The quantity γ can be also experimentally determined by fitting the above equation to the measured SPA. Following these considerations Nucciotti and coworkers performed the direct comparison of SPAs from muscle at rest and during contraction (Fig 4.9). Fig. 4.9c shows a clear difference in the SPA profiles between resting and active muscle yielding a dependence of γ on the physiological state: $\gamma_{rest} = 0.30 \pm 0.03$; $\gamma_{act} = 0.64 \pm 0.02$. These results indicate that the structural changes occurring in the active actin-binding site of myosin can be monitored by SPA. By

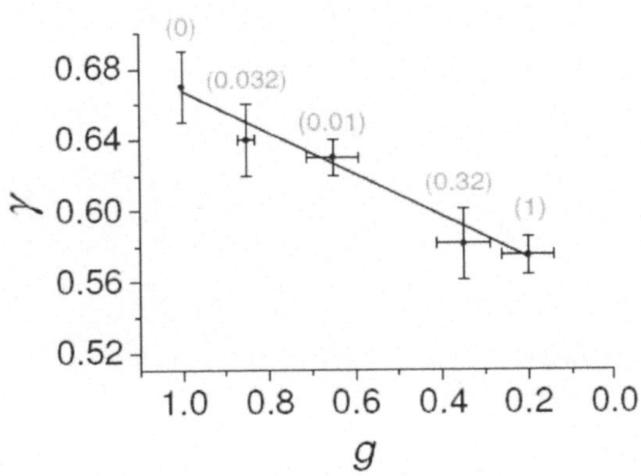

Figure 4.10: Effect of PPi on attached myosins: γ is measured as a function of the fraction of attached molecules g. The fraction was experimentally reduced by increasing PPi concentrations (reported in mM in parenthesis). The line represents a linear regression through the data ($R^2 = 0.97$). Figure modified from [33].

depleting ATP from the muscle fiber, it is possible to induce a static and structurally homogenous state (the rigor state) in which all myosin heads are attached to actin in a well characterized conformation [126, 128]. The measurement of SPA in rigor (Fig. 4.9) produced a value ($\gamma_{rig} = 0.74 \pm 0.02$) statistically different ($p < 0.001$) from γ_{act}, further demonstrating that SPA monitors the structural conformation of the active site of myosin. In this physiological state, the fraction of attached myosin (g) can be biochemically modulated by pyrophosphate (PPi) in a concentration-dependent manner [129, 130]. Fig. 4.10 shows the measurement of γ as a function of g: the data show that, as g diminishes, γ decreases linearly. This result shows the sensitivity of γ to partitioning of attached molecules into a mixture of different states.

As described in this chapter, in recent years, NLO microscopy has gained enormous momentum in life science by providing optical sectioning in deep tissues. Although a large array of morpho-functional applications have stemmed from this opportunity, further advantages will be gained from the capability of probing structural dynamics at the molecular level as shown in this last section.

Acknowledgment

The research leading to these results has received funding from the European Union Seventh Framework Programme (FP7/2007-2013) under grant agreements number 228334 and 241526. This research project has been also supported by the Human Frontier Science Program research grant (RGP0027/2009), and by the Italian Ministry for Education, University and Research in the framework of the Flagship Project Nanomax and by Italian Ministry of Health in the framework of the "Stem Cells Call for Proposals." This research has been carried out in the framework of the research activities of ICON Foundation supported by "Ente Cassa di Risparmio di Firenze."

References

[1] W.R. Zipfel, R.M. Williams, and W.W. Webb, "Nonlinear magic, multiphoton microscopy in the biosciences," *Nat. Biotechnol.* **21**, 1369–1377 (2003).

[2] F. Helmchen and W. Denk, "Deep tissue two-photon microscopy," *Nat. Methods* **2**, 932–940 (2005).

[3] V.E. Centonze and J.G. White, "Multiphoton excitation provides optical sections from deeper within scattering specimens than confocal imaging," *Biophys. J.* **75**, 2015–2022 (1998).

[4] M. Goppert-Mayer, "Uber elementarekte mit zwei Quantensprunger," *Ann. Phys.* **9**, 273 (1931).

[5] W. Kaiser and C.G.B. Garret, "Two-photon excitation in CaF_2, Eu^{2+}," *Phys. Rev. Lett.* **7**.229–231 (1961).

[6] W. Denk, H.J. Strickler, and W.W. Webb, "Two-photon laser scanning fluorescence microscope," *Science* **248**, 73–76 (1990).

[7] R.M. Williams, W.R. Zipfel, and W.W. Webb, "Multiphoton microscopy in biological research," *Curr. Opin. Chem. Biol.* **5**, 603–608 (2001).

[8] K. König, "Multiphoton microscopy in life sciences," *J. Microsc.* **200**, 83–104 (2000).

[9] S. Huang, A.A. Heikal, and W.W. Webb, "Two-photon fluorescence spectroscopy and microscopy of NAD(P)H and flavoprotein," *Biophys. J.* **82**, 2811–2825 (2002).

[10] A. Volkmer, V. Subramaniam, D.J.S. Birch, and T.M. Jovin, "One and two-photon excited fluorescence lifetimes and anisotropy decays of green fluorescent proteins," *Biophys. J.* **78**, 1589–1598 (2000).

[11] C. Xu, W. Zipfel, J.B. Shear, R.M. Williams, and W.W. Webb, "Multiphoton fluorescence excitation, New spectral windows for biological nonlinear microscopy," *Proc. Natl. Acad. Sci. U.S.A.* **93**, 10763–10768 (1996).

[12] M.Rubart, E.Wang, K.W. Dunn, and L.J. Field, "Two-photon molecular excitation imaging of Ca62+ transients in Langendorff-perfused mouse hearts," *Am. J. Physiol. Cell Physiol.* **284**, C1654–C1668 (2003).

[13] M. Oheim, E. Beaurepaire, E. Chaigneau, J. Mertz, and S. Charpak, "Two-photon microscopy in brain tissue, parameters influencing the imaging depth," *J. Neurosci. Methods* **111**, 29–37 (2001).

[14] A. Zoumi, A.T. Yeh, and B.J. Tromberg, "Imaging cells and extracellular matrix *in vivo* by using second-harmonic generation and two-photon excited fluorescence," *Proc. Natl. Acad. Sci. U.S.A.* **99**, 11014–11019 (2002).

[15] W.R. Zipfel et al., "Live tissue intrinsic emission microscopy using multiphoton-excited native fluorescence and second harmonic generation," *Proc. Natl. Acad. Sci. U.S.A.* **100**, 7075–7080 (2003).

[16] B.R. Masters, P.T.C. So, and E. Gratton, "Multi photon excitation fluorescence microscopy and spectroscopy of *in vivo* human skin," *Biophys. J.* **72**, 2405–2412 (1997).

[17] B.R. Masters, P.T.C. So, and E. Gratton, "Optical biopsy of in vivo human skin, multi-photon excitation microscopy," *Lasers Med. Sci.* **13**, 196–203 (1998).

[18] B.R. Masters and P.T.C. So, "Confocal microscopy and multi-photon excitation microscopy of human skin *in vivo*," *Opt. Express* **8**, 2–9 (2001).

[19] K. Konig and I. Riemann, "High-resolution multiphoton tomography of human skin with subcellular spatial resolution and picosecond time resolution," *J. Biomed. Opt.* **8**, 432–439 (2003).

[20] F. Helmchen and W. Denk, "Deep tissue two-photon microscopy," *Nat. Methods* **2**(12), 932–940 (2005).

[21] K. Svoboda and R. Yasuda, "Principles of two-photon excitation microscopy and its applications to neuroscience," *Neuron* **50**(6), 823–839 (2006).

[22] M.T. Myaing, D.J.MacDonald, and X. Li, "Fiber-optic scanning two-photon fluorescence endoscope," *Opt. Lett.* **31**, 1076–1078 (2006).

[23] J.N. Gannaway and C.J.R. Sheppard, "Second-harmonic imaging in the scanning optical microscope," *Opt. Quant. Elect.* **10**, 435–439 (1978).

[24] C.J.R. Sheppard, R. Kompfner, J. Gannaway, and D. Walsh, "Scanning harmonic optical microscope," *IEEE J. Quantum Electron.* **13E**, 100D (1977).

[25] S. Fine and W.P. Hansen, "Optical second harmonic generation in biological systems," *Appl. Opt.* **10**, 2350–2353 (1971).

[26] W.A. Mohler, A.C. Millard, and P.J. Campagnola, "Second harmonic generation imaging of endogenous structural proteins," *Methods* **29**, 97–109 (2003).

[27] S. Roth and I. Freund, "Second harmonic generation in collagen," *J. Chem. Phys.* **70**, 1637–1643 (1979).

[28] I. Freund, M. Deutsch, and A. Sprecher, "Optical second-harmonic microscopy, crossed-beam summation and small-angle scattering in rat-tail tendon," *Biophys. J.* **50**, 693–712 (1986).

[29] R. Cicchi et al., "From molecular structure to tissue architecture, collagen organization probed by SHG microscopy," *J. Biophoton.* (2012).

[30] M. Both et al., "Second harmonic imaging of intrinsic signals in muscle fiber *in situ*," *J. Biomed. Opt.* **87**, 882–892 (2004).

[31] T. Boulesteix, E. Beaurepaire, M.P. Sauviat, and M.C. Schanne-Klein, "Second-harmonic microscopy of unstained living cardiac myocytes, Measurements of sarcomere length with 20 nm accuracy," *Opt. Lett.* **29**, 2031–2033 (2004).

[32] M.E. Llewellyn, R.P.J. Barretto, S.L. Delp, and M.J. Schnitzer, "Minimally invasive high-speed imaging of sarcomere contractile dynamics in mice and humans," *Nat. Lett.* **454**, 784–788 (2008).

[33] V. Nucciotti et al., "Probing myosin structural conformation in vivo by second-harmonic generation microscopy," *Proc. Natl. Acad. Sci. U.S.A.* **107**, 7763–7768 (2010).

[34] S.V. Plotnikov, A.C. Millard, P.J. Campagnola, and W.A. Mohler, "Characterization of the myosin-based source for second-harmonic generation from muscle sarcomeres," *Biophys. J.* **90**, 693–703 (2006).

[35] F. Vanzi, L. Sacconi, R. Cicchi, and F.S. Pavone, "Protein conformation and molecular order probed by second-harmonic generation microscopy," *J. Biomed. Opt.* **17**, 060901 (2012).

[36] D.A. Dombeck et al., "Uniform polarity microtubule assemblies imaged in native brain tissue by second-harmonic generation microscopy," *Proc. Natl. Acad. Sci. U.S.A.* **100**, 7081–7086 (2003).

[37] P.J. Campagnola, M.D. Wei, A. Lewis, and L.M. Loew, "High-resolution nonlinear optical imaging of live cells by second harmonic generation," *Biophys. J.* **77**, 3341–3349 (1999).

[38] T. Pons, L. Moreaux, O. Mongin, M. Blanchard-Desce, and J. Mertz, "Mechanisms of membrane potential sensing with second-harmonic generation microscopy," *J. Biomed. Opt.* **8**, 428–431 (2003).

[39] A. Zoumi, A. Yeh, and B.J. Tromberg, "Imaging cells and extracellular matrix in vivo by using second harmonic generation and two-photon excited fluorescence," *Proc. Natl. Acad. Sci. U.S.A.* **99**, 11014–11019 (2002).

[40] P.J. Campagnola and L.M. Loew, "Second-harmonic imaging microscopy for visualizing biomolecular arrays in cells, tissues and organisms," *Nat. Biotechnol.* **21**, 1356–1360 (2003).

[41] J. Mertz and L. Moreaux, "Second-harmonic generation by focused excitation of inhomogeneously distributed scatterers," *Opt. Commun.* **196**, 325–330 (2001).

[42] L. Moreaux, O. Sandre, S. Charpak, M. Blanchard-Desce, and J. Mertz, "Coherent scattering in multi-harmonic light microscopy," *Biophys. J.* **80**, 1568–1574 (2001).

[43] L. Moreaux, O. Sandre, and J. Mertz, "Membrane imaging by second-harmonic generation microscopy," *J. Opt. Soc. Am. B* **17**, 1685–1694 (2000).

[44] L. Moreaux, O. Sandre, M. Blanchard-Desce, and J. Mertz, "Membrane imaging by simultaneous second-harmonic generation and two-photon microscopy," *Opt. Lett.* **25**, 320–322 (2000).

[45] P.J. Campagnola et al., "Three-dimensional high-resolution second-harmonic generation imaging of endogenous structural proteins in biological tissues," *Biophys. J.* **81**, 493–508 (2002).

[46] Y. Guo et al., "Second-harmonic tomography of tissues," *Opt. Lett.* **22**, 1323–1325 (1997).

[47] G. Cox et al., "Three dimensional imaging of collagen using second harmonic generation," *J. Struct. Biol.* **141**, 53–62 (2003).

[48] M. Han, G. Giese, and J.F. Bille, "Second harmonic generation imaging of collagen fibrils in cornea and sclera," *Opt. Express* **13**, 5791–5797 (2005).

[49] A. Yeh, N. Nassif, A. Zoumi, and B.J. Tromberg, "Selective corneal imaging using combined second harmonic generation and two-photon excited fluorescence," *Opt. Lett.* **27**, 2082–2084 (2002).

[50] P. Stoller, B.M. Kim, A.M. Rubenchik, K.M. Reiser, and L.B. Da Silva, "Polarization-dependent optical second-harmonic imaging of a rat-tail tendon," *J. Biomed. Opt.* **7**(2), 205–214 (2002).

[51] T. Theodossiou, C. Thrasivoulou, C. Ekwobi, and D. Becker, "Second harmonic generation confocal microscopy of collagen type I from rat tendon cryosections," *Biophys. J.* **91**, 4665–4677 (2006).

[52] A. Zoumi, X. Lu, G.S. Kassab, and B.J. Tromberg, "Imaging coronary artery microstructure using second-harmonic and two-photon fluorescence microscopy," *Biophys. J.* **87**, 2778–2786 (2004).

[53] M.J. Buehler, "Nature designs tough collagen, Explaining the nanostructure of collagen fibrils," *Proc. Natl. Acad. Sci. U.S.A.* **102**, 12285–12290 (2006).

[54] S. Roth and I. Freund, "Second-harmonic generation in collagen," *J. Chem. Phys.* **70**, 1637–1643 (1979.)

[55] R.M. Williams, W.R. Zipfel, and W.W. Webb, "Interpreting second-harmonic generation images of collagen I fibrils," *Biophys. J.* **88**, 1377–1386 (2005).

[56] S.V. Plotnikov et al., "Measurement of muscle disease by quantitative second-harmonic generation imaging," *J. Biomed. Opt.* **13**, 044018 (2008).

[57] O. Nadiarnykh et al. "Second harmonic generation imaging microscopy studies of osteogenesis imperfecta," *J. Biomed. Opt.* **12**, 051805 (2007).

[58] R. LaComb, O. Nadiarnykh, and P.J. Campagnola, "Quantitative second harmonic generation imaging of the diseased state osteogenesis imperfecta, experiment and simulation," *Biophys. J.* **94**, 4504–4514 (2008).

[59] K.M. Reiser et al., "Quantitative analysis of structural disorder in intervertebral disks using second harmonic generation imaging, comparison with morphometric analysis. *J. Biomed. Opt.* **12**, 064019 (2007).

[60] N. Tiwari et al., "Imaging of normal and pathologic joint synovium using nonlinear optical microscopy as a potential diagnostic tool," *J. Biomed. Opt.* **15**, 056001 (2010).

[61] O. Nakamura, "Fundamentals of two-photon microscopy," *Micr. Res. and Tech.* **47**, 165–172 (1999).

[62] C.J.R. Sheppard and M. Gu, "Image formation in two-photon fluorescence microscopy," *Optik* **3**, 104–110 (1990).

[63] Y. Barad, H. Eisenberg, M. Horowitz, and Y. Silberberg, "Nonlinear scanning laser microscopy by third harmonic generation," *Appl. Phys. Lett.* **70**, 922–924 (1997).

[64] D. Oron et al., "Depth-resolved structural imaging by third-harmonic generation microscopy," *J. Struct. Biol.* **147**, 3–11 (2004).

[65] D. Débarre et al., "Imaging lipid bodies in cells and tissues using third-harmonic generation microscopy," *Nat. Methods* **3**, 47–53 (2006).

[66] P. Theer, M.T. Hasan, and W. Denk, "Two-photon imaging to a depth of 1000 mm in living brains by use of a Ti, Al_2O_3 regenerative amplifier," *Opt. Lett.* **28**, 1022–1024 (2003).

[67] L. Qiao, J. Ni, Z. Mao, C. Wang, and Y. Cheng, "Two-color two-photon excitation of indole using a femtosecond laser regenerative amplifier," *Opt. Commun.* **282**(5), 1056–1061 (2008).

[68] A. Bullen, S.S. Patel, and P. Saggau, "High-speed, random-access fluorescence microscopy, I. High-resolution optical recording with voltage-sensitive dyes and ion indicators," *Biophys. J.* **73**, 477–491 (1997).

[69] L. Sacconi et al., "Optical recording of electrical activity in intact neuronal networks with random-access second-harmonic generation microscopy," *Opt. Express* **16**, 14910–14921 (2008).

[70] G.D. Reddy and P. Saggau, "Fast three-dimensional laser scanning scheme using acousto-optic deflectors," *J. Biomed. Opt.* **10**, 064038 (2005).

[71] P.T.C. So, H. Kim, and I.E. Kochevar, "Two-Photon deep tissue ex vivo imaging of mouse dermal and subcutaneous structures," *Opt. Express* **3**, 339–351 (1998).

[72] J.C. Malone et al., "Three-dimensional imaging of human skin and mucosa by two-photon laser scanning microscopy" *J. Cutan. Pathol.* **29**, 453–458 (2002).

[73] P. Stoller, K.M. Reiser, P.M. Celliers, and A.M. Rubenchik, "Polarization-modulated second harmonic generation in collagen," *Biophys. J.* **82**, 3330–3342 (2002).

[74] T. Yasui, Y. Tohno, and T. Araki, "Characterization of collagen orientation in human dermis by two-dimensional second-harmonic-generation polarimetry," *J. Biomed. Opt.* **9**, 259–264 (2004).

[75] Y. Sun et al., "Investigating mechanisms of collagen thermal denaturation by high resolution second-harmonic generation imaging," *Biophys. J.* **91**, 2620–2625 (2006).

[76] A. Pena et al., "Multiphoton microscopy of engineered dermal substitutes, assessment of 3-D collagen matrix remodeling induced by fibroblast contraction," *J. Biomed. Opt.* **15**, 056018 (2010).

[77] P. Matteini et al., "Photothermally-induced disordered patterns of corneal collagen revealed by SHG imaging," *Opt. Express* **17**(6), 4868–4878 (2009).

[78] E.B. Brown et al., "Dynamic imaging of collagen and its modulation in tumors in vivo using second-harmonic generation," *Nat. Med.* **9**, 796–800 (2003).

[79] S.J. Lin et al., "Discrimination of basal cell carcinoma from normal dermal stroma by quantitative multiphoton imaging," *Opt. Lett.* **31**, 2756–2758 (2006).

[80] P.P. Provenzano et al., "Collagen reorganization at the tumor-stromal interface facilitates local invasion," *BMC Med.* **4**, 38 (2006).

[81] X. Han, R.M. Burke, M.L. Zettel, P. Tang, and E.B. Brown, "Second harmonic properties of tumor collagen, determining the structural relationship between reactive stroma and healthy stroma," *Opt. Express* **16**, 1846–1859 (2008).

[82] R. Cicchi et al., "Nonlinear laser imaging of skin lesions," *Journal of Biophotonics* **1**(1), 62–73 (2008).

[83] Y. Guo et al., "Subsurface tumor progression investigated by noninvasive optical second harmonic tomography," *Proc. Natl. Acad. Sci. U.S.A.* **96**, 10854–10856 (1999).

[84] A.M. Raja et al., "Pulse-modulated second harmonic imaging microscope quantitatively demonstrates marked increase of collagen in tumor after chemotherapy," *J. Biomed. Opt.* **15**, 056016 (2010).

[85] O. Nadiarnykh, R.B. LaComb, M.A. Brewer, and P.J. Campagnola, "Alteration of the extracellular matrix in ovarian cancer studied by Second Harmonic Generation imaging microscopy," *BMC Cancer* **10**, 94 (2010).

[86] S.J. Lin et al., "Evaluating cutaneous photoaging by use of multiphoton fluorescence and second-harmonic generation microscopy," *Opt. Lett.* **30**, 2275–2277 (2005).

[87] M.J. Koehler, K. König, P. Elsner, R. Buckle, and M. Kaatz, "*In vivo* assessment of human skin aging by multiphoton laser scanning tomography," *Opt. Lett.* **31**, 2879–2881 (2006).

[88] M.J. Koehler et al., "Morphological skin ageing criteria by multiphoton laser scanning tomography, non-invasive *in-vivo* scoring of the dermal fibre network," *Exp. Dermatol.* **17**, 519–523 (2008).

[89] M.J. Koehler et al., "Intrinsic, solar and sunbed-induced skin aging measured in vivo by multiphoton laser tomography and biophysical methods," *Skin Res. Tech.* **15**, 357–363 (2009).

[90] R. Cicchi et al., "Scoring of collagen organization in healthy and diseased human dermis by multiphoton microscopy," *J. Biophoton.* **3**, 34–43 (2010).

[91] P.J. Su et al., "Discrimination of collagen in normal and pathological skin dermis through second-order susceptibility microscopy," *Opt. Express* **17**, 11161–11171 (2009).

[92] J. Chen et al., "Multiphoton microscopy study of the morphological and quantity changes of collagen and elastic fiber components in keloid disease," *J. Biomed. Opt.* **16**, 051305 (2011).

[93] A. Medyukhina et al., "Automated classification of healthy and keloidal collagen patterns based on processing of SHG images of human skin," *J. Biophoton.* **4**, 627–636 (2011).

[94] J. Paoli, M. Smedh, A.-M. Wennberg, and M.B. Ericson, "Multiphoton laser scanning microscopy on non-melanoma skin cancer, morphologic features for future non-invasive diagnostics," *Journal of Investigative Dermatology* **128**, 1248–1255 (2008).

[95] R. Cicchi et al., "Multidimensional non-linear laser imaging of basal cell carcinoma," *Opt. Express* **15**(16), 10135–10148 (2007).

[96] N. Vogler et al., "Towards multimodal nonlinear optical tomography - experimental methodology," *Laser Phys. Lett.* **8**, 617–624 (2011).

[97] E. Dimitrow et al., "Spectral fluorescence lifetime detection and selective melanin imaging by multiphoton laser tomography for melanoma diagnosis," *Exp. Dermatol.* **18**, 509–515 (2009).

[98] S.Y. Chen, H.Y. Wu, and C.K. Sun, "*In vivo* harmonic generation biopsy of human skin," *JBO Lett.* **14**, 060505 (2009).

[99] F. Fischer et al., "Risk estimation of skin damage due to ultrashort pulsed, focused near-infrared laser irradiation at 800 nm," *J. Biomed. Opt.* **13**, 04132 (2008).

[100] ACS http: //www.cancer.org/downloads/STT/CAFF2006PWSecured.pdf. in *Cancer Facts and Figures* (2006).

[101] D.R. Rivera et al., "Compact and flexible raster scanning multiphoton endoscope capable of imaging unstained tissue," *Proc. Natl. Acad. Sci. U.S.A.* **108**(43), 17598–17603 (2011).

[102] K. Steenkeste et al., "*Ex-vivo* fluorescence imaging of normal and malignant urothelial cells to enhance early diagnosis," *Photochem. Photobiol.* **83**, 1157–1166 (2007).

[103] R. Yadav et al., "Multiphoton microscopy of prostate and periprostatic neural tissue, a promising imaging technique for improving nerve-sparing prostatectomy," *J. Endourol.* **23**, 861–867 (2009).

[104] S.M. Zhuo, J.X. Chen, T. Luo, X.S. Jiang, and S.S. Xie, "Multiphoton microscopy of unstained bladder mucosa based on two-photon excited autofluorescence and second-harmonic generation," *Laser Phys. Lett.* **1**, 80–83 (2009).

[105] L.H. Laiho, S. Pelet, T.M. Hancewicz, P.D. Kaplan, and P.T.C. So, "Two-photon 3-D mapping of *ex vivo* human skin endogenous fluorescence species based on fluorescence emission spectra," *J. Biomed. Opt.* **10**, 024016 (2005).

[106] R. Cicchi et al., "Time- and spectral-resolved two photon imaging of healthy bladder mucosa and carcinoma *in situ*," *Opt. Express* **18**, 3840–3849 (2010).

[107] O. Warburg, *The metabolism of tumors*, Constabel, London (1930).

[108] E. Neher and B. Sakmann, "Single-channel currents recorded from membrane of denervated frog muscle fibres," *Nature* **260** (5554), 799–802 (1976).

[109] J. Mapelli and E. D'Angelo, "The spatial organization of long-term synaptic plasticity at the input stage of cerebellum," *J. Neurosci.* **27**(6), 1285–1296 (2007).

[110] U. Egert, D. Heck, and A. Aertsen, Two-dimensional monitoring of spiking networks in acute brain slices," *Exp. Brain Res.* **142**(2), 268–274 (2002).

[111] L.B. Cohen and B.M. Salzberg, "Optical measurement of membrane potential," *Rev. Physiol. Biochem. Pharmacol.* **83**, 35–88 (1978).

[112] D.S. Peterka, H. Takahashi, and R. Yuste, "Imaging voltage in neurons," *Neuron* **69**(1), 9–21 (2011).

[113] L. Sacconi et al., "Cell imaging and manipulation by nonlinear optical microscopy," *Cell Biochem. Biophys.* **45**(3), 289–302 (2006).

[114] F. Vanzi, L. Sacconi, R. Cicchi, and F.S. Pavone, "Protein conformation and molecular order probed by second-harmonic-generation microscopy," *J. Biomed. Opt.* **17**(6), 060901 (2012).

[115] T. Pons, L. Moreaux, O. Mongin, M. Blanchard-Desce, and J. Mertz, "Mechanisms of membrane potential sensing with second-harmonic generation microscopy," *J. Biomed. Opt.* **8**(3), 428–431 (2003).

[116] D.A. Dombeck, M. Blanchard-Desce, and W.W. Webb, "Optical recording of action potentials with second-harmonic generation microscopy," *J. Neurosci.* **24**(4), 999–1003 (2004).

[117] L. Sacconi, D.A. Dombeck, and W.W. Webb, "Overcoming photodamage in second-harmonic generation microscopy, real-time optical recording of neuronal action potentials," *Proc. Natl. Acad. Sci. U.S.A.* **103**(9), 3124–3129 (2006).

[118] D.A. Dombeck, L. Sacconi, M. Blanchard-Desce, and W.W. Webb, "Optical recording of fast neuronal membrane potential transients in acute mammalian brain slices by second-harmonic generation microscopy," *J. Neurophysiol.* **94**(5), 3628–3636 (2005).

[119] M. Nuriya, J. Jiang, B. Nemet, K.B. Eisenthal, and R. Yuste, "Imaging membrane potential in dendritic spines," *Proc. Natl. Acad. Sci. U.S.A.* **103**(3), 786–790 (2006).

[120] A. Bullen, S.S. Patel, and P. Saggau, "High-speed, random-access fluorescence microscopy, I. High-resolution optical recording with voltage-sensitive dyes and ion indicators," *Biophys. J.* **73**(1), 477–491 (1997).

[121] L. Sacconi et al., "Optical recording of electrical activity in intact neuronal networks with random access second-harmonic generation microscopy," *Opt. Express* **16**(19), 14910–14921 (2008).

[122] L. Sacconi et al., "Action potential propagation in transverse-axial tubular system is impaired in heart failure," *Proc. Natl. Acad. Sci. U.S.A.* **109**(15), 5815–5819 (2012).

[123] M. Both et al., "Second harmonic imaging of intrinsic signals in muscle fibers *in situ*," *J. Biomed. Opt.* **9**(5), 882–892 (2004).

[124] S.V. Plotnikov, A.C. Millard, P.J. Campagnola, and W.A. Mohler, "Characterization of the myosin-based source for second-harmonic generation from muscle sarcomeres," *Biophys. J.* **90**(2), 693–703 (2006).

[125] P. Stoller, K.M. Reiser, P.M. Celliers, and A.M. Rubenchik, "Polarization-modulated second harmonic generation in collagen," *Biophys. J.* **82**(6), 3330–3342(2002).

[126] M.A. Geeves and K.C. Holmes, "The molecular mechanism of muscle contraction," *Adv. Protein Chem.* **71**, 161–193 (2005).

[127] M.K. Reedy, K.C. Holmes, and R.T. Tregear, "Induced changes in orientation of the cross-bridges of glycerinated insect flight muscle," *Nature* **207**(5003), 1276–1280 (1965).

[128] I. Rayment et al., "Structure of the actin-myosin complex and its implications for muscle contraction," *Science* **261**(5117), 58–65 (1993).

[129] R. Cooke and E. Pate, "The effects of pyrophosphate on myosin heads and on fiber stiffness," *Adv. Exp. Med. Biol.* **226**, 255–265 (1988).

[130] P.G. Fajer, E.A. Fajer, N.J. Brunsvold, and D.D. Thomas, "Effects of AMPPNP on the orientation and rotational dynamics of spin-labeled muscle cross-bridges," *Biophys. J.* **53**(4), 513–524 (1988).

[131] R. Cicchi, D. Kapsokalyvas, D. Stambouli, V. De Giorgi, D. Massi, T. Lotti, and F. S. Pavone, "In-vivo tissue imaging using a compact mobile non-linear microscope," *SPIE Proceed.* **7569**, 756930 (2010).

5

Optical Coherence Tomography: Technical Aspect

Hrebesh M. Subhash
Division of Biomedical Engineering, School of Medicine, Oregon Health and Science University, 3303 SW Bond Ave, Portland, OR

Ruikang K. Wang
Biophotonics and Imaging Laboratory, Department of Bioengineering, University of Washington, Seattle, WA

This chapter describes the state of the art of optical coherence tomography (OCT), a low coherence interferometric imaging technique that provides cross-sectional depth resolved information from the subsurface microstructure of biological tissue. Following a discussion of the basic theory of OCT, an overview of the design aspect and different configuration of OCT in both time and frequency domain is presented. The chapter also includes various functional extensions of OCT and its potential clinical and non-clinical application.

Key words: imaging, interferometry, optical coherence tomography, biomedical imaging, functional imaging

5.1 Introduction

Optical coherence tomography (OCT) is a novel, non-invasive, optical imaging modality based on low coherence interferometry. It was first conceived in 1990 by Dr. Naohiro Tanno, a professor at Yamagata University [1, 2], and then perfected in 1991 by a Massachusetts Institute of Technology team headed by Prof. James Fujimoto [3]. OCT enables the non-invasive, non-contact imaging of cross-sectional structures in biological tissues and materials with high resolution. In principle, OCT is an optical analogue to clinical ultrasound. In OCT, the temporally gated optical pulse remitted from scattering sites within the sample is localized by low-coherence interferometry (LCI)

[4, 5, 6, 7, 8, 9]. This is typically achieved with a Michelson interferometer. The sample rests in one arm of the interferometer and a scanning reference optical delay line is in the other arm. In LCI, light interferes at the detector only when light reflected from the sample is matched in optical pathlength with that reflected from the scanning reference mirror. A single scan of the reference mirror thus provides a one-dimensional depth-reflectivity profile of the sample. Two-dimensional cross-sectional images are formed by laterally scanning the incident probe beam across the sample. The reconstructed OCT image is essentially a map of the changes of reflectivity that occurs at internal interfaces, similar to the discontinuities in acoustic impedance in ultrasound images.

The principle difference between ultrasound and optical imaging is that the velocity of light is approximately a million times faster than that of sound. For this reason, the distance within the materials or tissues with a resolution of 10 μm by measuring the echo time delay of back reflected or back-scattered light wave corresponds to a time resolution of 30 femto (10^{-15}) seconds, which is well beyond the limits of currently available electronic detection systems. But for ultrasound, the echo time delay is approximately 100 ns, which can be easily realized with modern electronic detection systems. Thus, in OCT, each time delay has to be measured indirectly, normally by correlation techniques, in which the backscattered light is compared to the reference light with known optical pathlength. OCT uses the low coherence interferometric method to measure this echo time delay with high dynamic range and sensitivity.

5.1.1 Advantages of OCT over other imaging modalities

Recently, OCT has attracted much attention in many clinical and basic research fields due to its high-sensitivity for non-invasive high-resolution imaging at cellular level. The diagnostic capability of OCT has revolutionized many fields such as ophthalmology, dermatology and cardiology, etc. In terms of other medical imaging devices, OCT is the best one offered currently. OCT has rapidly become an important biomedical tool for imaging tissues and engineered tissues [10]. OCT has critical advantages over other medical imaging systems. Microscopes work well for examining small tissue samples and cells but not for examining biological tissues inside the body [11]. The Ultrasound, CT, and MRI can peer inside the body however they do not have sufficient resolution to capture cellular detail [11]. Electron microscopy can pick up extremely fine details; however, it is not able to view living samples within the body [11]. Figure 5.1 shows the comparison of OCT with presently existing clinical imaging modalities [12]. The two major advancements which assist both scientists and medical physicians is the improvement in the depth and clarity at which they can view tissues. Current OCT systems have resolutions at 1–20 μm compared to 110 μm for high frequency ultrasound [13]. The advancement of medical imaging systems is illustrated by the technology inherent in OCT, which allows images of living tissue to become clearer and more defined in both structure and detail. Using information inherent to the returning photon signals, OCT can perform both spectroscopic and polarization imaging to better evaluate the composition of tissues and lesions. Moreover, the use of fiber optics and its ability to integrate with medical catheters, surgical guiding systems like endoscopes, and microscopes, makes OCT much easier to observe internal structures, widening its clinical application scope. With other technology to aid the development of OCT, doctors can actually use OCT not only on the body but within the body. Figure 5.1 shows that OCT fills the gap between the optical microscopy and the currently available clinical imaging modalities in terms of imaging depth and resolution.

There are many important advantages to OCT over other existing clinical imaging modalities, making it an important new complementary medical imaging tool. It is minimally invasive, non-contacting and non-ionizing, has very high spatial resolution, sensitivity and high speed and real-time data acquisition. The basic setup can be extended to obtain measurement based on the functional, polarization, spectroscopic and other tissue parameters.

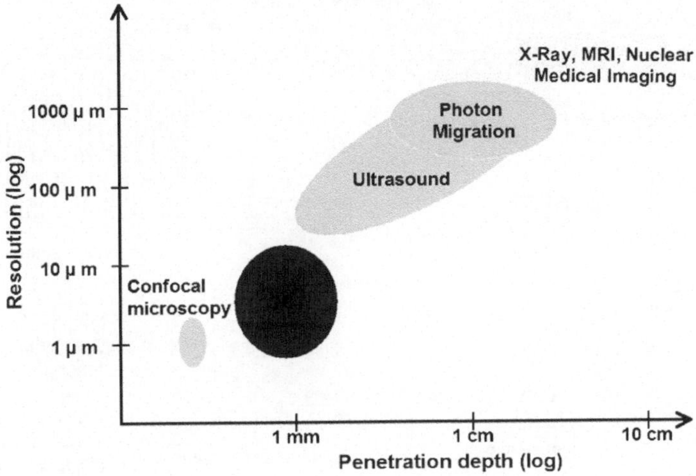

Figure 5.1: Comparison of OCT with other clinical imaging modalities in terms of their resolution and penetration depth.

5.2 Low Coherence Interferometry

As mentioned in Section 5.1, OCT uses the interferometric detection and correlation method to measure the echo time delay of backscattered light with high dynamic range and sensitivity [14]. The basic building block of OCT is based on a Michelson interferometer (or its variant) with a low coherence optical source, and this scheme is generally called low coherence interferometry or white light interferometry. In LCI, low coherence light reflected from the sample is used to provide information on the time-of-flight (echo time delay) from refractive boundaries and backscattered sites in the sample. LCI measures the delay and intensity of backscattered light by comparing it with the light that has traveled a known reference pathlength and delay through use of a Michelson interferometer. Another variant form of LCI called optical time domain reflectometry (OTDR) is used to determine the location of defects in optical fibers and characterization of optical wave-guides in the telecommunication industry [15, 16]. Figure 5.2(a) shows the schematic diagram of a simple free space implementation of a Michelson type interferometer.

The incident optical beam is directed on to a beamsplitter, which splits the beam into two, from where one beam leads to a sample mirror, while the other acts as a reference beam with variable pathlength. The sample beam $\mathbf{E}_S(t - L_S/c)$, which reflects from the sample mirror, is interfered with the reference beam $\mathbf{E}_R(t - L_R/c)$ at the output of the interferometer, where L_S and L_R are the corresponding optical path of the sample arm and reference arm respectively and c is the speed of light. According to the wave theory, interference is the superposition of two or more waves, resulting in a new wave pattern. If we consider wave as electromagnetic radiation, which can be described as [17]

$$\mathbf{E} = \mathbf{E}_0 e^{i(\mathbf{k}\cdot\mathbf{r} - \omega t + \phi)} \tag{5.1}$$

where $\mathbf{k}$ ($|\mathbf{k}| = k = 2\pi/\lambda$) is the propagation vector, $\mathbf{r}$ is the position vector, $\omega = 2\pi f$ is the angular frequency and ϕ is the initial phase. The resulting field of the beams at the output of the interferometer can be written as

$$\mathbf{E}_D(t) = \mathbf{E}_S(t - L_S/c) + \mathbf{E}_R(t - L_R/c) \tag{5.2}$$

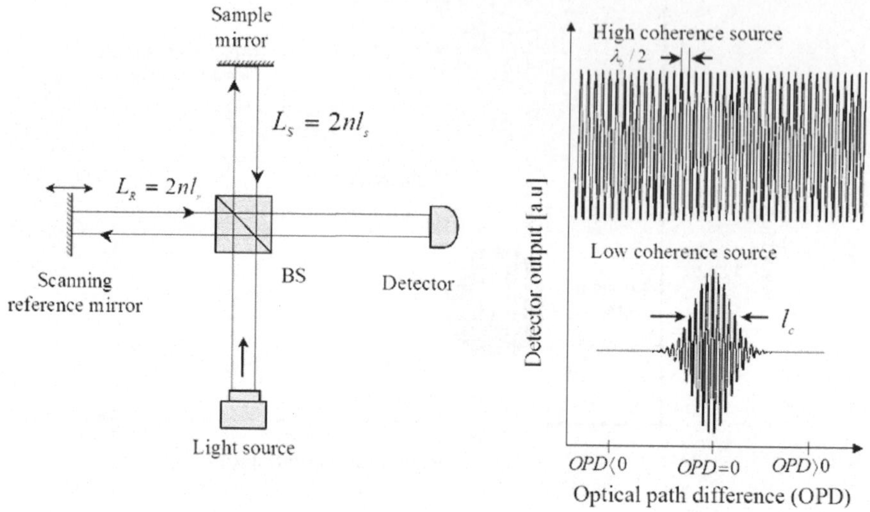

(a) (b)

Figure 5.2: (a) Free space Michelson interferometer setup (b) comparison between the photo detector output in cases when a high coherence source (top) or a low coherence source (bottom) is used.

using the principle of superposition. By applying Eq. (5.1) and putting $\mathbf{r}$ and ϕ to 0 for the convenience, Eq. (5.2) can be written as

$$\mathbf{E}_D(t) = \mathbf{E}_S e^{i(t-L_S/c)} + \mathbf{E}_R e^{i(t-L_R/c)} \tag{5.3}$$

The detector measures the intensity of the output beam, which is proportional to the square of the electromagnetic field. The irradiance (power per unit area) at the detector can be expressed in terms of the Poynting vector $\mathbf{S} = \varepsilon_0 c^2 \mathbf{E}_D \times \mathbf{B}_D$. The irradiance measured by the detector is the time average of the rapidly varying fields ($\sim 10^{14}$ Hz for near-infrared region), i.e., $I_D = \langle|\mathbf{S}|\rangle = \varepsilon_0 c^2 \langle|\mathbf{E}_D \times \mathbf{B}_D|\rangle$, since $|\mathbf{E}| = c|\mathbf{B}|$. The irradiance can be written as $I_D = \varepsilon_0 c^2 \langle|\mathbf{E}_D|^2\rangle$. Using Eq. (5.3) the resultant intensity I_D can be expressed as

$$I_D = \varepsilon_0 c \left\langle (\mathbf{E}_S(t) + \mathbf{E}_R(t+\tau)) \cdot (\overline{\mathbf{E}_S(t)} + \overline{\mathbf{E}_R(t+\tau)}) \right\rangle \tag{5.4}$$

where $\tau = \Delta L/c$ is the time delay corresponding to the roundtrip optical pathlength difference between the reference and sample arm, i.e.

$$\Delta L = L_S - L_R = 2n(l_S - l_R) \tag{5.5}$$

where l_S and l_R are the geometric lengths of the sample arm and reference arms, respectively, $n \sim 1$ corresponds to the refractive index of air, and the bar symbol denotes complex conjugate operation. The angle brackets denote the time average.

$$\langle f \rangle = \lim_{T\to\infty} \int_0^T f(t)dt \tag{5.6}$$

Then by omitting the constant term $\varepsilon_0 c$, the resulting intensity can be written as follows

$$I_D = \left\langle |\mathbf{E}_S(t)|^2 + |\mathbf{E}_R(t+\tau)|^2 + \mathrm{Re}[\mathbf{E}_S(t) \cdot \overline{\mathbf{E}_R(t+\tau)}] \right\rangle \tag{5.7}$$

By assuming that the optical fields of both reference and sample beam have the same polarization states, the dot product term $\left\langle \boldsymbol{E_S}(t)\cdot\overline{\boldsymbol{E_R}(t+\tau)}\right\rangle = \left\langle E_S(t)\overline{E_R(t+\tau)}\right\rangle$. By introducing the correlation function (mutual coherence function) of the two fields, $\Gamma_{SR}(\tau) = \left\langle E_S(t)\overline{E_R(t+\tau)}\right\rangle$, the interference Eq. (5.7) can be written as:

$$I_D = I_S + I_R + 2Re[\Gamma_{SR}(\tau)] \tag{5.8}$$

where $I_S = \langle|\mathbf{E}_S(t)|^2\rangle$ and $I_S = \langle|\mathbf{E}_S(t+\tau)|^2\rangle$. For convenience, a normalized correlation function is defined, which gives the degree to which the temporal and spatial characteristics of sample and reference beam matches, and it can be defined as

$$\gamma_{SR}(\tau) = \frac{\Gamma_{SR}(\tau)}{\sqrt{I_S I_R}} \tag{5.9}$$

Then the irradiance equation Eq. (5.8) can be expressed as follows:

$$I_D = I_S + I_R + 2\sqrt{I_S I_R}\,\mathbf{Re}[\gamma_{SR}(\tau)] \tag{5.10}$$

The normalized correction function $\gamma_{SR}(\tau)$ is a complex periodic function of τ, and the interference pattern results if $|\gamma_{SR}(\tau)|$ has a non-zero value. Depending upon the value of $|\gamma_{SR}(\tau)|$ the following type of coherence occurs:

$$\begin{aligned} |\gamma_{SR}(\tau)| &= 1, && \text{Complete coherence} \\ 0 < |\gamma_{SR}(\tau)| &< 1, && \text{Partial coherence} \\ |\gamma_{SR}(\tau)| &= 0, && \text{Complete incoherence} \end{aligned}$$

In an interference pattern, the fringe intensity varies between two limits I_{max} and I_{min}. From Eq. (5.10) this can be written as:

$$I_{\max} = I_S + I_R + 2\sqrt{I_S I_R}|\gamma_{SR}| \tag{5.11}$$

$$I_{\min} = I_S + I_R - 2\sqrt{I_S I_R}|\gamma_{SR}| \tag{5.12}$$

Thus the visibility of fringe V is defined as the ratio

$$V = \frac{I_{\max} - I_{\min}}{I_{\max} + I_{\min}} = \frac{2\sqrt{I_S I_R}|\gamma_{SR}|}{I_{\max} + I_{\min}} \tag{5.13}$$

If $I_{max}= I_{min}$, then $V = |\ \gamma_{SR}\ |$, i.e. the fringe visibility is equal to the modulus of degree of partial coherence. Thus depending upon the different cases of degree of partial coherence, the interference fringe visibility varies from maximum contrast of unity (in case of complete coherence, $|\ \gamma_{SR}(\tau)\ | = 1$) to zero contrast (complete incoherence, $|\ \gamma_{SR}(\tau)\ | = 0$; there are no interference fringes at all).

Depending upon the source, the light will have frequencies within a certain frequency spectrum. According to Fourier analysis this can be written as:

$$\Delta\omega = \frac{2\pi}{\tau_0} \tag{5.14}$$

where $\Delta\omega$ is the spectral line width of the source and τ_0 is the coherence time, which is the time interval in which the phase of the wave can be predictable. The coherence length, $l_c = c\tau_0$, is the propagation path difference where the beam can maintain a specified degree of coherence. Using Eq. (5.14) the coherence length can be written as:

$$l_c = \frac{2\pi c}{\Delta\omega} = \frac{c}{\Delta\nu} \tag{5.15}$$

According to the Wiener-Khintchine theorem, the complex degree of coherence $\gamma_{SR}(\tau)$ can be expressed as the Fourier transform of the power spectral density $S(\nu)$ of the source, which is fully characterized by its spectral width ($\Delta\lambda$), its central wavelength (λ_0) and its shape [18].

$$\gamma_{SR}(\tau) = \int_0^\infty S(\nu)e^{-i2\pi\nu\tau}d\nu \tag{5.16}$$

From the above relation, it reveals that the width of emission spectrum of light source and its shape are vital parameters, which influence the sensitivity of the LCI to the optical path difference of the sample and reference arms.

The normalized power spectral density of light source $S(\nu)$ is $\int S(\nu) = 1$, then the complex coherence can be written as,

$$\gamma_{SR}(\tau) = |\gamma_{SR}|(\tau)e^{-i2\pi\nu_0\tau} \tag{5.17}$$

where ν_0 is the center frequency of the light source. Eq. (5.10) can be rewritten by introducing Eq. (5.17) as follows

$$I_D = I_S + I_R + 2\sqrt{I_S I_R}|\gamma_{SR}(\tau)|\cos(2\pi\nu_0\tau) \tag{5.18}$$

The normalized correlation function for a quasi-monochromatic source can be given by

$$|\gamma_{SR}(\tau)| = (1 - \tau/\tau_0), \quad \tau < \tau_0 \tag{5.19}$$

then Eq. (5.18) becomes as follows:

$$I_D = I_S + I_R + 2\sqrt{I_S I_R}(1 - \tau/\tau_0)\cos(2\pi\nu_0\tau) \tag{5.20}$$

If the power spectrum of the light source is approximated by a Gaussian spectrum,

$$S(\nu) = \frac{2\sqrt{\ln 2}}{\Delta\nu\sqrt{\pi}}\exp\left[-4\ln 2\left(\frac{\nu - \nu_0}{\Delta\nu}\right)^2\right] \tag{5.21}$$

substituting Eq. (5.21) into Eq. (5.16) results in

$$\gamma_{SR}(\tau) = \exp\left[-\left(\frac{\pi\Delta\nu\tau}{2\sqrt{\ln 2}}\right)^2 e^{-i2\pi\nu_0\tau}\right] \tag{5.22}$$

From this equation the quantity $\Delta\nu$ represents the FWHM of the normalized spectral width of the source, then the corresponding free space correlation length can be obtained as follows

$$l_c = \frac{2\ln 2}{\pi}\frac{c}{\Delta\nu} = \frac{2\ln 2}{\pi}\frac{\lambda^2}{\Delta\lambda} \approx 0.44\frac{\lambda^2}{\Delta\lambda} \tag{5.23}$$

Since the coherence length gives the practical estimation of the width of the signal envelope, it is considered as the axial resolution in low coherence interferometry. Figure 5.2(b) shows the signal at the photo-detector for the case of high coherence source and low coherence source. If the light source is highly coherent with narrow line width (a laser with $\Delta\lambda \approx 0.01$ nm, in which case $l_c \approx 9$ cm) then the interference will occur for a wide range of relative pathlength delays of the reference and sample arms. But, when the optical source is low coherence with broad line width laser (a tungsten with $\Delta\lambda \approx 300$ nm, in which case $l_c \approx 3$ μm), then the interference occurs only when the pathlength in the reference and sample arms matches within the coherence length of the source of the light source. Thus in low coherence interferometry, the coherence length is the parameter that determines the resolving ability of backscattering or backreflecting sites in the sample.

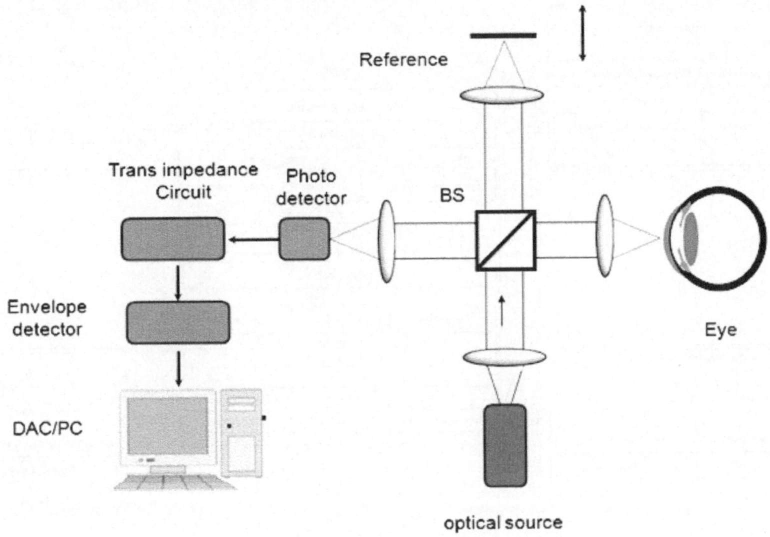

Figure 5.3: Schematic of a typical first generation free-space optics based optical coherence tomography setup with balanced heterodyne detection scheme.

5.3 OCT Principle of Operation

As described above, the interferometry is the core of the OCT imaging method. Different interferometric configurations can be used in OCT. One of the most common interferometric schemes used in the development of the OCT system is the Michelson interferometer, which can be implemented either with a free-space optic or fiber-optics configuration. The fiber-optics implementations of the OCT are seen as the most convenient for clinical applications because the fiber has the potential to be rugged, compact, and can be integrated with a wide range of medical instruments. However, there are also a few possible issues associated with the utilization of fiber. Fibers show absorption, although this will be negligible for the distances involved, but this limits the dispersion-free spectral width, resulting in degradation of longitudinal resolution. Figure 5.3 shows the schematics of a typical first generation time-domain free space OCT system based on heterodyne envelope detection scheme.

The beam from the low coherence optical source splits into two parts, a reference and sample beam. The reference beam reflects from a reference mirror mounted on the scanning reference optical delay and returns to the detector. The sample beam reflects off from the different layers within the sample. And at the output of the interferometer both the reference and sample beam recombines. Due to the broadband nature of the light source, the interference between the optical fields is only observed when the reference and sample arm optical path lengths are matched within the coherence length of the source. The light reflected from the sample and the reference mirror are mixed at a photodetector, and the resulting current signal corresponding to the interference signal is amplified and converted into a voltage signal by a transimpedance circuit. The amplified signal is demodulated by using sophisticated electronic envelope detection stages (e.g., lock in amplifier). Then the demodulated signal is fed into a data acquisition system that is interfaced with the computer. The data acquisition system is an integral part of the OCT setups that do all the timing and synchronization between different modular units of an OCT system. In OCT, the depth information can also be derived from frequency domain measurement by taking the Fourier transform of the output

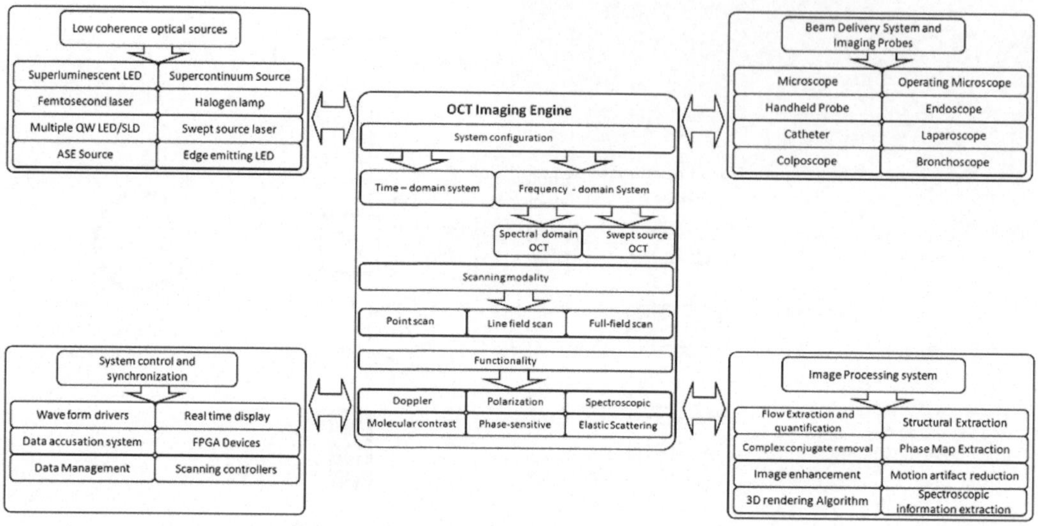

Figure 5.4: A modular overview of an OCT system with various peripheral components and schematic of a typical first generation free-space optics based optical coherence tomography setup with balanced heterodyne detection scheme.

spectrum of the interferogram, this alternative modality has better speed and sensitivity advantages than conventional time-domain detection scheme, which will be described later in this chapter.

In general, an OCT system can be considered from a modular viewpoint in terms of various integrated hardware and software functionalities such as imaging engine, low coherence light source, beam delivery and probes, computer control and image processing. Figure 5.4 shows the schematic of various modular components of a generic OCT system. Depending upon the applications there are many variant embodiments of the interferometer and imaging engines such as polarization sensitive, Doppler flow imaging, optical microangiography, spectroscopy, frequency scanning, spectral radar and parallel detection.

5.4 Practical Aspect of OCT System Design

5.4.1 Axial resolution

Unlike the conventional optical microscopy, the apparent advantage of OCT is that the axial resolution is completely de-coupled from the lateral resolution. The axial resolution of an OCT is an important specification of an OCT system and in many biomedical applications high axial resolution is often required to distinguish different cellular ultra-structures. As described in the preceding section, axial resolution is defined as the full width half maximum of the source coherence length l_c. For a source with a Gaussian spectral distribution, the axial resolution is given by,

$$\Delta z = \frac{2\ln 2}{\pi}\frac{c}{\Delta \nu} = \frac{2\ln 2}{\pi}\frac{\lambda^2}{\Delta\lambda} \approx 0.44\frac{\lambda^2}{\Delta\lambda} \tag{5.24}$$

where Δz and $\Delta\lambda$ are the full width at half maximum of the autocorrelation function and spectral width and λ_0 is the source center wavelength [19]. It can be seen that broadband light sources are required to achieve high axial resolution, as the axial resolution is inversely proportional to the

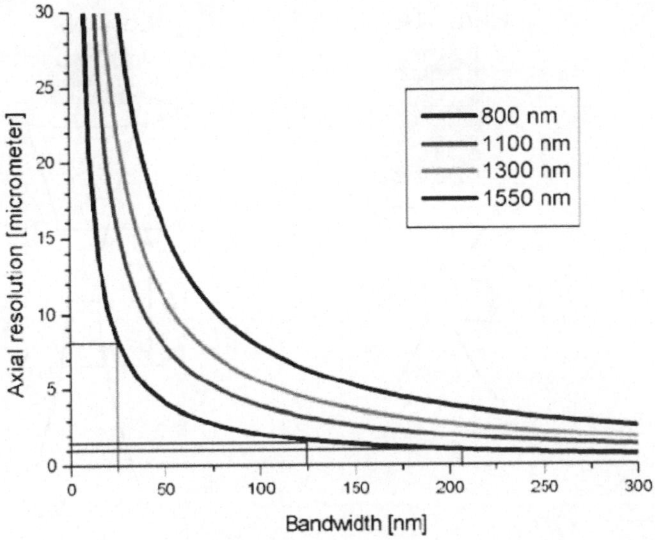

Figure 5.5: Axial resolution vs. bandwidth of light sources for center wavelengths of 800, 1100, 1300 nm and 1500 nm. Micrometer scale axial resolution requires extremely broad optical bandwidths and bandwidth requirements increase dramatically for longer wavelengths.

spectral width of the light source. The most popular light source currently used in OCT appears to be superluminescent diode (SLD). A typical SLD has a bandwidth $\Delta\lambda = 20$ nm centered at 830 nm, which corresponds to a coherence length of ~ 30 μm and since l_c is defined for a round trip, so this leads to a depth pixel size of 15 μm in air, and in tissue, by considering the refractive index of 1.4 gives ~ 11 μm. Modern sources for OCT use Kerr-lens mode-locked lasers and photonic crystal fibers to achieve submicron coherence length. Apart from the wide-line width, the sources for OCT have to exhibit a smooth Gaussian spectrum profile [20, 21]. Figure 5.5 shows a plot of axial resolution vs. bandwidth for light sources at different wavelengths. Since axial resolution is inversely proportional to the bandwidth of the light source, broadband width light sources are required to achieve high axial resolution.

5.4.2 Lateral resolution

As in conventional microscopy, the lateral resolution that may be achieved with OCT imaging is determined by the focus spot of the light beam and is completely decoupled from the axial resolution. Therefore, the optical design of the lateral scanning does not correlate with the axial resolution. The lateral resolution Δx can be written as:

$$\Delta x = \frac{4\lambda}{\pi}\left(\frac{f}{d}\right) \tag{5.25}$$

where f is the focal length of the objective lens and d is the $1/e^2$ Gaussian beam wrist at the objective lens. It can be seen from the above equation that high lateral resolution can be achieved by using a large numerical aperture (NA) to decrease the spot size. However, for the selection of optics there is a trade-off between the lateral resolution and the imaging depth. A higher lateral resolution leads to a decrease in the depth of focus, or confocal parameter b, which is twice the Rayleigh range,

$$2\Delta z_R = b = \frac{\pi \Delta x^2}{2\lambda} \tag{5.26}$$

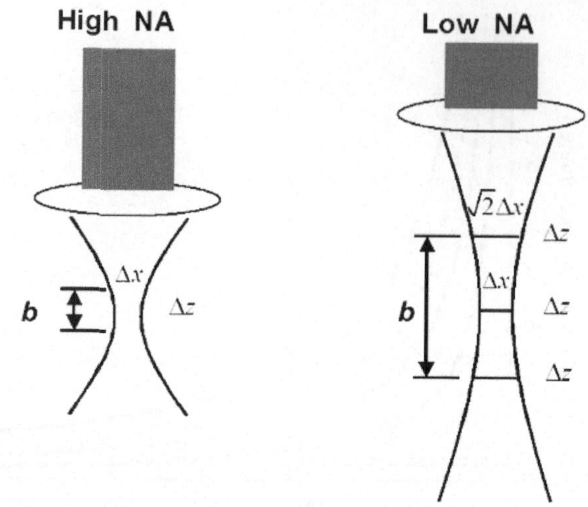

Figure 5.6: Relationship between focus spot size and depth of field for objective lens with high and low numerical aperture.

The Rayleigh range gives the distance from the focal point to the point where the light beam diameter has increased by a factor of $\sqrt{2}$. This effectively limits the scanning range of the OCT, quite apart from the working range of the scanning reference delay line, as it is the range over which lateral resolution is maintained. Figure 5.6 shows the relation between the depth of focus (confocal parameter) and the focused spot size for the objective lens with high and low numerical apertures.

5.4.3 Sensitivity

The sensitivity or the optical dynamic range of an OCT system can be defined as the ratio of the signal power generated by a perfectly reflecting mirror to the noise of the system and is given by the equation

$$SNR = \frac{I_{\mathrm{S}}^2}{I_{\mathrm{N}}^2} \tag{5.27}$$

where I_{S} is the photocurrent at the detector due to the interference term of Eq. (5.18) and which in the case of an ideal 50:50 beam splitter and perfectly reflecting sample is equal to the total source power P. Therefore, the signal photocurrent can be expressed as

$$I_{\mathrm{S}} = \frac{\eta q_e}{\hbar \nu_0} P \tag{5.28}$$

where η is the quantum efficiency of the detector, q_e is the electron charge, ω_0 is the source center angular frequency, $\hbar$ is the Planck's constant divided by 2π and P is the integral of the source power spectral density. I_{N} corresponds to the overall noise of the optical detection system and has three significant sources: shot noise (I_{SH}), optical intensity noise or relative intensity noise (I_{RIN}) and the thermal noise (I_{TH}). Therefore, the total noise current is the sum of squares of each of the noise contributions and can be expressed as

$$I_N^2 = I_{\mathrm{SH}}^2 + I_{\mathrm{RIN}}^2 + I_{\mathrm{TH}}^2 \tag{5.29}$$

However, in the OCT system the optical detection scheme employed is heterodyne. Therefore it can be arranged to achieve shot-noise limited optical detection whereby the reference arm optical field is much higher than that in the sample arm. This is often the case in OCT when imaging highly scattering and absorbing biological specimens. In the shot-noise limited case the relative intensity noise and the thermal noise become negligible. So the total noise can be expressed as:

$$I_N = I_{SH} = \sqrt{2q_e I_{DC} B} \tag{5.30}$$

where I_{SH} is the rms shot noise, B is the detection bandwidth and I_{DC} is the DC photo current and is assumed to be entirely due to the reference arm's optical power. In case of shot noise limit, the overall noise variance can be expressed as:

$$I_N = \sqrt{\frac{\eta q_e}{h\nu_0} 2PB} \tag{5.31}$$

Therefore, substituting the equations (5.28) and (5.31) into equation (5.27) yields

$$\text{SNR} = \frac{\eta P}{2h\nu_0 B} \tag{5.32}$$

Generally the SNR is quoted as a figure of merit in logarithmic unit and is related to the power SNR by

$$\text{SNR} = 10\log_{10}\left(\frac{\eta P}{2h\nu_0 B}\right) \tag{5.33}$$

For a single detector, the measurement bandwidth $B = 1/\tau$ is a function of the acquisition time τ detector. Therefore, this expression implies that to increase either image acquisition speed or image resolution, which increases the measurement bandwidth, higher source power is required to maintain the SNR performance of the system.

5.4.4 Selection of OCT wavelength

In OCT, the characteristics of the optical source determine the general performance of the system. For example, the shot coherence length of the optical source determines the axial resolution and the nominal wavelength determines the achievable penetration depth of the system. The broader the line-width $\Delta\lambda$ of the source, the smaller the coherence length l_c (Eq. (5.23)) of the source. There are four main criteria that need to be considered when choosing a light source for OCT. These parameters are wavelength, bandwidth, single transverse mode power, and stability. The depth of penetration in OCT is limited by both scattering and absorption of the sample. The absorption window for most biological tissues between 0.65 and 1.4 μm has a local minimum in the absorption of water and blood in the tissues. Absorption attenuates the light in the imaging subject and is wavelength dependent. Because more than 80% of biological tissue consists of water, the absorption of tissue is mostly attributed to the water. If we analyze the water absorption spectrum shown in Fig. 5.7, we can find a window with lower absorption, termed "therapeutic windows" for biomedical optics, existing around 600 nm to 800 nm. Absorption by melanin, as well as the scattering from structure protein such as collagen and elastin, exhibits a nearly monotonic decrease with increasing wavelength over this region. These optical properties of tissues have been investigated to some degree both experimentally and by a number of analytical and numerical models. Therefore the selection of wavelength is a very critical parameter in OCT.

Most of the conventional OCT systems utilize the near infrared to far infrared region of the optical spectrum, which ranges from 700 nm to 1600 nm. The exact choice of the central wavelength depends on the prospective applications, and is mostly determined by the absorption and scattering properties of the medium under investigation, though the expected resolution must also be taken into account. In general, imaging at shorter wavelengths around 800 nm delivers higher axial resolutions; however the depth of penetration is considerably degraded due to increased scattering at

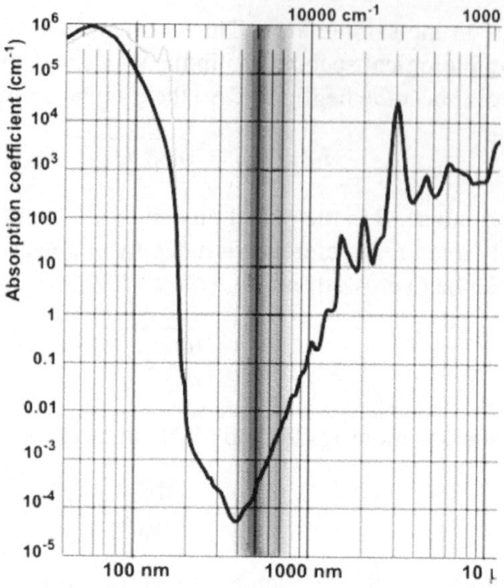

Figure 5.7: Water absorption spectrum. The original data consult from http://omlc.ogi.edu/spectra/water/index.html.

shorter wavelength. In the 700 to 1600 nm region, scattering decreases monotonically with wavelength, in particular the scattering behavior of light in a biological specimen shows significant degradation with longer wavelength. Thus OCT systems operating at center wavelengths around 1300 nm show an enhanced penetration depth due to less tissue scattering and absorption of endogenous chromophores like hemoglobin and melanin [22, 23]. Recently, OCT imaging in the 1050–1060 nm wavelength region is getting much attention in the field of ophthalmology, where imaging the deeper layers of retina is very crucial in diagnosing retinal pathologies [24, 25, 26, 27, 28]. In ocular imaging, the highly scattering and absorbing retinal pigment epithelium reduces the penetration depth for wavelengths at the 800 nm region commonly used today in retinal scanning OCT systems, while the application of long wavelength in retinal imaging is limited by the water absorption in the relative long path through the vitreous humor, which contains $> 95\%$ of water. However, in the 1050 to 1060 nm, a suitable compromise between water absorption, wavelength dispersion and scattering loss exists, where the water absorption profile has a local minimum ($\mu_a \sim 0.015$ mm^{-1} at $\lambda = 1060$ nm [24], as compared to $\mu_a \sim 0.0023$ mm^{-1} at $\lambda = 800$ nm [13]). This results in a reduction of the detectable light signal from the retina from $\sim 89.4\%$ at 800 nm to about 48.4% at 1060 nm.

5.4.5 Optical sources for OCT

In developing optical coherence tomography (OCT), the axial resolution has been one of the key issues. Because, as described in section 5.4.1, for the OCT, the axial and the transversal imaging resolutions are decoupled, i.e., the axial resolution is mainly determined by the coherence length of the light source and is decoupled from the beam focusing. Since the coherence length of a light source is inversely proportional to its bandwidth, broad bandwidth of optical sources is required to improve the OCT axial resolution. The axial resolution is inversely proportional to the spectral width of the used light source and the generation of broadband light sources has been a topic of great interest. So far, several approaches have been proposed to achieve high axial resolution, such as superluminescent diode, multiplexed superluminescent diode, femtosecond laser, continuum generation from photonic crystal fiber, amplified spontaneous emission (ASE), and xenon illuminator.

In general, these solutions either have high cost, exhibit bumpy spectrum, or both. The following section briefly reviews various state-of-the-art broad bandwidth light sources as potential light sources for the applications in OCT.

5.4.5.1 Superluminescent diodes (SLED)

In principle, operations of SLED are very similar to the laser diode (LD) with the lasing action based on amplified simulated emission. However, in SLED, lasing action cannot be built up due to insufficient feedback for oscillations. The unique property of SLED is the combination of laser diode-like output power and brightness with broad LED-like optical spectrum. Such a combination is allowed by high optical gain and wide gain spectrum in semiconductor laser materials. SLEDs are very compact, relatively cheap and very friendly to use. Current SLEDs operate at various wavelengths, such as 0.8 μm, 1 μm, 1.3 μm and 1.55 μm and all of these wavelengths have been used for OCT in different applications. At the 830 nm range, the SLEDs are based on AlGaAs emitters and single SLED with up to 70 nm bandwidths and 3–15 mW fiber pigtailed output power (corresponding to around 3.3 μm axial resolution in the tissue) are commercially available (Superlum Ltd, Russia). For ranges above 1 μm, the SLED emitters are based on InGaAs and the typical bandwidths are nearly from 50 nm to 60 nm, which limits the axial resolution to >10 μm in the tissue. However, using multiplexed SLED technology (synthesized optical source), SLEDs with a bandwidth more than 130 nm and optical power up to 15 mW are commercially available (Denselight Semiconductors, Singapore). While in some specific areas, like ultra-high resolution OCT, there are strong competitors to SLEDs, namely femtosecond lasers/supercontinuum sources, for most practical applications SLEDs are now considered the most attractive emitters due to their small size, easy use, and cost efficiency compared to alternative light sources.

5.4.5.2 Multiple quantum well semiconductor optical amplifiers

Multiple quantum well (MQW) optical amplifiers are another class of promising semiconductor sources widely used in OCT because of their inherently large saturation power and bandwidth. MQW are generally considered for the use in analogue and digital communication links, and are commercially available with wavelength ranges from 1300 nm to 1600 nm. Extremely broadband MQW optical amplifiers based on InGaAsP/InP ridge bent-waveguide semiconductor structures with several non-identical multiple quantum wells were designed and fabricated on InP substrate [29, 30, 31]. However there are a few potential disadvantages for these sources: most of the MQW sources operate at the far infrared region of the optical spectrum and the optical output is unpolarized, which limits its application in OCT where polarization-sensitive imaging is required.

5.4.5.3 Doped fiber based amplified spontaneous emission (ASE) sources

Doped fiber based optical sources can provide high power and high brightness broadband superfluorescent optical spectrum that has many applications in many areas including evaluation of fiber optical components by low coherence interferometry, rotation sensing, spectroscopy, and medical imaging [32]. One attractive way to generate broadband output is via the process of amplified spontaneous emission (ASE) in a rare-earth doped fiber. Over the last few years there has been very rapid progress in developing highly efficient output power from cladding-pumped fiber lasers and amplifiers. Rare-earth doped fluoride, telluride and silicon fibers realize broadband spectra ranges from 1300 nm to 1600 nm. One drawback with doped fiber based ASE is the need of a high power single-mode pump for optimal coupling into the doped single-mode core. Fiber coupled single mode semiconductor pump sources are commercially available; however they are typically very expensive.

5.4.5.4 Kerr lens mode-locked (KLM) lasers

As described earlier, SLEDs are easy to use and generate smooth and stable spectra; they can permit 20–7 μm resolution imaging at a fixed wavelength and are attractive because of their simplicity and low amplitude noise. However, achieving high-speed imaging with a high signal-to-noise ratio requires more than the mW-level power typically available from diode sources. Additionally, the limited optical bandwidth of diodes precludes cellular-level-resolution imaging. With the development of an ultrafast laser, it is possible to achieve broad band spectrum. Recently, Kerr-lens mode-locked (KLM) lasers are getting more attention in the field of OCT. The titanium:sapphire laser is tunable from 0.7 μm to 1.1 μm and can produce not only broad spectral bandwidths for high-resolution imaging, but also high output powers for fast image acquisition [33, 34]. Ti:Al_2O_3 lasers are optimized for short coherence length and was demonstrated to achieve sub-2-μm resolution with a power exceeding 100 mW. Although this source provided cellular-resolution imaging, comparative studies have shown that the 800 nm center wavelength of Ti:Al_2O_3 is not optimal for deeply penetrating biological tissue. An optimally penetrating optical source will take advantage of the diminishing scattering cross section with wavelength, while avoiding the resonant molecular absorption of common tissue constituents such as water and melanin. The chromium:forsterite laser has also been used to generate high output powers and broad spectral bandwidths (5 μm axial resolution) centered around 1,300 nm wavelength, for deeper imaging penetration in highly scattering tissue [35]. Both of these laser sources, however, are large, and require additional pump laser sources, water-cooling, and an experienced operator to align and maintain them. The ultrashort pulses from these lasers can be coupled into new tapered [36], microstructured [37], or ultrahigh numerical aperture fiber [38] to achieve even broader bandwidths and hence higher axial resolution imaging. The bandwidth and pulse duration of a mode locked laser can be calculated by

$$\Delta\lambda(nm) = 1.47 \times 10^{-3} \frac{\lambda_0^2(nm)}{\tau(fs)} \tag{5.34}$$

Figure 5.8 plots the relation between time and bandwidth. For achieving high axial resolution, the femtosecond laser should emit less than 20 fs pulses at 800 nm. Currently, the Ti:sapphire laser, with pulses down to 7 fs, has been commercialized. With a compact design and low cost, Ti:sapphire lasers at 800 nm with axial resolution up to 1.2 μm in the tissue have been utilized for corneal and retinal imaging [39]. However, at 1 μm and 1.3 μm, the available lasers can emit pulses only above 50 fs. Especially for the 1.3 μm laser, bulkiness and maintenance issues continue to be problematic, particularly outside of a research laboratory.

5.4.5.5 Supercontinuum light source

Supercontinuum (SC) lasers are a new type of light source based on a nonlinear optical phenomenon. Supercontinuum light is generated by invoking high optical nonlinearity in a material. Typically, mode-locked pulsed laser sources are used in the near infrared (1064 nm) in the nanosecond, picosecond, or femtosecond range, ensuring high peak powers to drive the nonlinear effect in a material, which "breaks" the pulse out into a SC spectrum. The supercontinuum combines high brightness with broad spectral coverage – a combination offered by no other technology. Figure 5.9 shows the comparison of supercontinuum with other broadband sources. The generation of supercontinuum is due to a plethora of nonlinear optical effects, which generate new frequencies which covers a broad band. Mathematically, the nonlinear effects can be described on the molecular scale by the following total polarization:

$$P = m + \varepsilon_0(\chi^{(1)}E + \chi^{(2)}E^2 + \chi^{(3)}E^3 + \ldots) \tag{5.35}$$

where P is the total polarization of the molecule; m is the permanent dipole moment; E represents the electric field; $\chi^{(1)}$is the linear polarization; $\chi^{(2)}$ and $\chi^{(3)}$ are the first and second hyperpolarizability coefficients. Here, the most noticeable terms are the second and third hyperpolarizabilities

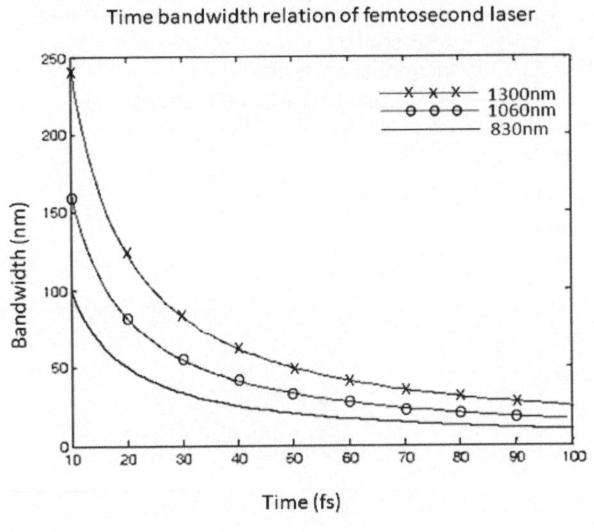

Figure 5.8: Pulse width vs. bandwidth of femtosecond lasers.

and the related phenomena are called second harmonic generation (SHG) and third order nonlinear effects, including self phase modulation (SPM), four-wave mixing (FWM), stimulated Raman scattering (SRS) and others. Broad band light sources can be generated through efficient non-linear effects. In order to enhance non-linear effects, two conditions must be satisfied: extremely high power and long walking distance for keeping such high power. Ultrafast lasers such as femtosecond lasers can produce very high peak power. In recent years, renewed interest in supercontinuum generation has been closely related to the remarkable progress in the development of photonic crystal fibers (PCF) as well as the development of robust, well-engineered single box ultrafast lasers. Coupling an ultrafast laser pulse directly out of an oscillator into a few centimeters of PCF produces more than one octave broad supercontinuum. The fact that only an oscillator with a few nJ of energy is required to generate a supercontinuum makes the PCF-based sources reliable, affordable and relatively simple to operate. These sources make use of optical nonlinear effects in specially designed PCF to create light with a wide spectrum that can span the visible and near-infrared, typically from around 400 to 2000 nm. Due to their spectral properties, they are suitable for OCT imaging with sub micrometer axial resolution [40]. SC light sources generating two separate spectral bands were also introduced into OCT allowing separate scanning at 800 nm and 1300 nm with axial resolutions of ~ 3 μm and ~ 5 μm, respectively [41, 42]. Commercially SC sources are available from Fianium and Koheras. Koheras A/S (NKT Photonics, Birkerod, Denmark) offers the SuperK Extreme, which it says is the brightest visible supercontinuum source available. The source, with the highest power the company offers, has a broad spectrum, from 460 to 2400 nm, and provides a spectral power density of more than 3 mW nm^{-1} in the visible wavelength range. Combining the source with a tunable filter allows a user to tune up to eight simultaneous laser lines independently across the visible spectrum. The SC500-FC supercontinuum source from Fianium (Southampton, UK) is a low-cost, mode-locked fiber laser generating supercontinuum radiation in the spectral band from 500 to 1700 nm, with an average power in excess of 250 mW. The feasibilities of the Fianium and Koheras SCs were demonstrated for both time-domain and frequency domain OCT configurations [43, 44, 45].

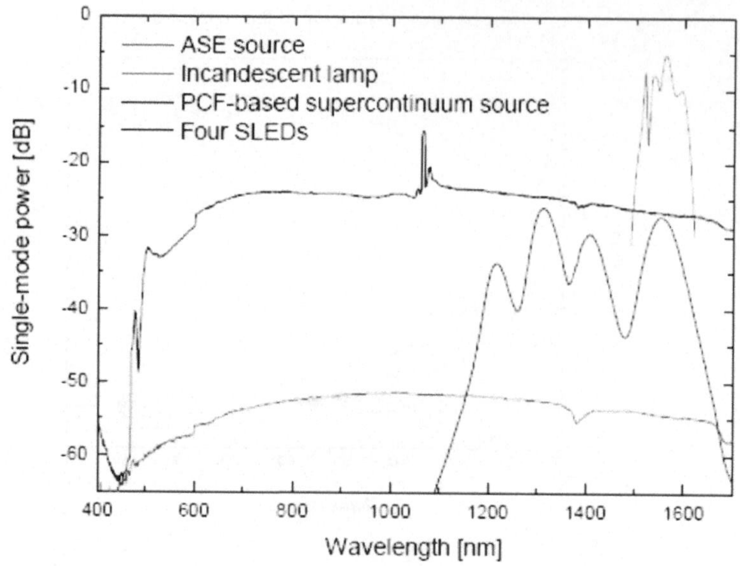

Figure 5.9: A comparison of supercontinuum with other broadband sources.

5.4.5.6 Swept source lasers

Swept-source lasers are a tunable light source emitting one wavelength at a time, rapidly swept over a broad spectral range. The promising capabilities of frequency swept light sources for OCT imaging have gained intense interest in their development and enabled a quantum leap in the speed and sensitivity of OCT technology development. There are three major concepts to achieve high speed tuning depending on the method used for wavelength selection inside the laser cavity of the wavelength swept source: one based on a fast rotating polygonal mirror [46, 47], the second based on a diffraction grating on a mechanically resonant galvo-scanner [48] and the third using a fiber Fabry-Perot tunable filter (FFP-TF) [49, 50]. For very high tuning speeds and to overcome limitations given by the buildup time of lasing in the cavity, the technique of Fourier Domain Mode Locking (FDML) has been introduced. High repetition rates up to 370 kHz have been already demonstrated for FDML swept sources [51, 52, 53, 54, 55]. Recent advancement in the field of ultrahigh speed swept-source optical source enables Fourier domain detection approach using frequency swept lasers and provides a powerful, complementary approach for spectral/Fourier domain detection.

Recently researchers from Praevium Research, Thorlabs, and the Massachusetts Institute of Technology reported on a high performance swept source laser running at 760 kHz axial scan rate at 1.3 μm with 100 nm tuning range [170]. The MEMS tunable vertical cavity surface emitting laser (VCSEL) used had a very long dynamic coherence length exceeding 25 mm at 150 kHz sweep rate. The laser used an optically pumped InP-based multi-quantum well gain region, a post amplifier, and is compact and potentially low cost. This laser promises to be the latest entry into the hot field of commercially available OCT sources for OCT system and subsystem vendors.

5.4.6 Scanning modalities in OCT

In conventional point scan OCT (flying spot OCT), various types of scanning modalities have been implemented for representing the cross-sectional information about the sample. Depending

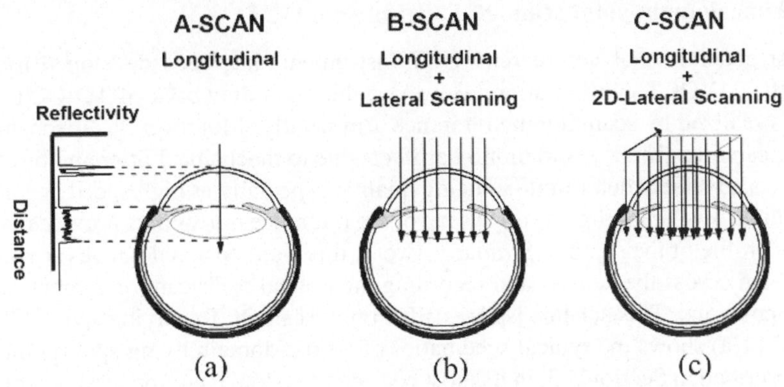

Figure 5.10: Different scanning modalities in flying spot optical coherence tomography. (a) A-Scan (b) B-Scan (c) C-Scan.

upon the priority of longitudinal (depth) and transverse direction, the scanning modalities can be mainly classified into three, A-scan, B-scan and C-scan [12]. As in an ultrasound instrument an A-scan (Axial-Scan) typically records the two fundamental parameters of an echo: how large it is (amplitude) and where it occurs in time with respect to zero time delay (pulse transit time). As explained in Section 5.3, in a TD-OCT system an A-scan is implemented by scanning the reference mirror throughout the entire depth to obtain a time domain interference pattern as shown in Figure 5.10(a); however, in a FD-OCT system the total distribution of an A-scan is measured at one time without any reference scan. Similarly, a B-scan can be generated by acquiring several A-scans for different adjacent transverse positions, as shown in Figure 5.10(b). In the case of a C-scan, the sample is scanned along many successive x and y directions at a fixed depth as shown in Figure 5.10(c), which can provide different transverse cross-sectional (*en-face*) images at different depths.

5.5 Different OCT Detection Schemes

In OCT the coherence-gated information about the elementary volume of the scatters within the obscuring scattering specimen can be obtained from either the time domain measurement principle (TD-OCT) or the frequency domain (FD-OCT) measurement principle.

5.5.1 Time domain OCT systems

The time-domain OCT operates as described in Section 5.2, the wavenumber-dependent photo detector current I_D in Eq. (5.10) is captured using a single or multiple detector where the reference mirror is scanned to match the optical path from reflections within the sample. Depending on the scanning modality and the signal detection scheme employed, the time-domain OCT can be further classified into three: 1) point-scan (flying-spot OCT), 2) line-field (linear-OCT) and full-field (wide-field) OCT.

5.5.1.1 Time domain point scan OCT (flying-spot OCT)

The first generation of commercial OCT instruments has been developed for ophthalmology based on the TD-OCT configuration. However, the main drawback of TD-OCT is that the depth scanning is realized by scanning the reference arm axially. Moreover, the mechanical scanner pair for lateral scanning gives rises to motion artifacts due to mechanical jitter and limited repeatability. These effects adversely deteriorate imaging quality, especially at high speed and at high resolution for sub-cellular level imaging. A single scan of the reference mirror thus provides a one-dimensional reflectivity profile of the sample. Similarly, two or three-dimensional images are produced by scanning the beam across the sample and recording the optical backscattering versus depth at different transverse positions. This scheme is also called point scan OCT or flying spot OCT.

Figure 5.11(a) shows the typical schematics of a time-domain flying spot (point scan) OCT system. As described in Section 5.3, in its most common version, it comprises a broadband light source emitting light of high spatial and low temporal coherence, which is coupled into a 2×2 fiber optics based Michelson interferometer. The Michelson interferometer divides the light beam and directs it into two arms of the interferometer. The sample arm beam directs into the object to be analyzed. It usually contains collimating optics enabling formation of a narrow beam, which penetrates the object. In order to reconstruct two-dimensional cross-sectional images of the object, the beam is galvanometrically scanned across the sample surface. Light backscattered or reflected from the various structures returns to the interferometer and is brought to interference with light reflected back from the reference arm mirror (RM), which scanned back and forth through the required depth of imaging. The standard fiber-optics Michelson interferometer is not the most efficient design for practical implementation, because a major disadvantage of this configuration is that the dc signal and intensity noise generated by the light from the reference arm add to the interference signal. In order to eliminate this problem, an alternative configuration called balanced heterodyne configurations as shown in Figure. 5.11(a) has been commonly used, in which these background noise components are cancelled by subtracting the photocurrents generated by two photodetectors. Then the resulting interfering light is detected by a photodiode (PD). Figure 5.11(b) shows the relative target positions in the eye and Figure 5.11(c) shows the raw interferograms (A-scan) which is obtained by scanning the reference arm mirror, and corresponds to the different structural features of the ocular medium. Figure 5.11(d) shows the reference arm signal subtracted interference signal from the output of the balanced detector. In the preceding step, the interferograms are amplified and backed up with a band pass filter tuned to the Doppler frequency, often called the "carrier frequency," which is related to the scanning speed of the reference mirror. This procedure helps to eliminate extraneous signals arising from background light. Then, for the next scan of the reference mirror, the probing beam is shifted to an adjacent position and so on, to yield a set of consecutive A-scans. These A-scans are then combined into a single picture to form a cross-sectional image of the object, the B-scan. Three-dimensional, volumetric data sets can be generated by acquiring sequential cross-sectional images by scanning the incident optical beam in a raster pattern.

5.5.1.2 Line-field OCT (linear OCT) and full-field OCT

Conventional point-scan optical coherence tomography (OCT) [56, 57, 58] can enable non-invasive, non-contact 3D cross-sectional imaging of structures in highly scattering specimens with very high resolution. However, for reconstructing the 3D image the conventional OCT system needs single pointer raster-scanning scheme, in which the focus of the probing beam scans across the sample surface and detects the back-scattered light with a single element photo-detector. Thus a fiber optics based point-scan time-domain OCT scheme requires at least three scans (one depth and two lateral scans) for acquiring three-dimensional images. The lateral scan addresses laterally adjacent sample positions whereas the depth scan detects longitudinal depth positions of light-reflected sites in the sample. A major limitation in the point scan OCT approach is the mechanical scanning system, giving rise to motion artifacts due to mechanical jitter and limited repeatability.

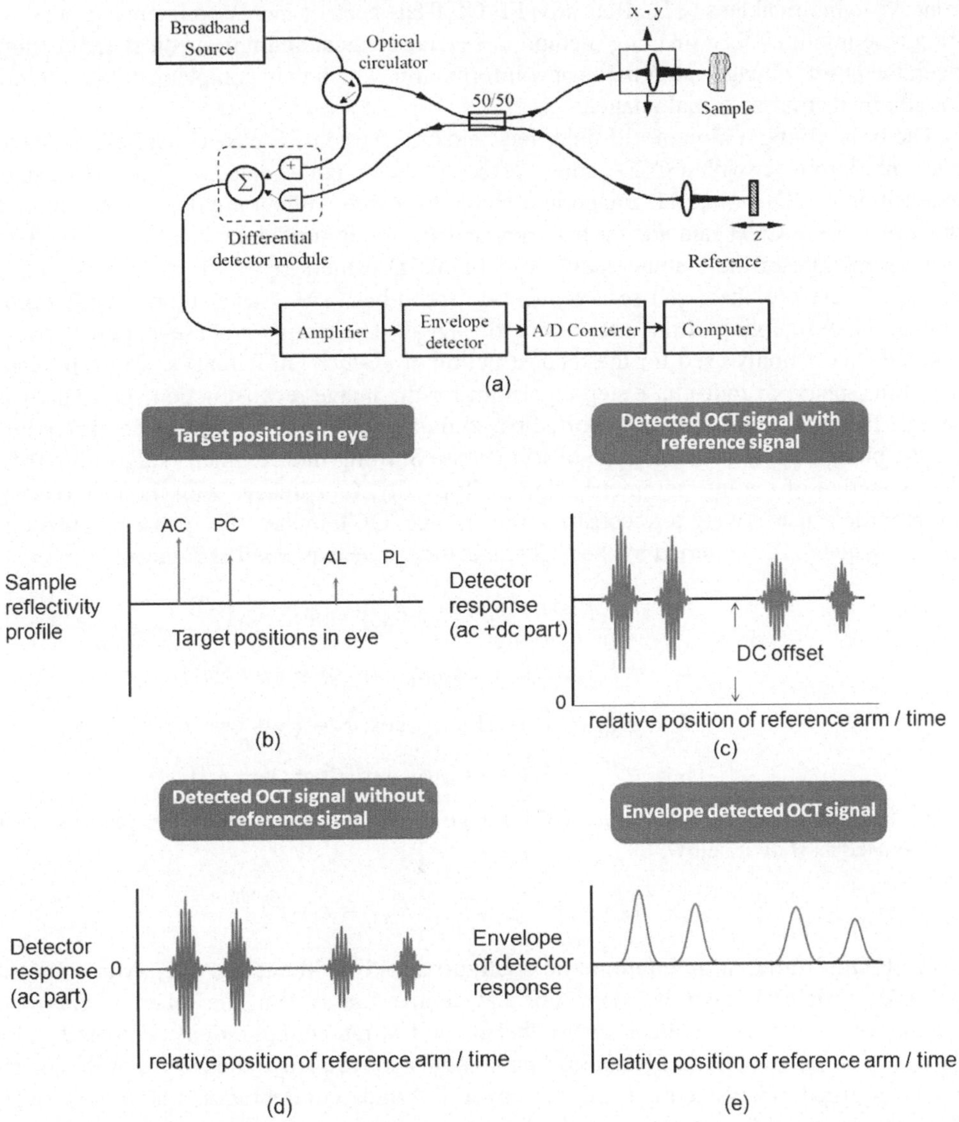

Figure 5.11: (a) Schematic of a typical fiber optics based time-domain OCT setup (b) Reflectivity profile of target position in the ocular medium (c) detected interference signal by the photodetector (d) detected signal with reference signal filtered out (e) demodulated and envelope detected OCT signal.

Line-field [59, 60, 61] and full-field OCT (FF-OCT or wide-field - WF-OCT) [62, 63] are alternative OCT concepts, which aim to improve the image acquisition speed and to simplify the optical setup of conventional point-scan OCT by realizing direct line field or full-field sample imaging onto an array or line detector such as CCD [62] or CMOS [64] camera. FF-OCT is based on bulk optics Linnik-type Michelson interferometer with relatively high numerical aperture (NA) microscopic objectives, but identical, on both arms of the interferometer. Whereas WF-OCT uses imaging optics with a single lens to image the large sample area, compromising the lateral resolution. In the case of line-field OCT, the line illumination was achieved with a spherical focusing lens and a plano-concave cylindrical lens (CL). Recently, FF-OCT has been of increased interest as a non-scanning, high resolution, *en-face* imaging method in several medical and non-medical applications. Moreover, the *en-face* image can provide new information, which may complement that provided by the longitudinal cross-sectional image.

The basic configuration of full-field/line-field OCT systems is based on a bulk optics low coherence interferometer with a CCD camera placed at the output as detector. The CCD can enable the acquisition of 2D *en-face*/1D image in a single exposure without any lateral scanning. However, the direct use of CCD cameras for heterodyne detection in time-domain is limited by the relatively slow frame rate of the commercially available CCD camera (typically $\approx$ 100 Hz for 512×512 pixels). Therefore, the depth-scan acquisition speed has to be drastically reduced in order to permit sufficient sampling of the interferometric signal. The temporal phase-stepping interferometric scheme is commonly used for the reconstruction of *en-face* OCT images. Conventional FF-OCT uses three-phase or four-phase step algorithm for the image reconstruction. Over the past decade several FF-OCT schemes were reported based on a wide variety of optical configurations to realize the phase stepping and the type of PSI (Phase Shifting Interferometry) algorithm [65] used for the extraction of the interferometric signal. Typically, four images with the different phase shift are recorded successively to reconstruct the *en-face* OCT image. The phase stepped interference images sequentially recorded by the CCD detector can be expressed as follows:

$$I_0 = E_{S0}^2 + E_{R0}^2 + 2E_{S0}E_{R0}\cos(\varphi_S - \varphi_R) \tag{5.36}$$

$$I_{\pi/2} = E_{S0}^2 + E_{R0}^2 + 2E_{S0}E_{R0}\cos(\varphi_S - \varphi_R + 90^\circ) \tag{5.37}$$

$$I_{\pi} = E_{S0}^2 + E_{R0}^2 + 2E_{S0}E_{R0}\cos(\varphi_S - \varphi_R + 180^\circ) \tag{5.38}$$

$$I_{3\pi/2} = E_{S0}^2 + E_{R0}^2 + 2E_{S0}E_{R0}\cos(\varphi_S - \varphi_R + 270^\circ) \tag{5.39}$$

Then, for reconstructing the *en-face* OCT image I_{OCT}, the conventional four phase shift algorithm can be used as shown below:

$$I_{\mathrm{OCT}} = \left[(I_0 - I_\pi)^2 + (I_{3\pi/2} - I_{\pi/2})^2\right]^{1/2} \tag{5.40}$$

In FF-OCT, different interferometric configurations like Michelson [62], Mirau [66] or Linnik [67, 68] configuration can be used. For a wide aperture system, the spherical aberration in the axial direction is very dominant for Michelson and Mirau configurations compared to Linnik. In the case of Linnik configuration, optical pathlength and focusing in both arms of the interferometer can be adjusted independently [12]. Moreover, in Linnik configuration a high numerical aperture (NA) objective can be used to obtain high spatial resolution. In general, the axial resolution of the tomographic image in FF-OCT depends on both coherence length of the source (coherence effect) and the NA of the objective (aperture effect). A variant scheme of FF-OCT that utilizes an objective with high NA (< 0.4) is called full-field optical coherence microscopy (FF-OCM) and which is used for obtaining very high resolution [69, 70]. In this scheme, the aperture effect is more dominant than the coherence effect. Figure 5.12 shows the basic setup of FF-OCT based on Michelson (Fig. 5.12(a)) and Linnik configuration (Fig. 5.12(b)).

An FF-OCT scheme can utilize a wide variety of optical sources, including either a source with spatially coherent illumination or spatially incoherent illumination. In FF-OCT, depending on the nature of illumination, the multiply scattered light from the specimen can result in strong cross-talk generated noise between parallel detection channels, thus each detector should ideally not detect light originating from outside its conjugate volume. To avoid cross-talk, one must prevent interference occurring between adjacent pixels at the detection plane [71]. This can be achieved by controlling the degree of spatial coherence of full-field illumination. FF-OCT utilizing spatially incoherent sources such as thermal sources can effectively suppress the effect of coherent cross-talk [72]. Moreover, thermal sources may provide high axial resolution due to its broad spectral

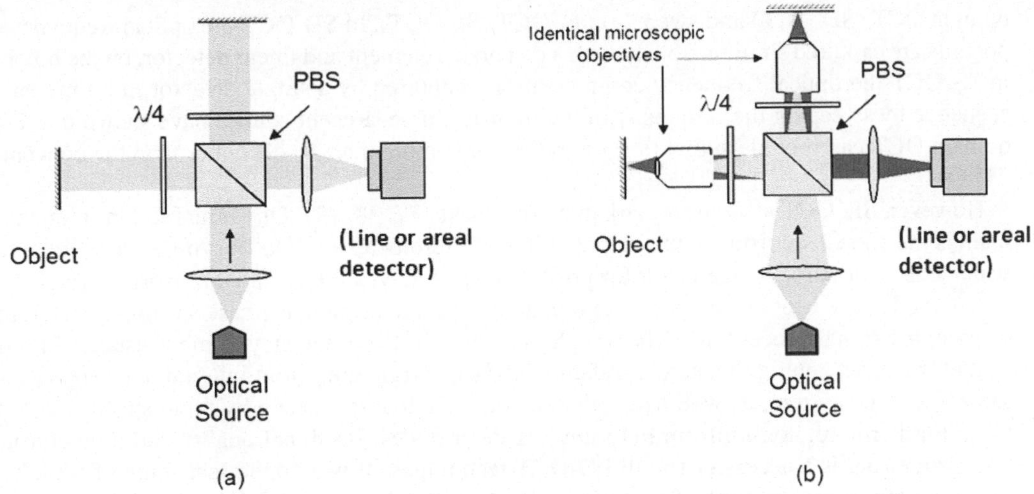

Figure 5.12: Typical full-field OCT configurations (a) Michelson geometry for wide field OCT (WF-OCT) (b) Linnik geometry for full-field OCT (FF-OCT).

bandwidth. However, the brightness per spatial mode of thermal sources often remains insufficient, requiring a trade-off between sensitivity and imaging speed. The major interest of spatially coherent illumination in FF-OCT resides in the possibility to use powerful pulsed lasers such as femtosecond lasers, allowing higher sensitivity and acquisition speed than with thermal light sources. In contrast, a spatially coherent source can generate a considerable amount of coherent cross-talk that degrades the image quality.

However, the temporal phase stepping method employed in FF-OCT for reconstruction of *en-face* image degrades the time resolution of the system. Over the last several years different techniques have been reported for improving the time resolution of FF-OCT. Single-shot FF-OCT (SS FF-OCT) is a relatively new concept, which aims to improve the time resolution of FF-OCT and extending the feasibility of FF-OCT for fast imaging application in biological application. The basic principle of SS FF-OCT is similar to the simultaneous phase-shifting interferometric method, which has been developed over the years for high speed vibration insensitive optical testing. Nevertheless, the optical configuration of the four-channel phase stepper optics is quite complex, which limits this system's performance for practical implementation. Any differences caused by image projections, optical aberration and response uniformity will directly influence the reconstruction accuracy. Recently, feasibility SS FF-OCT was reported for dynamic imaging of biological specimens [73] and materials [74, 75].

5.5.2 Frequency domain OCT

Frequency domain OCT (FD-OCT) [21, 76] is a variant interferometric imaging modality. It has been widely attracted in the biomedical imaging field due to its higher sensitivity and imaging speed compared to conventional TD-OCT. The principle of FD-OCT relies on the transformation of the OCT time varying signal along the optical axis, termed the A-scan, into the frequency domain. The basic physics behind FD-OCT is based on the inverse scattering theorem. According to the Wiener-Khintchine theorem the spectral power amplitude of the back scattered wave equals the Fourier transform of the axial distribution of the object scattering potential. FD-OCT has the advantage that the full sample depth information is obtained in a parallel manner such that no moving parts are necessary. Based on the implementation the FD-OCT can be divided into two classes, spectral domain OCT (SD-OCT) and swept-source OCT (SS-OCT). In SD-OCT the optical frequency components are captured simultaneously with a dispersive element and linear detector, on the other hand in SS-OCT the optical frequency components are captured by a single detector in a time encoded sequence by sweeping the frequency of the optical source. Recent studies have shown that Fourier domain OCT can provide signal to noise ratio that is more than 20 dB better than the conventional TD-OCT.

However, SD-OCT also has remarkable drawbacks [77, 78, 79]. One limitation in frequency domain is the optical spectrum at the output of the interferometer consists of symmetric spectral terms, which cause the same image result for positive and negative OPDs, called mirroring effect. Different methods have been developed to eliminate this problem, such as phase shifting interferometry, or complex signal processing. The simple detection in the frequency domain usually introduces spatial frequency ambiguity, autocorrelation artifacts, originating from internal interferences of the sample and the system, as well as depth dependent SNR loss, caused by finite spectral line width [11]. Furthermore, non-uniform FD sampling deteriorates TD signal quality and time consuming post-processing is a necessity for all FD-OCT techniques. It was found that some of these effects can be largely compensated for by multiple, phase shifted imaging of the same region (i.e., A-scan), followed by reconstruction of the complex phase of the FD-signal [80], re-sampling and transformation into the time domain. Moreover, for getting better lateral resolution, the technique such as dynamic focusing, which is generally used in time domain OCT, is not easily implemented in FD-OCT. In traditional FD-OCT the imaging optics are devised with large depth of focus, to accommodate the entire range of the A-scan, usually 1–2 mm, which limits the possibility of using high numerical aperture objective to enhance the transverse resolution. However, recently by employing Bessel beam with axicon lenses, the extended focal length FD-OCTs were demonstrated with cellular level resolution.

5.5.2.1 Spectral domain OCT (SD-OCT)

A typical implementation of fiber optics based SD-OCT setup is shown in Figure. 5.13(a). The back scattered low coherence light is mixed with a reference beam by the 2×2 fiber optics based Michelson interferometer, then the grating based spectrometer at the output of the interferometer separates each spectral components detected using a linear array detector. The interference signal detected by the linear detector is expressed as

$$I(k) = I_S(k) + I_R(k) + 2\sqrt{I_S(k) I_R(k)} \sum_n \alpha_n \cos(2kz_n) \quad (5.41)$$

where $I_R(k)$ and $I_S(k)$ are the wavelength dependent intensities reflected from the reference and sample arms, respectively, and k is the wave number. The third term on the right-hand side of Eq. (5.41) represents the interference between the back reflected lights from the sample and reference arm. α_n is the square root of the sample reflectivity at depth z_n. In order to reconstruct the depth information, the spectrum is inverse Fourier transformed, which yields the following convolution.

$$\left|FT^{-1}[I(k)]\right|^2 = \Gamma^2(z) \otimes \left[I_R \delta(z) + \sum_n I_{S,n} \delta(z) + \sum_n \alpha_n^2 \delta(z - z_n) + \sum_n \alpha_n^2 \delta(z + z_n) \right] \quad (5.42)$$

where $\Gamma(z)$ represents the envelope of the coherence function. The first and second terms in the right-hand side of the Eq. 5.42 describe the autocorrelation (or self-interference) of the reference signal and sample signal, respectively. The third and fourth terms are due to the interference of back reflected beam from reference and sample surfaces and its complex conjugates. The SD-OCT detects the spectrally resolved interference signal with a spectrometer that consists of a high efficiency diffraction grating and a high-speed line camera. Figure 5.13(b) shows the reflectivity profile of the different target positions in the ocular medium and Fig. 5.13(c) shows the detected intensity spectrum by the camera. In order to suppress autocorrelation, self-cross correlation, and camera noise artifacts, first, all the spectral interferogram in each slice along the x-direction (B-scan) were ensemble-averaged at each wavelength to obtain a reference spectrum, this background spectrum then subtracted from each A-scans. Since the Fourier transform relates the physical distance (z) with the wavenumber ($k = 2\pi/\lambda$), however, the spectra obtained with the SD-OCT spectrometer are not necessarily evenly spaced in k-space. In order to obtain a proper depth profile, the subtracted spectral interferograms are then remapped from λ-space to k-space by use of the spline interpolation method [81], as shown in Fig. 5.13(d). Due to the Fourier relation (Wiener-Khintchine theorem between the auto correlation and the spectral power density) the depth resolved information can be immediately reconstructed by a Fourier-transformation from the remapped spectra, without movement of the reference arm, as show in Fig. 5.13(e).

For a Gaussian source centered at k_0 with a full width at half maximum bandwidth Δk, the complex coherence function is described in Section 5.3. The depth range that can be probed with a SD-OCT is dependent on the spectrometer resolution and the detector size (number of pixels). For a conventional SD-OCT system, the maximum imaging depth is defined as

$$l_{\max} = \frac{1}{4n}\frac{\lambda_0^2}{\Delta\lambda_S}N, \tag{5.43}$$

where n is the refractive index of the medium, λ_0 is the center wavelength of the detected spectrum, $\Delta\lambda_S$ is the spectrometer bandwidth and N is the number of pixels of the camera. For ambiguity free image this depth range should be doubled. The term $(\Delta\lambda_s/N)^{-1}$ can be seen as the inverse of the spectral resolution power $\delta\lambda^{-1}$ of the detecting spectrometer and is proportional to the coherence length of the detected spectral channel, which is responsible for one of the main drawbacks of SD-OCT, which is the signal decay observed for structures far away from the relative zero-delay.

5.5.2.1.1 Line-field SD-OCT Line-field SD-OCT is an alternative implementation to improve imaging speed. To improve imaging speed, transversally multi-dimensional techniques have already been extensively investigated for TD-OCT imaging, as described in the above section, which profit the continued high-speed camera development with full frame acquisition in the multi kframe/s range as well as of the high stability due to the transversally static setup. Their major advantages found in almost isotropic high resolution sampling of microscopic specimen (within the depth of field), but suffers from low imaging speed and high power requirements because of very low signal to noise, limiting in vivo applications. SD-OCT based on the introduction of one transversal imaging dimension and detection by a highly parallel spectrometer have been investigated by multiple groups [82, 84]. These seem to have potential for high speed acquisition of cross-sectional scans, but involve a complicated mixture of geometrical imaging in one sensor axis and a spectrometer setup in the orthogonal direction, that confines area detectors to rather low pixel counts due to cross-talk in the "spatial" axis. For full volume acquisition they still need beam translation. Figure 5.14 shows the basic schematic of a line-field SD-OCT implementation.

5.5.2.2 Swept source OCT (SS-OCT)

The concept of FD-OCT can also be implemented using a tunable laser source over a broad spectral range in conjunction with a single detector. FD-OCT of this type has been called swept source OCT (SS-OCT) [84]. Despite the difference in system configuration, both SD-OCT and SS-OCT have a common net result: the OCT signal is sampled in spectral domain and a SNR improvement is gained because of the Fourier reconstruction. In SS-OCT the time required to tune the wavelength determines the time to produce an A-scan. Recently swept source with sweeping frequency of few hundreds of kHz has been achieved, which drastically improves the imaging speed of SS-OCT to compete with SD-OCT and TD-OCT in terms of imaging speed [85].

Figure 5.15 shows the typical implementation of SS-OCT systems, which employ a broadband, rapid frequency-swept laser source and InGaAs photodetectors to perform Fourier domain OCT

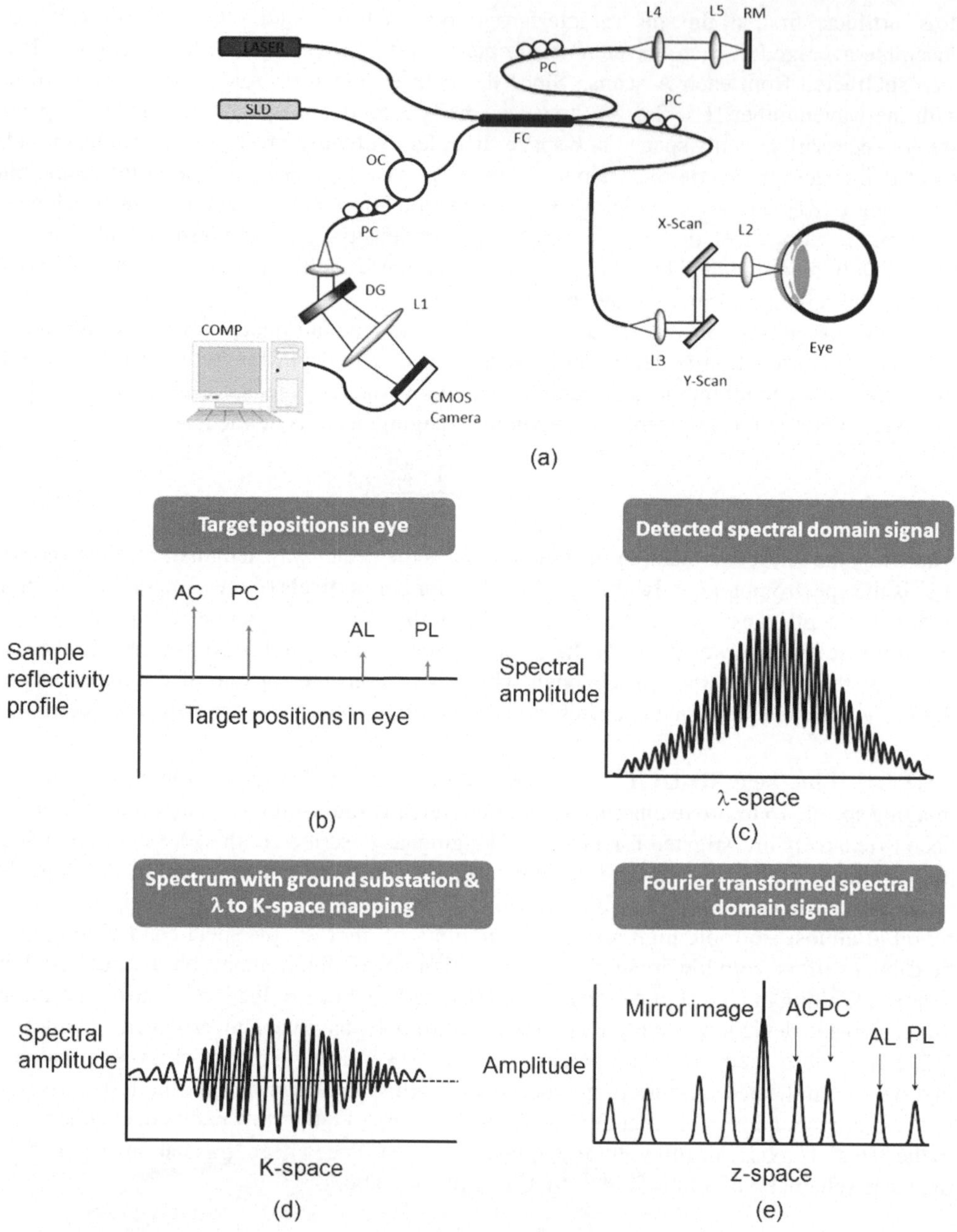

Figure 5.13: (a) Experimental schematic of a FD-OCT setup (b) reflectivity profile of anterior chamber of an eye (c) detected spectral interferogram by the camera (A-scan) (d) remapped spectral interferogram in *k*-space with back ground subtraction (e) Fourier transformed spectrum.

imaging without the use of a spectrometer [46, 51, 52, 53, 54, 55, 78]. With such a wavelength-swept source, interference signals at individual wavelengths can be measured sequentially with high spectral resolution. This spectrally resolved data acquisition is central to frequency-domain ranging. This method offers significantly higher sensitivity than the time-domain ranging method used in conventional OCT. Furthermore, frequency-domain ranging does not require reference delay

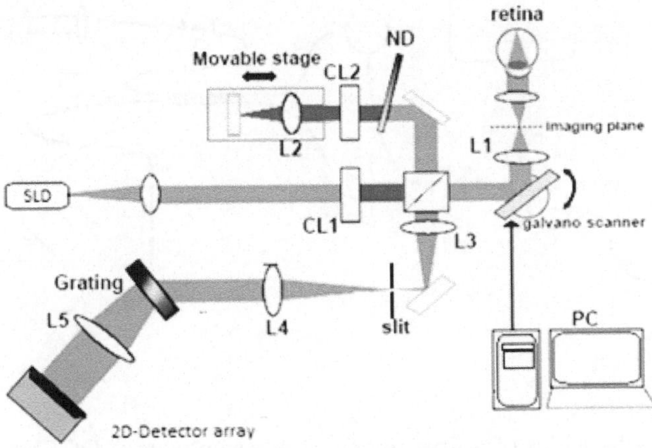

Figure 5.14: Optical scheme of line-field – spectral domain optical coherence tomography. CL – cylindrical lens, ND – neutral density filter, SLD – superluminescent diode, and PC – personal computer.

scanning and can therefore be applied to increase imaging speed. Since SD-OCT systems typically employ silicon-based CCD detectors, they cannot operate at wavelengths longer than $\sim$ 1000 nm, since the detector efficiency degrades rapidly beyond this point. Moreover the unavailability of relatively cheap spectrometer at 1300 nm, which is very essential for OCT imaging of epithelial tissues and many non-biological samples to achieve an image penetration depth of 1–3 mm. With a pressing need for high imaging speed at 1000–1300 nm in various applications, wavelength-swept sources, particularly rapidly tuned lasers, have developed substantially in recent years and have emerged as important and practical light sources for OCT. One particular advantage of SS-OCT over SD-OCT is worth mentioning, that is that a balanced detection scheme can be used in SS-OCT (see Fig. 5.15) to cancel out the strong background light in the interferometer, therefore enhancing the dynamic range of the system.

5.5.2.2.1 Line-field/full-field SS-OCT The schematics of line-field OCT system using frequency-sweeping source is similar to that of LF-SD-OCT, which is based on free space implementation of Michelson interferometer and instead of 2D detector array line-field SS-OCT uses a 1D linear detector at the spectrometer side. The irradiation is done by an elliptical beam onto the imaging sample through using a cylindrical lens; and then, the wavelength-resolved interference signal is detected by a line CCD camera [87]. Since the system uses the line CCD camera as a detector, the exposure time can be reduced (in the microsecond range); therefore, the images are influenced to a lesser extent by motion artifacts.

Instead, the full-field SS-OCT is a full-field version of swept-source optical coherence tomography. A set of 2D Fourier holograms are recorded at discrete wavenumbers spanning the swept-source tuning range. The resultant 3D data cube contains comprehensive information on 3D morphology of the sample that can be retrieved by software via 3D discrete Fourier-transform. This method of recording of the OCT signal confers signal-to-noise ratio improvement in comparison with "flying-spot" TD-OCT. The spatial resolution of the 3D reconstructed image, however, is degraded due to the presence of a phase cross-term, whose origin and effects are addressed below.

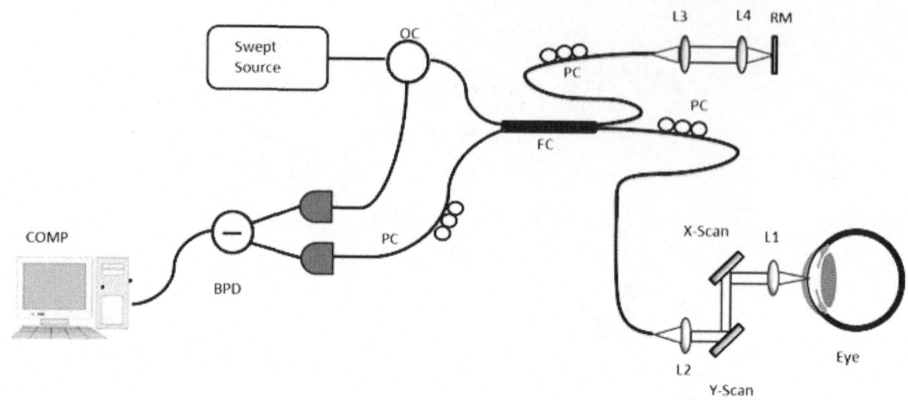

Figure 5.15: (a) Schematics of a fiber optics based swept-source OCT setup. OC – optical circulator, PC – polarization controller, RM – reference mirror, BPD – balanced photodetector, FC – fiber coupler.

5.5.2.3 Full range complex Fourier domain OCT

As described in the preceding section, one of the major drawbacks of FD-OCT that limits its practical application is the complex-conjugate ambiguity. This is because in FD-OCT the detected real valued spectral interferogram is Fourier transformed to localize the scatter within the sample. The Fourier transform of a real valued function is Hermitian, so the reconstructed image is symmetric with respect to the zero-phase delay of the interferometer, leading to ambiguity in interpretation of the resulted OCT images. In order to overcome this problem, one has to place the sample entirely within the positive or negative space. Consequently, only half of the imaging depth is available for imaging in practice. By resolving the complex conjugate artifact, the imaging depth range can be doubled that would in turn provide additional flexibility to explore the most sensible measurement range near the zero delay line [76].

To achieve the full-range complex imaging for FD-OCT, several methods have been proposed. Phase-shifting methods were among the first attempt to achieve the full-range imaging [80], however this limits the imaging speed and complex conjugate rejection ratio due to the requirements of several phase steps at the same sampling location and its accuracy. Another approach that uses a 3×3 optical coupler as phase shifting element was proposed, which allows simultaneous detection of two quadraturely phase shifted interferograms to obtain the complex ambiguity free images [88]. This technique requires two separate detectors for image acquisition, which adds additional cost and complexity, thus limiting its practical application. For high speed full-range complex imaging, an elegant, practical scheme is to introduce a constant modulation frequency into the spatial interferogram during transverse scanning of the sample [89]. In this way, the complex data can be obtained either by Fourier transform or Hilbert transform of the B-scan interferogram in transverse direction. By using this method, it is possible to achieve a full-range complex imaging with high speed. However, the original implementation requires a piezo-stage to provide modulation in the interferograms, which limits the full imaging speed due to the mechanical movement of the piezo-stage used.

Recently, the modulation of the spectral interferograms is achieved by the galvo-scanner [91], that is used for transversely (x-direction) scanning the sample. In doing so, the sample beam is offsetted from the pivot axis of the x-scanner, which causes a path length modulation during x-scanning, thus introduces a modulation frequency into the B-scan interferograms. The main advantage of this method is that it does not need any additional phase shifting elements to realize frequency modulation and the modulation frequency is inherently given by the system itself. Another important advantage of using frequency modulation in the interferogram to achieve a full-range complex FD-OCT image is that it is relatively insensitive to sample movement that is critical for *in vivo* application. These aspects render high speed full-range complex FD-OCT imaging without any restriction on additional hardware component, and without limitation on the imaging speed, which is critical for *in vivo* imaging applications.

5.6 Functional OCT

In conventional OCT, the contrast mechanism relies upon the spatial variation of the coherent back scatters within a cross-sectional plane or volume of tissue or materials. However, a number of other intrinsic properties of the tissue have been demonstrated to provide information about the morphological changes by altering the amplitude, phase or polarization states of the probing beam. Exploiting these properties, thus providing novel imaging contrast mechanisms, enhances the clinical and biomedical applications for OCT to achieve functional imaging that can reveal more details about the tissue dynamics and physiology. Some of the important functional modes of OCT are polarization sensitive OCT, Doppler OCT, spectrometric OCT and differential absorption OCT.

5.6.1 Polarization-sensitive OCT

Most of the body tissues such as muscle, tendons and nerve fibers contain collagen and elastin, which exhibit birefringence when they form a specific structure. Birefringence depicts a change in polarization state of light due to the refractive index difference for light polarized in two orthogonal planes. The propagation of light through such birefringence samples may alter the optical polarization state of reflected light. Therefore, polarization sensitive measurements at the output of the interferometer can provide depth-correlated information about the birefringence nature of the material or tissue specimen. As well as providing added contrast, changes in birefringence may indicate changes in functionality or structure of the tissue. Since the first report of functional polarization sensitive OCT (PS-OCT) system [92], a variety of PS-OCT configurations has been investigated [93, 94, 95, 96, 97, 98]. They all differ in complexity, capabilities and signal processing schemes. The most complete information about the polarization properties of a biological specimen is given by system capable of producing depth resolved Mueller matrix elements. These configurations can account for the depolarization as well as the changes in total, linear and circular degree of polarization of the probe beam during propagation in tissue.

The TD-OCT and FD-OCT configurations do not account for birefringence within a sample, treating the electromagnetic wave as a scalar quantity. However, light waves are transverse and, therefore, have extra degrees of freedom described by the polarization state. The PS-OCT measurement apparatus is similar to that of TD-OCT or FD-OCT, with the addition of a light polarizer after the source, and a polarizing beam-splitter (PBS) with an extra detector in the output arm (Fig. 5.3). Propagation of light through a sample may alter the optical polarization state of the reflected light. This can occur due to optical scattering and birefringence within the sample. Birefringence describes a change in the polarization state of light due to the refractive index difference for light polarized in two orthogonal planes. Therefore, polarization sensitive measurement of the output interferogram can resolve depth correlated information about the birefringence of the sample material. Mathematically, the two orthogonal polarization states can be treated separately as two electromagnetic waves propagating in separate interferometers.

The polarization state of light can be expressed in terms of Stokes vector S as:

$$S = \begin{bmatrix} I \\ Q \\ U \\ V \end{bmatrix} = \begin{bmatrix} a_x^2 + a_y^2 \\ a_x^2 - a_y^2 \\ 2a_x a_y \cos\varphi \\ 2a_x a_y \sin\varphi \end{bmatrix} \tag{5.44}$$

where I, Q, U, V are Stokes parameters, a_x and a_y are amplitudes of two orthogonal components of the electric vector and φ represents the phase difference between the two orthogonal components, By using a 4×4 Mueller matrix the effect of an optical device on the polarization of light can be expressed, and the matrix acts on the input state S_1 to give the output state S_2:

$$S_2 = \begin{bmatrix} I_2 \\ Q_2 \\ U_2 \\ V_2 \end{bmatrix} = MS_1 = \begin{bmatrix} M_{00} M_{01} M_{02} M_{03} \\ M_{10} M_{11} M_{12} M_{13} \\ M_{20} M_{21} M_{22} M_{23} \\ M_{30} M_{31} M_{32} M_{33} \end{bmatrix} \begin{bmatrix} I_1 \\ Q_1 \\ U_1 \\ V_1 \end{bmatrix} \tag{5.45}$$

If we consider the Poincaré sphere representation, a polarization state S can be represented by a point (Q, U, V). The Poincaré sphere representation provides a convenient method to evaluate changes of Stokes vector. By determining either the Stokes vector or the Mueller matrix, the full quantification of birefringence properties of the biological sample can be obtained. PS-OCT imaging of the Stokes vector and Mueller matrix has been demonstrated by several groups [99, 100, 101, 102]. It is attractive for medical applications, providing an extra contrast mechanism that could potentially lead to optical diagnosis of certain pathologies [103, 104].

5.6.2 Doppler OCT

Doppler OCT (DOCT) or optical Doppler tomography (ODT) is another functional mode, which can permit quantitative imaging of fluid flow in highly scattering specimens [105, 106, 107, 108, 109, 110]. The technique is similar to Doppler velocimetry. Doppler velocimetry suffers from imprecise imaging due to the long coherence length of the light source used, which results in the interference of the static and Doppler shifted components of light occurring over a long optical path. The low coherence gating property of OCT overcomes this problem, permitting quantitative imaging of fluid flow in highly scattering media, such as monitoring *in vivo* blood flow beneath the skin. In DOCT the velocity resolution depends upon detection electronics, scan angle and acquisition time. Reported flow velocity resolutions are in the region 10–100 μms^{-1}; however recent development in Fourier Domain Doppler OCT (FD-DOCT) has shown that a velocity resolution of just a few micrometers per second may be achieved [111, 112, 113, 114, 115, 116, 117, 118]. The DOCT can provide 3D-tomographic map and velocity profile of blood flow in tissue, which attracted a number of biomedical applications, e.g., determination of the depth of burns; determining tissue perfusion to ensure adequate oxygenation of the tissue after injury, wound closure, grafting, etc. Other applications include distinguishing between arterial and venous blockages in tissue after injury; or monitoring the effect of pharmaceuticals on blood transport in the tissues.

The Doppler effect describes the shift in frequency of waves reflected from moving objects. This frequency shift can be used to determine object-moving velocity. For electromagnetic waves such as light, derivation of the Doppler shifted frequency from a moving object requires the application of special relativity. The result for a Doppler shifted frequency f_d is,

$$f_d = \sqrt{\frac{c+u}{c-u}} f_0 \tag{5.46}$$

where f_0 is the initial frequency of the electromagnetic wave, c the speed of light and u is the speed of the moving object. Here it is assumed that u is positive when the object is moving towards the

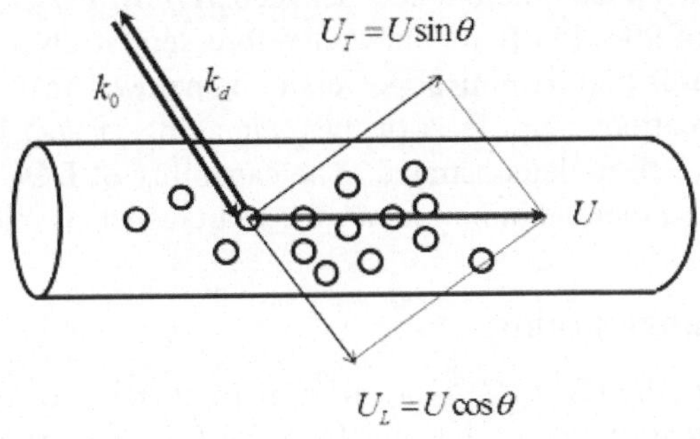

Figure 5.16: Schematic for optical Doppler tomography. The sample arm beam is held at some angle θ to the direction of flow. Therefore, an optical signal with wave-vector $\mathbf{k}_0$ falls on a particle moving with velocity $\mathbf{u}$. The light scattered back into the sample objective is Doppler shifted and has wave-vector $\mathbf{k}_d$.

observer. In this case, it is seen that the Doppler shifted frequency, Δf, must be greater than the initial frequency:

$$\Delta f = f_d - f_0 \tag{5.47}$$

It can be shown that when u is much less than c, the velocity of the moving sample is given by

$$\Delta f = \frac{u}{c} f_d \tag{5.48}$$

In the practical DOCT system, Fig. 5.16, the interferometer sample arm is angled relative to the direction of flow by an amount θ. Detected light is scattered from a moving particle in the sample, undergoing a double Doppler shift—once from the source to the particle, and once again from the particle back to the objective. These two factors are taken into account by expressing equation (5.48) in terms of initial source and scattered wave-vectors $\mathbf{k}_0$ and $\mathbf{k}_d$, respectively. The Doppler shift can then be written as

$$\Delta f = \frac{1}{2\pi}(\mathbf{k}_d - \mathbf{k}_0) \cdot \mathbf{u} \tag{5.49}$$

Therefore, the velocity of moving particles can be determined from the measurement of the Doppler shift and knowledge of the relative angle between the optical signal and the flow [114].

$$u = \lambda_0 \frac{\Delta f}{2\cos\theta} \tag{5.50}$$

Structural information about the sample is obtained by either conventional TD-OCT or more recently FD-OCT [113]. However, to retrieve data regarding the flow of particles within submerged capillary, extra measurements of the Doppler shifted frequency must be made. To do this in the time domain the reference mirror of the interferometer is scanned to match the path length within the capillary. At each spatial point within the capillary the detector intensity is sampled at a rate not less than two samples per time period of the source. The time varying result is then Fourier transformed to give the Doppler frequency shift due to moving particles within the capillary. By doing this at a number of points within the capillary, a profile of particle flow is determined.

The axial resolution of DOCT is again dependent on the source temporal coherence length, and the lateral scan resolution on the beam spot size. Velocity resolution depends upon the detection electronics, scan angle and the acquisition time. Reported flow velocity resolutions are in the region

10–100 μms^{-1}; however, recent developments in Fourier domain DOCT (FD-DOCT) have shown a velocity resolution of just a few micrometers per second [86]. FD-DOCT has also shown greater sensitivity in the region of 90–115 dB and may, therefore, lend itself to ocular flow imaging where ANSI laser safety standards require optical powers to be below 1 mW. DOCT has been applied to a number of medical situations. Not least of these, imaging *in vivo* blood flow in both the skin [119] and retina [112] has been demonstrated. The capability of DOCT to measure flow within a scattering sample also has potential in new areas of research such as micro-fluidics [120].

5.6.3 Optical microangiography

Optical micro-angiography (OMAG) is a functional extension to FD-OCT imaging modality, capable of resolving 3D distribution of dynamic blood perfusion at the capillary level within micro-circulatory beds *in vivo*. Unlike Doppler OCT to image blood flow, OMAG explores implicitly the phase information embedded in the OCT spectral interferograms. By using heterodyne technology, OMAG method effectively separates the scattering signals caused by the moving scatters, for example moving blood cells, from the scattering signals backscattered by the static tissue background, i.e., by the tissue microstructures, to achieve imaging of blood perfusion. In essence, OMAG mathematically maps the backscattered optical signals from the moving particles into one image – that is, the blood flow image – while it simultaneously maps the backscattered optical signals from the static particles into a second image, which is the microstructural image, identical to the conventional OCT image. In OMAG, the spatial interferogram in the lateral direction (B-scan) is modulated with a Doppler frequency feasible to separate the moving and static scattering components within sample. This Doppler modulation frequency can be introduced either by mounting the reference mirror in the reference arm onto a linear piezo-translation stage, that moves the mirror at a constant velocity across the B scan (i.e., *x*-direction scan) or simply by the inherent scattering fluid flow within sample. In the earlier version of the OMAG system [121, 122], this is achieved by mounting the reference mirror in the reference arm onto a linear piezo-translation stage that moved the mirror at a constant velocity across the B scan (i.e., *x*-direction scan). However, the latest version of OMAG utilizes the spatial modulation frequency provided by the inherent blood flow modulation rather than reference arm modulation [123]. OMAG is an emerging imaging modality with clear potential applications in many basic research and medical imaging applications. Because of its exceptionally high spatial resolution and velocity sensitivity, OMAG can provide useful information regarding microcirculation in a number of applications, both in clinical [124, 125] and basic research [126].

5.6.4 Spectroscopic OCT

Spectroscopic OCT is an alternative mode of OCT, which provides further access to the composition and functional state of the specimen. Spectroscopic OCT can be implemented in a variety of ways. One approach is based on spectral ratio imaging of OCT images using two or more spectral bands with wavelength division multiplexer, which combine lights with different wavelength and then electronically distinguish the resulting signal by their different Doppler shift resulting from the reference arm scan [127, 128]. By use of state-of-the-art ultra-broadband femtosecond Ti:Al_2O_3 lasers, spectroscopic imaging over the wavelength range from 650 to 1000 nm has been reported by Morgner et. al [129]. Another implementation is based on estimation of depth resolved spectral of the source spectrum, in which the modification of the source spectrum caused by the sample can be measured directly from the Fourier domain processing of cross-correlation interferometric data [130, 131].

5.6.5 Second harmonic OCT

Second harmonic OCT incorporates the uses coherence gating of second-order nonlinear optical response of biological tissues for imaging of tissue structure with molecular contrast [132, 133]. Optical second harmonic generation (SHG) is the lowest order nonlinear optical process where the second order nonlinear optical susceptibility is responsible for the generation of light at second harmonic frequency. Femtosecond laser pulses were usually used to excite second harmonic waves from biological specimens in conjunction with a reference nonlinear crystal. Second harmonic interference fringe signals were detected and used for image construction. Because of the strong dependence of second harmonic generation on molecular and tissue structures, this technique offers contrast and resolution enhancement to conventional optical coherence tomography. The second order nonlinear optical susceptibility is sensitive to electron configurations, molecular structure and symmetry, local morphology, and ultra-structures, thus, SHG provides molecular contrast for the coherence image.

5.7 Applications and New Trends in OCT

5.7.1 Medical applications

OCT has recently emerged as a promising imaging technique, mainly for medical applications. It has a number of features that make it attractive for a broad range of biological, clinical and material investigations. First, the imaging can be performed *in situ* and nondestructively. The image resolution of the order 10–15 μm is now routine using standard technology, and high resolution of the order of 1 μm may be achieved using state-of-the-art laser systems. High speed, real-time imaging is possible with more than video rate acquisition. OCT can be interfaced with a wide range of imaging delivery systems and imaging probes. The specific features of OCT compare with alternative optical techniques such as the depth resolution which is independent of the sample beam aperture and that the coherence gate can substantially improve the probing depth in scattering medium and make this technique a unique place in clinical imaging.

So far, the most successful medical application of OCT that has been identified and developed is in the field of ophthalmology due to the low scattering found in the optical materials of the eye [134, 135]. OCT has provided ophthalmologists with depth resolution in imaging the posterior and anterior of the eye previously only achievable with histology. OCT can detect subtle changes to the eye caused during early stages of ocular disease, such as age-related macular degeneration [136, 137], diabetic retinopathy [138, 139], macular holes [140, 141], intraocular tumors [142] and glaucoma [143, 144, 145]. Other than ophthalmology, imaging studies using OCT have been performed in a wide range of biological, medical and surgical specialties including developmental biology [146], cardiology [147], gastroenterology [148], urology [149] and neurosurgery [150].

Fiber-based OCT can be integrated into different imaging delivery systems including catheters and forward imaging devices to enable internal body OCT imaging [151]. More recently, an OCT catheter has been combined with endoscope based delivery to perform *in vivo* imaging in animal models and human patients. Endoscopic OCT can increase the functionality, detecting the sub-surface margins of lesions and quantifying tumor volumes. The feasibility of OCT to perform image guided surgical intervention has been investigated. OCT has been used to monitor laser ablation therapy in real-time and may enable more precise control of laser delivery [152].

Apart from the more immediate medical applications of OCT, it has been demonstrated in the field of developmental biology and cell research as a method to perform high resolution, high speed imaging of developing morphology and function [146, 153]. The ability of OCT to identify the mitotic activity, the nuclear to cytoplasmic ratio, and the migration of cells has the potential to not only impact cell and developmental biology, but also impact medical and surgical disciplines for early diagnostics of diseases such as cancer [154].

5.7.2 Non-medical applications

While the majority of OCT applications have been in the field of biology and medicine. OCT has also been demonstrated in the non-biological areas of materials investigation [155, 156], optical data storage [157], and microfluidic devices [158]. OCT has been used to identify subsurface defects in ceramic and polymer composites. The optical ranging capability of OCT through scattering materials has been utilized for increasing the data storage capability by assembling multiple layers of optically accessible data. The advancement of micro-fabrication techniques has led to increasing complex and bioMEM (biological micro-electro-mechanical) systems. Microstructures within the microfluidic systems range from 10–1000 μm, which is within both imaging depth and resolution of OCT. In addition, microfluidic systems are typically fabricated from transparent or semi-transparent substrates, facilitating imaging penetration to deeper 3D features [12].

5.7.3 New trends in OCT

Although already being applied to a number of medical and non-medical problems, the OCT technology itself is still evolving and there have also been further developments in the refinement of OCT. The threshold of a new era in OCT imaging with the transformation of technology from the current "time-domain" OCT to the "spectral domain" or "frequency domain" OCT. FD-OCT will allow much faster image capture because it does not require the reference mirror movement that is necessary in current "time-domain" systems [159]. It appears that FD-OCT can result in as many as 60,000,000 A-scans per second [160]. The major benefit of FD-OCT is that it permits point-to-point registration and can give accurate volumetric analysis. Not only has technology already improved upon OCT, but it has also made imaging scans easier and clearer than ever before. Ultra-high speed FD-OCT allows imaging of large areas of the retina and rapid three-dimensional volume rendering of optic nerve head and fovea [161]. Scientists and researchers have already begun refining the technique of OCT to view biological tissues as they are in the body. This represents a transition in technology from two-dimensional imaging to three-dimensional screening of large retinal volumes that is also an achievement in the efficiency of three-dimensional imaging [161]. Furthermore, OCT has been improved upon to speed up imaging scans and increase clarity of the image. This new technology is definitely a more efficient method compared to standard procedures [161]. Every photon that is emitted is detected, thus increasing efficiency by a factor of a hundred and fifty. This is extremely beneficial because the imaging speed is increased without decreasing the quality of the image. This new progress made in OCT is going to make it easier for medical practitioners to perform quick and easy non-invasive procedures.

Research and development concerned with the improvement of fundamental characteristics such as imaging resolution, speed and sensitivity are very active. Some of the technology and application areas currently having great impact on the field are ultra-high resolution system [162], polarization sensitive imaging, high-speed, high-sensitive optical spectral-domain systems such as SS-OCT and FD-OCT, and novel approaches like full-field or wide-field OCT [163, 164, 165, 166]. Another active area of research involved the use of external contrast agents to enhance both penetration, through reduced scattering (optical clearing), and contrast through enhanced refractive index variation, which can enable the enhanced visualization of selected futures such as abnormal tissues, microvasculature, etc. [167, 168, 169]. There are numerous research applications of this technology in a broad range of fields. In addition advances in technology are continuing. More research remains to be done, and numerous clinical studies must be performed in order to determine where OCT can play a role in clinical medicine, apart from ophthalmology. However, unique capabilities of OCT imaging suggest that it will have significant impact on fundamental research as well as on medicine.

5.8 Conclusion

OCT is a high resolution, non-invasive, 3D-imaging technique with great potential in both clinical and fundamental research application in many areas. Its wide range of current applications ranges from medical diagnosis and surgical guidance to the characterization of polymer micro-structures and reading of multi-layered storage media etc., which indicate that OCT will play a major role in practical scientific innovation and research in years to come. Therefore, it is essential that OCT technologies are developed further as an enabling measurement technology. The exceptionally high spatial resolution and velocity sensitivity, the functional extension of the OCT technique, could simultaneously provide tissue structure, blood perfusion, birefringence, and other physiological information; thus it has great potential for basic biomedical research and clinical medicine. OCT has the far reaching potential to be a quantitative imaging technique that could impact many as yet unexplored areas, and should therefore be considered a vital measurement tool. Important emerging fields already impacted by OCT are those of tissue engineering and polymer composite manufacture. To realize true optical biopsy, and full optical diagnosis and grading of malignant tumors by OCT will require a great number of clinical trials, and solid experimental demonstration of the robustness of the technique. To enable such developments, the measurement technique must also be quantitatively validated. In particular, the clinical potential and reliability of OCT will be greatly enhanced by validated measurements of volume, structural dimensions and flow. These stringent requirements present new and exciting challenges for optical medical metrology. Clearly it will not be possible to fulfill all of these criteria immediately. However, as these issues are addressed, the applicability of OCT can only grow.

Acknowledgments

We thank many of our colleagues who have contributed to the OCT/OMAG project at the Wang laboratory, particularly the graduate students and postdoctoral fellows. Dr. Wang also acknowledges grant supports from the National Heart, Lung, and Blood Institute (R01 HL093140, R01HL093140S), National Institute of Biomedical Imaging and Bioengineering (R01EB009682), National Institute on Deafness and Other Communication Disorders (R01DC010201, R01DC010201S) and the American Heart Association Grant-in-Aid (0855733G).

References

[1] N. Tanno, T. Ichikawa, A. Saeki, "Lightwave Reflection Measurement," *Japanese Patent* No. 2010042 (1990) (Japanese Language).

[2] S. Chiba, N. Tanno "Backscattering Optical Heterodyne Tomography," prepared for the *14th Laser Sensing Symposium* (1991) (Japanese language).

[3] D. Huang, E.A. Swanson, C.P. Lin, J.S. Shuman, W.G. Stinson, W. Chang, M.R. Hee, T. Flotte, K. Gregory, C.A. Puliafito, and J.G. Fujimoto, "Optical coherence tomography," *Science* **254**, 1178–1181 (1991).

[4] A.F. Fercher, K. Mengedoht, and W. Werner, "Eye-length measurement by interferometry with partially coherent light," *Opt. Lett.* **13**, 1867–1869 (1988).

[5] C.K. Hitzenberger, W. Drexler, and A.F. Fercher, "Measurement of corneal thickness by laser doppler interferometry," *Invest. Ophthalmol. Vis. Sci.* **33**, 98–103 (1992).

[6] J.A. Izatt, M.R. Hee, E.A. Swanson, C.P. Lin, D. Huang, J.S. Schuman, C.A. Puliafito, and J.G. Fujimoto, "Micrometer-scale resolution imaging of the anterior eye with optical coherence tomography," *Arch. Ophthalmol.* **112**, 1584–1589 (1994).

[7] W. Clivaz, F. Marquis-Weible, R.P. Salathe, R.P. Novak, and H.H. Gilgen, "High-resolution reflectometry in biological tissue," *Opt. Lett.* **17**, 4–6 (1992).

[8] J.M. Schmitt, A. Knüttel, and R.F. Bonner, "Measurement of optical properties of biological tissues by low-coherence reflectometry," *Appl. Opt.* **32**, 6032–6042 (1993).

[9] X. Clivaz, F. Marquis-Weible, R.P. Salathé, R.P. Novak, and H.H. Gilgen, "High resolution reflectometry in biological tissues," *Optics Letters* **17**, 4–6 (1992).

[10] J.O. Schenk and M.E. Brezinski, "Ultrasound induced improvement in optical coherence tomography (OCT) resolution," *PNAS* **99**, 9761–9764 (2002).

[11] A.M Rollins, "Another way to peer inside the body: optical coherence tomography combines interferometry and high-tech light sources to capture images of living tissue," *Machine Design* (2005) [online]. Available from: http://www.machinedesign.com/ASP/viewSelectedArticle.asp?strArticleId=57768&strSite=MDSite&catId=0 [Accessed 11 January 2007].

[12] B.E. Bouma and G.J. Tearney (eds.) *Handbook of Optical Coherence Tomography*, Marcel Dekker, Inc. (2003).

[13] P. Latkany, "Retinal Disease: Evolving Treatment Approaches," *Medscape Medical News* (2006) [online]. Available from: http://www.medscape.com/viewarticle/549001 [Accessed 11 Jan. 2007].

[14] P.H. Tomlins and R.K. Wang, "Theory, developments and applications of optical coherence tomography," *Journal of Physics D: Applied Physics* **38**(15), 2519–2535 (2005).

[15] R.C. Youngquist, S. Carr, and D.E.N. Davies, "Optical coherence-domain reflectometry — a new optical evaluation technique," *Opt. Lett.* **12**, 158–160 (1987).

[16] K. Takada, I. Yokohama, K. Chida, and J. Noda, "New measurement system for fault location in optical waveguide devices based on an interferometric technique," *Appl. Opt.* **26**, 1603–1606 (1987).

[17] E. Hecht, *Optics*, 3rd Ed, Addison Wesley (1998).

[18] J.W. Goodman, *Statistical Optics*, John Wiley & Sons (1985).

[19] E.A. Swanson, D. Huang, M.R. Hee, J.G. Fujimoto, C.P. Lin, and C.A. Puliafito, *Opt. Lett.* **17**, 151 (1992).

[20] A. Fercher, W. Drexler, C.K. Hitzenberger, and T. Lasser, "Optical coherence tomography — principles and applications," *Rep. Progr. Phys.* **66**, 239–303 (2003).

[21] A.F. Fercher, C.K. Hitzenberger, G. Kamp, and S.Y. Elzaiat, "Measurement of intraocular distances by backscattering spectral interferometry," *Opt. Commun.* **117**, 43–48 (1995).

[22] J.M. Schmitt and G. Kumar, "Optical scattering properties of soft tissue: A discrete particle model," *Appl. Opt.* **37**, 2788–2797 (1998).

[23] J.M. Schmitt, A. Knuttel, M. Yadlowsky, and M.A. Eckhaus, "Optical-coherence tomography of a dense tissue: statistics of attenuation and backscattering," *Phys. Med. Biol.* **39**, 1705 (1994)

[24] B. Povaay, K. Bizheva, B. Hermann, A. Unterhuber, H. Sattmann, A.F. Fercher, W. Drexler, C. Schubert, P.K. Ahnelt, M. Mei, R. Holzwarth, W.J. Wadsworth, J.C. Knight, and P.S. Russel, "Enhanced visualization ofchoroidal vessels using ultrahigh resolution ophthalmic OCT at 1050 nm," *Opt. Express* **11**, 1980–1986 (2003).

[25] A. Unterhuber, B. Povaay, B. Hermann, H. Sattmann, A. Chavez-Pirson, and W. Drexler, "In vivo retinaloptical coherence tomography at 1040 nm-enhanced penetration into the choroid," *Opt. Express* **13**, 3252–3258 (2005).

[26] B. Povaay, B. Hermann, A. Unterhuber, B. Hofer, H. Sattmann, F. Zeiler, J.E. Morgan, C. Falkner-Radler, C. Glittenberg, S. Binder, and W. Drexler, "Three-dimensional optical coherence tomography at 1050 nm versus 800 nm in retinal pathologies: enhanced performance and choroidal penetration in cataract patients," *J. Biomed. Opt.* **12**, 041211 (2007).

[27] D.M. de Bruin, D.L. Burnes, J. Loewenstein, Y. Chen, S. Chang, T.C. Chen, D.D. Esmaili, and J.F. de Boer, "*In vivo* three-dimensional imaging of neovascular age-related macular degeneration using optical frequency domain imaging at 1050 nm," *Invest. Ophthalmol. Vis. Sci.* **49**, 4545–4552 (2008).

[28] R. Huber, D. Adler, V. Srinivasan, and J.G. Fujimoto, "Fourier domain mode locking at 1050 nm for ultrahigh-speed optical coherence tomography of the human retina at 236000 axial scans per second," *Opt. Lett.* **32**, 2049–2051 (2007).

[29] C.F. Lin and B.L. Lee, "Extremely broadband AlGaAs/GaAs superluminescent diodes," *Appl. Phys. Lett.* **71**, 1598–1600 (1997).

[30] C.F. Lin, B.R. Wu, L.W. Laih, and T.T. Shih, "Sequence influence of nonidentical InGaAsP quantum wells on broadband characteristics of semiconductor optical amplifiers superluminescent diodes," *Opt. Lett.* **26**, 1099–1101 (2001).

[31] P.J. Poole, M. Davies, M. Dion, Y. Feng, S. Charbonneau, R. D.Goldberg, and I.V. Mitchell, "The fabrication of a broad-spectrum light-emitting diode using high-energy ion implantation," *IEEE Photon.Technol. Lett* **8**, 1145–1147 (1996).

[32] J.R. Digonnet, *Rare Earth Doped Fiber Lasers and Amplifiers*, New York: Marcel Dekker (1993).

[33] B.E. Bouma, G.J. Tearney, S.A. Boppart, M.R. Hee, M.E. Brezinski, and J.G. Fujimoto, "High-resolution optical coherence tomographic imaging using a mode-locked Ti:Al_2O_3 laser source," *Opt. Lett.* **20**, 1486–1489 (1995).

[34] X. Clivaz, F. Marquis-Weible, and R.P. Salathe, "Optical low-coherence reflectometry with 1.9 mm spatial resolution," *Electronics Lett.* **28**, 1553–1555 (1992).

[35] B.E. Bouma, G.J. Tearney, I.P. Biliinski, B. Golubovic, J.G. Fujimoto, "Self-phase-modulated Kerr-lens mode-locked Cr: foorsterite laser source for optical coherence tomography," *Opt. Lett.* **21**, 1839–1842 (1996).

[36] T.A. Birks, W.J. Wadsworth, and P.S.J. Russell, "Supercontinuum generation in tapered fibers," *Opt. Lett.* **25**, 1415–1417 (2000).

[37] A.L. Gaeta, "Nonlinear propagation and continuum generationin microstructured optical fibers," *Opt. Lett.* **27**, 924–926 (2002).

[38] D.L. Marks, A.L. Oldenburg, J.J. Reynolds, and S.A. Boppart, "Digital algorithm for dispersion correction in optical coherence tomography for homogeneous and stratified media," *Appl. Opt.* **42**, 204–217 (2003).

[39] A. Unterhuber, B. Povazay, B. Hermann, H. Sattmann, W. Drexler, V. Yakovlev, G. Tempea, C. Schubert, E.M. Anger, P.K. Ahnelt, M. Stur, J.E. Morgan, A. Cowey, G. Jung, and A.S.T. Le, "Compact, low-cost $TiAl_2O_3$ laser for *in vivo* ultrahigh-resolution optical coherence tomography," *Opt. Lett.* **28**, 905–907 (2003).

[40] B. Povazay, K. Bizheva, A. Unterhuber, B. Hermann, H. Sattmann, A. F. Fercher, W. Drexler, A. Apolonski, W.J. Wadsworth, J.C. Knight, P.St.J. Russell, M. Vetterlein, and E. Scherzer, "Submicrometer axial resolutionoptical coherence tomography," *Opt. Lett.* **27**, 1800–1802 (2002).

[41] A. Aguirre, N. Nishizawa, J. Fujimoto, W. Seitz, M. Lederer, and D. Kopf, "Continuum generation in a novelphotonic crystal fiber for ultrahigh resolution optical coherence tomography at 800 nm and 1300 nm," *Opt. Express* **14**, 1145–1160 (2006).

[42] H. Wang, and A.M. Rollins, "Optimization of dual-band continuum light source for ultrahigh-resolution optical coherence tomography," *Appl. Opt.* **46**, 1787–1794 (2007).

[43] P. Cimalla, J. Walther, M. Mehner, M. Cuevas, and E. Koch, "Simultaneous dual-band optical coherence tomography in the spectral domain for high resolution *in vivo* imaging," *Opt. Express* **17**, 19486-19500 (2009).

[44] F. Spöler, S. Kray, P. Grychtol, B. Hermes, J. Bornemann, M. Först, and H. Kurz, "Simultaneous dual-band ultra-high resolution optical coherence tomography," *Opt. Express* **15**, 10832–10841 (2007).

[45] S. Kray, F. Spöler, M. Först, and H. Kurz, "High-resolution simultaneous dual-band spectral domain optical coherence tomography," *Opt. Lett.* **34**, 1970–1972 (2009).

[46] S.H. Yun, C. Boudoux, G.J. Tearney, and B.E. Bouma, "High-speed wavelength-swept semiconductor laser with a polygon-scanner-based wavelength filter," *Opt. Lett.* **28**, 1981–1983 (2003).

[47] S. Yun, G. Tearney, J. de Boer, N. Iftimia, and B. Bouma, "High-speed optical frequency-domain imaging," *Opt. Express* **11**, 2953–2963 (2003).

[48] R. Huber, M. Wojtkowski, J.G. Fujimoto, J.Y. Jiang, and A.E. Cable, "Three-dimensional and C-mode OCT imaging with a compact, frequency swept laser source at 1300 nm," *Opt. Express* **13**, 10523–10538 (2005).

[49] M.A. Choma, K. Hsu, and J.A. Izatt, "Swept source optical coherence tomography using an all-fiber 1300-nm ring laser source," *J. Biomed. Opt.* **10**, 044009 (2005).

[50] R. Huber, M. Wojtkowski, K. Taira, J. Fujimoto, and K. Hsu, "Amplified, frequency swept lasers for frequency domain reflectometry and OCT imaging: design and scaling principles," *Opt. Express* **13**, 3513–3528 (2005).

[51] R. Huber, M. Wojtkowski, and J.G. Fujimoto, "Fourier Domain Mode Locking (FDML): A new laser operating regime and applications for optical coherence tomography," *Opt. Express* **14**, 3225–3237 (2006).

[52] R. Huber, D.C. Adler, and J.G. Fujimoto, "Buffered Fourier domain mode locking: Unidirectional swept laser sources for optical coherence tomography imaging at 370,000 lines/s," *Opt. Lett.* **31**, 2975–2977 (2006).

[53] M.Y. Jeon, J. Zhang, and Z. Chen, "Characterization of Fourier domain mode-locked wavelength swept laser for optical coherence tomography imaging," *Opt. Express* **16**, 3727–3737 (2008).

[54] G.Y. Liu, A. Mariampillai, B.A. Standish, N.R. Munce, X. Gu, and I. A. Vitkin, "High power wavelength linearly swept mode locked fiber laser for OCT imaging," *Opt. Express* **16**, 14095–14105 (2008).

[55] Y. Mao, C. Flueraru, S. Sherif, and S. Chang, "High performance wavelength-swept laser with mode-locking technique for optical coherence tomography," *Opt. Commun.* **282**, 88–92 (2009).

[56] J. G. Fujimoto, "Optical coherence tomography for ultrahigh resolution *in vivo* imaging," *Nature Biotechnology* **21**, 1361-1367 (2003).

[57] M.E. Brezinski, G.J. Tearney, S.A. Boppart, B.E. Bouma, E.A. Swanson, J.F. Southern, and J.G. Fujimoto, "High speed catheter based OCT imaging of coronary microstructure," *Circulation* **94**, 1494–1494 (1996).

[58] W. Drexler, U. Morgner, F.X. Kartner, C. Pitris, S.A. Boppart, X.D. Li, E.P. Ippen, and J.G. Fujimoto, "*In vivo* ultrahigh-resolution optical coherence tomography," *Opt. Lett.* **24**, 1221–1223 (1999).

[59] Yu Chen, Shu-Wei Huang, Aaron D. Aguirre, and James G. Fujimoto, "High-resolution line-scanning optical coherence microscopy," *Opt. Lett.* **32**, 1971–1973 (2007).

[60] Y. Watanabe, K. Yamada, and M. Sato, "*In vivo* nonmechanical scanning grating-generated optical coherence tomography using an InGaAs digital camera," *Opt. Commun.* **261**, 376–380 (2006).

[61] Y. Watanabe, K. Yamada, and M. Sato, "Three-dimensional imaging by ultrahigh-speed axial-lateral parallel time domain optical coherence tomography," *Opt. Express* **14**, 5201–5209 (2006).

[62] E. Beaurepaire, A.C. Boccara, M. Lebec, L. Blanchot, and H. Saint-Jalmes, "Full-field optical coherence tomography," *Opt. Lett.* **23**, 244–246 (1998).

[63] E. Bordenave, E. Abraham, G. Jonusauskas, N. Tsurumachi, J. Oberl, C. Rulliére, P. Minot, M. Lasségues, J. Bazeille, "Wide-field optical coherence tomography: imaging of biological tissues," *Appl. Opt.* **41**, 2059–2064 (2002).

[64] S. Bourquin, V. Monterosso, P. Seitz, and R. P. Salathe, "Video-rate optical low-coherence reflectometry based on a linear smart detector array," *Opt. Lett.* **25**, 102–104 (2000).

[65] K. Creath, "Phase measurement interferometry techniques," in: *Progress in Optics*, E. Wolf (ed.), Vol. 24, Elsevier Science Publishers, Amsterdam, 349–393 (1988).

[66] G.S. Kino and S.S.C. Chim, "Mirau correlation microscope," *Appl. Opt.* **29**, 3775–3783 (1990).

[67] M. Davidson, K. Kaufman, I. Mazor, and F. Cohen, "An application of interference microscope to integrated circuit inspection and metrology," *SPIE*, **775**, 233–247 (1987).

[68] A. Dubois, A.C. Boccara, and M. Lebec, "Real-time reflectivity and topography imagery of depth-resolved microscopic surfaces," *Opt. Lett.* **24**, 309–311 (1999).

[69] A. Dubois, L. Vabre, A.C. Boccara, and E. Beaurepaire, "High-resolution full-field optical coherence tomography with a Linnik microscope," *Appl. Opt.* **41**, 805–812 (2002).

[70] W.Y. Oh, B.E. Bouma, N. Iftimia, S.H. Yun, R. Yelin, and G.J. Tearney, "Ultrahigh-resolution full-field optical coherence microscopy using InGaAs camera," *Opt. Express* **14**, 726–735 (2006).

[71] A.F. Fercher, C.K. Hitzenberger, M. Sticker, E. Moreno-Barriuso, R. Leitgeb, W. Drexler, and H. Sattmann, "A thermal light source technique for optical coherence tomography," *Opt. Commun.* **185**, 57–64 (2000).

[72] B. Karamata, P. Lambelet, M. Laubscher, R.P. Salathé, and T. Lasser, "Spatially incoherent illumination as a mechanism for cross-talk suppression in wide-field optical coherence tomography," *Opt. Lett..* **29**, 736–738 (2004).

[73] M.S. Hrebesh, R. Dabu, and M. Sato, "*In vivo* imaging of dynamic biological specimen by real-time single-shot full-field optical coherence tomography," *Opt. Commun.* **282**, 674–683 (2009).

[74] M.S. Hrebesh, Y. Watanabe, M. Sato, "Spatial phase-shifting interferometer using paired wedge prism and combined wave plate," *Japanese J. of Appl. Phys., Part 2: Letters*, **46**, L369–L371 (2007).

[75] M.S. Hrebesh, Y. Watanabe, and M. Sato, "Profilometry with compact single-shot low-coherence time-domain interferometry," *Opt. Commun.* **281**, 4566–4571 (2008).

[76] G. Hausler and M.W. Lindner, "Coherence radar and spectral radar: new tools for dermatological diagnosis," *J. Biomed. Opt.* **3**, 21–31 (1998).

[77] R. Leitgeb, C.K. Hitzenberger, and A.F. Fercher, "Performance of Fourier domain vs. time domain optical coherence tomography," *Opt. Express* **11,** 889–894 (2003).

[78] M.A. Choma, M.V. Sarunic, C.H. Yang, and J.A. Izatt, "Sensitivity advantage of swept source and Fourier domain optical coherence tomography," *Opt. Express* **11**, 2183–2189 (2003).

[79] J.F. de Boer, B. Cense, B.H. Park, M.C. Pierce, G.J. Tearney, and B.E. Bouma, "Improved signal-to-noise ratio in spectral-domain compared with time-domain optical coherence tomography," *Opt. Lett.* **28**, 2067–2069 (2003).

[80] M. Wojtkowski, A. Kowalczyk, R. Leitgeb, and A.F. Fercher, "Full range complex spectral optical coherencetomography technique in eye imaging," *Opt. Lett.* **27**, 1415–1417 (2002).

[81] R.K. Wang and Z. Ma, "A practical approach to eliminate autocorrelation artefacts for volume-rate spectral domain optical coherence tomography," *Physics in Medicine and Biology* **51**(12), 3231 (2006).

[82] B. Grajciar, M. Pircher, A.F. Fercher, and R.A. Leitgeb, "Parallel Fourier domain optical coherence tomographyfor *in vivo* measurement of the human eye," *Opt. Express* **13**, 1131–1137 (2005).

[83] T. Endo, Y. Yasuno, F. Truffer, G. Aoki, S. Makita, M. Itoh, and T. Yatagai, "Line-field Fourier-domain optical coherence tomography," *Proc. SPIE* **5690**, 168–173 (2005).

[84] S.R. Chinn, E.A. Swanson, and J.G. Fujimoto, "Optical coherence tomography using a frequency-tunable optical source," *Opt. Lett.* **22**, 340–342 (1997).

[85] R. Huber, M. Wojtkowski, and J.G. Fujimoto, "Fourier Domain Mode Locking (FDML): A new laser operating regime and applications for optical coherence tomography," *Opt. Express* **14**, 3225–3237 (2006).

[86] R.K.Wang and Z. Ma, "Real-time flow imaging by removing texture attern artifacts in spectral-domain optical Doppler tomography," *Optics Letters* **31**(20), 3001–3003 (2006).

[87] Lee, S.-W. Kim, B.-M. "Line-field optical coherence tomography using frequency-sweeping source," *IEEE J. Sel. Top. Quantum Electron*, **14**, 50–55 (2008).

[88] M. Sarunic, M.A. Choma, C. Yang, and J.A. Izatt, "Instantaneous complex conjugate resolved spectral domain and swept-source OCT using 3×3 fiber couplers," *Opt. Express* **13**, 957–967 (2005).

[89] R.K. Wang, "*In vivo* full range complex Fourier domain optical coherence tomography," *Appl. Phys. Lett.* **90**, 054103 (2007).

[90] Y. Yasuno, S. Makita, T.Endo, M. Itoh, and T. Yatagai, "Simultaneous B-M-mode scanning method for real time Fourier domain optical coherence tomography," *Appl. Opt.* **45**, 1861–1865 (2006).

[91] L. An and R.K. Wang, "Use of a scanner to modulate spatial interferograms for *in vivo* full-range Fourier-domain optical coherence tomography," *Opt. Lett.* **32**, 3423–3425 (2007).

[92] M.R. Hee, D. Huang, E.A. Swanson, and J.G. Fujimoto, "Polarization sensitive low-coherence reflectometer for birefringence characterization and ranging," *JOSA B* **9**, 903–908 (1992).

[93] E. Gotzinger, M. Pircher, and C.K. Hitzenberger, "High speed spectral domain polarization sensitive optical coherence tomography of the human retina," *Opt. Express* **13**, 10217–10229 (2005).

[94] Y. Yasuno, S. Makita, Y. Sutoh, M. Itoh, and T. Yatagai, "Birefringence imaging of human skin by polarization-sensitive spectral interferometric optical coherence tomography," Opt. Lett. **27**, 1803-1805 (2002).

[95] B.H. Park, M.C. Pierce, B. Cense, S.H. Yun, M. Mujat, G.J. Tearney, B.E. Bouma, and J.F. de Boer, "Real-time fiber-based multi-functional spectral-domain optical coherence tomography at 1.3 μm," *Opt. Express* **13**, 3931–3944 (2005).

[96] S. Makita, Y. Yasuno, T. Endo, M. Itoh, and T. Yatagai, "Polarization contrast imaging of biological tissues by polarization-sensitive Fourier-domain optical coherence tomography," *Appl. Opt.* **45**, 1142–1147 (2006).

[97] M. Yamanari, S. Makita, V.D. Madjarova, T. Yatagai, and Y. Yasuno, "Fiber-based polarization-sensitive Fourier domain optical coherence tomography using B-scan-oriented polarization modulation method," *Opt. Express* **14**, 6502–6515 (2006).

[98] M. Yamanari, S. Makita, and Y. Yasuno, "Polarization-sensitive swept-source optical coherence tomography with continuous source polarization modulation," *Opt. Express* **16**, 5892–5906 (2008).

[99] J.F. de Boer, S.M. Srinivas, A. Malekafzali, Z. Chen, and J.S. Nelson, "Imaging thermally damaged tissue by polarization sensitive optical coherence tomography," *Opt. Express* **3**, 212–218 (1998).

[100] C.E. Saxer, J.F. de Boer, B.H. Park, Y. Zhao, Z. Chen, and J.S. Nelson, "High-speed fiber-based polarization-sensitive optical coherence tomography of *in vivo* human skin," *Opt. Lett.* **25**, 1355–1357 (2000).

[101] J. Shuliang and L.V. Wang, "Two-dimensional depth-resolved Mueller matrix of biological tissue measured with double-beam polarization-sensitive optical coherence tomography," *Opt. Lett.* **27**, 101–103 (2002).

[102] J. Shuliang, Y. Gang, and L.V. Wang, "Depth-resolved two-dimensional Stokes vectors of backscattered light and Mueller matrices of biological tissue measured with optical coherence tomography," *Appl. Opt.* **39**, 6318–6324 (2000).

[103] J.F. de Boer, T.E. Milner, M.J.C. van Gemert, and J.S. Nelson, "Two-dimensional birefringence imaging in biological tissue by polarization-sensitive optical coherence tomography," *Opt. Lett.* **22**, 934–936 (1997).

[104] S.J. Matcher, M. Cope, and D.T. Delpy, "*In vivo* measurements of the wavelength dependence of tissue-scattering coefficients between 760 and 900 nm measured with time-resolved spectroscopy," *Appl. Opt.* **36**, 386–396 (1997).

[105] Z.P. Chen, T.E. Milner, D. Dave, and J.S. Nelson, "Optical Doppler tomographic imaging of fluid flow velocity in highly scattering media," *Opt. Lett.* **22**, 64–66 (1997).

[106] Z.P. Chen, T.E. Milner, S. Srinivas, X.J. Wang, A. Malekafzali, M.J.C. van Gemert, and J.S. Nelson, "Noninvasive imaging of *in vivo* blood flow velocity using optical Doppler tomography," *Opt. Lett.* **22**, 1–3 (1997).

[107] J.A. Izatt, M.D. Kulkarni, S. Yazdanfar, J.K. Barton, and A.J. Welsh, "*In vivo* color Doppler imaging of picoliter blood volumes using optical coherence tomography," *Opt. Lett.* **22**, 1439–1441 (1997).

[108] S. Yazdanfar, M.D. Kulkarni, and J.A. Izatt, "High-resolution of *in-vivo* cardiac dynamics using color Doppler optical coherence tomography," *Opt. Express* **1**, 424–431 (1997).

[109] M.D. Kulkarni, T.G. van Leeuwen, S. Yazdanfar, and J.A. Izatt, "Velocity-estimation accuracy and frame-rate limitations in color Doppler optical coherence tomography," *Opt. Lett.* **23**, 1057–1059 (1997).

[110] Z. Ding, Y. Zhao, H. Ren, J. Nelson, and Z. Chen, "Real-time phase-resolved optical coherence tomography and optical Doppler tomography," *Opt. Express* **10**, 236–245 (2002).

[111] B.R. White, M.C. Pierce, N. Nassif, B. Cense, B.H. Park, G.J. Tearney, B.E. Bouma, T.C. Chen, and J.F. de Boer, "*In vivo* dynamic human retinal blood flow imaging using ultra-high-speed spectral domain optical Doppler tomography," *Opt. Express* **11**, 3490–3497 (2003).

[112] R.A. Leitgeb, L. Schmetterer, W. Drexler, A.F. Fercher, R.J. Zawadzki, and T. Bajraszewski, "Real-time assessment of retinal blood flow with ultrafast acquisition by color Doppler Fourier domain optical coherence tomography," *Opt. Express* **11**, 3116–3121 (2003).

[113] R.A. Leitgeb, L. Schmetterer, C.K. Hitzenberger, A.F. Fercher, F. Berisha, M. Wojtkowski, and T. Bajraszewski, "Real-time measurement of in vitro flow by Fourier-domain color Doppler optical coherence tomography," *Opt. Lett.* **29**, 171–173 (2004).

[114] Z. Chen, Y. Zhao, S.M. Srinivas, J.S. Nelson, N. Prakash, and R.D. Frostig, "Optical Doppler tomography," *IEEE J. Sel. Top. Quantum Electron.* **5**, 1134–1141 (1999).

[115] S. Makita, Y. Hong, M. Yamanari, T. Yatagai, and Y. Yasuno, "Optical coherence angiography," *Opt. Express* **14**, 7821–7840 (2006).

[116] M.A. Choma, A.K. Ellerbee, S. Yazdanfar, and J.A. Izatt, "Doppler flow imaging of cytoplasmic streaming using spectral domain phase microscopy," *J. Biomed. Opt.* **11**, 024014 (2006).

[117] A. Mariampillai, B.A. Standish, N.R. Munce, C. Randall, G. Liu, J. Y. Jiang, A.E. Cable, I.A. Vitkin, and V.X.D. Yang, "Doppler optical cardiogram gated 2D color flow imaging at 1000 fps and 4D *in vivo* visualization of embryonic heart at 45 fps on a swept source OCT system," *Opt. Express* **15**, 1627–1638 (2007).

[118] H. Wehbe, M. Ruggeri, S. Jiao, G. Gregori, C.A. Puliafito, and W. Zhao, "Automatic retinal blood flow calculation using spectral domain optical coherence tomography," *Opt. Express* **15**, 15193–15206 (2007).

[119] Y. Zhao, Z. Chen, C. Saxer, S. Xiang, J.F. de Boer, and J.S. Nelson, "Phase-resolved optical coherence tomography and optical Doppler tomography for imaging blood flow in human skin with fast scanning speed and high velocity sensitivity," *Opt. Lett.* **25**, 114–116 (2000).

[120] R.K. Wang, "High resolution visualisation of fluid dynamics with Doppler Optical Coherence Tomography," *Measurement Sci. and Tech.* **15**, 725–733 (2004).

[121] R.K. Wang, S.L. Jacques, Z. Ma, S. Hurst, S. Hanson, and A. Gruber, "Three dimensional optical angiography," *Opt. Express* **15**, 4083–4097 (2007).

[122] R.K. Wang, and S. Hurst, "Mapping of cerebro-vascular blood perfusion in mice with skin and skull intact by Optical Micro-Angiography at 1.3 μm wavelength," *Opt. Express* **15**, 11402–11412 (2007).

[123] R.K. Wang and L. An, "Doppler optical micro-angiography for volumetric imaging of vascular perfusion *in vivo*," *Opt. Express* **17**, 8926–8940 (2009).

[124] L. An, H.M. Subhash, D.J. Wilson, and R.K. Wang, "High resolution wide-field imaging of retinal and choroidal blood perfusion with optical micro-angiography," *J. Biomed. Opt.* **15**, 026011 (2010).

[125] R.K. Wang, L. An, S. Saunders, and D. Wilson, "Optical microangiography provides depth resolved images of directional ocular blood perfusion in posterior eye segment," *J. Biomed. Opt.* **15**, 020502 (2010).

[126] Y.L. Jia, and R.K. Wang, "Optical micro-angiography images structural and functional cerebral blood perfusion in mice with cranium left intact," *J. Biophotonics* **4**, 57-63 (2011).

[127] J.M. Schmitt, S.H. Xiang, and K.M. Yung, "Differential absorption imaging with optical coherence tomography," *J. Opt. Soc. Am. A* **15**, 2288–2296 (1998).

[128] Y. Pan and D. Farkas, "Non-invasive imaging of living human skin with dual-wavelength optical coherence tomography in two and three dimensions," *J. Biomed. Opt.* **3**, 446–455 (1998).

[129] U. Morgner, W. Drexler, F.X. Krtner, X.D. Li, C. Pitris, E.P. Ippen, and J.G. Fujimoto, "Spectroscopic optical coherence tomography," *Opt. Lett.* **25**, 111–113 (2000).

[130] R. Leitgeb, M. Wojtkowski, A. Kowalczyk, C.K. Hitzenberger, M. Sticker, and A.F. Fercher, "Spectral measurement of absorption by spectroscopic frequency-domain optical coherence tomography," *Opt. Lett.* **25**, 820–822 (2000).

[131] R. Leitgeb, M. Wojtkowski, C. Hitzenberger, A. Fercher, and H. Sattmann, "Spectroscopic analysis of substances by frequency domain optical coherence tomography," in *Coherence Domain Optical Methods In Biomedical Science And Clinica Applications V*, SPIE, Bellingham, 123-127 (2001).

[132] J. Su, I.V. Tomov, Y. Jiang, and Z. Chen, "High-resolution frequency-domain second-harmonic optical coherence tomography," *Appl. Opt.* **46**, 1770–1775 (2007).

[133] M.V. Sarunic, B.E. Applegate, and J.A. Izatt, "Spectral domain second-harmonic optical coherence tomography," *Opt. Lett.* **30**, 2391–2393 (2005).

[134] J.A. Izatt, M.R. Hee, E.A. Swanson, C.P. Lin, D. Huang, J.S. Schuman, C.A. Puliafito, and J.G. Fujimoto, "Micrometer-scale resolution imaging of the anterior eye *in vivo* with optical coherence tomography," *Arch. Ophthalmol.* **112**, 1584–1589 (1994).

[135] E.A. Swanson, J.A. Izatt, M.R. Hee, D. Huang, C.P. Lin, J.S. Schuman, C.A. Puliafito, and J.G. Fujimoto, "*In vivo* retinal imaging by optical coherence tomography," *Opt. Lett.* **18**, 1864–1866 (1993).

[136] H. Ozdemir, S.A. Karacorlu, and M. Karacorlu, "Early optical coherence tomography changes after photodynamic therapy in patients with age-related macular degeneration," *Am. J. Ophthalmol.* **141**, 574–576 (2006).

[137] A. Salinas-Alaman, A. Garcia-Layana, M.J. Maldonado, C. Sainz-Gomez, and A. Alvarez-Vidal, "Using optical coherence tomography to monitor photodynamic therapy in age related macular degeneration," *Am. J. Ophthalmol.* **140**, 23–28 (2005).

[138] W. Goebel and R. Franke, "Retinal thickness in diabetic retinopathy - Comparison of optical coherence tomography, the retinal thickness analyzer, and fundus photography," *Retina*, **26**, 49-57 (2006).

[139] A. Polito, M. Del Borrello, G. Polini, F. Furlan, M. Isola, and F. Bandello, "Diurnal variation in clinically significant diabetic macular edema measured by the stratus OCT," *Retina*, **26**, 14–20 (2006).

[140] A.J. Witkin, T.H. Ko, J.G. Fujimoto, J.S. Schuman, C.R. Baumal, A.H. Rogers, E. Reichel, and J.S. Duker, "Redefining lamellar holes and the vitreomacular interface: An ultrahigh-resolution optical coherence tomography study," *Ophthalmol.* **113**, 388–397 (2006).

[141] M.L. Subramanian, S.N. Truong, A.H. Rogers, J.S. Duker, E. Reichel, and C.R. Baumal, "Vitrectomy for stage 1 macular holes identified by optical coherence tomography," *Ophthalmic Surg. Lasers* **37**, 42–46 (2006).

[142] C.L. Shields, M.A. Materin, and J.A. Shields, "Review of optical coherence tomography for intraocular tumors," *Curr. Opin. Ophthalmol.* **16**, 141–154 (2005).

[143] B. Cense, T.C. Chen, B.H. Park, M.C. Pierce, and J.F. de Boer, "Thickness and birefringence of healthy retinal nerve fiber layer tissue measured with polarization sensitive optical coherence tomography," *Invest. Ophthalmol. Visual Sci.* **45**, 2606–2612, (2004).

[144] G. Wollstein, J.S. Schuman, L.L. Price, A. Aydin, P.C. Stark, E. Hertzmark, E. Lai, H. Ishikawa, C. Mattox, J.G. Fujimoto, and L.A. Paunescu, "Optical coherence tomography longitudinal evaluation of retinal nerve fiber layer thickness in glaucoma," *Arch. Ophthalmol.* **123**, 464–470 (2005).

[145] F.A. Medeiros, L.M. Zangwill, C. Bowd, R.M. Vessani, R. Susanna, and R.N. Weinreb, "Evaluation of retinal nerve fiber layer, optic nerve head, and macular thickness measurements for glaucoma detection using optical coherence tomography," *Am. J. Ophthalmol.* **139**, 44–55 (2005).

[146] S.A. Boppart, M.E. Brezinski, J.G. Fujimoto, "Optical coherence tomography imaging in developmental biology," *Methods Mol. Biol.* **135**, 217–33 (1999).

[147] N. Burris, K. Schwartz, C. Tang, M. Jafri, J. Schmitt, M. Kwon, O. Toshinaga, J. Gu, J. Brown, E. Brown, R. Pierson, R. Poston, "Catheter-based infrared light scanner as a tool to assess conduit quality in coronary artery bypass surgery," *J. Thorac. Cardiovasc. Surg.* **133**, 419–427 (2007).

[148] P. Testoni, A. Mariani, B. Mangiavillano, P. Arcidiacono, S. Pietro, and E. Masci, "Intraductal optical coherence tomography for investigating main pancreatic duct strictures," *Am. J. Gastroenterol.* **101**, 1–6 (2006).

[149] G.J. Tearney, M.E. Brezinski, J.F. Southern, B.E. Bouma, S.A. Boppart, J.G. Fujimoto, "Optical biopsy in human urologic tissue using optical coherence tomography," *J. Urol.* **157**, 1915–1919 (1997).

[150] S.A. Boppart, M.E. Brezinski, C. Pitris, J.G. Fujimoto, "Optical coherence tomography for neurosurgical imaging of human intracortical melanoma," *Neurosurgery* **43**, 834–841 (1998).

[151] G.J. Tearney, M.E. Brezinski, B.E. Bouma, S.A. Boppart, S. Pitris, J.H. Southern et al., "*In vivo* endoscopic optical biopsy with optical coherence tomography," *Science* **276**, 2037–2039 (1997).

[152] S.A. Boppart, J.M. Herrmann, C. Pitris, D.L. Stamper, M.E. Brezinski, J.G. Fujimoto, "Real-time optical coherence tomography for minimally-invasive imaging of prostate ablation," *Computer Aided Surgery* **6**, 94–103 (2001).

[153] C. Mason, J.F. Markusen, M.A. Town, P. Dunnill, and R.K. Wang, "The potential of optical coherence tomography in the engineering of living tissue," *Phys. Med. Biol.* **49**, 1097–1115 (2004).

[154] S.A. Boppart, W. Luo, D.L. Marks, K.W. Singletary, "Optical coherence tomography: feasibility for basic research and image-guided surgery of breast cancer," *Breast Cancer Research and Treatment* **84**, 85–97 (2004).

[155] J.P. Dunkers, F.R. Phelan, C.G. Zimba, K.M. Flynn, D.P. Sanders, R.C. Peterson, R.S. Parnas, "The prediction of permeability for an epoxy/E-glass composite using optical coherence tomographic images," *Polymer Composites*, **22**, 803 (2001).

[156] M.D. Duncan, M. Bashkansky, and J. Reintjes, "Subsurface defect detection in materials using optical coherence tomography," *Opt. Express* **13**, 540–545 (1998).

[157] Shin Yongjin, Jung Woonggyu, Chen Zhongping, S. Nelson John, Kim Hyunjin, and Park Jinseong, "Investigation of pit formation in multilayer optical storage disk using optical coherence tomography," *Proc SPIE* **5604**, 38–43 (2004).

[158] C. Xi, D.L. Marks, D.S. Parikh, L. Raskin, S.A. Boppart, "Structural and functional imaging of three-dimensional microfluidic mixers using optical coherence tomography," *Proc. Natl. Acad. Sci.* **101**, 7516–7521 (2004).

[159] B.E. Bouma, S.-H. Yun, B.J. Vakoc, M.J. Suter, and G.J. Tearney, "Fourier-domain optical coherence tomography: recent advances toward clinical utility," *Curr. Opin. Biotechnol.* **20**, 111-118 (2009).

[160] D. Choi, H. Hiro-Oka, H. Furukawa, R. Yoshimura, M. Nakanishi, K. Shimizu, and K. Ohbayashi, "Fourier domain optical coherence tomography using optical demultiplexers imaging at 60,000,000 lines/s," *Opt. Lett.* **33**, 1318–1320 (2008).

[161] E. Hitt, "New optical coherence tomography allows rapid three-dimensional volume rendering of the retina," *Medscape Medical News* [online]. Available from: http://www.medscape.com/viewarticle/474656 [Accessed 9 January 2007].

[162] W. Drexler, "Ultrahigh resolution optical coherence tomography," *J. Biomed. Opt.* **9**, 47–74 (2004).

[163] A. Dubois, K. Grieve, G. Moneron, R. Lecaque, L. Vabre, and C. Boccara, "Ultrahigh-resolution full-field optical coherence tomography," *Appl. Opt.* **43**, 2874–2883 (2004).

[164] M. Akiba, N. Maeda, K. Yumikake, T. Soma, K. Nishida, Y. Tano, and K.P. Chan, "Ultrahigh-resolution imaging of human donor cornea using full-field optical coherence tomography," *J. Biomed. Opt.* **14**, 041202 (2007).

[165] Y. Watanabe, Y. Takasugi, and M. Sato, "Quasi-single shot axial-lateral parallel time domain OCT," *Opt. Express* **15**, 5208–5217 (2008)

[166] C. Dunsby, Y. Gu, and P. French, "Single-shot phase-stepped wide-field coherence gated imaging," *Opt. Express* **11**, 105–115 (2003).

[167] T. Man, A.L. Oldenburg, S. Sitafalwalla, D.L. Marks, W. Luo, F.J. Toublan, K.S. Suslick, S.A. Boppart, "Engineered microsphere contrast agents for optical coherence tomography," *Opt. Lett.* **28**, 1546–1548. (2003)

[168] Y. He, R.K. Wang, "Dynamic optical clearing effect of tissue impregnated with hyperosmotic agents and studied with optical coherence tomography," *J. Biomed. Opt.* **9**, 200–206 (2004).

[169] D.C. Adler, S.-W. Huang, R. Huber, and J.G. Fujimoto, "Photothermal detection of gold nanoparticles using phase-sensitive optical coherence tomography," *Opt. Express* **16**, 4376–4393 (2008).

[170] V. Jayaraman, J. Jiang, H. Li, P. Heim, G. Cole, B. Potsaid, J.G. Fujimoto, and A. Cable, "OCT imaging up to 760 kHz axial scan rate using single-mode 1310 nm MEMs-tunable VCSELs with $>$ 100 nm tuning range," in *CLEO:2011 - Laser Applications to Photonic Applications, OSA Technical Digest (CD)*, Optical Society of America, paper PDPB2 (2011).

6

Speckle in Optical Coherence Tomography

Andrea Curatolo, Brendan F. Kennedy

Optical+Biomedical Engineering Laboratory (OBEL), School of Electrical, Electronic and Computer Engineering, The University of Western Australia, 35 Stirling Highway, Crawley, Western Australia, Australia

David D. Sampson

Optical+Biomedical Engineering Laboratory (OBEL), School of Electrical, Electronic and Computer Engineering, and Centre for Microscopy, Characterisation and Analysis, The University of Western Australia, 35 Stirling Highway, Crawley, Western Australia, Australia

Timothy R. Hillman

Optical+Biomedical Engineering Laboratory (OBEL), School of Electrical, Electronic and Computer Engineering, The University of Western Australia, 35 Stirling Highway, Crawley, Western Australia 6009, Australia

Optical coherence tomography (OCT) is a biomedical imaging modality that produces high-resolution cross-sectional images of tissues, using infrared light and low-coherence interferometry. For a thorough discussion of OCT, please refer to Chapter 5. As OCT is a coherent modality, its images are corrupted by speckle, giving them a grainy or mottled appearance.

In this chapter, we discuss OCT speckle in detail. In Section 6.1, we start with a brief overview of speckle and its main characteristics, as discussed in the copious literature on the phenomenon.

In Section 6.2, we introduce a simple model of OCT image formation in the single-backscattering regime. This permits us to define speckle and to understand its most important properties as a fundamental characteristic of coherent imaging.

In Section 6.3, classification of different types of speckle are provided based on situations for which the model of Section 6.2 is not applicable, leading to different statistics of speckle when treated as a stochastic phenomenon. Both first- and second-order statistics are described in order to quantify the extent to which speckle is a corrupting influence on the image. In the former case, the magnitude of the speckle fluctuations is assessed using the *contrast ratio*. In the latter case, speckle size is assessed by virtue of the speckle *correlation coefficient*. To calculate the speckle correlation coefficient (a normalized autocorrelation function), a more detailed theory of OCT image formation is needed.

In Section 6.4, we therefore introduce a linear, spatially variant (in the axial dimension) system framework for OCT. The sample's scattering potential is the input to the imaging system, and the output response is determined by the local point spread function (PSF) of the OCT system. The Fourier equivalent of the local PSF in the spatial frequency domain, the local (coherent) transfer function (TF), is used for the correlation-coefficient calculation. Based on this formalism, we demonstrate that speckle size is (almost) invariant over an A-scan, that is, as the scan axial position varies with respect to the illumination-beam focal plane.

In Section 6.5, we extend our discussion to additional light-tissue interaction mechanisms relevant to OCT, in particular, multiple scattering, and how they affect the specific speckle realization (the image) and the statistics of speckle (calculated over an ensemble of image points). Even when the effects of multiply scattered light are included in the OCT detection model, both the speckle contrast ratio and the correlation coefficient will be, in general, sample-independent, given the OCT system parameters.

In Section 6.6, we focus on scenarios for which analysis of speckle statistics *can* be used to either: extract sample-specific information, or to assess the validity of the image-formation process, at progressively greater sample depths. In the first method, for sparsely distributed scatterers within the OCT resolution volume, the speckle contrast ratio is dependent on scatterer density. In the second, the correlation between multiple speckle patterns for a static sample under different illumination conditions can be used to assess the degree to which the recorded OCT images are corrupted by multiple scattering. Also, the correlation between multiple speckle patterns acquired from a dynamic sample, recorded at different times, can be used to extract useful sample-specific information, e.g., to quantify the extent to which scatterers at different spatial locations in the sample have moved between the images.

Finally, in Section 6.7, we discuss both experimental and post-processing methods to improve OCT image quality by reducing the impact of speckle.

Experimental validation of the main theoretical results and of speckle reduction methods is provided throughout the chapter using tissue-simulating phantoms, for which fine control of the sample structural and optical properties is possible. Additionally, we present a number of examples from the literature on biological samples showing the relevance of speckle, its analysis and exploitation, and the mitigation of its image-corrupting effects in OCT imaging.

Key words: optical coherence tomography, speckle

6.1 Introduction

Speckle is an intrinsic feature of images acquired with any imaging system employing coherent wavefields [1, 2]. The phenomenon is present, and has been studied extensively, in narrowband imaging modalities, such as ultrasound, astronomy, synthetic aperture radar and optical holography. It appears as a rapid fluctuation of the detected intensity (or field envelope) over the spatial extent of the image, conveying a granular texture.

In optical coherence tomography (OCT) [3], speckle is generated by the summation of multiple optical wavefields, backscattered from the sample arm of an interferometer. The wavefields must return to the detector within the temporal coherence gate, so that an interference signal is generated with the light returning from the reference arm. They must also retain their spatial "coherence," so that they are focused onto the optical detector (a confocal pinhole, or an optical fiber). They are represented by complex phasors, the sum of which determines the intensity and phase of the detected signal at a given depth in the sample. An OCT image of a human fingertip, clearly illustrating speckle, is presented in Fig. 6.1 [4].

Coherent, in the context of imaging modalities such as OCT, implies that the detected signal is linear with respect to the complex amplitude of the resultant back-propagating wavefield. An imaging technique that is linear with intensity (or the squared modulus of the complex amplitude) is termed *incoherent* [1]. The large number of backscattered waves (treated as random variables) included in the summation at the detector leads to two very different results in the incoherent and coherent cases. In the incoherent case, where the wavefields are added on a positive intensity basis, the standard deviation of the sum will be much less than its mean, so the "random" fluctuations will be negligible. In the coherent case, where the wavefields are added on a complex amplitude basis, the mean will be zero, and the complex-valued fluctuations about it will constitute the entirety of the signal. (The fluctuations are preserved when the modulus of the signal is taken.) For this reason, speckle is present only in coherent techniques [1].

Although speckle is often regarded as a source of noise, it is distinct from system noise components such as intensity, shot, phase and electrical noises that depend only upon the properties of the source and detection scheme. In fact, its realization is highly sample dependent and time invariant, if the sample is stationary with respect to the probing beam. In this sense, speckle is fundamental to OCT image formation, to the extent that its complete removal would leave us with no image at all [5].

A specific speckle realization depends on the sample structure down to length scales on the order of fractions of the wavelength. Besides the sample structure or motion of its scattering components, the realization is also affected by the temporal and spatial characteristics of the light, multiple scattering and phase aberrations of the propagating beam and the aperture of the detector [5].

OCT speckle has been discussed in detail in the literature, e.g., Refs. [5–18], and in several reviews of the modality as a whole [19–21]. As in most of these cases speckle is perceived as a corrupting influence on the ability to resolve microstructure in the image, the majority of this literature is devoted to methods to suppress or overcome speckle. This often involves a form of "incoherent" averaging of images of the same target featuring different speckle patterns (realizations), acquired with different system hardware configurations [5]. An alternative is to apply image post-processing techniques. In both cases, there is an inherent trade-off between the reduction in speckle contrast and the image resolution: ameliorating one comes at the expense of the other.

Another perspective is to regard speckle as a source of sample information and devise approaches to extract this information. We dwell extensively on this, as we believe it is an important perspective that deserves more space in the literature. In other areas of optical metrology [1, 2], such approaches are common. In considering its information content, a "missing frequency" characterization of speckle [5, 22] is valuable. This interprets the phenomenon as arising from the band-pass filtering properties of the OCT point-spread function. The speckled OCT signal is a reconstruction of only a small subset of the entire range of sample spatial frequencies; speckle only conveys information in the specific frequency range. If described in statistical terms, it is possible in some instances to extract sample-dependent information from the speckle's temporal or spatial characteristics. Dynamic speckle is also used to determine tissue motion, by speckle tracking or cross-correlation methods, and finds application in functional imaging such as optical coherence elastography (OCE) [11, 23], the measurement of displacement resulting from compression to extract a local strain map of the sample, and micro-angiography [24], the imaging of blood flow.

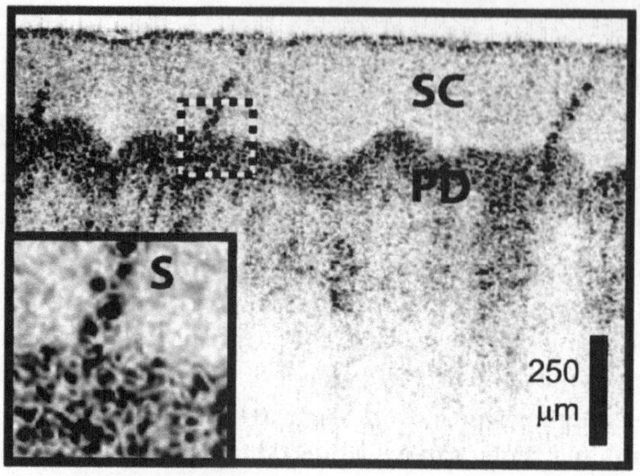

Figure 6.1: OCT image of a human fingertip with high contrast speckle pattern plotted on a logarithmic grayscale. The transverse extension of the image is 7 mm. Sweat duct (S) extending from the papillary dermis (PD) to the stratum corneum (SC). Reproduced from [4] with permission.

6.2 OCT Speckle Characteristics in the Single Scattering Regime

In this section, we describe a simple model for image formation in both coherent and incoherent imaging systems, and utilize it to describe some of the key characteristics of OCT speckle arising from light which has been singly backscattered from a static sample. We use a time-domain (TD-) approach in our formalism. By doing so, there is no loss of generality, as the Fourier-domain (FD-) and time-domain OCT signals are related by the Fourier transform operation.

6.2.1 OCT speckle: one-dimensional case

We proceed with a one-dimensional example showing how speckle can effectively "mask" the structure of the sample we would like to image. Figure 6.2(a) contains a representation of the axial OCT *point-spread function* (PSF) Ψ in the z (depth) direction. It can be represented as a complex sinusoidal "carrier" modulated by a Gaussian envelope (also plotted),

$$\Psi(z) \triangleq \exp\left[-jk_{\lambda,c}(2z)\right] \exp\left[-\frac{\pi}{2}\left(\frac{2z}{\ell_c}\right)^2\right], \tag{6.1}$$

where we assume that the source has a near-Gaussian spectrum (in optical-frequency, or wavenumber space) and establish the following notation:

c: speed of light in the sample;
λ: wavelength in the sample;
$\Delta\lambda$: full-width-at-half-maximum (FWHM) spectral bandwidth;
$k_\lambda = 2\pi/\lambda$: wavenumber in the sample;
$k_{\lambda,c}$: center wavenumber of the source spectrum (with corresponding wavelength λ_c);
Δk_λ: FWHM spectral bandwidth (wavenumber space);
$\Delta v = \Delta k_\lambda c/(2\pi)$: FWHM spectral bandwidth (optical frequency space);
$\ell_c = \sqrt{8\pi \ln 2}/\Delta k_\lambda$: coherence length of the source.[1]

[1] We utilize the definition of coherence length consistent with that for coherence time given in Ref. [25].

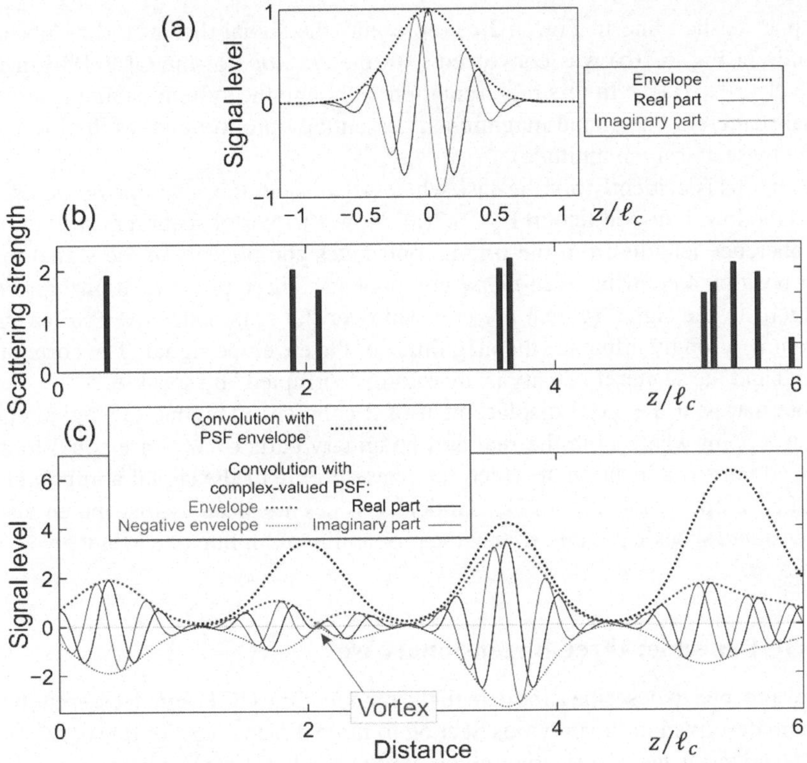

Figure 6.2: Simulation of the axial distortion of an OCT A-scan caused by the coherent detection process. (a) OCT one-dimensional complex point-spread function (PSF) $\Psi(z)$ (real & imaginary parts, and envelope); (b) Sample scatterer distribution $H(z)$; (c) Convolution of scatterer distribution with both PSF envelope $|\Psi(z)|$ and complex PSF $\Psi(z)$. Units on both axes are consistent over the three parts. (The distance units are scaled by the coherence length ℓ_c.)

The depth z corresponds to *physical* distance in the sample, since the medium's average refractive index is taken into account by scaling c and λ.[2] The factor $2z$ is utilized in each exponent of Eq. (6.1) to explicitly describe the *double-pass* of the light through the sample (in reflection mode).

Next, we consider a one-dimensional profile $H(z)$ of the sample's scatterer distribution, as indicated in Fig. 6.2(b). The OCT signal we record (as a function of scan position z) will be equal to the convolution of this profile with the PSF,

$$S(z) = \Psi(z) \otimes H(z). \tag{6.2}$$

The scatterers in Fig. 6.2(b) are assumed to have identical (zero) phase responses, so that $H(z) = \sum_{i=1}^{N} h_i \delta(z - z_i)$, where δ is the Dirac delta function and h_i is the magnitude of the response of the i-th scatterer. (The delta functions are represented as bars of different heights in the figure.) Thus, the phase difference between different scatterers' contributions to the final signal is dependent only on their relative displacement (as a fraction of wavelength).

[2]We note that Eq. (6.1) represents the OCT response to a point scatterer as the reference arm is scanned in the axial direction. For the purpose of this chapter, we deal with non-unity sample average refractive index by scaling the "actual" reference-arm scan distance so that z corresponds to physical distance in the sample.

The upper dashed line in Fig. 6.2(c) represents the signal that would be observed if the scatterer profile in Fig. 6.2(b) was convolved with the *envelope* of the OCT PSF in Fig. 6.2(a), i.e., $S_{\text{env}}(z) = |\Psi(z)| \otimes H(z)$. In this representation, although the system cannot resolve closely spaced individual scatterers, the signal magnitude is essentially proportional to the local scatterer density (weighted by scattering magnitude).

However, this is evidently *not* the case when we consider the envelope of the OCT signal, $|S(z)|$, plotted as the lower dashed line in Fig. 6.2(c). Now, the pair of scatterers with axial displacements near 2 coherence lengths from the origin contributes components to the signal in *anti*-phase; the pair near position 4 contributes *in-phase* components. These phase relationships between scatterer contributions to the signal (which are constant over the scan, since the PSF carrier is sinusoidal, without chirp) strongly influence the magnitude of the envelope signal. The correlation between the final signal and the scatterer density is, therefore, "corrupted" by speckle.

We note that near the axial displacement of 2 coherence lengths, the signal envelope vanishes entirely at a point where both the real and imaginary parts of $S(z)$ are equal to zero. This point is an optical vortex, a location at which the phase profile of the signal abruptly changes by π and the signal envelope is not smooth [1]. Optical vortices are sparsely distributed discrete points in a *two-dimensional* speckle pattern, so that the probability of finding one in any given one-dimensional profile is zero.[3]

6.2.2 OCT speckle: three-dimensional case

We now proceed to describe a more realistic model of the OCT signal, essentially the extension of the scenario described in the previous Section to three dimensions. To do so, we note that a sample may be described using a refractive-index continuum [26], $n(\mathbf{r})$, where $\mathbf{r}$ is a three-dimensional spatial location vector. An optical wave is scattered when it encounters variations in this profile.

At this point, we consider only the signal arising due to "single scattering," in particular, "first-order-Born-approximation scattering" [27], for which the sample may be represented as a superposition of non-interacting phase gratings. Then, for monochromatic light, the scattered wave, for any incident wave, depends linearly on the sample's scattering potential, $F_S(\mathbf{r}, k_\lambda) = k_\lambda^2 \left(n^2(\mathbf{r}) - 1\right)/(4\pi)$. The magnitudes and phases of the gratings are recoverable from the sample's scattering potential function $F_S(\mathbf{r})$ via the Fourier transform. In the case of OCT imaging with a broadband source, we must consider that $F_S(\mathbf{r})$ is dependent on k_λ. If it is assumed that the *refractive index* is wavenumber-independent (the sample is non-dispersive[4]), this dependence will be removed if we utilize the sample susceptibility $\chi(\mathbf{r}) = n^2(\mathbf{r}) - 1 = F_S(\mathbf{r})/\left[k_\lambda^2/(4\pi)\right]$ instead [28]. For our purposes, we shall utilize $\chi(\mathbf{r})$ throughout the manuscript, and absorb the effect of the factor $\left[k_\lambda^2/(4\pi)\right]$ into the local PSF as required.

Now we describe the form of a sample scattering distribution for which the "speckle" component of the generated OCT image will be clear. In particular, we assume that the scattering potential takes the form $\chi(\mathbf{r}) = A(\mathbf{r})R(\mathbf{r})$, where A is a slowly varying non-negative function describing the large-scale (macroscopic) variations in the sample, and R is a rapidly varying complex function describing the microscopic scatterer distribution within the macroscopically locally homogeneous regions. "Slowly" and "rapidly" varying in this context is with respect to the spatial scale of the OCT PSF envelope. The function A should be regarded as deterministic; *the purpose of the imaging system is to determine its form.* On the other hand, R is better regarded as a particular realization of an ergodic random process, such that, at each point in space, its phase is random (reflecting the

[3]Even in this case, for which the two scatterers at an axial displacement near 2 coherence lengths give anti-phased signal contributions, the point would only be a true optical vortex if all the other scatterers have exactly zero contribution at this location, which would not hold precisely for our Gaussian (infinite-tailed) PSF envelope.

[4]This assumption permits us to simplify the sample description and it is also legitimate as dispersion has negligible effect on the description of speckle, as we shall see in Section 6.4.2.

random phase responses of the individual microscopic scatterers), and its autocorrelation function,

$$\Gamma_R(\mathbf{r}+\Delta\mathbf{r},\mathbf{r}) \equiv \Gamma_R(\Delta\mathbf{r}) \equiv \overline{R(\mathbf{r}+\Delta\mathbf{r})R^*(\mathbf{r})} \tag{6.3}$$

is extremely narrow. The asterisk ($*$) represents complex conjugate and the overline represents an ensemble-average operation (over the possible realizations of R). Indeed, we may assume that $\Gamma_R(\Delta\mathbf{r})$ is delta-correlated, so that it may be replaced with the Dirac delta function, $\delta(\Delta\mathbf{r})$, when convolved with another function.

Under single backscattering satisfying the first-order-Born approximation, the OCT signal is linear with respect to the sample's susceptibility $\chi(\mathbf{r})$. That is, the detected OCT signal, as a function of scan position, is given by the superposition integral:

$$S(\mathbf{r}) = \iiint_{-\infty}^{\infty} \chi(\mathbf{r}')\,\Psi(\mathbf{r}-\mathbf{r}';\mathbf{r})\,\mathrm{d}^3\mathbf{r}', \tag{6.4}$$

where $\Psi(\mathbf{s};\mathbf{r})$ is the local system PSF corresponding to the point $\mathbf{r}$. As an aside, if the imaging system is spatially invariant, as we implicitly assumed in the one-dimensional case, then Eq. (6.4) is a convolution integral, $S(\mathbf{r}) = \chi(\mathbf{r}) \otimes \Psi(\mathbf{r})$, so that $\Psi(\mathbf{s};\mathbf{r}) \equiv \Psi(\mathbf{s})$. For OCT in general, we cannot make this assumption, but the spatial variance can be assumed to be only *axial-position* variance, that is, $\Psi(\mathbf{s};\mathbf{r})$ depends on $\mathbf{r}=(x,y,z)$ only through the axial position z. This dependence is due to the diffraction of the illumination beam (which is assumed to be stationary throughout a scan) and the confocal gating effect. We address this point in more detail in Section 6.4. It means, for example, that the OCT PSF can be assumed to be spatially invariant when performing *en-face* imaging.

Following our assumption of R being delta-correlated, the integral of R over its entire domain is equal to 1; any other constant can be absorbed into the function A. The ensemble-average mean value $\overline{S(\mathbf{r})} = 0$, due to the random phase of R. This simple fact is an "explanation" for the speckle phenomenon. The entirety of the OCT signal is due to "fluctuations" about this zero-mean point. The mean-squared value of $S(\mathbf{r})$ is:

$$\begin{aligned}\overline{|S(\mathbf{r})|^2} &= \iiint_{-\infty}^{\infty}\iiint_{-\infty}^{\infty} \overline{\chi(\mathbf{r}')\chi^*(\mathbf{p}')}\,\Psi(\mathbf{r}-\mathbf{r}';\mathbf{r})\;\Psi^*(\mathbf{r}-\mathbf{p}';\mathbf{r})\,\mathrm{d}^3\mathbf{r}'\mathrm{d}^3\mathbf{p}' \\ &\cong |A(\mathbf{r})|^2 \iiint_{-\infty}^{\infty} |\Psi(\mathbf{r}';\mathbf{r})|^2 \mathrm{d}^3\mathbf{r}',\end{aligned} \tag{6.5}$$

by the sifting property of the delta function. The factor $|A(\mathbf{r})|^2$ can be brought outside the integral due to the assumption that it is slowly varying (in comparison with the size scale of $|\Psi(\mathbf{r}';\mathbf{r})|^2$).

Now consider a hypothetical equivalent *incoherent* imaging system, that is, linear with respect to optical *intensity* instead of optical *field*. Its detected signal could be described by the convolution integral

$$I(\mathbf{r}) = \iiint_{-\infty}^{\infty} |\chi(\mathbf{r}')|^2 |\Psi(\mathbf{r}-\mathbf{r}';\mathbf{r})|^2 \mathrm{d}^3\mathbf{r}'. \tag{6.6}$$

Due to the narrowness of the function Γ_R, many independent statistical samples contribute to the integral, and so I is extremely close to its expected value with near-certainty. (It may be verified formally that the variance of I is equal to zero under the delta-function limit.) Thus, up to a constant factor, $I(\mathbf{r})$ is given by

$$I(\mathbf{r}) = \overline{I(\mathbf{r})} = |A(\mathbf{r})|^2 \iiint_{-\infty}^{\infty} |\Psi(\mathbf{r}';\mathbf{r})|^2 \mathrm{d}^3\mathbf{r}'. \tag{6.7}$$

Equations (6.5) and (6.7) demonstrate the speckle effect in coherent imaging. The incoherent image $I(\mathbf{r})$ is a "perfect" reconstruction of $|A(\mathbf{r})|^2$, equal to its mean (deterministic), and completely insensitive to the small-scale fluctuations represented by the factor $R(\mathbf{r})$. The squared modulus of the coherent complex amplitude distribution has the same mean as the incoherent intensity distribution. However, $|S(\mathbf{r})|^2 \neq \overline{|S(\mathbf{r})|^2}$ in general; the signal is subject to apparently-random fluctuations that are dependent on the precise scattering behavior of the small-scale microstructure. We describe the statistics of these fluctuations in more detail in Section 6.3.

Based on the preceding analysis, speckle can be defined as the difference between a "coherent" image $|S(\mathbf{r})|^2$ *and the corresponding "incoherent" image* $I(\mathbf{r})$. Provided that the imaging process can be described using a superposition integral, this definition will be valid even if (as in OCT), there is no incoherent analog of the imaging process.

Figure 6.3 presents the comparison between experimental "coherent" (OCT) and "incoherent" (non-OCT) images. The experimental sample was a structured 3D phantom for use in OCT, fabricated from a transparent PDMS silicone (n = 1.41) matrix and different concentrations of optical scatterers (1-μm-mean-diameter titanium dioxide (TiO_2) particles (n = 2.71) in a two-stage soft-lithography casting process [29]). The dimensions and optical properties of the features within the phantom are representative of those found in tissue [30]. The large-scale structure $A(\mathbf{r})$ in this case is the text "OBEL" (the acronym for the authors' research group). The letters are part of the structured casting with a TiO_2 scatterer concentration of 3 mg/mL, corresponding to a scattering coefficient at 1325 nm, calculated using Mie theory [31], of 4.3 mm^{-1}. The letters are encased by the embedding casting with a TiO_2 scatterer concentration of 0.5 mg/mL of silicone, corresponding to a scattering coefficient of 1.4 mm^{-1}.

The image of the phantom in Fig. 6.3(a) was recorded using a swept-source OCT system (Thorlabs OCS1300SS) with a central wavelength of $\lambda_c = 1325$ nm and a bandwidth $\Delta\lambda = 100$ nm. The theoretical *axial resolution*[5] is 7.7 μm in air and the theoretical *lateral resolution*[6] (at focus) is 15 μm; the numerical aperture (NA) is 0.056. The phantom is imaged with light incident from above in Fig. 6.3(a), in free space, with the beam focus set to the middle of the letters. The image in (a) is displayed on a linear grayscale, with the white level corresponding to a signal strength of approximately 200 times that of the noise floor.

Corruption of the text image by speckle effects is clearly evident in Fig. 6.3(a). However, such effects are not present in Fig. 6.3(b), recorded using white-light bright-field microscopy on the partially fabricated sample, before the embedding silicone was cast. This image is strictly only *representative* of the "incoherent" image $I(\mathbf{r})$, as it was acquired from a different orientation and with different source and optics. Nevertheless, it shows a more realistic profile of the large-scale structure $A(\mathbf{r})$.

To further illustrate the concepts discussed so far, we present a numerical simulation based on the sample structure shown in Fig. 6.3(c). We model the effect of the small-scale structure, $R(\mathbf{r})$, by utilizing $A(\mathbf{r})$ as a *local density map* for a large collection of individual point scatterers. The point scatterers are represented in two dimensions in the figure as small identical spheres. Each such scatterer is assumed to have an identical *amplitude* response, but a *phase response* (associated with its angular-scattering phase function, in the backward direction) that is uniformly distributed over $(-\pi, \pi]$. This gives rise to a random-phasor sum that we shall discuss further in Section 6.3.1.1.[7]

Incoherent and coherent images are displayed in Fig. 6.4, in which Eqs. (6.4) and Eq. (6.6) are graphically represented as convolution operations. (Both images are plotted on an "intensity" basis.) We assume a spatially invariant convolution kernel, or PSF. The random phase assigned to each

[5]The OCT axial resolution is conventionally expressed as $2\ln 2\ \lambda_c^2/(\pi\ \Delta\lambda) = 4\ln 2/(\Delta k_\lambda) = \sqrt{2\ln 2/\pi}\ \ell_c$.

[6]The OCT lateral resolution is conventionally expressed as twice the Gaussian beam waist radius ($2W_0$) at the center wavenumber. It is $\sqrt{2}$ times larger than the full $1/e$ width of the lateral PSF, as we demonstrate in Section 6.4, due to the benefit of the system confocal detection ability. The former and the latter full widths are shown in Fig. 6.8(a), (b), respectively, bound between the dashed lines.

[7]Note that even if this phase condition is not satisfied for a given sample, the phase responses of the individual scatterers are effectively randomized by their precise position on the scale of half of a wavelength due to the sinusoidal carrier component of the PSF. We discuss this point further in Section 6.3.1.1.

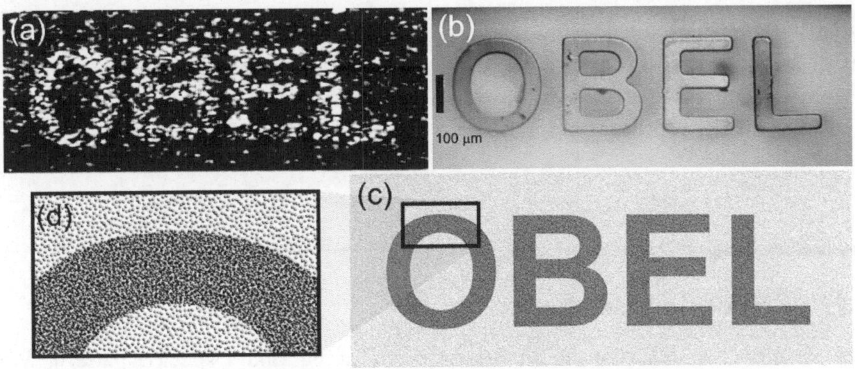

Figure 6.3: Comparison between images of a structured phantom acquired using a coherent OCT system (a) and a bright-field microscope, i.e., an incoherent system (b). Part (c) (partially magnified in (d)) shows a representation of the sample microscopic scatterer distribution utilized to simulate the coherent/incoherent image formation process.

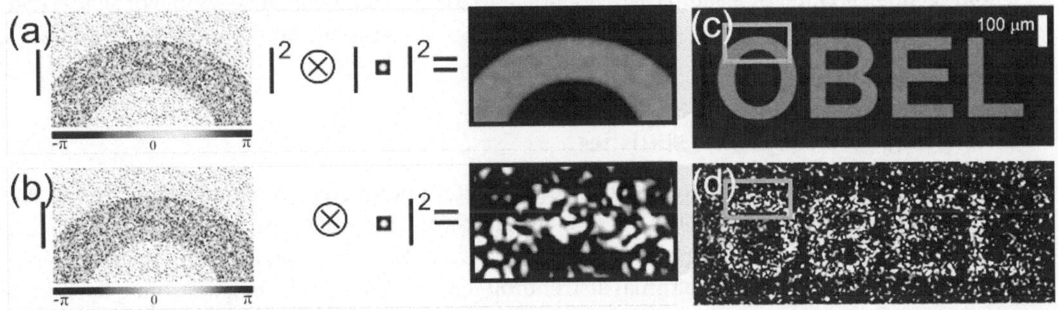

Figure 6.4: Simulation of (a) a hypothetical incoherent and (b) a coherent OCT image formation process, according to the simple model presented in this section. The resultant images of the scatterer distribution [of Fig. 6.3(c)] displayed in (c), (d), correspond to the incoherent and coherent cases, respectively. The spatially invariant convolution kernel (PSF envelope) is shown in the small square black box in both (a) and (b).

scatterer in the distribution is indicated using a color scale. Because of this random assignment, we did not need to incorporate the high-frequency spatial carrier factor into the PSF in order to effectively simulate the speckle pattern. Direct comparison of Figs. 6.4(c) and 6.4(d) shows that the incoherent imaging modality is a clear reconstruction of the distribution $A(\mathbf{r})$, almost unaffected by the particular scatterer distribution $R(\mathbf{r})$ we generated. (The random variation in the observed intensity $I(\mathbf{r})$ is much smaller than its expected value.) By contrast, since the expected value of the complex quantity $S(\mathbf{r})$ is zero, then the random variation in the coherent image *is* the image![8]

We note that Figs. 6.3(a) and 6.4(d) show similar characteristics, except perhaps at large sample depths (near the bottom of the figures), for which the observed signal in the experimental image exhibits some decline due to attenuation of light. This effect is not taken into account in our simple model.

To summarize, in this section we have presented a simple model that has permitted us to define

[8]Of course, the expected value of the plotted intensity distribution $|S(\mathbf{r})|^2$ is not zero. It may be described using exponential statistics, as we shall see in Section 6.3.1.1.

speckle in the singly backscattering scenario, as the difference between the coherent and incoherent images of a highly random microstructure modulated by a slowly varying "mean" function. The latter represents the large-scale variations in a stationary sample's structure (susceptibility map) that we want to faithfully represent in an image.

6.3 OCT Speckle Statistics

In this section, we describe the characteristics of a stationary speckle pattern. We focus on the first-order statistics, that is, the marginal distribution of a *single-point* signal value for a speckle realization. This distribution may be measured as the value of the OCT point signal over an ensemble of scan positions, sample scatterer distributions, or times. We note that in Section 6.2, we explicitly dealt with only an ensemble of scatterer distributions. In practice, it is usually much easier to evaluate the statistics over, say, regions within a 2D image. This is permissible under the assumption that the speckle realization process is ergodic [25]: statistics taken over a range of scan positions (over a homogeneous region of a sample) are identical to those taken over an ensemble of scatterer distributions (at a single "scan location"). In this section, we also focus on the second-order (size-scale) statistics of the speckle.

6.3.1 First-order speckle statistics

The *first-order* spatial statistics of the speckle pattern permit us to quantify the extent of the corrupting effect of speckle at a point. We also use the term "marginal" speckle statistics to distinguish them from the joint distributions of the speckle realizations at different locations (or points in time). A key parameter of a speckle marginal distribution that is highly useful in quantifying the magnitude of its fluctuations is the *contrast ratio*, equal to the standard deviation divided by the mean.

6.3.1.1 OCT speckle with degenerate (Rayleigh) statistics

In Section 6.2, we developed a model for a sample which gives rise to a speckle pattern when imaged with OCT: "random" microstructure is modulated by a slowly varying "mean" function. When performing numerical simulations, we represented the fine microstructure by a distribution of point scatterers, whose local density corresponded to the large-scale structures of interest. This latter representation of the sample as a collection of point scatterers corresponds directly to the "random-phasor sum" mathematical formalism [25], which has been previously applied to speckle in general [32] and OCT [33] in particular. We now briefly summarize it.

We express the OCT signal $S \equiv S(\mathbf{r})$ as the sum:

$$S = |S|\exp(j\theta_S) = \sum_{i=1}^{N} S_i = \sum_{i=1}^{N} a_i \exp(j\phi_i), \tag{6.8}$$

where S_i is the phasor contribution of the i-th scatterer (of N total) to the signal, and both the sum and the individual summands are expressed in terms of their moduli and phases. We refer to $|S|$ as the speckle *envelope*, which forms the basis for which images are commonly displayed. However, in OCT, the modulus and phase of S are generally detected directly.

Now, we assume that the a_is are identically distributed with finite mean and variance[9], the ϕ_is are uniformly distributed on $(-\pi, \pi]$, and all of the a_is and ϕ_is are independent [1]. Then the sum S is

[9]If the scatterers are identical, then the distribution of a_i depends only on the shape of the local PSF.

asymptotically *circularly complex Gaussian* as $N \to \infty$; its real and imaginary parts are zero-mean independent Gaussian variables with variance σ^2. If N itself is a random variable, then provided its standard deviation is much less than its mean (as is generally the case for large numbers of scatterers), S will maintain the same distribution.

The envelope $|S|$ will be *Rayleigh*-distributed with parameter σ. This result can be formally demonstrated under our model of Section 6.2.2 by noting that the even moments[10] of $|S(\mathbf{r})|$ (such as the second moment, in Eq. (6.5)) match those of the Rayleigh distribution. Its probability density function (PDF) is:

$$p_{|S|}(s) = \frac{s}{\sigma^2}\exp\left\{-\frac{s^2}{2\sigma^2}\right\}, \quad (s>0), \tag{6.9}$$

with mean $\mu'_{1,|S|} = \sqrt{\pi/2}\sigma$, and variance $\mu_{2,|S|} = (2-\pi/2)\sigma^2$. The phase of S, θ_S, is *uniformly-distributed* over $(-\pi, \pi]$.

In conventional laser speckle images (for example, the image obtained by reflecting a laser-pointer light from a wall), the *intensity* pattern, proportional to $|S|^2$, is viewed directly. At any point, the signal will follow an *exponential* distribution[11] with mean $\overline{I_n} = 2\sigma^2$ equal to its standard deviation, and PDF:

$$p_{|S|^2}(t) = \frac{1}{2\sigma^2}\exp\left\{-\frac{t}{2\sigma^2}\right\}, \quad (t>0). \tag{6.10}$$

We have already plotted Figs. 6.3(a) and 6.4(d) on an $|S|^2$ basis.

The contrast ratio is:

$$\mathrm{CR} = \frac{\sqrt{\mu_{2,|S|}}}{\mu'_{1,|S|}}, \tag{6.11}$$

so for the Rayleigh distribution, it is:

$$\mathrm{CR}_{\mathrm{Rayleigh}} = \sqrt{4/\pi - 1} \approx 0.52. \tag{6.12}$$

For the exponential distribution,

$$\mathrm{CR}_{\mathrm{Exponential}} = \frac{2\sigma^2}{2\sigma^2} = 1. \tag{6.13}$$

This means that the observed fluctuations of speckle displayed on an *intensity* basis are approximately twice as "severe" as those of speckle displayed on a *envelope (amplitude)* basis, as is evidenced in the comparison of the forthcoming Fig. 6.6(a), for example. Of course, one distribution is obtained from the other by a squaring operation, so the "comparison" has limited meaning. Instead, it is more useful to compare speckle patterns plotted on the *same* basis.

6.3.1.2 OCT speckle with non-degenerate statistics

The speckle definition we have given in Section 6.2.2, that is, the difference between a coherent and an incoherent image, may be strictly applicable only to our stated sample model, namely, highly random microstructure modulated by a slowly varying "mean" function.

Significantly, it is inadequate for situations for which the signal cannot be described in terms of a random-phasor sum. (For example, in OCT, imaging the specular reflection from a planar interface.) In such cases, the image will not be characterized by rapid fluctuations of constructive

[10] We use the following notation for the moments $\mu'_{n,|S|}$ of a distribution $|S(\mathbf{r})|$: the "prime" ($'$) denotes a statistical moment centered about zero (its absence denotes a statistical moment about the mean), the numbered subscript denotes the order of the moment. For example, the second moment about the mean $\mu_{2,|S|}$ is the variance of the envelope signal $|S(\mathbf{r})|$.

[11] We note that this distribution is only applicable for fully polarized laser speckle [1]. We consider the issue of polarization diversity as it applies to OCT in Section 6.7.1.1.

and destructive interference. However, it is arguably only meaningful to speak of "speckle" to the extent that the sample can be described according to the model, and the intensity fluctuations observed as "pure speckle," exhibiting "degenerate"[12] (Rayleigh) statistics. Under this model, the sample image is viewed as a realization of an ergodic random process.[13]

In this Section, we consider a number of ways in which pure speckle would *not* be observed in a coherent imaging system, and examine how the observed statistics differ from the degenerate case. A list of some circumstances in which non-pure speckle would be observed follows:

1. *Small number of scatterers in the resolution volume*:

   If only a few scatterers are present within the OCT resolution volume sample, then the central limit theorem cannot be invoked, yielding non-Rayleigh marginal statistics [34]. This observation suggests that it may be possible to extract sample-dependent information from first-order speckle statistics. We explore this possibility in Section 6.6.1.

2. *Phasor sum with a non-zero bias*:

   If the phases of the individual contributors to the random-phasor sum are not uniformly distributed over $(-\pi, \pi]$, but are biased towards a particular value, then the speckle is said to be *partially developed* [1], and its envelope will have a contrast ratio substantially less than the Rayleigh limit of 0.52. It would seem that this scenario would be rare in OCT, at least when the technique is performed in *reflection mode* (as is usually the case), because of the bandpass filtering characteristic [5] in the axial direction. As is evident in Eq. (6.1), the imaging system effectively applies to the sample an axial phase "ramp" whose period is equal to one-half of the mean wavelength. Even if all of the scatterers within the sample had *identical* phase responses when backscattering an incoming illumination beam, this uniformity would be thoroughly randomized by the ramp (because of the dependence on the scatterers' precise relative positions). An exception would occur when imaging scattering surfaces with roughness on the scale of a wavelength, or less. However, when one speaks of "speckle" in OCT, one is almost inevitably referring to imaging thick samples with minimum depths in the hundreds of micrometers range.

   A more likely scenario of non-zero bias would be the case of random-phase scatterers in the presence of a single dominant scatterer/reflector, such as a sample interface or boundary. This dominant contributor constitutes a single large phasor, which may dwarf the signal arising from the surrounding back-scatterers. In this case the speckle statistics will be altered to those of the *Rician* distribution (assuming the magnitude of the dominant phasor can be regarded as deterministic [1]).

3. *Medium-scale sample structure*:

   In order to observe a pure speckle pattern, we require that the sample be composed of large-scale structure (much greater than the system resolution) and small-scale structure (much smaller). If moderate-size structure exists on the scale of the speckles themselves, then it will be partially resolvable, primarily through the way in which it *modifies* the local speckle first- and second-order statistics (taken over an ensemble of points in a single OCT image). Sample structures of this type are amenable to being characterized by a texture-analysis method such as that of Gossage et al. [17, 35].

4. *Non-uniform illumination*:

---

[12] We introduce the terminology ("*pure*"-"*degenerate*" versus "*non-pure*"-"*non-degenerate*") as distinct from *fully developed* versus *partially developed* [1] speckle (see Case 2 below). *Partially developed* speckle is a subset of "*non-degenerate*" speckle.

[13] That is, to the degree that $A(\mathbf{r})$ is actually *constant* over the area of interest.

When performing OCT in scattering media, we must expect that the detected signal strength will decay as a function of depth. If this rate of decay is uniform over all axial scans (A-scans) in the OCT image, then speckle statistics, calculated over an ensemble of positions in a lateral plane, should be describable according to the analysis of Section 6.3.1.1. However, sample inhomogeneities in the overlying layers may result in lateral-position-dependent illumination attenuation, over both the input and output paths. Shadowing artifacts, for example, will generate spurious "dark" regions in an *en-face* image plane. Especially if the size scale of these effects is comparable with the speckle size, then they will appear to modify the speckle statistics, as in the previous case. Outside of OCT, one well-known case of speckle statistics being altered by non-uniform illumination is so-called "speckled speckle" [1]. An input speckle illumination pattern becomes the intensity distribution for a secondary speckle generation process.

5. *"Incoherent" averaging*:

   If the speckle intensity or envelope pattern is subject to spatial averaging (subsequent to detection), either in hardware or software (depending on the system application), then the fluctuations will be, to a large degree, washed out. This is the most natural method of eliminating the granularity of the speckle pattern within the images, although it comes at the price of degrading the image resolution. (We will consider this concept further in our discussion of speckle reduction techniques in Section 6.7.)

If at least one of Conditions 1–3 holds, then sample-specific information may indeed be obtained merely from the statistics of a stationary speckle pattern. (In principle, the same is true for Condition 4, provided that the non-uniform illumination is generated by the sample itself.)

Utilizing the same simple model of coherent image formation presented in Section 6.2, we present, in Fig. 6.5, an image of a sample composed of the structured phantom of Figs. 6.3 and 6.4 with an overlayer of different scatterer concentration. The figure shows graphical examples of the resulting speckle patterns, which exhibits both degenerate and non-degenerate speckle statistics. Inset (i) features a part of the sample structure for which $A(\mathbf{r})$ is actually *constant* over the area of interest (degenerate case). Inset (ii) shows a close-up on the boundary between the overlayer and the structured phantom, which is represented by a strong constant phasor (non-degenerate Case 2). Inset (iii) shows an area where there are medium-scale sample structure variations (non-degenerate Case 3). Insets (iv), (v), and (vi) are the observed speckle patterns corresponding to Insets (i), (ii), and (iii), respectively; they are plotted on an intensity $|S|^2$ basis.

Figure 6.6 shows representative probability distribution functions for the cases highlighted in Insets (i) and (ii) of Fig. 6.5. Fig. 6.6(a) refers to the degenerate case, and Figs. 6.6(b)–(c) refer to the non-degenerate Case 2. In Fig. 6.6(c), the magnitude of the phasor representing the boundary is around 2.5 times stronger than in (b). All speckle patterns are plotted on an amplitude $|S|$ basis on the left and on an intensity $|S|^2$ basis on the right. For comparison purposes, the dynamic ranges are both clipped to the 95-th percentile.

The OCT signal in the vicinity of a tissue boundary (non-degenerate speckle Case 2) of Fig. 6.6(b) corresponds to the case modeled by a random phasor sum S_n plus a known constant phasor s_0. The modulus $|S|$ will be *Rician*-distributed with parameters s_0, σ. Its PDF is:

$$p_{|S|}(s) = \frac{s}{\sigma^2}\exp\left\{-\frac{s^2+{s_0}^2}{2\sigma^2}\right\} I_0\left(\frac{s s_0}{\sigma^2}\right), \qquad (s>0), \tag{6.14}$$

where I_0 is a modified Bessel function of the first kind, zeroth order. In the case where the interface signal is strong and the surrounding signal weak, as in Fig. 6.6(c), the modulus $|S|$ is approximately *Gaussian*-distributed, that is, for $s_0/\sigma \to \infty$, the probability density function is approximated by

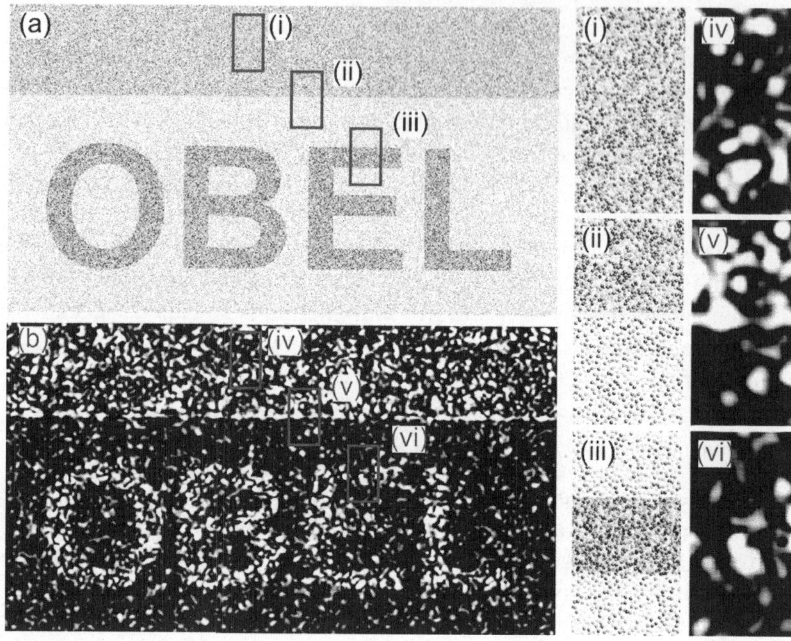

Figure 6.5: (a) Microscopic scatterer distribution representing a sample composed of the structured phantom and an overlayer of different scatterer concentration. (b) Simulated OCT image of the scatterer distribution in (a). Insets (i) and (iv) show scatterer distributions and corresponding speckle patterns for the degenerate case. Insets (ii), (iii) and (v), (vi) show scatterer distribution and corresponding speckle pattern for two non-degenerate cases (2 and 3).

$$p_{|S|}(s) \approx \frac{1}{\sqrt{2\pi}\sigma}\exp\left\{-\frac{(s-s_0)^2}{2\sigma^2}\right\}. \tag{6.15}$$

In the general case (not assuming $s_0/\sigma \to \infty$), the intensity signal $|S|^2$ follows a *modified Rician-*distribution [1]. If the average intensity of the random phasor sum alone is $\overline{I_n} = \overline{|S_n|^2} = 2\sigma^2$, the intensity of the constant phasor alone $t_0 = s_0{}^2$, and their ratio $r = t_0/\overline{I_n}$; then the expression for the PDF is:

$$p_{|S|^2}(t) = \frac{1}{\overline{I_n}}\exp\left\{-\frac{t+t_0}{\overline{I_n}}\right\} I_0\left(2\sqrt{\frac{t}{\overline{I_n}}r}\right), \qquad (t>0). \tag{6.16}$$

As was the case for $r = 0$, the intensity distribution has a much greater contrast ratio than the corresponding envelope distribution.

In summary, the probability distribution of the amplitude (or the intensity) in a point of an OCT image degenerates to the Rayleigh (or the exponential) distribution under the sample-structure model presented in Section 6.2. The contrast ratio is a valuable tool for describing the magnitude of the speckle fluctuations, when the speckle's probability distribution function departs from this degenerate case, as in Cases 1–4. In some cases, it can be used to extract sample-specific information solely from the speckle statistics, as we shall see in Section 6.6.

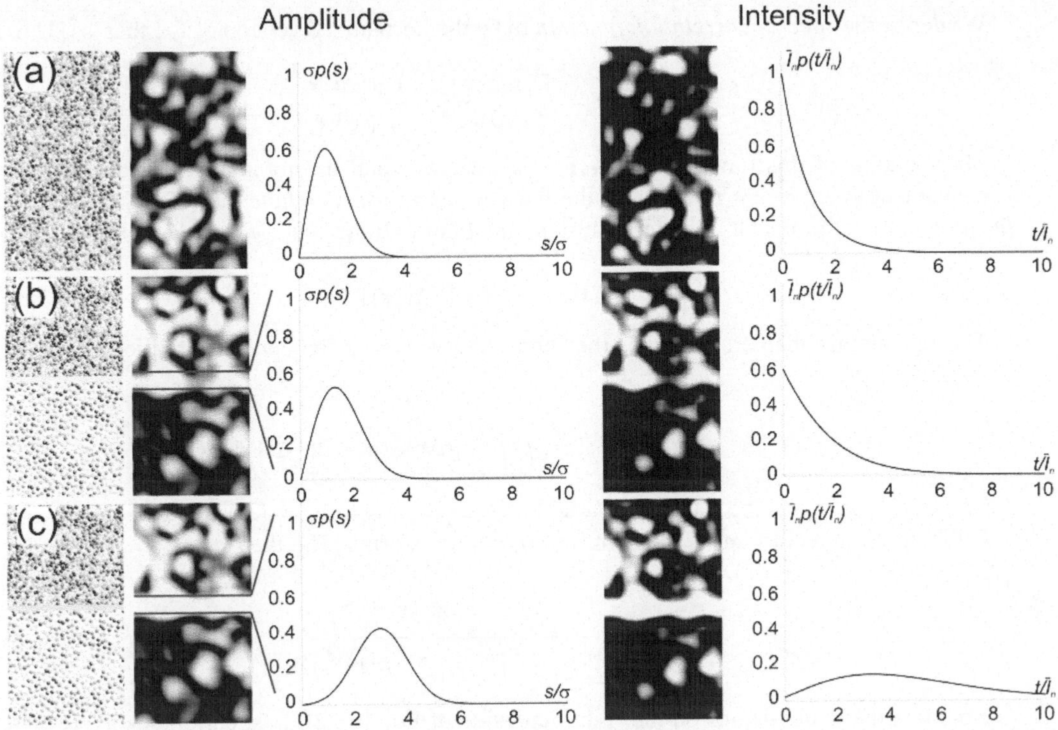

Figure 6.6: Scatterer distribution, corresponding amplitude $|S|$ and intensity $|S|^2$ speckle pattern and representative probability distribution function for the (a) degenerate case of Fig. 6.5(i); and (b), (c) non-degenerate Case 2. Part (b) refers to Fig. 6.5(ii) and (c) represents the same scatterer distribution as in (b) but with the magnitude of the phasor s_0 representing the boundary around 2.5 times stronger. The PDFs shown for (b) and (c) refer to the area around the tissue interface, bound by the thin lines. For comparison purposes, the dynamic ranges of the amplitude and intensity images are both clipped to the 95-th percentile.

6.3.2 Second-order speckle statistics

The *second-order* spatial statistics (joint, at two points) permit us to quantify the size of the speckle grains in the axial and lateral dimensions. Specifically, starting from Eq. (6.4), we calculate the *autocorrelation function* of the speckle signal:

$$\Gamma_S(\Delta\mathbf{r};\mathbf{r}) = \overline{S\left(\mathbf{r}+\frac{\Delta\mathbf{r}}{2}\right) S^*\left(\mathbf{r}-\frac{\Delta\mathbf{r}}{2}\right)}$$

$$= \iiint_{-\infty}^{\infty}\iiint_{-\infty}^{\infty} \overline{\chi(\mathbf{r}')\chi^*(\mathbf{p}')}\Psi\left(\mathbf{r}+\frac{\Delta\mathbf{r}}{2}-\mathbf{r}';\mathbf{r}+\frac{\Delta\mathbf{r}}{2}\right)\Psi^*\left(\mathbf{r}-\frac{\Delta\mathbf{r}}{2}-\mathbf{p}';\mathbf{r}-\frac{\Delta\mathbf{r}}{2}\right)d^3\mathbf{r}'d^3\mathbf{p}'. \quad (6.17)$$

We can treat this equation in the same manner as Eq. (6.5), provided we make the assumptions that for the small values of $\Delta\mathbf{r}$ for which Γ_S is significant (i.e., over the length scale of the PSF), $A(\mathbf{r})$ is nearly constant, i.e., $A(\mathbf{r}) \cong A(\mathbf{r}\pm\Delta\mathbf{r}/2)$ and the PSF is spatially invariant over that same length scale, i.e., $\Psi(\cdot;\mathbf{r}) \cong \Psi(\cdot;\mathbf{r}\pm\Delta\mathbf{r}/2)$. Then we find:

$$\Gamma_S(\Delta\mathbf{r};\mathbf{r}) = |A(\mathbf{r})|^2\,\Gamma_\Psi(\Delta\mathbf{r};\mathbf{r}) \triangleq |A(\mathbf{r})|^2 \iiint_{-\infty}^{\infty}\Psi\left(\mathbf{s}+\frac{\Delta\mathbf{r}}{2};\mathbf{r}\right)\Psi^*\left(\mathbf{s}-\frac{\Delta\mathbf{r}}{2};\mathbf{r}\right)d^3\mathbf{s}. \quad (6.18)$$

We define the *speckle correlation function* to be the normalized version of Γ_S, that is ([1] p. 64),

$$\gamma(\Delta\mathbf{r};\mathbf{r}) \triangleq \frac{\Gamma_S(\Delta\mathbf{r};\mathbf{r})}{\Gamma_S(0;\mathbf{r})} = \frac{\Gamma_\Psi(\Delta\mathbf{r};\mathbf{r})}{\Gamma_\Psi(0;\mathbf{r})}. \tag{6.19}$$

The modulus of this function, $|\gamma(\Delta\mathbf{r};\mathbf{r})|$, is what we shall use to characterize speckle size. It is convenient to express it in terms of the local *coherent transfer function* (CTF), or just *transfer function* (TF) $\mathscr{H}$ of the OCT imaging system, the Fourier transform ($\mathscr{F}$) of the local PSF, that is,

$$\mathscr{H}(\mathbf{k};\mathbf{r}) = \mathscr{F}\{\Psi(\Delta\mathbf{r};\mathbf{r})\}. \tag{6.20}$$

Throughout this chapter, we utilize the "non-unitary angular frequency" definition of the Fourier transform, so that:

$$U(\mathbf{k}) = \mathscr{F}\{u(\Delta\mathbf{r})\} \triangleq \iiint_{-\infty}^{\infty} u(\Delta\mathbf{r})\exp[-j\mathbf{k}\cdot\Delta\mathbf{r}]\ \mathrm{d}^3\Delta\mathbf{r}, \tag{6.21}$$

where $\mathbf{k} = (k_x, k_y, k_z)$ is the transform variable corresponding to $\Delta\mathbf{r} = (\Delta x, \Delta y, \Delta z)$.

Utilizing the autocorrelation theorem for Fourier transforms [36], then

$$\gamma(\Delta\mathbf{r};\mathbf{r}) = \frac{\mathscr{F}^{-1}\left\{|\mathscr{H}(\mathbf{k};\mathbf{r})|^2\right\}}{\left[\left(\frac{1}{2\pi}\right)^3 \iiint_{-\infty}^{\infty} |\mathscr{H}(\mathbf{k};\mathbf{r})|^2 \mathrm{d}^3\mathbf{k}\right]}. \tag{6.22}$$

Note that the denominator on the right-hand side of Eq. (6.22), in square brackets, is merely a scaling constant, equal to $\Gamma_\Psi(0;\mathbf{r})$ from Eq. (6.19). Thus, Eq. (6.22) states that [1] up to this scaling constant, *the speckle correlation function and the squared-modulus (local) transfer function are a Fourier-transform pair*. We can derive a number of conclusions about speckle size from this important result. For example, if $\mathscr{H}(\mathbf{k};\mathbf{r})$ is separable with respect to the k_x, k_y and k_z coordinates, with a Gaussian profile in each direction, then the squaring operation will essentially decrease the three Gaussian-function widths by a factor of $\sqrt{2}$. In other words, the function $\gamma(\Delta\mathbf{r};\mathbf{r})$ is $\sqrt{2}$ times *broader* than the local PSF $\Psi(\Delta\mathbf{r};\mathbf{r})$ in each of the $\Delta x, \Delta y$ and Δz directions: this factor links speckle "size" to system resolution. *However*, this statement only applies for an aberration-free imaging system (in focus). If the optical imaging system *does* contain aberrations, so that $\mathscr{H}(\mathbf{k};\mathbf{r})$ contains complex-valued modulations [1], then the image resolution *will* degrade, but the speckle size will be unchanged [because of the modulus operation in Eq. (6.22)]. For the purposes of OCT, this includes the effect of diffraction and dispersion, a fact we will consider again in Section 6.4.

To this point, all of our discussion of speckle has been limited to the "single backscattering" scenario. In Section 6.4, we derive an explicit form of the OCT-system local TF. That permits us to evaluate the speckle correlation function numerically, and verify the aforementioned claim about the average speckle size in relation to the system resolution. Then, in Section 6.5, we extend our analysis to the characteristics of speckle due to multiply scattered light, including its effect on speckle size.

6.4 OCT Image Formation Using Singly Backscattered Light: Linear System Framework

In Section 6.2.2, we described the OCT system in the single scattering model, as a scalar, spatially *variant* linear system. Linear-systems representations of OCT in the literature include a representation of the 3D PSF of an OCT scanner by Schmitt [37]. Fercher et al. adopted an inverse scattering formalism to describe the OCT signal, identifying the accessible regions of the spatial-frequency spectrum of the sample [21, 38]. Coupland and Lobera [39] derive and plot "in-focus" (spatially invariant) forms of the OCT PSF and TF.

A depth-dependent lateral point-spread function was derived by Yasuno et al. [40] in order to apply a numerical deconvolution to the acquired signal. Ralston et al. developed "interferometric synthetic aperture microscopy" (ISAM) [41], which utilizes the fact that the system local TF has identical spatial-frequency-space coverage (support) over the entire length of an A-scan. For this technique, full 3D signal acquisition and digital correction can overcome (under some circumstances) the problem of "out-of-focus" transverse resolution degradation.

Villiger and Lasser [28] utilized the principle of a three-dimensional generalized aperture [42] to describe the illumination and detection operations in OCT, in order to calculate the CTF of the individual wavelength components of the OCT system. Both Gaussian and Bessel-type beams were modeled in the approach, which was based on theory developed by Sheppard, Gu and their colleagues [43, 44, 45]. A recent paper by Sheppard et al. [46] presents a generic model based on the 3D CTF and investigates the effect of different system configurations and of different pupils on the image formation.

In this section, we utilize similar methods to those of the preceding references to generate specific forms of the OCT local PSF and TF. It is necessary for us to avoid the simplification that OCT PSF is spatially invariant, because we would like to investigate how speckle size varies with axial scan position (relative to the focal plane).

We adopt an intuitive approach, and do not specify a "generalized aperture" pupil function to describe the system optics. Instead, we begin with the focal-plane complex amplitude (field) distribution for a focused illumination beam, and then determine an expression for its 3D angular spectrum (of plane waves). Next, we utilize the symmetry of the system's illumination and collection processes to determine the monochromatic (or single-wavenumber) contribution to the OCT TF. Finally, we incorporate the effect of the full "broadband" optical source spectrum in order to generate an expression for the local TF $\mathscr{H}(\mathbf{k};\mathbf{r})$.

6.4.1 Point spread function and coherent transfer function

The PSF of an imaging system describes its response to a point source. In order to obtain an expression for the system's local PSF Ψ, or its frequency-domain equivalent, the local TF $\mathscr{H}$, we make the following assumptions:

1. Each wavelength component of the (broadband) sample illumination beam, the output of a single-mode optical fiber focused by the sample arm optics, may be described as a scalar Gaussian propagating beam. The components share a common axis of propagation (z), their waists are co-located, and their far-field divergence angles θ_0 are equal.[14]
2. A confocal sectioning ability is provided by the fact that, in order to be detected, backscattered light from the sample must be coupled into the same optical fiber that provided the illumination.[15] This is illustrated in Fig. 6.7(a).

We reiterate that the illumination and detection paths share the same optics and the corresponding beams are assumed to be stationary throughout an OCT axial scan. Assumption 2 permits us to consider the axial sectioning ability provided by the confocal gate alone, at a single wavelength. The confocal gate is fixed at a particular position ($z = 0$) in the axial scan, the beam waist, according to Assumption 1.

Therefore, we consider a monochromatic (wavelength λ, wavenumber $|k_\lambda| = 2\pi/\lambda$) propagating

[14]This means, for example, that they do *not* share equal beam widths at the waist.

[15]In a free-space system this could be achieved equivalently by focusing the collected light through a confocal "pinhole."

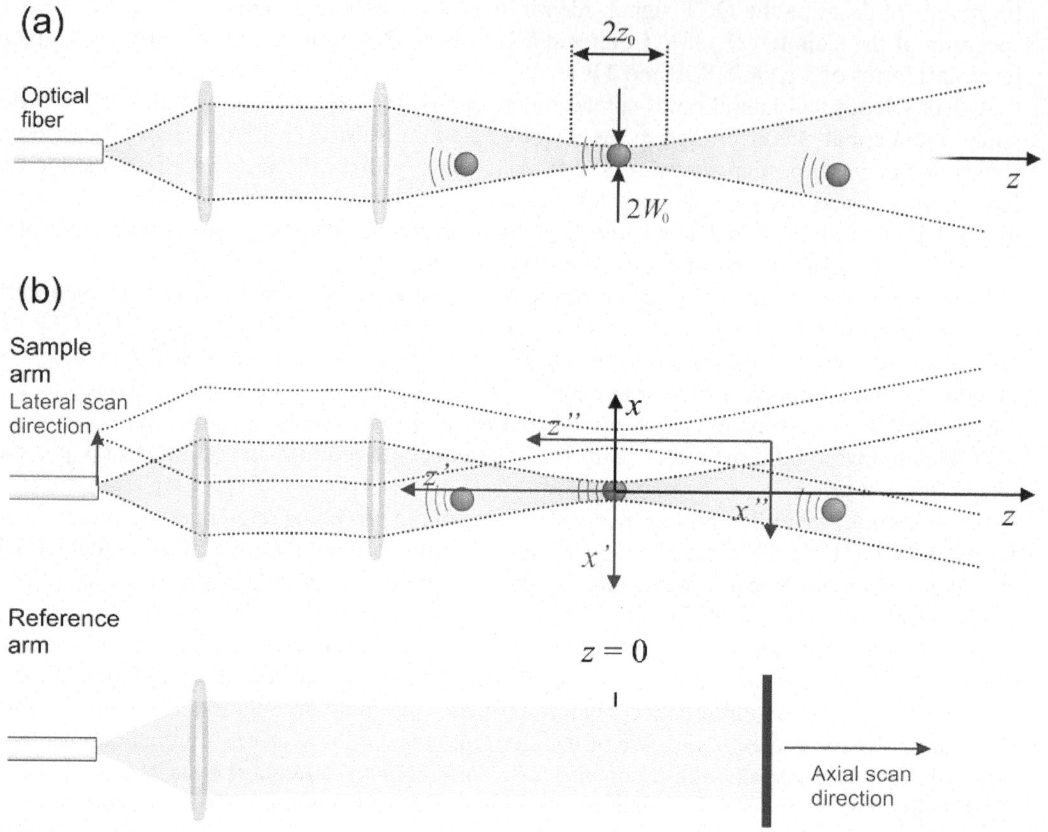

Figure 6.7: (a) Confocal sectioning ability of OCT. The same optical system is used for illumination and collection. Light backscattered from near the focused illumination beam waist will tend to be coupled back into the optical fiber, whereas light backscattered from elsewhere will not. The beam half-width at the waist is equal to W_0 and the Rayleigh range is $2z_0$. (b) Depiction of the coordinate systems used in the analysis, particularly subsequent to Eq. (6.26). The (x,z) coordinates represent absolute position in space, relative to the optical axis and the beam waist. The (x',z') coordinates represent the position of the (x,z)-*origin* with respect to a scatterer, so that they will be *positive* when the *scatterer* position is in the directions indicated by the arrows. The (x'',z'') coordinates (translated with respect to the (x',z') coordinates) indicate the current (axial and lateral) *scan position* relative to a scatterer, suitable for defining the local PSF.

Gaussian beam, with far-field divergence angle θ_0.[16] The numerical aperture (NA) of the beam is equal to $\sin\theta_0$, and the beam width at the waist is equal to $W_0 = \lambda/(\pi\theta_0)$.

In Fig. 6.7(b), we depict the three different spatial coordinate systems that will be used in the subsequent analysis. They are represented by the vectors $\mathbf{r}$, $\mathbf{r}'$, $\mathbf{r}''$. The first, $\mathbf{r} = (x,y,z)$ indicates (absolute) position in space, in particular the OCT scan position in Eq. (6.29). [The origin is set by the beam waist location and the optical axis at the (central) lateral scan position.] The vector $\mathbf{r}' = (x',y',z')$ indicates the position of the *origin* (in absolute $\mathbf{r}$-space) relative to the position of an individual scatterer. In the figure, the directions of the axes' arrows are reversed (compared

[16] As we shall explain later, following Eq. (6.28), we utilize "negative" wavenumber values k_λ in defining the source spectrum in this section, hence the need for the modulus sign in $|k_\lambda|$.

with the absolute-position case) so that they indicate the *scatterer-position* directions for which the coordinates will be more *positive*. Vector $\mathbf{r}'' = (x'', y'', z'')$ indicates the *scan position* relative to the scatterer, appropriate for a local-PSF formalism.

The Gaussian profile at the waist has scalar, complex amplitude:

$$U(x,y) = \frac{\sqrt{2}}{\sqrt{\pi}W_0} \exp\left[-\left(x^2+y^2\right)/W_0^2\right]. \tag{6.23}$$

It has been normalized so the total power is unity, i.e., $\iint_{-\infty}^{\infty} |U(x,y)|^2 \mathrm{d}x\mathrm{d}y = 1$. Its Fourier transform is:

$$\mathscr{F}_U(k_x, k_y; k_\lambda, \theta_0) \triangleq \mathscr{F}[U(x,y)] = \sqrt{2\pi}\, W_0 \exp\left[-(W_0/2)^2\left(k_x^2 + k_y^2\right)\right]. \tag{6.24}$$

Let the corresponding propagating wave (in the $+z$ direction), be represented by $U(x,y,z)$, for which $U(x,y)$ is the beam profile at the waist ($z = 0$), that is, $U(x,y) \equiv U(x,y,0)$. Note that this complex-amplitude representation suppresses the time-dependent factor $\exp(-jk_\lambda ct)$. The Fourier transform of $U(x,y,z)$ can be obtained from $\mathscr{F}_U$ by associating each two-dimensional Fourier component of the latter with a three-dimensional component of magnitude k_λ, projecting the distribution onto a hemispherical sphere cap according to the rule:

$$\mathscr{F}_{U,3}(\mathbf{k}; k_\lambda, \theta_0)$$
$$= \begin{cases} \mathscr{F}_U(k_x, k_y; k_\lambda, \theta_0)\left[2\pi\, \delta(k_r - |k_\lambda|)\right] \sqrt{1 - \frac{k_x^2 + k_y^2}{k_\lambda^2}}, & \text{if } k_x^2 + k_y^2 < k_\lambda^2 \text{ and } k_z > 0; \\ 0 & \text{otherwise,} \end{cases} \tag{6.25}$$

where $k_r = \|\mathbf{k}\| = \left[k_x^2 + k_y^2 + k_z^2\right]^{1/2}$ and δ is the one-dimensional Dirac delta function. Only propagating plane-wave components (as opposed to evanescent waves) are permitted. The square-root reduction factor arises through the necessity to keep the integral of the function over any region of (k_x, k_y)-space constant despite the fact that it is spread from a plane to a hemisphere. That is, it guarantees that $\int_{-\infty}^{\infty} \mathscr{F}_{U,3}(k_x, k_y, k_z)\mathrm{d}k_z = 2\pi\, \mathscr{F}_U(k_x, k_y)$. Equation (6.25) represents the Gaussian beam's plane-wave angular spectrum [36]. We note that the Gaussian beam is normally defined for paraxial optics [47], in which case the hemisphere in spatial-frequency space is approximated with a paraboloid. Additionally, the restriction $k_x^2 + k_y^2 < k_\lambda^2$ amounts to aperturing or cropping the Gaussian spectral profile. For our purposes, these issues are of minor consequence: we are of course free to utilize any arbitrary focal-plane illumination distribution in Eq. (6.23). Its Fourier transform can then be projected onto the sphere as in Eq. (6.25). For our primary objective of calculating speckle size, we do not need to inverse-Fourier transform the latter equation to generate an expression for the "Gaussian" or other beam profile in 3D space. The spatial-frequency representation is sufficient.

According to the first-order Born approximation, the detectable sample three-dimensional spatial-frequency components $\mathbf{K}$ are given by the difference between the scattered ($\mathbf{k}_s$) and incident ($\mathbf{k}_i$) wave-vectors, $\mathbf{K}=\mathbf{k}_s-\mathbf{k}_i$ [27]. Thus, the contribution of one wavenumber to the local TF can be represented as the *convolution* between the angular spectrum of $\mathbf{k}_s$ and the angular spectrum of $-\mathbf{k}_i$ (that is, the respective distributions of plane-wave components of the two beams). *Both of these spectra are the same*, due to the confocal gate effect of Assumption 2. That is, the collectable backscattered angular spectrum is identical to that of the reverse-propagating incident wave. We note that complex-conjugate operation must be applied to the propagating wave profile $U(x,y,z)$ to effect a reversal in direction, and that $\mathscr{F}\{U^*(x,y,z)\} = \mathscr{F}_{U,3}^*(-\mathbf{k}; k_\lambda, \theta_0)$. Thus, the Fourier transform of the single-wavelength contribution to the OCT PSF may be obtained by convolving the Gaussian sphere cap $\mathscr{F}_{U,3}^*(-\mathbf{k}; k_\lambda, \theta_0)$ with itself. Since $\mathscr{F}_{U,3}$ is strictly real, then, the single-wavenumber contribution to the TF:

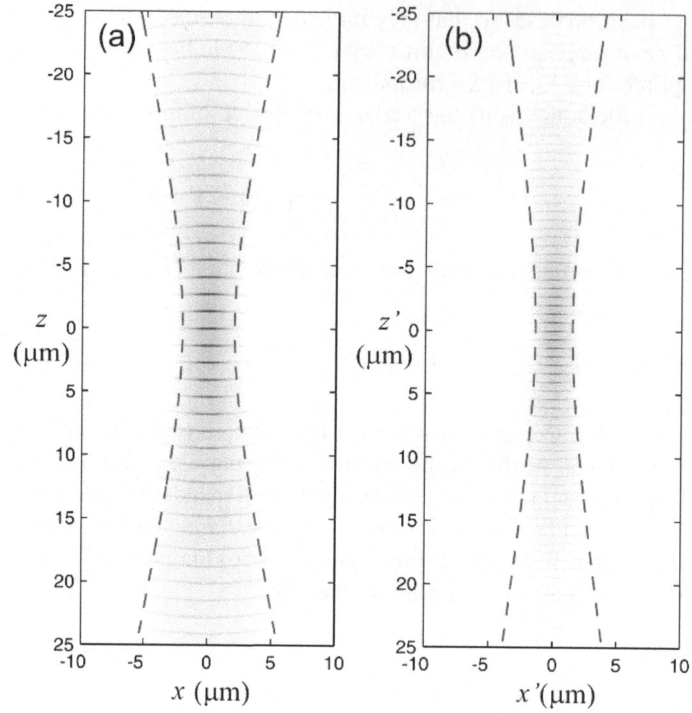

Figure 6.8: (a) Gaussian beam (field) profile in space (1325-nm wavelength, 0.2 NA). The phase fronts corresponding to zero phase are highlighted; (b) Single-wavelength contribution to the OCT PSF, exhibiting the confocal sectioning (gating) effect, obtained by squaring the complex conjugate of the profile in (a). The dashed lines indicate $1/e$ widths.

$$\mathscr{K}(\mathbf{k};k_\lambda,\theta_0) = \iiint_{-\infty}^{\infty} \mathscr{F}_{U,3}(\mathbf{m})\,\mathscr{F}_{U,3}(-\mathbf{k}-\mathbf{m})\,\mathrm{d}^3\mathbf{m}. \tag{6.26}$$

The single-wavelength contribution in **r***-space is, thus, the square of the complex conjugate of the original propagating Gaussian beam complex amplitude profile*, as we use the same aperture for illumination and collection (otherwise, this "squaring" operation becomes the product of two distinct beam profiles). This fact is illustrated in Fig. 6.8. In Fig. 6.8(a), the Gaussian-beam complex amplitude profile is depicted, for a wavelength of 1325 nm and an NA of 0.2. The total beam power is the same in each lateral plane. The single-wavelength contribution to the OCT PSF, $\mathscr{F}^{-1}\{\mathscr{K}\}$, is depicted in Fig. 6.8(b). Now, if we use the inverse Fourier transform operation $\mathscr{F}^{-1}$ to map between the **k** and the $\mathbf{r}'$ domains, then $\mathscr{F}^{-1}\{\mathscr{K}\}$ represents the system response to a point scatterer at location $-\mathbf{r}' = (-x', -y', -z')$ when the system scan position is at the origin.[17] In Fig. 6.8(b), the spacing between phase fronts has halved [as compared with those of Fig. 6.8(a)], and the profile $\mathscr{F}^{-1}\{\mathscr{K}\}$ exhibits a confocal sectioning effect – its signal power is more concentrated near the origin.

This overlap integral of Eq. (6.26), between two sphere caps, is represented in Fig. 6.9(a) in **m**-space[18], $\mathbf{m}=(m_x, m_y, m_z)$. The case NA $= 0.5$ is represented, to clearly depict the effect of the curvature of the sphere caps $\mathscr{F}_{U,3}$. (Other figures in this section, with the exception of Fig. 6.15,

[17]Thus, the position of the origin relative to the scatterer is $\mathbf{r}'$; see Fig. 6.7(b).

[18]The dummy vector **m** represents wavenumber in order to perform the convolution operation.

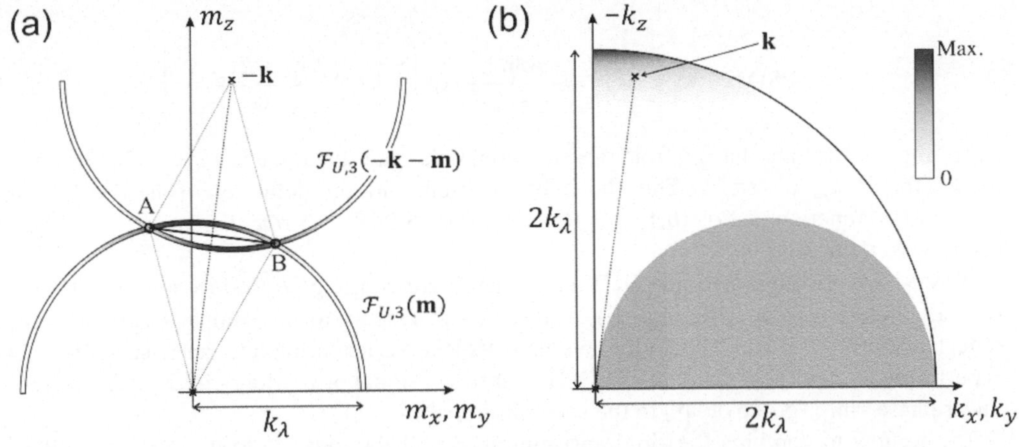

Figure 6.9: (a) Depiction of the integral of Eq. (6.26) for the case NA $= 0.5$, the convolution of two sphere caps with radius k_λ (k_λ is depicted as a positive quantity); (b) The result of the convolution, the single-wavenumber contribution to the OCT TF $\mathscr{K}(\mathbf{k}; k_\lambda, \theta_0)$. The grayed-out region corresponds to the area for which Eq. (6.27) is not applicable.

are plotted with NA $= 0.2$.) The plane of the page contains the m_z-axis and the center of the second sphere (at point $-\mathbf{k}$). The circle of intersection between the two hemispheres is orthogonal to this plane; its diameter is the line segment AB. $\mathscr{K}$, is represented in Fig. 6.9(b). Note that its spatial-frequency range of support is a "solid" sphere cap, with some depth in the k_z direction, corresponding to the confocal axial sectioning ability evident in Fig. 6.8(b).

Based on the preceding expressions, we obtain the following result (after some calculation):

$$|k_\lambda|\mathscr{K}(\mathbf{k}; k_\lambda, \theta_0) = \frac{8\pi^4}{R\theta_0^2}\exp\left[\frac{Q^2+2Z^2-8}{4\theta_0^2}\right]\left[(2Z^2-Q^2)I_0\left(\frac{Q^2}{4\theta_0^2}\right) - Q^2 I_1\left(\frac{Q^2}{4\theta_0^2}\right)\right], \quad (6.27)$$

where I_0 and I_1 are modified Bessel functions of the first kind, zeroth- and first-order, respectively, and the scaled parameters are $X = k_x/|k_\lambda|$, $Y = k_y/|k_\lambda|$, $Z = k_z/|k_\lambda|$, and $\rho = \sqrt{X^2+Y^2}$, $R = \sqrt{\rho^2+Z^2}$, $Q^2 = \left(4/R^2-1\right)\rho^2$. The expression on the right-hand side of Eq. (6.27) depends on the *five* arguments of $\mathscr{K}$ only through the *three* parameters ρ, Z, and θ_0.

The expression of Eq. (6.27) is only valid when $k_z < 0$ and $||\mathbf{k}|| \leq 2|k_\lambda|$. If either of these conditions is not satisfied, then $\mathscr{K}(\mathbf{k}; k_\lambda, \theta_0) = 0$. However, there is another case for which $\mathscr{K} \neq 0$, but Eq. (6.27) is not valid. This is when the intersection of the hemispherical shells does not constitute an entire circle, but only a partial circle, which will occur when $\left(\sqrt{k_x^2+k_y^2} - |k_\lambda|\right)^2 + k_z^2 < k_\lambda^2$. This region is grayed out in Fig. 6.9(b). However, as can be seen in the image, the value of $\mathscr{K}$ is negligible in this region when compared with the maximum value (darkest gray), at $\mathbf{k} = (0, 0, -2|k_\lambda|)$. This is true for the low-to-moderate NAs used in OCT (certainly, if NA < 0.3, say), in which case the value of $\mathscr{K}$ in this region may be ignored.

We now combine multiple wavelengths to generate the OCT local TF. This will permit us to describe the coherence gate, whose axial position is varied to perform an axial scan. When the coherence gate is aligned with the confocal gate ($z = 0$), the imaging system is described by an "in-focus" local PSF. Otherwise, it is described by an "out-of-focus" local PSF. Recalling our assumption from Section 6.2 that the source power spectral density (PSD) is Gaussian in the k_λ -domain, with center wavenumber $k_{\lambda,c}$ and FWHM bandwidth Δk_λ , then its PSD is given by:

$$\mathrm{PSD}\left(k_\lambda;k_{\lambda,c},\Delta k_\lambda\right)=\frac{4\ \ln 2}{\pi(\Delta k_\lambda)^2}\exp\left[-4\ \ln 2\left(\frac{k_\lambda+k_{\lambda,c}}{\Delta k_\lambda}\right)^2\right]. \tag{6.28}$$

Note, importantly, that starting from this equation, we explicitly utilize *negative* values for wavenumber k_λ, that is, $k_\lambda = -2\pi/\lambda$. This choice is consistent with our definition of the Fourier transform and analytic function of Eq. (6.1) (cf. Ref. [1], Eq. (6-24)). We maintain a positive value for the center wavenumber $k_{\lambda,c}$.

As we have already noted, the OCT TF is merely *local*, not *global*, since although the modality (in the single backscattering regime) is linear (with respect to the sample's complex amplitude reflectance profile) it is *not* spatially invariant. Its PSF varies throughout an A-scan. The scanning is performed (either physically in TD-OCT or through signal processing in FD-OCT) by applying a linear phase ramp (group delay) to the spectral-domain signal.

To see how to combine the single-wavenumber contributions $\mathscr{K}$ to generate the full TF, note that $\mathscr{K}$ is non-zero only for negative values of k_z. Thus, the phase of its inverse Fourier transform, $\mathscr{F}^{-1}\{\mathscr{K}\}$, tends to become more *negative* as z' (the origin position relative to the scatterer position) increases.[19] This phase variation will increase in proportion to $|k_\lambda|$, so that in order to "target" a location $z' \neq 0$ on the axis of $\mathscr{F}^{-1}\{\mathscr{K}\}$ [see Fig. 6.8(b)] by equalizing the phases of each spectral contribution to the OCT signal, we would need to multiply each such spectral component by the factor $\exp[-jk_\lambda(2z')]$, noting that $|k_\lambda| = -k_\lambda$. This is equivalent to scanning the reference arm. We recall that it still corresponds to targeting a scatterer at depth $-z'$, so the reference-arm axial scan position is $z = -z'$. Also, as in Eq. (6.1), the factor 2 is due to the double-pass. The phase factor corresponds exactly to the scanning operation mentioned in the previous paragraph.

So the detected signal (as a function of $\mathbf{r}'$), in response to a scatterer located at position $-\mathbf{r}'$, when the reference-arm scan position is z, has Fourier transform:

$$\mathscr{R}\left(\mathbf{k};z,k_{\lambda,c},\Delta k_\lambda,\theta_0\right)=\int_{-\infty}^{0}\mathscr{K}\left(\mathbf{k};k_\lambda,\theta_0\right)\left(\frac{k_\lambda^2}{4\pi}\right)\mathrm{PSD}\left(k_\lambda;k_{\lambda,c},\Delta k_\lambda\right)\exp\left[+jk_\lambda(2z)\right]\,dk_\lambda. \tag{6.29}$$

The Fourier transform in this case is still from the $\mathbf{r}'$ to $\mathbf{k}$ coordinates, and the correction factor $k_\lambda^2/(4\pi)$ takes into account the wavenumber dependence of F_S, as described in Section 6.2.1.

The exponential factor in the integrand on the right-hand side of Eq. (6.29) is equal to unity when $z = 0$. This represents the fact that the focal-plane complex amplitude distribution $U(x,y,z=0)$, was originally defined to have uniform phase, constant (zero) over all wavenumbers. This is also true for the *square* of the complex conjugate of U, so that the in-focus TF may be generated without applying a wavenumber-dependent phase correction factor to the individual solid sphere cap ($\mathscr{K}$) components. The different-wavenumber contributions to $\mathscr{R}$ will add in phase to give the strongest possible accumulation. This is illustrated in Fig. 6.10(a), for which solid caps are generated assuming $\mathrm{NA} = 0.2$, $\lambda_c = 1325$ nm, and $\Delta k_\lambda = 0.36\ \mu\mathrm{m}^{-1}$.[20] The uniform shading over the caps indicates constant phase. However, for non-zero values of z, the single-wavenumber solid sphere caps will be assigned a different phase (constant over the extent of the cap); the rate at which the phase varies with k_λ will depend on z. To the extent that the solid sphere caps overlap, they will not add in phase, and therefore partially cancel each other (when compared to the $z = 0$ case). This will diminish the relative strength of the "out-of-focus" TF. This point is illustrated graphically in Fig. 6.10(b), where the phase factors are indicated with different colors over a continuum from red to blue (represented as gray scale).

[19] As z' increases, or as scatterer position decreases with respect to the scan position, the detected sample-arm signal will appear to be delayed less, or be emitted later in time ([36], Section 4.2.1, pp. 67-68).

[20] The system FWHM bandwidth in wavelength space is 100 nm.

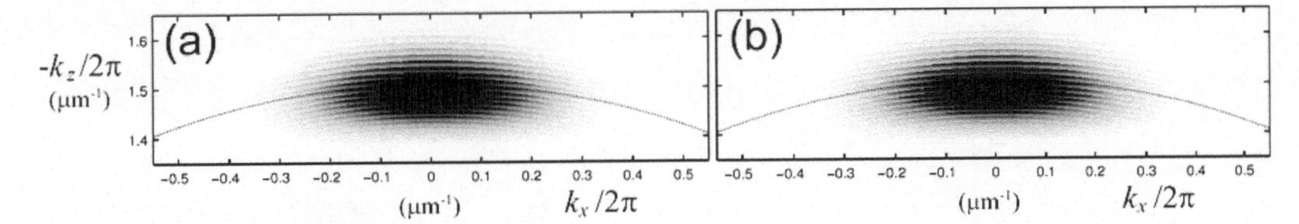

Figure 6.10: Demonstration of the construction of the OCT local TF by combining the single-wavenumber contributions, following Eq. (6.29). (a) Generation of the "in-focus" local TF ($z = 0$) by combining the solid sphere caps $\mathscr{K}$ (associated with different wavenumbers k_λ, depicted discretely every 36 μm^{-1}) "in phase"; (b) Generation of the "out-of-focus" local TF ($z \neq 0$) by applying a k_λ-dependent phase factor to the different solid sphere caps. The OCT system parameters are NA $= 0.2$, $\lambda_c = 1325$ nm, and $\Delta k_\lambda = 0.36\ \mu\text{m}^{-1}$, and the dashed line is a circle of radius $2k_{\lambda,c}$, similar to the circle in Fig. 6.9(b).

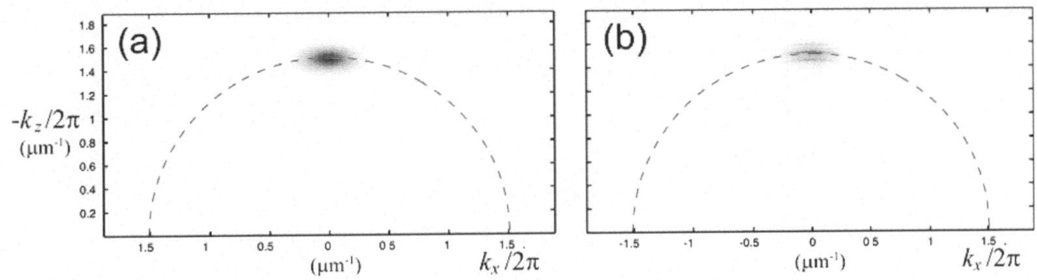

Figure 6.11: OCT local TFs [before the correction of Eq. (6.30): (a) "in-focus", $z = 0$; (b) "out-of-focus", $z = 15\ \mu$m. The system parameters are the same as for Fig. 6.10 (NA $= 0.2$, $\lambda_c = 1325$ nm, and $\Delta k_\lambda = 0.36\ \mu\text{m}^{-1}$), and the dashed line is the circle of radius $2k_{\lambda,c}$. The linear color scales are consistent between the plots; zero-phase fringes are depicted in (b).

Figure 6.11 depicts the form of the function $\mathscr{R}\left(\mathbf{k}; z, k_{\lambda,c}, \Delta k_\lambda, \theta_0\right)$ for the two cases: (a) $z = 0$; and (b) $z \neq 0$. The OCT system parameters are the same as those used to generate Fig. 6.10; in Fig. 6.11(b)the scan distance $z = 15\ \mu$m. The two curves are plotted using the same scale, indicating the relative weakness of the "out-of-focus" local TF. It contains a strong phase ramp component (indicated with fringes in the figure), due to the k_λ-dependent phase factor illustrated in Fig. 6.11(b).

The expression for $\mathscr{R}$ in Eq. (6.29) is not yet the local TF. This is because its inverse Fourier transform will be centered at the point $z' = -z$ rather than the origin. To correct for this, we must multiply the entire expression by the phase ramp $\exp[-jk_z z]$, yielding the final expression for the OCT local TF:

$$\mathscr{H}\left(\mathbf{k}; z, k_{\lambda,c}, \Delta k_\lambda, \theta_0\right) = \int_{-\infty}^{0} \mathscr{K}\left(\mathbf{k}; k_\lambda, \theta_0\right) \left(\frac{k_\lambda^2}{4\pi}\right) \mathrm{PSD}\left(k_\lambda; k_{\lambda,c}, \Delta k_\lambda\right) \exp\left[jz(2k_\lambda - k_z)\right] \, \mathrm{d}k_\lambda . \tag{6.30}$$

The Fourier transform $\mathscr{F}$ can now be viewed as mapping between the $\mathbf{r}''$ and the $\mathbf{k}$ domains, where $\mathbf{r}'' = \mathbf{r}' + \mathbf{r}$ indicates the *scan* position with respect to the scatterer, as is appropriate for a PSF [refer again to Fig. 6.7(b)]. The effect of the factor $\exp[-jk_z z]$ is to remove the linear component of the k_z-phase ramp in the local TF of Fig. 6.11(b). (The residual phase curvature remains.) We also note that $\mathscr{H}$ depends on $\mathbf{r}$ only through the z coordinate. As shown, it is a function of seven arguments. By appropriate parameter scaling, they may be reduced to five: $\hat{Z} = k_z/k_{\lambda,c}$, $\widehat{\rho} = \sqrt{k_x^2 + k_y^2}/k_{\lambda,c}$, $\Delta\beta = \Delta k_\lambda / k_{\lambda,c}$, $\hat{z} = k_{\lambda,c} z$, and θ_0. The function can be evaluated numerically.

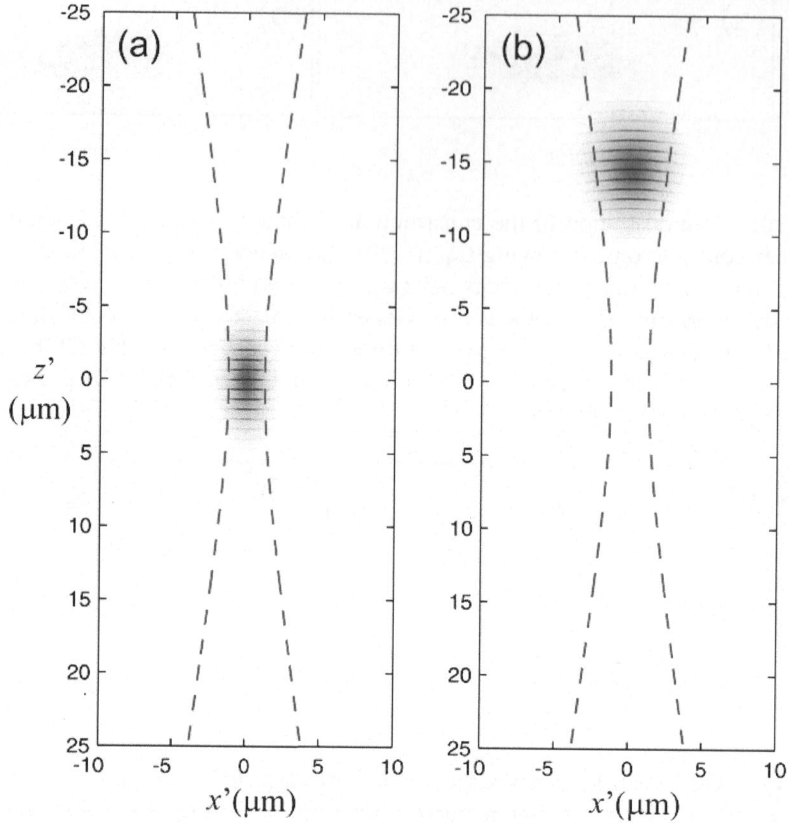

Figure 6.12: Representation of the OCT local PSFs at different axial scan positions: (a) "in-focus", $z = 0$; (b) "out-of-focus", $z = 15\ \mu$m. (In the latter case, we are targeting a scatterer at position $z = -z' = 15\ \mu$m, and we do not include the translation to the origin represented by Eq. (6.30).) Both distributions have been plotted on a gray color scale (after normalization to their respective peak values) and zero-phase fringes are indicated.

The inverse Fourier transforms of the functions $\mathscr{R}(\mathbf{k})$ corresponding to the cases of Fig. 6.11 are plotted in Fig. 6.12. Both PSFs are normalized (to their respective peaks) so that their relative widths and fringe patterns can be easily compared. (Their relative magnitudes can be gleaned by inspecting the relative on-axis signal strengths in Fig. 6.8(b) corresponding to their respective peak positions.) In the out-of-focus case [Fig. 6.11(b)], the PSF broadening and phase front curvature are clearly evident.

The OCT system's low-pass-filter transverse characteristics and band-pass-filter axial characteristics are clearly evident from Fig. 6.11. The speckle distortion introduced by coherent imaging systems can be explained in terms of this limited spatial-frequency coverage of the OCT TF $\mathscr{H}$ [5]. As a comparison, for incoherent imaging systems, both the relevant sample information [$A(\mathbf{r})$ from Section 6.2.2] and the *optical* transfer function are "baseband." For the coherent case, the useful sample information is diffused over a broad range of 3D spatial frequencies, due to the rapidly fluctuating phase distribution $R(\mathbf{r})$. (Reconstructions from each spatial-frequency subrange give different speckled realizations of the structure, accessible to the incoherent image.)

It is difficult to put a size scale on the relevant range of possible spatial sample frequencies over which useful information could be obtained. Schmitt et al. [5] have proposed that the length scales of useful variations in tissue are set by the scales of the continuous structures, with the smallest

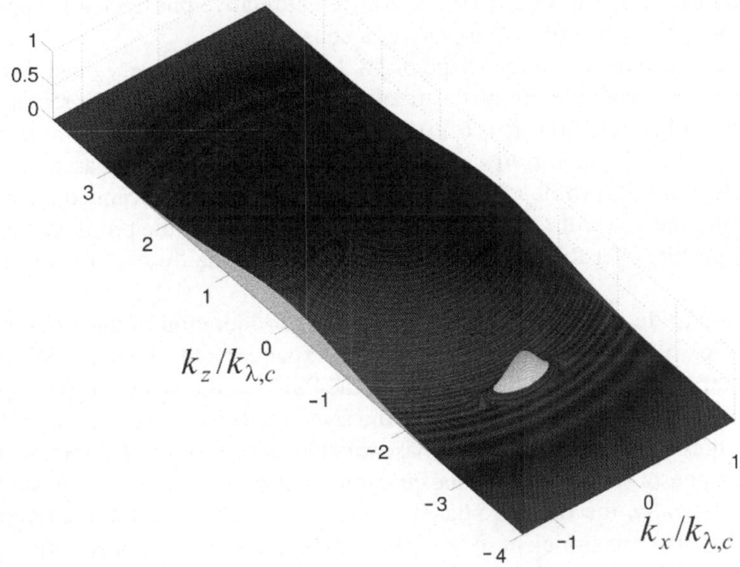

Figure 6.13: Representation of the spatial frequency content of biological tissue $\overline{|\mathrm{X}(\mathbf{k})|}$ (broad Gaussian function centered at the origin) compared with the spatial frequency response of OCT $\mathscr{H}(\mathbf{k})$ (small peak at $k_x = 0,\ k_z = -k_{\lambda,c}$). In this representation, $\Delta\beta = 0.075$, and NA = 0.2.

being a protein macromolecule.

If we assume a circularly Gaussian-profiled sample spatial frequency spectrum (say, in expected modulus) $\overline{|\mathrm{X}(\mathbf{k})|} = \overline{|\mathscr{F}\{\chi(\mathbf{r})\}|}$, then we can plot representative values for the expected magnitudes of the sample's spatial frequency spectrum $\mathrm{X}(\mathbf{k})$ and the TF $\mathscr{H}(\mathbf{k})$, as shown in Fig. 6.13. The figure further demonstrates graphically the "missing"-frequency [5] interpretation of OCT image formation (and speckle).

This "missing"-frequency interpretation is particularly relevant to OCT as it is a coherent imaging modality performed in reflection mode. In transmission mode, the speckle pattern depends almost entirely on the phase responses of the sample scatterers. In reflection mode, it depends also on their relative axial positions; the total distance travelled by the backscattered light will determine its phase contribution to the final signal. Equivalently, this is due to the fact that reflection-mode coherent imaging is band-pass (in the axial direction), but transmission-mode imaging is low-pass. (Because of the possibly different phase responses of the scatterers, both coherent imaging modes will be affected by speckle.)

6.4.2 Speckle size: single backscattering case

What implications can we draw for second-order speckle statistics? As noted in Section 6.3.2, the speckle correlation function is given by the inverse Fourier transform of $|\mathscr{H}|^2$ (after normalization). So how does this vary with scan position z?

To answer this question, recall from Section 6.3.2 that the speckle correlation function is the Fourier transform of a scaled version of $|\mathscr{H}(\mathbf{k})|^2$ (or alternatively, $|\mathscr{R}(\mathbf{k})|^2$). And, indeed, the shape of $|\mathscr{H}(\mathbf{k})|^2$ depends on z. To examine this dependence, consider Eq. (6.29). In the integrand, the solid cap $\mathscr{K}(\mathbf{k};k_\lambda,\theta_0)$ is multiplied by a k_λ-dependent phase factor $\exp[+jk_\lambda(2z)]$. Because the solid caps $\mathscr{K}$ have non-zero spatial extent in the k_z-direction, then they will overlap for different wavenumbers k_λ. (Refer to Fig. 6.10.) The different relative phase factors applied to the caps as z varies will cause the shape of $|\mathscr{H}|$ to vary as a consequence.

However, it is also true that the shape of $|\mathscr{H}|$ will not change very much for common values of the parameters. For example, its spatial-frequency region of support will remain approximately the same. (Refer to Figs. 6.11(a) versus 6.11(b).) Thus, we can infer that *speckle size will remain almost constant over the entire scan range.* This may seem counterintuitive, based on an inspection of the single-wavelength PSF profile of Fig. 6.8. If the beam focus is scanned laterally, then we might assume that the speckle will remain correlated to the extent that the profile remains overlapped with the original profile. Yet the profile is much narrower at the "waist" ($z=0$) than anywhere else ($z\neq 0$).

The solution to this apparent paradox lies in the consideration of the phase fronts of the profile. As seen in Fig. 6.12(b), the phase fronts of the expanded out-of-focus PSF are curved. Speckle spatial correlation arises due to the fact that as the PSF[21] is translated in space (generating the OCT scan), it continues to "see" at least some of the same scatterers in each region of coverage. Equally importantly, they must retain the same phase relationship (or phase difference) in their contribution to the random phasor sum. However, the curvature of the PSF phase fronts ensures that as the profile is translated laterally, the relative phases applied to different sample scatterers will vary. These relative phase shifts are sufficient to maintain almost the same lateral speckle correlation length as for the in-focus PSF, despite the fact that the out-of-focus profile is broader. That is, away from the focus, OCT lateral resolution will degrade, but speckle size will remain almost constant. From an alternative standpoint, the information content of the OCT signal remains constant along the z axis. Thus, as demonstrated in the previously mentioned ISAM technique, it is possible in some instances to utilize this information to synthesize an OCT signal with in-focus lateral resolution over a large scan range [41].

To quantify the (small) increase in speckle size due to z-defocus, we firstly define two quantities, the speckle *characteristic length* in the axial direction, ℓ_a, and the *characteristic area* in the transverse direction A_t, in terms of the speckle correlation function $\gamma(\Delta\mathbf{r})\equiv\gamma(\Delta x,\Delta y,\Delta z)$, defined in Eq. (6.19), as follows:

$$\ell_a\left(z,k_{\lambda,c},\Delta k_\lambda,\theta_0\right)=\int_{-\infty}^{\infty}|\gamma(0,0,\Delta z)|^2\,\mathrm{d}(\Delta z); \tag{6.31}$$

$$A_t\left(z,k_{\lambda,c},\Delta k_\lambda,\theta_0\right)=\iint_{-\infty}^{\infty}|\gamma(\Delta x,\Delta y,0)|^2\,\mathrm{d}(\Delta x)\,\mathrm{d}(\Delta y). \tag{6.32}$$

Using Parseval's theorem [36], we can express these quantities in terms of $|\mathscr{H}|$. Thus, using Eq. (6.30), we plot speckle *relative size* for $z\neq 0$, specifically the ratios $\ell_a(z)/\ell_a(0)$, $A_t(z)/A_t(0)$ for different OCT system parameters in Fig. 6.14.

In each case, it is observed that the speckle size tends to increase with defocus distance, reaching an asymptote for large values after only a few Rayleigh lengths. The effect in the axial direction is much stronger than that in the transverse direction, unsurprisingly because the $\mathscr{K}$-contributions of each wavelength to the local TF $\mathscr{H}$ are displaced with respect to each other primarily in the axial direction. For the axial case, values that are significantly greater than 1 are observed for either high NAs (in which case the axial scanning range will be very limited), or low system bandwidths (in which case the axial resolution will be very broad). Neither case is relevant to conventional OCT imaging over a significant depth range. Thus, we may conclude that speckle size is constant over the extent of an A-scan.

[21] Strictly speaking, we mean a mirrored version of the PSF in all three directions.

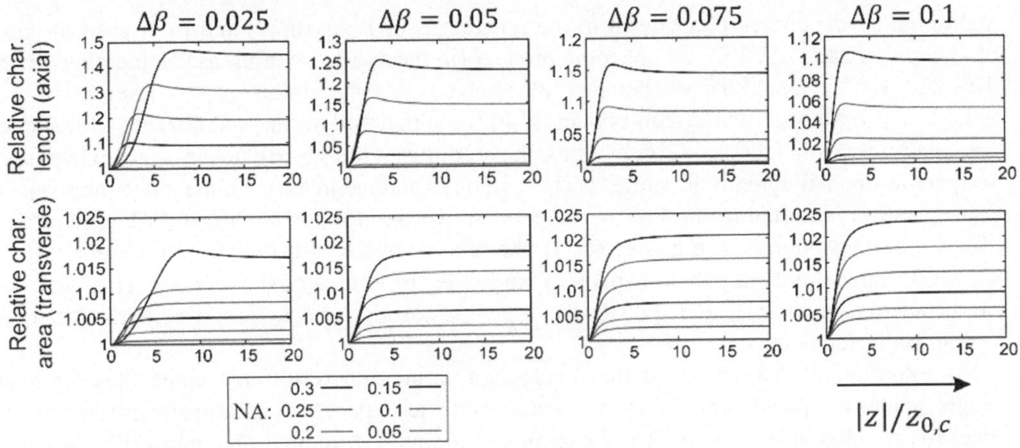

Figure 6.14: Plots of relative characteristic length (axial) $\ell_a(z)/\ell_a(0)$, and area (transverse) $A_t(z)/\ell_a(0)$ for OCT speckle versus $|z|/z_{0,c}$, where $z_{0,c}$ is the Rayleigh length of the beam at the center wavenumber. The curves are plotted for a range of relative bandwidths $\Delta\beta = \Delta k_\lambda / k_{\lambda,c}$ and NAs.

For low system NAs, it is often convenient to ignore the curvature of the sphere cap of $\mathscr{F}_{U,3}$, essentially disregarding the diffraction of the beam. Under this assumption, the preceding expressions become particularly simple. We have, up to k_λ-independent scaling constants:

$$\mathscr{F}_{U,3}(\mathbf{k};k_\lambda,\theta_0) = \left(\frac{1}{|k_\lambda|}\right)\exp\left[-\left(\frac{1}{k_\lambda\theta_0}\right)^2 (k_x^2+k_y^2)\right]\delta(k_z-|k_\lambda|); \tag{6.33}$$

$$\mathscr{K}(\mathbf{k};k_\lambda,\theta_0) = \left(\frac{1}{k_\lambda}\right)^2\exp\left[-\frac{1}{2}\left(\frac{1}{k_\lambda\theta_0}\right)^2 (k_x^2+k_y^2)\right]\delta(k_z+2|k_\lambda|); \tag{6.34}$$

$$\mathscr{H}(\mathbf{k};k_{\lambda,c},\Delta k_\lambda,\theta_0) = \exp\left[-\frac{1}{2}\left(\frac{2}{k_z\theta_0}\right)^2 (k_x^2+k_y^2)\right]\exp\left[-\ln 2\left(\frac{k_z+2k_{\lambda,c}}{\Delta k_\lambda}\right)^2\right]. \tag{6.35}$$

For this case, the TF $\mathscr{H}$ is global. It is not quite of the separable (with respect to k_x, k_y, k_z) Gaussian form described in Section 6.3.2, but it is close. The approximation $k_z = -2k_{\lambda,c}$ inside the first exponential factor on the right-hand side of Eq. (6.35) would suffice to make it so. Under this approximation,

$$\ell_a(z,k_{\lambda,c},\Delta k_\lambda,\theta_0) = \frac{2\sqrt{\pi \ln 2}}{\Delta k_\lambda}; \tag{6.36}$$

$$A_t(z,k_{\lambda,c},\Delta k_\lambda,\theta_0) = \frac{2\pi}{k_{\lambda,c}^2\theta_0^2}. \tag{6.37}$$

These expressions represent good approximations for the (full-width) speckle size parameters using conventional OCT. Recalling Section 6.3.2, then, if equations like Eqs. (6.31) and (6.32) are used with the in-focus PSF in place of γ, then the speckle size parameter in the axial direction, ℓ_a, is $\sqrt{2}$ times *broader* than the full-width axial resolution ℓ_c; and the speckle size parameter in the transverse directions, A_t, is 2 times *greater* than the lateral resolution area $\pi W_0^2/4$ (where W_0 corresponds to the center-wavenumber beam waist in this case).

We next briefly consider the issue of dispersion, which arises when the sample (average) refractive index contains quadratic and/or higher-order dependence on wavelength. This would result in an additional k_λ-dependent phase term in the integrands of Eqs. (6.29) and (6.30). In the presence of dispersion, the OCT PSF will become broader (in the axial direction) as sample depth increases. This will result in axial PSF broadening [48]. However, at least for the low-NA assumption provided in Eqs. (6.33)–(6.35), each k_λ component $\mathcal{K}$ of the signal will occupy a different k_z-slice of spatial-frequency spectrum (at $k_z = -2|k_\lambda|$). Thus, the modulus of the TF will not be affected by dispersion, so speckle size will remain the same.[22] This can be explained in terms of the *chirp* (non-linear axial phase profile) imparted to the PSF by dispersion. Unlike for the unchirped PSF generated in the absence of dispersion (see, e.g., Eq. (6.1)), the relative phase contribution of different scatterers to the OCT signal (random phasor sum) will vary over the course of the A-scan. This variation will be sufficient to maintain the dispersion-free speckle correlation function, despite the fact that axial resolution is degraded.

An experimental validation of the theory and simulation results presented thus far regarding single-scattering speckle first- and second-order statistics (speckle fluctuation magnitude and speckle size) is provided in Fig. 6.15. The imaging target was a structured phantom [29], similar to that presented in Section 6.2.2. In this case the letters are part of the structured casting (with a TiO_2 scatterer concentration of 10 mg/mL of silicone) and are encased by a transparent embedding silicone casting.

Three FD-OCT systems were used to image the phantom. They had respective center wavelengths of 1325 nm, 835 nm, and 835 nm; bandwidths of 100 nm, 50 nm, and 50 nm; NAs of 0.056, 0.033, and 0.056; theoretical axial resolutions of 7.7 μm, 6.1 μm, and 6.1 μm in air; and theoretical lateral PSF $1/e$ resolutions of 10 μm, 11 μm, and 7 μm.

The images are displayed on a logarithmic scale with the white level corresponding to a signal strength of approximately 60 dB above the noise floor of each image. Different signal-to-noise ratios (SNR) are evident due to the different wavelengths and other system parameters (e.g., sample power, reference reflectivity, shot and intensity noise). Different signal attenuations (attenuation coefficients) are experienced, mainly as a function of wavelength. Once these effects are accounted for, a fair comparison of the speckle patterns can be performed. Their contrast ratio is very close to the exponential limit (or the Rayleigh) if the intensity (or the amplitude), instead of its logarithm, is considered.

The speckle patterns reflect the coarseness as imparted by the respective resolutions (at focus). This means that for the 1325 nm system (Fig. 6.15(a)) the speckle size is relatively isotropic and nearly twice as big as that for the second 835 nm system (Fig. 6.15(c)), while the speckle size for the first 835 nm system (Fig. 6.15(b)) is quite elongated in the lateral direction. Although the resolution changes slightly (small NAs) through the depth (height) of the letters (it could be assessed by the sharpness of the letter edges), the speckle size stays constant both in the axial and the lateral directions.

Inspection of Fig. 6.15 confirms the results presented in Fig. 6.14 by the lower curve (NA = 0.05) for the cases of $\Delta\beta = 0.075$ (approximating the 1325-nm system) and $\Delta\beta = 0.05$ (approximating the second 835-nm system). In both cases the axial speckle size is practically constant and the lateral speckle size varies less than 0.5%.

6.5 OCT Image Formation: Multiple Scattering

A turbid biological sample is composed of many constituents of varying shape, size and refractive index, such as cells and connective structures [49]. As light propagates in tissue it is attenuated, due

[22] This is analogous to the previous observation that the "defocused" and "focused" lateral speckle sizes are nearly the same.

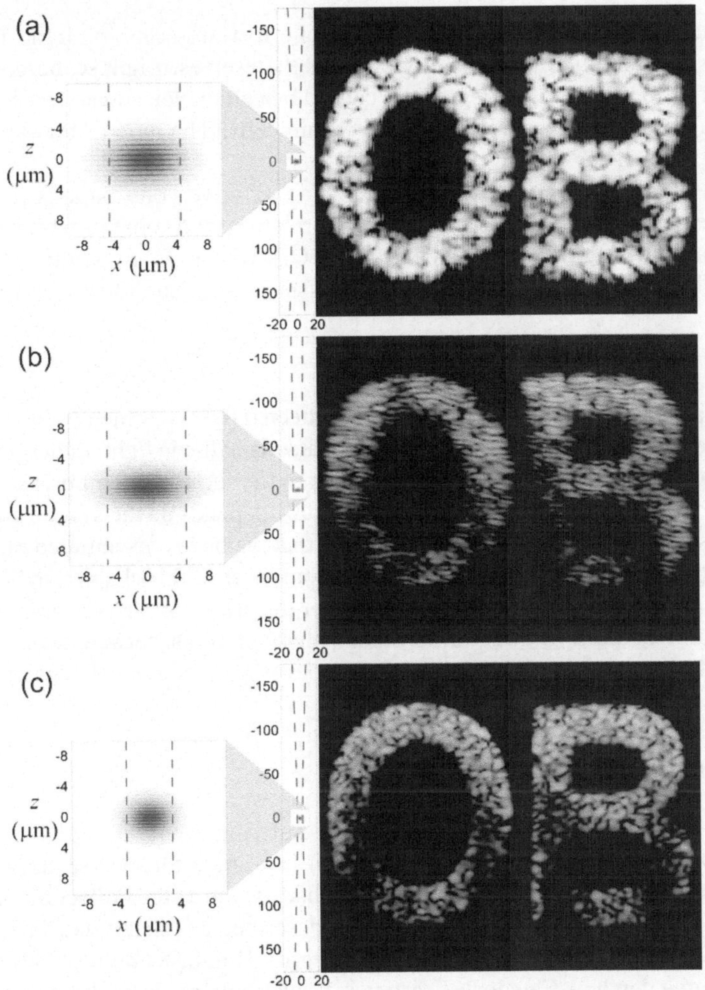

Figure 6.15: Speckled images of a structured phantom acquired with three FD-OCT systems with respective center wavelengths of (a) 1325 nm, (b) 835 nm, and (c) 835 nm; bandwidths of (a) 100 nm, (b) 50 nm, and (c) 50 nm; NAs of (a) 0.056, (b) 0.033, and (c) 0.056; theoretical axial resolutions of (a) 7.7 μm, (b) 6.1 μm, and (c) 6.1 μm in air; and theoretical lateral PSF 1/e resolutions of (a) 10 μm, (b) 11 μm, and (c) 7 μm. Visual inspection indicates that the speckle size changes according to the size of the resolution volume, but does not change with defocus.

to both absorption and scattering. In OCT, the effects of absorption are usually minor as near-infrared light represents a low-absorption window in tissue [30]. Scattering describes the deviation of light waves from a straight trajectory caused by the variation in refractive index of the medium through which they pass.

Tissue may be described as a spatially varying refractive index continuum [26, 50]. The strength and directionality of scattering depend on the gradient of the refractive index. More conveniently, we regard the scattered field contributing to the OCT signal as having undergone only a discrete number of scattering events, the result of light interacting with a finite number of particles that are randomly distributed throughout a scattering sample [26, 51].

The majority of studies directed towards the understanding of light scattering from tissues have been conducted *in vitro* on cell suspensions [26, 50, 52–61]. These studies have broadly confirmed the expectations from Mie theory [49]. Low-angle forward-scattered light in tissues is primarily caused by large spheroid objects, i.e., by the cells themselves. Light scattered at slightly larger angles, perhaps up to a few tens of degrees, is caused by cell nuclei, and at very large angles, including backscattering, is caused by small structures within cells. The ratio of forward to backscattering is typically in excess of 10^3 [62].

Speckle is the result of the coherent summation of wave contributions backscattered from the sample, some of which contain useful image information, and some of which do not, depending on the amount of scattering they have undergone [5, 60]. It is useful to partition the detected light into three categories accordingly. The categories are listed below, and illustrated in Fig. 6.16.

I. Singly backscattered light

Light that propagates through the sample undeflected [63] is termed *ballistic*. In reflection-mode imaging, Category I includes all light that propagates as ballistic light, undergoes a single back scattering event and then propagates undeflected back to the surface. It comprises light scattered within a narrow solid angle around the optic axis. This angle depends on the system collection aperture. Of course, this is the contribution to the OCT signal that we have concentrated on up to this point. We have explicitly defined "single scattering" for the purposes of this chapter, in Section 6.2.2, as "first-order-Born-approximation scattering" [27]. Under this assumption, the sample can be described as the superposition of multiple three-dimensional, phase gratings, between which there are no interaction effects. The assumption has permitted us to develop the previously described transfer-function approach for modelling the imaging system.

II. Low-angle forward-scattered light

The deeper within the sample the single backscattering event takes place, the higher the likelihood of the wave being subjected to a number of low-angle forward-scattering events both in the direction towards the ultimate backscatterer and back towards the collection optics. The trajectory of the scattered wave in both directions is often described as "snake-like," because of the winding paths determined by these scattering events. Category-II light with the backscattering event taking place at the same depth as Category-I carries a greater optical delay, due to its non-direct propagation paths.

III. Wide-angle multiply scattered light

Category-III light has undergone several wide-angle multiple scattering events. For such light, the optical delay travelled does not correspond to a specific depth in the sample. In the limiting case of a great number of scattering events (diffuse light), precise determination of the optical delay will be lost owing to sample dispersion and wavelength-dependent scattering.

We reiterate that the contributions to the OCT signal described in previous sections of the manuscript all correspond to Category-I light, which best represents the sample structure. There is an important distinction between the *multiple instances of singly backscattered light* contributing to the random-phasor sum, and a *multiply scattered wave(let)*, which can be treated as a single phasor.

Category-II scattering implies wavefront distortion of the incident and backscattered beams, resulting in loss of transverse spatial coherence and beam spreading, i.e., resolution degradation and contrast reduction [9], but the detected signal maintains some relation with the sample structure. The backscattering event appears to be deeper than the actual optical depth of the backscattering center, due to the additional pathlength accumulated in its "snake-like" trajectory.

Category-III light does not represent the sample structure, as the signal arises from several scattering events with a complicated trajectory. It degrades contrast without affecting resolution significantly [9]. Multiply scattered light can lead to wide variations in the apparent value of the

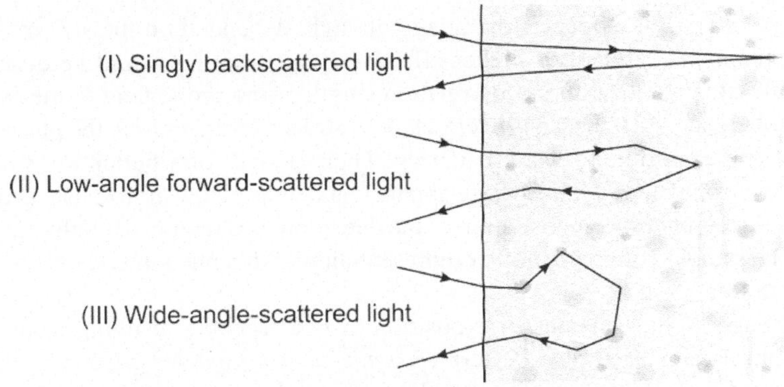

Figure 6.16: Scattering interaction in tissue classified into three categories.

attenuation coefficient μ_t, and a dependence of the measured value on the experimental setup [22, 64–66].

In early work, Schmitt et al. [64] showed that the measured attenuation coefficient depended strongly on beam diameter in the sample and to a slightly lesser degree on wavelength. In their experiment, increasing the beam diameter in the sample by shifting the focal point of the objective to a greater depth, with all else equal, increased the measured attenuation of rat artery. The main effect of shifting the focal point was to increase the transverse cross-section of the medium probed by the beam. The authors supposed that this in turn increased the size range of structures contributing to Category-II low-angle forward-scattering, which led to a greater degradation of the transverse spatial coherence of the beam. As a result, mixing with the reference beam was less efficient and so produced a higher attenuation. Pan et al. [22] showed that the OCT signal was significantly enhanced above what was to be expected based on separately performed narrow-beam, angle-gated backscattering measurements. In their experiment, the higher numerical aperture of the OCT system compared with the angle-gated measurement led to the capture of a greater proportion of all types of multiply scattered light, thus, increasing the overall signal and producing a lower attenuation than expected.

The relative fractions of the three categories of light generated depend on the optical properties of the medium. For illustrative purposes, consider transmission in a homogeneous medium in which absorption can be neglected. We define the optical depth $\mathrm{OD} = \mu_t z_0$, where μ_t is the total attenuation coefficient (assumed equal in this case to the scattering coefficient μ_s, i.e., no absorption), and z_0 is the thickness of the medium. Assuming $\mathrm{OD} = 3$, a Henyey-Greenstein scattering function with anisotropy parameter $g = \langle \cos\theta \rangle$ of 0.85, and that the trajectory of "snake light" does not deviate from the optical axis by more than an angle of $\theta = 10°$, gives 5, 20, and 75%, respectively for the proportions of ballistic, low-angle forward-scattered, and diffuse light. In reflection mode, the proportions of the three categories will be different, but the OCT gating mechanisms also serve to preferentially select the Category-I signal.

The relative contribution of multiple scattering was examined by Yadlowsky et al. [65], commencing with the observation that the signal strength in the OCT image of a fingernail viewed through the 300-μm-thick cuticle was much less than expected based on the signal strength for direct viewing of the nail, and the more or less constant signal strength of the underlying dermis when viewed through either region. This same effect can be observed in subsequently published images [67]. The authors of Ref. [65] conducted a series of experiments in which A-scan signals were detected from small isotropic scatterers overlaid by suspensions of varying concentrations and particle sizes. They concluded that multiple low-angle forward scattering increased the strength of the probe field at depth, and the probe field increased with particle size, consistent with a higher anisotropy parameter. The effect on the image, though, depended on the size of the structures in the sample volume. They claimed higher effective backscattering would be observed only from structures smaller than the transverse correlation length of the probe field (a measure of the transverse spatial coherence [68]), because in effect these structures did not see the phase front distortion caused by low-angle multiple forward scattering. Their second contribution was to demonstrate the presence of an isotropic non-localized haze apparent at depths below high densities of isotropic scatterers, which is an emphatic demonstration of the detection of Category-III light, multiple scattering from outside the sample volume. Another representation of this phenomenon in an OCT image was demonstrated in Ref. [69].

The OCT image is the coherent superposition of both speckle resulting from a small sample resolution volume (Categories I and II), termed *signal-bearing speckle* [5], and speckle representing "noise" associated with light from Category III, termed *signal-degrading speckle* [5]. Category I, as in the example above, is generally the smallest contribution to the light exiting the sample, yet is preferentially selected at detection by the combination of the OCT coherence and confocal gates [3]. As the depth in tissue increases, Category-I light is extinguished exponentially, due to both scattering and absorption [49], and eventually the other categories start to dominate the detected signal. The other multiple scattering mechanisms of low-angle forward scattering (Category II) and wide-angle scattering (Category III) further modify the specific realization of the speckle pattern, such as that shown in the simulation of Fig. 6.4(d).

6.5.1 Speckle size: multiple scattering case

For multiply scattered illumination, the first-order-Born approximation breaks down, and there is no longer a direct dependence between each wavevector illumination/collection pair and a sample spatial frequency component. We consider the extreme case of highly diffuse light, in which there is no direct relationship between the signal associated with any different wavevector pairs. Recognizing that the plane-wave angular spectrum of the light both emitted and collected by the optical system remains the same as in the single-scattering case, and describable in terms of the function $\mathscr{F}_{U,3}$ of Eq. (6.25), then for each wavenumber k_λ, let $\mathscr{G}(\mathbf{k}_{t,\text{in}}, \mathbf{k}_{t,\text{out}};\ k_\lambda)$ be the multiply scattered sample response function, where the transverse wavevector components $\mathbf{k}_{t,\text{in}}=(k_{x,\text{in}}, k_{y,\text{in}})$ and $\mathbf{k}_{t,\text{out}}=(k_{x,\text{out}}, k_{y,\text{out}})$. That is, it is the ratio of the complex amplitude of the plane-wave component of the scattered wave with wavevector $\mathbf{k}_{\text{out}}=\left(k_{x,\text{out}}, k_{y,\text{out}}, -\left[k_\lambda^2 - \|\mathbf{k}_{t,\text{out}}\|^2\right]^{1/2}\right)$ in response to a unit-amplitude plane wave with wavevector $\mathbf{k}_{\text{in}}=\left(k_{x,\text{in}}, k_{y,\text{in}}, \left[k_\lambda^2 - \|\mathbf{k}_{t,\text{in}}\|^2\right]^{1/2}\right)$. The distribution $\mathscr{G}$ is related in a complicated way to the sample refractive index profile. The multiply scattered component of the OCT signal is

$$\begin{aligned} S_{\text{ms}}(\mathbf{r}; k_{\lambda,c}, \Delta k_\lambda, \theta_0) = {} & \tfrac{1}{2\pi}\int_{-\infty}^{0} \mathrm{d}k_\lambda\ \text{PSD}(k_\lambda; k_{\lambda,c}, \Delta k_\lambda)\ \exp[j2k_\lambda z]\ \times \\ & \tfrac{1}{(2\pi)^4}\int\iint_{-\infty}^{\infty}\int \mathrm{d}^2\mathbf{k}_{t,\text{in}}\ \mathrm{d}^2\mathbf{k}_{t,\text{out}}\ \exp[j\mathbf{r}_t\cdot(\mathbf{k}_{t,\text{out}}-\mathbf{k}_{t,\text{in}})]\ \times \\ & \mathscr{G}(\mathbf{k}_{t,\text{in}}, \mathbf{k}_{t,\text{out}};\ k_\lambda)\,\mathscr{F}_U(\mathbf{k}_{t,\text{in}}; k_\lambda, \theta_0)\,\mathscr{F}_U(\mathbf{k}_{t,\text{out}}; k_\lambda, \theta_0). \end{aligned} \tag{6.38}$$

Using the overline notation, as in Section 6.2.2, to represent an ensemble average over possible "microstructure" distributions, then under the highly-diffuse-light assumption, $\mathscr{G}$ is delta-correlated with respect to all of its arguments. Thus, up to a scaling constant:

$$\begin{aligned} & \overline{\mathscr{G}(\mathbf{k}_{t,\text{in}}, \mathbf{k}_{t,\text{out}};\ k_\lambda)\,\mathscr{G}(\mathbf{k}_{t,\text{in}}-\Delta\mathbf{k}_{t,\text{in}}, \mathbf{k}_{t,\text{out}}-\Delta\mathbf{k}_{t,\text{out}};\ k_\lambda-\Delta k_\lambda)} \\ & = (2\pi)^5\,\delta(\Delta\mathbf{k}_{t,\text{in}})\,\delta(\Delta\mathbf{k}_{t,\text{out}})\,\delta(\Delta k_\lambda)\left[1-\left(\|\mathbf{k}_{t,\text{in}}\|/k_\lambda\right)^2\right]\left[1-\left(\|\mathbf{k}_{t,\text{out}}\|/k_\lambda\right)^2\right]. \end{aligned} \tag{6.39}$$

The terms in square brackets arise due to the fact that the random process $\mathscr{G}$ should be regarded as stationary with respect to three-dimensional (3D) wavevectors. These terms are correction factors for the 2D transverse-wavevector case. Then, the multiple-scattering autocorrelation function is, up to a scaling constant:

$$\Gamma_{S,\mathrm{ms}}\left(\Delta\mathbf{r};k_{\lambda,c},\Delta k_\lambda,\theta_0\right) = \int_{-\infty}^{0} \mathrm{d}k_\lambda \left[\mathrm{PSD}\left(k_\lambda;k_{\lambda,c},\Delta k_\lambda\right)\right]^2 \exp\left[j2k_\lambda z\right] \times \left|\iint_{-\infty}^{\infty} \mathrm{d}^2\mathbf{k}_t \exp\left[j\Delta\mathbf{r}_t\cdot\mathbf{k}_t\right]\left[1-\left(\frac{\|\mathbf{k}_t\|}{k_\lambda}\right)^2\right]\left|\mathscr{F}_U\left(\mathbf{k}_t;k_\lambda,\theta_0\right)\right|^2\right|^2. \tag{6.40}$$

For this multiple-scattering case, the axial characteristic length and transverse characteristic area can be defined in an analogous way to their single-scattering counterparts. Based on the preceding equations,

$$\ell_{a,\mathrm{ms}}\left(k_{\lambda,c},\Delta k_\lambda,\theta_0\right) = \frac{2\sqrt{\pi\ln 2}}{\Delta k_\lambda}; \tag{6.41}$$

$$A_{t,\mathrm{ms}}\left(k_{\lambda,c},\Delta k_\lambda,\theta_0\right) = \frac{\pi\left(2-2\theta_0^2+\theta_0^4\right)}{k_{\lambda,c}^2\theta_0^2\left(1-2\theta_0^2+\theta_0^4\right)} \approx \frac{2\pi}{k_{\lambda,c}^2\theta_0^2}\left(1+\theta_0^2\right). \tag{6.42}$$

Equation (6.41) is exact; Eq. (6.42) is valid in the limit $\Delta\beta \to 0$. However, provided $\Delta\beta < 0.2$ (apart from which the Gaussian spectrum assumption is invalid), its error is less than 0.5%. From these equations, it is evident that the *speckle size due to the multiply scattered signal is almost identical to that due to the singly backscattered signal*, the general conclusion of this section. The result is not surprising, given that the angular spectra of the illumination and collected light are the same in each case. This observation is true for the intermediate Category-II contribution to the signal in addition to Category-I and Category-III contributions treated explicitly in this chapter. Indeed, the assumption of Eq. (6.39), that $\mathscr{G}$ is delta-correlated, is probably valid even for the Category-II light. Note finally that the factor $1+\theta_0^2$ in Eq. (6.42) would be absent if the terms in square brackets were not included in Eq. (6.39). In practice, we would need to correct both equations according to the angular backscattering distribution of the diffuse light.

To experimentally validate these observations we use a constrained phantom model that allows us to view *signal-degrading speckle* independently from any *signal-bearing speckle*. The phantom we use is a combination of a series of scattering layers of known constant depth (300 μm) but different scatterer concentrations overlaid on top of the structured phantom reported in Section 6.4.2. The letters in the structured casting have a TiO_2 scatterer concentration of 10 mg/mL of silicone, corresponding to a calculated scattering coefficient at 1325 nm of 13.4 mm^{-1}. Three overlayers were used to demonstrate the effect of multiple scattering on the speckle realization and the speckle size. The overlayers were made with silicone and a homogeneous distribution of TiO_2 particles (1-μm mean diameter), in the following concentrations: 0 mg/mL; 6.5 mg/mL; and 13 mg/mL.

The phantom model was imaged using a swept-source OCT system (Thorlabs OCS1300SS), the specifications of which were reported in Section 6.2.2. The phantom was imaged with light coming from the top of Fig. 6.17, in free space, with the beam focus set to the middle of the letters. The various overlayers were interchanged keeping the structured phantom in the exact same position with respect to the illumination beam. The images are displayed on a logarithmic grayscale with the white level corresponding to a signal strength of approximately 50 dB above the noise floor. As the structured phantom is transparent around the letters, no signal contribution should arise from that sample area. This is the case for the lower concentration overlayers (Fig. 6.17(a) and Fig. 6.17(b)). Another important observation is that the speckle realization within the letters changes very moderately (e.g., the signal-envelope correlation coefficient within the letter L between (a) and (b) is 0.7), even though the preceding structure is clearly different, meaning that these two different overlayers introduce a limited amount of phase front aberration.

On the other hand, Fig. 6.17(c) shows a "tail" of signal extending from the overlayer into the embedding casting of the structured phantom. At the top of the overlayer there is predominance

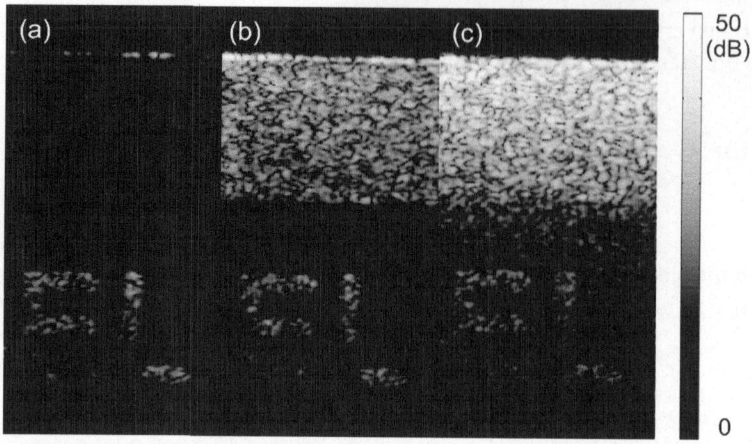

Figure 6.17: Experimental validation of speckle size for different OCT images, where the contribution from different signal categories can be independently identified in different regions of the image. Different overlayers: (a) 0 mg/mL TiO_2/Silicone; (b) 6.5 mg/mL TiO_2/Silicone; (c) 13 mg/mL TiO_2/Silicone are placed on top of the structured phantom. Multiple scattering "tails" can be seen in (c). The speckle size does not change from (a) to (c).

of Category-I signal; as depth increases, there is an increasing contribution of multiply scattered Category-II and III signal. The detected signal will feature only Category-II and III contributions as we move to the embedding casting of the structured phantom.

It is interesting to observe in the letters of the structured phantom, that the speckle realization has changed more significantly in going from the case of Fig. 6.17(a) to Fig. 6.17(c) (the signal-envelope correlation coefficient within the letter L between (a) and (c) is 0.5). The contribution from Categories I, II and III add on an amplitude basis, as expected, modifying the position of peaks and troughs in the speckle realization. Nevertheless, the speckle size is consistently the same, within the experimental error, at every depth of the image, across all three parts of Fig. 6.17(a–c), before noise dominates. This result is consistent with Eqs. (6.31), (6.32), (6.41), and (6.42), with $\Delta\beta = 0.075$ and NA $= 0.056$. As expected from our constrained phantom model, the grainy pattern similar to speckle seen under close inspection at the bottom of the image derives only from system noise and, as such, is completely uncorrelated between the images.

In summary, the second-order speckle statistics give us information on the coarseness of a speckle pattern and on the physical properties that influence it. It turns out that both the axial and lateral speckle size are dependent only upon the source lateral resolution: sample dispersion, beam divergence, or multiple scattering have no effect. This directly contradicts the common claim in the OCT speckle literature that the characteristic size of signal-degrading speckle is much less than that of signal-bearing speckle [5].

6.6 Retrieving Information from Speckle

In this section, we demonstrate that a correlation exists between OCT speckle statistics and sample properties.

Initially, we review the case of static speckle patterns. A first approach is that of Gossage et al. [17, 35], in which quantitative texture analysis methods were used to extract information from the first- and second-order spatial speckle statistics. Some preliminary success, particularly for the purpose of distinguishing between gelatin/microsphere tissue phantoms [35], has been reported. To the extent that such discrimination is possible, it represents acquiring information at an intermediate point on the structural size-scale continuum for which large-scale macrostructure is at one extreme, and unresolvable microstructure is at the other (as mentioned in Section 6.3.1.2, non-degenerate Case 3).

Two approaches to acquiring information on the unresolvable microstructure scale have been put forward by our research group [18, 71], and are explicitly presented in Sections 6.6.1 and 6.6.2, respectively. In the first, using first-order speckle statistics, theoretical calculations and experimental verification showed that the OCT speckle contrast ratio is dependent on the local density of scattering particles in a sample, provided that the effective number of scatterers in the probed volume is less than about five. The observed contrast ratios vary significantly from the Rayleigh limit of 0.52, suggesting that speckle contrast ratio could be a useful sample characterization mechanism in OCT, particularly when imaging in ultrahigh-resolution regimes.

In the second, using second-order (spatial) speckle statistics, angle-dependent detection can be used to distinguish between the singly backscattered (Category-I) and multiply scattered (Category-III) signal components. The technique requires acquisition of several speckle patterns of the same sample by varying the detection over a range of angles. Single backscattering (predominant at shallower depths) is highly correlated over a large range of detection angles; multiple scattering rapidly decorrelates as the angle is varied.

Second-order (temporal) speckle statistics are also very useful in extracting information from dynamic speckle patterns. In this case, images are acquired over time, during which the distribution of scatterers with respect to the probing beam changes, either due to an endogenous mechanism, e.g., blood flow, or an exogenous mechanism, e.g., an external force applied to the tissue. Temporally-dynamic OCT speckle has been used to determine spatially resolved diffusion [66] and flow [71–73] in liquids, including blood *in vivo*, and choroidal perfusion in the outer retina [75]. Whole vasculature maps have been presented using speckle variance [24], and tissue elasticity mapping techniques have been proposed using speckle tracking [11].

6.6.1 Sample discrimination by scatterer density

In this Section, based on Refs. [18, 76], we demonstrate that when the density of scatterers in the sample is sufficiently low, the central limit theorem (that yielded the result, in Section 6.3.1, that the distribution of $|S|$ was Rayleigh) no longer applies. Thus, speckle contrast ratio is dependent upon the local density of scattering particles in a sample. We confirm theoretical predictions with experiments on suspensions of microspheres, and consider the scattering coefficients and OCT parameters for which a measurement of the contrast ratio could be used to infer properties of the sample composition.

We briefly describe the theoretical model utilized in this Section. More detail is provided in Ref. [62]. The starting point is Eq. (6.8), in the case for which the number of phasors N contributing to the signal is small. For simplicity, we assume that the sample is composed of identical particles (i.e., with the same backscattering profile), which may be treated as point scatterers. This means that the random variables a_i that constitute the magnitudes of the random phasors depend only on the shape of the OCT PSF. We preserve the assumptions that they are independent and identically distributed, and that ϕ_i is uniformly distributed on $(-\pi, \pi]$, and independent of a_i.

We also assume that N is stochastic, with the *expected* number of scatterers in a region of volume V being equal to $\rho_v V$, where ρ_v is the volume density of scatterers. In the simple model, we assume that the scatterers' positions are independent[23], so the number of scatterers in any region is *Poisson-*

[23] This assumption is clearly false when the scatterers have a non-zero volume, but it is an adequate approximation for our

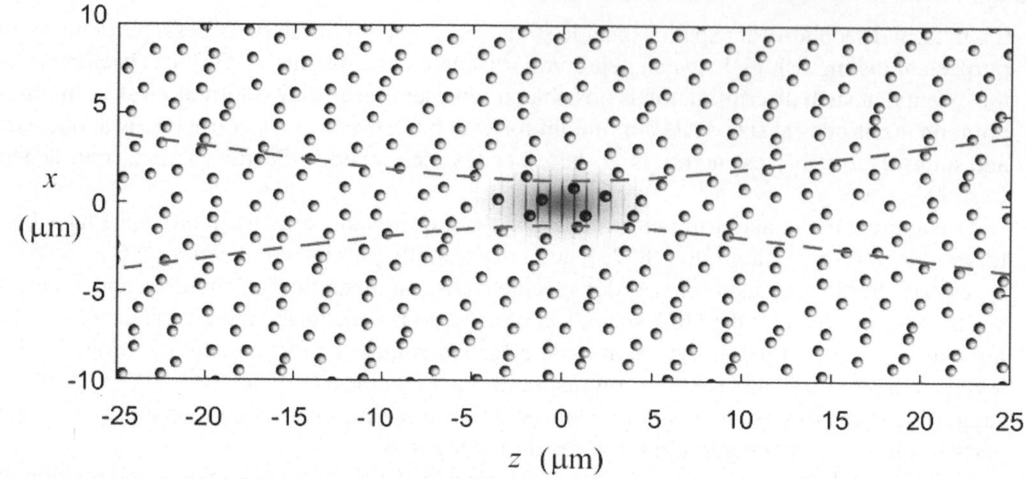

Figure 6.18: Graphical representation of the case for which there are few scatterers in the sample volume (ENS ≈ 5).

distributed.

Finally, we performed our calculations using the "in-focus" PSF obtained by inverse-Fourier-transforming the three-dimensional Gaussian approximation of the global TF given in Eq. (6.35):

$$\Psi(\mathbf{r}) = \exp\left\{-\left[\frac{x^2+y^2}{(D/2)^2} + \frac{2\pi z^2}{\ell_c^2}\right]\right\}, \tag{6.43}$$

where diameter $D = \sqrt{2}W_0$, and W_0 is the beam waist corresponding to the center wavenumber of the source in this case.

We define the "effective number of scatterers" within the sample volume to be ENS $= D^2\ell_c\rho_v$. Figure 6.18 provides a graphical representation of the sample's scatterer distribution for the case ENS ≈ 5.

Within the model, we also account for the possibility of both noise and multiple scattering effects that are inevitably present when the signal is measured, assuming them to be additive, with circular Gaussian statistics. The multiple-scattering effects refer to the detected signal from the minor categories (II and III), and the noise refers to, for example, system electrical noise. There is no difference between signal components, with regards to their first-order statistics. The second-order statistics will be different, since, as highlighted in Section 6.5.1, the size of the speckle due to multiply scattered light will depend on the system parameters. In fact, denoting the random phasor associated with these effects by $E_{\mathrm{MS+N}}$, then the observed signal $S_{\mathrm{SB+MS+N}}{=}S+E_{\mathrm{MS+N}}$ is the net phasor sum of them and the singly backscattered signal.

If the noise contribution to the signal is assumed to be much less than that due to multiply scattered light, then we may define the *degree of multiple scattering* (DOMS),

$$\mathrm{DOMS} = \frac{\mu'_{2,|S+E_{\mathrm{MS}}|} - \mu'_{2,|S|}}{\mu'_{2,|S+E_{\mathrm{MS}}|}}, \tag{6.44}$$

where $\mu'_{2,|S|}$, $\mu'_{2,|S+E_{\mathrm{MS}}|}$ indicate the second moments (about zero) of $|S|$, $|S+E_{\mathrm{MS}}|$ respectively (excluding the "+N" in the subscript of the latter). A similar factor has been invoked in previous

purposes.

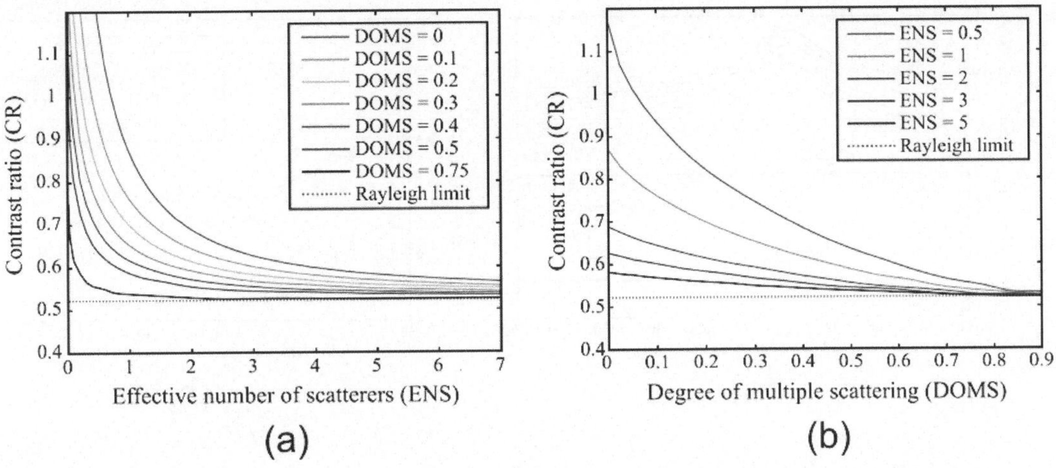

Figure 6.19: Dependence of contrast ratio (CR) on: (a) the effective number of scatterers in the sample volume (ENS); and (b) the degree of multiple scattering (DOMS). Reproduced from [62].

studies of the effects of multiple scattering in OCT [9].

We utilize the contrast ratio to distinguish between the speckle patterns observed for different values of ENS and DOMS. Plots of the contrast ratio of Eq. (6.11) as a function of both DOMS (with ENS held constant) and ENS (with DOMS held constant) are presented in Fig. 6.19.

The curves show the strong dependence of CR upon ENS. Under this model, CR is a strictly decreasing function of ENS. In the absence of multiply scattered signal (or noise), CR exceeds 0.58 when ENS = 5, a quantity over 10% greater than its value in the Rayleigh limit. It is also clear that the presence of multiple scattering greatly mitigates the signal contrast ratio when there are few scatterers in the FWHM sample volume, so that it is a serious confounding factor when attempting to utilize contrast ratio measurements to determine sample scatterer density.

Experimental contrast-ratio measurements on sample suspensions of polystyrene microspheres ($n = 1.34$) in water confirmed these theoretical predictions. The microspheres that were used had two different mean diameters: 0.51 μm and 1.01 μm. The microsphere sample concentrations ranged from 5.8×10^{10} to 2.8×10^{8} particles/mL, obtained by performing successive dilutions of the stock solution. Brownian motion of the particles, together with lateral scanning over 120 μm, ensured that a large ensemble of speckle states was probed. Figure 6.20(a) shows plots of the mean voltage signal and CR versus axial position corresponding to the measurements of 0.51-μm spheres. Each point is calculated using the data in its corresponding position over all A-scans. The mean curves show that the relative signal strength is strictly increasing with sphere concentration. Each CR curve shows a sharp peak at the center of the confocal gate. As the beam diverges away from its focal point, the contrast ratio rapidly decreases as large numbers of scatterers begin to contribute to the signal.

Figure 6.20(b) shows a plot of the CR at the peak signal location versus ENS, for both 0.51-μm and 1.01-μm spheres. In both cases, the experimental results support the theoretical predictions. For ENS values of 5 or less, Fig. 6.20(b) shows that there is a rapid increase in CR, with a maximum measured value in excess of 2.

According to Mie theory [31], if ENS = 5, then for our cases of 0.51-μm and 1.01-μm microspheres, the scattering coefficient is 0.37 mm^{-1} and 7.8 mm^{-1}, respectively. If one reduces the refractive index contrast to 1.06, a value more typical of tissue [26], and considers sphere sizes ranging from 1 to 3 μm (corresponding to volume fractions from 0.01 to 0.2), then the same calculation yields scattering coefficients ranging from 1.0 to 50.0 mm^{-1}. These values cover a range which

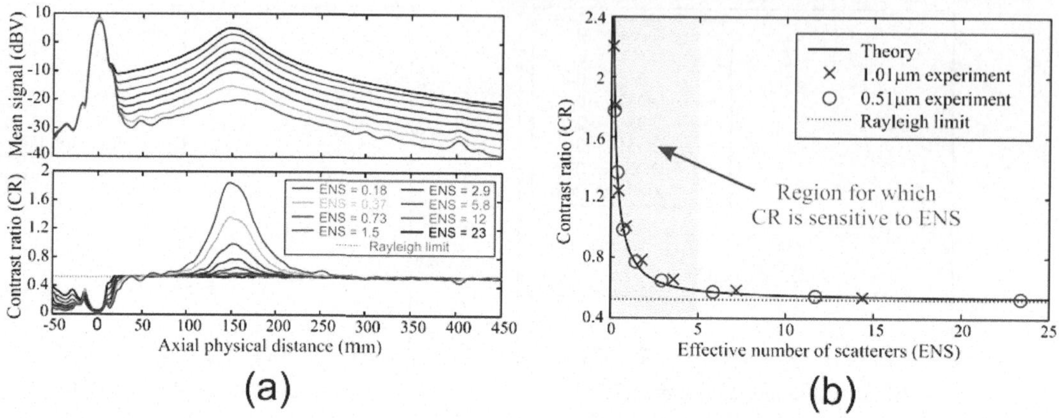

Figure 6.20: (a) Plot of mean detected signal (upper) and contrast ratio (lower) versus axial position (referenced to the sample-glass interface), for 0.51-μm microspheres; (b) Plot of contrast ratio versus effective number of scatterers for 0.51-μm and 1.01-μm spheres. Reproduced from [62].

includes many typical scattering coefficients reported for various tissue types [49]. This suggests that speckle contrast ratio is a potentially feasible means of discriminating between different sample regions. Its effectiveness would be increased if higher bandwidth sources and/or higher resolution objective lenses were utilized in order to decrease the sample volume (the size of the PSF).

To experimentally determine the effects of multiple scattering, the contrast ratio was measured versus depth for a solution of polystyrene microspheres in 1:2 glycerol to water ratio. The group refractive index of the medium was 1.38, and the concentration of the microspheres was 3.9×10^8 particles/mL. The scattering coefficient, the scattering component of the attenuation coefficient μ_t, can be determined using Mie theory. It is $\mu_s = 4.8$ mm^{-1}, corresponding to a mean-free path MFP $= 1/\mu_s = 210$ μm. The scattering coefficient calculated by performing a fit versus physical depth (from optical depths 100 μm to 420 μm, or physical depths 70 μm to 300 μm from the surface) to the peaks of the OCT datasets is $\mu_s = 3.9$ mm^{-1} (MFP = 260 μm).

Both spatial and temporal variation in the sample state were utilized to generate an ensemble of speckle realizations. In order to circumvent the problem of beam width variation with depth, the confocal gate was successively advanced deeper in the solution and different measurements taken. This process of dynamic focusing allowed the contrast ratio peak to be measured as a function of depth, always at the beam focus.

The peaks of the averaged A-scan signals in Fig. 6.21(a) show a log-linear dependence. The contrast ratios measured for each dataset show a peak value significantly above the Rayleigh-limited value of 0.52 corresponding to the center of the confocal gate then consistently equal to 0.52 outside the beam focus. The peaks of the contrast ratios show a linear drop-off with increasing depth, from 2 near the surface to less than 1 at the greatest depth. Given the relatively good SNR, the reduction in CR with depth can be attributed to the increasing effects of multiple scattering rather than the influence of the noise floor. Measurements such as this could be used to estimate DOMS, noting that ENS can be determined from the value of CR near the surface (or that it may be known by some other means). Alternatively, to accurately calculate ENS in the presence of multiple scattering, DOMS must be known in addition to CR.

Other issues must be considered when utilizing CR to determine useful information about the sample. Accurate CR measurement relies on independent sampling of many speckle states from the same distribution. In biological tissue, this can be accomplished by acquiring a 3D dataset, however, the inhomogeneity of biological tissue limits the spatial range over which independent and identically distributed speckle states may be sampled. The condition of independent measurements

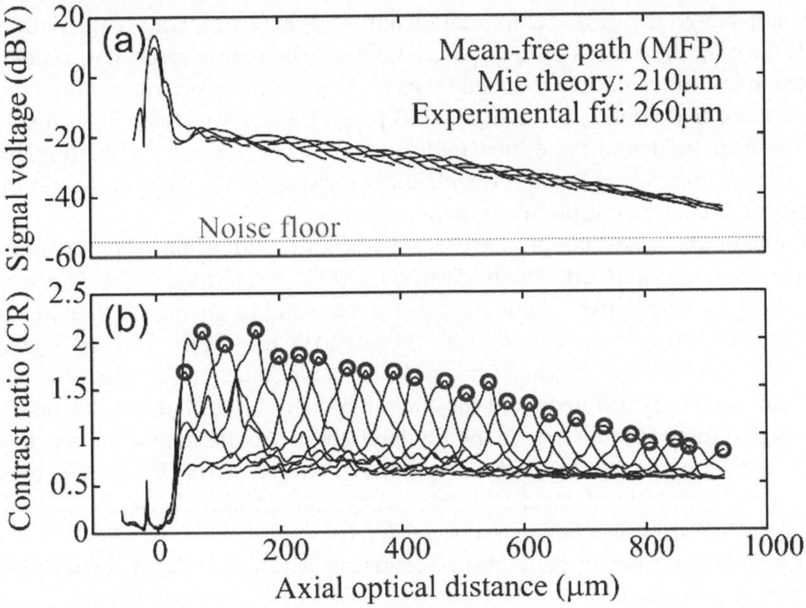

Figure 6.21: Measurement of 2.5-μm microspheres in water-glycerol solution. (a) OCT signal strength; (b) contrast ratio at a set of discrete confocal gate positions. The circles in the lower plot denote the peak CR at each position. Reproduced from [62].

is equivalent to ensuring that the sample volumes of the two measurements do not overlap. To obtain a contrast ratio accuracy of 0.02 [62] in a 3D sample, this corresponds to a measurement range (and thus a homogeneous region) of size approximately 7 times a resolution element in each direction. For layered or stratified samples, the measurement range may be increased in the lateral direction, with a consequent reduction in the axial direction. Alternatively, angular compounding approaches [77, 78], discussed further in Section 6.7.1.2, can probe multiple independent speckle states within the same resolution volume (up to 40), which should substantially reduce the size of the sample volume which needs to be probed to estimate CR.

6.6.2 Testing OCT image fidelity: detection of multiple scattering

We can infer image information from the OCT signal only if the detected backscattered light belongs to Category I (or to a lesser extent, to Category II), as mentioned in Section 6.5. Thus, the problem of Category-III "multiple scattering" [9, 79, 80] remains a serious corrupting influence on image quality. Because, at its most severe, the optical delay undergone by the signal component from Category III cannot be directly associated with structure at a particular depth, it serves only to mask the singly scattered component, or provide spurious sample information [Refer to Fig. 6.17(c)].

Quantification of the contributions of multiple scattering to OCT images remains a difficult problem. For homogeneous suspensions of varying turbidity, observations of the distinct change in slope of the measured signal versus depth, quantifying the transition from the ballistic to the diffuse scattering regime, have been made [69, 81, 82].

There is perhaps surprisingly little unequivocal data on the impact of multiple scattering on image quality. Izatt et al. [81] show *en-face* OCT trans-illumination images of a standard target imaged through a latex-sphere suspension corresponding to the first emergence of multiple scattering. However, translating these results to a detailed understanding of reflectance imaging in heterogeneous tissues is not straightforward. Schmitt and Knüttel [9] have produced a simulation which partially takes into account the effects of multiple scattering. Their simulated images show the lack of improvement in lateral resolution obtained by increasing the numerical aperture of the objective when multiple scattering dominates. Pan et al. [69] present a series of three OCT images of a 100-μm-thick razor blade hidden in three Intralipid solutions with increasing scattering coefficient of μ_s = 1.6, 6.4, and 12.7 mm^{-1} (at a center wavelength of 830 nm). The images show how feature contrast is seriously affected by multiple scattering.

Depending on the scattering properties of the sample, and/or the system parameters, the effects of multiple scattering may effectively destroy an OCT image long before the signal is attenuated to below the system sensitivity limit. It is therefore useful to quantify the degree to which the signal corresponding to each image point has been corrupted in this way. In Section 6.6.1 (e.g., in Fig. 6.21) we saw how the marginal (first-order) speckle statistics for relatively sparse distributions of near-point scatterers differed from the Rayleigh distribution, but that the detection of multiply scattered signal forced them towards the Rayleigh limit. An alternative approach for DOMS quantification adopted by our group [82], using polarization-sensitive (PS-) OCT, is based on the fact that the polarization state of incident light will be randomized after a large number of scattering events, a point we mention again in Section 6.7.1.1.

The approach we adopt in the current Section, based on Ref. [71], is to use the second-order speckle statistics to quantify the OCT speckle cross-correlation coefficient at various depths in a homogenous sample recorded with angularly diverse detection. That is, we separately detect the light backscattered in different directions in multiple OCT recordings using the same sample and illumination. The speckle decorrelation between recordings at a given angular separation increases with image depth, indicating the increasing contribution of multiply scattered light to the signal.

Consider illumination of the sample by a unit-amplitude plane wave with wavevector $\mathbf{k}_{\text{in}}$. The complex amplitude of the scattered field plane-wave component with wavevector $\mathbf{k}_{\text{out}}$ is equal to exactly one Fourier component of the scattering potential F_S, as defined in Section 6.2, at angular spatial frequency $\mathbf{K} = \mathbf{k}_{\text{out}} - \mathbf{k}_{\text{in}}$. For each wavenumber, as described in Section 6.4.1, the OCT system both illuminates the sample and collects (detects) the scattered light over a range of different plane-wave components, depending on the system NA. Within these ranges, there are multiple pairs $(\mathbf{k}_{\text{in}}, \mathbf{k}_{\text{out}})$ whose resultants (differences) $\mathbf{K}$ are identical; the sample's singly backscattered response is the same for all.

For multiply scattered light in the diffuse limit, this property does not hold, as described in Section 6.5.1. (The sample cannot be represented as a superposition of non-interacting phase gratings, as in the first-order Born approximation, so there is no such correspondence between the scattering responses for different wavevector pairs.)

Now, for the angularly diverse detection approach, each image accesses a *different* range of scattered wavevector components, although the scattered light originates from the same spatial location. To the extent that we probe the same wavevector differences $\mathbf{K}$, but different wavevector pairs $(\mathbf{k}_{\text{in}}, \mathbf{k}_{\text{out}})$, in separate recordings, the singly backscattered signal (or signal-bearing speckle) will remain highly correlated between them; however, the multiply scattered signal (signal-degrading speckle) will be almost uncorrelated. (This point is clarified in Fig. 6.22.)

We achieve angularly diverse detection by passing the returning expanded and collimated backscattered beam through an iris with opening narrower than the spatial extent of the beam. Only a subset of the far-field scattered-wave angular spectrum will contribute to the interferometric signal. The iris position is varied along a plane normal to the propagation axis, so we term it "detector lateral position" P.

In the singly backscattering regime, the correspondence between wavevector resultants and Fourier components of $F_S(\mathbf{r})$ permits us to utilize the transfer-function approach described in Section 6.4. The system is spatially invariant provided that the objective-lens NA is small. The complex-scalar OCT signal, $S(\mathbf{r})$, is given by the 3D-convolution $S(\mathbf{r}) = \chi(\mathbf{r}) \otimes \Psi(\mathbf{r})$, as in Eq. (6.4), where $\Psi(\mathbf{r})$ is the system PSF. We maintain the assumptions from Section 6.4.1, that all Gaussian-profiled

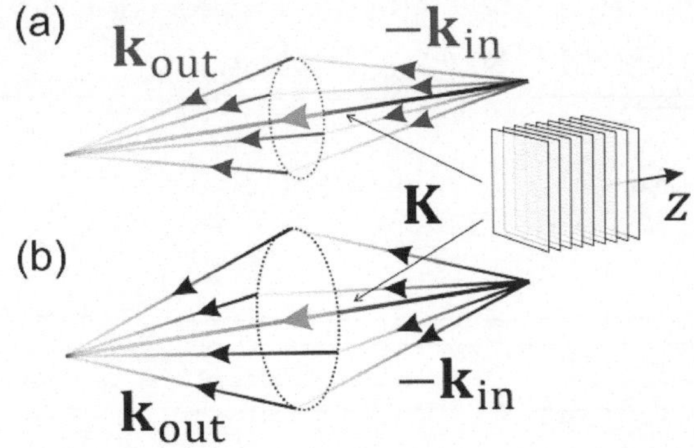

Figure 6.22: For the first-order Born approximation scenario (single backscattering), there are multiple pairs of illumination ($\mathbf{k}_{\text{in}}$) and scattered ($\mathbf{k}_{\text{out}}$) wavevectors which yield the same difference $\mathbf{K}$. That is, they are sensitive to exactly the same sample spatial-frequency component. For a single value of $\mathbf{K}$, several such pairs are shown for two different wavenumbers (in (a) and (b)). A representation of the sample "grating" component corresponding to $\mathbf{K}$ is shown on the right-hand side of the figure.

wavenumber components k_λ of the illumination beam have co-located waists and the same divergence angle, θ_0. Then we consider the system TF, as a function of the added variable P, which can be expressed in the manner of Eq. (6.30):

$$\mathscr{H}\left(\mathbf{k};z,k_{\lambda,c},\Delta k_\lambda,\theta_0,P\right)=\int_{-\infty}^{0}\mathscr{K}\left(\mathbf{k};k_\lambda,\theta_0,P\right)\left(\frac{k_\lambda^2}{4\pi}\right)\text{PSD}\left(k_\lambda;k_{\lambda,c},\Delta k_\lambda\right)\,\exp\left[jz(2k_\lambda-k_z)\right]\,\mathrm{d}k_\lambda. \tag{6.45}$$

The single-wavenumber contributions $\mathscr{K}\left(\mathbf{k};k_\lambda,\theta_0,P\right)$ are derived from the system illumination and collection functions (wavevector distributions), $\mathscr{F}^*_{U,3,\text{in}}\left(-\mathbf{k};k_\lambda,\theta_0\right)$ and $\mathscr{F}^*_{U,3,\text{ out}}\left(-\mathbf{k};k_\lambda,\theta_0\right)$, respectively. The former is based on Eq. (6.4); it represents the angular spectrum of the Gaussian illumination beam.

For the low-NA case, the hemisphere can be approximated by a plane, $|k_\lambda|=-k_z$. This is the scenario which yielded Eq. (6.33); the following expression (for which equality holds up to a constant factor) is equivalent:

$$\mathscr{F}^*_{U,3,\text{in}}\left(-\mathbf{k};k_\lambda,\theta_0\right)=\left(\frac{1}{|k_\lambda|}\right)\exp\left[-\left(\frac{1}{k_\lambda\,\theta_0}\right)^2\left(k_x^2+k_y^2\right)\right]\delta\left(k_z+|k_\lambda|\right). \tag{6.46}$$

If the illumination and collection apertures are identical in the absence of the iris then the iris is taken into account by writing $\mathscr{F}^*_{U,3,\text{out}}\left(-\mathbf{k};k_\lambda,\theta_0,P\right)=\mathscr{F}^*_{U,3,\text{in}}\left(-\mathbf{k};k_\lambda,\theta_0\right)\,\text{circ}\left[\|\mathbf{k}_t-\mathbf{k}_{P,t}\|/k_{P,r}\right]$. The "circ" function describes the circular iris aperture profile, with center $\mathbf{k}_{P,t}=\left(k_{P,x},k_{P,y}\right)$ and radius $k_{P,r}$. The single-wavenumber contribution to the OCT TF, $\mathscr{K}\left(\mathbf{k};k_\lambda,\theta_0,P\right)$, is given by the convolution of the two (flattened) sphere caps. Figure 6.23 shows the derivation of the single-wavenumber TFs as the convolutions of the angular spectra of the illumination and collection for various detection angles.

We now calculate the complex correlation coefficient, $\gamma_{1,2}$, between the singly scattered complex-amplitude OCT signals $S_1(\mathbf{r})$, $S_2(\mathbf{r})$, recorded at respective iris positions, P_1, P_2. In general, this represents the degree of correlation measured between two OCT signals recorded using the *same* sample, but using different imaging systems. In general, the cross-correlation function:

$$\Gamma_{1,2}\left(\Delta\mathbf{r};\mathbf{r}\right)=\overline{S_1\left(\mathbf{r}\right)S_2^*\left(\mathbf{r}-\Delta\mathbf{r}\right)}, \tag{6.47}$$

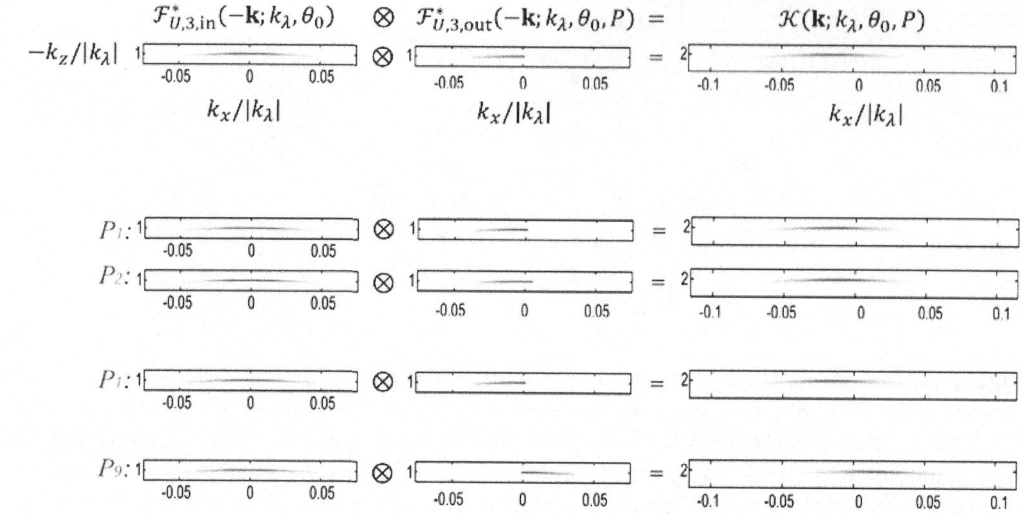

Figure 6.23: Derivation of the single-wavenumber TFs as a convolution of the angular spectra of the illumination and collection for various detection angles (iris positions P_1, P_2 and P_9, shown in Fig 6.24(b) as (i),(ii), and (iii)). In the single-backscattering case, the complex correlation coefficient $\gamma_{1,2}$ depends on the overlap region of the $\mathcal{K}$ functions; for the multiple-scattering case, it depends on the overlap region of the collection angular spectrum.

is calculated over the ensemble of sample scatterer distributions as in Section 6.2. Utilizing the local TFs, we have, for the singly backscattered signal (Category-I light):

$$\Gamma_{1,2}(\Delta\mathbf{r};\mathbf{r}) = \frac{1}{(2\pi)^6}\iiint_{-\infty}^{\infty}\iiint_{-\infty}^{\infty}\mathcal{H}_1(\mathbf{k})\mathcal{H}_2^*(\mathbf{k}')\overline{\mathrm{X}(\mathbf{k})\mathrm{X}^*(\mathbf{k}')}\exp\left[j\left(\mathbf{k}\cdot\mathbf{r}-\mathbf{k}'\cdot(\mathbf{r}-\Delta\mathbf{r})\right)\right]\mathrm{d}^3\mathbf{k}\mathrm{d}^3\mathbf{k}' \tag{6.48}$$

where $\mathrm{X}(\mathbf{k}) = \mathcal{F}\{\chi(\mathbf{r})\}$. We assume that, over the ensemble, the sample's spatial frequency spectrum $\mathrm{X}(\mathbf{k})$ has a delta-function autocorrelation, with uniform magnitude over the OCT TF's region of support, similar to the case depicted for $\overline{|\mathrm{X}(\mathbf{k})|}$ in Fig. 6.13. Then, for the single-backscattering (SB) case,

$$\gamma_{1,2,\mathrm{SB}}(\Delta\mathbf{r};\mathbf{r}) \triangleq \frac{\Gamma_{1,2}(\Delta\mathbf{r};\mathbf{r})}{\sqrt{\Gamma_{1,1}(0;\mathbf{r})\Gamma_{2,2}(0;\mathbf{r})}} = \frac{\iiint_{-\infty}^{\infty}\mathcal{H}_1(\mathbf{k})\mathcal{H}_2^*(\mathbf{k})\exp\left[j\mathbf{k}\cdot\Delta\mathbf{r}\right]\mathrm{d}^3\mathbf{k}}{\sqrt{\left[\iiint_{-\infty}^{\infty}|\mathcal{H}_1(\mathbf{k})|^2\mathrm{d}^3\mathbf{k}\right]\left[\iiint_{-\infty}^{\infty}|\mathcal{H}_2(\mathbf{k})|^2\mathrm{d}^3\mathbf{k}\right]}}. \tag{6.49}$$

We consider this cross-correlation coefficient between the signals recorded at the same spatial location, i.e., for $\Delta\mathbf{r} = 0$, for different iris positions. The exponential factor in the integrand of the denominator is, therefore, set to zero, and the cross-correlation coefficient becomes a normalized Fourier-domain overlap integral. In the low-NA approximation, it may be calculated with respect to the single-wavenumber contributions $\mathcal{K}_1$, $\mathcal{K}_2$ rather than the full TFs $\mathcal{H}_1$, $\mathcal{H}_2$.

For the Category-I-signal case mentioned so far, the acquisition of different wavevector pairs with the same resultant ensures that the speckle patterns remain highly correlated even when the iris positions are well separated. This correspondence breaks down for highly multiply scattered light; the speckle patterns remain correlated only to the extent that the iris positions overlap. If the iris physical diameter, d_i, is much smaller than the beam width, then the multiply scattered correlation

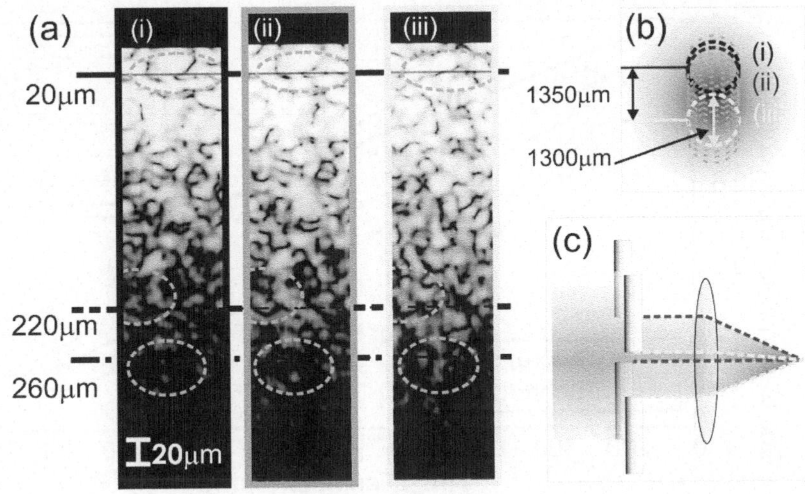

Figure 6.24: (a) Portions of B-scans for a scattering sample at three iris positions (i)-(iii), displayed using a logarithmic grayscale. The horizontal lines indicate the three optical depths chosen for Fig. 6.25. The ellipses highlight prominent features (speckle), which may be used as a visual guide for interpreting the correlation magnitudes. (b) Transverse- and (c) axial-plane views of iris positions with respect to the backscattered beam. Positions (i)–(iii) represent the iris-position corresponding to three B-scans shown in (a). Adapted from [71] with permission.

coefficient, $\gamma_{1,2,\mathrm{MS}}$, is given by the normalized overlap area of the relatively displaced circular iris openings:

$$\gamma_{1,2,\mathrm{MS}} = \frac{2\theta - \sin(2\theta)}{\pi}, \tag{6.50}$$

where $\theta = \mathrm{acos}\,(s/d_i)$, and s is the distance between the iris positions. Note that in Fig. 6.23, completely non-overlapping iris positions (P_1 and P_9) would correspond to $\mu_{1,2,\mathrm{MS}} = 0$, but $\gamma_{1,2,\mathrm{SB}} \neq 0$ since there is still some overlap between the $\mathscr{K}$ functions.

Multiple scattering is negligible close to the sample surface; its influence is progressively greater for increasing depths. Thus, $\gamma_{1,2}$, for any pair of detector positions, calculated over an ensemble of lateral scan positions, should decrease with depth, varying from the $\gamma_{1,2,\mathrm{SB}}$ to the $\gamma_{1,2,\mathrm{MS}}$ limits. We provide some experimental evidence in support of this claim.

Two room-temperature vulcanizing silicone phantoms ($n = 1.42$), containing 1-μm-mean-diameter TiO_2 particles in different concentrations, were utilized. Figure 6.24 shows three representative B-scans for the higher-scattering sample (H): (i) and (ii) correspond to consecutive iris displacements (P_1 and P_2); (i) and (iii) to non-overlapping iris positions (P_1 and P_9). The regions within the ellipses were chosen to highlight speckle, which correlates most strongly between adjacent iris positions and at shallow depths.

The correlation coefficient modulus, $|\gamma_{1,2}|$, was calculated for each depth position of the homogeneous sample, regarding the multiple A-scans as an "ensemble" of measurements. Figure 6.25 shows the experimental $|\gamma_{1,2}|$, versus iris displacement for both samples at three optical depths: within 30 μm; 220 μm; and 260 μm. The minimum probing depth was chosen to avoid surface-reflection correlation artifacts; the maximum depth was limited by system sensitivity. (The electronic noise floor was reached before the multiply scattered contribution to the signal could dominate.) Each experimental point in Fig. 6.25 is averaged over the multiple pairs. Theoretical curves, corresponding to the single backscattered (Eq. (6.49)) and highly multiply scattered (Eq. (6.50)) extremes, are also plotted. As expected, the theoretical curves bound the experimental ones, which

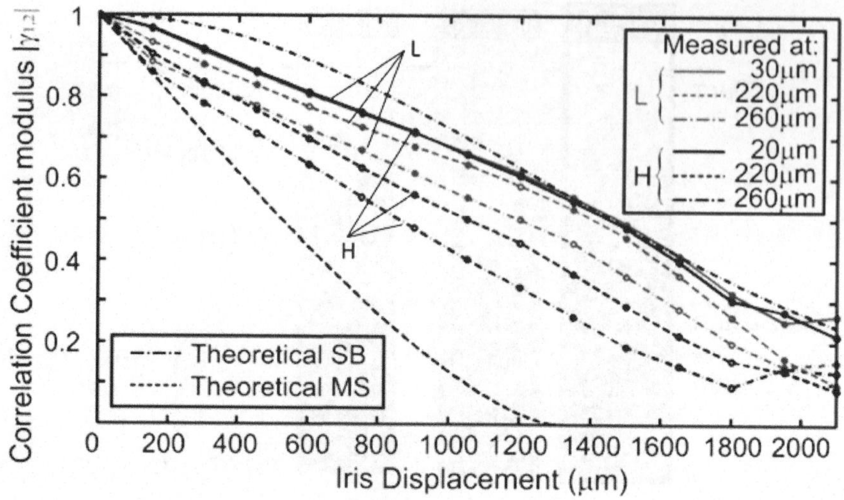

Figure 6.25: Measured correlation coefficient moduli versus iris displacement, for the samples with low (L) and high (H) scatterer concentrations, at the depths indicated in the legend. The theoretical curves represent the singly backscattered (SB) and multiply scattered (MS) extremes. Reproduced from [71] with permission.

show the expected progression as the prevalence of multiple scattering increases with depth. Moreover, the higher-scattering-sample (blue) curves show more pronounced decorrelation at depths of 220 μm and 260 μm than the lower-scattering-sample (red) curves. For both samples, the increase in multiple scattering versus depth over the probed depth range is consistent with the phantoms' scattering parameters.

We note that the results of this Section serve to illustrate the possibility that the correlation between speckle patterns can be used to determine the degree to which multiple scattering affects the OCT signal. The use of an iris in the manner we have described is generally counterproductive, since it reduces system resolution and also increases the relative proportion of multiply scattered light that constitutes the OCT signal. (The single backscattered contribution tends to be reinforced over the full extent of the aperture; the multiply scattered contribution does not, i.e., confocal gating assists in suppressing multiple scattering.) Ideally, this method could be utilized in an angularly diverse detection mode, as discussed in Section 6.7.1.2, which involves collection over multiple non-overlapping apertures over a wide-collection solid angle rather than over different sub-regions of the conventional system aperture.

6.6.3 Functional imaging using dynamic OCT speckle

The view of OCT speckle as a useful source of information can be extended most emphatically to dynamic, i.e., temporally varying speckle. Indeed, dynamic speckle has been widely applied and studied in optical metrology [1, 2]. Its utility is based on the fact that a particular speckle realization is highly dependent upon the precise locations (on the optical-wavelength scale) of the backscatterers within the sample. The inverse problem of determining the microscopic backscatterer distribution from an observed speckle pattern is, of course, grossly underdetermined. However, by treating speckle as a stochastic phenomenon, its variation between successive scans (or images), that is, its second-order temporal statistics, can provide quantitative information about microstructure motion, making functional imaging possible.

In applications probing endogenous changes in the sample microstructure, flow imaging is the main area where dynamic speckle has been used to extract quantities of interest. To extract flow velocity and direction, for example, Imai et al. [72] used the autocorrelation function of the TD-OCT A-scan signal. In this case the correlation length, during the course of the scan, becomes shorter as the flow velocity increases. A similar approach has been adopted by Barton et al. [74] as an alternative to Doppler optical coherence tomography (DOCT) for extracting flow information. It has the advantage of insensitivity to flow in the direction normal to the imaging beam and no requirement for knowledge of the phase. The speckle pattern changes over the time scale at which the TD-OCT image is acquired. Alternatively, the spatial frequency content of the acquired image is modified according to flow velocity. Specifically, the ratio of high to low OCT image spatial frequencies was shown to bear a linear relation to flow velocity.

Amongst those techniques insensitive to flow velocity and direction, Wu et al. [75] proposed a speckle imaging algorithm to analyse sequential axial depth scans to obtain an indicator of choroidal perfusion in a rat's eye. This indicator is calibrated by correlating its results with the known changes in choroidal blood flow in response to increased intraocular pressure. More recently, several other techniques have been introduced: logarithmic intensity and speckle-based motion contrast [83]; and intensity-based Doppler variance [84]. By using a temporal or spatial window, measured temporal speckle fluctuations are used to perform vasculature imaging (angiography). More on this subject and on correlation mapping [85, 86] methods, introduced by Leahy's group, is presented in detail in Chapter 9 of this volume.

The primary focus of this Section is speckle variance, another interesting technique for flow imaging, proposed by Mariampillai et al. [24, 87]. The technique has enabled the visualization of vessel-size dependent vascular shutdown and transient vascular occlusion. The algorithm calculates interframe speckle variance in two-dimensional and three-dimensional OCT data sets and shows little dependence on the Doppler angle when this parameter varies from 75° to 90°. Interframe speckle variance images $SV_i(x,z)$ of the structural OCT intensity $S_i(x,z)$ are calculated across $N=3$ OCT B-scans as follows:

$$SV_i(x,z) = \frac{1}{N}\sum_{i=1}^{N}\left(S_i(x,z) - \overline{S}_i(x,z)\right)^2, \tag{6.51}$$

where i denotes the OCT B-scan index with $\overline{S}_i(x,z)$ as the average over the set of B-scans. Figure 26(d) shows an *en-face* projection image of the speckle variance 3D map extracted from the dorsal skinfold window chamber applied to an athymic nude mouse.

A parallel research area is based on making use of changes in a speckle pattern due to exogenous mechanisms, for example, derived from different mechanical loads on a sample, or different and unknown lateral scanning speed. Ahmad et al. [88] have described a cross-correlation based approach for image acquisition utilizing the structural and speckle information from the acquired A-scans. They demonstrated the successful implementation of this technique to assemble manually scanned images of several phantom samples and biological tissues.

Schmitt [11] demonstrated the use of two-dimensional cross-correlation of speckle to track the local motion in a sample undergoing compression. The motivation was the use of the elastic or shear modulus of a tissue as a contrast mechanism for detecting lesions in soft tissue. OCE based on speckle-tracking techniques has also been reported by Kirkpatrick et al. [23], with different methods utilized to track small and large speckle motions. The approach for small speckle motion estimation is essentially a two-dimensional implementation of a one-dimensional maximum-likelihood estimator [89, 90] based on the concept of "optical flow This concept relies on the assumption that the brightness, $g(x,z,t)$, is conserved over an image (only its spatial distribution changes with time) so that the total time derivative, dg/dt, is zero, i.e.,

$$\frac{dg}{dt} = (\nabla g)\cdot\mathbf{f} + g_t = 0, \tag{6.52}$$

where $\mathbf{f} = (f_x, f_z)$ is the optical flow, an estimate of local velocity, and g_t is the central difference

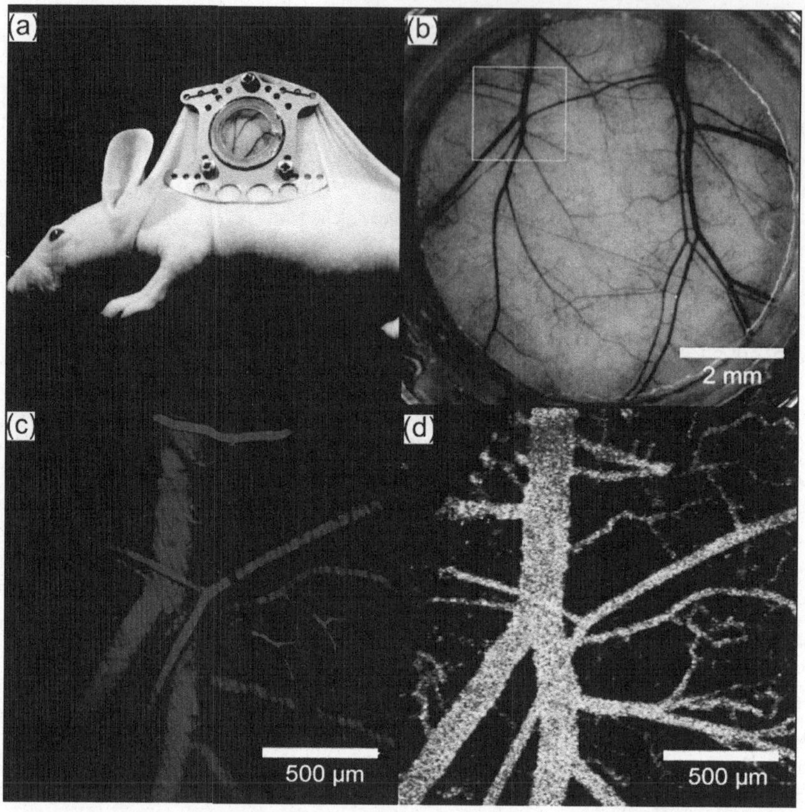

Figure 6.26: (a) Dorsal skinfold window chamber model in an athymic nude mouse. (b) White light microscopy of the entire window. The white box represents the approximate location of confocal and OCT imaging. (c) Maximum intensity projection image of a fluorescence confocal z stack obtained using 500 kD fluorescein-labeled dextran (1.8 mm $\times$ 1.8 mm). (d) Speckle-variance OCT *en-face* projection image of vasculature without the use of external contrast agents (1.8 mm $\times$ 1.8 mm). Reproduced from [24] with permission.

approximation to the temporal gradient. Once the velocities (f_x, f_z) are estimated, they can be integrated over time and mapped on a pixel-by-pixel basis to create an image whose gray values encode displacements in either the x or z direction. Normalizing these displacement maps by the initial dimensions of the sample yields elastograms that encode strain in the limit of small deformations. Figure 6.27(a) shows the structural OCT image of a bi-layered tissue phantom and Fig. 6.27(b) the corresponding elastogram obtained by tracking motion and velocity via this estimator.

The other method, presented in Ref. [23], is devised for large compressions, and conveniently only requires that the speckle patterns retain some correlation between successive A-scans. (Previously developed OCE approaches required that the speckle be correlated between successive OCT *B-scans* [11, 91].) The calculation of tissue motion and strain maps from the phase information is straightforward and rapid.

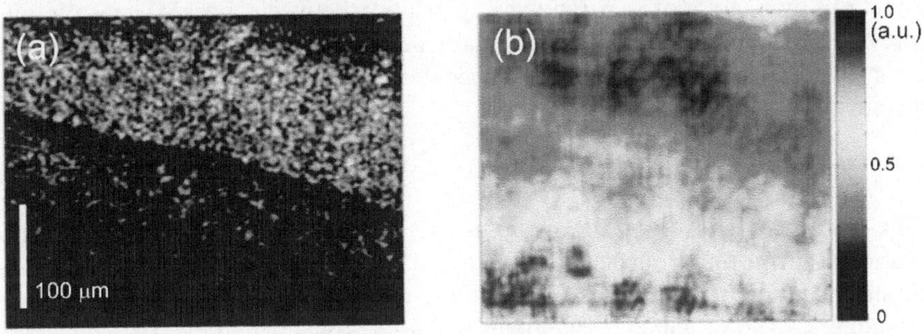

Figure 6.27: (a) Portion of OCT image of a bi-layered tissue phantom under compression. (b) Corresponding feature-based elastogram encoded to display the relative cumulative strains in the different layers of the tissue phantom. The highest strain was normalized to unity. Reproduced from [23] with permission.

6.7 Mitigation of OCT Speckle

Speckle is often regarded as a form of "noise," in the sense that it impedes one's ability to extract information from an OCT image, such as a sample's structure or its local optical properties. Consequently, there is a body of literature devoted to trying to mitigate its effects by reducing speckle contrast ratio in the image. The task is hindered by the fact that "speckle" and "structure" cannot be easily dissociated. The distinction is only clear when the sample can be described using a model such as that of Section 6.2.2, in which $A(\mathbf{r})$ represents the structure and $R(\mathbf{r})$ the underlying "speckle-generating" mechanism. One method for speckle reduction is to simply apply a low-pass spatial filter (averaging kernel) to the detected envelope (or squared envelope) signal. This will certainly reduce the speckle contrast, but at a severe spatial resolution cost. Indeed, speckle reduction almost inevitably involves a corresponding resolution deterioration, either spatial or temporal.

OCT speckle reduction methods have been reviewed in Refs. [1, 5, 38, 92]. Broadly speaking, they may be classified into those involving modifications to the experimental apparatus and those involving post-processing of the recorded images. We treat these cases in Sections 6.7.1 and 6.7.2, respectively.

Experimental methods involve taking multiple image acquisitions under different illumination or detection conditions, with the aim to access uncorrelated speckle-pattern realizations corresponding to the same local region. Such methods include varying: the illumination or detection polarization states [5, 82]; the illumination center wavelength [33]; the detection angle [4, 10, 77, 78, 93]; the beam focal position [94, 95] and strain induced in the sample [96, 97].

Signal post-processing methods have been applied to the problem of speckle reduction, for the most part in an attempt to extract useful sample information from speckle-corrupted images and suppress image-distorting effects. Many methods have been proposed, including: averaging filters [5]; I-divergence regularization [98]; wavelet transforms [14]; and anisotropic diffusion [99].

6.7.1 Experimental methods

To achieve speckle reduction experimentally, it is generally necessary to sample multiple realizations of the speckle fluctuations, while preserving the structural information captured within each OCT scan. Averaging M independent speckle (envelope) states reduces the standard deviation of the fluctuations by a factor of $\sqrt{M}$ (and any correlation between speckle states diminishes this factor). However, the sample resolution is potentially degraded by a factor of M, or greater. In this Section, we consider the possibility of effecting speckle reduction through modification to the experimental apparatus.

6.7.1.1 Polarization diversity

The first approach we consider is *polarization diversity* [5]. The principle is based on the observation that if a rough surface is illuminated by unpolarized monochromatic light, the observed intensity pattern is the sum of two potentially uncorrelated speckle patterns (corresponding to orthogonal polarization states), reducing the observed speckle contrast ratio by a factor of $\sqrt{2}$. However, OCT speckle contrast cannot be reduced merely by replacing the polarized source with an unpolarized one, because even though the signals from the detected orthogonal states would add on an intensity basis, in OCT the optical fields are encoded into the intensity cross term and, thus, the speckle patterns would add on a *field* basis, which will not reduce the observed speckle contrast. Instead, the individual polarization state envelopes must be detected separately [as in polarization-sensitive (PS)-OCT] and the OCT signals added on an envelope basis [100]. If the speckle patterns in each are uncorrelated, the sum of the envelopes would effectively double both the speckle mean and variance, yielding the required $\sqrt{2}$ contrast-ratio improvement. (As noted by Goodman [1], the use of both orthogonal illumination and detection states could permit a contrast-ratio improvement by a factor of up to $\sqrt{4} = 2$.)

However, for most samples, it is likely that the speckle patterns would be highly correlated, so the actual improvement achieved would be much less. Moreover, it is likely that the improvement would be most pronounced with respect to the "signal-degrading" speckle component, offering little benefit.[24] For "signal-bearing speckle," under the single-scattering, first-order-Born-approximation model, all illumination/detection polarization states probe the same range of sample spatial frequency components; decorrelation between the signals relies on the scattering profile being polarization-dependent. Indeed, our group has utilized decorrelation between the signals in PS-OCT as a mechanism for detecting the degree to which multiply scattered light contributes to the OCT signal [82].

Employing unpolarized light in OCT would also require engineering the OCT system to be free from polarization-dependent loss, birefringence and polarization-mode dispersion in order not to introduce distortions into the axial response function.

6.7.1.2 Spatial and angular compounding

Spatial compounding, or spatial diversity, is another hardware implementation to achieve speckle reduction. It involves taking multiple measurements of the sample, for which the illumination or detection methods are altered in order to probe multiple speckle states.

Schmitt et al. [10, 77] implemented a spatial diversity method by employing a segmented detector and summing incoherently the resulting interference signals. This approach, which may be described as angular diversity or angular compounding, is indicated schematically in Fig. 6.28. The authors investigated equal weighting in the summations as well as an adaptive weighting scheme. Their free-space system performed averaging of the backscattered signals from different angular apertures. Although only a quadrant photodetector ($M = 4$) was used, implying a maximum improvement in the contrast ratio of $\sqrt{M} = 2$, the visual impact of the consequent reduction in speckle from images of human skin taken *in vivo* is substantial. We reiterate that the maximum improvement would only occur if the detected signals are uncorrelated; in Ref. [10], the lack of correla-

[24] This is why imaging incoherently with crossed polarizers for illumination and collection permits one to suppress surface scattering and see deeper into a tissue sample.

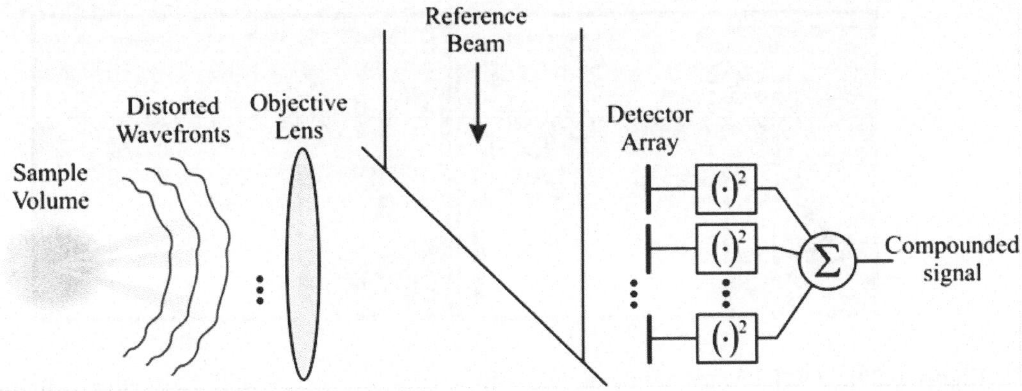

Figure 6.28: Principle of the angular compounding method for speckle reduction. Each detector receives light backscattered from a different angle. The detected signals are squared prior to summation. Adapted from [10] with permission.

tion was tentatively attributed to the detected Category-II signal rather than the Category-I signal. This is consistent with our statements in Section 6.6.2. As we noted there, the different collection angles ensure that the range of sample 3D spatial frequencies accessible to the image-formation system varies with aperture position. Accordingly, there will be some decorrelation even between the detected singly scattered contribution to the OCT signal, but not so much as between the highly multiply scattered contributions.

Even though the combined image represents a distinct improvement over the image obtained from an individual quadrant aperture, it would not be superior to the OCT image generated if all quadrants could be combined "coherently" in a single "super-aperture".[25] Nonetheless, using multiple detectors circumvents some of the engineering difficulties associated with high-NA imaging. Another technical difficulty associated with this method is that the shot noise-limited signal-to-noise ratio scales as $1/\sqrt{M}$, and the sampling rate for real-time operation scales with M.

The first approach to angular compounding that is compatible with optical-fiber-based systems was published in 2003, by Iftimia et al. [16]. Termed "path length encoded" angular compounding, it involves the insertion of a glass optical element in the sample arm beam path which imparts different optical group delays to different parts of the sample beam. These so-called beamlets illuminate the sample at different angles, providing the angle-compounding effect. A novelty of this approach is that the separate images can be captured in the same OCT A-scan; they are axially separated due to the different optical group delays associated with either propagating, or not propagating, through the optical element. It is convenient for use with catheter-based OCT probes; the instrument modification requires only a minimal increase in complexity. However, the fact that the illumination beam is partitioned into separate sub-beams immediately invokes a resolution and sensitivity trade-off.

Another approach to angular compounding for speckle reduction extends the earlier approach of Schmitt et al. to the case of $M = 400$ detectors [78]. Termed "massively-parallel" detection, it utilizes a swept-source OCT setup to record time-resolved frequency measurements, and a line-scan camera detector array to record the output signal at the 400 angular positions. This means that the lateral resolution of the system is provided by the focusing power of the illumination beam alone, not by the extent of the full detection aperture.

The resulting compounded images show an effective suppression of speckle contrast equivalent

[25] The result of such a combination would be a "pure" (Rayleigh-distributed) speckle pattern, but with very fine speckle grains consistent with the improvement in system resolution.

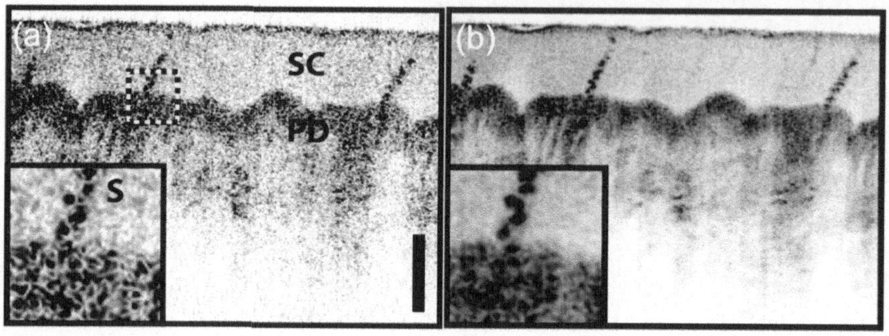

Figure 6.29: OCT images of human fingertip acquired *in vivo* (a) with no angular compounding; (b) with 32 angular samples. The scale bar corresponds to 250 μm. Reproduced from [4] with permission.

to that of about 40 independent measurements, with startling visual impact and little or no apparent resolution degradation, compared with an image from a single detector. Like the earlier approach, this is due to the fact that the individual speckle recordings access multiple non-overlapping regions of spatial-frequency space (under the single backscattering assumption). Also, like the earlier approach, it provides a partial benefit of accessing the range of backscattering angles associated with a large-NA aperture, but avoids the technical challenges associated with utilizing high-NA optics. (These would include, for example, a limited depth of field.)

When considering spatial/angular compounding approaches, one must distinguish between setups that detect multiple speckle states simultaneously, as do those described above, and those that utilize successive sample recordings. An example of the latter is the method presented in Ref. [4]. In this method, a galvanometer mirror is incorporated in a transmissive sample arm, allowing light from different backscattering angles to be detected selectively. The images presented in Fig. 6.29, extracted from [4], seem to indicate an increased ability to delineate between sample regions. Another example is the angular compounding scheme of Bashkansky and Reintjes [12], who make multiple recordings by varying the sample illumination angle by translating a right-angle prism.

An example of a spatial (not angular) compounding scheme is the proposal by Popescu et al. [94], for which the sample position is shifted (axially) with respect to the focused illumination beam. A similar method has been presented to improve OCT imaging of basal cell carcinomas [101]. The method has also been demonstrated by our group in a recently proposed 3D-structured phantom, as shown in Fig. 6.30 [29]. The variation in phase curvature over the length of the beam ensures that multiple speckle states (relative scatterer phases) are probed at the same sample location. There is a corresponding loss of resolution due to beam diffraction, when comparing the in-focus PSF to the largest out-of-focus PSF used in the scheme. This resolution trade-off perhaps has a minor effect on perceptible image quality, but it is unavoidable (unlike the angular compounding schemes) because the separate recordings do *not* access different regions of the sample's spatial frequency spectrum. A disadvantage of these approaches is the increased signal acquisition time associated with the multiple recordings. (There is also a loss of temporal resolution; such a scheme is most beneficial for static samples.) We mention in passing that if the ISAM procedure [41] is applied to the acquired OCT images, it seems plausible that the "in-focus" speckle realization would be observed over the length of the axial scan, so that this technique would not be useful.

Angular compounding continues to be the most popular hardware approach, with several extensions presented [102–105]. A novel approach for spatial compounding was recently presented for retinal imaging. This method takes advantage of motion artefacts occurring between B-scan acquisitions to obtain images with decorrelated speckle patterns. Although this inevitably results in loss of resolution, incoherent averaging leads to a significant reduction in speckle and a notable

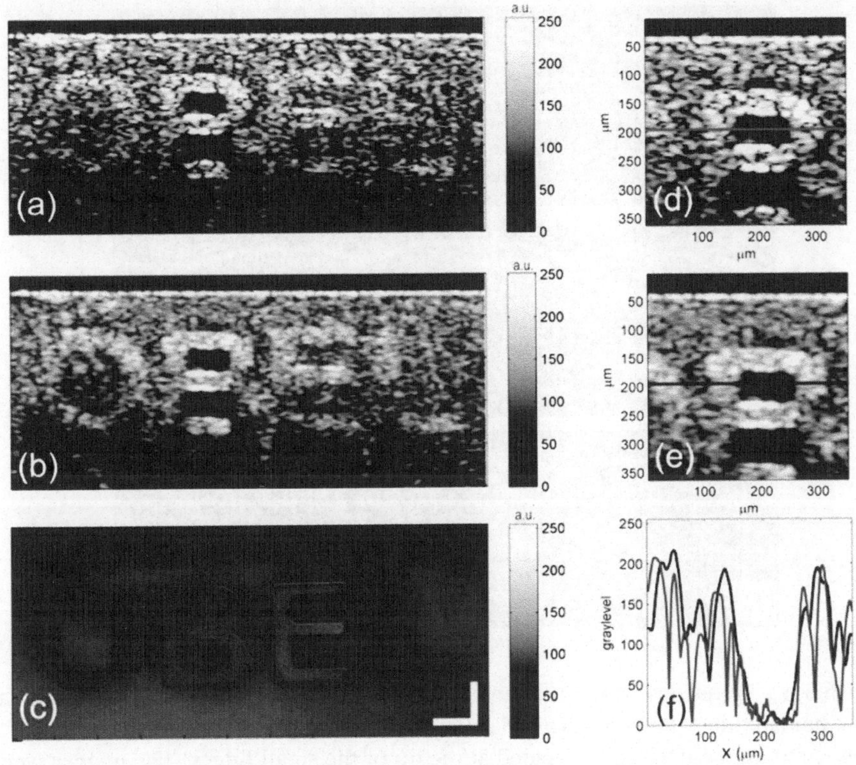

Figure 6.30: Spatial compounding speckle reduction performed on images of a 3D-structured phantom: (a) Single B-scan; (b) Incoherent average of 20 co-registered offset B-scans; (c) Microscope image of the lettering from the front (x-z plane) (Scale bar: 100 μm). Close-up of a portion of the letter "B" for: (d) a single B-scan; and (e) the speckle-reduced image; and (f) pixel logarithmic intensities plotted as a function of the lateral position (x axis) for the horizontal lines shown in (d) (lower curve) and (e) (upper curve), respectively. Reproduced from [29] with permission.

improvement in image quality [106]. In a related method, also developed for retinal imaging, several B-scans are averaged together causing a resolution degradation in the y-direction rather than in the plane of a B-scan [107]. For the particular symmetry of the imaged structure (e.g., laminar structures such as the cornea or retina) this corresponds to preserving the in-plane resolution.

6.7.1.3 Frequency compounding

Just as angular diversity schemes partition the detection aperture into separate sub-apertures, each of which generates a distinct signal, frequency diversity schemes divide the bandwidth of the light source into separate optical bands. The signal envelopes from each are added "incoherently" [5]. Clearly, the speckle contrast/resolution trade-off is manifested in the fact that the OCT system resolution is inversely proportional to bandwidth. It is unclear that such schemes would, in general, have any benefit over merely performing spatial averaging along the axial direction. However, a scheme by Pircher et al. [33] combines (on an envelope basis) the sample OCT signals acquired with two different (well-separated) center wavelengths. It thereby accesses two different regions of the sample's spatial frequency spectrum (which cannot meaningfully be combined on a "coherent" basis). In performing speckle reduction, the authors expected a decrease in contrast ratio by 1.4, but observed instead 1.25, which they attributed to residual correlation between the images due to

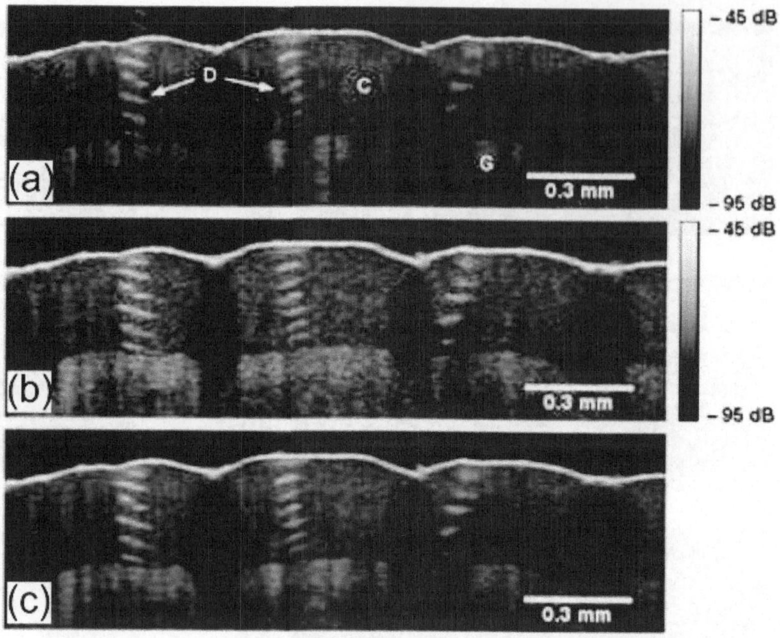

Figure 6.31: Frequency compounding combined with spatial compounding. Simultaneous *in vivo* scans of human skin at 800 nm (a) and 1250 nm (b) showing the stratum corneum, C, sweat ducts, D, and the stratum granulosum, G, located at the tip of the small finger. The images were obtained by averaging five adjacent B-scans of a three-dimensional stack resulting in a displayed cross-section thickness of 20 μm. (c) Frequency compounded image of (a) and (b). Adapted from [108] with permission.

large structures. [It seems that, in this case, the statistics were not measurements of "pure" speckle, as defined in this chapter; the individual contrasts measured were 0.625 and 0.637, greater than the expected 0.52 (see Section 6.3).] It should be noted that the expected reduction of the coherence length (and speckle size) if the two signals could be added on a *coherent* basis would still be equal to 2, so that a speckle contrast/resolution trade-off still applies.

Frequency compounding has also been implemented using a dual-band spectral-domain OCT system designed for high-resolution *in vivo* imaging [108]. This system employed a supercontinuum source, the emission spectrum of which was filtered to achieve a double-peak spectrum containing the bands 700–900 nm and 1100–1400 nm. These bands were detected separately using two spectrometers. The two OCT images were averaged to significantly reduce the speckle present in murine arteries and human skin images (Fig. 6.31).

Another recently proposed frequency compounding method takes advantage of Fourier-domain detection by subdividing the digitized spectrum into a number of narrower windows each at a different central frequency [109]. Speckle reduction is achieved by averaging the corresponding patterns, with the associated resolution decrease. The authors demonstrated their method using an intravascular optical-frequency domain imaging system on data acquired *in vivo*.

6.7.1.4 Strain compounding

Speckle reduction by strain compounding is achieved by imparting strain to a sample to achieve speckle decorrelation between B-scans. Strain is defined as the ratio of change in sample thickness to its original thickness. The method is related to speckle tracking used in OCE: strain is measured by measuring speckle motion as the sample is compressed [11]. However, unlike the large-scale structure of the sample, the speckle pattern is not merely spatially distorted through sample deformation. Instead, a different speckle realization is obtained, only partially correlated with the first. To explain this, note that compressing the sample actually stretches its **k**-space representation (spatial frequency spectrum) about the origin. Thus, different information is accessible to the OCT TF (the small peak in Fig. 6.13). Because the TF is bandpass in the k_z direction, only a small "stretch" factor in this direction (corresponding to an equivalently small sample compression factor) is necessary to achieve significant speckle decorrelation. This fact is exploited in strain compounding for speckle reduction, by incoherently averaging B-scans for different sample strains, correcting for the spatial distortion due to compression. (We reiterate that the large-scale structure in the corrected images is the same, but the speckle patterns are different.) Strain compounding has also been employed in ultrasound [110]. In OCT, our group demonstrated a 1.5-fold reduction in speckle CR by varying the strain by 0.027 in a silicone phantom.

A closely related method our group proposed takes advantage of the "creep strain" in a viscoelastic sample under constant load in order to achieve speckle reduction [111]. The method, creep compounding, simplifies the loading element required in the OCT system sample arm (compared with strain compounding) because no increment in stress is required. Creep compounding is also better suited to being used with soft tissues, which are generally viscoelastic, not purely elastic.

Correction for compression-induced relative spatial distortions between any two B-scans is achieved by applying a coordinate-system transformation to one of them. Affine transformations are used to account for sample dilation, shearing and translation in the imaging plane. Co-registering an entire sequence of B-scans in this way prior to incoherent averaging minimizes the loss in resolution due to blurring. This procedure for creep compounding is illustrated in Fig. 6.32.

Figure 6.33(a) shows an OCT B-scan of a human breast lymph node, and a comparison of two speckle reduction methods: creep compounding in Figs. 6.33(e) and 6.33(f) and Gaussian smoothing in Figs. 6.33(c) and 6.33(d). Both methods attain the same contrast ratio reduction but creep compounding proves to be more efficient in maintaining high resolution.

A related method which also co-registers images using a spatial diversity approach has been applied to retinal imaging [112].

6.7.2 Post-processing methods

Post-processing methods to reduce speckle in OCT do not require any modification to the system hardware. This is a significant advantage for several reasons. Firstly, commercial OCT systems are now widely used in both clinical and research environments. Manipulation of the hardware is generally not possible with these systems. Secondly, new application areas for OCT, e.g., in cardiology and breast cancer, require the use of endoscopic and interstitial probes, making the implementation of experimental speckle reduction methods far more challenging. In these situations, post-processing methods are the only speckle-reduction mechanism possible. Despite the disadvantage of not being able to access "new" sample-specific information, they have the advantage of being generally applicable to a wide range of OCT recordings. In this Section, we describe the most prominent post-processing methods presented in the literature to date.

6.7.2.1 Filtering methods

As noted at the beginning of this section, the most straightforward method to reduce speckle in post-processing is simply to apply an averaging filter to the recorded data. This approach has the significant disadvantage that it necessarily degrades the spatial resolution. The resolution sacrifice may be worthwhile if it permits quasi-homogeneous optical properties of the sample to be accurately measured. Thus, a common means to reduce the effect of speckle is simply to average multiple A-scans, recorded at different times (in a non-static sample) [113, 114] or lateral positions [65, 69,

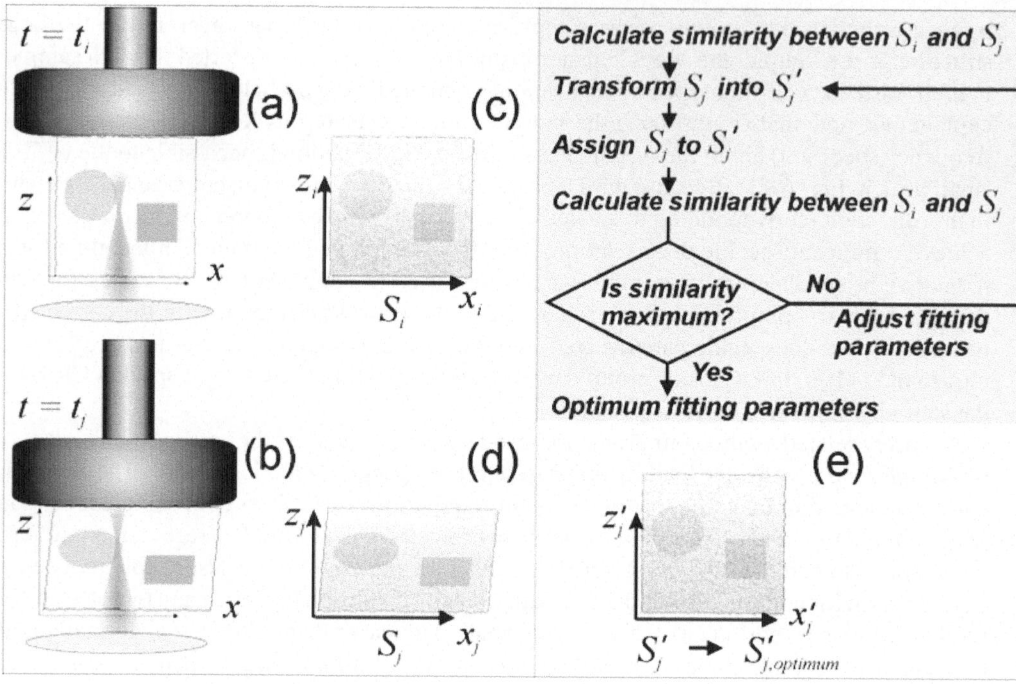

Figure 6.32: Illustration of the sample arm geometry unloaded (a) and loaded (b) and corresponding OCT image representations, before (c) and after (d) creep strain. The flow chart illustrates the processing steps required for co-registration leading to a distortion-corrected OCT image, represented in (e). Reproduced from [97] with permission.

115]. Another straightforward method is median filtering [5]. Again, the simplicity of this method is offset by the resolution degradation. Improved performance has been achieved using adaptive Wiener filtering [92]. Another example in this class is the locally adaptive *rotating kernel transform* method utilized by Rogowska et al. [15, 116] for the purpose of edge-enhancement in speckled images. The OCT images are convolved with a series of two-dimensional binary kernels, in which the non-zero regions resemble narrow slits, one pixel wide, at different angles. For each pixel, the maximum signal, obtained using these kernels, is selected to generate the processed image. This method also represents a trade-off between speckle contrast and image resolution; its usefulness lies in the fact that the resolution decrease occurs exactly in the direction of the image boundaries (that is, exactly in the direction for which high resolution is unnecessary).

6.7.2.2 Complex-signal methods

In general, access to both the full envelope and phase information provides enhanced opportunities for post-processing over those from the envelope alone. For the full interferometric signal, it is possible to alter the shape of the response function, and compensate for dispersion as well as to reduce speckle.

The first application of a phase-domain method specifically to reduce speckle noise was the so-called zero adjustment procedure (ZAP) [7]. ZAP was originally developed to reduce speckle in ultrasound images [117]. Its goal is to “fill in” the dark speckles in an image, which it does by detecting the spikes of the instantaneous spatial frequency associated with dark speckles. As a trade-off, it tends to blur feature boundaries.

Another method, based on an adaptation of the so-called iterative point deconvolution CLEAN

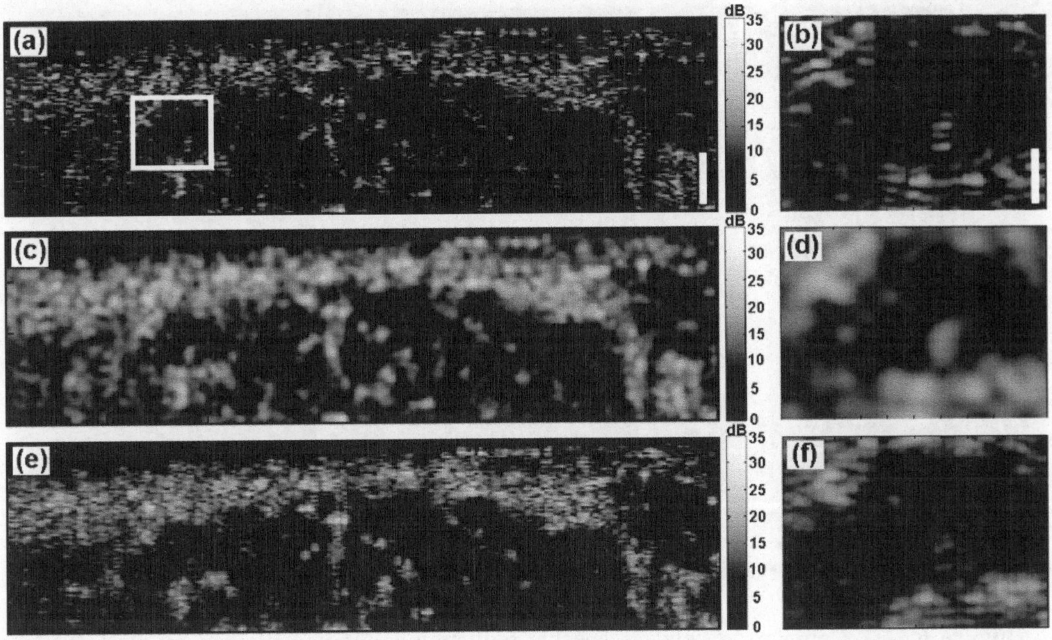

Figure 6.33: B-scans of human lymph node tissue with: (a) no speckle reduction; (c) speckle reduction using post-processing spatial averaging; and (e) after creep compounding, plotted on a logarithmic scale. Images (b), (d) and (f) are magnifications of (a), (c) and (e), respectively, corresponding to the indicated region in (a). Identical CR reduction is achieved in (c) and (e), and (d) and (f), although higher resolution is maintained in (e) and (f). The scale bar in (a) represents 100 μm and in (b) 40 μm. Reproduced from [97] with permission.

algorithm, used to enhance weak scattering signals in the presence of nearby strong signals, has also been proposed [37]. However, it works best when the scatterers within the sample are separated by at least the width of the PSF envelope, so that the sample does not conform to the highly turbid model considered throughout this chapter. The performance of the method degrades steeply as the number of scatterers increases.

A post-processing method for speckle reduction based on I-divergence regularization [98] operates by determining the optimal sample scattering distribution that is both: consistent with the detected speckled image, assuming the latter is obtained by convolving the optimal scattering distribution with the coherent PSF (subject to noise); and has a modulus distribution that matches a low-pass-filtered version of the original image [$A(\mathbf{r})$ in the notation of this chapter]. A metric is defined which incorporates the two conditions, and must be minimized to generate the corrected image.

Recently, a speckle reduction method based on this divergence technique has been presented, specifically for endovascular OCT [118]. In this paper, the authors used a generalized divergence measure and claimed its superiority over the I-divergence measure when processing porcine artery images acquired in an *in vivo* scenario. In Fig. 6.34, it can be seen that the generalized divergence measure achieves greater speckle reduction, while maintaining feature edges. The results are significant as they demonstrate a practical implementation of speckle reduction in a commercial OCT scanner. Furthermore, they highlight a key advantage of post-processing methods, i.e., that they can readily be applied to any acquired OCT image. Hardware methods to reduce speckle in the scenario presented in [118] would be far more challenging.

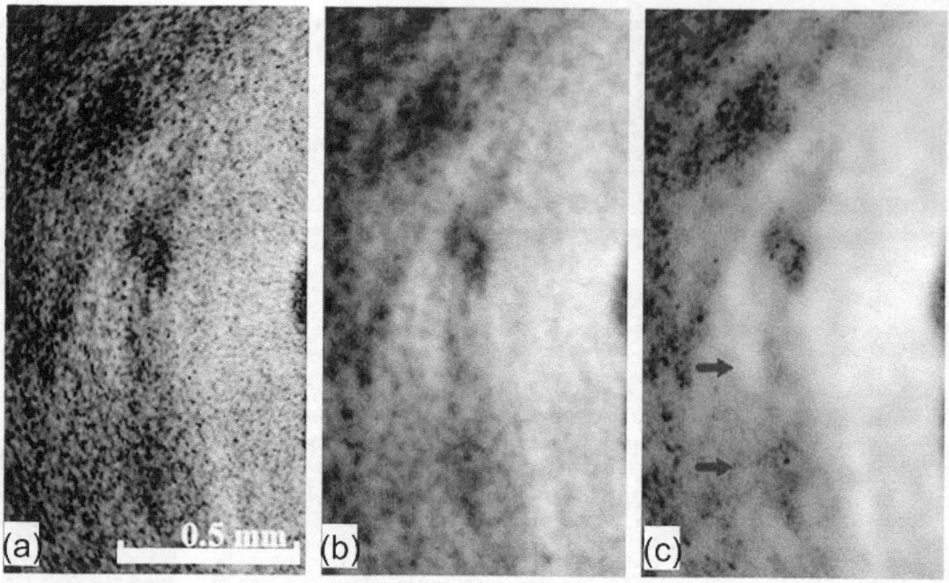

Figure 6.34: Comparison between speckle reduction methods applied to an OCT B-scan of a region of porcine arterial wall. (a) Original image; (b) Image processed with I-divergence algorithm; (c) Image processed using the generalized divergence method; the arrows indicate structures that are rendered more visible using the approach. Reproduced from [118] with permission.

6.7.2.3 Transform-domain methods

Wavelet filtering methods to reduce speckle have been used widely in ultrasound and synthetic aperture radar imaging. More recently, they have also been applied to OCT [14]. These methods work by transforming the detected OCT signal into the wavelet domain. This involves representing the OCT data as scaled and translated copies of a finite-length oscillating waveform, which allows the signal to be analyzed at multiple scales. The signal is decomposed into wavelet coefficients. Those coefficients associated with "features" tend to cluster spatially, whereas those from "speckle noise" do not. By comparing the correlation of each wavelet coefficient to its immediate neighbours, a spatially adaptive estimate of whether a coefficient is "signal" or "noise" can be made. Thus, wavelet filters can differentiate between signal discontinuities caused by speckle or features, and the thresholds can be adapted to strongly reduce speckle while leaving edges intact. The threshold conveniently represents a single parameter that can be used to control the inherent trade-off between speckle reduction and loss of spatial resolution. We note the implicit assumption that the sample is composed of quasi-homogeneous, contiguous regions separated by well-defined edges.

Initially, wavelet filtering in OCT was performed using the discrete wavelet transform, providing the most compact coefficient-based representation of the signal [14]. Recent work has presented a more sophisticated filter based on the dual-tree complex wavelet transform [119]. An example of this method on OCT images of a rat cavernous nerve is shown in Fig. 6.35. The method is shift-invariant and allows orientation in 2D. It has been demonstrated on a prostate sample and compared with corresponding histology images. Puvanathasan et al. presented a variation on the wavelet method, implementing a novel thresholding strategy [120]. Another method specifically designed for visualization of OCT data in 3D has been implemented in a scheme called optimized non-orthogonal wavelet (ONW) denoising [121]. The transform was implemented in 2D but its effect was assessed in 3D.

A related method based on operating on the OCT signal in the "curvelet" (as opposed to wavelet)

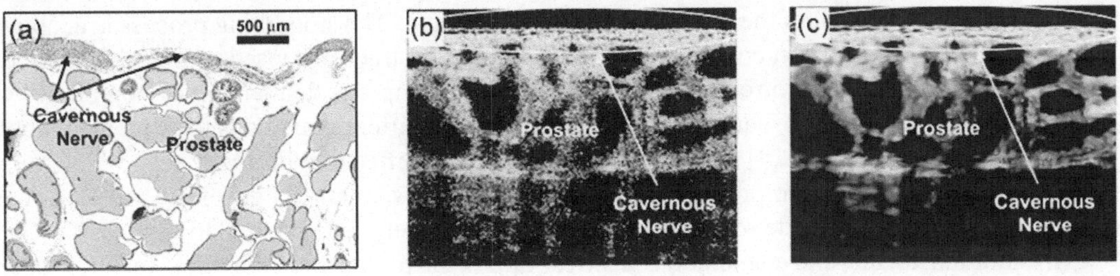

Figure 6.35: (See color insert.) Longitudinal section of a rat cavernous nerve: (a) histology; (b) OCT; and (c) OCT after wavelet denoising. The cavernous nerve corresponds to a relatively high signal intensity (shown in red) and lies superficial to the prostate. Adapted from [119] with permission.

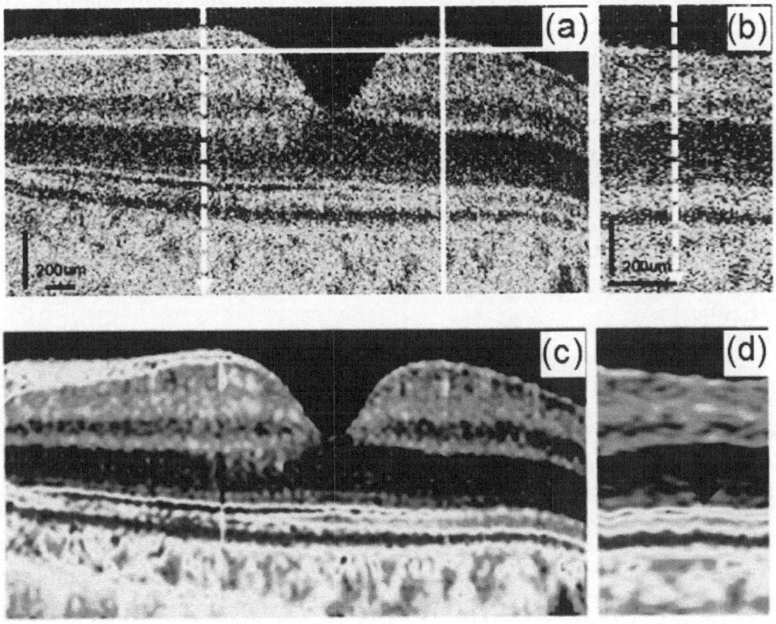

Figure 6.36: (See color insert.) Acquired cross-sectional retinal images: (a) before; (b) after 3D curvelet denoising. Adapted from [123] with permission.

transform domain has also been presented [122]. Wavelet and curvelet methods differ mainly in the choice of basis function. The premise for this method is that curvelets better describe the edge discontinuities (rather than point discontinuities) that are associated with OCT. The authors extended the curvelet method to implement the first 3D post-processing speckle reduction method [123], fully exploiting the recorded OCT signal in a region surrounding each image point. This is a powerful extension, which utilizes more information in the acquired OCT volume. An example of 3D curvelet denoising on OCT images of the human retina is shown in Fig. 6.36.

6.7.2.4 Diffusion methods

Diffusion methods are common in signal processing. They come about from an analogy with fluid diffusion: the image intensity distribution is considered as a fluid concentration. A diffusion equation is used to smooth the grayscale levels in an image. The smoothing process is adaptive and is controlled by a diffusion coefficient. The first diffusion filter proposed for speckle reduction in OCT was a nonlinear anisotropic diffusion filter used to improve delineation of boundaries within the human retina [99]. Subsequent papers have compared different methods to implement nonlinear diffusion filters in OCT [124] and combined anisotropic diffusion with fuzzy sets to determine the uncertainty in the diffusion process [120, 125]. Whilst these methods generally preserve features, they provide limited speckle reduction and require a relatively long computation time.

In addition to the above methods, a novel approach to speckle reduction in OCT based on Bayesian least squares estimation has been presented [126]. This method is unique in that it learns the underlying noise distribution of the observed data dynamically. The authors claim that it provides significant speckle noise suppression while preserving image details.

A 2007 paper compared the performance of a number of software methods to achieve speckle reduction in OCT [92]. The authors concluded that the combination of wavelet-transform, Lee and adaptive Wiener filters significantly reduced speckle whilst preserving strong edges. The authors also compared these methods to the hardware method of angular compounding. Such comparisons are an important step in arriving at optimum speckle reduction. Further work is required to comprehensively compare and contrast the most prominent experimental and post-processing methods. An important aspect of this is the need for a suitable calibration phantom that gives rise to 3D speckled features and a standard protocol for quantitative image quality assessment. The parameters to be used would include speckle contrast ratio (CR), signal to noise ratio (SNR), contrast to noise ratio (CNR), and feature resolution, in a similar way to the protocol used in image processing of computational standard phantoms, e.g., the Shepp-Logan phantom [127] for X-ray computed tomography and magnetic resonance imaging. A first step towards this standardization is the phantom recently demonstrated by our group [29] and used in the focus-compounding experimental method described above (Fig. 6.30).

6.8 Conclusions

Speckle is a feature of any coherent optical system and, as such, appears prominently in OCT images. It represents the apparently random but highly sample-dependent fluctuations in the detected OCT envelope signal. OCT speckle is strongly affected by the precise position relationship between the sample scatterers.

We have described the OCT image formation process using a spatially variant linear-system framework, allowing us, under the first-order Born approximation, to express the OCT signal in terms of the sample's scattering potential and the local system point spread function, or equivalently in the spatial frequency domain, the sample's spectrum and the local (coherent) transfer function. The transfer function is of great importance when considering second-order speckle statistics. The normalized inverse Fourier transform of its squared modulus yields the speckle correlation function, from which we can deduce speckle size.

The various light-tissue interaction mechanisms that contribute to the image formation process in OCT can be classified according to their relative value in constructing a sample representation and their associated artifacts. Category-I (singly-backscattered) light generates the image of highest fidelity to the sample structure. Both Category-I and the Category-II (low-angle forward-scattered) light provide useful image information. Category-III (wide-angle multiply scattered) light gives rise to signal-degrading speckle. Contributions from all three categories are combined on a "coherent" basis to yield the detected OCT signal.

With regard to second-order speckle statistics, we have demonstrated that both axial and lateral speckle size are dependent only on the optical source employed and the focal spot size (i.e., lateral resolution): sample dispersion, beam divergence, and multiple scattering have almost no effect.

We have also described how information can be retrieved from OCT speckle. We have demonstrated, for low density of scatterers, that the speckle contrast ratio is correlated with the concentration of scatterers in the OCT coherence volume, and shown good agreement between experimental results and the predictions of a theoretical random phasor sum model. A simple Mie-theoretical analysis suggests that, particularly in ultrahigh-resolution regimes, where the effective number of scatterers within the resolution volume is small, OCT speckle contrast ratio could be used to distinguish regions of a sample with different microscopic properties.

The speckle correlation coefficient can be used to discriminate between different categories of light contributing to the OCT signal, providing a metric to quantify the deleterious structure-masking contribution of Category-III light. This is possible if applied in combination with angularly diverse detection scheme (as is already utilized for speckle reduction).

Speckle cross-correlation may also be used to track motion within tissue, e.g., tissue deformation and blood flow. OCT angiography based upon dynamic speckle is a rapidly emerging area, by far the most promising utilisation of OCT speckle. Cross-correlation methods are gathering great momentum in retinal imaging and are likely to displace Doppler methods in many instances. They are also likely to impact on imaging animal models of tumor growth, and in dermatology and plastic surgery, e.g., wound healing.

By far the topic of most widespread interest and potential impact is the improvement of OCT image quality through speckle mitigation. Here, the promise is much more mixed. Firstly, many images show "improvement" without actually demonstrating additional information content – such enhancements are aesthetically appealing while being of limited intrinsic value. The principal exceptions occur when multiple speckle realizations are acquired for different hardware configurations and the results are "incoherently" averaged, particularly when (according to the linear-system framework) a different range of 3D sample spatial frequencies is accessible to each recording. Even in such cases, the results fall short of the improvement in image quality that would be expected if the realizations could be combined "coherently," although often this would not be technically feasible.

Secondly, regardless of the method used, speckle reduction techniques are onerous, computationally or otherwise, and so require a commensurate benefit, often not in evidence. In all likelihood, what will emerge are methods highly specialised for specific applications, such as preserving layer edges in the retina, or adapting to vascular dimensions in angiography or in cardiovascular OCT. In these instances, small benefits will accumulate to drive commercial advantage and make an overall impact on clinical applications.

Acknowledgments

We gratefully acknowledge Dr. Martin Villiger of the Wellman Center for Photomedicine, Massachusetts General Hospital, for valuable discussions relating to the linear-systems model for OCT image formation, and his great help in reviewing and proofreading the chapter as a whole. We also acknowledge early collaboration on speckle with Prof. Steven Jacques, Oregon Health and Science University, useful discussions with Prof. Maciej Wojtkowski, Nicolaus Copernicus University, Poland, and the contributions of our co-worker Dr. Steven Adie. Funding for this work has been received from the Australian Research Council's Discovery program.

References

[1] J. W. Goodman, *Speckle Phenomena in Optics* (Roberts and Company, Englewood, Colorado, 2007).

[2] J. C. Dainty, ed. *Laser Speckle and Related Phenomena* (Springer-Verlag, Berlin, 1984).

[3] W. Drexler and J. G. Fujimoto, eds. *Optical Coherence Tomography: Technology and Applications* (Springer, Berlin, 2008).

[4] A. E. Desjardins, B. J. Vakoc, W. Y. Oh, S. M. R. Motaghiannezam, G. J. Tearney, and B. E. Bouma, "Angle-resolved Optical Coherence Tomography with sequential angular selectivity for speckle reduction," *Optics Express* **15**, 6200–6209 (2007).

[5] J. M. Schmitt, S. H. Xiang, and K. M. Yung, "Speckle in optical coherence tomography," *Journal of Biomedical Optics* **4**, 95–105 (1999).

[6] D. A. Boas, K. K. Bizheva, and A. M. Siegel, "Using dynamic low-coherence interferometry to image Brownian motion within highly scattering media," *Optics Letters* **23**, 319–321 (1998).

[7] K. M. Yung, S. L. Lee, and J. M. Schmitt, "Phase-domain processing of optical coherence tomography images," *Journal of Biomedical Optics* **4**, 125–136 (1999).

[8] G. Hausler, J. M. Herrmann, R. Kummer, and M. W. Lindner, "Observation of light propagation in volume scatterers with 10(11)-fold slow motion," *Optics Letters* **21**, 1087–1089 (1996).

[9] J. M. Schmitt and A. Knüttel, "Model of optical coherence tomography of heterogeneous tissue," *Journal of the Optical Society of America A* **14**, 1231–1242 (1997).

[10] J. M. Schmitt, "Array detection for speckle reduction in optical coherence microscopy," *Physics in Medicine and Biology* **42**, 1427–1439 (1997).

[11] J. M. Schmitt, "OCT elastography: imaging microscopic deformation and strain of tissue," *Optics Express* **3**, 199–211 (1998).

[12] M. Bashkansky and J. Reintjes, "Statistics and reduction of speckle in optical coherence tomography," *Optics Letters* **25**, 545–547 (2000).

[13] S. J. Kirkpatrick and D. D. Duncan, "Optical assessment of tissue mechanics," in *Handbook of Optical Biomedical Diagnostics*, V. V. Tuchin, ed. (SPIE Press, Bellingham, Washington, 2002), pp. 1037–1084.

[14] D. C. Adler, T. H. Ko, and J. G. Fujimoto, "Speckle reduction in optical coherence tomography images by use of a spatially adaptive wavelet filter," *Optics Letters* **29**, 2878–2880 (2004).

[15] J. Rogowska and M. E. Brezinski, "Evaluation of the adaptive speckle suppression filter for coronary optical coherence tomography imaging," *IEEE Transactions on Medical Imaging* **19**, 1261–1266 (2000).

[16] N. Iftimia, B. E. Bouma, and G. J. Tearney, "Speckle reduction in optical coherence tomography by 'path length encoded' angular compounding," *Journal of Biomedical Optics* **8**, 260–263 (2003).

[17] K. W. Gossage, T. S. Tkaczyk, J. J. Rodriguez, and J. K. Barton, "Texture, analysis of optical coherence tomography images: feasibility for tissue classification," *Journal of Biomedical Optics* **8**, 570–575 (2003).

[18] T. R. Hillman, S. G. Adie, V. Seemann, J. J. Armstrong, S. L. Jacques, and D. D. Sampson, "Correlation of static speckle with sample properties in optical coherence tomography," *Optics Letters* **31**, 190–192 (2006).

[19] J. M. Schmitt, "Optical coherence tomography (OCT): a review," *IEEE Journal of Selected Topics in Quantum Electronics* **5**, 1205–1215 (1999).

[20] A. F. Fercher and C. K. Hitzenberger, "Optical coherence tomography," in *Progress in Optics*, E. Wolf, ed. (Elsevier Science, Vienna, 2002), pp. 215–302.

[21] A. F. Fercher, W. Drexler, C. K. Hitzenberger, and T. Lasser, "Optical coherence tomography - principles and applications," *Reports on Progress in Physics* **66**, 239–303 (2003).

[22] Y. T. Pan, R. Birngruber, J. Rosperich, and R. Engelhardt, "Low-coherence optical tomography in turbid tissue: theoretical analysis," *Applied Optics* **34**, 6564–6574 (1995).

[23] S. J. Kirkpatrick, R. K. Wang, and D. D. Duncan, "OCT-based elastography for large and small deformations," *Optics Express* **14**, 11585–11597 (2006).

[24] A. Mariampillai, B. A. Standish, E. H. Moriyama, M. Khurana, N. R. Munce, M. K. K. Leung, J. Jiang, A. Cable, B. C. Wilson, I. A. Vitkin, and V. X. D. Yang, "Speckle variance detection of microvasculature using swept-source optical coherence tomography," *Optics Letters* **33**, 1530–1532 (2008).

[25] J. W. Goodman, *Statistical Optics* (John Wiley and Sons, New York, 1985).

[26] J. M. Schmitt and G. Kumar, "Optical scattering properties of soft tissue: A discrete particle model," *Applied Optics* **37**, 2788–2797 (1998).

[27] M. Born and E. Wolf, *Principles of Optics: Electromagnetic Theory of Propagation, Interference and Diffraction of Light* (Cambridge University Press, 1999).

[28] M. Villiger and T. Lasser, "Image formation and tomogram reconstruction in optical coherence microscopy," *Journal of the Optical Society of America A* **27**, 2216–2228 (2010).

[29] A. Curatolo, B. F. Kennedy, and D. D. Sampson, "Structured three-dimensional optical phantom for optical coherence tomography," *Optics Express* **19**, 19480–19485 (2011).

[30] W. F. Cheong, S. A. Prahl, and A. J. Welch, "A review of the optical properties of biological tissues," *IEEE Journal of Selected Topics in Quantum Electronics* **26**, 2166–2185 (1990).

[31] A. Ishimaru, *Wave Propagation and Scattering in Random Media, Volume 1, Single Scattering and Transport Theory* (Academic Press, New York, 1978).

[32] J. W. Goodman, "Some fundamental properties of speckle," *Journal of the Optical Society of America A* **66**, 1145–1150 (1976).

[33] M. Pircher, E. Gotzinger, R. Leitgeb, A. F. Fercher, and C. K. Hitzenberger, "Speckle reduction in optical coherence tomography by frequency compounding," *Journal of Biomedical Optics* **8**, 565–569 (2003).

[34] J. W. Goodman, "Speckle with a finite number of steps," *Applied Optics* **47**, A111–A118 (2008).

[35] K. W. Gossage, C. M. Smith, E. M. Kanter, L. P. Hariri, A. L. Stone, J. J. Rodriguez, S. K. Williams, and J. K. Barton, "Texture analysis of speckle in optical coherence tomography images of tissue phantoms," *Physics in Medicine and Biology* **51**, 1563–1575 (2006).

[36] J. W. Goodman, *Introduction to Fourier Optics* (McGraw-Hill Book Co., 2004).

[37] J. M. Schmitt, "Restoration of optical coherence images of living tissue using the CLEAN algorithm," *Journal of Biomedical Optics* **3**, 66–75 (1998).

[38] A. F. Fercher, "Inverse scattering, dispersion, and speckle in optical coherence tomography," in *Optical Coherence Tomography: Technology and Applications*, W. Drexler and J. G. Fujimoto, eds. (Springer, Berlin, 2008), pp. 119–146.

[39] J. M. Coupland and J. Lobera, "Holography, tomography and 3D microscopy as linear filtering operations," *Measurement Science and Technology* **19**, 074012 (2008).

[40] Y. Yasuno, J.-I. Sugisaka, Y. Sando, Y. Nakamura, S. Makita, M. Itoh, and T. Yatagai, "Non-iterative numerical method for laterally superresolving Fourier domain optical coherence tomography," *Optics Express* **14**, 1006–1020 (2006).

[41] T. S. Ralston, D. L. Marks, C. P. Scott, and S. A. Boppart, "Interferometric synthetic aperture microscopy," *Nature Physics* **3**, 129–134 (2007).

[42] C. W. McCutchen, "Generalized aperture and the three-dimensional diffraction image," *Journal of the Optical Society of America A* **54**, 240–242 (1964).

[43] C. J. R. Sheppard, M. Gu, Y. Kawata, and S. Kawata, "Three-dimensional transfer functions for high-aperture systems," *Journal of the Optical Society of America A* **11**, 593–598 (1994).

[44] M. Gu, *Advanced Optical Imaging Theory* (Springer, Berlin, 2000).

[45] C. J. R. Sheppard, M. Roy, and M. D. Sharma, "Image formation in low-coherence and confocal interference microscopes," *Applied Optics* **43**, 1493–1502 (2004).

[46] C. J. R. Sheppard, S. S. Kou, and C. Depeursinge, "Reconstruction in interferometric synthetic aperture microscopy: comparison with optical coherence tomography and digital holographic microscopy," *Journal of the Optical Society of America A* **29**, 244–250 (2012).

[47] B. E. A. Saleh and M. C. Teich, "Beam Optics," in *Fundamentals of Photonics* (John Wiley & Sons, Inc., 1991), pp. 80–107.

[48] T. R. Hillman and D. D. Sampson, "The effect of water dispersion and absorption on axial resolution in ultrahigh-resolution optical coherence tomography," *Optics Express* **13**, 1860–1874 (2005).

[49] V. V. Tuchin, *Tissue Optics: Light Scattering Methods and Instruments for Medical Diagnosis* (SPIE Press, Bellingham, Washington, 2007).

[50] R. A. Meyer, "Light scattering from biological cells: dependence of backscatter radiation on membrane thickness and refractive index," *Applied Optics* **18**, 585–588 (1979).

[51] D. H. P. Schneiderheinze, T. R. Hillman, and D. D. Sampson, "Modified discrete particle model of optical scattering in skin tissue accounting for multiparticle scattering," *Optics Express* **15**, 15002–15010 (2007).

[52] N. N. Boustany, S. A. Boppart, and V. Backman, "Microscopic imaging and spectroscopy with scattered light," *Annual Review of Biomedical Engineering* **12**, 285 (2010).

[53] J. Beuthan, O. Minet, J. Helfmann, M. Herrig, and G. Müller, "The spatial variation of the refractive index in biological cells," *Physics in Medicine and Biology* **41**, 369 (1996).

[54] J. R. Mourant, J. P. Freyer, A. H. Hielscher, A. A. Eick, D. Shen, and T. Johnson, "Mechanisms of light scattering from biological cells relevant to noninvasive optical-tissue diagnostics," *Applied Optics* **37**, 3586-3593 (1998).

[55] R. Drezek, A. K. Dunn, and R. Richards-Kortum, "Light scattering from cells: finite-difference time-domain simulations and goniometric measurements," *Applied Optics* **38**, 3651-3661 (1999).

[56] C. Smithpeter, A. K. Dunn, R. Drezek, T. Collier, and R. Richards-Kortum, "Near real time confocal microscopy of cultured amelanotic cells: sources of signal, contrast agents and limits of contrast," *Journal of Biomedical Optics* **3**, 429-436 (1998).

[57] A. P. Wax, C. Yang, V. Backman, K. Badizadegan, C. W. Boone, R. R. Dasari, and M. S. Feld, "Cellular organization and substructure measured using angle-resolved low-coherence interferometry," *Biophysical Journal* **82**, 2256-2264 (2002).

[58] J. M. Steinke and A. P. Shepherd, "Comparison of Mie theory and the light scattering of red blood cells," *Applied Optics* **27**, 4027-4033 (1988).

[59] J. D. Wilson, and T. H. Foster, "Mie theory interpretations of light scattering from intact cells," *Optics Letters* **30**, 2442-2444 (2005).

[60] B. Karamata, M. Laubscher, M. Leutenegger, S. Bourquin, T. Lasser, and P. Lambelet, "Multiple scattering in optical coherence tomography. I. Investigation and modeling," *Journal of the Optical Society of America A* **22**, 1369-1379 (2005).

[61] E. A. Vitol, T. P. Kurzweg, and B. Nabet, "Light scattering properties of kidney epithelial cells and nuclei," in *Optical Biopsy VI* (SPIE, 2006), pp. 609108–609108.

[62] T. R. Hillman, "Microstructural information beyond the resolution limit: studies in two coherent, wide-field biomedical imaging systems," Ph. D. dissertation, The University of Western Australia, 2007.

[63] L. Wang, P. P. Ho, C. Liu, G. Zhang, and R. R. Alfano, "Ballistic 2-D imaging through scattering walls using an ultrafast optical Kerr gate," *Science* **253**, 769–771 (1991).

[64] J. M. Schmitt, A. Knuttel, M. Yadlowsky, and M. A. Eckhaus, "Optical-coherence tomography of a dense tissue: statistics of attenuation and backscattering," *Physics in Medicine and Biology* **39**, 1705 (1994).

[65] M. J. Yadlowsky, J. M. Schmitt, and R. F. Bonner, "Multiple-scattering in optical coherence microscopy," *Applied Optics* **34**, 5699–5707 (1995).

[66] D. A. Boas, K. K. Bizheva, and A. M. Siegel, "Using dynamic low-coherence interferometry to image Brownian motion within highly scattering media," *Optics Letters* **23**, 319–321 (1998).

[67] B. H. Park, M. C. Pierce, B. Cense, and J. F. de Boer, "Real-time multi-functional optical coherence tomography," *Optics Express* **11**, 782–793 (2003).

[68] L. Thrane, H. T. Yura, and P. E. Andersen, "Analysis of optical coherence tomography systems based on the extended Huygens-Fresnel principle," *Journal of the Optical Society of America A* **17**, 484–490 (2000).

[69] Y. T. Pan, R. Birngruber, and R. Engelhardt, "Contrast limits of coherence-gated imaging in scattering media," *Applied Optics* **36**, 2979–2983 (1997).

[70] T. R. Hillman, A. Curatolo, B. F. Kennedy, and D. D. Sampson, "Detection of multiple scattering in optical coherence tomography by speckle correlation of angle-dependent B-scans," *Optics Letters* **35**, 1998–2000 (2010).

[71] Y. Imai and K. Tanaka, "Direct velocity sensing of flow distribution based on low-coherence interferometry," *Journal of the Optical Society of America A* **16**, 2007–2012 (1999).

[72] Y. H. Zhao, Z. P. Chen, C. Saxer, S. H. Xiang, J. F. de Boer, and J. S. Nelson, "Phase-resolved optical coherence tomography and optical Doppler tomography for imaging blood flow in human skin with fast scanning speed and high velocity sensitivity," *Optics Letters* **25**, 114–116 (2000).

[73] J. K. Barton and S. Stromski, "Flow measurement without phase information in optical coherence tomography images," *Optics Express* **13**, 5234–5239 (2005).

[74] F. I. Wu and M. R. Glucksberg, "Choroidal perfusion measurements made with optical coherence tomography," *Applied Optics* **44**, 1426–1433 (2005).

[75] S. G. Adie, T. R. Hillman, and D. D. Sampson, "Investigation of speckle contrast ratio in optical coherence tomography," in *Proceedings of SPIE, Photonics West* **6085**, 608506 (2006).

[76] J. M. Schmitt, S. L. Lee, and K. M. Yung, "An optical coherence microscope with enhanced resolving power in thick tissue," *Optics Communications* **142**, 203–207 (1997).

[77] A. E. Desjardins, B. J. Vakoc, G. J. Tearney, and B. E. Bouma, "Speckle reduction in OCT using massively-parallel detection and frequency-domain ranging," *Optics Express* **14**, 4736–4745 (2006).

[78] B. Karamata, M. Laubscher, M. Leutenegger, S. Bourquin, T. Lasser, and P. Lambelet, "Multiple scattering in optical coherence tomography. I. Investigation and modeling," *Journal of the Optical Society of America A* **22**, 1369–1379 (2005).

[79] P. E. Andersen, T. M. Jørgensen, L. Thrane, A. Tycho, and H. T. Yura, "Modeling light-tissue interaction in optical coherence tomography systems," in *Optical Coherence Tomography: Technology and Applications*, W. Drexler, and J. G. Fujimoto, eds. (Springer, Berlin, 2008), pp. 73–115.

[80] J. A. Izatt, M. R. Hee, D. Huang, J. G. Fujimoto, E. A. Swanson, C. P. Lin, J. S. Schuman, and C. A. Puliafito, "Optical coherence tomography for medical diagnostics," in *Medical Optical Tomography: Functional Imaging and Monitoring*, G. J. Muller, ed. (SPIE, Bellingham, WA, 1993), pp. 450–472.

[81] J. S. Derek, L. Tore, Z. Chen, J. S. Nelson, and E. M. Thomas, "Signal attenuation and localization in optical coherence tomography studied by Monte Carlo simulation," *Physics in Medicine and Biology* **43**, 3025 (1998).

[82] S. G. Adie, T. R. Hillman, and D. D. Sampson, "Detection of multiple scattering in optical coherence tomography using the spatial distribution of Stokes vectors," *Optics Express* **15**, 18033–18049 (2007).

[83] R. Motaghiannezam and S. Fraser, "Logarithmic intensity and speckle-based motion contrast methods for human retinal vasculature visualization using swept source optical coherence tomography," *Biomedical Optics Express* **3**, 503–521 (2012).

[84] G. Liu, W. Jia, V. Sun, B. Choi, and Z. Chen, "High-resolution imaging of microvasculature in human skin in-vivo with optical coherence tomography," *Optics Express* **20**, 7694–7705 (2012).

[85] J. Enfield, E. Jonathan, and M. J. Leahy, "In vivo imaging of the microcirculation of the volar forearm using correlation mapping optical coherence tomography (cmOCT)," *Biomedical Optics Express* **2**, 1184–1193 (2011).

[86] E. Jonathan, J. Enfield, and M. J. Leahy, "Correlation mapping method for generating microcirculation morphology from optical coherence tomography (OCT) intensity images," *Journal of Biophotonics* **4**, 583–587 (2011).

[87] A. Mariampillai, M. K. K. Leung, M. Jarvi, B. A. Standish, K. Lee, B. C. Wilson, A. Vitkin, and V. X. D. Yang, "Optimized speckle variance OCT imaging of microvasculature," *Optics Letters* **35**, 1257–1259 (2010).

[88] A. Ahmad, S. G. Adie, E. J. Chaney, U. Sharma, and S. A. Boppart, "Cross-correlation-based image acquisition technique for manually-scanned optical coherence tomography," *Optics Express* **17**, 8125–8136 (2009).

[89] D. D. Duncan and S. J. Kirkpatrick, "Processing algorithms for tracking speckle shifts in optical elastography of biological tissues," *Journal of Biomedical Optics* **6**, 418–426 (2001).

[90] D. D. Duncan and S. J. Kirkpatrick, "Performance analysis of a maximum-likelihood speckle motion estimator," *Optics Express* **10**, 927–941 (2002).

[91] R. Chan, A. Chau, W. Karl, S. Nadkarni, A. Khalil, N. Iftimia, M. Shishkov, G. J. Tearney, M. Kaazempur-Mofrad, and B. E. Bouma, "OCT-based arterial elastography: robust estimation exploiting tissue biomechanics," *Optics Express* **12**, 4558–4572 (2004).

[92] A. Ozcan, A. Bilenca, A. E. Desjardins, B. E. Bouma, and G. J. Tearney, "Speckle reduction in optical coherence tomography images using digital filtering," *Journal of the Optical Society of America A* **24**, 1901–1910 (2007).

[93] L. Ramrath, G. Moreno, H. Mueller, T. Bonin, G. Huettmann, and A. Schweikard, "Towards multi-directional OCT for speckle noise reduction," *Proceedings of Medical Image Computing Computer Assisted Intervention (MICCAI)* **5241**, 657–664 (2009).

[94] D. P. Popescu, M. D. Hewko, and M. G. Sowa, "Speckle noise attenuation in optical coherence tomography by compounding images acquired at different positions of the sample," *Optics Communications* **269**, 247–251 (2007).

[95] T. M. Jørgensen, L. Thrane, M. Mogensen, F. Pedersen, and P. E. Andersen, "Speckle reduction in optical coherence tomography images of human skin by a spatial diversity method," *Proceedings of SPIE* **6627**, 6627–6620P (2007).

[96] B. F. Kennedy, T. R. Hillman, A. Curatolo, and D. D. Sampson, "Speckle reduction in optical coherence tomography by strain compounding," *Optics Letters* **35**, 2445–2447 (2010).

[97] B. F. Kennedy, A. Curatolo, T. R. Hillman, C. M. Saunders, and D. D. Sampson, "Speckle reduction in optical coherence tomography images using tissue viscoelasticity," *Journal of Biomedical Optics* **16**, 020506 (2011).

[98] D. L. Marks, T. S. Ralston, and S. A. Boppart, "Speckle reduction by I-divergence regularization in optical coherence tomography," *Journal of the Optical Society of America A* **22**, 2366–2371 (2005).

[99] D. C. Fernandez, "Delineating fluid-filled region boundaries in optical coherence tomography images of the retina," *IEEE Transactions on Medical Imaging* **24**, 929–945 (2005).

[100] B. Cense, T. C. Chen, B. H. Park, M. C. Pierce, and J. F. de Boer, "In vivo depth-resolved birefringence measurements of the human retinal nerve fiber layer by polarization-sensitive optical coherence tomography," *Optics Letters* **27**, 1610–1612 (2002).

[101] M. Mogensen, T. M. Jørgensen, L. Thrane, B. M. Nürnberg, and G. B. E. Jemec, "Improved quality of optical coherence tomography imaging of basal cell carcinomas using speckle reduction," *Experimental Dermatology* **19**, 293–295 (2010).

[102] M. Hughes, M. Spring, and A. Podoleanu, "Speckle noise reduction in optical coherence tomography of paint layers," *Applied Optics* **49**, 99–107 (2010).

[103] Y. Watanabe, H. Hasegawa, and S. Maeno, "Angular high-speed massively parallel detection spectral-domain optical coherence tomography for speckle reduction," *Journal of Biomedical Optics* **16**, 060504 (2011).

[104] H. Wang and A. M. Rollins, "Speckle reduction in optical coherence tomography using angular compounding by B-scan Doppler-shift encoding," *Journal of Biomedical Optics* **14**, 030512 (2009).

[105] A. E. Desjardins, B. J. Vakoc, G. J. Tearney, and B. E. Bouma, "Backscattering spectroscopic contrast with angle-resolved optical coherence tomography," *Optics Letters* **32**, 3158–3160 (2007).

[106] E. Gotzinger, M. Pircher, B. Baumann, T. Schmoll, H. Sattmann, R. A. Leitgeb, and C. K. Hitzenberger, "Speckle noise reduction in high speed polarization sensitive spectral domain optical coherence tomography," *Optics Express* **19**, 14568–14584 (2011).

[107] M. Szkulmowski, I. Gorczynska, D. Szlag, M. Sylwestrzak, A. Kowalczyk, and M. Wojtkowski, "Efficient reduction of speckle noise in optical coherence tomography," *Optics Express* **20**, 1337–1359 (2012).

[108] P. Cimalla, J. Walther, M. Mehner, M. Cuevas, and E. Koch, "Simultaneous dual-band optical coherence tomography in the spectral domain for high resolution in vivo imaging," *Optics Express* **17**, 19486–19500 (2009).

[109] G. van Soest, M. Villiger, E. Regar, G. J. Tearney, B. E. Bouma, and A. F. W. van der Steen, "Frequency domain multiplexing for speckle reduction in optical coherence tomography," *Journal of Biomedical Optics* **17**, 076018 (2012).

[110] P. C. Li and C. L. Wu, "Strain compounding: spatial resolution and performance on human images," *Ultrasound in Medicine & Biology* **27**, 1535–1541 (2001).

[111] B. F. Kennedy, A. Curatolo, T. R. Hillman, C. M. Saunders, and D. D. Sampson, "Speckle reduction in optical coherence tomography images using tissue viscoelasticity," *Journal of Biomedical Optics* **16**, 020506 (2011).

[112] D. Alonso-Caneiro, S. A. Read, and M. J. Collins, "Speckle reduction in optical coherence tomography imaging by affine-motion image registration," *Journal of Biomedical Optics* **16**, 116027 (2011).

[113] Y. T. Pan and D. L. Farkas, "Noninvasive imaging of living human skin with dual-wavelength optical coherence tomography in two and three dimensions," *Journal of Biomedical Optics* **3**, 446–455 (1998).

[114] A. M. Rollins, M. D. Kulkarni, S. Yazdanfar, R. Ung-arunyawee, and J. A. Izatt, "In vivo video rate optical coherence tomography," *Optics Express* **3**, 219–229 (1998).

[115] A. I. Kholodnykh, I. Y. Petrova, K. V. Larin, M. Motamedi, and R. O. Esenaliev, "Precision of measurement of tissue optical properties with optical coherence tomography," *Applied Optics* **42**, 3027–3037 (2003).

[116] J. Rogowska, C. M. Bryant, and M. E. Brezinski, "Cartilage thickness measurements from optical coherence tomography," *Journal of the Optical Society of America A* **20**, 357–367 (2003).

[117] A. J. Healey and S. Leeman, "Speckle reduction methods in ultrasound pulse-echo imaging," in *International Conference on Acoustic Sensing and Imaging*, 1993, pp. 68–76.

[118] K. H. Y. Cheng, E. Y. Lam, B. A. Standish, and V. X. D. Yang, "Speckle reduction of endovascular optical coherence tomography using a generalized divergence measure," *Optics Letters* **37**, 2871–2873 (2012).

[119] S. Chitchian, M. A. Fiddy, and N. M. Fried, "Denoising during optical coherence tomography of the prostate nerves via wavelet shrinkage using dual-tree complex wavelet transform," *Journal of Biomedical Optics* **14**, 014031 (2009).

[120] P. Puvanathasan and K. Bizheva, "Speckle noise reduction algorithm for optical coherence tomography based on interval type II fuzzy set," *Optics Express* **15**, 15747–15758 (2007).

[121] M. Gargesha, M. W. Jenkins, A. M. Rollins, and D. L. Wilson, "Denoising and 4D visualization of OCT images," *Optics Express* **16**, 12313–12333 (2008).

[122] Z. P. Jian, Z. X. Yu, L. F. Yu, B. Rao, Z. P. Chen, and B. J. Tromberg, "Speckle attenuation in optical coherence tomography by curvelet shrinkage," *Optics Letters* **34**, 1516–1518 (2009).

[123] Z. P. Jian, L. F. Yu, B. Rao, B. J. Tromberg, and Z. P. Chen, "Three-dimensional speckle suppression in optical coherence tomography based on the curvelet transform," *Optics Express* **18**, 1024–1032 (2010).

[124] H. M. Salinas and D. C. Fernandez, "Comparison of PDE-based nonlinear diffusion approaches for image enhancement and denoising in optical coherence tomography," *IEEE Transactions on Medical Imaging* **26**, 761–771 (2007).

[125] P. Puvanathasan and K. Bizheva, "Interval type-II fuzzy anisotropic diffusion algorithm for speckle noise reduction in optical coherence tomography images," *Optics Express* **17**, 733–746 (2009).

[126] A. Wong, A. Mishra, K. Bizheva, and D. A. Clausi, "General Bayesian estimation for speckle noise reduction in optical coherence tomography retinal imagery," *Optics Express* **18**, 8338–8352 (2010).

[127] L. A. Shepp and B. F. Logan, "Reconstructing interior head tissue from X-ray transmissions," *IEEE Transactions on Nuclear Science* **21**, 228–236 (1974).

7

Optical Coherence Tomography and Light-Induced Fluorescence: Optical Slicing Plus Biochemical Probing

Jennifer Kehlet Barton

Department of Biomedical Engineering, The University of Arizona

This chapter describes the combination of optical coherence tomography (most commonly used to visualize the microstructure of tissue) with light-induced fluorescence (which probes the biochemical composition of tissue). This combination has synergistic potential to accurately identify disease, or to elucidate the basic structure and function of tissue. Because the two imaging modalities have very different capabilities and technical requirements, combination into a dual-modality instrument can be challenging, yet can be accomplished in many different configurations. This chapter will examine the motivation for combined systems, several different instrumentation implementations, and example successful applications.

Key words: colon, detectors, eye, fluorescence, imaging instrumentation, light sources, optical coherence tomography, optical fibers, skin

7.1 Introduction

Optical coherence tomography (OCT) is a non-destructive imaging modality that obtains micron-scale resolution, depth-resolved images of scattering tissue. Near-infrared light backscattered by tissue is interfered with light reflected from a reference mirror to provide depth ranging. Light-induced fluorescence (LIF) is the emission of light by a substance after stimulation by incident excitation light. Usually the emitted light is of a longer wavelength than the excitation source, although in two photon excited fluorescence, the simultaneous absorption of two excitation photons leads to emission of light at a shorter wavelength. As explained in more detail below, these two imaging modalities have different contrast mechanisms, and thus are complementary in the type of information they provide about tissue. Therefore, there exists the potential for substantial synergy in basic research studies and clinical diagnostics when using a dual modality imaging system.

7.1.1 Optical Coherence Tomography

The interferometric portion of the OCT signal contains amplitude and phase information. For time-domain OCT, this information is provided as a function of time, or equivalently for a constant known index of refraction material, depth into the sample. For Fourier domain systems, this information is initially provided as a function of wavelength, which, knowing the optical properties of the tissue, can be converted into depth information by resampling and a Fourier transform [1]. Most usually, only the amplitude of the depth-resolved signal is considered, mapped to grayscale, and presented as a typical OCT image. This amplitude image provides information about the local backscattering properties of the tissue. Backscattering can be examined quantitatively [2], or simply visualized qualitatively as a map of tissue microstructure. Backscattering occurs at changes in index of refraction, which occur at all size scales, from the macroscopic (interface between tissue layers, e.g. between the aqueous humor and the lens of the eye) to the nanoscopic (interfaces of structural proteins, membranes). The ability of amplitude OCT to visualize tissue microstructure is extremely powerful and has been utilized in nearly all tissues of the body. OCT can be implemented to have submicron resolution, but often the ability to visualize features is limited by lack of inherent tissue backscattering contrast, rather than instrument resolution.

OCT has available other contrast mechanisms. The phase of the signal is sensitive to moving scatterers, e.g. red blood cells, so Doppler OCT can be used to visualize blood vessels, even though there is little contrast between blood and tissue at many OCT wavelengths [3]. Exquisite maps of microvasculature have been obtained, though careful processing of the phase-resolved signal, e.g. [4, 5]. If the amplitude and phase of the signal is recorded as a function of polarization state in a polarization-sensitive OCT system, tissue diattenuation, birefringence, and orientation of the fast axis can be extracted [6]. These factors are sensitive to parameters such as collagen fiber thickness, abundance, and orientation, which cannot usually be visualized with amplitude OCT.

OCT is a interferometric imaging technique, dependent upon coherent detection of scattered light. Therefore, OCT is not sensitive to fluorescence emission. However, there are methods whereby OCT can be sensitive to particular molecules, either endogenous (naturally occurring in the tissue) or exogenous (added targeted or untargeted molecular probes). Reviews of these molecular OCT methods are available [7, 8, 9]. One method relies on detecting the absorption of light as a function of wavelength, within the bandwidth of the OCT source. This method is referred to as spectroscopic OCT [10]. The most abundant tissue absorbers with distinctive spectral signatures in the near infrared are oxyhemoglobin and deoxyhemoglobin. Absorbing substances can be added to tissue, or alternatively, agents which increase light backscattering can be added. Ideally such exogenous agents passively or actively target sites of interest, and have a strong wavelength-dependent signature. One example of a backscattering contrast agent is plasmon resonant nanoparticles. Since tissue is highly scattering and usually heterogeneous, OCT has significant speckle noise, and the concentration of contrast agent which can be achieved in a living system is practically limited, simple integrated intensity changes may not be sufficient to detect the presence of the agent. Measurement of the wavelength-dependent changes can be more sensitive. A variety of scattering and absorbing agents have been used *in vivo* or in whole organisms, such as nanoshells [11], titanium dioxide nanoparticles [12], gold-coated protein microspheres [13], and indocyanine green [14]. These agents have all been shown to increase image contrast, although sensitivity is generally limited.

A variation on this technique, which can provide some background rejection and thus greater sensitivity, is pump-probe OCT, whereby the absorption spectra of a dye is dynamically changed, and this differential signal is used to localize and estimate the concentration of the dye [15, 16]. A differential approach is also used in magnitomotive OCT, which utilizes magnetic particles that are displaced under an oscillating magnetic field. The magnetomotive signal can be obtained by a Fourier transform of the OCT data in the transverse time direction at the magnetic modulation frequency [17]. In another technique, called photothermal OCT, absorbing particles are exposed to short-pulsed or modulated light, which causes them to launch an acoustic wave that is detected by phase-sensitive OCT [18].

Coherent non-linear effects can also be utilized with OCT. One example is second harmonic OCT [19]. In this system, a short-pulsed OCT source is used, which can elicit the generation of light at the second-harmonic frequency in some media (in tissue, notably collagen). Second harmonic waves are also produced in the reference arm through a nonlinear crystal, to interfere with the signal from tissue. This technique can be useful to detect small changes in tissue molecular structure and symmetry. Another coherent non-linear effect measured with OCT is coherent anti-Stokes Raman scattering (CARS); this technique is called non-linear inteferometric vibrational imaging (NIVI). NIVI provides background suppression not present in conventional CARS, a signal orders of magnitude higher than spontaneous Raman imaging, and can create high resolution and sensitivity maps of molecule-specific spectral profiles. Various substances have been examined including *ex vivo* skin [20].

While exciting and under rapid development, molecular contrast OCT has some limitations and drawbacks. The sensitivity of many of the absorptive and scattering contrast techniques is low compared to fluorescence. Operation is limited to the wavelength range of broadband OCT sources, typically near infrared, whereas biological molecules are often optically active in the ultraviolet and visible range. The high performance of coherent non-linear OCT techniques comes at the expense of system complexity and cost. Therefore, it is interesting to combine simple, low-cost amplitude OCT with sensitive, flexible molecular imaging LIF.

7.1.2 Light-induced fluorescence

The simplest LIF system consists of a narrow-band light source illuminating tissue, a filter to block this excitation light, and a single-element detector to measure the fluorescence emission light. The detected light is proportional to the concentration of fluorophores in the tissue, although it is also proportional to many other factors, including the tissue optical properties, the position distribution of the fluorophores, their quantum yield, and the geometry of the excitation and emission collection channels.

LIF systems can be considerably more sophisticated. Fluorescence spectroscopy systems incorporate a spectrometer to measure the intensity of the emission light as a function of wavelength. For measurement of endogenous fluorescence, changes in spectral shape have been shown to be useful for differentiating normal from diseased tissue [21]. Also, rather than measuring at only a single point, one- or two-dimensional images of tissue fluorescence emission light can be obtained.

For the LIF systems described thus far, the signal is a depth-weighted integrated measurement, rather than depth-resolved. Depth resolution is possible through spatial gating (confocal fluorescence microscopy) or non-linear effects (two photon excited fluorescence [TPEF]). In confocal fluorescence microscopy, a point source (e.g., laser) is imaged into the tissue, and the focal point is imaged back to a pinhole-covered detector [22]. Fluorescence emission from the focal volume is preferentially admitted through the pinhole and detected. The imaging depth limit of confocal fluorescence microscopy occurs when tissue attenuation leads to the amount of light detected from the focal volume to decrease below the level of the small amount of out-of-focus surface light which can pass through the detector pinhole.

In TPEF a tightly focused, short pulsed laser source is used. The simultaneous absorption of two photons by a fluorophore in one quantum event is unlikely to occur except at the focus [23], so depth sectioning can be achieve without the need for a pinhole. The fluorescence emission light is at shorter wavelengths than the excitation light. TPEF systems can typically image deeper than confocal systems due to the use of longer excitation wavelengths and less generated out-of-focus fluorescence emission light.

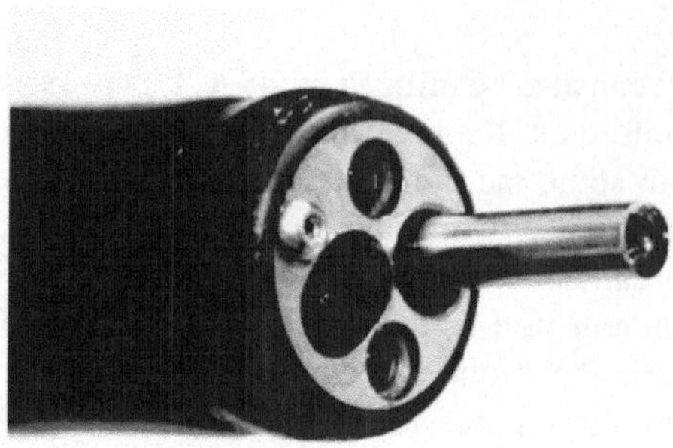

Figure 7.1: An OCT probe integrated through the surgical channel of a gastroscope. White light or ALA-enhanced fluorescence imaging, with its wide field of view, can be used to guide positioning of OCT probe [from 25].

7.1.3 Motivation for dual-modality systems

The natural synergy of OCT and LIF has been recognized for some time. As mentioned above, OCT is primarily a structural imaging modality, and LIF primarily a molecular imaging modality. Each one has limitations. For example, in OCT, cancer may appear homogeneous, lacking the typical organized structure. However abnormal but benign conditions, such as scar tissue or hyperplasia, may have a similar appearance. On the other hand, in LIF, contrast agents may localize not only in areas with dysplasia and cancer, but also in areas of inflammation. One of the first published examples of dual-modality imaging was the sequential imaging of the cervix with separate OCT and LIF systems, with systemic administration of the fluorescence sensitizer 5-aminolevulinic acid (ALA) [24]. These investigators found that the combination of OCT and LIF produced fewer false positive results: increased ALA-fluorescence due to inflammatory reactions was clearly differentiated from cancer by OCT since structure was preserved; conversely, a lack of structure in OCT due to a mature scar was clarified as a benign condition using LIF, since there was strong collagen presence and lack of ALA uptake. The disadvantage of using two separate OCT and LIF systems was the size and complexity of two instruments, and also the difficulties in co-registering data from the two devices.

An intermediate step in creating a dual modality OCT/LIF system can be the use of an OCT daughter probe in a fluorescence endoscope. This type of system takes advantage of the large field of view of fluorescence endoscopes to guide positioning of an OCT probe, for a closer look at a suspicious area. An example is given in Figure 7.1. The positive predictive value (PVV) of some diagnostic procedures can be greatly increased with this combination. One study [25] found that the PPV of fluorescence cystoscopy of flat bladder lesions was only 16%, which could be increased to 43% with in addition of OCT. The data suggest that 78% of biopsies based on fluorescent positive findings could be avoided, if areas were classified as normal when OCT imaging revealed a regular layered structure. A larger study with hexaminolevulinate (HAL) fluorescence cystoscopy plus OCT confirmed impressive improvement in diagnostic accuracy though dual-modality imaging [26]. On a per-lesion basis, sensitivity and specificity were respectively 97.5% and 78.6% for HAL cystoscopy alone, but 97.5% and 97.9% for HAL combined with OCT.

A challenge with OCT is the small field of view and additional time required to evaluate the OCT images. Three dimensional OCT with automated image analysis to detect bladder carcinoma *in situ* (CIS) may mitigate this problem. Another study showed that OCT can greatly increase the sensitivity and specificity of CIS detection to 93% and 94%, respectively, much better than white light, narrow band, or fluorescence imaging, and potentially in a rapid, automated fashion [27].

Integrating an OCT probe into a larger fluorescence-enabled endoscope is a relatively straightforward process; the endoscope and probe remain essentially separate systems, mechanically coupled at their distal ends. Co-registration can be facilitated by endoscopic visualization of the OCT probe, and images can be presented simultaneously to the operator. Little consideration need be given to dual-use of system components. In the remainder of this chapter, integrated systems that share optical components will be considered. These systems generally acquire images of the target tissue simultaneously or in close sequence, are co-registered by design, and have similarly-sized fields of view. The goal with these systems is to acquire additional information about tissue, taking advantage of the different mechanisms of contrast for OCT and LIF imaging.

7.2 Dual-Modality System Design

Combining OCT and LIF functionality into an integrated system presents several challenges, since each subsystem has different, and sometimes seemingly incompatible specifications. Separate OCT and LIF systems can simply be concurrently directed at a sample, to provide complimentary information on sample properties. However, to be considered "dual-modality" the two subsystems should be mechanically coupled, share at least one optical component, and allow integrated operation.

7.2.1 Light sources

Challenges facing shared used of components for OCT and LIF is immediately evident when considering requirements for light sources. For greatest depth of imaging, OCT sources normally operate in the near infrared, most typically from 800–1300 nm. Wavelengths on the longer end of this range are optimum for highly scattering tissues, while the shorter end of the range offers potentially higher resolution and less water absorption. Single photon LIF, on the other hand, is generally performed with shorter wavelengths. Efficient excitation of naturally-occurring fluorophores (amino acids, structural proteins, and metabolic co-factors) is performed with ultraviolet to blue (about 250–500 nm) light. Most available exogenous fluorophores are excited in the visible wavelength range, with a paucity of fluorophores available with peak excitation wavelengths above 700 nm. Indocyanine green (ICG), a clinically-utilized indicator dye, is a notable exception, with peak excitation around 800 nm. Table 7.1 provides approximate peak excitation and emission wavelengths of common endogenous and exogenous fluorophores.

Notable from Table 7.1 is the relatively small Stokes shift (difference between peak excitation and emission wavelengths) of most fluorophores. Therefore, LIF systems typically utilize narrowband sources, which ease filter requirements and minimize signal loss due to overlap between the excitation and emission wavelengths. On the contrary, for high axial resolution, OCT by necessity requires a broadband (or broadly tunable) light source. For a Gaussian source spectrum, the coherence length, and hence axial resolution is given by:

$$l_c = \frac{2\ln 2}{\pi} \frac{\lambda_0^2}{\Delta\lambda} \tag{7.1}$$

where λ_0 is the center wavelength of the source and $\Delta\lambda$ is the bandwidth. One possible compromise can be seen from this equation — if the center wavelength is short, good resolution can be achieved with relatively narrow bandwidth sources. A short center wavelength also provides more opportunity for utilization of common fluorophores. This approach has been utilized by Podoleanu group to develop a combined OCT/ ICG angiography [28] and OCT/ ICG/ scanning laser ophthalmoscopy (SLO) device [29]. A superluminescent diode with center wavelength 792 nm and bandwidth 21 nm is sufficient for both good axial OCT resolution (9 μm), efficient excitation of ICG, and collection of the majority of ICG emission, with careful choice of filters.

TABLE 7.1: Approximate single-photon excitation and emissions wavelengths of common endogenous and exogenous fluorophores.

Fluorophore	Excitation wavelength (nm)	Emission wavelength (nm)
Tryptophan	275	355
Elastin	290	340
Reduced Nicotinamide adenine dinucleotide (NADH)	290, 350	440,460
Collagen	325	400
Flavin adenine dinucleotide (FAD)	450	535
Fluorescein isothiocyanate	495	521
Cy3	550	570
Cy5	650	670
Methylene blue	668	680
Cy7	743	767
Indocyanine green	800	830

Superluminescent diodes are now available in the visible (red) wavelength range, and broadband visible light can also be obtained through other means, such as frequency doubled broadband Titanium:Sapphire (Ti:Sapp) lasers or supercontinuum generation sources. In the blue wavelength range, a bandwidth of only about 10 nm is sufficient for good resolution OCT. This bandwidth is comparable to that used in fluorescence microscopes with filtered lamp excitation. Therefore this single source will function well for both modalities. The trade-off in this situation will be limited depth of imaging of the OCT system, due to strong scattering and absorption of the light in tissue at the short visible wavelengths.

While sources for OCT and single photon excited fluorescence are at best marginally compatible, those for OCT and TPEF are better matched. In TPEF, efficient excitation may be obtained at wavelengths approximately twice those used for single photon excited fluorescence, meaning that excitation of endogenous fluorophores is possible in the near infrared wavelength region. Also, fluorescence emission is at wavelengths considerably shorter than the excitation wavelength, so source bandwidth is less of an issue. Femtosecond pulsed sources such as Ti:Sapp lasers produce broadband light needed for high axial resolution OCT as well as the ultrashort pulses needed for efficient TPEF [30]. In one example, a 12-fs, 100 nm bandwidth laser was used in a scanning microscope configuration to obtain simultaneous OCT, TPEF, and second harmonic generation images of cells in matrix with no added contrast agent [31]. This laser source was at a fixed center wavelength of 800 nm, and represented a trade-off of the pulse duration and bandwidth requirements for OCT and TPEF. A more flexible source has been created from a tunable, $\sim$100 fs pulse Ti:Sapp laser, a portion of the output which is spectrally broadened via continuum generation in a photonic crystal fiber [32]. The original $\sim$10 nm bandwidth Ti:Sapp laser pulse, tunable from about 730–1000 nm, can optimally excite a variety of fluorophores, while the spectrally broadened pulse (52–86 nm bandwidth), provides good axial resolution in the OCT images.

7.2.2 Fiber delivery

Fiber optics are typically used in OCT and LIF systems for convenience, safety (avoiding open beams), and ease of alignment. They are a necessity in flexible endoscopes. However, the requirements for fiber optics appear to be incompatible between OCT and LIF. Single-mode fibers are used in OCT systems, since the transit time must be the same for all light travelling in the fiber. Single-mode fibers have a normalized frequency parameter, or V number, of less than 2.405. The V number is determined as

$$V = 2\pi \mathrm{NA} \frac{a}{\lambda}, \tag{7.2}$$

where NA is the numerical aperture of the fiber, a is the fiber core radius, and λ is the wavelength of the propagating light. Typical parameters (Corning SMF-28) are NA $= 0.14$ and $a = 4.1$ μm at 1310 nm. The small NA is compatible with most OCT systems operating at relatively low NA for large depth of focus (if desired lens systems can be used to adjust the system NA), and the small radius is a minor nuisance for efficient coupling of partially coherent light. Single mode fibers can be made with high NA, but at the cost of requiring a very small radius. Single-mode fibers can be used for fluorescence excitation light delivery, provide the source is a laser or other tightly focusable light source (not a filtered lamp), and the fiber is designed to transmit the wavelength of the LIF excitation source. On the other hand, fibers desired for collection of LIF emission have a large NA, since fluorescence emission is isotropic, and also usually have a large radius, for greater collection of weak emission light. In most situations, single-mode fibers cannot collect adequate LIF emission signal to be practically useful.

Most fiber-based dual-modality systems utilize separate fibers for OCT and LIF channels, e.g. [33]. However, in some circumstances, a single fiber optic can be used for both OCT and LIF. One example is use of a dual-cladding fiber (DCF). DCF are designed with a small core, surrounded by two concentric cladding layers. The core can be design to operate in single mode, whereas the inner cladding can have a large radius and high NA (multimode) for efficient light capture. Such a fiber was designed and used in an OCT/LIF (fluorescence spectroscopy) system [34]. Separate 1310 nm superluminescent OCT, and 488 nm Argon-ion LIF laser, sources were first combined using a single mode wavelength division multiplexor (WDM). The combined sources were coupled into the dual clad fiber in the sample arm of the OCT system. OCT and laser light were efficiently confined to the core of the DCF on the outbound trip to the tissue. OCT, laser excitation, and fluorescence emission light remitted from the tissue were collected by both core and inner cladding. Core light only was coupled back into the OCT systems single mode fiber, and cladding light was selected using a DCF coupler, bandpass filtered to remove OCT and excitation laser light, and analyzed with a spectrometer. The coupling components in this system were lossy, but improvements are possible.

DCF can also be used in OCT/TPEF systems [35, 36]. In one system [36], light from a 1310 superluminescent diode was combined with a 1550 nm femtosecond pulsed light source using a single mode WDM, then free-space coupled into the core of the DCF. As with the above OCT/LIF system, light remitted from the tissue is collected by the inner cladding and core of the DCF. Fluorescence emission light was separated out in free space using a dichroic filter at the proximal end of the DCF, and only OCT light from the core of the DCF was efficiently coupled back into the single mode, 1310 nm WDM channel. A diagram of the system is given in Fig. 7.2. Utilizing wavelengths of 1550 nm and 1310 nm mitigated dispersion in the fibers, focal shifts in the endoscope optics, and enabled the use of an efficient WDM, although the number of fluorophores with efficient two-photon excitation cross sections at 1550 nm is relatively limited (ICG can be used).

7.2.3 Focusing optics

The great advantage of a DCF system is the smallness of the fiber probe that can be created. The concentric arrangement of the core and inner cladding also simplifies scanning, for example rotary optical coupling is more practical with one DCF fiber than 2 or more single and multimode fibers, potentially enabling rotational- and spiral-scanning dual modality endoscopic systems. A disadvantage of DCF systems is the possible detection of unwanted OCT light that was initially coupled into the inner cladding and subsequently propagated into the core, potentially decreasing OCT image contrast.

Fluorescence imaging endoscopes and confocal microendoscopes frequently utilize fiber bundles.

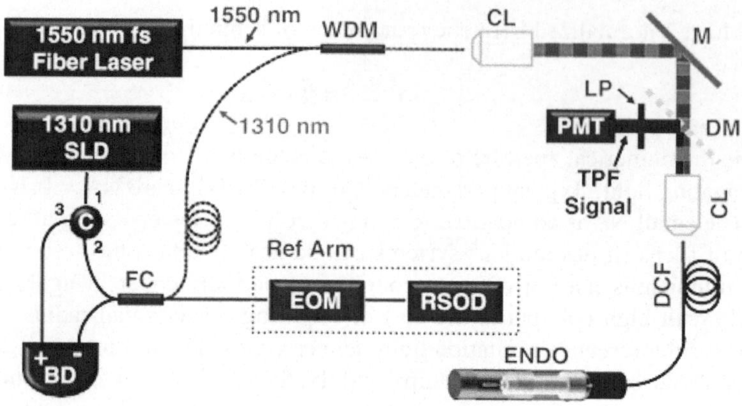

Figure 7.2: Dual-modality OCT-TPEF system utilizing a dual-cladding fiber (DCF). BD, balanced detector; C, circulator; CL, coupling lens; DM, dichroic mirror; ENDO, endoscope; EOM, electro-optic modulator; FC, fiber coupler; LP, long pass filter; M, mirror; PMT, photo-multiplier tube; RSOD, rapid scanning optical delay line; WDM, wavelength division multiplexer (from [36]).

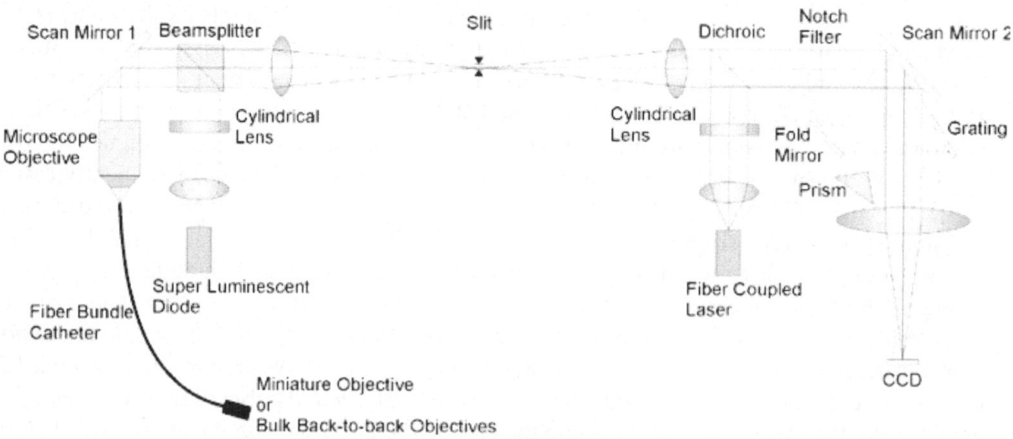

Figure 7.3: Combined line-scanning spectral domain OCT and fluorescence confocal microendoscope using a fiber bundle. Scan mirror 2 selects between modes: confocal, spectral confocal (utilizing prism) and OCT (utilizing grating). (From [37]).

Keen interest has arisen in using fiber bundles for OCT imaging. While single mode fiber bundles can be manufactured, the mode confinement in such bundles is generally poor when reasonably small core-to-core distances are used. Commercial fiber bundles have high V numbers and semi-random core arrangement to minimize core-to-core light coupling. Typical parameters (Sumitomo IGN-08/30) are NA=0.35, core radius=1.5 μm, core-to-core distance $\sim$4 μm. The multimode nature of the fiber bundle, in principle, can be accommodated by utilizing a common-path interferometer. In this case, any instabilities generated in light propagating through the fiber bundle are common to both the sample and reference. A fluorescence confocal/OCT system based on a fiber bundle has been demonstrated [37]. For OCT, the system utilized a superluminescent diode focused to a line and scanned across the proximal face of the fiber bundle. A cover slip at the distal end provided a reference reflection. The spectral interferogram was recorded on a 2D CCD array (one spatial and one spectral dimension), enabling cross-sectional imaging with no scanning, or 3D imaging with a single sweep. For confocal imaging, a laser focused to a line was swept through the same fiber bundle, and fluorescence recorded through separate proximal optics onto the same CCD array. The advantage of this system was minimization of scanning (elimination of scanning in the distal optics). Light loss through the fiber bundle and pixelation of the acquired image are limitations of fiber bundle-based OCT-LIF systems. A schematic of this system is given in Fig. 7.3.

Challenges facing dual-modality operation of distal focusing optics generally fall under two categories: 1) different optical material properties needed at the different wavelengths used in OCT and LIF, and 2) varying desired image orientation and resolution for the two systems.

While systems that operate only in the visible (VIS) to near-infrared (NIR) wavelength range usually face little materials challenges, optical materials needed for ultraviolet (UV) applications need to be chosen carefully. For example, BK7 glass is inexpensive, commonly available, and has excellent transmission in the VIS-NIR, but it is not appropriate for applications utilizing wavelengths below about 350 nm. Fused silica and magnesium fluoride are excellent materials choices for high broadband transmission from at least 200–2000 nm, albeit at higher cost. Depending on the materials used and method of manufacture, gradient index of refraction (GRIN) lenses may exhibit very strong autofluorescence with UV excitation. GRIN material in a cylindrical shape is a convenient choice for focusing lenses in microendoscopes, in part due to ease of assembly, but they may not be appropriate if UV wavelengths are used. In the dual modality endoscope shown in Fig. 7.4, the LIF fibers bypass the GRIN lens used to focus the OCT channel [33]. In this configuration, UV LIF excitation wavelengths can be used with minimal autofluorescence from the endoscope.

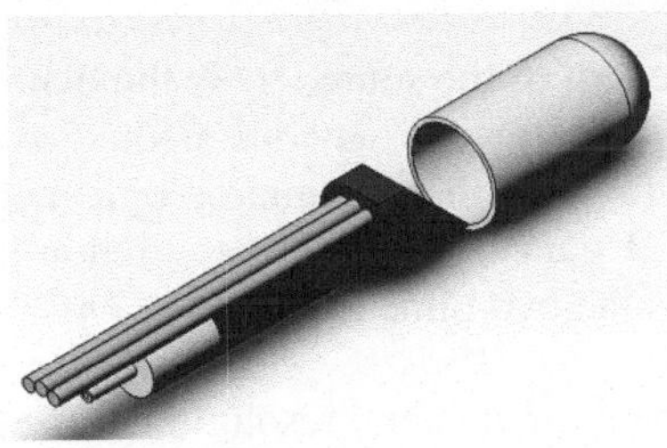

Figure 7.4: Example configuration of a dual-modality endoscope. The single fiber abutting the spacer (below) carries the OCT light, which is focused by the GRIN lens (darkened). Three LIF fibers (above) bypass the GRIN lens and abut the rod prism (gray), which directs light from both modalities out the side of the fused silica envelope (white).

UV operation also limits the types of polymer materials used; materials such as polycarbonate and polyimides have poor UV transmission, polymethyl methacrylate may be acceptable for wavelengths above 300 nm, and fluoropolymers such as Teflon©may have excellent UV transmission characteristics. Adhesive choice also needs to be considered. UV-curing epoxies will, by nature, absorb light in the UV and typically suffer from autofluorescence. Two-part epoxies with low fluorescence are available. In practice, the thickness of the material, transmission requirements, and sensitivity of the optical system to autofluorescence contamination need to be considered. For example, the effect of a small thickness of UV-absorbing and fluorescent adhesive on overall system performance may be practically negligible.

One notable optical aberration that must be considered in dual-modality systems is chromatic aberration, originating with the varying index of refraction of materials as a function of wavelength (material dispersion), and typically leading to a focus shift as a function of wavelength. Chromatic aberration may be an issue even in single-modality OCT systems that utilize very broadband light sources, but it is especially challenging in OCT/LIF systems that can operate with a thousand nanometers of wavelength difference between the UV LIF excitation and NIR OCT sources. Chromatic aberration correction can be accomplished in refractive systems at the expense of optical system complexity, and this is often accomplished in microscope objectives, where size is not a limiting factor, and micron-scale co-registration of OCT and fluorescence images is required. Reflective systems do not suffer from chromatic aberration; one published miniature endoscope utilized a reflective lens to enable operation over the UV-NIR wavelength range [38]. Focal shift can be limited by minimizing the difference in wavelengths between the OCT and LIF channels. In fact, for limited wavelength separation, chromatic aberration can be used to advantage. For example one OCT/ fluorescence surface imaging system utilized natural chromatic aberration present in a GRIN lens to focus 635 nm LIF excitation light at the surface of a tissue, while the same lens focused 890 nm OCT source light 190 μm deep into the tissue, enabling a greater depth of focus and imaging for OCT [39].

Another challenge with focusing optics in dual modality systems is a disparity in the conventional orientation of images, and in the resolution requirements for the two systems. Most microscopy techniques provide *en face* images, whereas OCT images are typically cross-sectional. Conventional OCT systems typically have modest lateral resolution (given by the focusing optics), to enable a good depth of focus. This is particularly true of Fourier domain systems, where the advantage of being able to simultaneously acquire information at all depths can be lost if high numerical aperture, low depth of focus optics are used. The lateral resolution according to the Rayleigh criterion is:

$$R_l = 0.61\frac{\lambda}{\mathrm{NA}}; \quad \mathrm{NA} \approx n\frac{D}{2f} \tag{7.3}$$

where λ is the center wavelength of the source, D is the diameter of the beam, and f is the focal length of the focusing lens. Therefore, an obvious method of achieving different resolutions is to use a smaller beam diameter for OCT than the microscopic modality. This case is illustrated in Fig. 7.5. A three-dimensional OCT data set might be acquired in the same time period, with the same two-dimensional scanning, as the two-dimensional, e.g., *en face* fluorescence confocal microscopy image.

In some cases, however, the desired lateral resolution of the fluorescence imaging modality may actually be larger than the OCT system, for example in an OCT/ fluorescence lifetime imaging microscopy (FLIM) system [40], with an OCT resolution of 13 μm and a FLIM resolution of 100 μm.

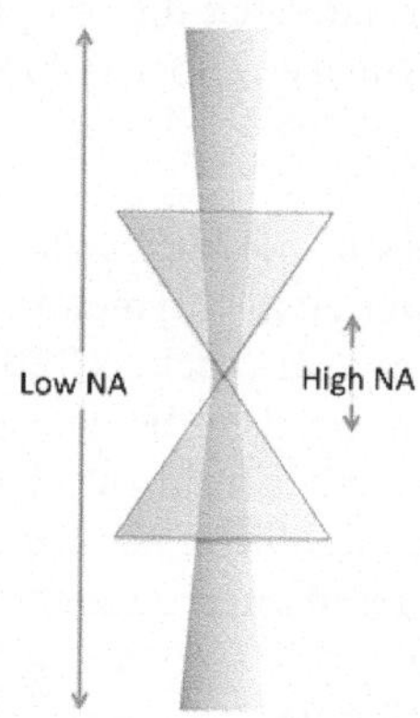

Figure 7.5: Depth of focus (identified by arrow length) and spot size for low and high NA systems. Typically, OCT is a low NA system, with large depth of focus and modest lateral resolution, whereas microscopic techniques such as fluorescence confocal microscopy are high NA systems with limited depth of focus and high lateral resolution.

When an extended source is imaged into the tissue, the focused spot is a convolution of the Rayleigh resolution and the source dimension. Therefore, for fiber optic-based systems, the fiber core size must be considered. While OCT systems normally use single mode fibers with small core diameters, the resolution of an LIF system can be limited by the large core diameter of the multimode fiber used.

7.2.4 Detectors

Conventional time domain, as well as swept-source Fourier domain, OCT systems typically use single element detectors. Spectral domain OCT systems generally utilize a one-dimensional detector array, and full field OCT systems utilize a two-dimensional detector array, typically a CCD or CMOS array. Fluorescence systems may use photomultiplier tubes for point-scanning systems or sensitive CCDs for full field or spectroscopic systems. Often, there is little ability to use the same detector, due to differences in signal wavelength, detector dimensionality, or necessary detection sensitivity between the two subsystems. Most published dual modality systems incorporate separate detectors.

One interesting design sharing the same CCD is the line-scanning, OCT/fluorescence confocal microendoscope shown in Fig. 7.3 [37]. In this instrument, both subsystems map one lateral tissue dimension to one axis of the CCD array, and the spectral component of the signal (corresponding to the fluorescence emission wavelength for the confocal subsystem, or encoding the depth information for the OCT subsystem) to the second axis of the CCD array. Because of the difference in wavelength range, separate dispersive elements were used in the detection assembly, and the system was sequentially switched between confocal and OCT mode.

7.2.5 Multiplexing data acquisition

Sharing of system components, the wavelengths employed in each subsystem, and properties of the acquired signal determine the method of multiplexing OCT and LIF data acquisition. There are several possible methods:

Wavelength multiplexing. The most commonly-implemented method of multiplexing OCT/LIF systems is wavelength multiplexing. A common or separate light source, and some common optics may be used, but the detected OCT signal is at a different wavelength than the detected LIF emission signal. Separate detectors are normally used, with wavelength filtering of the returned signal such that only the signal of interest is acquired at each detector.

Time multiplexing. If the signals cannot be separated by wavelength alone, system components need to be utilized in an incompatible fashion, or signal characteristics make simultaneous acquisition impractical, time multiplexing (i.e. sequential acquisition) may be appropriate. If the object to be imaged is not rapidly changing, the OCT and LIF signals may be considered co-registered. One situation where time multiplexing is practical is when a rapid-acquisition OCT is utilized with a LIF system that requires long integration times. In this case simultaneous acquisition would lead to either insufficient LIF signal or excessive oversampling of OCT.

Two additional potential multiplexing options are:

Spatial multiplexing. If the OCT and LIF channels are interrogating different regions of tissue, overlapping wavelengths may be acceptable since cross-talk between the two subsystems can be negligible. This might be implemented, for example, in a rotationally-scanning endoscope with the OCT and LIF systems pointing 180° apart.

Frequency multiplexing. A single detector, as well as overlapping wavelengths, can be used if the signals are frequency encoded. OCT signals typically have both DC/low and high frequency components, so the LIF signal would need to be modulated at an intermediate or very high frequency.

7.3 Applications

Dual modality OCT/LIF systems have been used for a variety of diagnostic purposes, in a variety of tissues. Three examples are given below.

7.3.1 Imaging of the retina

Fluorescence imaging, through fluorescence angiography or confocal scanning laser ophthalmoscopy (SLO), is an established technique to evaluate the circulation of the retina. Optical coherence tomography has been rapidly adopted for retinal imaging, due to its ability to obtain very high axial resolution images. Therefore, it is not surprising that combined LIF/OCT systems for retinal imaging have also been developed. Both research and commercial (Heidelberg Engineering; Heidelberg, Germany) units have been providing comprehensive evaluation of retinal disorders.

In the combined systems discussed previously [29], *en face* OCT, *en face* SLO, and ICG fluorescence (not depth resolved) images can be obtained simultaneously and presented separately or superimposed. The high resolution OCT images enable correlations to be made between late fluorescence accumulation, visualized in the ICG channel, with abnormal structures deep to the retinal surface at the retina–choroid interface, visualized with OCT. For example, in Figure 7.6, the OCT images clearly show areas of retinal pigment epithelium in the same region as abnormal ICG fluorescence accumulation [29]. Utilizing these two modalities, the structure of the retina can be visualized and quantified, and these anatomical changes registered with functional changes (leakiness of the vasculature) obtained from fluorescence imaging.

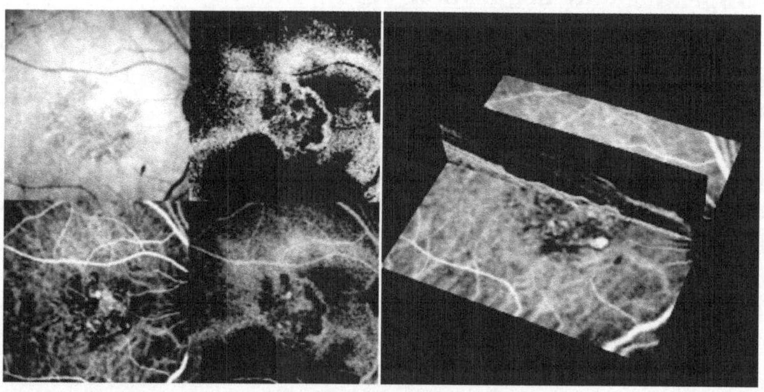

Figure 7.6: (See color insert.) Combined OCT/LIF images of a retina with choroidal neovascularization. Left panel: upper left, scanning laser ophthalmoscope image, bottom left, ICG angiography, upper right, *en face* OCT, bottom right, superimposed image. Right panel: ICG angiography image with cross sectional OCT image, showing correspondence between areas of ICG leakage and retinal pigment epithelium elevation. Lateral size $12^{\circ} \times 12^{\circ}$. (From [29]).

7.3.2 Imaging of the colon

The combination of structural imaging and molecular information is of interest in the colon. The endogenous fluorophores collagen and NADH dominate the emission signal when unstained colon

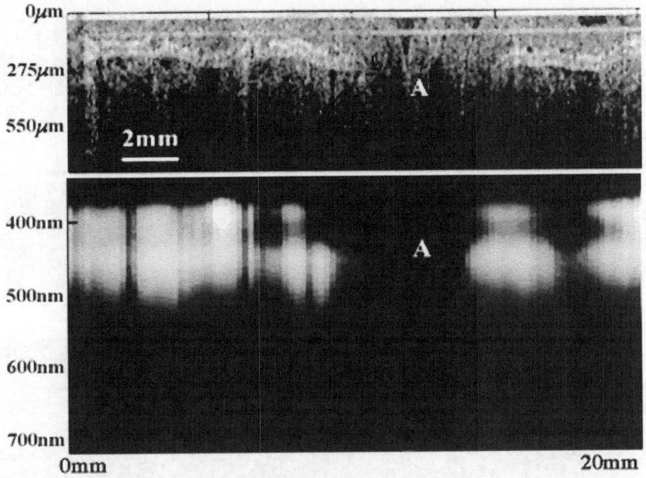

Figure 7.7: (See color insert.) Example OCT image and autofluorescence spectra of mouse colon. At an excitation wavelength of 325 nm, fluorescence from collagen and metabolic co-factors dominates the signal. At the adenoma (A), the autofluorescence decreases and shifts to higher wavelengths, also long wavelengths fluorescence emission is visible.

tissue is illuminated with UV light. It is well established that colon disease alters the distribution and quantity of endogenous fluorophores, and thus the fluorescence emission spectrum [41]. Alternatively, exogenous fluorophores can be administered, either to highlight tumors or to target specific molecules. OCT/LIF imaging has been performed in the mouse colon and small intestine, where imaging of the entire, relatively small, volume at microscopic resolution is practical. In humans, dual modality imaging is more likely to be performed using wide-field fluorescence imaging to guide OCT, or with another wide field imaging technique to guide the combination of OCT and narrow-field fluorescence imaging or spectroscopy.

Autofluorescence imaging of the mouse colon has been performed using the dual-modality endoscope shown in Fig. 7.4. The excitation source was a 325 nm He:Cd laser. Cross sectional OCT images and depth-weighted fluorescence spectra were obtained for 10–30 mm longitudinal images. As shown in Fig. 7.7, the fluorescence emission spectra showed two peaks, at 390 and 450 nm, with a dip at 420 nm from oxyhemoglobin absorption. Over the region of the adenoma, the overall fluorescence emission decreased, and the ratio of 450:390 nm light increased [42]. Occasionally, fluorescence at 680 nm was also seen in the region of the adenoma. However, this fluorescence was attributed to chlorophyll metabolites from mouse chow. The combination of OCT and LIF was successful in identifying adenoma. Strong variation in the LIF signal meant that it alone was at best 81% sensitive and 80% specific to disease. The loss of layered structure in the OCT image was a very sensitive indicator of adenoma, however OCT could be confounded by lymphoid aggregates or fecal contamination. The former did not illustrate abnormal fluorescence emission and the later had a distinct emission spectra, so both confounders were easy to identify with LIF, increasing overall specificity.

Use of targeted exogenous fluorophores offers potentially greater sensitivity to disease, and also visualization of specific receptors upregulated during carcinogenesis. Fig. 7.8 illustrates an OCT/fluorescence spectra image pair taken with the same system used for autofluorescence detection. An *ex vivo* image taken with a fluorescence surgical microscope is also presented. In this case, the colon was lavaged with Cy5.5 dye conjugated to a vascular endothelial growth factor (VEGF) fragment, and a 633 nm He:Ne laser was used for LIF excitation. The dye preferentially attached to VEGF receptor-2, typically overexpressed in adenoma. A large variation in fluorescence emis-

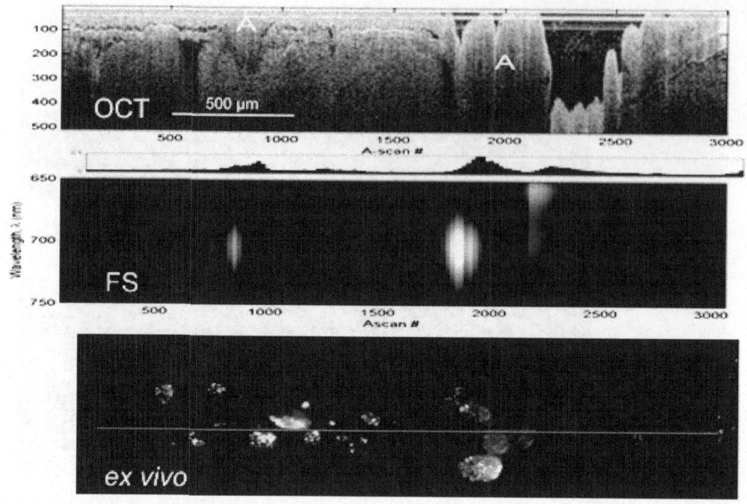

Figure 7.8: OCT and fluorescence images of mouse colon stained with Cy5.5 conjugated to a vascular endothelial growth factor fragment. Top: *in vivo* endoscopic OCT image showing a small and large adenoma (A). Middle: simultaneously acquired fluorescence spectroscopy image, y axis is wavelength. Bottom: *ex vivo, en face* fluorescence image. Line shows approximate location where the cross sectional OCT image, and fluorescence spectroscopy information, was obtained *in vivo*.

sion exists, however, suggesting that expression of VEGF receptor-2 is not homogeneous in disease [43]. Time-serial imaging might be performed to determine if adenomas with high levels of VEGF receptor-2 expression have more aggressive growth patterns.

Many possible contrast agents exist. In another study, an OCT system was combined in free space with a fluorescence system, and galvo scanning used to simultaneously image *ex vivo* mouse intestine [44]. The fluorescence system utilized 532 nm excitation, and detected both reflected light as well as fluorescence emission between 590–610 nm. The tissue was incubated with Lissamine Rhodamine PE conjugated to legume lectin Ulex europaeus agglutinin I, which binds to the surface of adenomas. The fluorescence emission was seen to be significantly greater in regions of adenoma than in normal tissue. The authors also presented a model for correcting the LIF signal using depth and bulk tissue attenuation measurements obtained from OCT. Although in the mouse tissue the fluorophore was located primarily on the surface and thus correction was unnecessary, the presented correction could be useful for tissues where a fluorophore is known to be confined to a deep layer (e.g., collagen in epithelial tissues).

7.3.3 Imaging of skin-equivalent models

Skin equivalent models are *in vitro* constructs that closely resemble human skin in structure and many functions. Typically they are made from a layer of collagen with embedded fibroblasts, topped with keratinocytes. If the epithelial layer is raised out of culture medium, a keratinized surface layer can be developed [45]. Skin equivalents are useful for visualizing the effect of drugs. In one study, an optical coherence microscopy (OCM)/multiphoton microscopy (MPM) system was used to study the effect of dimethyl sulfoxide (DMSO) on a skin equivalent model [46]. The system was similar to that described earlier [31], using a 12-fs, 100 nm bandwidth laser centered at 800 nm to obtain simultaneous OCM, TPEF, and second harmonic generation (SHG) microscopy images. The measured resolution was 0.5 μm transverse and 1.5 μm axial for all three modalities, and each was obtained in an *en face* manner, using a 0.95 NA, 63x objective.

The skin equivalents were stained with Hoechst 33343 or rhodamine 123. Figure 7.9 shows two OCM/TPEF image pairs, taken at the top of the keratinocyte layer, showing how the cells become smaller and more numerous with depth, as in human skin epithelium. When DMSO was applied to the skin equivalent models, the OCM signal strength greatly reduced, as expected since DMSO visibly "clears" tissue. Because the cells were stained with a fluorophore, the TPEF signal remained strong. It showed distortion of cells, with both cell types shrinking in volume and undergoing alterations in cell shape. The SHG signal also decreased, suggesting alterations in the collagen structure. Since histological processing of the skin equivalents would necessarily alter their structure. Understanding of the effects of DMSO on tissue can only be performed with an in situ, non-invasive imaging system. Therefore, this study illustrates how dual modality systems are critical for basic science studies.

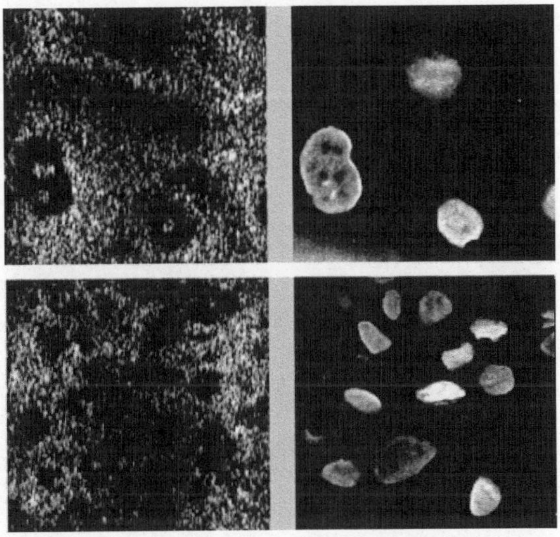

Figure 7.9: Optical coherence microscopy (OCM)/ two photon excited fluorescence (TPEF) image pairs of a skin equivalent model stained with Hoechst 33342. Top: image pair taken at the surface of the epithelial layer, bottom: image pair taken at the bottom of the epithelial layer. Left: OCM image, right: TPEF image. Cell nuclei become smaller and more numerous with depth.

7.4 Conclusion

Combining OCT and LIF functionality into an integrated system presents several challenges, since each subsystem has different, and sometimes incompatible specifications. However, the combination of structural imaging with OCT and molecular information obtained with LIF can be very powerful for disease detection as well as basic science research. Future instrument improvements should include: development of miniature (< 1 mm diameter) combined endoscopes to enable access to additional tissue types, new light sources with single or multiple outputs suitable for OCT and LIF, speed improvements particularly in LIF, and improved user interfaces that flexibly display the multimodality information.

Acknowledgment

The author acknowledges the assistance of Dr. Garret Bonnema, Mr. James McNally, and Dr. Amy Winkler in the preparation of figures for this chapter.

References

[1] J.G. Fujimoto and M.E. Brezinski, "Optical coherence tomography imaging," Ch. 13 in *Biomedical Photonics Handbook,* Tuan Vo-Dinh (ed.), CRC Press, Boca Raton, Florida, 13.1–13.29 (2003).

[2] J.M. Schmitt, A. Knttel, M. Yadlowsky, and M.A. Eckhaus, "Optical-coherence tomography of a dense tissue: statistics of attenuation and backscattering," *Phys. Med. Biol.* **39** (10), 1705–1720 (1994).

[3] J.A. Izatt, M.D. Kulkarni, S. Yazdanfar, J.K. Barton, and A.J. Welch, "*In vivo* bidirectional Doppler flow imaging of picoliter blood volumes using optical coherence tomography," *Opt. Lett.* **22** (18), 1439–1441 (1997).

[4] L. An, T.T. Shen, and R.K. Wang, "Using ultrahigh sensitive optical microangiography to achieve comprehensive depth resolved microvasculature mapping for human retina," *J. Biomed. Opt.* **16** (10), 106013 (2011).

[5] G. Liu, W. Jia, V. Sun, B. Choi, and Z. Chen, "High-resolution imaging of microvasculature in human skin in-vivo with optical coherence tomography," *Opt. Express* **20** (7), 7694–7705 (2012).

[6] J.F. de Boer and T.E. Milner, "Review of polarization sensitive optical coherence tomography and Stokes vector determination," *J. Biomed. Opt.* **7** (3), 359–371 (2002).

[7] B.E. Applegate, C. Yang, and J.A. Izatt, "Theoretical comparison of the sensitivity of molecular contrast optical coherence tomography techniques," *Opt. Express* **13** (20), 8146–8163 (2005).

[8] S,A. Boppart, A.L. Oldenburg, C.Xu, and D.L. Marks, "Optical probes and techniques for molecular contrast enhancement in coherence imaging," *J. Biomed. Opt.* **10** (4), 041208 (2005).

[9] C. Yang, "Molecular contrast optical coherence tomography: A review," *Photochem. Photobiol.* **81** (2), 215–237 (2005).

[10] U. Morgner, W.Drexler, F.X. Krtner, X.D. Li, C.Pitris, E.P. Ippen, and J.G. Fujimoto, "Spectroscopic optical coherence tomography," *Opt. Lett.* **25** (2), 111–113 (2000).

[11] A.M. Winkler, P.F. Rice, R.A. Drezek, and J.K. Barton, "Quantitative tool for rapid disease mapping using optical coherence tomography images of azoxymethane treated mouse colon," *J. Biomed. Opt.* **15** (4), 041512 (2010).

[12] M. Kirillin, M. Shirmanova, M. Sirotkina, M. Bugrova, B. Khlebtsov, and E. Zagaynova, "Contrasting properties of gold nanoshells and titanium dioxide nanoparticles for optical coherence tomography imaging of skin: Monte Carlo simulations and in vivo study," *J. Biomed. Opt.* **14** (2), 021017 (2009).

[13] T. M. Lee, A. L. Oldenburg, S. Sitafalwalla, D. L. Marks, W. Luo, F. Jean-Jacques Toublan, K. S. Suslick, and S. A. Boppart, "Engineered microsphere contrast agents for optical coherence tomography," *Opt. Lett.* **28** (17), 1546–1548 (2003).

[14] Y. Changhuei, L.E.L. McGuckin, J.D. Simon, M.A. Choma, B.E. Applegate, and J.A. Izatt, "Spectral triangulation molecular contrast optical coherence tomography with indocyanine green as the contrast agent," *Opt. Lett.* **29** (17), 2016–2018 (2004).

[15] B.E. Applegate and J.A. Izatt, "Molecular imaging of endogenous and exogenous chromophores using ground state recovery pump-probe optical coherence tomography," *Opt. Express* **14** (20), 9142–9155 (2006).

[16] Z. Yaqoob, E. McDowell, J. Wu, X. Heng, J. Fingler, and C. Yang, "Molecular contrast optical coherence tomography: a pump-probe scheme using indocyanine green as a contrast agent," *J. Biomed. Opt.* **11** (5), 054017 (2006).

[17] R. John, R. Rezaeipoor, S.G. Adie, E.J. Chaney, A.L. Oldenburg, M. Marjanovic, J.P. Haldar, B.P. Sutton, and S.A. Boppart, "In vivo magnetomotive optical molecular imaging using targeted magnetic nanoprobes," *P. Natl Acad. Sci.* **107** (18), 8085–8090 (2010).

[18] D.C. Adler, S.W. Huang, R. Huber, and J.G. Fujimoto, "Photothermal detection of gold nanoparticles using phase-sensitive optical coherence tomography," *Opt. Express* **16** (7), 4376–4393 (2008).

[19] Y. Jiang, I. Tomov, Y. Wang, and Z. Chen, "Second-harmonic optical coherence tomography," *Opt. Lett.* **29** (10), 1090–1092 (2004).

[20] W.A. Benalcazar and S.A. Boppart, "Nonlinear interferometric vibrational imaging for fast label-free visualization of molecular domains in skin," *Anal. Bioanal. Chem.* **400** (9), 2817–2825 (2011).

[21] S. Andersson-Engels, J. Johansson, K. Svanberg, and S. Svanberg, "Fluorescence imaging and point measurements of tissue: applications to the demarcation of malignant tumors and atherosclerotic lesions from normal tissue," *Photochem. Photobiol.* **53** (6), 807–814 (1991).

[22] T. Wilson, "Confocal Microscopy, " Ch. 10 in *Biomedical Photonics Handbook,* Tuan Vo-Dinh (ed.), CRC Press, Boca Raton, Florida, (2003).

[23] P.T.C. So, C.Y. Dong, and B.R. Masters, "Two-Photon Excitation Fluorescence Microscopy," Ch. 11 in *Biomedical Photonics Handbook,* Tuan Vo-Dinh (ed.), CRC Press, Boca Raton, Florida, (2003).

[24] R.V. Kuranov, V.V. Sapozhnikova, H.M. Shakhova, V.M. Gelikonov, E.V. Zagainova, and S.A. Petrova, "Combined application of optical methods to increase the information content of optical coherent tomography in diagnostics of neoplastic processes," *Quantum Electron+* **32** (11), 993–998 (2002).

[25] E. Zagaynova, N. Gladkova, N. Shakhova, G. Gelikonov, and V. Gelikonov, "Endoscopic OCT with forward-looking probe: clinical studies in urology and gastroenterology," *J. Biophotonics* **1** (2), 114–128 (2008).

[26] J. Schmidbauer, M. Remzi, T. Klatte, M. Waldert, J. Mauermann, M. Susani, and M. Marberger, "Fluorescence cystoscopy with high-resolution optical coherence tomography imaging as an adjunct reduces false-positive findings in the diagnosis of urothelial carcinoma of the bladder," *Eur. Urol.* **56** (6), 914–919 (2009).

[27] H. Ren, K.C. Park, R. Pan, W.C. Waltzer, K.R. Shroyer, and Y. Pan, "Early detection of carcinoma in situ of the bladder: A comparative study of white light cystoscopy, narrow band imaging, 5-ALA fluorescence cstoscopy and 3-dimensional optical coherence tomography," *J. Urol.* **187** (3), 1063–1070 (2012).

[28] G.M. Dobre, A.Gh. Podoleanu, and R.B. Rosen, "Simultaneous optical coherence tomography–indocyanine green dye fluorescence imaging system for investigations of the eye's fundus," *Opt. Lett.* **30** (1), 58–60 (2005).

[29] R.B. Rosen, M. Hathaway, J. Rogers, J. Pedro, P. Garcia, G.M. Dobre, and A.Gh. Podoleanu, "Simultaneous OCT/SLO/ICG imaging," *Invest. Ophth. Vis. Sci.* **50** (2), 851–860 (2009).

[30] E. Beaurepaire, L. Moreaux, F. Amblard, and J. Mertz, "Combined scanning optical coherence and two-photon excited fluorescence microscopy," *Opt. Lett.* **24** (14), 969–971 (1999).

[31] S. Tang, T.B. Krasieva, Z. Chen, and B.J. Tromberg, "Combined multiphoton microscopy and optical coherence tomography using a 12-fs broadband source," *J. Biomed. Opt.* **11** (2), 020502 (2006).

[32] B.W. Graf, Z. Jiang, H. Tu, and S.A. Boppart, "Dual-spectrum laser source based on fiber continuum generation for integrated optical coherence and multiphoton microscopy," *J. Biomed. Opt.* **14** (3), 034019 (2009).

[33] A.R. Tumlinson, L.P. Hariri, U. Utzinger, and J.K. Barton, "A miniature endoscope for simultaneous OCT-LIF measurement," *Appl. Opt.* **43** (1), 113–121 (2004).

[34] S.Y. Ryu, H.Y. Choi, J. Na, E.S. Choi, and B.H. Lee, "Combined system of optical coherence tomography and fluorescence spectroscopy based on double-cladding fiber," *Opt. Lett.* **33** (20), 2347–2349 (2008).

[35] G. Liu and Z. Chen, "Fiber-based combined optical coherence and multiphoton endomicroscopy," *J. Biomed. Opt.* **16** (3), 036010 (2011).

[36] J. Xi, Y. Chen, Y. Zhang, K. Murari, M. Li, and X. Li, "Integrated multimodal endomicroscopy platform for simultaneous en face optical coherence and two-photon fluorescence imaging," *Opt. Lett.* **37** (2), 362–364 (2012).

[37] H. Makhlouf, A.R. Rouse, and A.F. Gmitro, "Dual modality fluorescence confocal and spectral-domain optical coherence tomography microendoscope," *Biomed. Opt. Express* **2** (3), 634–644 (2011).

[38] R.A. Wall, G.T. Bonnema, and J.K. Barton, "Novel focused OCT-LIF endoscope," *Biomed. Opt. Express* **2** (3), 421–430 (2011).

[39] R.A. Wall and J.K. Barton, "Fluorescence-based surface magnifying chromoendoscopy and optical coherence tomography endoscope," *Proc. SPIE* **8217**, 821703 (2012).

[40] J. Park, J.A. Jo, S. Shrestha, P. Pande, Q. Wan, and B.E. Applegate, "A dual-modality optical coherence tomography and fluorescence lifetime imaging microscopy system for simultaneous morphological and biochemical tissue characterization," *Biomed. Opt. Express* **1** (1), 186–200, (2010).

[41] R. Richards-Kortum, R.P. Rava, R.E. Petras, M. Fitzmaurice, M. Sivak, and M.S. Feld, "Spectroscopic diagnosis of colonic dysplasia," *Photochem. Photobiol.* **53** (6), 777–786 (1991).

[42] J. McNally, N. Kirkpatrick, L.P. Hariri, A.R. Tumlinson, D. Besselsen, E. Gerner, U. Utzinger, and J. Barton, "Task based imaging of colon cancer in a mouse model (ApcMin/+)," *Appl. Opt.* **45** (13), 3049–3062 (2006).

[43] A.M. Winkler, P.F. Rice, J. Weichsel, J. Watson, M. Backer, J. Backer, and J.K. Barton, "In vivo, dual modality OCT/LIF imaging using a novel VEGF receptor targeted NIR fluorescent probe in the AOM-treated mouse model," *Mol. Imaging Biol.* **13** (6), 1173–1182 (2011).

[44] S. Yuan, C.A. Roney, J. Wierwille, C. Chen, B. Xu, J. Jiang, H. Ma, A. Cable, R.M. Summers, and Y. Chen, "Combining optical coherence tomography with fluorescence molecular imaging: Towards simultaneous morphology and molecular imaging," *Phys. Med. Biol.* **55** (1), 191–206 (2010).

[45] E. Bell, H.P. Ehrlich, D.J. Buttle, and T. Nakatsuji, "Living tissue formed in vitro and accepted as skin-equivalent tissue of full thickness," *Science* **211**(4486), 1052–1054 (1981).

[46] J.K. Barton, S. Tang, R. Lim, and B.J. Tromberg, "Simultaneous optical coherence and multiphoton microscopy of skin-equivalent tissue models," *Proc. SPIE* **6627**, 66270X (2007).

8

Multi-Modal Tomography Combining Optical Coherence Tomography (OCT) with Fluorescence Laminar Optical Tomography (FLOT)

Chao-Wei Chen
Department of Electrical and Computer Engineering, University of Maryland, College Park, MD

Yu Chen
Fischell Department of Bioengineering, University of Maryland, College Park, MD

This chapter describes multi-modal optical imaging techniques combining OCT with FLOT for depth-resolved imaging of tissue morphology and molecular function. OCT provides high-resolution, cross-sectional imaging of tissue microstructure. Depth-resolved FLOT provides highly-sensitive molecular information through fluorescence contrast agents. Multi-modal OCT/FLOT provides more comprehensive information for biomedical applications. This chapter will describe the theoretical modeling, instrumentation, as well as biomedical applications of this new multi-modal imaging modality.

Key words: optical coherence tomography (OCT), laminar optical tomography (LOT), fluorescence laminar optical tomography (FLOT), tissue engineering, breast cancer

8.1 Introduction

Optical coherence tomography (OCT) is an emerging imaging technology which can provide subsurface imaging of biological tissues [1]. OCT images are similar to ultrasound images, but with significantly higher resolution (5–10 times) than clinical ultrasound. OCT enables imaging of tissue microstructure with high resolution, approaching that of standard excisional biopsy and histopathology, except that imaging can be performed in real time without the removal of a tissue specimen. OCT has been successfully translated to various clinical applications including ophthalmology [2], cardiology [3], gastroenterology [4–7], dermatology [8], dentistry [9], urology [10], among others [1, 11–15]. Typical OCT systems provide a resolution of 1–10 μm with a penetration depth of 1–2 mm [1, 15, 16]. OCT is primarily based on contrasts from the linear characteristics of the tissue such as scattering, birefringence, and refractive index variations. Therefore, it is well-suited for high resolution imaging of tissue microstructures, as well as tissue functions based on the scattering (such as Doppler OCT [17–20]) or birefringence (such as polarization-sensitive OCT [21–25]). Different approaches have been pursued to enhance the scattering contrast though exogenous contrast agents [26–35], or exploit other contrast mechanisms including absorption [36–41], fluorescence [42–44], second-harmonics [45–47], and coherent anti-Stokes Raman scattering (CARS) [48, 49]. Alternatively, OCT can be combined with other imaging modalities with complementary contrast mechanisms to obtain more comprehensive information of tissue.

Since OCT provides high-resolution imaging of tissue microstructure, and fluorescence imaging provides the complementary biochemical, molecular, and metabolic information, there are great interests to combine these two modalities to provide the structural and functional information of the tissues simultaneously to enhance the disease detection capability. Pan et al. [50] suggested that ALA fluorescence-guided endoscopic OCT could enhance the efficiency and sensitivity of early bladder cancer diagnosis [50]. In the animal model studies, they demonstrated that the specificity of fluorescence detection of transitional cell carcinoma was significantly enhanced by fluorescence-guided OCT (53% vs. 93%), and the sensitivity of fluorescence detection also improved by combination with OCT (79% vs. 100%) [51]. Tumlinson et al. have developed a combined OCT and laser-induced fluorescence (LIF) spectroscopy imaging catheter for *in vivo* mouse colon imaging [52, 53]. An extensive overview of combining OCT with fluorescence spectroscopy is provided in previous chapter.

In this chapter, we focus on the combination of OCT and fluorescence tomography. Laminar optical tomography (LOT) has been developed to perform depth-resolved functional imaging with ~100 μm resolution and up to 2.5 mm depth [54–60]. LOT is an extension of confocal microscopy by using multiple-displaced-confocal-pinhole design to capture the photons traveling through different depths, and the image is obtained through transport-based reconstruction [54]. Fluorescence LOT (FLOT) has been demonstrated [61, 62]. The comparable imaging scale (1–2 mm in depth) of OCT and FLOT as well as their complementary contrast mechanisms motivate the integration of OCT and FLOT as a multimodality imaging platform to provide tissue structural and molecular information in 3D in millimeter imaging scale.

8.2 Combined OCT and FLOT: Instrumentation

Figure 8.1 shows the schematic of the co-registered OCT and line-scan FLOT imaging system. The left portion is the OCT subsystem, which utilizes a wavelength-swept laser as the light source. It generates a broadband spectrum of 100 nm at 1310 nm, which provides an axial resolution of ~10 μm in the tissue. The laser operates at a sweep rate of 16 kHz (equivalent to an imaging speed of 30 frames per second for a 512 axial-line image) with an average output power of 12 mW. A Michelson interferometer composed of one circulator and a fiber-optic 50/50 splitter is used to generate the Fourier-domain OCT signal. The reference arm consists of a stationary mirror (M) and a polarization controller (PC). The light from the sample arm passes through a collimator (C) and is steered by a pair of galvanometer mirrors (X and Y) then focused by an objective lens. The power on the sample is 4 mW with a spot size of 15 μm. The OCT interference signal returned from both the sample and reference arms is detected by a balanced photodetector (BD). A Mach-Zehnder interferometer (MZI) with a fixed path difference is used to generate an optical frequency clock.

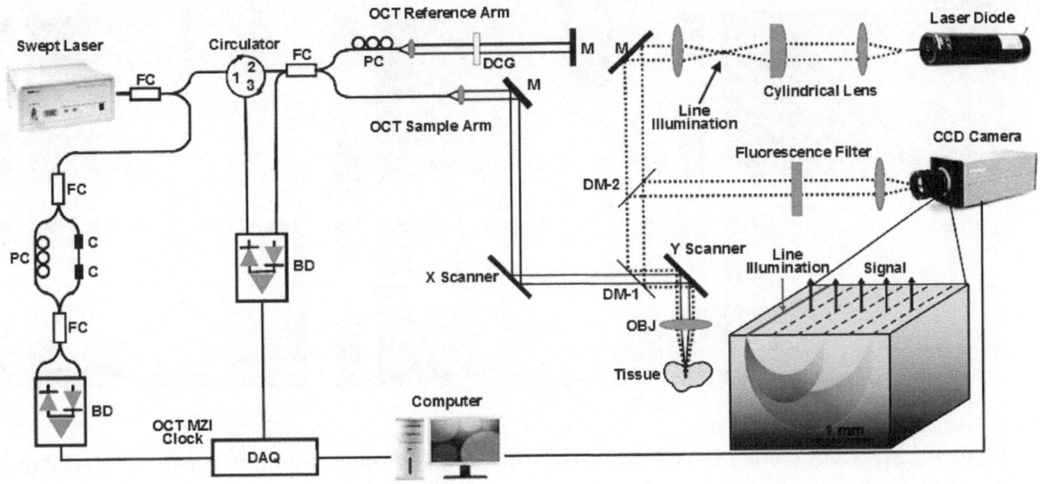

Figure 8.1: Schematic of the combined OCT and line-scan FLOT system. From [64].

Data acquisition is triggered by the zero-crossings of the MZI fringes, which are evenly spaced in optical frequency. Discrete Fourier transform (DFT) is performed on the data to generate an axial depth profile of the sample (A-line) with 3 mm imaging depth and 512 pixels [63]. The system sensitivity is 95 dB.

The line-scan FLOT system is shown in the right portion. The excitation source is either a laser diode at various wavelength or a mode-locked Ti:Sapphire laser. A cylindrical lens is used to expand the point illumination into a line. The excitation light is combined with the OCT sample arm by a dichroic mirror (DM-1). The reflectance and fluorescence light is separated by another dichroic mirror (DM-2), and the fluorescence signal is detected by an electron-multiplying CCD (EM-CCD) camera (Cooke Corp.) with an emission filter. The excitation/emission wavelengths are chosen based on the optical properties of specific fluorescent dye used in a particular study. The line illuminated on the sample measures 2.2 mm in length and 25 μm in width with <20 mW power. The OCT and line-scan FLOT imaging are synchronized by scanning with the same galvanometer (Y). The OCT beam is scanned in two axes (fast axis X and slow axis Y). The scanning speed for X is 25 Hz (with 624 samples in 2.5 mm), and the scanning speed for Y is 0.1 Hz (with 256 samples in 2.5 mm). Line-scan FLOT scans in Y only at the same speed as OCT, with 256 frames acquired by CCD (acquisition speed of 25 Hz with 30 ms exposure time). The resulting OCT 3D volume size is 624 (X) by 256 (Y) by 512 (Z) pixels (with voxel size of 4 μm $\times$ 10 μm $\times$ 4.4 μm), and FLOT image raw data is 501 (X) by 1024 (Y) (2.2 mm $\times$ 2.2 mm) by 256 (T) frames. The total acquisition time for each 3D volume is approximately 10 s. The rate-limiting factors are the FLOT CCD frame rate, and the high number of OCT images acquired in the Y dimension. The 3D imaging time can be significantly reduced by binning the CCD camera.

8.3 FLOT Theory and Image Reconstruction

Depth-resolved FLOT image is obtained through image reconstruction process similar to those used in X-ray computerized tomography (CT) or diffuse optical tomography (DOT) [65]. In scattering media, the fluorescence signal can be expressed as [61, 66]:

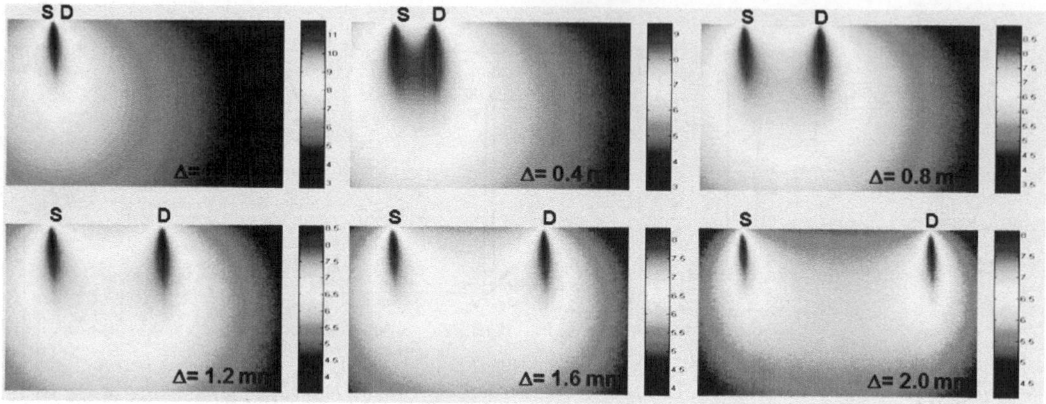

Figure 8.2: (See color insert.) Monte-Carlo simulated measurement sensitivity distribution of FLOT measurements (log scale). Tissue geometry is 3 mm (lateral) by 2 mm (depth) with scattering coefficient μ_s = 8 mm^{-1} for excitation and 7 mm^{-1} for emission (g = 0.9). From [64].

$$F_0(\vec{r}_d,\widehat{\Omega}_d) = \frac{\sigma_{ex}\cdot\gamma}{4\pi}\int \psi_{ex}(\vec{r}-\vec{r}_s)\cdot C_f(\vec{r})\cdot\psi_{em}(\vec{r}_d-\vec{r})\cdot d^3\vec{r}, \tag{8.1}$$

where $\sigma_{ex}$is the absorption cross-section of the fluorophores at the excitation wavelength, γ is the fluorescence quantum yield, $\psi_{ex}(\vec{r}-\vec{r}_s)$ is the excitation fluence distribution calculated from the excitation photon radiance from a source located at $\vec{r}_s$, $C_f(\vec{r})$ is the fluorophore concentration at position $\vec{r}$, and $\psi_{em}(\vec{r}_d-\vec{r})$ is the probability that a photon emitted by a source at position $\vec{r}$ will be detected by a detector located at $\vec{r}_d$. Eq. (8.1) can be discretized into voxels, which yields a matrix equation:

$$F = JC, \tag{8.2}$$

where F is the fluorescence measurements, C is the spatially-distributed fluorophores concentration, and J is the weight matrix that represent the sensitivity of each measurement to the fluorophore concentration at each voxel, and can be expressed as:

$$J_{s,m}(\vec{r}_s,\vec{r}_d,\vec{r}) = D_0\cdot\psi_{ex}(\vec{r}-\vec{r}_s)\cdot\psi_{em}(\vec{r}_d-\vec{r}), \tag{8.3}$$

where D_0 is a constant. The sensitivity distribution of FLOT can be calculated using Monte-Carlo simulation (see Fig. 8.2). The sensitivity profile varied as the source-detector separation increased. Therefore, depth-dependent information is encoded in the multiple detector measurement, and can be recovered through image reconstruction.

Image reconstruction is performed within individual planes (YZ) perpendicular to the illumination line (X). Two main approaches have been used for FLOT image reconstruction, including: 1) Simultaneous iterative reconstruction technique approach (SIRT) [67], with iteration number N = 1000 to make sure the change between iterations is <0.1%; 2) Tikhonov regularization [55]:

$$C = [J^T\times J+\lambda^2\text{Max}(SV)^2\times I]^{-1}\times J^T\times F, \tag{8.4}$$

where $\text{Max}(SV)$ is the largest singular value in J and λ is the regularization factor that leverages the signal level and noise level. Typically, we choose $\lambda = 3\times10^{-4}$.

8.4 Results: Phantom Experiments and Subsurface Cancer Imaging

The performance of the OCT/FLOT system was first demonstrated by imaging a tissue phantom, which consisted of a capillary tube with an inner diameter of $\sim$110 μm and outer diameter of $\sim$130μm, suspended in a scattering medium consisting of 2% Intralipid mixed with Indian ink (μ_a= 0.2 mm^{-1} and μ_s = 7.2 mm^{-1} at 670 nm, anisotropy factor g = 0.9, similar to those of human skin tissue). The tube was filled with 10 μM fluorescent dye Cy5.5.

Figure 8.3 shows the comparison of OCT and FLOT images of the capillary tube phantom. OCT readily images the 3D structure of the tube as shown in Fig. 8.3(A). Figure 8.3(B) shows the comparison of OCT cross-sectional image (YZ) and FLOT image at location "1" denoted in (A). Cross-sectional OCT reveals the capillary tube (indicated by the arrow) with approximately 0.6 mm beneath the surface. FLOT cross-sectional image shows a fluorescence object at the same location, with slightly larger size due to the relatively larger FLOT resolution compared to OCT. Cross-sectional OCT and FLOT images at location "2" also show good agreement with the tube depth approximately 0.9 mm (Figure 8.3(C)). Compared to 8.3(B), the FLOT image for the deeper object shows slight enlargement in size. In addition, the peak values are slightly reduced when object gets deeper due to the enlargement of the reconstructed object size. Figure 8.3(D) shows the OCT cross-sectional image along the tube longitudinal dimension (XZ). The tube is placed with an angle with respect to the horizontal axis, and slightly bends flat. The FLOT image (XZ) reveals similar contour of the capillary tube as shown by OCT. Also, this image is averaged over a range of 150 m in Y dimension along the center of the tube, and the results indicated nearly constant fluorophore concentration. Here the OCT image provides the structural information of the phantom and the FLOT reconstructed image provides the fluorescence dye distribution information. In biomedical applications, FLOT would provide fluorescence-dye-targeted molecular information. Together, the hybrid OCT/FLOT system can be used for concurrent depth-resolved tissue-structural and molecular imaging.

Next, we imaged an animal model of breast cancer using OCT/FLOT [64]. A triple negative human breast cancer cell line, MDA-MB-231, originally expanded from a pleural effusion, was obtained from the American Type Culture Collection (ATCC). Plasmid DNA encoding tdTomato (pRSETB-tdTomato) was kindly donated by Professor Roger Tsien (University of California, San Diego) [68], cloned into the mammalian expression vector pEF-1α-myc/his (Invitrogen, Carlsbad, CA) generating pEF-1α-tdTomato [69]. pEF-1α-tdTomato was stably transfected into MDA-MB-231 cells using the Amaxa Nucleofector II instrument (Amaxa Biosystems, Gaithersburg, MD), followed by fluorescence activated cell sorting (FACS) of tdTomato-fluorescing cells, and further expansion without antibiotics, which was performed by Winnard Jr. et al as previously described [69]. Prior to inoculation, MDA-MB-231-tdTomato cells displayed intense tdTomato fluorescence in cell culture as tested with live cell fluorescence microscopy [69].

One hundred thousand to two million MDA-MB-231-tdTomato cells were orthotopically inoculated in the mammary fat pad of anesthetized female athymic nude mice as previously described [70]. Tumor xenografts reached their final experimental size of about 5 mm^3 within 4 weeks. *In vivo* whole-body fluorescence imaging of MDA-MB-231-tdTomato tumor xenografts was confirmed using a commercially available optical imaging system, the Xenogen IVIS 200 Spectrum (Caliper Life Sciences, Hopkinton, MA) before *in vivo* OCT-FLOT imaging under anesthesia.

Figure 8.4 shows OCT/FLOT imaging of human breast cancer xenograft model *in vivo*. Figure 8.4(A) shows an OCT cross-sectional image of the breast tumor. Mouse skin layer is highly scattering therefore limiting the penetration depth. However, the boundary between the skin and the tumor is clearly visible (arrow). Figure 8.4(B) shows the co-registered FLOT image revealing the subcutaneous tumor (which is transfected with red fluorescence protein). Figure 8.4(C) is the fused OCT-FLOT image which shows the relative position and distribution of tumor regions underneath

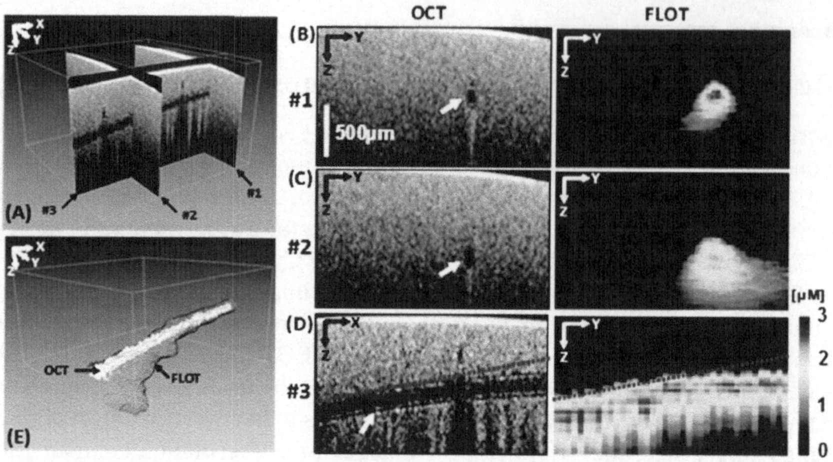

Figure 8.3: (See color insert.) Co-registration of OCT and line-scan FLOT of a capillary tube filled with fluorescence dye. (A) 3D OCT imaging showing three representative slices. (B) Left, OCT image (slice #1) of the capillary tube (arrow); right, FLOT image reconstruction of the fluorescence object. (C) OCT and FLOT images of different position (slice #2). (D) OCT and FLOT image (slice #3) reveal the curvature of the capillary tube (two identical dotted lines serve as the reference slopes). (E) 3D isosurface of FLOT image shows good co-localization with OCT. From [53].

the skin. Figure 8.4(D) shows the corresponding histology confirming the presence of tumor. Figure 8.4(E) shows the OCT cross-sectional image of another region of the breast tumor. The boundary between skin and tumor is less well-defined (arrow) indicating tumor invasion. Figure 8.4(F) shows the co-registered FLOT image revealing a larger tumor volume than that shown in (B). Figure 8.4(G) shows the fused OCT-FLOT image. The corresponding histology 7(H) confirms the larger tumor size than Fig. 8.4(D). The estimated tumor sizes from FLOT images are: 2.17 mm$\times$0.92 mm for the smaller tumor region (B) and 2.50 mm$\times$1.11 mm for the larger tumor region (F) (the dimensions are estimated using the FWHM of the long and short axes assuming an oval shape tumor). The histology findings indicate the tumor sizes of 2.30 mm$\times$0.83 mm for the smaller tumor region (D) and 2.33 mm$\times$1.25 mm for the larger tumor region (H). These results indicate FLOT can visualize the difference in subsurface tumor sizes. Figure 8.5 shows the 3D view of mouse skin (from OCT) and subsurface tumor (from FLOT).

8.5 Improvement of FLOT Resolution Using Angled Configuration

One of the limitations for our current FLOT system is the point spread function (PSF) enlarges while the object locates deeper [55, 64]. Our previous measurement (see Fig 8.3E) indicates that the axial PSF is $\sim$100–200 μm at $\sim$0.6 mm depth and increases to $\sim$300–400 μm at $\sim$1 mm depth [64]. To overcome this limitation, we investigated the effects of the source and detector angles upon the imaging performance [71]. Previous work in optical spectroscopy suggests that using angled illumination-collection fiber design (oblique illumination/collection) will enhance the depth selectivity of epithelium tissues [72–76]. This novel approach can be implemented in FLOT imaging to vary the depth selectivity, and potentially enhance the depth resolution of image reconstruction.

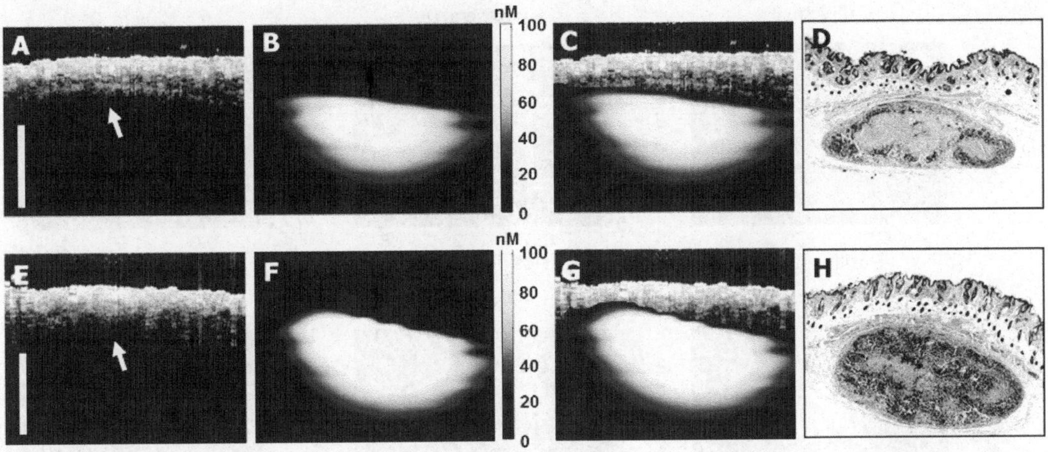

Figure 8.4: (See color insert.) OCT/FLOT of subcutaneous human breast tumor xenograft on mouse model *in vivo*. Breast cancer cells (MDA-MB-231) are constitutively labeled with tdTomato red fluorescence protein. (A) OCT cross-sectional image of breast tumor. Mouse skin layer shows highly scattering, and the boundary between skin and tumor is clearly visible (arrow). (B) Co-registered FLOT image revealing subsurface tumor. (C) Fused OCT-FLOT image, and (D) the corresponding histology. (E) OCT cross-sectional image of another region of the breast tumor. The boundary between skin and tumor is less well-defined (arrow). (F) Co-registered FLOT image revealing a larger tumor volume than (B). (G) Fused OCT-FLOT image. The corresponding histology (H) confirms the larger tumor size than (D). Bar: 1 mm. From [64].

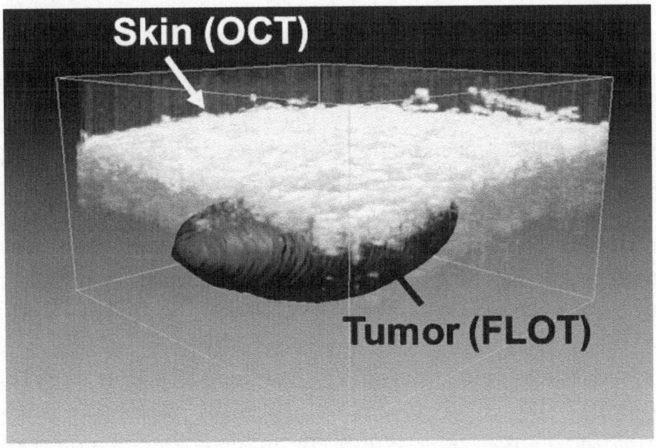

Figure 8.5: (See color insert.) Combined OCT and depth-resolved FLOT reveals subcutaneous breast tumor xenograft *in vivo* in 3D. Tumor cells are transfected with red fluorescence protein (RFP), and displayed as isosurface of 30 nM of calibration dye Rhodamine 6G. Tumor size: 2.2 mm×2.3 mm×0.9 mm.

8.5.1 Theoretical analysis and simulation

The matrix inversion in Eq. (8.4) is ill-posed so that the reconstructed image C is underdetermined and as a result non-unique. Optimization of the sensitivity matrix J (determined by source-detector configuration and tissue optical properties) is therefore critical to the reconstruction process and overall image performance. Singular-value analysis (SVA) is a method to decompose the sensitivity

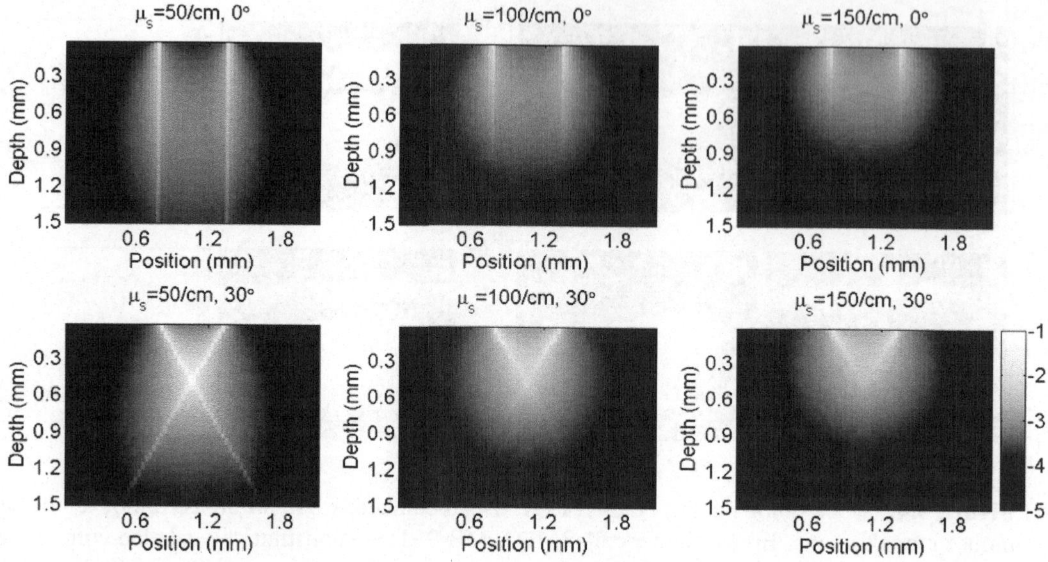

Figure 8.6: Sensitivity maps (in log10 scale) for source-detector pair with 0° (top row) and 30° (bottom row) incidence/detection angles. For each configuration, different scattering coefficient is specified for the medium (left to right). The sensitivity map (plotted in log10 scale) indicates the probability density of photons delivered to the location by the source and captured at the location by the detector. From [71].

matrix (J) into an eigenvalue spectrum, and has been demonstrated in the optimization of DOT to achieve a favorable image resolution [77, 78]. SVD of the sensitivity matrix J yields a triplet of matrices: $J = USV^T$. The magnitude of the singular values of S provides a measure of the relative effects of these image-space modes on the detected signal. The singular values are ordered to decrease in magnitude with increasing image-space mode indices [2].

In this study, we used SVA to investigate the optimization of resolution and sensitivity by varying the FLOT source incidence angle and detector detecting angle. For convenience, we began with cases where both angles are equal. Figure 8.6 shows the sensitivity profiles of FLOT for a representative source-detector pair based on Monte Carlo simulation. Configurations with 0° (top row) and 30° (bottom row) incidence and detection angles show distinct sensitivity pattern. For each configuration, different scattering coefficients (μ_s= 50, 100, and 150 cm^{-1}) is chosen as the background medium (left to right). The sensitivity map indicates the probability density of photons delivered to each location by the source and captured by the detector. Photon paths appear more ballistic for low-scattering medium (μ_s= 50 cm^{-1}) while become more scattered in high-scattering medium (μ_s= 150 cm^{-1}). A set of singular values (SVs) of $J$are generated for each angle from 0° to 50° with 10° increment and plotted in Fig. 8.7. Figure 8.7(A-C) correspond to different background scattering coefficients (μ_s= 50, 100, 150 cm^{-1}, respectively). The threshold for the singular value analysis is set to $10^{-3.6}$ (corresponding to the dynamic range of detector). The number of SVs above the threshold represents a measure of the useful information contained in that data for image reconstruction. Figure 8.7(D) plots of the number of useful SVs above the threshold for different scattering coefficients. From this figure, 30° configuration excels among other angles in the sense of having the highest number of useful SVs, especially in low scattering medium (μ_s= 50 cm^{-1}).

To validate the results from singular value analysis, we performed image reconstruction of a point object (with intensity equal to 1) under different configurations, using simulated measurement data (with 1.5% Gaussian noise added). The point spread function along axial (z) direction through the

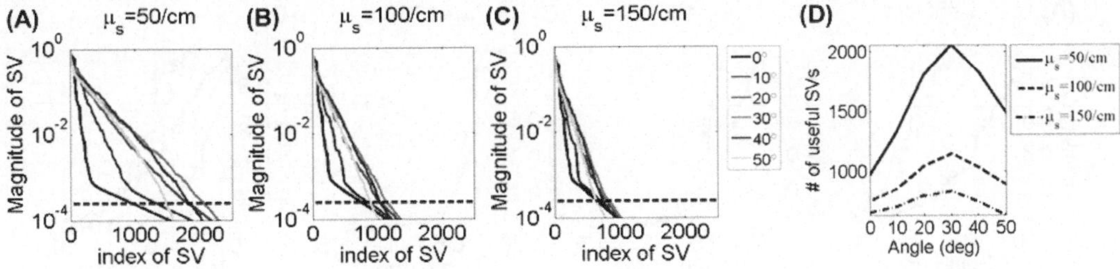

Figure 8.7: Comparison of singular value (SV) distributions among different incidence/detection angles. For convenience, same incidence and detection angles are specified. (A) SV distribution for μ_s= 50 cm^{-1}; (B) SV distribution for μ_s= 100 cm^{-1}; and (C) SV distribution for μ_s= 150 cm^{-1}. Detection threshold is specified as $10^{-3.6}$(dotted horizontal lines in A-C). Only SV above the threshold carries useful information for image reconstruction. (D) Plot of the number of useful SV (above the threshold). From [71].

position of point object was quantified at every depth of the object. As expected, axial point spread function (PSF_z) broadens and its peak intensity decreases as the object goes deeper. The details of PSF_z were further analyzed using two parameters: 1) the reconstructed peak intensity (or depth sensitivity); and 2) the interquartile range (IQR). IQR represents the range that bounds an area of 50% centered around the median value under the PSF curve. IQR is a more stable estimate of spread than full-width-at-half-maximum (FWHM) in the presence of long tail distribution [79]. Figure 8.8(A-D) shows the PSF_z peak intensity (or depth sensitivity) versus depth for different configurations. In general, at a given depth, 30° incidence /detection angle configuration has higher peak intensity (sensitivity) than 0° configuration, especially in the shallower depth region. The difference becomes less prominent for high scattering medium (μ_s= 150 cm^{-1}). It is interesting, however, that when normalizing these sensitivity curves to mean free path (MFP) ($1/\mu_s$) (i.e., replacing d with $\mu_s d$ in x-axis of the plot), only 30° configurations grouped together, as shown in Fig. 8.8(D). The fact that normal configurations are not unified indicates that the underlying mechanisms between angled and normal configurations are different as photons significantly rely on backscattering to travel from source to detector in normal configurations, while the incidence and detection paths overlap in angled configurations. When normalized to MFP, the backscattering factor (as in 0° configuration) might not be linearly scaled.

Figure 8.8(E-H) plot the IQR of PSF_z versus depth for different configurations. In general 30° configuration has smaller IQR (higher axial resolution) than 0° configuration. Especially, in low scattering medium (μ_s= 50 cm^{-1}), IQR for 30° configuration remains ~30 μm up to 1 mm, and remains <100 μm up to 1.5 mm. In contrast, IQR for 0° configuration increases rapidly to ~400 μm at 1 mm. However, the difference between these two configurations becomes less prominent as the background scattering increase, and the IQRs for both configurations are almost identical for high scattering medium (μ_s= 150 cm^{-1}). Again, when normalized to MFP as shown in Figure 13.8(H), the grouping of the curves was observed. However, different from the sensitivity, the grouping (unifying) of IQR curves occurred at both normal and angled configurations, which is expected because both IQR and MFP are in terms of distance. This result also indicates IQR and sensitivity provide inherently different measures.

In previous analysis, we set both the source incidence and detector collection angles the same. In practice, both angles may vary independently. We also analyzed the number of useful SVs versus the incidence and detection angels, respectively, for different $\mu_s$values. Our results indicate that the combination of source incidence angle of $\leq 20°$ and detection angel of $\geq 30°$ yields the optimal number of useful SVs, therefore suggesting a better imaging performance. However, the

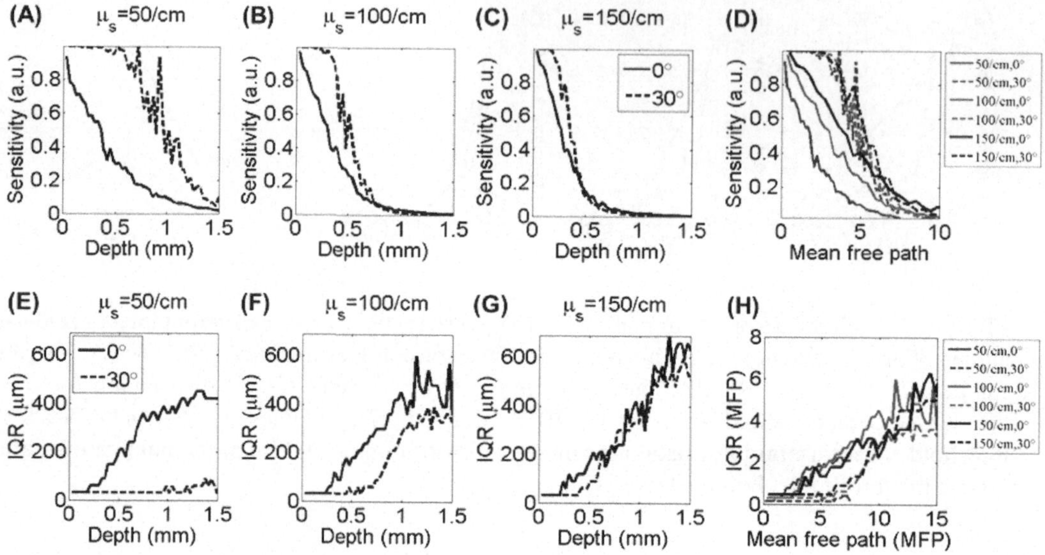

Figure 8.8: A-D: PSFz peak intensity versus depth for different source/detector angle configurations and background scattering. E-H: PSFz interquartile range (IQR) versus depth for different source/detector angle configurations and background scattering. From [71].

enhancement from 0° configuration degrades when the background scattering coefficient increases. These results suggest the enhancement via angled incidence/detection is more significant in lower scattering medium (μ_s= 150 cm^{-1}).

8.5.2 Experimental validation

Figure 8.9 shows the schematic diagram and the photo of the angled FLOT (aFLOT) system. The excitation light source was expanded into line-field illumination using a cylindrical lens (CL). An emission filter (F) was placed in the detection axis to select only the fluorescence signal, which was recorded by a 12-bit electron-multiplying CCD (EM-CCD, CooKe). Another CCD (CCD2) was placed vertically to record the reflected light distribution to determine the reduced scattering coefficient of the sample using oblique-incidence reflectometry [80]. When acquiring aFLOT measurement, the translating stage was moved in Y-direction (perpendicular to the line-illumination along X) with a speed of 50 μm/s. One raw measurement dataset has a format of XYT where EM-CCD recorded each XY frame with 0.4 s exposure time and the total recording time was 170 s for one 3D dataset. Image reconstruction converted each YZ plane (2D) from YT measurements using Tikhonov regularization. In this study, 70 source-detector (SD) pairs with 70 scanning positions were used to determine a single YZ field of view (FOV) of 3 mm$\times$3 mm. Local YZ frames were then pieced together longitudinally to form a global FOV.

We then validated aFLOT imaging experimentally using a capillary tube phantom. The capillary tube (110 μm in diameter) was filled with 1 μm fluorescent dye Rodamine 6G and embedded at 1.2 mm deep inside 1% Intralipid. The excitation wavelength was set to 532 nm and the filter was set to 605$\pm$15 nm, based on the spectrum of Rodamine 6G. Figure 8.10(A) shows the cross-section of the reconstructed capillary tube phantom using aFLOT. The position of the capillary from the reconstructed image ($\sim$1.14 mm) was close to the position independently measured using optical coherence tomography ($\sim$1.2 mm) (data not shown). As a comparison between angled and conventional FLOT systems, Figure 8.10(B) shows the reconstruction using FLOT with normal in-

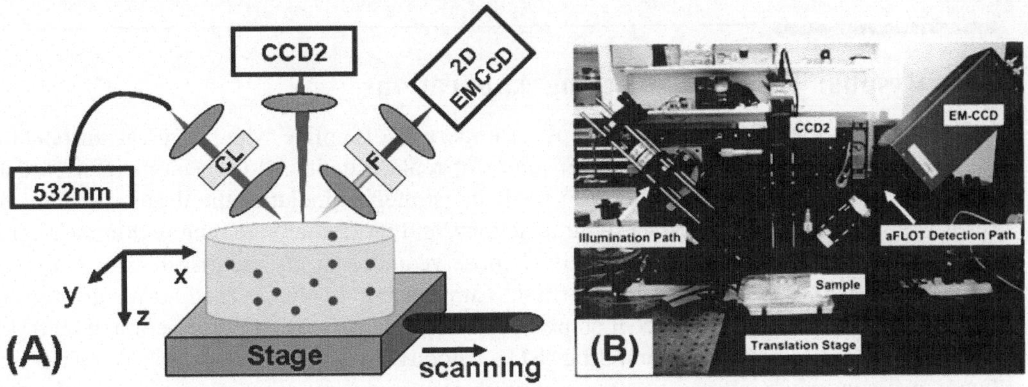

Figure 8.9: (A) Schematic of the aFLOT system. CL: cylindrical lens. F: filter. (B) Photo of the $45° - 45°$ aFLOT system. The illumination/detection arms are arranged at 45° in air (or 30° inside the sample assuming an index of refraction of 1.4).

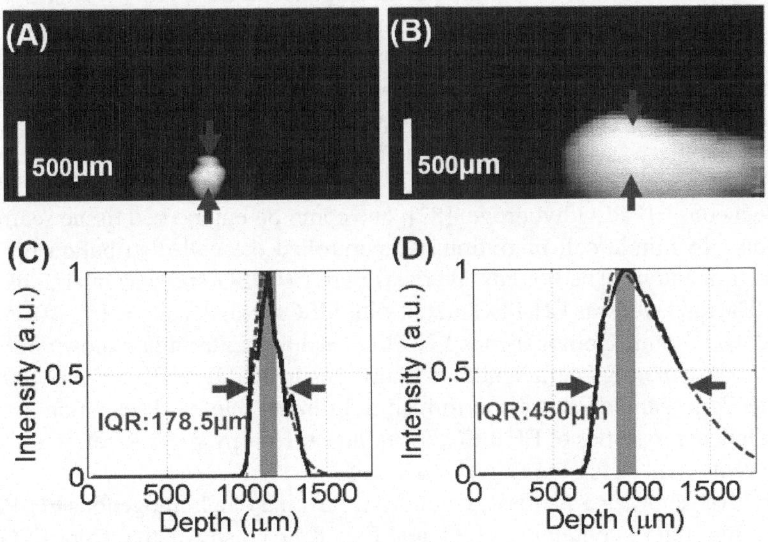

Figure 8.10: Comparison of aFLOT (A,C) and conventional FLOT (B,D). A,B: cross-sectional reconstruction; C,D: axial profile through the center of the object. Gray area denotes the true dimension of the capillary tube. IQR: Inter-quartile range.

cidence/detection. Figure 8.10(C-D) illustrate the center axial profiles of the reconstructed capillary tube shown in Figure 8.10(A-B), respectively. Quantitatively, interquartile range (IQR) was measured and compared. The measured IQR was 178.5 μm for the aFLOT system and was 450 μm for the conventional FLOT. This represents approximately 2.5-fold improvement in axial resolution.

8.6 Results: Tissue Engineering Applications

Regenerative medicine has emerged as an important discipline which aims at introducing living cells or functioning tissues to repair injury or replace damaged tissues or organs which lose functions. Optimization of regenerative medicine strategies includes the design of biomaterials, cell-seeding methods, cell-biomaterial interactions, and molecular signaling within the engineered tissue. One challenge is to non-destructively observe and quantify the distribution and migration of seeded cells throughout the bulk scaffold. Current state-of-the-art method for quantifying 3D cell distribution involves fluorescent confocal microscopy imaging of cryo-sectioned scaffolds followed by digital 3D image recompiling [81]. Although robust, this approach is destructive and time-consuming, thereby may become a concern in longitudinal inspection of massive amount of samples.

FLOT (and aFLOT) overcomes the depth-limitation of confocal microscopy by using multiple detectors to collect photon travelling through different depths. In this study, we experimentally demonstrated two configurations of aFLOT on two types of engineered tissues respectively. Mesenchymal stem cells (MSCs) embedded in homogeneous EH-PEG hydrogels [82], which is low scattering ($\mu_s = 10$ cm^{-1}), was imaged through an incidence-detection angle of $45° - 45°$ aFLOT (as shown in Fig. 8.9). In the other experiment, a capillary (100 μm in diameter) containing 1 mM Rhodamine 6G was embedded in a heterogeneous macroporous EH-PEG hydrogel [83, 84], which is high scattering ($\mu_s = 110$ cm^{-1}). This phantom was imaged through $45° - 0°$ aFLOT. The tomography of capillary was reconstructed and co-registered with that from OCT.

In the first experiment, we used the aFLOT system to image MSC distribution inside transparent, homogeneous EH-PEG hyodrogel [82], one common engineered tissue scaffold used for bone regeneration. To mimic cell migration, we controlled the cell distribution thickness by preparing a bi-layer phantom. The bottom layer was pure EH-PEG and was intentionally prepared thick (>6 mm). The top layer was EH-PEG mixed with MSCs (cell density = 10^4–10^5 /ml) with thickness of 0.5, 1, 2, and 3 mm. Homogeneous EH-PEG has low scattering as shown in Fig. 8.11(A), with typical reduced scattering coefficient of $\sim$1 cm^{-1}, estimated by reflectometry [80]. For reconstruction, Monte-Carlo simulation was performed to estimate photon distribution inside homogeneous EH-PEG. Optical properties of EH-PEG, including anisotropy $g = 0.9$, refractive index of 1.33, and absorption coefficient of 0.1 cm^{-1}, were assumed.

Figure 8.11(B) shows a YZ cross-section from stacking of a homogenous EH-PEG phantom with top layer (2-mm thick) containing MSC, and Fig. 8.11(C) shows that from FLOT reconstruction. Stacking (as used in conventional 3D digital microscopy) provides a blurred yet quick 3D view of the sample due to the weak but non-zero scattering of the sample. FLOT image reconstruction using proper modeling improves the image quality as shown in Fig. 8.11(C). Figure 8.11(D) is the composite 3D reconstruction of the same phantom. The FOV is $6.5 \times 7.6 \times 2.9$ mm^3. Figure 8.11(E) renders together the phantoms with 0.5, 1, 2, and 3-mm thick MSC distributions on the top layer. Lastly, we show the histogram of stem cell depth distribution of all four samples. The estimated cell distribution depths are distinct and consistent with the nominal thickness of each sample during fabrication. One interesting point is that all the cell-distribution patterns peaked at the bottom surface, which may be attributed to the condensation of cells. Further research is needed to confirm this finding. In addition, from Fig. 8.8, the detection sensitivity drops toward a deeper region so that the histogram also shows the peaks declining toward a deeper region. In summary, Fig. 8.11 demonstrates that aFLOT can resolve the depth-dependent distribution of cell clusters in weakly scattering EH-PEG hydrogel.

In the second set of experiments where heterogeneous macroporous EH-PEG is of interest, the advantage of the $45° - 45°$ configuration is diminished as the sample scattering coefficient is higher. Moreover, if the camera was placed at 45°, because the imaging area is of a few millimeters, raw

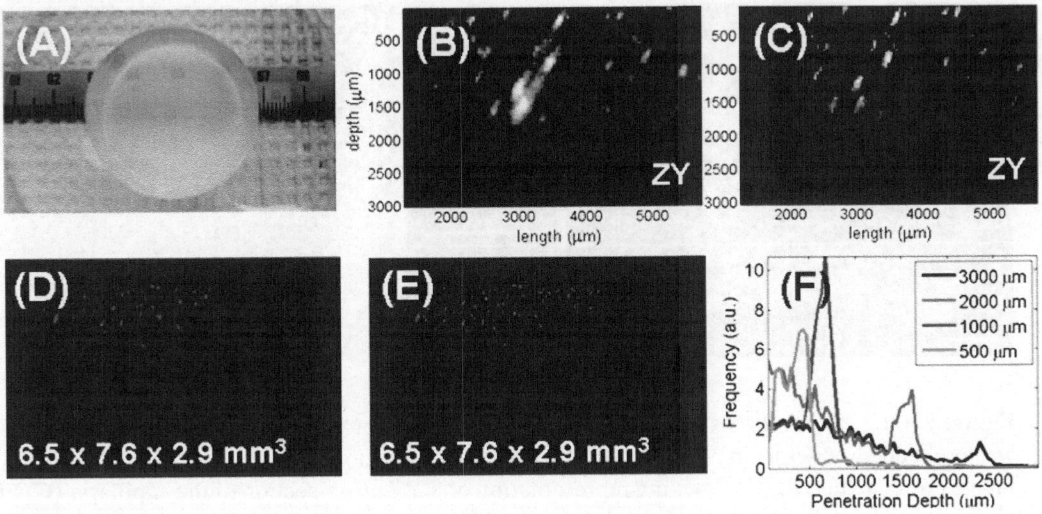

Figure 8.11: (See color insert.) 3D aFLOT imaging of EH-PEG hydrogels with stem cells embedded at top layers. (A) Photo of a sample. Transparency indicates low scattering. (B) Stacking representation of a YZ cross-section of the hydrogel with 2-mm thick top layer containing MSC. (C) Reconstruction of the same YZ cross-section. Image reconstruction (PSF-deconvolution) through Tikhonov regularization makes MSC clearer. (D) 3D reconstruction of the same sample. (E) Combined view of four samples with different stem-cell-laden layer thickness: 0.5-mm (cyan), 1-mm (red), 2-mm (green), and 3-mm (blue). (F) Histogram of cell distribution.

CCD images were not able to maintain in-focus across the entire FOV as the sample is now opaque. We therefore changed the illumination-detection angles to $45^\circ - 0^\circ$ configuration. We embedded a capillary tube (100 μm in diameter) containing 50 μm fluorescent dye Indocyanine Green (ICG) in a macroporous EH-PEG hydrogel, which is highly scattering at visible wavelength ($\mu_s = 110$ cm^{-1} at 530 nm). The scattering coefficient was reduced at near infrared (NIR) wavelength ($\mu_s = 50$ cm^{-1} at 780 nm). This phantom was imaged through FLOT with 780 nm excitation. The FLOT tomography of the capillary was reconstructed and co-registered with that from OCT. Figure 8.12(A) shows the photo of the opaque scaffold. Figure 8.12(B) is the stacking representation of a capillary cross-section from raw data. Both the unwanted vertical and oblique long tails are resulted from the scattering background. FLOT reconstruction deconvoluted the capillary to a localized position as shown in Fig. 8.12(C). To validate the reconstruction, co-registered OCT images of the same sample was acquired. Figures 8.12(D-G) show the co-registered XZ and YZ cross-sections. Figure 8.12(H) shows 3D FLOT image of the fluorescent capillary co-registered with macroporous EH-PEG hydrogel obtained by OCT. In this experiment, we demonstrated the capability of aFLOT imaging in heterogeneous macroporous scaffolds. These results indicate that OCT/FLOT represents a promising imaging technique to quantify the depth-resolved fluorophore distribution information in engineered tissue scaffold for investigating cell-scaffold cellular and molecular interactions in situ.

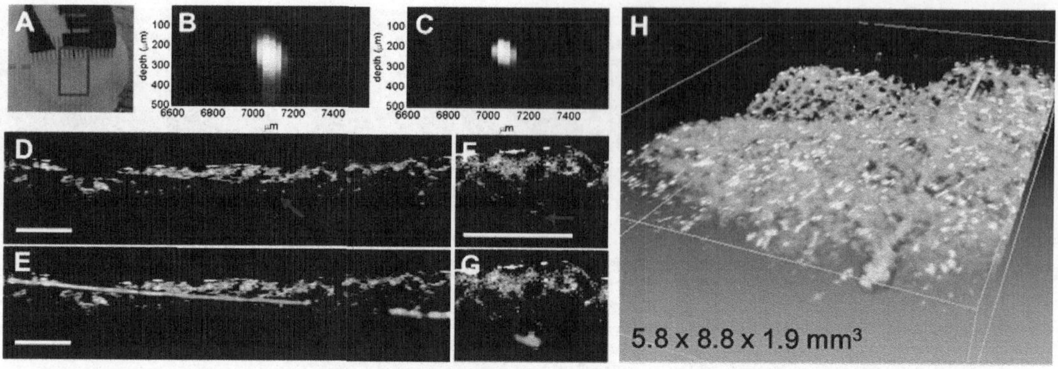

Figure 8.12: (See color insert.) (A) Photo of the macroporous EH-PEG hydrogel. A capillary tube was embedded underneath. The red quotation indicates region of interest where FLOT and OCT images were acquired. (B) Stacking representation of a YZ cross-section of the capillary. (C) FLOT reconstruction of the same cross-section. (D) XZ cross-sectional OCT image (gray colormap), where capillary tube can be visualized (arrow). (E) Co-registered OCT/FLOT image of the same cross-section. FLOT highlights the fluorescent signals in the capillary (green colormap). Scale bar: 1 mm. (F) YZ cross-sectional OCT image, where capillary tube can be visualized (arrow). (G) Co-registered OCT/FLOT image of the same cross-section. FLOT highlights the fluorescent signals in the capillary (green colormap). Scale bar: 1 mm. (H) 3D view of co-registered OCT/FLOT. Capillary tube can be visualized by FLOT while not visible in conventional microscopy (A).

8.7 Conclusion

In this chapter, we provided a summary of the instrument and algorithm for combined OCT/FLOT system for biomedical applications. Co-registered OCT morphology and FLOT molecular information can be resolved at millimeter imaging scale, which has strong potential to provide depth-resolved tissue structural and molecular imaging. This unique multi-modality platform represents a new multi-modal imaging regime that bridges the macroscopic and microscopic imaging regimes. By varying the source incidence and/or detector collection angles, angled FLOT promises to enhance the imaging resolution and depth sensitivity, especially for low-scattering medium. Examples of OCT/FLOT imaging of subsurface tumor and stem-cell-laden hydrogels are presented. OCT/FLOT could be a useful tool for investigating tissue structural and functional relationship in mesoscopic (mm) scales. Future work will focus on the utilization of OCT structural image as the a priori information to improve FLOT reconstruction, and incorporation of line-scan OCT to co-register with line-scan FLOT for endoscopic imaging.

Acknowledgment

We acknowledge Dr. David Boas from Massachusetts General Hospital (MGH) for providing the Monte Carlo simulation code (tmcimg), and Drs. Heng Lian (Nan Yang Technological University, Singapore), Quan Zhang (MGH), and Qianqian Fang (MGH) for technical assistance in modifying the code. We also acknowledge the collaboration with Dr. James Jiang and Alex Cable

(Thorlabs, Inc.) on OCT imaging, Drs. Kristine Glunde and Venu Raman (Johns Hopkins University) for breast cancer imaging, and Dr. John Fisher (University of Maryland) on tissue engineering and stem cell imaging. This work is supported in part by the Nano-Biotechnology Award of the State of Maryland, the Minta Martin Foundation, the General Research Board (GRB) Award of the University of Maryland, the University of Maryland Baltimore (UMB) and College Park (UMCP) Seed Grant Program, the Prevent Cancer Foundation, the American Society for Laser Medicine and Surgery (ASLMS)'s A. Ward Ford Memorial Institute Research Grant, the National Institutes of Health grant (R21 AR059325-01A1, R21 EB012215-01A1, R21 DK088066-01A1), and the National Science Foundation grant (CBET-1135514).

References

[1] D. Huang, E.A. Swanson, C.P. Lin, J.S. Schuman, W.G. Stinson, W. Chang, M.R. Hee, T. Flotte, K. Gregory, C.A. Puliafito, and J.G. Fujimoto, "Optical coherence tomography," *Science* **254**, 1178-1181 (1991).

[2] M.R. Hee, C.R. Baumal, C.A. Puliafito, J.S. Duker, E. Reichel, J.R. Wilkins, J.G. Coker, J.S. Schuman, E.A. Swanson, and J.G. Fujimoto, "Optical coherence tomography of age-related macular degeneration and choroidal neovascularization," *Ophthalmology* **103**, 1260-1270 (1996).

[3] I.K. Jang, B. Bouma, B. MacNeill, M. Takano, M. Shishkov, N. Iftima, and G.J. Tearney, "In-vivo coronary plaque characteristics in patients with various clinical presentations using Optical Coherence Tomography," *Circulation* **108**, 373-373 (2003).

[4] B.E. Bouma, G.J. Tearney, C.C. Compton, and N.S. Nishioka, "High-resolution imaging of the human esophagus and stomach in vivo using optical coherence tomography," *Gastrointestinal Endoscopy* **51**, 467-474 (2000).

[5] M.V. Sivak, Jr., K. Kobayashi, J.A. Izatt, A.M. Rollins, R. Ung-Runyawee, A. Chak, R.C. Wong, G.A. Isenberg, and J. Willis, "High-resolution endoscopic imaging of the GI tract using optical coherence tomography," *Gastrointestinal Endoscopy* **51**, 474-479 (2000).

[6] X.D. Li, S.A. Boppart, J. Van Dam, H. Mashimo, M. Mutinga, W. Drexler, M. Klein, C. Pitris, M.L. Krinsky, M.E. Brezinski, and J.G. Fujimoto, "Optical coherence tomography: advanced technology for the endoscopic imaging of Barrett's esophagus," *Endoscopy* **32**, 921-930 (2000).

[7] Y. Chen, A.D. Aguirre, P.L. Hsiung, S. Desai, P.R. Herz, M. Pedrosa, Q. Huang, M. Figueiredo, S.W. Huang, A. Koski, J.M. Schmitt, J.G. Fujimoto, and H. Mashimo, "Ultrahigh resolution optical coherence tomography of Barrett's esophagus: preliminary descriptive clinical study correlating images with histology," *Endoscopy* **39**, 599-605 (2007).

[8] J. Welzel, C. Reinhardt, E. Lankenau, C. Winter, and H.H. Wolff, "Changes in function and morphology of normal human skin: evaluation using optical coherence tomography," *Br J Dermatol* **150**, 220-225 (2004).

[9] L.L. Otis, M.J. Everett, U.S. Sathyam, and B.W. Colston, Jr., "Optical coherence tomography: a new imaging technology for dentistry," *The Journal of the American Dental Association* **131**, 511-514 (2000).

[10] A.V. D'Amico, M. Weinstein, X. Li, J.P. Richie, and J. Fujimoto, "Optical coherence tomography as a method for identifying benign and malignant microscopic structures in the prostate gland," *Urology* **55**, 783-787 (2000).

[11] J.G. Fujimoto, M.E. Brezinski, G.J. Tearney, S.A. Boppart, B. Bouma, M.R. Hee, J.F. Southern, and E.A. Swanson, "Optical biopsy and imaging using optical coherence tomography," *Nature Medicine* **1**, 970-972 (1995).

[12] M.E. Brezinski, G.J. Tearney, B.E. Bouma, J.A. Izatt, M.R. Hee, E.A. Swanson, J.F. Southern, and J.G. Fujimoto, "Optical coherence tomography for optical biopsy. Properties and demonstration of vascular pathology," *Circulation* **93**, 1206-1213 (1996).

[13] G.J. Tearney, M.E. Brezinski, B.E. Bouma, S.A. Boppart, C. Pitvis, J.F. Southern, and J.G. Fujimoto, "In vivo endoscopic optical biopsy with optical coherence tomography," *Science* **276**, 2037-2039 (1997).

[14] J.G. Fujimoto, C. Pitris, S.A. Boppart, and M.E. Brezinski, "Optical coherence tomography: an emerging technology for biomedical imaging and optical biopsy," *Neoplasia* **2**, 9-25 (2000).

[15] J.G. Fujimoto, "Optical coherence tomography for ultrahigh resolution in vivo imaging," *Nature Biotechnology* **21**, 1361-1367 (2003).

[16] B.E. Bouma, S.H. Yun, B.J. Vakoc, M.J. Suter, and G.J. Tearney, "Fourier-domain optical coherence tomography: recent advances toward clinical utility," *Curr Opin Biotechnol* **20**, 111-118 (2009).

[17] Z. Chen, T.E. Milner, S. Srinivas, X. Wang, A. Malekafzali, M.J.C. van Gemert, and J.S. Nelson, "Noninvasive imaging of in vivo blood flow velocity using optical Doppler tomography," *Optics Letters* **22**, 1119-1121 (1997).

[18] J.A. Izatt, M.D. Kulkami, S. Yazdanfar, J.K. Barton, and A.J. Welch, "In vivo bidirectional color Doppler flow imaging of picoliter blood volumes using optical coherence tomography," *Optics Letters* **22**, 1439-1441 (1997).

[19] Y. Zhao, Z. Chen, C. Saxer, S. Xiang, J.F. de Boer, and J.S. Nelson, "Phase-resolved optical coherence tomography and optical Doppler tomography for imaging blood flow in human skin with fast scanning speed and high velocity sensitivity," *Optics Letters* **25**, 114-116 (2000).

[20] V.X.D. Yang, M.L. Gordon, E. Seng-Yue, S. Lo, B. Qi, J. Pekar, A. Mok, B.C. Wilson, and I.A. Vitkin, "High speed, wide velocity dynamic range Doppler optical coherence tomography (Part II): imaging in vivo cardiac dynamics of Xenopus laevis," *Optics Express* **11** (2003).

[21] J.F. De Boer, T.E. Milner, M.J.C. van Gemert, and J.S. Nelson, "Two-dimensional birefringence imaging in biological tissue by polarization-sensitive optical coherence tomography," *Optics Letters* **22**, 934-936 (1997).

[22] C.K. Hitzenberger, E. Gotzinger, M. Sticker, M. Pircher, and A.F. Fercher, "Measurement and imaging of birefringence and optic axis orientation by phase resolved polarization sensitive optical coherence tomography," *Optics Express* **9** (2001).

[23] S. Jiao and L.V. Wang, "Two-dimensional depth-resolved Mueller matrix of biological tissue measured with double-beam polarization-sensitive optical coherence tomography," *Optics Letters* **27**, 101-103 (2002).

[24] B. Cense, H.C. Chen, B.H. Park, M.C. Pierce, and J.F. de Boer, "In vivo birefringence and thickness measurements of the human retinal nerve fiber layer using polarization-sensitive optical coherence tomography," *Journal of Biomedical Optics* **9**, 121-125 (2004).

[25] Y. Yasuno, S. Makita, T. Endo, M. Itoh, T. Yatagai, M. Takahashi, C. Katada, and M. Mutoh, "Polarization-sensitive complex Fourier domain optical coherence tomography for jones matrix imaging of biological samples," *Applied Physics Letters* **85**, 3023-3025 (2004).

[26] S.A. Boppart, A.L. Oldenburg, C.Y. Xu, and D.L. Marks, "Optical probes and techniques for molecular contrast enhancement in coherence imaging," *Journal of Biomedical Optics* **10**, - (2005).

[27] A.L. Oldenburg, M.N. Hansen, D.A. Zweifel, A. Wei, and S.A. Boppart, "Plasmon-resonant gold nanorods as low backscattering albedo contrast agents for optical coherence tomography," *Optics Express* **14**, 6724-6738 (2006).

[28] A.L. Oldenburg, J.R. Gunther, and S.A. Boppart, "Imaging magnetically labeled cells with magnetomotive optical coherence tomography," *Optics Letters* **30**, 747-749 (2005).

[29] A. Agrawal, S. Huang, A.W.H. Lin, M.H. Lee, J.K. Barton, R.A. Drezek, and T.J. Pfefer, "Quantitative evaluation of optical coherence tomography signal enhancement with gold nanoshells," *Journal of Biomedical Optics* **11**, 041121 (2006).

[30] T.S. Troutman, J.K. Barton, and M. Romanowski, "Optical coherence tomography with plasmon resonant nanorods of gold," *Optics Letters* **32**, 1438-1440 (2007).

[31] D.C. Adler, S.W. Huang, R. Huber, and J.G. Fujimoto, "Photothermal detection of gold nanoparticles using phase-sensitive optical coherence tomography," *Opt Express* **16**, 4376-4393 (2008).

[32] M.C. Skala, M.J. Crow, A. Wax, and J.A. Izatt, "Photothermal Optical Coherence Tomography of Epidermal Growth Factor Receptor in Live Cells Using Immunotargeted Gold Nanospheres," *Nano Letters* **8**, 3461-3467 (2008).

[33] E.V. Zagaynova, M.V. Shirmanova, M.Y. Kirillin, B.N. Khlebtsov, A.G. Orlova, I.V. Balalaeva, M.A. Sirotkina, M.L. Bugrova, P.D. Agrba, and V.A. Kamensky, "Contrasting properties of gold nanoparticles for optical coherence tomography: phantom, in vivo studies and Monte Carlo simulation," *Physics in Medicine and Biology* **53**, 4995-5009 (2008).

[34] J.C.Y. Kah, T.H. Chow, B.K. Ng, S.G. Razul, M. Olivo, and C.J.R. Sheppard, "Concentration dependence of gold nanoshells on the enhancement of optical coherence tomography images: a quantitative study," *Applied Optics* **48**, D96-D108 (2009).

[35] M. Kirillin, M. Shirmanova, M. Sirotkina, M. Bugrova, B. Khlebtsov, and E. Zagaynova, "Contrasting properties of gold nanoshells and titanium dioxide nanoparticles for optical coherence tomography imaging of skin: Monte Carlo simulations and in vivo study," *Journal of Biomedical Optics* **14**, 021017 (2009).

[36] H. Cang, T. Sun, Z.Y. Li, J.Y. Chen, B.J. Wiley, Y.N. Xia, and X.D. Li, "Gold nanocages as contrast agents for spectroscopic optical coherence tomography," *Optics Letters* **30**, 3048-3050 (2005).

[37] K.D. Rao, M.A. Choma, S. Yazdanfar, A.M. Rollins, and J.A. Izatt, "Molecular contrast in optical coherence tomography by use of a pump-probe technique," *Optics Letters* **28**, 340-342 (2003).

[38] C.H. Yang, M.A. Choma, L.E. Lamb, J.D. Simon, and J.A. Izatt, "Protein-based molecular contrast optical coherence tomography with phytochrome as the contrast agent," *Optics Letters* **29**, 1396-1398 (2004).

[39] C.H. Yang, L.E.L. McGuckin, J.D. Simon, M.A. Choma, B.E. Applegate, and J.A. Izatt, "Spectral triangulation molecular contrast optical coherence tomography with indocyanine green as the contrast agent," *Optics Letters* **29**, 2016-2018 (2004).

[40] C.H. Yang, "Molecular contrast optical coherence tomography: A review," *Photochemistry and Photobiology* **81**, 215-237 (2005).

[41] B.E. Applegate and J.A. Izatt, "Molecular imaging of endogenous and exogenous chromophores using ground state recovery pump-probe optical coherence tomography," *Optics Express* **14**, 9142-9155 (2006).

[42] A. Bilenca, J. Cao, M. Colice, A. Ozcan, B. Bouma, L. Raftery, and G. Tearney, "Fluorescence interferometry - Principles and applications in biology," *Fluorescence Methods and Applications: Spectroscopy, Imaging, and Probes* **1130**, 68-77 (2008).

[43] A. Bilenca, T. Lasser, A. Ozcan, R.A. Leitgeb, B.E. Bouma, and G.J. Tearney, "Image formation in fluorescence coherence-gated imaging through scattering media," *Optics Express* **15**, 2810-2821 (2007).

[44] A. Bilenca, A. Ozcan, B. Bouma, and G. Tearney, "Fluorescence coherence tomography," *Optics Express* **14**, 7134-7143 (2006).

[45] B.E. Applegate, C. Yang, A.M. Rollins, and J.A. Izatt, "Polarization-resolved second-harmonic-generation optical coherence tomography in collagen," *Optics Letters* **29**, 2252-2254 (2004).

[46] Y. Jiang, I. Tomov, Y.M. Wang, and Z.P. Chen, "Second-harmonic optical coherence tomography," *Optics Letters* **29**, 1090-1092 (2004).

[47] Y. Jiang, I.V. Tomov, Y. Wang, and Z. Chen, "High-resolution second-harmonic optical coherence tomography of collagen in rat-tail tendon," *Applied Physics Letters* **86**, 133901 (2005).

[48] C. Vinegoni, J.S. Bredfeldt, D.L. Marks, and S.A. Boppart, "Nonlinear optical contrast enhancement for optical coherence tomography," *Optics Express* **12**, 331-341 (2004).

[49] D.L. Marks and S.A. Boppart, "Nonlinear interferometric vibrational imaging," *Physical Review Letters* **92**, 123905 (2004).

[50] Y.T. Pan, T.Q. Xie, C.W. Du, S. Bastacky, S. Meyers, and M.L. Zeidel, "Enhancing early bladder cancer detection with fluorescence-guided endoscopic optical coherence tomography," *Optics Letters* **28**, 2485-2487 (2003).

[51] Z.G. Wang, D.B. Durand, M. Schoenberg, and Y.T. Pan, "Fluorescence guided optical coherence tomography for the diagnosis of early bladder cancer in a rat model," *Journal of Urology* **174**, 2376-2381 (2005).

[52] A.R. Tumlinson, L.P. Hariri, U. Utzinger, and J.K. Barton, "Miniature endoscope for simultaneous optical coherence tomography and laser-induced fluorescence measurement," *Applied Optics* **43**, 113-121 (2004).

[53] J.B. McNally, N.D. Kirkpatrick, L.P. Hariri, A.R. Tumlinson, D.G. Besselsen, E.W. Gerner, U. Utzinger, and J.K. Barton, "Task-based imaging of colon cancer in the Apc(Min/+) mouse model," *Applied Optics* **45**, 3049-3062 (2006).

[54] A. Dunn and D. Boas, "Transport-based image reconstruction in turbid media with small source-detector separations," *Optics Letters* **25**, 1777-1779 (2000).

[55] E.M. Hillman, D.A. Boas, A.M. Dale, and A.K. Dunn, "Laminar optical tomography: demonstration of millimeter-scale depth-resolved imaging in turbid media," *Opt Lett* **29**, 1650-1652 (2004).

[56] E.M.C. Hillman and S.A. Burgess, "Sub-millimeter resolution 3D optical imaging of living tissue using laminar optical tomography," *Laser & Photonics Reviews* **3**, 159-179 (2009).

[57] E.M. Hillman, A. Devor, M.B. Bouchard, A.K. Dunn, G.W. Krauss, J. Skoch, B.J. Bacskai, A.M. Dale, and D.A. Boas, "Depth-resolved optical imaging and microscopy of vascular compartment dynamics during somatosensory stimulation," *Neuroimage* **35**, 89-104 (2007).

[58] B.H. Yuan, "Radiative transport in the Delta-P1 approximation for laminar optical tomography," *Journal of Innovative Optical Health Sciences* **2**, 149-163 (2009).

[59] S.A. Burgess, M.B. Bouchard, B.H. Yuan, and E.M.C. Hillman, "Simultaneous multiwavelength laminar optical tomography," *Optics Letters* **33**, 2710-2712 (2008).

[60] N. Ouakli, E. Guevara, S. Dubeau, E. Beaumont, and F. Lesage, "Laminar optical tomography of the hemodynamic response in the lumbar spinal cord of rats," *Opt. Express* **18**, 10068-10077 (2010).

[61] E.M.C. Hillman, O. Bernus, E. Pease, M.B. Bouchard, and A. Pertsov, "Depth-resolved optical imaging of transmural electrical propagation in perfused heart," *Opt. Express* **15**, 17827-17841 (2007).

[62] B.H. Yuan, S.A. Burgess, A. Iranmahboob, M.B. Bouchard, N. Lehrer, C. Bordier, and E.M.C. Hillman, "A system for high-resolution depth-resolved optical imaging of fluorescence and absorption contrast," *Review of Scientific Instruments* **80**, 043706 (2009).

[63] P.M. Andrews, Y. Chen, M.L. Onozato, S.W. Huang, D.C. Adler, R.A. Huber, J. Jiang, S.E. Barry, A.E. Cable, and J.G. Fujimoto, "High-resolution optical coherence tomography imaging of the living kidney," *Lab Invest* **88**, 441-449 (2008).

[64] Y. Chen, S. Yuan, J. Wierwille, R. Naphas, Q. Li, T.R. Blackwell, P.T.W. Jr., V. Raman, and K. Glunde, "Integrated optical coherence tomography (OCT) and fluorescence laminar optical tomography (FLOT)," *IEEE Journal of Selected Topics in Quantum Electronics* **16**, 755-766 (2010).

[65] S.R. Arridge, "Optical tomography in medical imaging," *Inverse Problems* **15**, R41-R93 (1999).

[66] R.J. Crilly, W.F. Cheong, B. Wilson, and J.R. Spears, "Forward-adjoint fluorescence model: Monte Carlo integration and experimental validation," *Applied Optics* **36**, 6513-6519 (1997).

[67] A.C. Kak, M. Slaney, and IEEE Engineering in Medicine and Biology Society, *Principles of computerized tomographic imaging*. New York: IEEE Press, 1987.

[68] N.C. Shaner, R.E. Campbell, P.A. Steinbach, B.N. Giepmans, A.E. Palmer, and R.Y. Tsien, "Improved monomeric red, orange and yellow fluorescent proteins derived from Discosoma sp. red fluorescent protein," *Nat Biotechnol* **22**, 1567-1572 (2004).

[69] P.T. Winnard, Jr., J.B. Kluth, and V. Raman, "Noninvasive optical tracking of red fluorescent protein-expressing cancer cells in a model of metastatic breast cancer," *Neoplasia* **8**, 796-806 (2006).

[70] K. Glunde, C.A. Foss, T. Takagi, F. Wildes, and Z.M. Bhujwalla, "Synthesis of 6'-O-lissamine-rhodamine B-glucosamine as a novel probe for fluorescence imaging of lysosomes in breast tumors," *Bioconjug Chem* **16**, 843-851 (2005).

[71] C.W. Chen and Y. Chen, "Optimization of Design Parameters for Fluorescence Laminar Optical Tomography," *Journal of Innovation in Optical Health Sciences* **4**, 309-323 (2011).

[72] C.F. Zhu, Q. Liu, and N. Ramanujam, "Effect of fiber optic probe geometry on depth-resolved fluorescence measurements from epithelial tissues: a Monte Carlo simulation," *Journal of Biomedical Optics* **8**, 237-247 (2003).

[73] T.J. Pfefer, A. Agrawal, and R.A. Drezek, "Oblique-incidence illumination and collection for depth-selective fluorescence spectroscopy," *Journal of Biomedical Optics* **10**, 044016 (2005).

[74] L. Nieman, A. Myakov, J. Aaron, and K. Sokolov, "Optical sectioning using a fiber probe with an angled illumination-collection geometry: evaluation in engineered tissue phantoms," *Applied Optics* **43**, 1308-1319 (2004).

[75] Q. Liu and N. Ramanujam, "Experimental proof of the feasibility of using an angled fiber-optic probe for depth-sensitive fluorescence spectroscopy of turbid media," *Opt Lett* **29**, 2034-2036 (2004).

[76] M.C. Skala, G.M. Palmer, C.F. Zhu, Q. Liu, K.M. Vrotsos, C.L. Marshek-Stone, A. Gendron-Fitzpatrick, and N. Ramanujam, "Investigation of fiber-optic probe designs for optical spectroscopic diagnosis of epithelial pre-cancers," *Lasers in Surgery and Medicine* **34**, 25-38 (2004).

[77] J.P. Culver, V. Ntziachristos, M.J. Holboke, and A.G. Yodh, "Optimization of optode arrangements for diffuse optical tomography: A singular-value analysis," *Optics Letters* **26**, 701-703 (2001).

[78] E.E. Graves, J.P. Culver, J. Ripoll, R. Weissleder, and V. Ntziachristos, "Singular-value analysis and optimization of experimental parameters in fluorescence molecular tomography," *Journal of the Optical Society of America a-Optics Image Science and Vision* **21**, 231-241 (2004).

[79] A.A. Tanbakuchi, A.R. Rouse, and A.F. Gmitro, "Monte Carlo characterization of parallelized fluorescence confocal systems imaging in turbid media," *J Biomed Opt* **14**, 044024 (2009).

[80] L. Wang and S.L. Jacques, "Use of a laser beam with an oblique angle of incidence to measure the reduced scattering coefficient of a turbid medium," *Appl Opt* **34**, 2362-2366 (1995).

[81] P. Thevenot, A. Nair, J. Dey, J. Yang, and L. Tang, "Method to analyze three-dimensional cell distribution and infiltration in degradable scaffolds," *Tissue Eng Part C Methods* **14**, 319-331 (2008).

[82] M.W. Betz, P.C. Modi, J.F. Caccamese, D.P. Coletti, J.J. Sauk, and J.P. Fisher, "Cyclic acetal hydrogel system for bone marrow stromal cell encapsulation and osteodifferentiation," *Journal of Biomedical Materials Research Part A* **86A**, 662-670 (2008).

[83] M.W. Betz, A.B. Yeatts, W.J. Richbourg, J.F. Caccamese, D.P. Coletti, E.E. Falco, and J.P. Fisher, "Macroporous hydrogels upregulate osteogenic signal expression and promote bone regeneration," *Biomacromolecules* **11**, 1160-1168 (2010).

[84] C.W. Chen, M.W. Betz, J.P. Fisher, A. Paek, and Y. Chen, "Macroporous hydrogel scaffolds and their characterization by optical coherence tomography," *Tissue Engineering: Part C* **17**, 101-112 (2011)

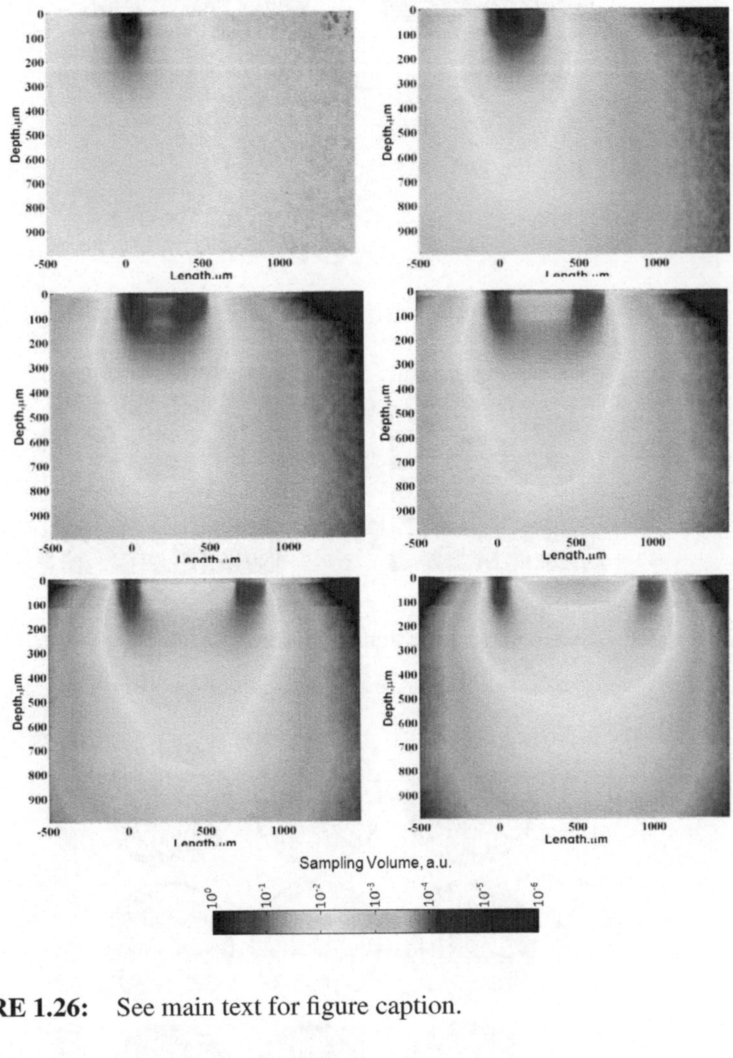

FIGURE 1.26: See main text for figure caption.

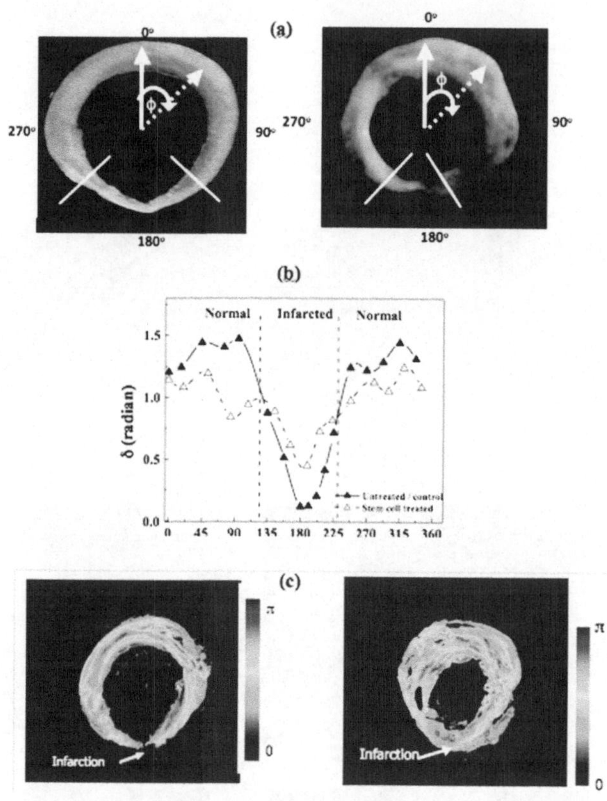

FIGURE 2.9: See main text for figure caption.

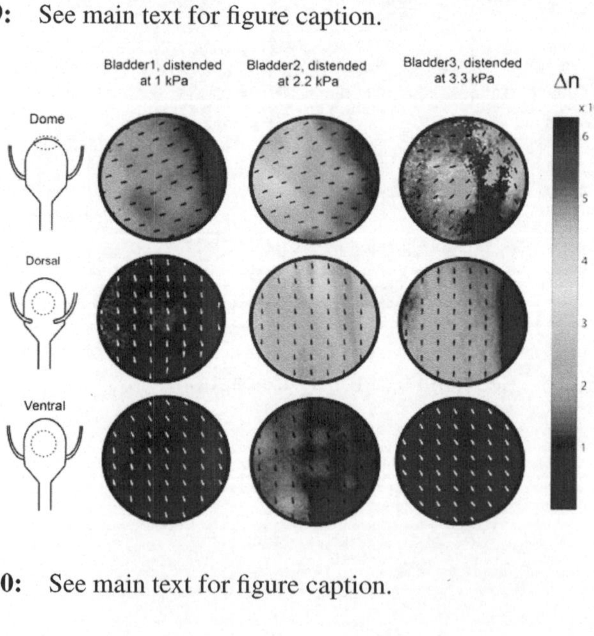

FIGURE 2.10: See main text for figure caption.

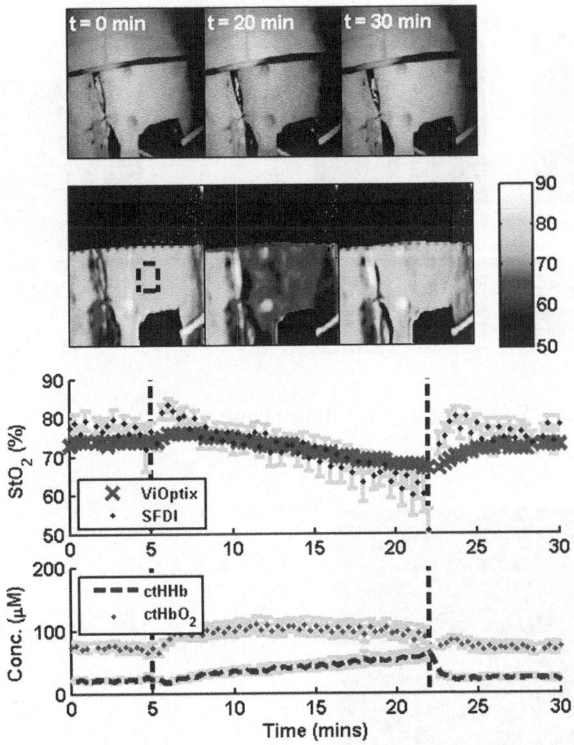

FIGURE 3.7: See main text for figure caption.

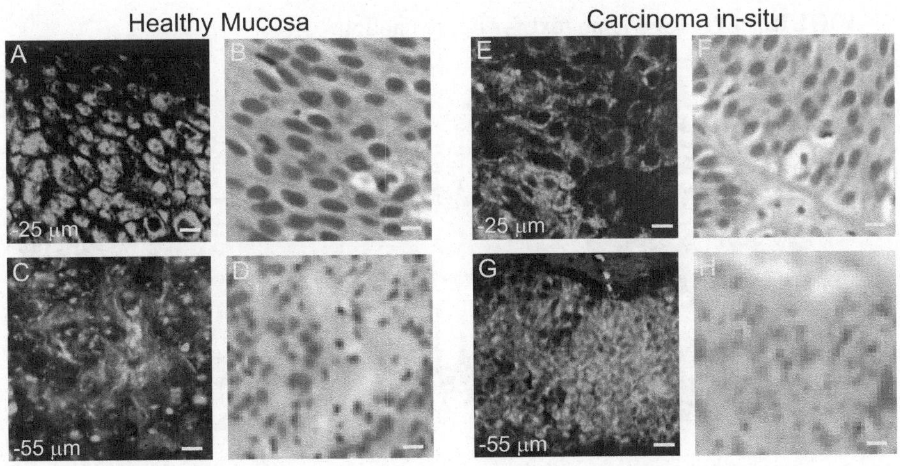

FIGURE 4.4: See main text for figure caption.

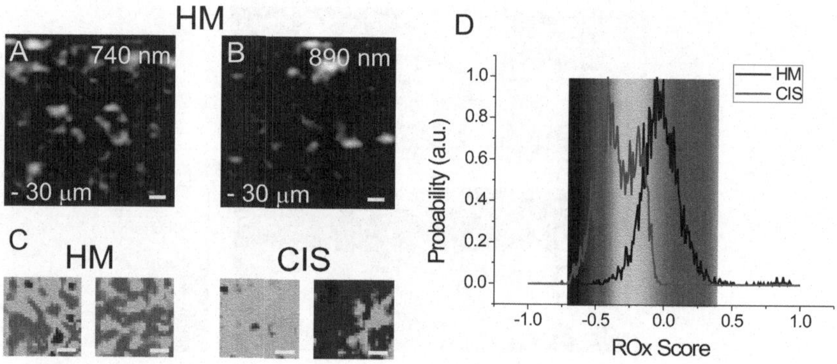

FIGURE 4.6: See main text for figure caption.

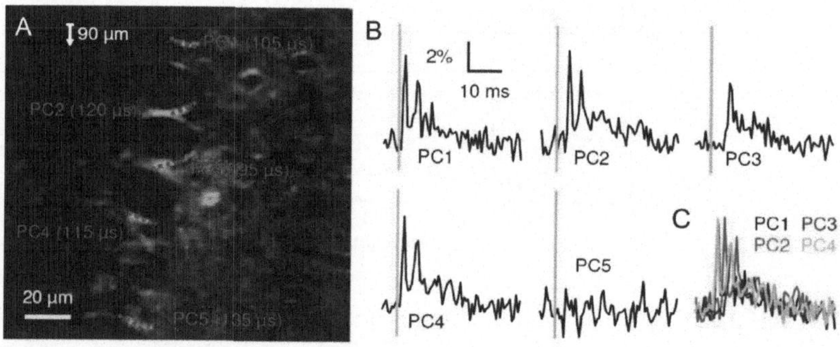

FIGURE 4.7: See main text for figure caption.

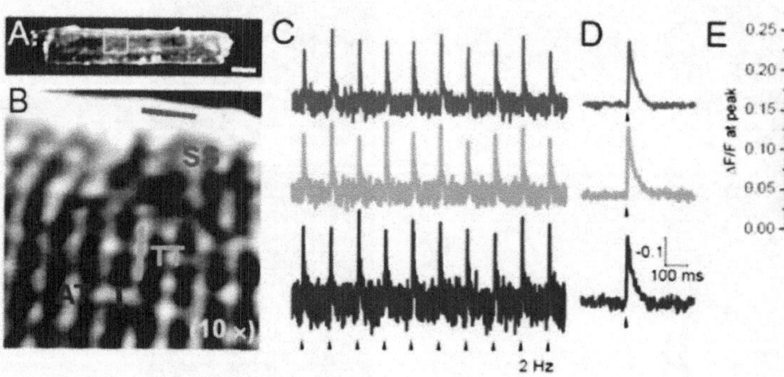

FIGURE 4.8: See main text for figure caption.

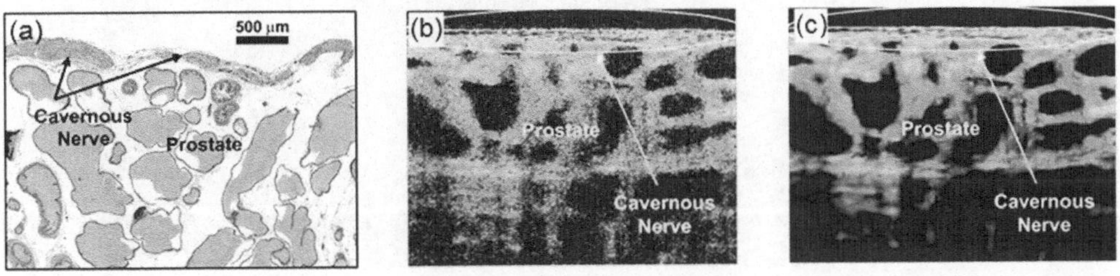

FIGURE 6.35: See main text for figure caption.

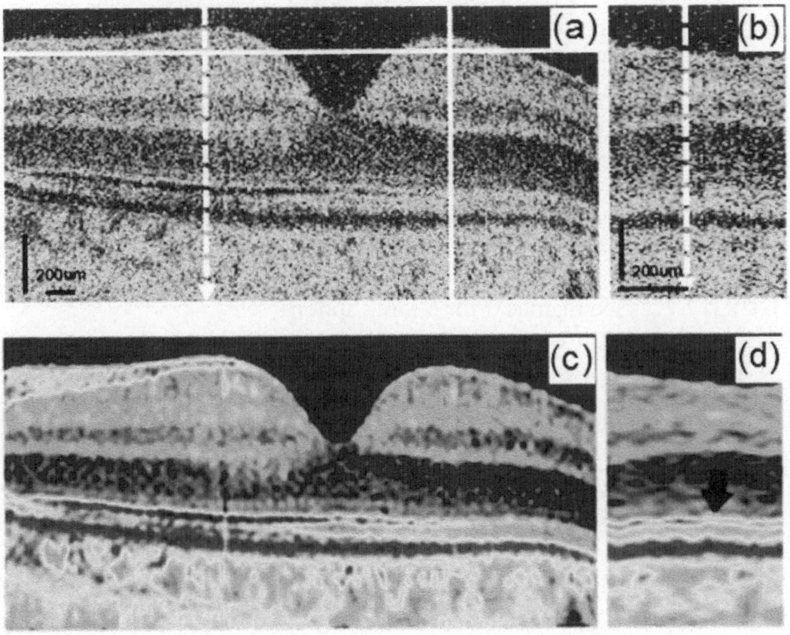

FIGURE 6.36: Acquired cross-sectional retinal images: (a) before; (b) after 3D curvelet denoising. Adapted from [123] with permission.

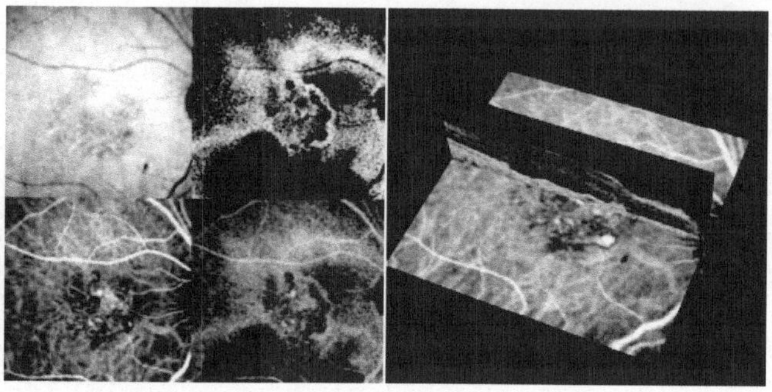

FIGURE 7.6: See main text for figure caption.

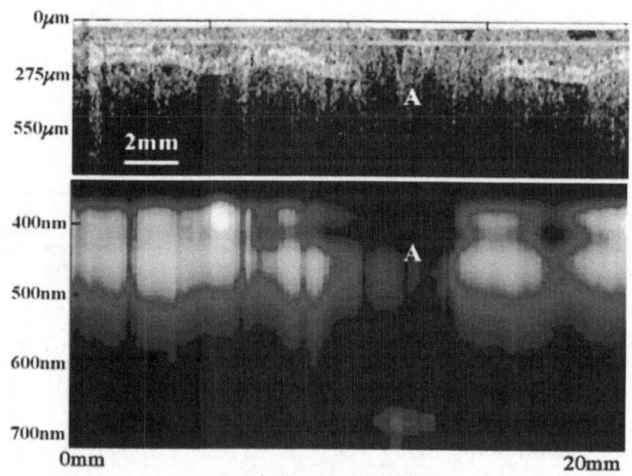

FIGURE 7.7: See main text for figure caption.

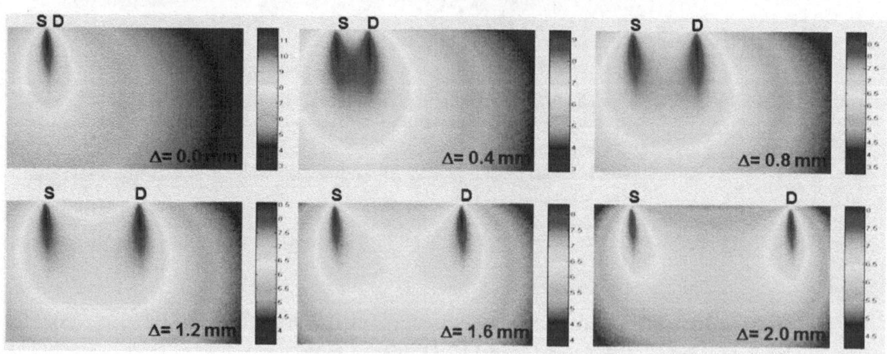

FIGURE 8.2: See main text for figure caption.

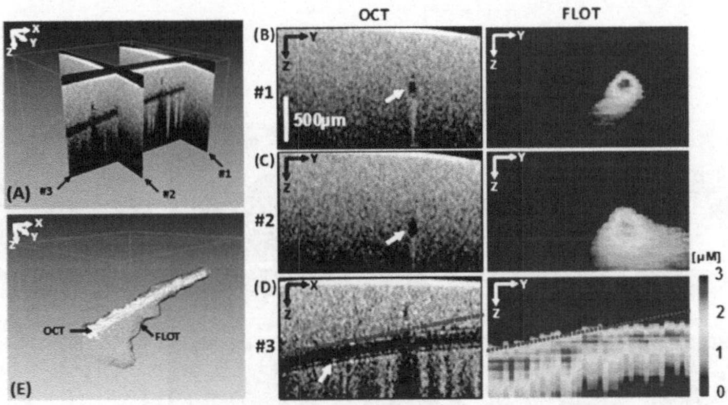

FIGURE 8.3: See main text for figure caption.

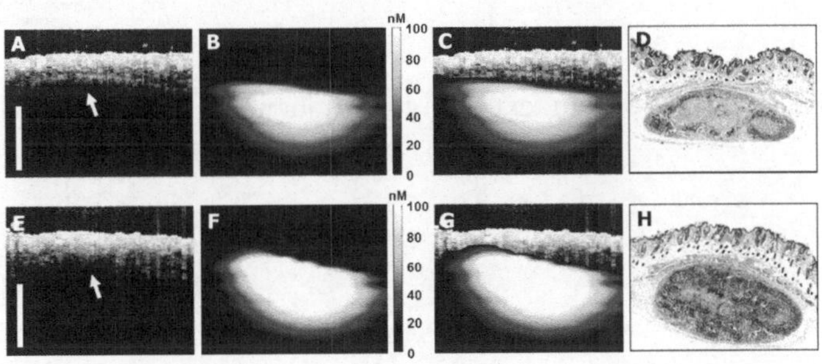

FIGURE 8.4: See main text for figure caption.

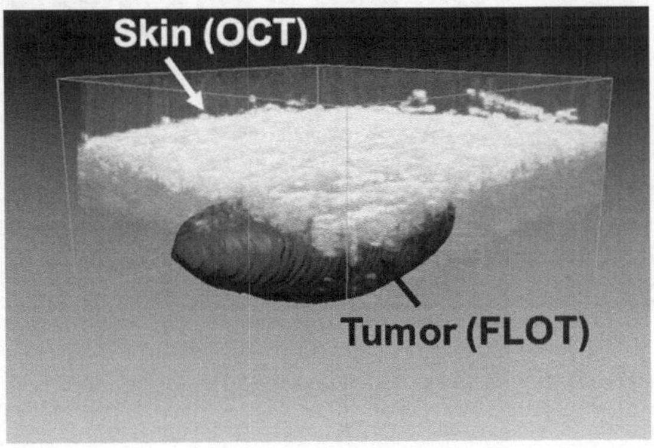

FIGURE 8.5: See main text for figure caption.

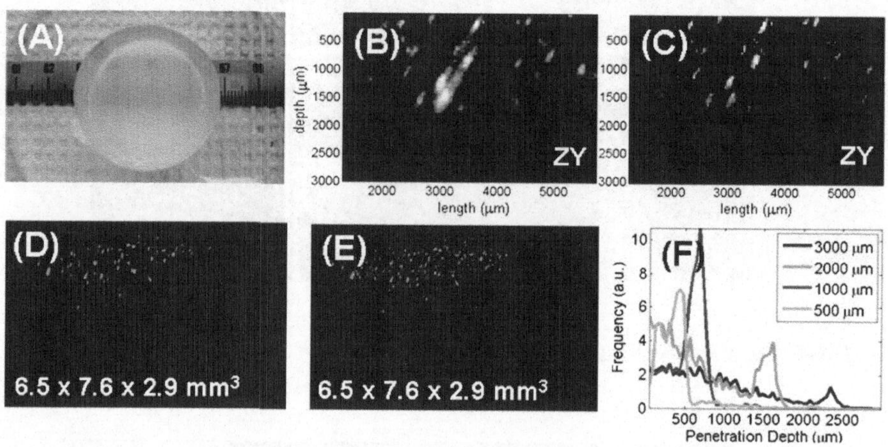

FIGURE 8.11: See main text for figure caption.

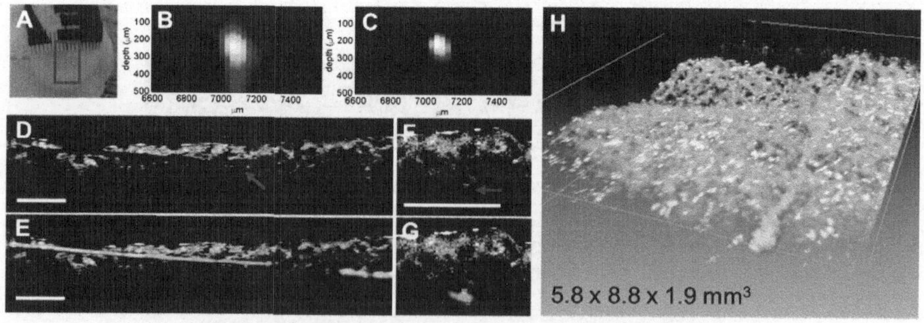

FIGURE 8.12: See main text for figure caption.

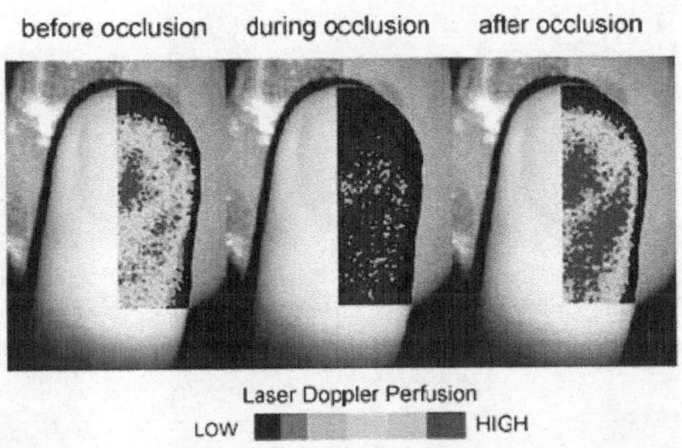

FIGURE 9.6: See main text for figure caption.

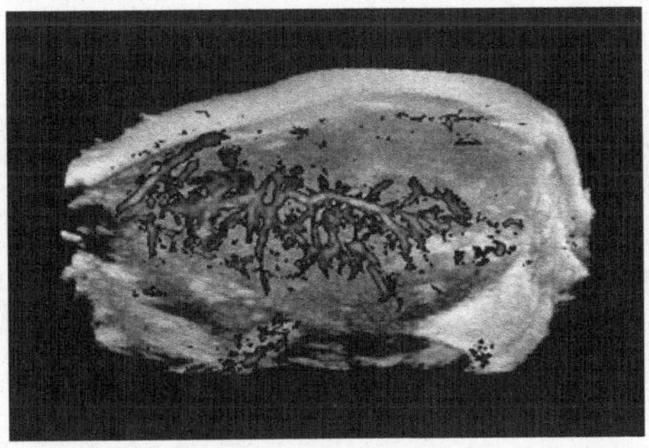

FIGURE 9.11: See main text for figure caption.

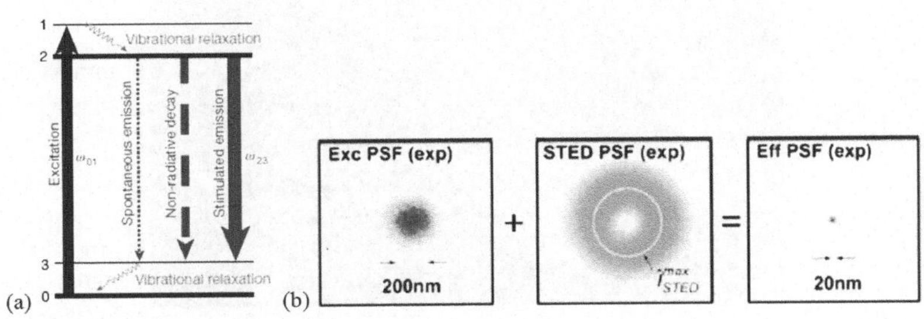

FIGURE 9.16: See main text for figure caption.

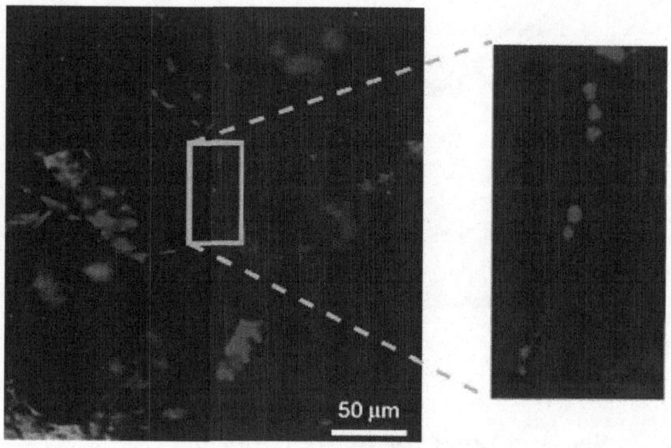

FIGURE 9.17: See main text for figure caption.

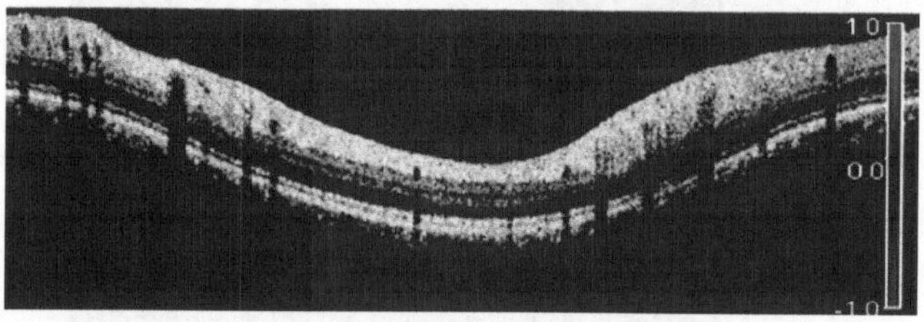

FIGURE 9.24: See main text for figure caption.

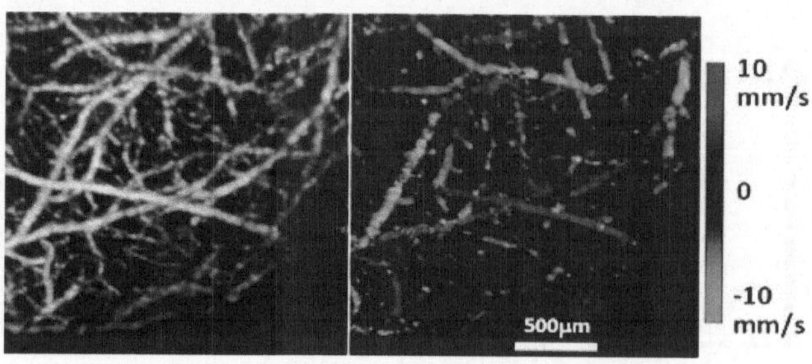

FIGURE 9.26: See main text for figure caption.

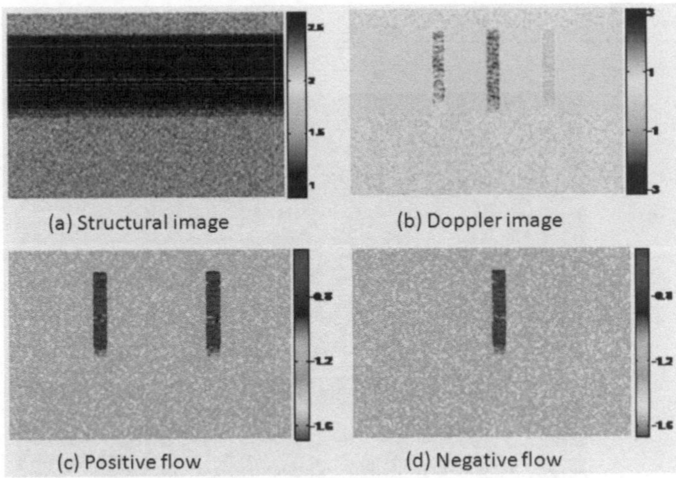

FIGURE 10.4: See main text for figure caption.

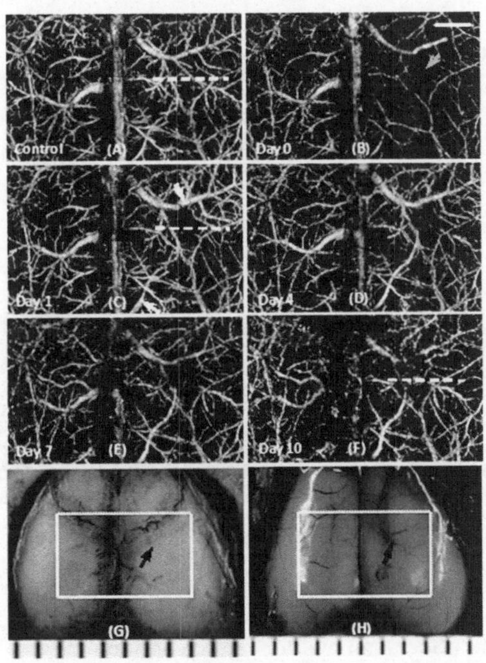

FIGURE 10.9: See main text for figure caption.

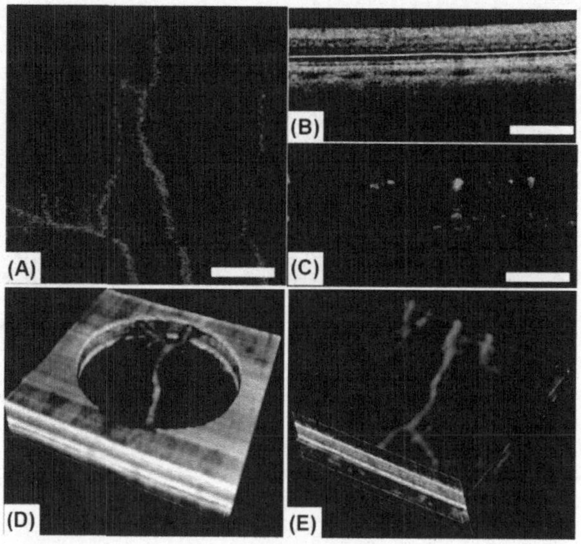

FIGURE 10.11: See main text for figure caption.

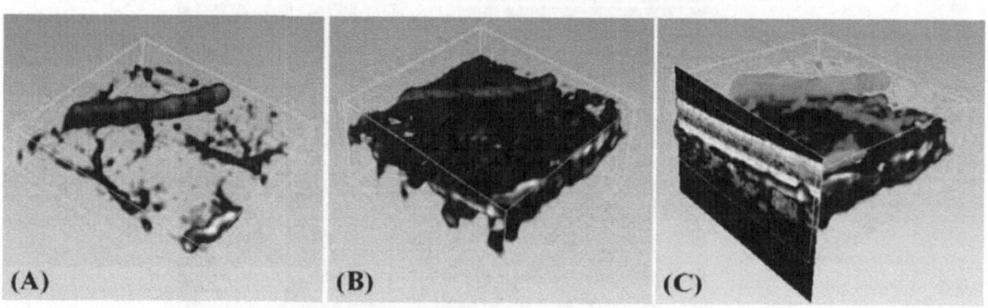

FIGURE 10.12: See main text for figure caption.

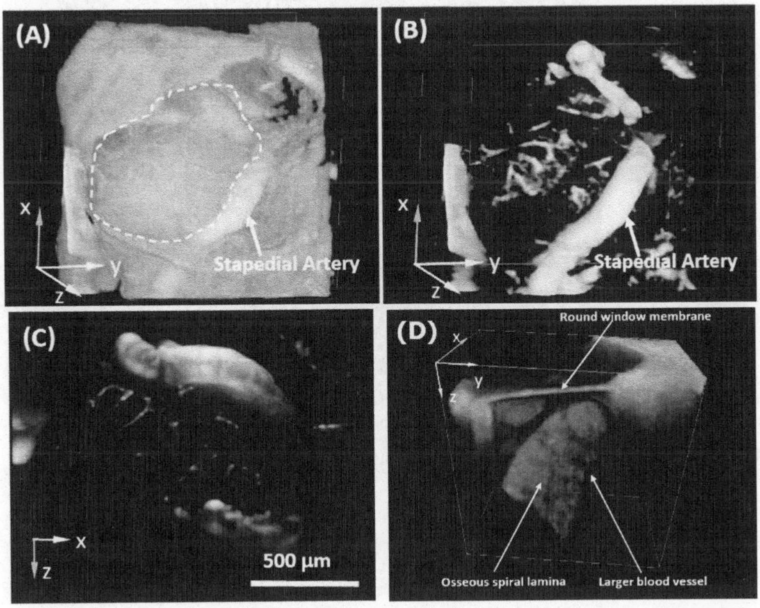

FIGURE 10.14: See main text for figure caption.

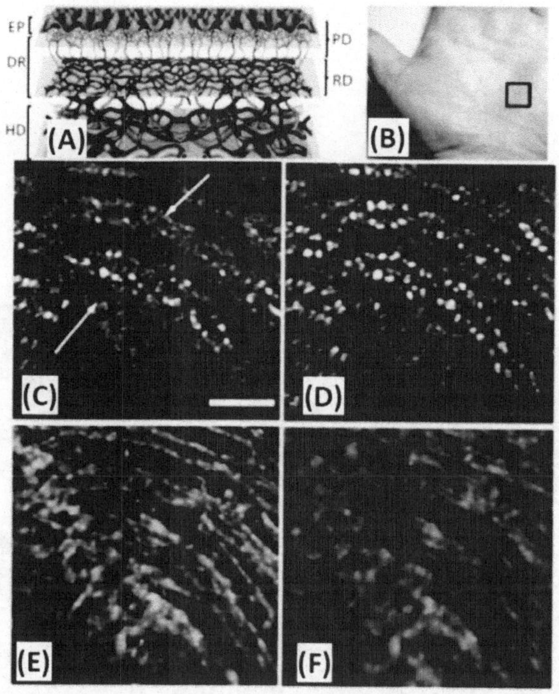

FIGURE 10.16: See main text for figure caption.

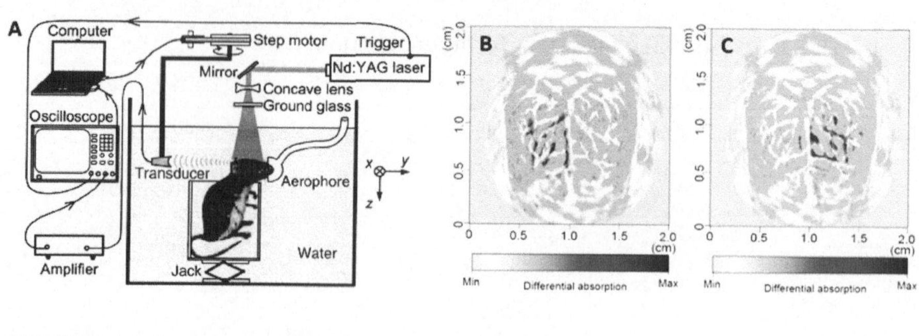

FIGURE 11.1: See main text for figure caption.

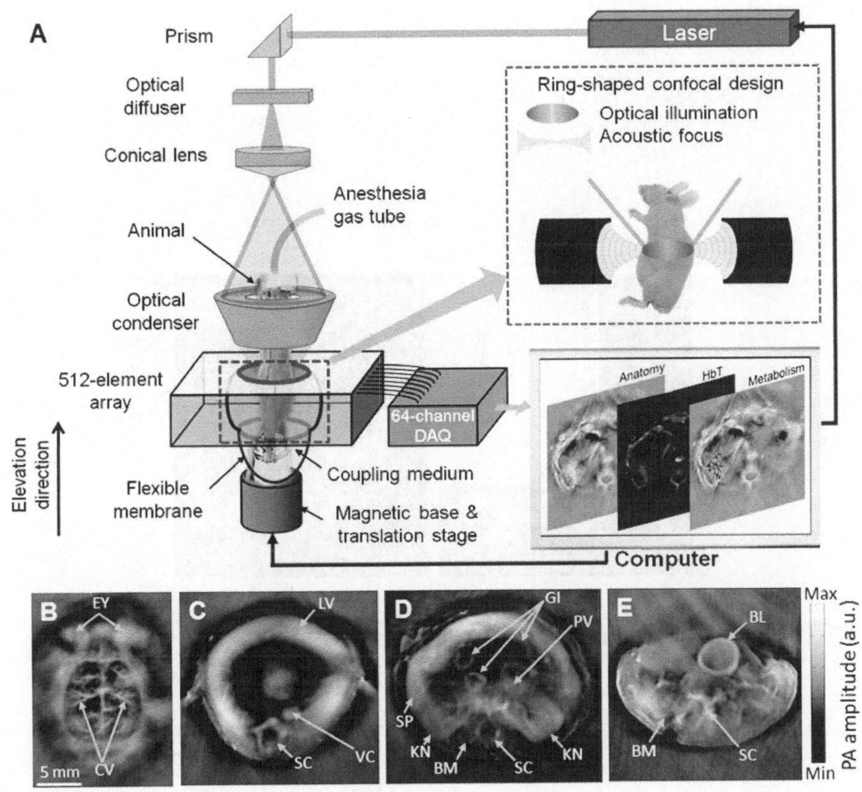

FIGURE 11.4: See main text for figure caption.

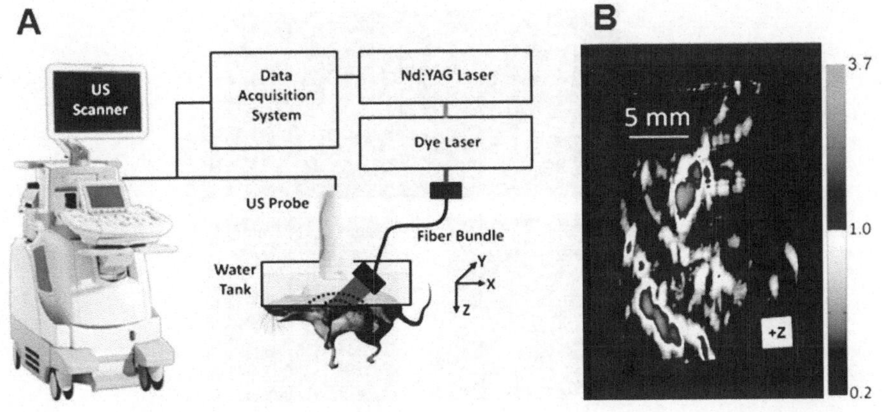

FIGURE 11.6: See main text for figure caption.

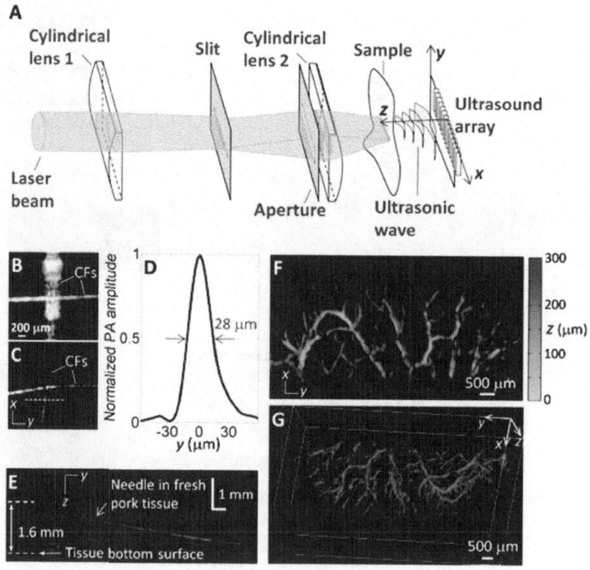

FIGURE 11.9: See main text for figure caption.

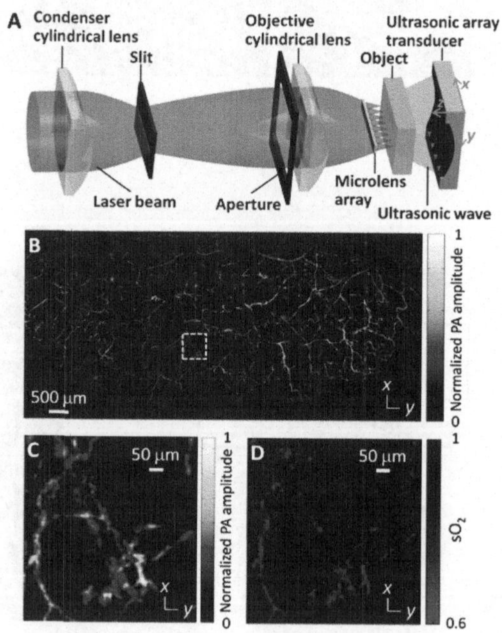

FIGURE 11.10: See main text for figure caption.

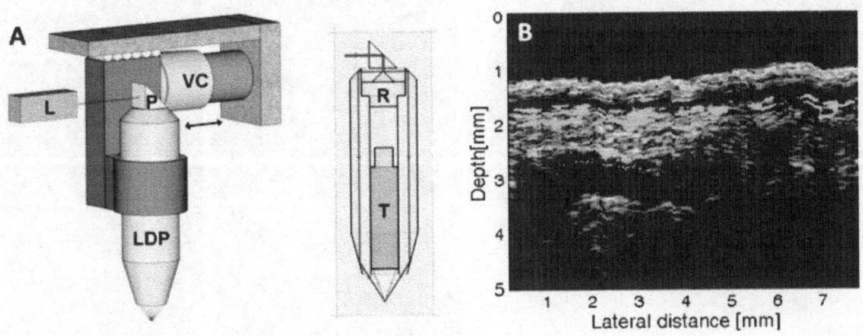

FIGURE 11.11: See main text for figure caption.

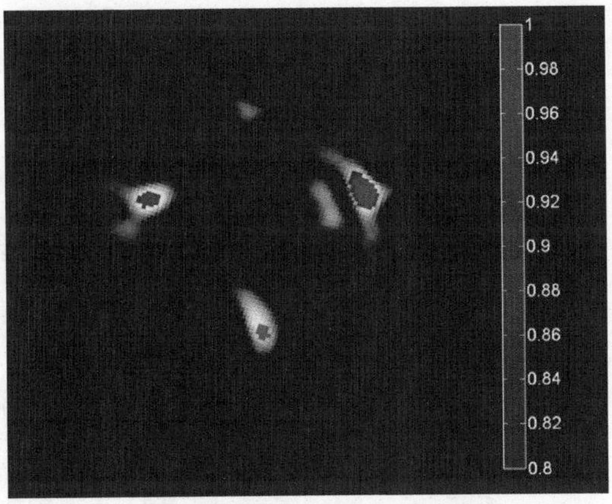

FIGURE 12.7: See main text for figure caption.

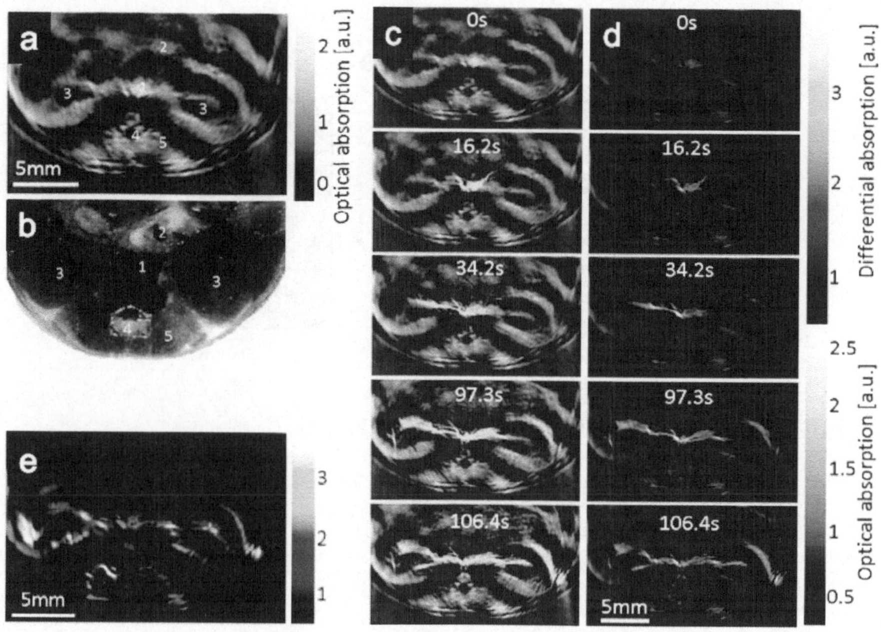

FIGURE 12.13: See main text for figure caption.

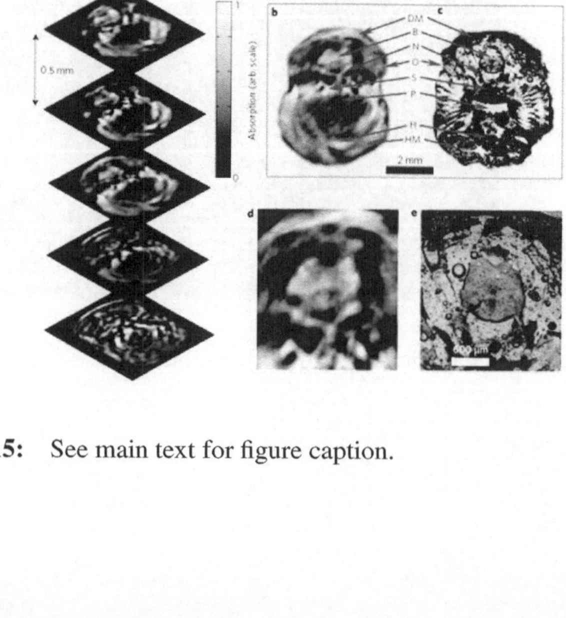

FIGURE 12.15: See main text for figure caption.

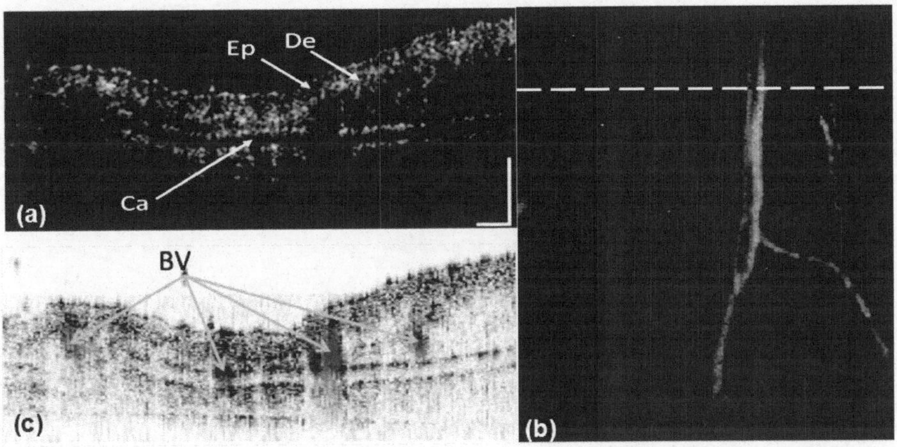

FIGURE 13.5: See main text for figure caption.

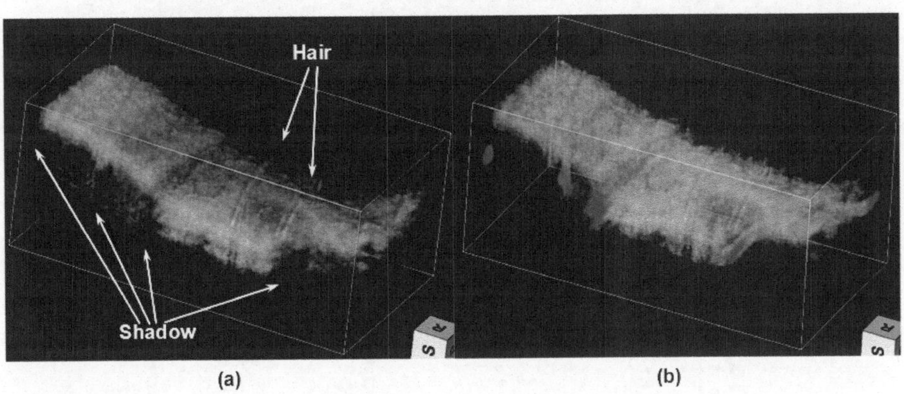

FIGURE 13.6: See main text for figure caption.

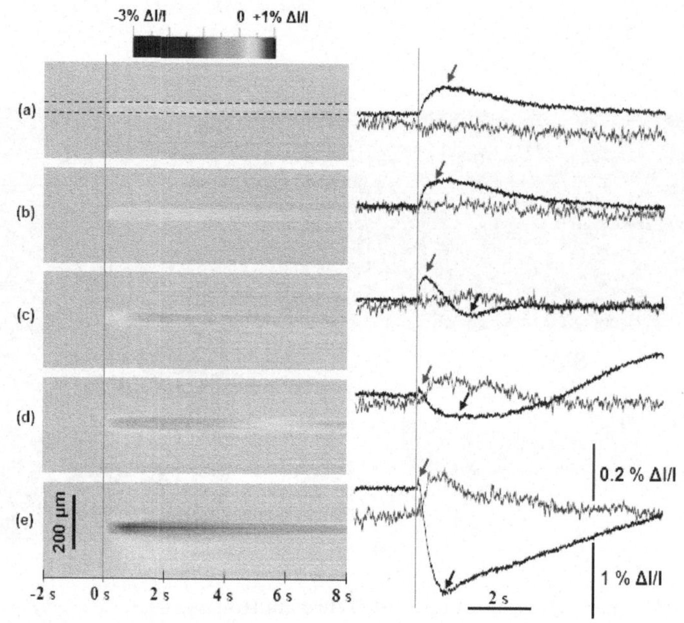

FIGURE 15.5: See main text for figure caption.

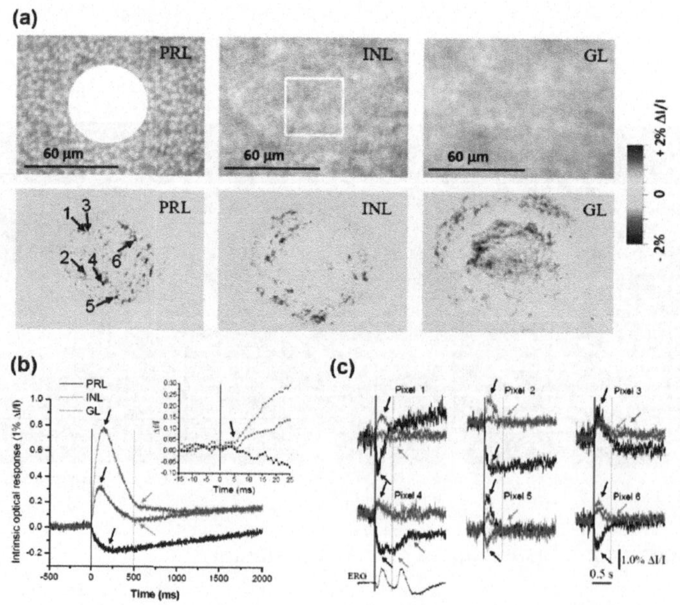

FIGURE 15.6: See main text for figure caption.

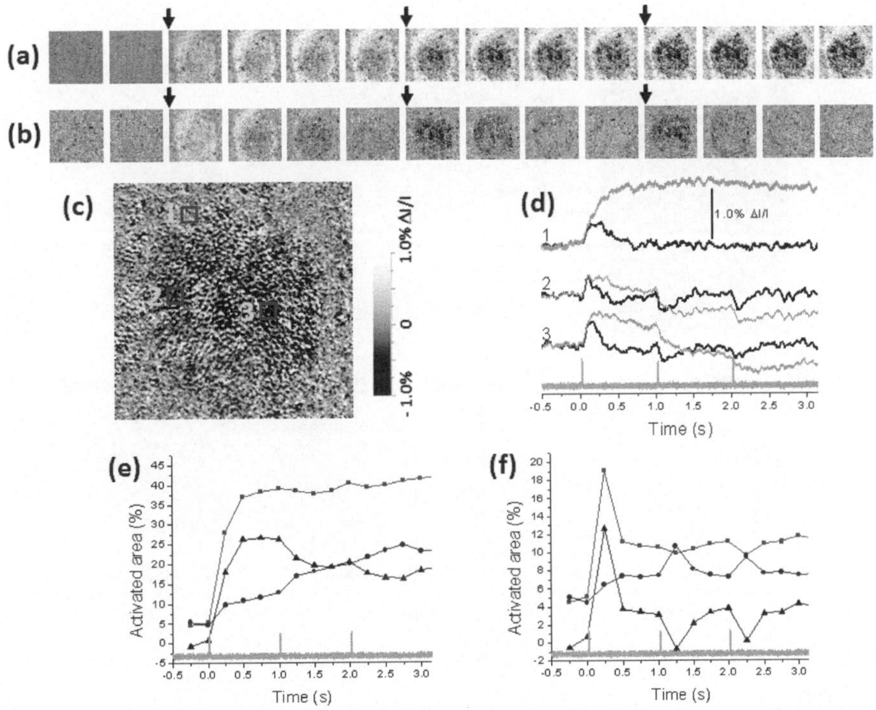

FIGURE 15.7: See main text for figure caption.

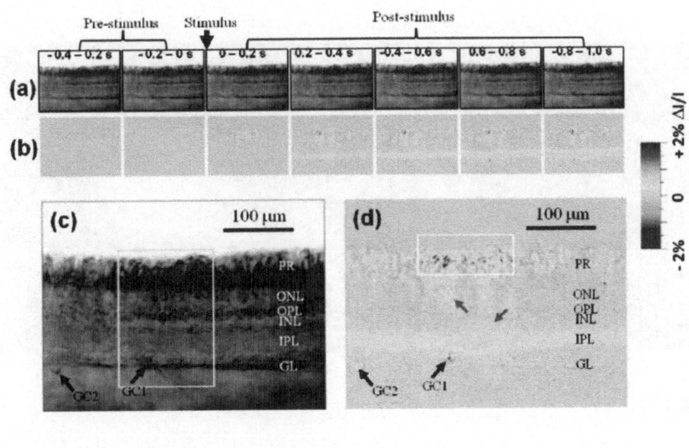

FIGURE 15.10: See main text for figure caption.

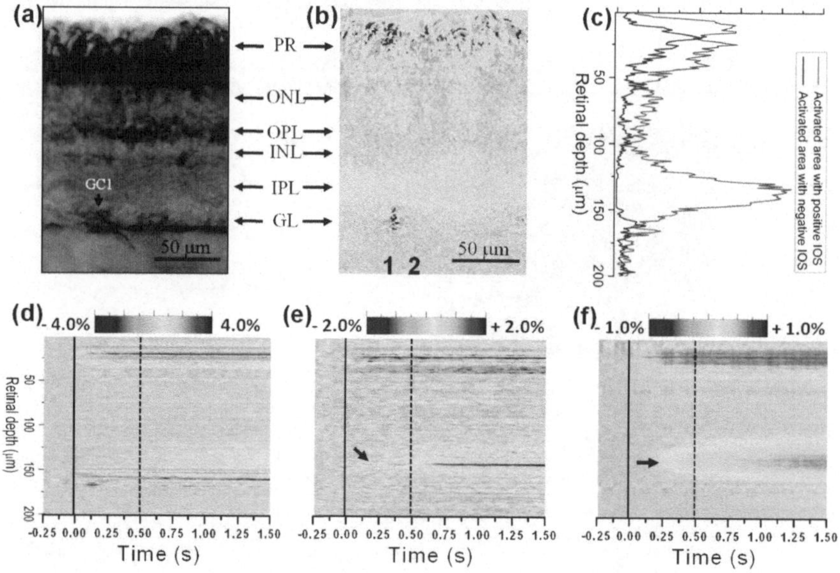

FIGURE 15.11: See main text for figure caption.

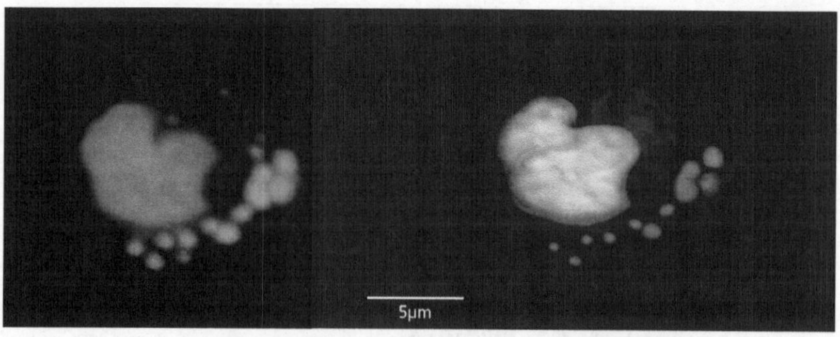

FIGURE 16.11: See main text for figure caption.

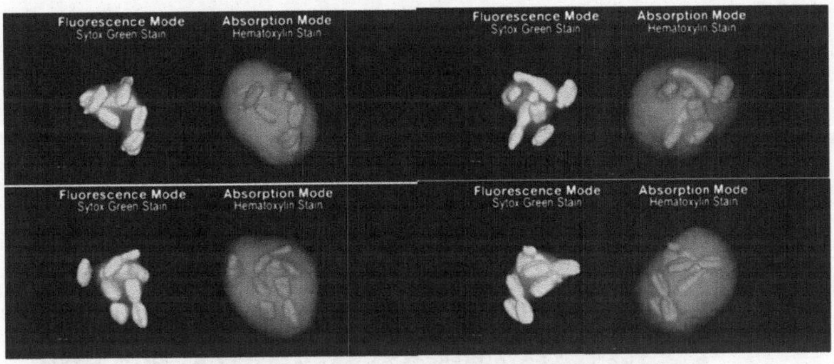

FIGURE 16.14: See main text for figure caption.

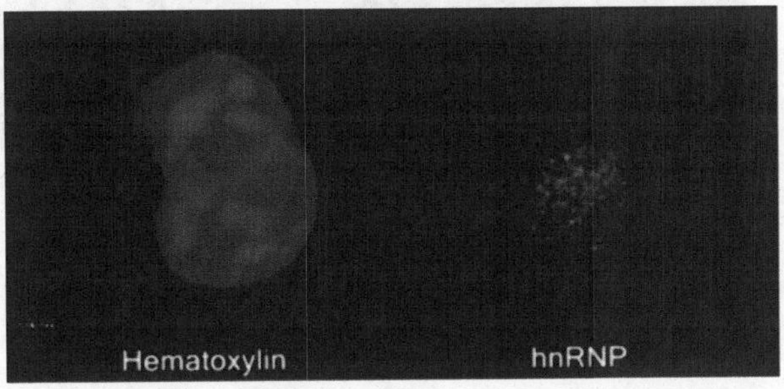

FIGURE 16.15: See main text for figure caption.

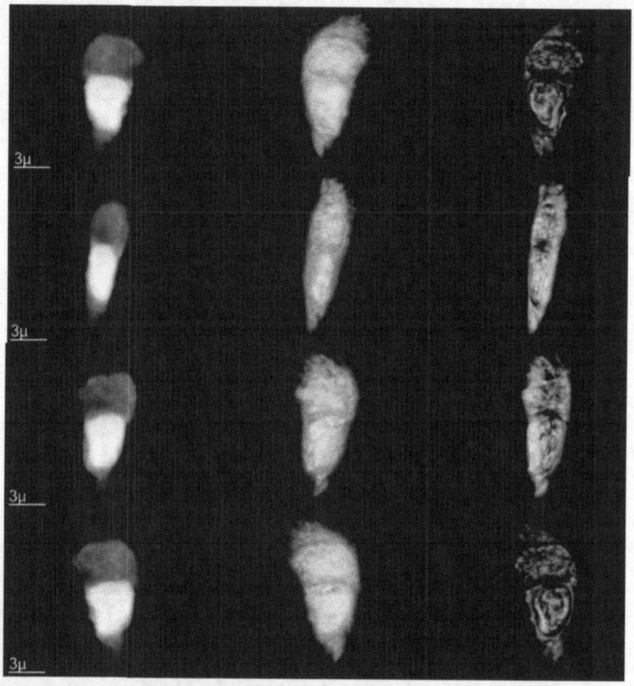

FIGURE 16.16: See main text for figure caption.

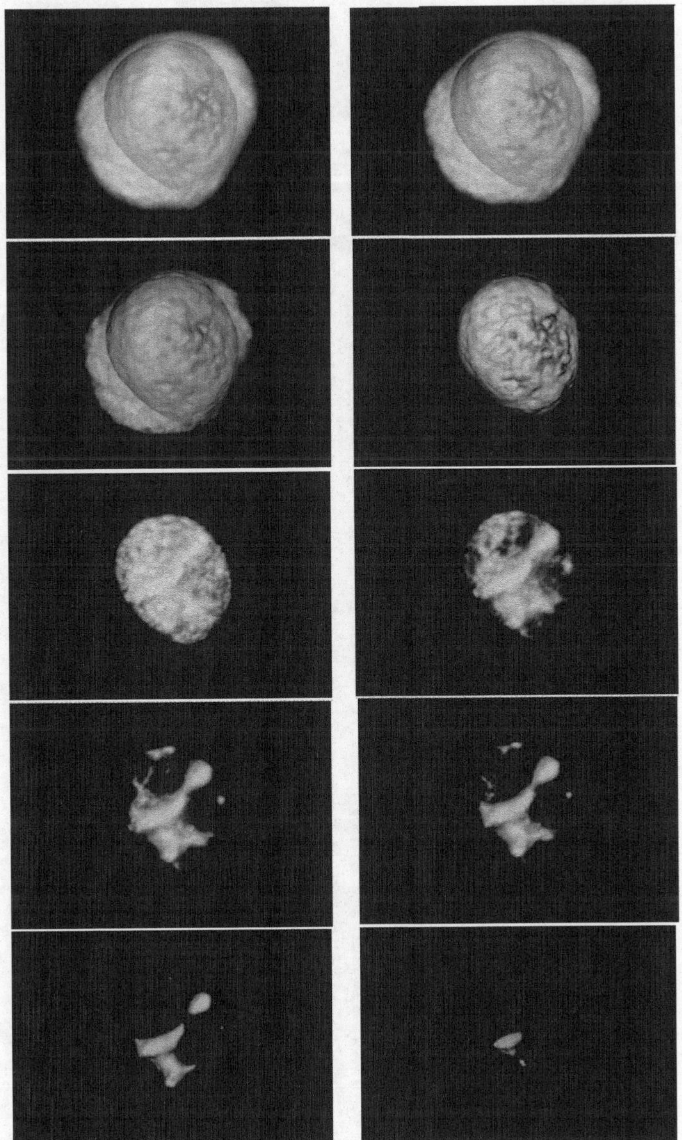

FIGURE 16.17: See main text for figure caption.

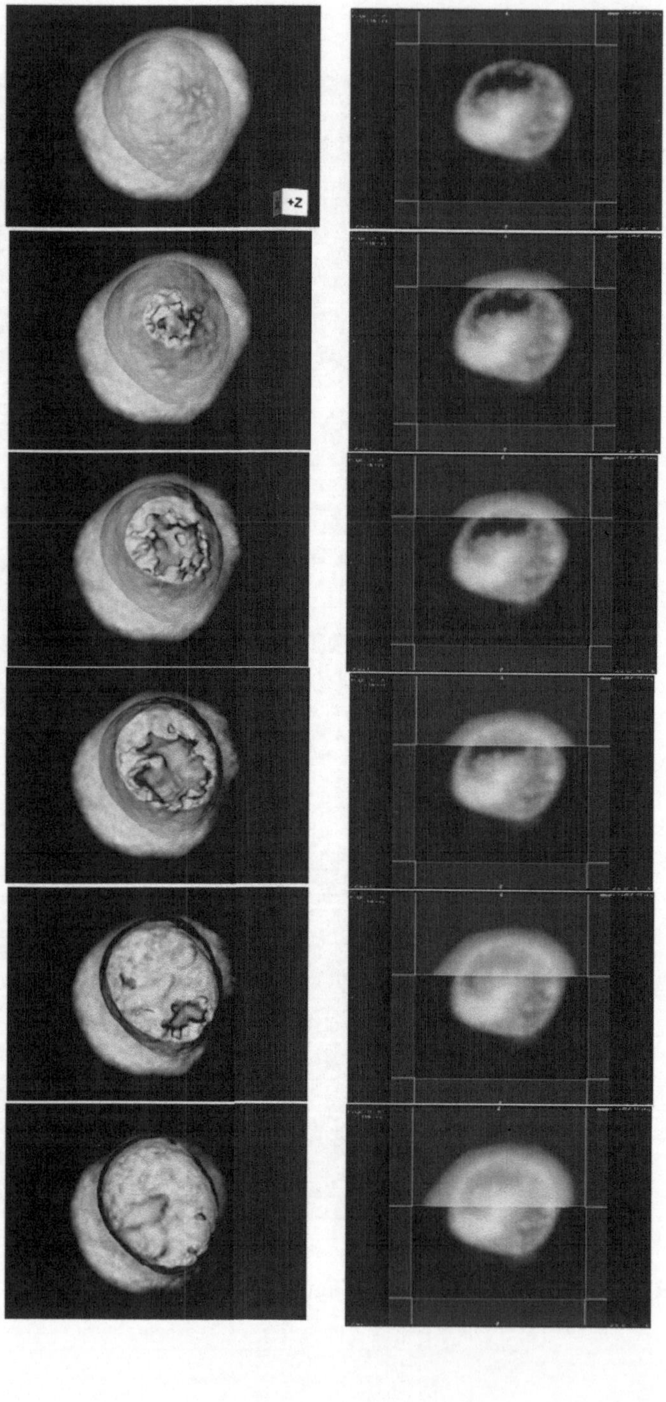
+Z

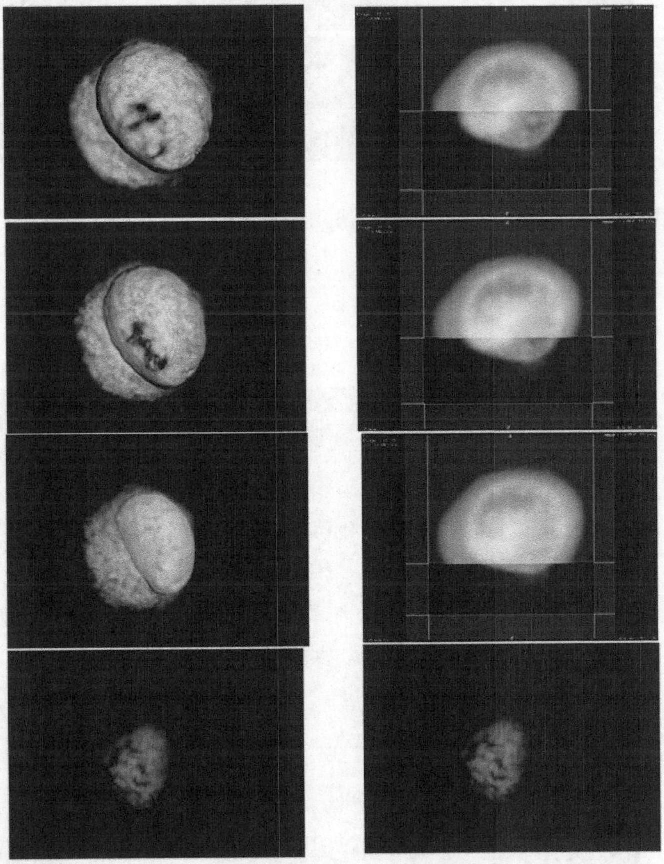

FIGURE 16.18: See main text for figure caption.

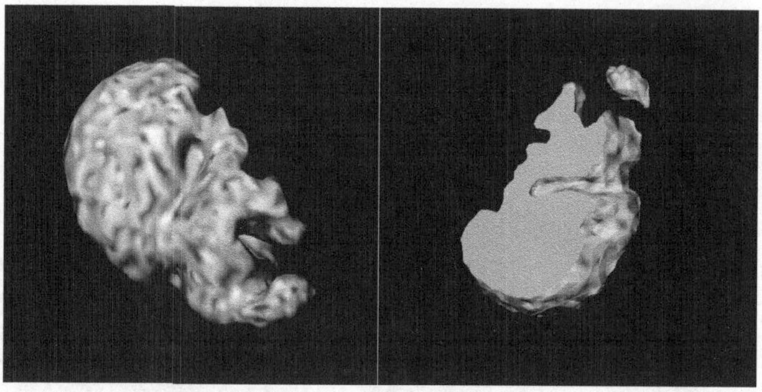

FIGURE 16.19: See main text for figure caption.

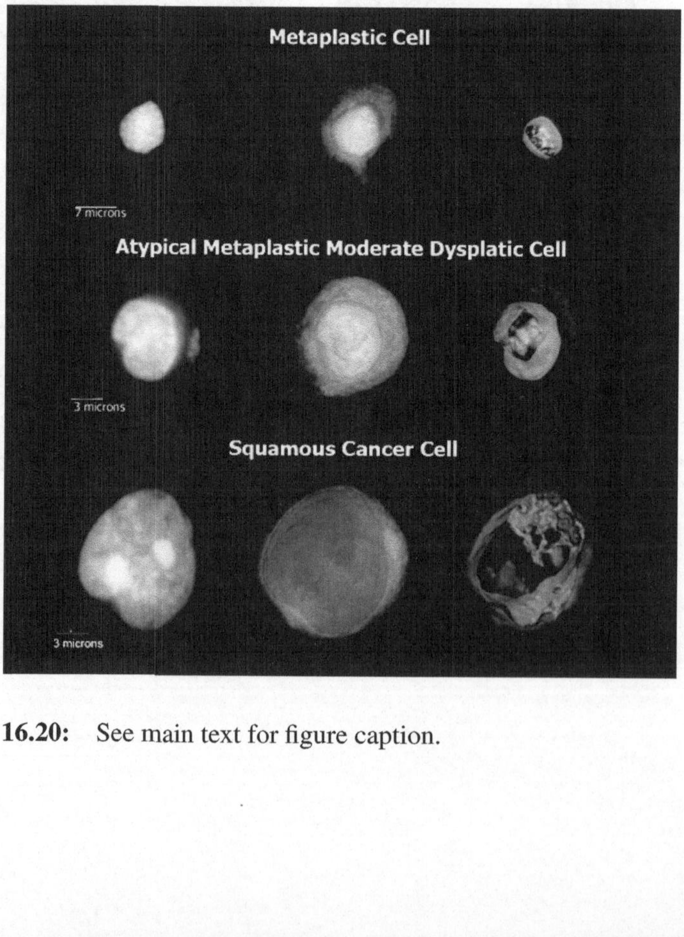

FIGURE 16.20: See main text for figure caption.

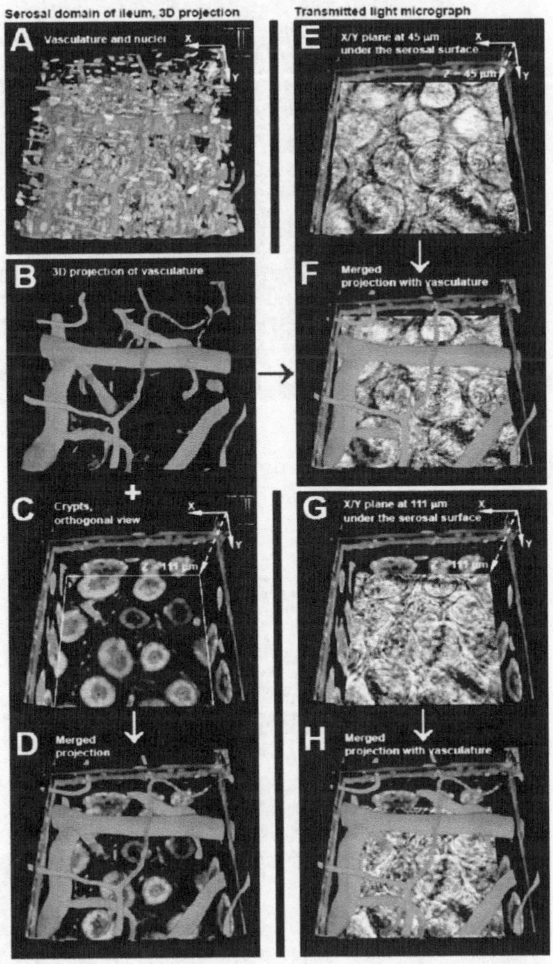

FIGURE 17.22: See main text for figure caption.

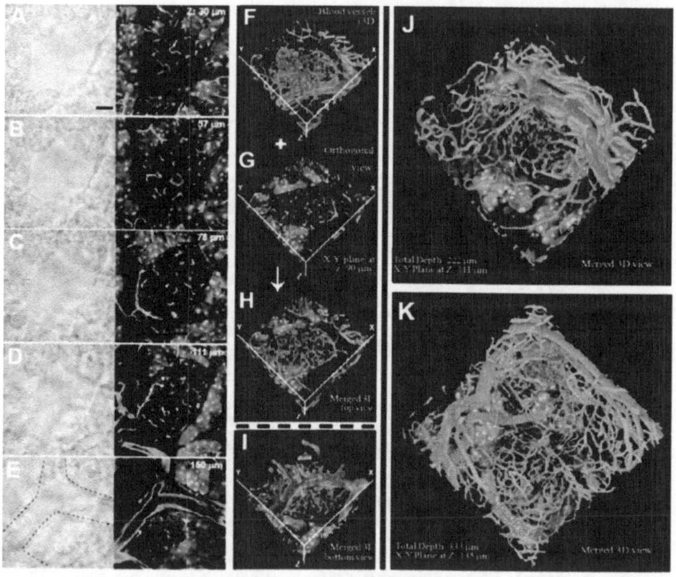

FIGURE 17.23: See main text for figure caption.

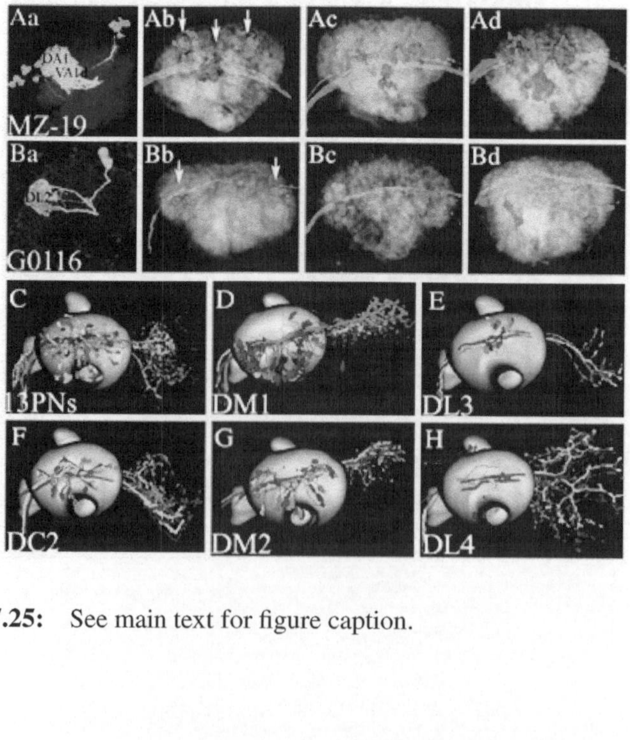

FIGURE 17.25: See main text for figure caption.

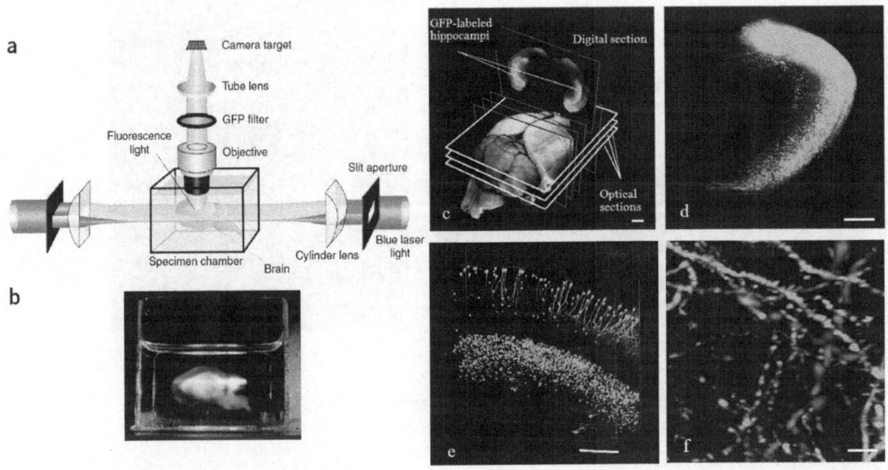

FIGURE 17.26: See main text for figure caption.

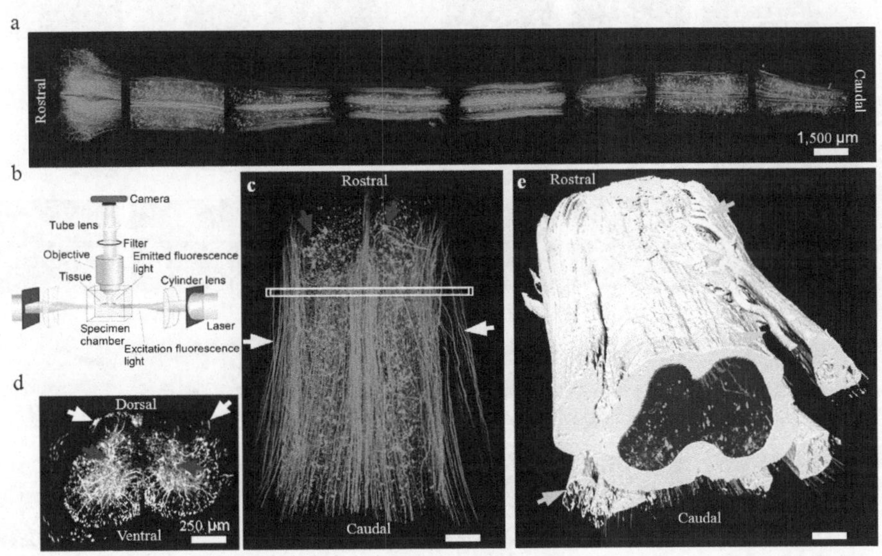

FIGURE 17.27: See main text for figure caption.

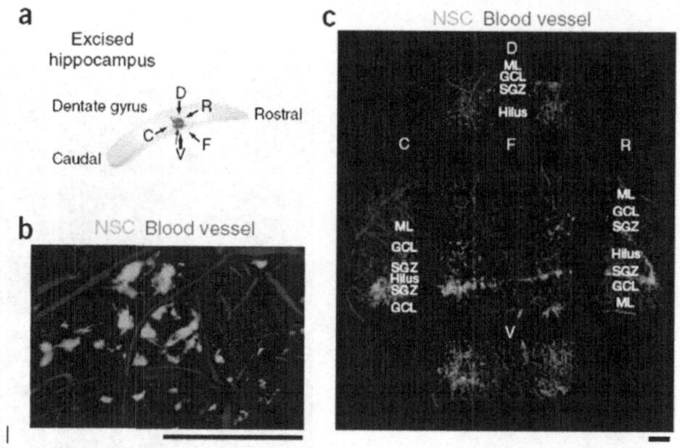

FIGURE 17.30: See main text for figure caption.

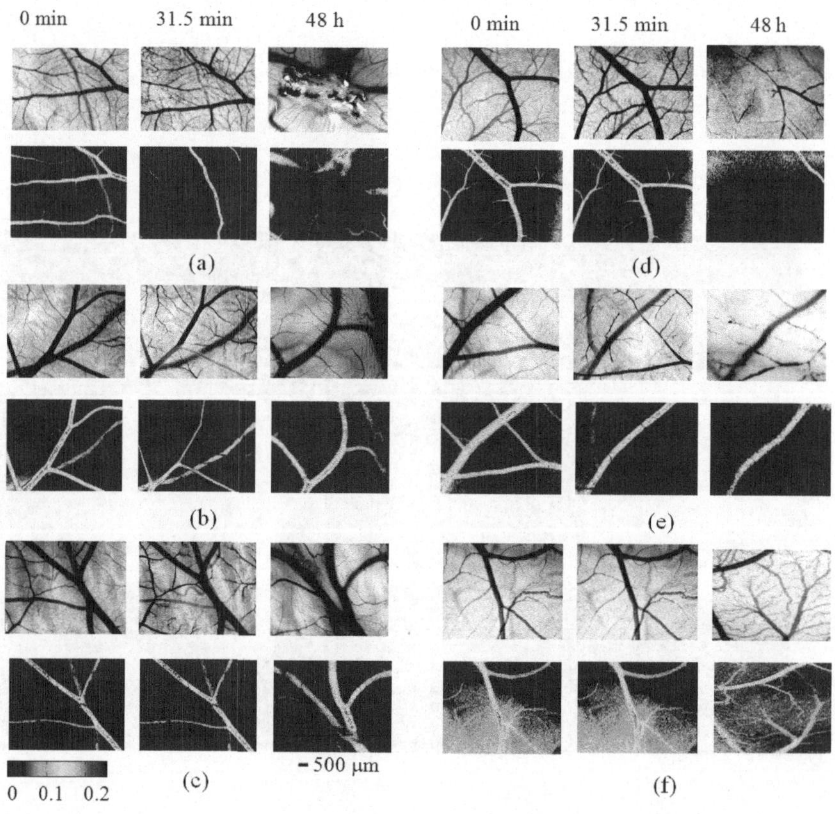

FIGURE 17.38: See main text for figure caption.

9

Advances in Blood Flow Imaging

Susan M. Daly

Department of Physics & Energy, University of Limerick, Ireland

Martin J. Leahy

Tissue Optics and Microcirculation Imaging Group, School of Physics, National University of Ireland, Galway, Ireland

This chapter describes the application of optical imaging techniques to biological tissue, to yield both qualitative and quantitative metrics of morphological and functional information. An in-depth narrative proffers reasoning for the diagnostic and prognostic value of such techniques via comparable descriptions of its invasive predecessors. Optical sectioning techniques of both the scattering and absorption based variety are described. The inherent need for non-invasive imaging modalities in modern medicine is discussed, in addition to the advantageous applications of their use and current limitations affecting performance.

Key words: biophotonics, circulation, correlation, flow, microvasculature, optical imaging, optical sectioning

9.1 Introduction

The analysis of light interactions with biological tissue facilitates a non-invasive morphological and functional "optical biopsy" [1], both of which are of outward importance diagnostically and prognostically. A biopsy of this form may be juxtaposed to its *core* or *excisional* biopsy precursor, wherein the procedure involves the surgical removal of a sampling of cells or tissues for examination *via* microscopy or chemical analysis. The medical removal of tissue from a living subject to determine the presence or extent of a disease is a commonplace procedure in clinical practice.

In addition to gleaning structural data, vascular imaging makes it possible to quantify the number and spacing of blood vessels, assess blood flow and permeability [2, 3], analyse cellular and molecular abnormalities and vessel wall shear stresses [4]. Structural and functional parameters may be elucidated by methods ranging from fluorescence to confocal and multiphoton microscopy. Magnetic resonance imaging, computed tomography, positron emission tomography, ultrasonography and optical imaging have been shown to provide non-invasive, functionally relevant images of

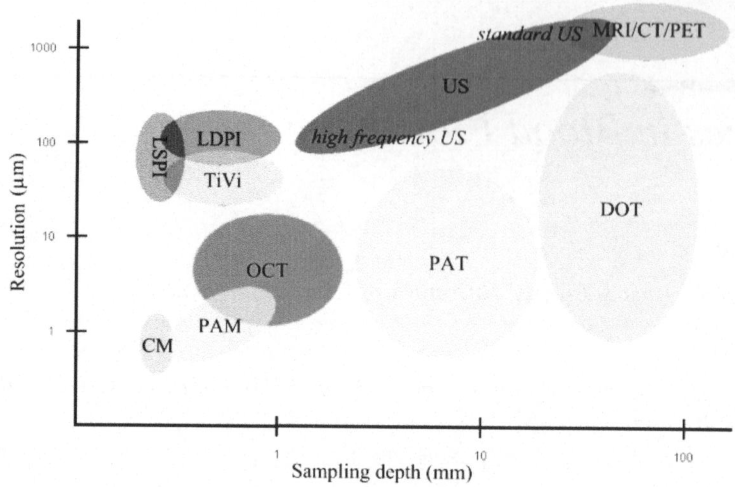

Figure 9.1: Illustration of the relative domains occupied by various imaging modalities in terms of resolution and sampling depth. DOT: diffuse optical tomography; CM: confocal microscopy; TiVi: tissue viability; LSPI: laser speckle perfusion imaging

angiogenesis[1] in animals and humans [5–10]. The principles upon which such methods are based vary widely, as does the suitability (e.g., resolution, imaging depth, etc.) and the relative technology and costs involved [11].

Great attention has been paid in the past two decades to the measurement of flow velocity on the micrometer scale and many techniques for assessing the blood supply have been investigated. This is borne out of recognition of the vitally important role that blood flow plays in the health of the individual. There are a myriad of (biological) reasons for this importance; for example, the onset of atheroma, a degeneration of the arterial wall which leads to arteriosclerosis or "artery hardening" [12, 13] manifests in disruption of localized flow patterns. In particular, there is growing clinical evidence that goal-directed intervention based on functional capillary density and heterogeneity of microcirculatory blood flow, in critically ill patients with septic and cardiogenic shock, led to improved outcomes [14]. However, the clinical applicability of optical methods is not solely confined to assessment of localized tissue regions. For instance, full-field skin perfusion techniques can assess the extent and aid in the diagnosis of burn depth [4, 15, 16] by visualizing the velocity distribution as a scalar velocity map. Assessing flow pattern disturbances is not of interest uniquely to the biomedical community; similar methods have been used in the field of chemical analysis, for example, in efforts to improve fluidic system performance [17]. There appears to be an ever-increasing emphasis being placed upon knowledge of precise distribution of flow velocities and the relative dynamics.

To meet this need, a wide variety of methods aimed towards measuring values of flow velocity within media have come into existence. However, every technique contains limitations or restrictions which must be minimised or compensated for in order to utilize the technique in a practical manner (see Fig. 9.1). In general, microscopic methods provide the highest resolution in terms of preserved tissue specimens, whereas clinical methods provide images of living tissues deep within the body, but at much lower resolution and specificity [5]. These constraints throw down the gauntlet of developing new imaging methods that can bridge this resolution dilemma.

Non-invasive *in vivo* imaging modalities have obvious advantages for the clinical realm; note-

[1] Angiogenesis: the formation and development of blood vessels

worthy are their ability to provide clinically relevant information without disturbing the normal biological environment. Methods which would allow the routine clinical assessment and monitoring at the microcirculatory level could greatly improve early detection and improve patient recovery rate. Furthermore, *ex vivo* tissue is not representative of the natural biological environment. Thus, non-invasive optical imaging techniques have filled this niche, garnering a reputation for fulfilling patient comfort during clinical assessment. Nonetheless, difficulties remain in obtaining accurate data in an environment which is subject to such large biological variability.

The present chapter will provide a number of examples of imaging techniques aimed at providing both qualitative and quantitative metrics of morphological and functional information. The first section will focus on providing a framework of the functional aspects of the (micro-) vasculature and will review the ailments associated with vascular irregularities and/or deformities. The second section will serve as an historical review of pioneering methods of imaging, utilizing both exogenous and endogenous contrast mechanisms. The third section will provide a summary of up-to-date high resolution optical sectioning techniques and the differing means by which each yields dynamic data. The final section will provide an examination of current correlation based mechanisms, capable of yielding information on both the static and dynamic aspects of the vasculature through statistical means. Furthermore, the inherent need for non-invasive imaging modalities in modern medicine is discussed, in addition to the advantageous aspects of their use in a clinical setting.

9.1.1 The microvasculature and related tissue optics

The *Ebers Papyrus*, an ancient Egyptian medical papyrus (16th BCE), outlined some of the earliest known acknowledgement of the connection between the heart to the surrounding arterial vessels. The Arabian physician, Ibn al-Nafis, provided the first accurate description of the process of pulmonary circulation [18], and did so more than 2700 years after the initial accounts of scientific thought on the subject by the Egyptians. It was not until the 17th CE that William Harvey deduced that the beating heart produced a continuous circulation through minute connections at the extremities of the body [19] (the Greek anatomist Erasistratus had previously postulated the existence of capillaries, 4th BCE). However, it is the Italian physician Marcello Malpighi who is credited with the discovery of the capillary interconnects between the arterial and venous vasculature, and ever since insights into the biophysical mechanisms that govern the hemodynamics of the microcirculation have been pursued.

The main constituents of blood are the liquid component "plasma" and blood cells. White blood cells (or leukocytes) play an active part in the defence system of the body. Red blood corpuscles (RBCs) are specialised to transport respiratory gases. They are roughly 8 μm in diameter at their widest point with a volume of approximately 90 μm^3 [20], have a biconcave shape and possess no nucleus [21, 22] (implying that the cell cannot repair itself and has limited lifespan). They produce one protein, the oxygen-carrying molecule hemoglobin and are one of the main chromophores (i.e., absorbers of light).

Microcirculation, the distal functional unit of the cardiovascular system, is the movement of blood or lymph through the vasculature via arterioles, venules, capillaries and arteriovenous anastomoses (AVAs) [23, 24]. Capillaries and the smallest venules are formed from a single layer of endothelial cells supported externally by a collagen rich basal laminar layer [21]. Blood perfusion through the capillaries serves several key functions within the body including regulation of blood pressure, supplying oxygen and nutrients to tissue, and removal of carbon dioxide and waste metabolites [25]. The heart is unique among organs in the cardiovascular system in that coronary arterial flow is exclusively diastolic and venous outflow is systolic. Furthermore, coronary vessels function as a highly organized hierarchical system of microvessel flow regulators matching local blood flows with myocardial energy demands to support the viability of the heart [26]. The transport of blood is by no means trivial [23]; complex boundary conditions, pulsatile flow patterns, and deformable, elastic vessel walls all interact with this non-Newtonian fluid, thus increasing the complexity of

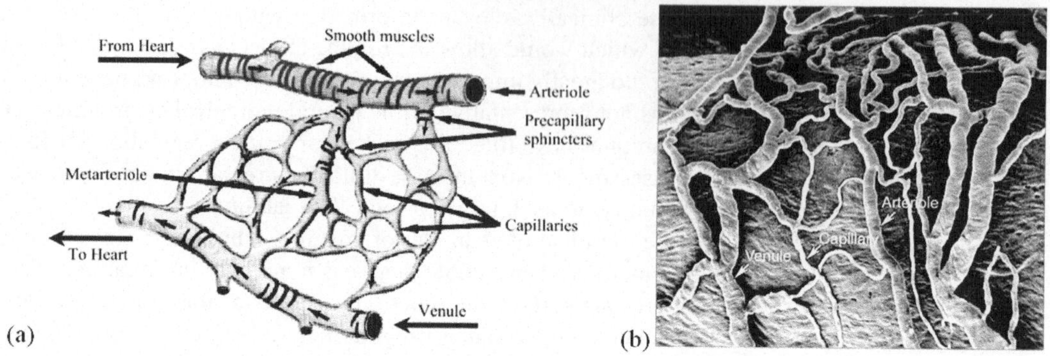

Figure 9.2: Illustration of the microcirculation including arterioles, capillaries and venules [22]; displays the extensive branching of capillaries (a); Scanning electron microscopic image of the vasa vasorum of rat carotid sinus, showing the organized arrangement of vessels [5] (b).

TABLE 9.1: Reference values for mean velocity ($\bar{v}$), diameter (d), Reynolds number (Re) and Womersley number (α); adapted from [4, 28].

Vessel type	$\bar{v}$ (m s^{-1})	d (mm)	Re (-)	α (-)
Artery	0.45	4	450	40
Arteriole	0.05	0.05	0.5	0.5
Capillary	0.001	0.008	0.002	0.1
Venule	0.002	0.02	0.01	0.2
Vein	0.1	5	125	50

analysis.

The scale of the cardiovascular system geometry spans several orders of magnitude (see Table 9.1), from the size of a minute capillary to the aorta (approximate diameter, 2 cm). In addition, these characteristic lengths are not consistent throughout the entire body; capillaries found in the skin have comparatively thicker walls (2–3 μm) [27] when compared with the rest of the body (0.1 μm) [22]. Furthermore, the type of flow experienced in these vessels varies greatly from strongly pulsatile (e.g. in arteries) to being almost stationary.

Flow is characterized by two dimensionless quantities: the Reynolds number (Re) and the Womersley number (α), defined as:

$$\mathrm{Re} = \frac{d \cdot \bar{v} \cdot \rho}{\vartheta}, \qquad \alpha = d\sqrt{\frac{2\pi f \cdot \rho}{\vartheta}}, \tag{9.1}$$

where d is the vessel diameter; $\bar{v}$, bulk velocity; ρ, density; ϑ, dynamic viscosity; and f is the characteristic frequency. Generally, Reynolds numbers below 2000 imply laminar flow rates, whereas for low Womersley values, pulsatile flow is dominated by viscous effects [4].

In the skin, the structure of vessels is arranged into superficial and deep horizontal plexuses [30] and serves a number of vital functions such as nutritional support for tissues and homeostasis [23, 31]. AVAs serve as low resistance channels for large volumes of blood to pass directly from arterioles to venules (i.e. bypasses the capillaries) [23] and play an important role in the thermoregulation of the body [32]. Assessment of AVAs in the acral regions of the body has shown them to be implicated in diabetes, where the volume of blood transferred by AVAs increases and is thought to be the cause of neuropathic ulcerations [33] (see Section 9.1.2).

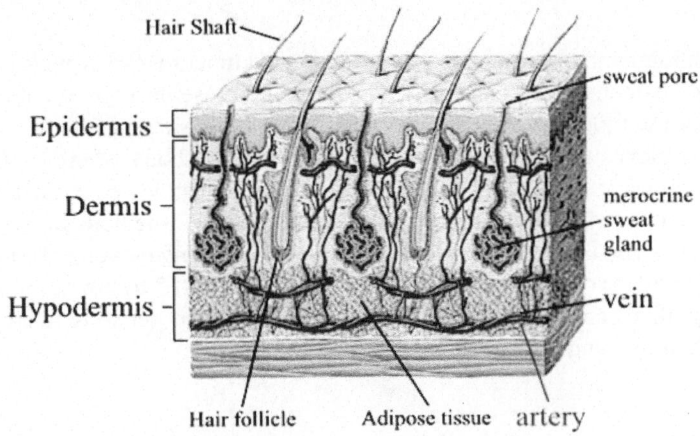

Figure 9.3: Illustration of dermal and epidermal strata and the arrangement of blood vessels in the skin. Adapted from [29].

Biological tissues are absorbing media and are optically inhomogeneous [20]. Light microscopy and direct visual inspection of the skin is hampered by scattering, regular surficial reflections and absorption by superficial chromophores. Light interaction with a multilayer and multicomponent substance such as skin is a highly complicated process [20, 34]. Light propagation within tissues depends on the scattering and absorbing of its cells and the size, shape and density of these structures, relative refractive indices and polarization states [35, 36]. For instance, the stratum corneum layer of the skin reflects 5–7% of incident light and a collimated beam may be transformed into a diffuse beam by interfacial microscopic inhomogeneities. A collimated beam attenuated in a thin tissue layer of thickness d, may be described by the Bouguer-Beer-Lambert exponential law [37]:

$$I(d) = (1 - R_F)I_0 \exp(-\mu_t d) \tag{9.2}$$

where I_0 is the incident light intensity; μ_t, extinction or total attenuation coefficient ($\mu_a + \mu_s$); and R_F, coefficient of Fresnel reflection, where at normal incidence:

$$R_F = \left[\frac{(\eta - 1)}{(\eta + 1)}\right]^2 \tag{9.3}$$

where η is the relative mean refractive index of tissue and surrounding media. At a microscopic scale, tissue components have no pronounced boundaries and appear to merge into a continuous structure with spatial variations in the refractive index. Quantitative models [38] assist in the comprehension of such complex morphologies by predicting the absolute magnitudes of optical coefficients, and wavelength and angular dependencies. One such model is the discrete particle model of tissue [20, 39].

9.1.2 Clinical implications of blood flow assessments

Aberrant microcirculatory morphology and hemodynamics are signatures of many human diseases such as cancer, macular degeneration, and many others. The skin is easily accessible and any compromise in nutritional support [40] and/or impairment in tissue viability can lead to disease manifestation [41]. Skin blood flow measurements are used to study clinical conditions which either intrinsically affect skin blood [27] or where measurement of skin blood flow is affected by the underlying pathology. Assessment of skin structure and function can provide evidence of a disorder, the dysfunction extent, serve as an early indication of disease onset or as a means of post-operative assessment, for example skin flap viability following plastic surgery [40].

The nailfold plexus is one of only a few location on the body where capillaries advance close enough to the skin surface (within 200 μm) to be naturally visible i.e., without the use of specialised optical equipment or optical clearing agents. This makes the methods of examining them simple. Moreover, the fingernail is easily fixed in position, free from any movement due to arterial pulsations or respirations, and the capillaries run in hairpin-like loops (6–15 μm in diameter) parallel to the skin surface. Initial microscopy techniques for capillaroscopic purposes were reliant on epi-illumination, with a magnification range of between 15 and 100 [23].

(a)

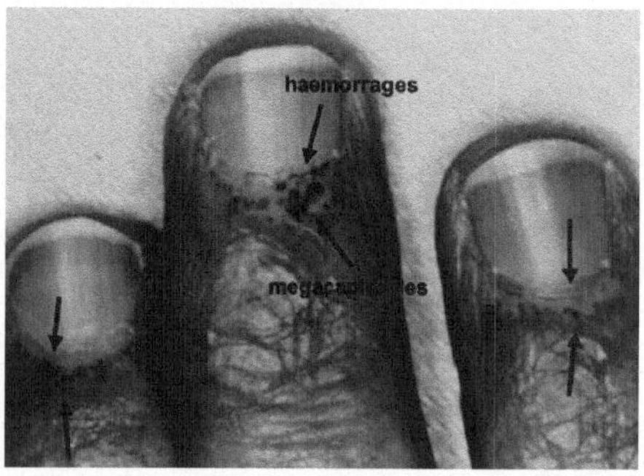

(b)

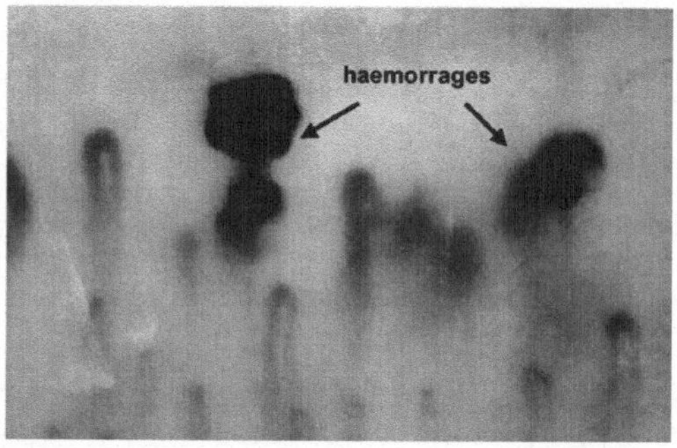

Figure 9.4: (a) Irregularly sized and shaped capillaries, representing one of the most striking early indications of secondary Raynauds phenomenon; (b) Typical capillary hemorrhaging prevalent in connective tissue disease [42].

The ease with which capillaries may be imaged does not imply that the range of ailments is by any means limited. Chronic illnesses such as systemic lupus erythematosus, scleroderma [43], systemic sclerosis [44], antiphospholipid syndrome [45], connective tissue disease [46], diabetes mellitus [47] and Raynaud's phenomenon [44] have been readily identified via specific physiological markers at the capillary level such as increased vessel permeability (hemorrhaging) [2, 3], the presence of avascular areas, enlarged loops, poor circulation, and increased tortuosity [23]. In addition, the identification of such ailments has not been limited to solely systemic diseases. Physiological irregularities have manifested in the nailfold plexus, stemming from localized areas of discomfort and have revealed the presence of conditions such as rheumatoid arthritis [48], vasculitis, psoriasis and psoriatic arthritis [49], and migraine, in addition to psychiatric disorders such as schizophrenia [50].

A brief list of ailments and the respective techniques used in their detection and identification are outlined on Table 9.2 Although the quoted imaging techniques do not proffer a clinical solution to such ailments, their value and the justification for their use may be understood from their potential to characterize disease progression and determine response to therapy, enabling timely modifications to therapeutic strategies. This is particularly pertinent from the perspective of preventative medicine and patient management, as the manifestation of vascular aberrations can occur initially in the peripheral areas of the body prior to clinical suspicion. Such early diagnoses and subsequent early intervention may offer the patient a decreased degree of suffering, a welcome measure for those who suffer habitually from such ailments.

TABLE 9.2 : Compilation of ailments which manifest in the acral regions and the respective technique used in their detection. OPS, Orthogonal Polarization Spectral; SDF, Sidestream Dark Field; LDF, Laser Doppler Flowmetry [11, 42, 43, 45, 47, 48, 51–63].

Ailment \ **Technique**	Wide-field microscopy	Capillaroscopy	OPS imaging	SDF Illumination	Fluorescence videomicroscopy	LDF
Systemic Lupus Erythematosus	■	■				
Osteoarthritis		■				
Scleroderma		■				
Reflex Sympathetic Dystrophy						■
Acrocyanosis		■				
Polymyositis		■				
Rheumatoid Arthritis	■	■				
Diabetes Mellitus		■				
Migraine		■				
Antiphospholipid Syndrome		■			■	
Hypertension		■				
Acromegaly		■				
Pre-eclampsia			■			■
Menopause		■				
Sjogren's Syndrome		■				
General Microcirculation			■	■		
Mixed Cryoglobulinaemia		■				
Psoriasis & Psoriatic Arthritis		■				
Raynaud's Phenomenon (primary and secondary)	■	■				
Dermatomyositis		■				
(mixed) Connective Tissue Disease		■				
Peripheral Arterial Obliterative Disease		■				■
Systemic Sclerosis		■				
Rheumatoid Vasculitis		■				
Pediatric Rheumatism		■				

9.2 Review of Pioneering Modalities towards Dynamic Data

9.2.1 Exogenous contrast mechanisms

9.2.1.1 Radionuclide techniques

Historically, the first means of measuring flow and perfusion were performed through invasive procedures. Examples of such procedures include direct measurements of capillary blood pressure [64], transcutaneous oxygen measurements [27, 65] and radionuclide techniques. Xenon clearance is the "gold standard" choice of radionuclide and subcutaneous injections of such are used to evaluate skin blood flow [66, 67] by measurement of the rate of isotope clearance (activity) from the injected area by the local blood supply [68]. Tissue blood flow (Q) may be calculated from the half-life ($t_{1/2}$) of the isotopic tracer involved [27]:

$$Q = \frac{100 \cdot \ln 2 \cdot \lambda}{t_{1/2}} \tag{9.4}$$

Although many other tracers have been used for these purposes (e.g. ^{22}Na, ^{24}Na, ^{125}I), difficulties arise with regard the choice of tracer as each has a different degree of diffusibility upon injection. The choice of an apt tracer and use of a suitable detector is crucial for measurement success, in addition to assessment of skin type for biological variation. The measurements of blood flow by these methods have been proven to be disadvantageous, however, by being very much a point measurement modality whose results may not bear any relationship to regional blood flow metrics. A poor choice in measurement site would therefore lead to inaccurate results.

9.2.1.2 Thermodilution

Cardiac output (CO) is regarded one of the most important hemodynamic variables for the assessment of cardiac function [69] and guidance of therapy in the intensive care setting. Thermodilution is a method of measuring blood flow based on the premise that when an indicator substance is added to circulating blood, the rate of blood flow is inversely proportional to the indicator concentration change over time. A fluid miscible with blood (e.g. a dextrose or saline solution) and at a lower temperature is injected into the coronary sinus at a constant rate and the resulting change in temperature is detected a short distance downstream [70]. The cold fluid mixes with blood in the right heart chambers, is ejected into the pulmonary artery and flows past a thermistor positioned on the distal end of the catheter which records temporal changes in blood temperature. CO is determined from the following equation [71]:

$$CO = \frac{V_i(T_B - T_i)K_1K_2}{\int_0^\infty \Delta T_B(t)dt} \tag{9.5}$$

where V_i is injectate volume; T_B and T_i are the blood and injectate temperature, respectively; K_1 is a density factor; and K_2 is a computation constant.

The method of thermodilution is gainful from the perspective that it permits measurements to be repeated in short intervals and allows rapid changes in coronary circulation to be studied since the body acts as a large heat sink. Detrimental and possibly harmful aspects of the method include the requirement of catheterisation of the coronary sinus and relatively large amounts of fluid are injected. Additionally, CO determination by thermodilution may be unreliable or impossible in patients with low CO states [72], and studies have shown that the thermodilution method overestimates true cardiac output in the low output range [73].

9.2.1.3 Iontophoresis

Iontophoresis is defined as the facilitatory motion of ions across a membrane, permitting the transdermal delivery of vasoactive drugs [23, 74]. The technique examines the relationship between pharmacological provocation and physiological responses of the vascular bed. Active agents capable of holding an electric charge are applied topically to the skin in a gel form. Depending on whether it is anodal (agent: atropine, acetylcholine) or cathodal (agent: L-arginine, sodium nitroprusside) iontophoresis, an electrode oppositely charged with respect to the active agent repels the ions down towards the anode/cathode via an electrical gradient, thus penetrating the skin. As the skin generally possesses a net negative charge, positively charged drugs are generally easier to deliver [33]. Although the iontophoretic method does not cause localized pain or swelling, it is a time consuming exercise and must be repeated at regular intervals.

9.2.2 Endogenous contrast mechanisms

9.2.2.1 Thermography

In thermography, two-dimensional (2D) maps of radiation differences are constructed of regional temperature distributions across the skin and are used as a direct measure of blood perfusion [27, 75]. There are contact and non-contact thermographic devices; the former utilizes liquid crystal technology directly on the skin surface, and the latter employs the infrared (IR) portion of the electromagnetic spectrum. The energy flux emitted by the skin is given by Stefan-Boltzmann's law,

$$R = \theta_S T_S^4 \tag{9.6}$$

where θ_S is the Stefan-Boltzmann constant and T_S is the temperature at the skin surface. Although thermography has good spatial resolution and is relatively easy to use [76], it provides details of surface temperature only and has poor responsiveness. However, microwave radiometry can penetrate to subcutaneous tissue depth (1–2 cm) and has been used in studies to assess peripheral vascular disease [77].

9.2.2.2 Laser Doppler imaging

If a system is composed of both stationary and mobile scatterers and illuminated with coherent light, some photons undergo a frequency change. This phenomenon is known as the Doppler Effect, named for its discoverer, Austrian physicist Christian Andreas Doppler. The effect occurs when photons are scattered from particles which are moving and the change in frequency is determined by the frequency of the emitting source and the velocity relative to the observer. As the reflected portion of the incident beam is found to be spectrally broadened [78, 79], this frequency shift can be used to determine the velocity of the moving object. Laser Doppler Flowmetry (LDF) refers to a general class of non-invasive techniques which utilize the optical Doppler effect to measure changes in microcirculatory blood perfusion for both *in vitro* [80] and *in vivo* [81] purposes. Perfusion is defined as the product of the local speed and concentration of blood cells [36, 82].

Of the incident coherent light that irradiates the tissue surface, only a fraction propagates through the tissue randomly interacting with different components. Within the vasculature, these components may be static or dynamic (such as RBCs); the moving portions will undergo a frequency shift, whereas the static components will not. These frequency shifts are allowed to impinge on the surface of a photodetector, producing beat frequencies from which it is possible to determine the product of the average speed and concentration (i.e. perfusion) of the moving components within the tissue volume in question. The scattering angle, the wavelength of the light in tissue (λ_T) and the velocity of the moving scattering object ($\vec{v}_S$) determine the frequency shift produced by Doppler scattering.

If an incident photon is described by the propagation vector $\vec{k}_i$ and is scattered by a moving

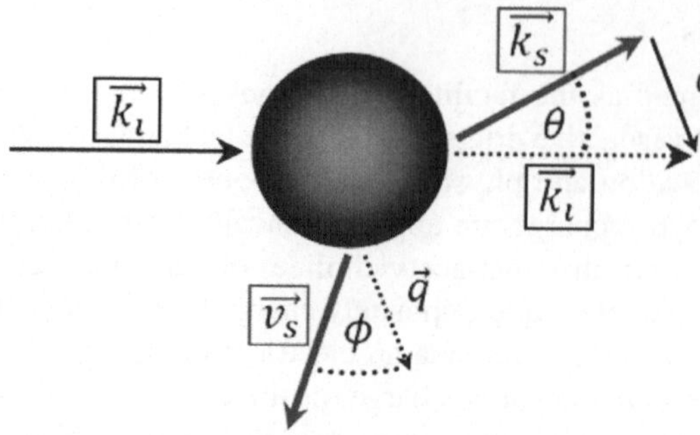

Figure 9.5: Illustration of single Doppler shift event; θ , scattering angle; ϕ , azimuthal angle.

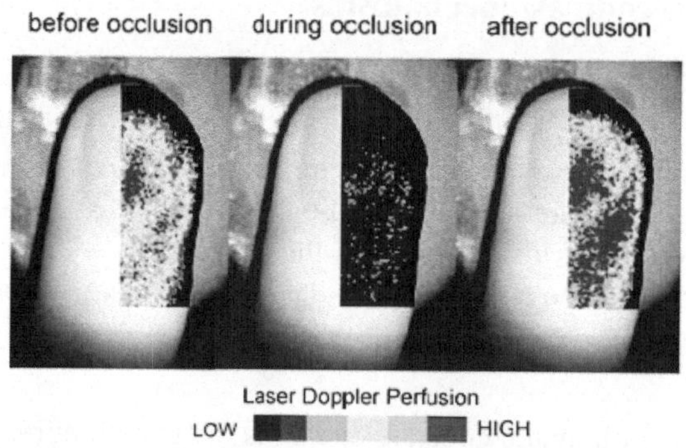

Figure 9.6: (See color insert.) Perfusion images of the finger obtained before, during, and after occlusion of the upper arm using LDPI (128×256 pixels) [85].

particle (see Fig. 9.5) in the direction $\vec{k}_S$, the scattering vector $\vec{q}$ (invariable with elastic scattering) is given by:

$$|\vec{q}| = \vec{k}_i - \vec{k}_S = 2k\sin\left(\frac{\theta}{2}\right) \tag{9.7}$$

The Doppler frequency shift (f_{Ds}) for a single scattering event may be given by [20]:

$$f_{Ds} = \frac{2v_S\eta\cos\theta}{\lambda_T} \tag{9.8}$$

The measurement depth in tissue depends on the source wavelength used; near IR light ($\lambda_T \cong 1$ μm) penetrates several mm, red light ($\lambda_T \cong 650$ nm) up to about 2 mm and green light ($\lambda_T \cong 540$ nm) hardly at all [4, 83]. In a system of moving particles such as RBCs in tissue, a more realistic scenario would involve a single photon undergoing multiple Doppler-shifts. In this case f_{Ds} would be the sum of the individual scattering events. The velocity of RBCs in cutaneous circulation is of the order of mm s^{-1} and correspondingly produces a Doppler shift of several kHz. Since this is very small, optical heterodyning techniques are utilized to obtain Doppler shifts [27].

Laser Doppler Perfusion Monitoring (LDPM) and Laser Doppler Perfusion Imaging (LDPI) were developed for point-wise monitoring and imaging of skin perfusion, respectively. In the case of LDPI, the laser beam illuminates the tissue by way of a single scanning point (Point Raster Scanning), a scanning line (Line Scanning) or static uniform illumination over the entire surface (Full-field) [84] and therefore can access flux across a region.

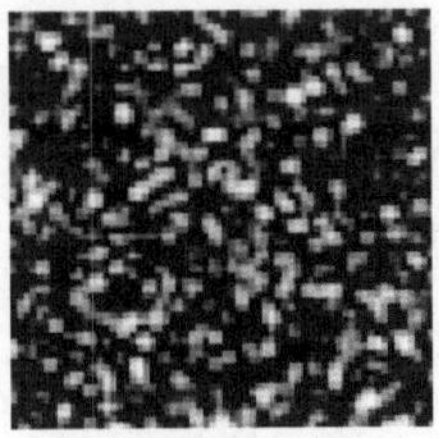

Figure 9.7: Illustration of a simulated speckle pattern with an exposure time of 1 ms [99].

LDPI techniques have good spatial resolution due to the wide field of vision and ability to record fluctuation patterns across a large area of the skin [30]. The first portable clinical instrument was developed by Holloway and Watkins although it had some practical limitations due to poor signal to noise ratio [27, 86]. Although Laser Doppler technology has many potential applications, it has yet to become integrated into clinical settings [87]. Angular limitations, the stochastic nature of the Doppler signal from a highly scattering medium [88, 89], phase wrapping, and interferometric fringe washout effects, prevent accurate assessment of the detected Doppler signal [90] causing measurement ambiguities as well as loss of information. Additionally, disturbances of the fluid refractive index resulting from large temperature fluctuations have caused the incident laser beam to wander and defocus [91]. In spite of this, LDPI technology has been demonstrated and used in the assessment of a plethora of clinical situations; for instance, assessment of burn extent [15, 16] and relative perfusion [36, 92, 93], post-operative malignant skin tumor assessment [94], and in the study of arthritis and joint inflammation [95].

9.2.2.3 Laser speckle imaging

Image speckle refers to the pattern observed on a surface [83]. As outlined in Section 9.2.2.2, analysis of the Doppler shift of the photon or the distribution of Doppler shifts from a distribution of photons, enables the discernment of the dynamics of scattering particles. *In vivo* experiments have shown a strong correlation between Doppler and speckle modalities [96]. A speckle pattern is formed either by the reflection of coherent light from a rough surface, or by transmitting the light through a transparent medium having a randomly fluctuating refractive index distribution and by subsequent 3D multiple beam interference [97]. The speckle pattern is a granular variation of light intensity (see Fig. 9.7) obtained from any rough surface such as skin (rough or randomly undulated on a scale comparable with the light wavelength) and is characterized by a random intensity distribution that may be described by statistical means [11, 98].

Scattering inhomogeneities within the skin can be considered as point sources and small differences in distances traversed, to the photodiode detector used, result in dark and bright speckles dispersed at all points in space. If scatterers (e.g. RBCs) within the vasculature are in motion, this results in temporal fluctuations in the laser speckle pattern, analogous to the intensity fluctuations that arise from Doppler shifts. This motion results in a speckle pattern that appears decorrelated or "blurred" [100]. The amount of decorrelation depends on the speed and volume of the scatterers in the tissue. To quantify the blurring of the speckles, the speckle contrast is computed as the ratio [101, 102]:

$$K_S = \frac{\sigma_S}{\langle I \rangle} \leq 1 \tag{9.9}$$

where σ_S is the standard deviation; and $\langle I \rangle$ is the mean intensity. A fluctuation in light intensity is recorded each time a scatterer moves through a distance of 0.5λ. Thus variations in speckle contrast are dependent on the velocity distribution of scatterers and determinations of velocity may be obtained by temporally assessing the statistical behaviour of speckles. The time-varying component of speckle may be quantified by comparisons of like pixel intensities recorded in successive scans

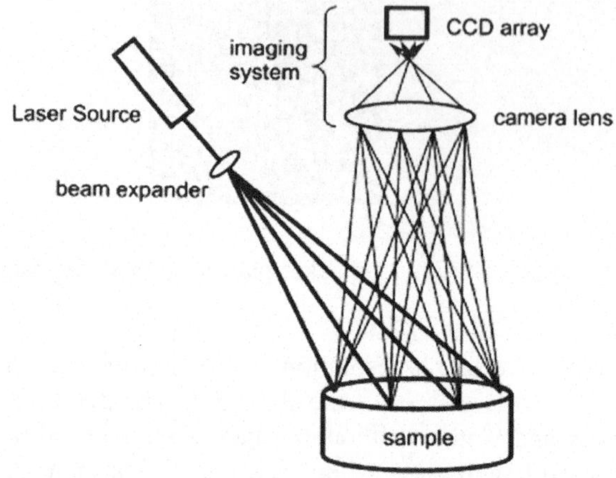

Figure 9.8: Full-field laser speckle contrast imaging. Tissue is illuminated by a laser, the speckle pattern is then recorded by a CCD camera and the speckle contrast, K, computed [11].

of the subject, thus forming 2D maps of flow across the region of interest. A successful approach was developed using laser speckle contrast analysis (LASCA), which assumes that (considering a Lorenztian flow profile) the speckle contrast could be related to correlation time τ_C (and hence RBC_V) [101, 103]:

$$K = \beta^{0.5}\left\{\frac{\tau_C}{T} + \frac{\tau_C^2}{2T^2}\left[\exp\left(-\frac{2T}{\tau_C}\right) - 1\right]\right\}^{0.5} \tag{9.10}$$

where β^2 accounts for loss of correlation related to the ratio of the detector size to the speckle size and polarization; τ_C, the correlation time; and T is the exposure time of the camera.

In full-field measurements, tissue is illuminated by an expanded laser beam and the resulting image speckle is recorded by a CCD camera (see Fig. 9.8).

Speckle techniques have the advantage of being able to acquire images in real-time, making it possible to measure blood flow response to occlusion and hyperemia, for instance. Although specular reflection effects may be disregarded with the addition of polarizing filters, static tissue reduces the signal-to-noise (SNR) ratio [104-106]. Additionally, the laser speckle signal is not frequency weighted implying that moving scatterers in deeper vessels cannot be isolated. These factors contribute to the confinement of the speckle technique to superficial measurements, with deeper measurements requiring the necessity of being performed on surgically exposed tissue.

Progress has been made in establishing a flow decorrelation time using laser speckle contrast techniques [107]; however, issues still remain of how to relate this time constant to the flow velocity [108]. Although accurate absolute measurements RBC_V cannot be calculated, perfusion changes can be successively monitored and tracked. Laser speckle imaging has been demonstrated on the rodent skin fold model [109, 110], assessed the vasodilation responses of intestinal tissues [111], analysed retinal blood flow and cerebral perfusion [112, 113], and stroke [101].

9.2.2.4 Polarisation spectroscopy

If polyvinyl alcohol (PVA) chains are stretched, they form an array of aligned, linear molecules. An iodine dopant attached to the PVA molecules makes these chains conducting along their length and thus light polarized parallel to these chains is absorbed whilst perpendicularly polarized light

[2] If the source is polarized and the detector is not, then $\beta = 0.5$

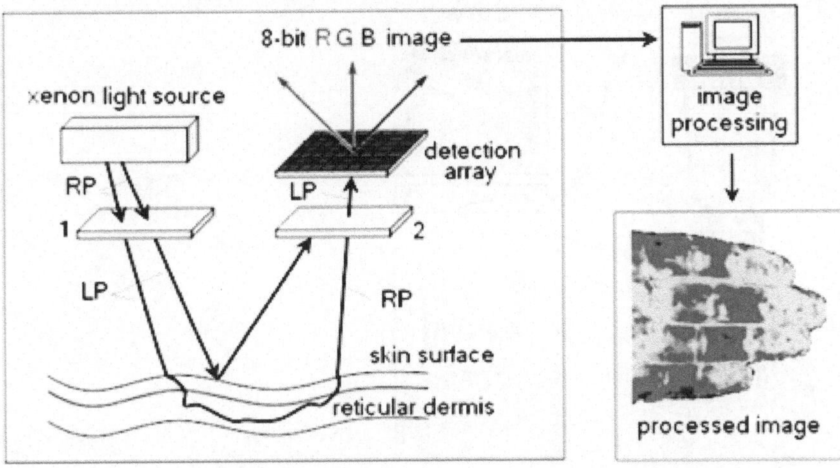

Figure 9.9: Illustration of the operating principle of PS using polarization gating method. Polarisation filters (1,2) are arranged so that their pass-directions are perpendicular, thus creating a cross-polarized image [119].

is transmitted. The technique of polarization spectroscopy (PS) makes use of this phenomenon for imaging purposes by gating photons returning from different skin tissue compartments [114].

Light from the superficial skin layers can be differentiated from light backscattered from the dermal tissue matrix by use of simple polarization filters. When monochromatic or white incoherent light is linearly polarized by a filter and is subsequently incident on the skin surface, 5% of the light is specularly reflected by Fresnel reflection as surface glare and a further 2% is reflected from the superficial *stratum corneum* layers. These two light fractions retain their original polarization state, dictated by the orientation of the first polarizer (see Fig. 9.9). The remaining portion penetrates through the epidermal layers, where it is absorbed or backreflected. The backscattered portion is exponentially depolarized by chromophore scattering [115] and tissue birefringence [116]; it has been suggested that more than 10 scattering events are required to sufficiently depolarize light [117, 118].

Light remerging from tissue structure is now diffusely reflected, consisting of equal (approx. 22%) divisions of parallel and perpendicular polarizations with respect to the original filter direction. By placing another polarizing filter over the detector, surficial [120] and subdermal [121] light fractions (i.e., co-polarized (CO) and cross-polarized (CR)) may be discriminated.

Image processing of PS techniques employ an algorithm which generates a normalised difference between CO and CR images [11]:

$$P = \frac{\mathrm{CO} - \mathrm{CR}}{\mathrm{CO} + \mathrm{CR}} \tag{9.11}$$

where P represents a composite image observing surface histology. The denominator cancels any non-uniform illumination. Using polarization imaging and Kubelka-Munk theories, an algorithm was developed [122] to produce an output variable ($\mathrm{TiVi}_{\mathrm{index}}$) capable of relaying information regarding RBC concentration:

$$\mathrm{TiVi}_{\mathrm{index}} = \frac{M_{\mathrm{red}} - M_{\mathrm{green}}}{M_{\mathrm{red}}} \cdot \exp\left[-p\left(\frac{M_{\mathrm{red}} - M_{\mathrm{green}}}{M_{\mathrm{red}}}\right)\right] \tag{9.12}$$

where M_{red} and M_{green} represent the red and green image color planes; and p is an empirical factor which produces the best linear fit between $\mathrm{TiVi}_{\mathrm{index}}$ and RBC concentration. The technique has high temporal and spatial aspects, with lateral resolution estimated at 50 μm [119].

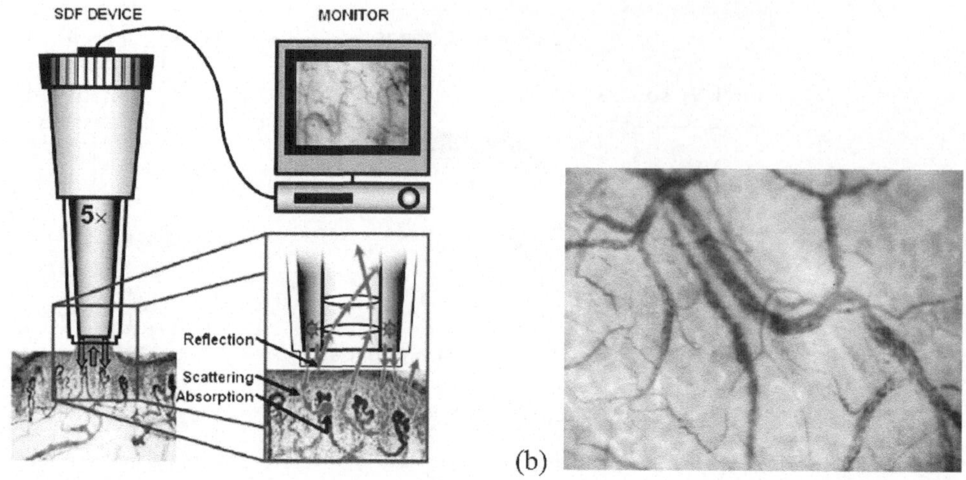

(a) (b)

Figure 9.10: (a) Hand-held SDF imaging device, imaging the tissue-embedded microcirculation [54]; (b) SDF image of the sublingual microcirculation (area = 0.98×0.73 mm^2) [127].

P images have been shown to be comparable to histopathology examination, the invasive "gold standard" of skin examination [11]. Polarisation filtering has been applied in specular reflection elimination in LSI [100] and in LDPI, which otherwise would have resulted in an overestimation of readings [123]; to provide chemical signatures to generate Raman spectra of the superficial layers [124]; and it has been applied in studies of burn depth [11, 15, 16, 125, 126]. The PS method has some limitations, however. A prominent error relates to the measurement inaccuracies obtained on persons with dark skin, due to the high absorption of melanin. Nonetheless, owing to its low cost, ease-of-use and portability, PS imaging systems are an attractive alternative for imaging purposes.

9.2.2.5 Side-stream dark field illumination

The computation of a $\text{TiVi}_{\text{index}}$ value relaying information regarding RBC concentration was discussed in Section 9.2.2.4 This methodology took advantage of the physiological fact that green light ensures optimal optical absorption by the hemoglobin in the RBCs (independent of oxygenation state) with respect to the lack of absorption by the tissue embedding the microcirculation [54]. This use of green light illumination thus acts as a contrast mechanism, where RBCs are visualized as dark moving globules and tissue is visualized as white/gray. Side-stream dark field illumination imaging was introduced as the successor of Optical Polarisation Spectroscopy (OPS) [127].

The SDF imaging device consists of a central light guide, surrounded by concentrically placed light emitting diodes that emit green light. In OPS imaging, the tissue embedding the microcirculation is illuminated with polarized green light [54, 121, 128-130]. As in the case of PS imaging, backscattered (and thus depolarized) light is projected onto a CCD camera after it passes an analyzer. Polarised light reflected by the tissue surface is not detected. Several shortcomings of SDF imaging have been reported [131]; the most prominent of which is the suboptimal imaging of the capillaries due to motion-induced image blurring. In order to overcome this motion-induced artifact, intravital stroboscopic illumination of the green light emitting diodes [54], i.e., providing pulsed illumination in synchrony with the CCD frame rate, (partially) prevents smearing of moving features and motion-induced blurring of capillaries due to the short illumination intervals.

OPS imaging has had an important clinical impact by observation of the microcirculation during sepsis, shock, and resuscitation [131-134]. In fact, results have shown that OPS observation of sublingual microcirculatory alterations provided more sensitive information about patient outcome

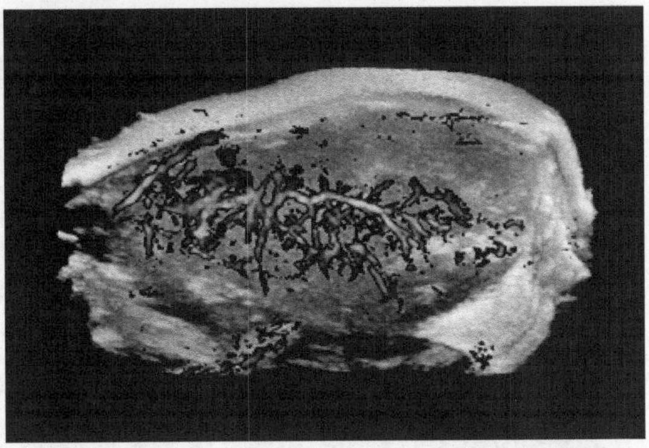

Figure 9.11: (See color insert.) 3D image of an experimental tumor growing in a mouse [139, 140].

from sepsis and shock than conventional clinical parameters. OPS imaging as well as SDF imaging are both validated techniques to investigate the microcirculation; reported investigations include that of the hamster dorsal nailfold [135], the human nailfold plexus [54, 136], the liver [126] and the sublingual tissues [54].

9.2.3 Ultrasound

Ultrasound (US) imaging systems rely on the propagation of mechanical (ultrasonic) waves from a transducer into tissue and the subsequent interactions of these waves with mechanical discontinuities in the tissue. Upon interaction with these discontinuities, a small reflected "echo" wave (scatter) is created and is detectable by the transmitting transducer. Payne *et al.* were the first to report on the topic of Doppler US and the potential the technique held for user defined preselection of measurement depths [137, 138]. The range, z, of the scattering structure is determined by the time of flight of the US to and from the target,

$$z = \frac{c \cdot t}{2} \tag{9.13}$$

where c is the speed of sound; and t is the time taken from initial emission to subsequent scatter remission. The frequency dependent attenuation of US within biological media limits the maximum depth to 300 wavelengths, suggesting that minimum wavelengths of 33 m (45 MHz) to 100 m (15 MHz) imaging 10 to 30 mm tissue depths, respectively, is apt for small animal studies.

US is a well established means of measuring blood velocity using the Doppler principle (see Section 9.2.2.2). Analogous to its optical counterpart, scattering of US waves from moving RBCs leads to a shift in the frequency relative to the initial sonification pulse. The expression for velocity of blood flow, v, is given by:

$$v = \frac{f_{Ds} c}{2 f_0 \cos\theta} \tag{9.14}$$

where f_{Ds} is the Doppler frequency shift, f_0, the sonification frequency, c, the local speed of sound, and θ, the angle between the axis of beam propagation and the flow velocity vector.

Recent work has been undertaken to examine the potential of US Doppler findings of tumor stage and/or patient prognosis [141-143]. It is, however, clear that these methods are sensitive only to large vessel flow, i.e. arterioles and venules larger than about 50 μm. Despite this, the development of high frequency micro-US [144, 145] and Doppler, has facilitated the non-invasive imaging of microscopic structure and blood flow with improved spatial resolution. The intensity

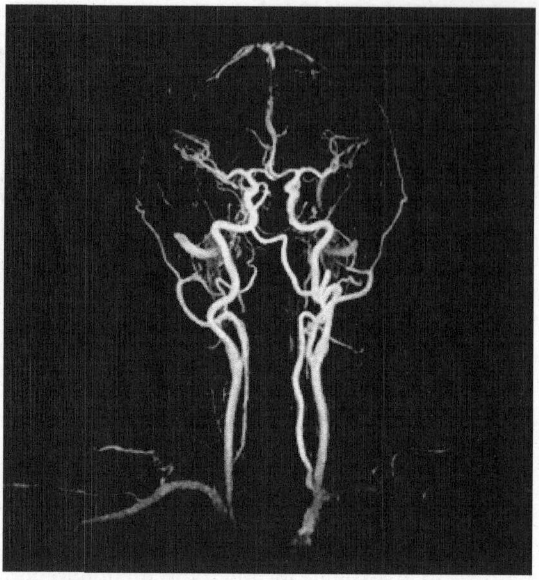

Figure 9.12: Maximum intensity projection of the whole data-set showing normal appearance of the head and neck arteries on contrast-enhanced MR-angiography [159].

of scatter echoes depends on the reflective property of the tracers [4]. The introduction of US microbubble contrast agents (diameter less than 1 to 5 μm) has created a significant opportunity for visualization of the microcirculation [146, 147] by enabling anatomical and functional aspects to be visualized and quantified. Due to these improvements in US imaging, the modality is now ripe to be exploited in a plethora of clinical applications. Efforts are underway to use the US technology in prostate imaging [148], neonatal imaging [149], skin and ocular imaging [150] and a wide range of intraluminal imaging applications [151]. The extensive applicability of US in the clinical domain may be seen from its qualitative and prognostic assessment of cardiovascular disease [152], developmental biology [153], musculoskeletal disease [154], arteriosclerosis [152] and a wide variety of other manifestations of human disease.

9.2.4 Magnetic resonance imaging

Magnetic Resonance Imaging (MRI) was first suggested by Lauterbur [155] and, independently, by Mansfield and Grannell [156]. Nuclei with an odd number of protons, neutrons or both, have an intrinsic nuclear spin [157, 158]. Ordinarily, nuclei spin with their axes randomly aligned. The potential energy of the magnetic momentum in a homogeneous external magnetic field depends on the direction of momentum. The magnetic momentum of a proton (e.g., hydrogen atom) of low potential energy (i.e., parallel momentum and field vectors) can be flipped to a higher energy state (anti-parallel vectors) by absorption of a photon of exactly the missing energy difference between these two states [4] — this is referred to as nuclear magnetic resonance. The nucleus reverts/realigns to its normal state via emission of a photon, whose frequency is dependent on the energy difference between the normal and excited spin states. It is this motion that is used to construct a 3D image composed of information from the strata of the object; this depth information is obtained by transmitting multiple radio waves at differing frequencies in space [157].

Contrast agents [160] are frequently used in MRI studies as a means of improving the visibility of internal body structures by contrast enhancement, the most common of which are gadolinium-based [161]. As tissue is approximately diamagnetic, a paramagnetic vascular contrast agent would change the environment and alter the relaxation times of tissues and body cavities in which they are present. Barium sulfate is commonly used as a means of signal enhancement in the gastrointestinal tract, but natural products high in manganese (e.g., green tea) serve the same purpose [162].

In the days of MRI's infancy, signals from dynamic tissue constituents (e.g., RBCs) were considered an insidious nuisance as it generated frequent artifacts which detracted from image quality. In due course, it was realised that these apparently errant signals could be exploited to generate diagnostic quality images of blood vessels. For example, phase contrast velocity MRI [163] estimates the phase shift of hydrogen nuclei as they pass through a magnetic field and this phase change is proportional to velocity [164]. Other methods of time-resolved contrast-enhanced functional assessment have since been introduced, for example, time-of-flight MR angiography (TOF MRA) [165] and contrast-enhanced MR-angiography (CEMRA) [166]. Contrast-enhanced techniques such as MRI offer unrivalled spatial and temporal resolution, in addition to having good soft tissue contrast and depth of penetration without any loss in sensitivity or resolution [23, 167]. However, it is an expensive research tool in terms of initial purchase and subsequent maintenance, requiring experienced operators. Image rendering is very time consuming, implying the technique is more suited to recordings of steady state conditions rather than transient phenomena. Moreover, MRI has not been well validated in terms of the microcirculation [168]. Nevertheless, functional MRI has become a most important tool for cognitive research since the latter part of the 20th century, with some of its most important applications being found in oncological studies [169, 170], cardiac perfusion and monitoring [171, 172] and neurological imaging [173, 174].

9.2.5 Positron emission tomography

Functional imaging with positron-emitting isotopes was first proposed as an imaging technique that could offer greater sensitivity with single photon-emitting isotopes than conventional nuclear medicine techniques [175]. It was recognized that high-energy photons produced by the annihilation of positron-emitting isotopes could be used to describe the physiological distribution of "tagged" chemical compounds [176]. Positron emission tomography (PET) is a nuclear medicine imaging technique which utilizes exogenous and endogenous contrast mechanisms (i.e., "tracers") to yield a 3D image of intrinsic functional processes and/or changes of regional blood flow in various anatomic structures.

The PET process is multifaceted. Imaging begins with a biological molecule that carries a positron-emitting isotope (a "tracer") injected into the patient. ^{15}O, ^{13}N, ^{11}C and ^{18}F are considered among the most important radionuclides for medical applications of PET [177]. Over time, this isotope accumulates in an area of the body for which the attached molecule has an affinity; e.g. ^{11}C accumulates in the brain or tumors where glucose is the primary source of energy [176]. The radioactive nuclei decay by positron emission and the emitted positron undergoes annihilation with an electron from the surroundings. The energy associated with this process divides equally between two photons (i.e. high energy γ-rays) which fly from each other at a 180° angle. An array of detectors surrounding the patient senses the γ-ray radiation (provided the line of coincidence is correct) and distribution of the positron-emitting tracer is computed via tomographic reconstruction procedures from the recorded projection data.

PET images qualitatively assess sites of unusual tracer accumulations (tumor sites) and quantitatively measure the tracer uptake for an assessment of the staging of a disease [176]. However, the use of radionuclides is not only invasive, as outlined in Section 9.2.1.1, but the use of such may induce patient-specific complications. Furthermore, PET utilizes ionizing radiation in its operation, and resulting images tend to be of poor resolution (in the order of mm [180]) in comparison to other methods. In spite of this, the ability of PET to analyse disease progression is well documented, for example, in Alzheimer's disease [179, 181] (see Fig. 9.13); Parkinson's disease [182, 183]; epilepsy [184-186]; visualization of the heart [187] and afflictions such as coronary artery disease [188]. PET has also been shown to be effective in locating metastatic disease in the breast [180],

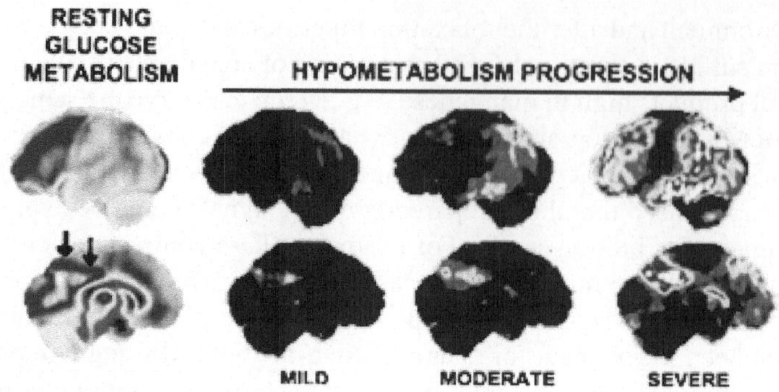

Figure 9.13: PET image of progressive reduction in glucose metabolism in Alzheimer's disease. Adapted from [178, 179].

lung [189] and lower gastrointestinal tract [190], in addition to distinguishing between both benign and malignant cancer [191, 192].

Micro positron emission tomography (micro-PET) is an advanced form of current PET technology [193]. It provides information pertaining to the function of living organisms with very high sensitivity, high signal-to-noise ratio, and requires minimal use of radioisotopes (e.g., nanoparticles) for detecting physiological characteristics. Nowadays, PET is always combined with CT to put the function in a structural context.

9.3 Optical Sectioning Techniques

9.3.1 Histology: staining

An essential tool of biology and medicine, histology is the study of the anatomy of cells and tissues via examination by microscopy, subsequent to sectioning and apt staining. As biological tissue has little inherent contrast in either light or electron microscopy, staining is employed to provide contrast and to highlight particular features of interest. Micro-Computed Tomography is one of the most common microscopy methods which employs histology (see Section 9.3.3).

Tissue processing initially involves ethanol dehydration to remove water, addition of an infiltration agent (e.g. paraffin wax or a resin) which solidifies the medium and then embedding in an external medium (e.g. agar, gelatine) to harden. The hardened blocks containing the tissue samples are then ready to be sectioned. Freezing a tissue section or applying chemical fixatives (e.g. formalin) can also preserve samples from degradation [194]. Depending on the section thicknesses involved, a steel or diamond knife mounted in a microtome is used to cut tissue into sections. Post-sectioning, specimens are mounted on a slide and treated with an apt stain. Hematoxylin and eosin is the most commonly used microscopy stain in histology and histopathology (see Fig. 9.14). Different tissue classifications such as blood cells (connective tissue) and the endothelial lining of blood and lymphatic vessels are subject to selective staining [22].

Processing of tissue samples in this manner can cause shrinkage and alterations in tissue pigments and structure, rendering it unrepresentative of *in vivo* morphology. Information on functional (perfused) capillary density is lost along with any dynamic data. Additionally, naturally occurring melanin within the skin can alter tissue appearance and obscure structures in histopathological examination [195]. However, live tissues may be stored indefinitely at room temperature, and nucleic

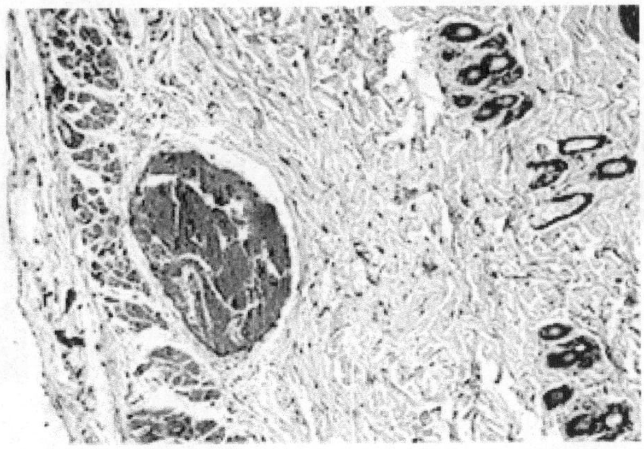

Figure 9.14: Hematoxylin and eosin stained sections (×100) of rodent dorsal skin flap [110].

acids may be recovered decades after fixation.

Given the extensive clinical reliance the value of histopathological findings, the application of its use is very broad. Reported studies have shown it to be used in the quantitative analysis of cancer metastatic growth [196, 197] and in the detection of hypoxic cells [198]; it has provided contrast in ocular surgery [199]; qualitative assessment of its use in esophageal lesions has been reported [200]; and analysis of irregular pigmentation, for example, port wine stains [201–203]. Histology has also been employed for flow purposes, for example, in the observation of novel threadlike structures on organ surfaces [204] and has been used in conjunction with LSI (see Section 9.2.2.3) to visualize blood vessel density [110].

9.3.2 High resolution sectioning

9.3.2.1 Optical projection tomography

Previously, the standard technique for mapping 3D gene and protein expression patterns involved serial sectioning [205]. However, reconstruction of images by these means was not only time consuming but also induced distortion. The wide range of optical methods which exist at present are optimised for the differing levels of scattering of various sized specimens within tissue. Small, non-scattering samples (through which photons will travel with a "ballistic trajectory") can be imaged with Optical Projection Tomography (OPT). OPT provides molecular specificity, resolution on the order of microns to tens of microns, and is suitable for imaging of transparent specimens whose thicknesses in the imaging direction lie in the 1–15 mm range [206]. With reference to Figure 9.1, OPT occupies the same imaging domain as that of Optical Coherence Tomography.

OPT is capable of producing very high resolution images and reconstructions due to the optical clearing process prior to imaging [205]. The clearing process matches the index of refraction of the sample tissue with that of the surrounding medium and renders samples transparent [207]. The raw data obtained in OPT must be then be mathematically transformed to recreate the original object [208, 209]. OPT imaging is performed in both transmission and emission modes; transmission is used for studies of anatomy, whereas emission mode is used to image the distribution of fluorescently labeled samples. In transmission mode, a wide field (diffuse or non-diffuse) light source illuminates a sample which is angularly rotated stepwise; the light transmitted in this stepwise fashion is captured using a CCD microscope (see Fig. 9.15). Similarly, in emission mode, wide field illumination of apt wavelength excites the same rotating sample and the emitted fluorescence is captured using in the same manner as transmission mode.

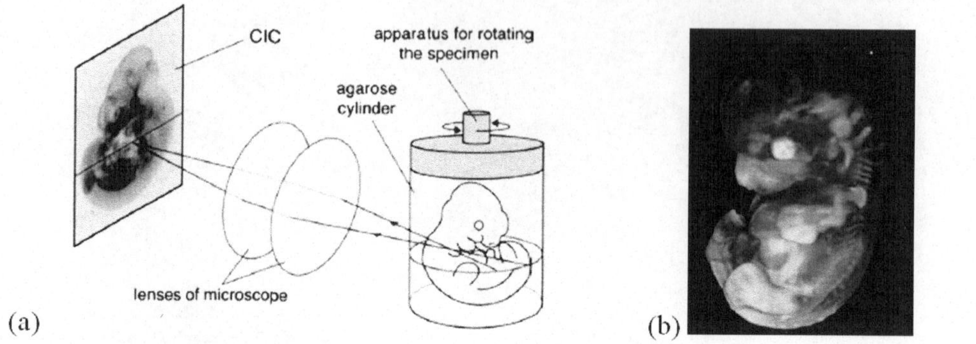

Figure 9.15: (a) Schematic of OPT microscopy setup [208]; (b) False-color images of a mouse embryo, stained with alcian blue and then scanned by OPT [210].

Generally, transmission and emission modes are used concurrently to render fluorescent visualizations against a morphological backdrop. As is the case with many optical imaging techniques, tradeoffs exist in their operation in terms of resolution and depth of field. For instance, partially closing the iris of the system in both transmission and emission modes of OPT increases the depth of field of the system, thus degrading the image resolution [205]:

$$\mathrm{DOF}_{\mathrm{max}} = \eta_{\mathrm{bath}} \left(\frac{1.305\lambda}{\mathrm{NA}^2} \right) \tag{9.15}$$

where $\mathrm{DOF}_{\mathrm{max}}$ is the maximum depth of field achievable by the system; NA is the system numerical aperture; η_{bath}, the refractive index of the material in which samples are suspended. Organic solvents which act as index-matching agents are, however, generally toxic. Resultantly, analysis of live specimens is restricted to those that are already adequately transparent, e.g. small embryonic tissue. Use of a wide-field CCD in OPT operation causes some of the pixel noise to be generated by multiply scattered photons that were emitted from regions of the tissue that do not lie on the intended projection for that pixel. Use of a laser scanning approach renders less noise at a given pixel, in a manner analogous to the use of laser scanning in confocal imaging [211].

In addition to its use in developmental biology, OPT microscopy has the potential for use in medical applications for which knowledge of the 3D structure may be useful, but not readily accessible from histopathological sections (see Section 9.3.1). Given OPT's versatility in its ability to simultaneously record both absorption and emission profiles, it is particularly useful in performing gene expression analysis [210–212].

OPT has been shown to reveal superb sectioning ability, useful for reconstructing vertebrate embryos and in the examination of the 3D anatomy of developing organs [210, 212, 213] (see Fig. 9.15); modelling of early human brain development [214]; 3D imaging of isolated cell nuclei [215]. With regard to contributions this technique has made to the knowledge of flow and related dynamics, OPT has been shown to be applicable in studies of gas-solids flow to analyse particle concentration [216]; general flow rate analyses [217, 218]; cell tracing [219]; and the spatiotemporal analysis of zebrafish [220].

9.3.2.2 Stimulated emission depletion microscopy

Since the research of Abbé, it has been considered that the resolution limit of light microscopy based on focusing optics had been reached [221]. Einstein's notion of de-exciting a quantum system by stimulated emission has not only facilitated the invention of the laser but also of stimulated emission depletion (STED), a super-resolution microscopy technique which utilizes the non-linear

(a) 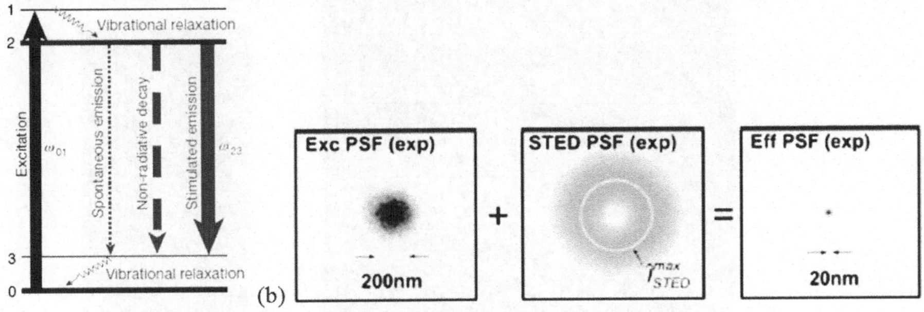

(b)

Figure 9.16: (See color insert.) (a) Energy diagram of spontaneous emission, non-radiative decay and stimulated emission processes for a typical four-level energy system [228]; (b) Measured focal spots for excitation (left: 470 nm; blue), STED (center: 603 nm, orange) and effective spot (right: 22 nm, green) [224]

de-excitation of fluorescent dyes to overcome the resolution limit imposed by diffraction. This has resulted in resolution improvements by a factor of 10–12 [222–224] with a focal plane resolution greater than 6 nm achievable [225], surpassing that of current high-end x-ray microscopy [226].

The intensity distribution of the excitation light in the focal plane of the lens is determined by diffraction and described by the point-spread function (PSF) [227],

$$h_{\text{exc}}(\nu) = \text{const} \cdot \left| \frac{2J_1(\nu)}{\nu} \right|^2 \tag{9.16}$$

where J_1 is the first-order Bessel function; $\nu = 2\pi r \text{NA}/\lambda_{\text{exc}}$; r is the distance from the focal point; NA, numerical aperture; and λ_{exc} is the excitation wavelength. One possible way to reduce the spatial extent of $h_{\text{exc}}(\nu)$) is to inhibit the fluorescence in its outer regions; this is equivalent to an increase in resolution [222]. Employment of an additional STED laser beam (see Fig. 9.16(b, center)) inhibits fluorescence by being focused with small lateral offsets $\pm\Delta\nu$ with respect to the excitation beam and overlaps with the excitation beam on either side. Thus, the STED beam depletes the excited state before fluorescence takes place via stimulated emission (see Fig. 9.16(a)) and only the innermost region of $h_{\text{exc}}(\nu)$ remains which contributes to the fluorescence signal (see Fig. 9.16(b, right)).

The first experimental confirmation of the superior lateral resolution of this non-invasive STED technique was demonstrated by separation of adjacent Pyridine nanocrystals [229] that are otherwise indiscernible.

Chromophores, such as hemoglobin, absorb but have undetectable fluorescence because the spontaneous emission is dominated by their fast non-radiative decay. STED competes effectively with this non-radioactive decay, providing a new contrast mechanism which has been investigated in the vascular network of a nude mouse ear [228]. In addition, STED has been implemented in nanofluidic studies [230, 231] with reported spatial resolutions better than 70 nm; and in protein flow cytometry research [232].

9.3.3 Micro-computed tomography

The basis of all computed tomography techniques is the ordered collection of x-ray projected data from multiple angles in space [233]. Many comparisons may be drawn between the working principles of micro-computed tomography (micro-CT) and those of OPT (see Section 9.3.2.1). 3D images of vasculature are obtainable by micro-CT imaging, with resolution on the micron scale.

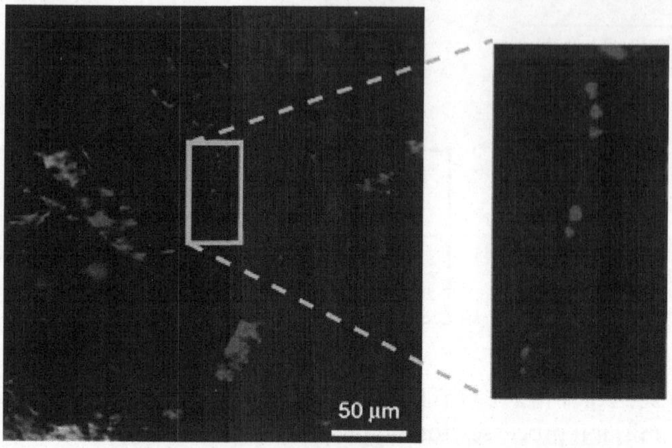

Figure 9.17: (See color insert.) Maximum intensity projection (red channel) stimulated emission *ex vivo* imaging of mouse ear microvasculature based on endogenous hemoglobin contrast. In the magnified image, individual RBC rouleaux are visible within a single capillary [228].

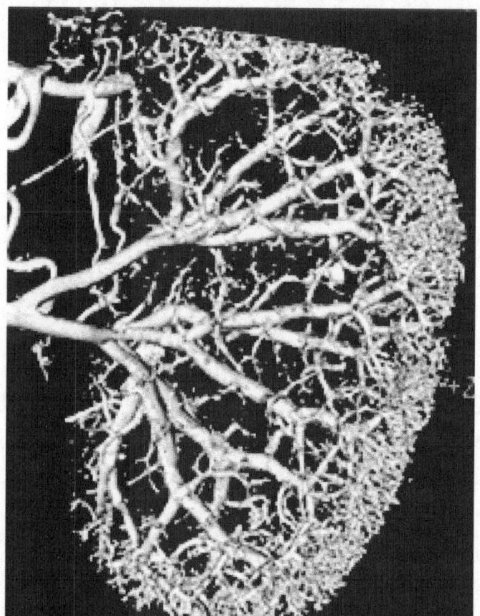

Figure 9.18: Micro-CT image of vascular tree of a mouse kidney [235].

A micro-CT system comprises three basic elements: an x-ray source; the conversion electronics; and a method for either rotating the specimen or rotating the scanner around the specimen. This experimental setup is very similar to that of Fig. 9.15(a), substituting bright-field illumination with an x-ray source. To generate 3D volume data, methods such as cone beam reconstruction [234] are used to convert the projection data into a stack of slices [233]; this may be further extended into filtered back projection methods, as is the case in OPT.

As an x-ray penetrates an object in transmission mode, it is exponentially attenuated by the material along its path in the same manner as described by the Beer-Lambert law in Eq. (9.2). However, the main limitation of micro-CT relates to contrast; as the absorption of x-rays by soft tissues or optical colored stains is low, this causes difficulties in the simultaneous imaging tissue structure and analysis of gene expression, respectively [236]. In addition, image quality is inherently related to x-ray dose, a concern that is particularly relevant for *in vivo* studies (e.g., the potential for radiation damage to the specimen, thereby altering the physiology). High spatial resolution requires high doses, and a reduction in dose causes higher image noise and reduced image contrast [237].

The modulation transfer function (MTF) of an imaging system is a common comparator for micro-CT spatial resolution [233, 238]:

$$\mathrm{MTF}(\rho) = \left| \int_{-\infty}^{+\infty} \exp(-j2\pi\rho x)[\mathrm{LSF}(x)]dx \right| \quad (9.17)$$

where ρ represents spatial frequency; and LSF is the integral of the point spread function. In any real imaging system, the MTF is non-ideal and values drop progressively at higher spatial frequencies. Resultantly, small vessel diameters appear to broaden and this causes inaccuracies in CT-values. However, improvements in scanner components have made bench-top nano-CT units feasible, having the ability to image at cellular and subcellular levels with voxel resolutions on the order of 500 nm [237].

Micro-CT provides high resolution 3D volumetric data, suitable for analysis, quantification, validation and visualization of vasculature. Reported studies for the use of micro-CT include the assessment of induced or implanted disease models [239, 240]; screening for anatomical abnormalities and/or changes in live animals [241]; assessing angiogenesis during fracture healing [242]; in morphological studies, for example, the rodent renal vasculature [243, 244]; and the assessment of cancer staging for predictions of metastatic relapse [245]. Micro-CT has also branched into the realm of fluid dynamic simulations in, for instance, the mouse aorta [246, 247] and assessment of coronary artery disease [248]. Although *in vivo* micro-CT imaging is still in its infancy, the possible implications and applications of its use in biomedical research is potentially far-reaching.

9.3.4 Confocal and two-photon imaging

The previously described methods of optical projection tomography and stimulated emission depletion microscopy (Section 9.3.2.1, Section 9.3.2.2) both utilize fluorescence in their operation. However, a severe problem with epi-fluorescence is the unwanted contribution of signals from structures above and below the focal plane; this can produce a background glow that can cause image degradation [249]. This is surmounted by employing the principles of confocal imaging.

Geometrically speaking, confocal means having the same foci. In the confocal rgime, an object is illuminated with a small (diffraction limited) spot, usually derived from a focused laser beam. An objective lens replaces that of the conventional microscope condenser and the field of illumination is limited by a pinhole positioned on the microscope axis. This spatially restricts the optical system so that only signals emanating from the focal point are detected. Both the intensity of illumination and the sensitivity of the detector fall rapidly with distance away from the focal plane. Thus, light scattered from parts other than the illuminated point on the specimen is rejected from the optical system (by the exit pinhole) resulting in reduced blurring from light scattering, improved effective resolution and signal-to-noise ratio [250]. This technique may be used in both transmitting and epi-illuminating modes, and an image of the complete specimen is built up by a raster scanning. Reported resolutions have been of the order of 100 nm [5]; however, with 4-Pi methods an axial resolution of 100 nm and a localization accuracy of < 10 nm in fixed and immune-labeled specimens [251].

As described above, confocal microscopy dramatically reduces the contribution of fluorescence from the out-of-focus regions of a specimen. However, regions above and below the focal plane are still exposed to the full intensity of the excitation light and "parasitic" fluorescence in every direction, converging and diverging from the illuminated spot in the focal plane. Resultantly, biological specimens still succumb to photon-induced damage and rapid fluorescent bleaching. These

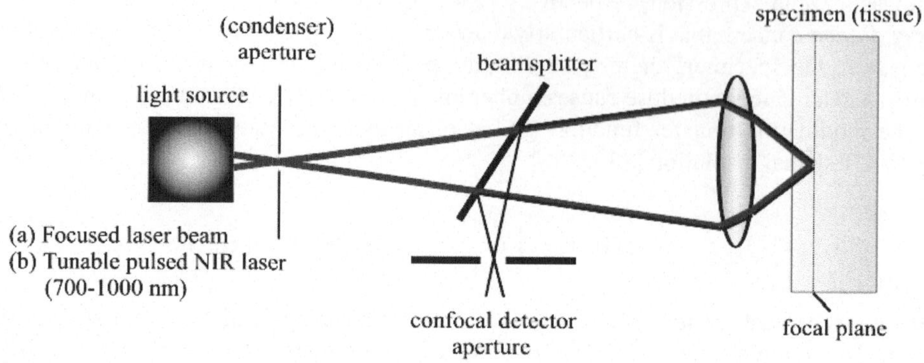

Figure 9.19: Microscope schematic for (a) confocal and (b) two-photon methods.

shortcomings are circumvented by two-photon microscopy [252, 253], and has been extended to the practice of multiphoton (i.e., more than 2) fluorescence microscopy [250].

The challenges posed by the confocal methods may be surmounted by outputting an intense IR laser pulse which induces fluorescence in the blue or UV excitable fluorophore at the focal spot of the system only. At this position, the coherent electromagnetic field strength is so high that its acts non-linearly to excite chromophores at twice the frequency of the IR pulse, inducing an electronic transition equivalent to the absorption of a single photon, possessing twice as much energy [254]. The excited fluorophore can then emit a single photon of fluorescence. As a result, fluorophores above and below the focus do not experience the fluorescence effects of the two-photon methods and are therefore neither excited nor damaged. Additionally, two-photon microscopy permits confocal imaging of planes much deeper in the tissue (new approaches have led to depths of almost 1 mm [255]) with considerably higher light coupling efficiency, with less bleaching and damage outside of the focal plane [252, 256, 257]. For very thin objects such as isolated cells, confocal microscopy produces images with higher optical resolution due to the shorter excitation wavelengths. Nonetheless, the superior optical sectioning and light detection capabilities of the two-photon modality results in better performance in highly scattering tissue.

The biggest advantage of 3D optical sectioning approaches such as confocal microscopy and two-photon microscopy [258], is their ability to visualize biologically significant molecular distributions within a single specimen. However both techniques do suffer some shortcomings. Although the confocal principle allows clear imaging within semitransparent tissue, turbid media causes scattering and absorption of light thus diminishing the ability to image with depth. This limits the actual useful depth of confocal imaging to around 100–200 μm [250] even with the use of near IR illumination which is more penetrating than visible light [259–261]. Moreover, use of IR illumination for imaging itself reduces image resolution, due to the longer wavelength for a given numerical aperture [259]. The pulsed lasers required for two-photon excitation are much more expensive than the continuous wave versions used in confocal microscopy. In addition, despite the fact that the *in vivo* resolution provided by multiphoton imaging is reportedly superior to that offered by MRI and PET, the necessity of either thinning or removing a portion of the skull for imaging the brain surface impedes the potential clinical applicability of this technique [262].

Yet, despite these limiting factors, confocal and two-photon imaging have been used in a wide variety of applications: rodent cerebral microcirculation investigations [263–266]; used in conjunction with particle image velocimetry (see Section 9.4.1) to investigate micro-channel blood flow [267]; as a quantitative method in the study of embryonic vasculature dynamics [268, 269]; dynamic studies of Alzheimer's disease and epilepsy [262]; and in cytometric studies of the relationships between stem cells [270], tumor cells [271] and their tissue environments [272, 273].

9.3.5 Photoacoustic tomography and microscopy

Purely optical imaging in biological media is hampered with the either imaging depth or spatial resolution trade-offs, owing to strong optical scattering. Purely ultrasonic (USn) imaging may improve upon these limiting factors in the optical (quasi-) diffusive rgime, due to the fact that USn scattering is 2–3 orders of magnitude weaker than optical scattering [238]. Photoacoustic tomography (PAT) refers to imaging based upon the tenets of the photoacoustic effect. If an object is irradiated with a short-pulsed laser beam, some of radiation is absorbed and partially converted into heat. This heat causes a pressure rise via localized thermoelastic expansion, and this pressure rise propagates as a USn or photoacoustic (or optoacoustic) wave. Detection of these signals by an array of transducers allows reconstruction of the light absorption distribution and deduction of information on the distribution of absorbing inclusions in tissue. A typical PAT system uses an unfocused US detector to acquire the photoacoustic (PA) signals, and the image is reconstructed by inversely solving the photoacoustic equations (e.g. backprojection algorithms based on time-reversal methods [274–277]).

PAT is an optical absorption based modality, with contrast and resolution based on the PA excitation phase and PA emission phase (derived from the USn detection), respectively. In PAT, NIR light is used as it is in this wavelength range (and that of the visible wavelengths) that hemoglobin dominates soft tissue optical absorption, producing functional network maps of hemoglobin oxygen saturation in the vasculature [278]. If an isosbestic point is selected for imaging, the PA signal represents total hemoglobin concentration, irrespective of oxygenation.

The generation and propagation of a PA wave in an inviscid medium may be described by the following [238],

$$\left(\nabla^2 - \frac{1}{v_S^2}\frac{\partial^2}{\partial t^2}\right) p(\vec{r},t) = -\frac{\beta}{\kappa v_S^2}\frac{\partial^2 T(\vec{r},t)}{\partial t^2} \tag{9.18}$$

where v_S is the speed of sound; t, time; $p(\vec{r},t)$, the acoustic pressure at location $\vec{r}$ and time t; β, thermal coefficient of volume expansion; κ, isothermal compressibility; and T, temperature rise. The spatial resolution (Δx) of a PAT system is determined by the frequency bandwidth of the PA signal detectors (Δf) [274]:

$$\Delta x \sim \frac{v_S}{\Delta f} \tag{9.19}$$

PAT combines the advantageous aspects of optical diffusion tomography and conventional US imaging, with achievable spatial resolutions on the order of 0.1–10 mm (frequency bandwidth dependent) and imaging depths of several cm.

Intravital microscopy is the current "gold standard" for imaging of dynamic microvascular regulation [279]; however, it is generally invasive and lacks crucial morphological parameters such as depth information. PA microscopy (PAM) overcomes these limitations by being reliant on endogenous optical contrast, working non-invasively in reflection mode with time-resolved depth detection.

In contrast to the PAT technique, a PAM system uses a spherically focused ultrasound detector with 2D point-by-point scanning, requiring no reconstruction algorithm. Conventional reflection-mode confocal PAM is implemented using both dark-field pulsed-laser illumination [282, 283] and high-NA USn detection. A pulsed laser beam (e.g., from a Q-switched pulsed Nd:YAG laser[3]) delivered by a multimode optical fiber passes through a conical lens forming annular illumination and is then weakly focused into biological tissues. Due to this illumination type, the PA signal is greatly minimised. A concave acoustic lens is attached to the transducer, which in turn is immersed in a water container for added USn coupling efficiency. Light from the optical fiber is expanded by a

[3]Nd:YAG: neodymium yttrium aluminium garnet

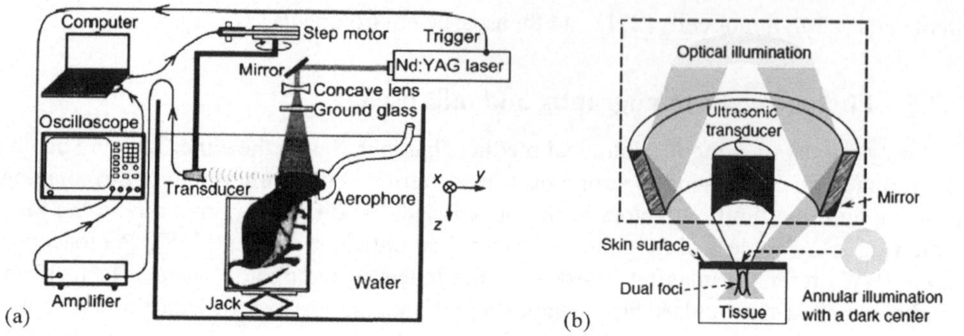

Figure 9.20: PAT setup for non-invasive transdermal and transcranial imaging of the rat brain *in vivo* [280]; (b) Annular illumination of functional PAM system [281].

conical lens and focused through an optical condenser. The optical dark-field illumination and USn detection are confocal, as the optical and USn transducer foci are overlapped. On each laser-pulse excitation, the emitted PA wave is recorded as a function of time (thus forming an A-scan[4]); raster scanning of the PAM probe head yields 3D volume data sets. The lateral resolution (Δr) depends on the USn parameters, the source center wavelength (λ_0) and the transducer numerical aperture (NA):

$$\Delta r = 0.71 \frac{\lambda_0}{\text{NA}} \tag{9.20}$$

In order to resolve fine structures, spatial resolutions of 10 μm or higher are desired. Applying this to the dark-field methodology, a USn transducer with center frequency of 400 MHz is required; however, this limits the penetration depth to <100 μm. Spatial resolution in dark-field PAM is limited by USn parameters (<50 μm), and is thus unable to resolve artifacts on the arteriole, venule and capillary scale [281, 284]. By employing techniques such as diffraction-limited optical focusing (OR-PAM) [285] (see Fig. 9.21 (b)), resolution improvements on the order of 5 μm or greater are obtainable.

The PA Doppler (PAD) effect [287–289] is the combination of the production of an acoustic wave from a light-absorbing medium and the shifting of this wave when it has a motion relative to a detector. Consider a light absorbing-particle suspended in a liquid is moving at a velocity $\vec{v}$ and an intensity-modulated laser beam illuminates the particle at an angle α. The particle undergoes the PA process and results in the formation of an acoustic wave which are collected in a solid angle Ω by a USn transducer. Doppler shifts values depend on θ, the angle between the flow path of the particle and the transducer. The PAD shift (f_{PAD}) of the PA wave along a typical angle θ may be expressed as [289]:

$$f_{\text{PAD}} = f_{\text{M}} \frac{v \cos\theta}{v_S} \tag{9.21}$$

where f_{M} is the modulation frequency; and v_S is the velocity of the moving scattering object. In Section 9.2.2.2, the method of laser Doppler flowmetry was outlined; a principle disadvantage of this method is its limited measuring depth and loss of flow directional information due to multiple light scattering. With the PAD methods, however, this is no longer an issue. Additionally, as light-absorbing particles are used as flow tracers, lower background noise and higher detection contrast result.

PA techniques are frequently used in cerebral microvascular imaging [280] (see Fig. 9.21 (a)) and cancer detection. Enhanced angiogenesis is typical for malignant tumors from onset and therefore

[4]A-scan: 1D depth-resolved image

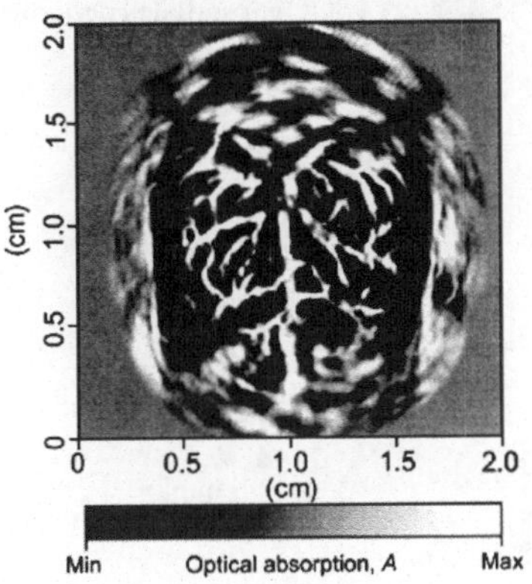

(a)

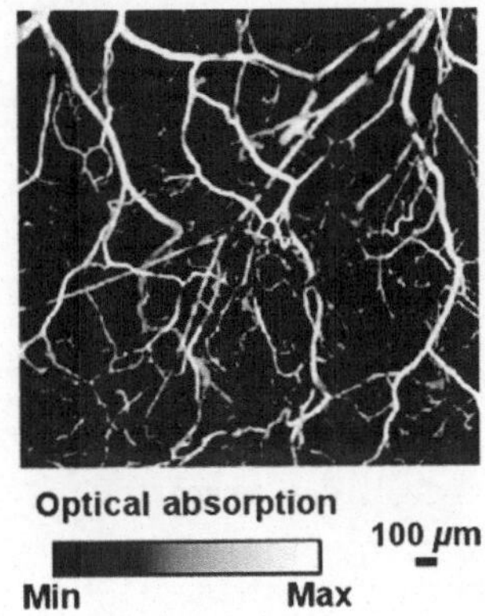

(b)

Figure 9.21: (a) Non-invasive PAT image of the vascular pattern in the superficial layer of the rat cortex acquired with intact skin and skull (2 cm×2 cm) [280]; (b) A representative microvascular network in a nude mouse ear imaged *in vivo* by OR-PAM [286].

PAT allows for early tumor detection and diagnosis [290, 291]. These methods have also been utilized in the assessment of absorption contrast differentiation between metastatic and normal breast tissue [292, 293]. In addition, PA techniques have been used alongside complementary multimodal modalities such as fluorescence imaging to yield *in vivo* functional molecular information [294, 295].

9.3.6 Optical coherence tomography (OCT)

Many of the aforementioned optical techniques (Polarisation Spectroscopy, Optical Projection Tomography and Photoacoustic Imaging) are based on the diffuse scattering of light with turbid media. Optical Coherence Tomography (OCT), on the other hand, falls into the category of *ballistic* (and *quasi-ballistic*) optical imaging. OCT is analogous to ultrasound pulse-echo imaging [296], employing coherence gating. The intensity of singly backscattered light is given by [238]:

$$I(z) = I_0 \exp(-2\mu_t z) R_B \tag{9.22}$$

where R_B denotes the portion of backscattered light received by the detector; the factor of two in the exponent results from the round-trip propagation. Ballistic imaging rejects non-ballistic photons; the retained ballistic photons have better collimation, a more well-defined wavefront, and retain their incident polarization state (in a non-birefringent medium). OCT detection is based on the principles of interferometry as the speed of light is 5 orders of magnitude larger than that of sound. It can provide clear visual boundaries between different vessel wall layers and is a non-contact modality.

OCT is based in Michelson interferometry, using low coherence light sources (e.g. superluminescent diodes) and may be implemented in free-space or (single-mode) fiber-based systems. In interferometry, if a monochromatic light source beam is emitted towards a beamsplitter it is split into two, with one half backreflected from a reference mirror and the remaining backreflected by an object surface. These split beams are then recombined by the original beamsplitter and received by a detector. The intensity received by a the detector may be written as [297],

$$I(t) = E_{R0}^2 + E_{S0}^2 + 2E_{R0}E_{S0}\cos(\underbrace{2(k_S l_S - k_R l_R)}_{\Delta\phi}) \tag{9.23}$$

where R and S denote the reference and sample arms, respectively; E_0 is the incident electric field; k, the propagation constant; and l is the arm length from beamsplitter to the back reflection surfaces.

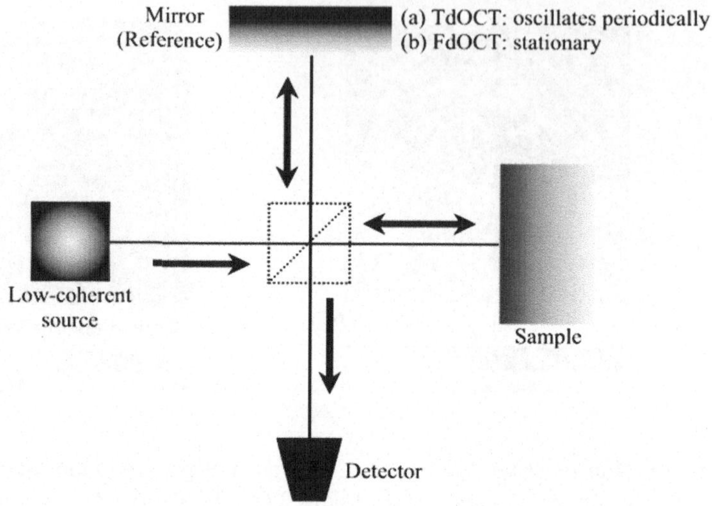

Figure 9.22: Schematic of free-space TdOCT (a) and FdOCT (b) systems.

The time-varying phase difference $\Delta\phi$ results in the interference term becoming an alternating current which produces interference fringes. Thus, the recorded I is referred to an as interferogram, varying periodically with optical pathlength difference (or mismatch) $2\eta(l_S - l_R)$.

The first generation OCT systems were based on time-domain principles (TdOCT) [296, 298]. In TdOCT systems, while the reference beam is reflected from a mirror as is in the traditional interferometric setup, the sample beam is backscattered from various depths in a biological tissue sample. The movement of the reference arm induces a Doppler frequency shift in the reflected reference beam. Detection of beams of this type may be categorised as heterodyne detection owing to the Doppler shift. However, the principle which enables OCT to resolve the back-scattered distribution of the backscattered light is coherence gating; beams will only interfere when their optical pathlength difference is within the coherence length of the light source. The coherence length (l_C) of light is defined as the spatial extent along the propagation direction over which the electric field is substantially correlated [299]:

$$l_C = \frac{4\ln 2}{\pi}\frac{\lambda_0^2}{\Delta\lambda} \tag{9.24}$$

where λ_0, the source center wavelength; and $\Delta\lambda$ is the full-width at half maximum (FWHM) bandwidth. Therefore, the axial resolution may be determined by the source coherence length (i.e. the arrival of time echoes), or more accurately, $l_C/2$. Although the above expression for l_C is for a Gaussian lineshape, it is the most common definition in OCT literature [300]. In contrast to convention microscopy, the axial and transverse resolutions in OCT are decoupled from each other. However, as is the case in traditional microscopic methods, the transverse resolution in the OCT imaging system is determined by the focused spot size [301]:

$$\Delta x = \frac{4\lambda}{\pi}\frac{f}{d} \tag{9.25}$$

where d is the spot size on the objective lens and f is its focal length; the transverse resolution results from the confocal mechanism. The path length distribution of ballistic light may be directly converted into a physical depth distribution; this conversion breaks down if diffuse light is considered.

The Fourier domain equivalent of TdOCT (FdOCT), which encompasses both spectral and swept-source variants [302], avoids the varying of the reference optical path by considering all multiple

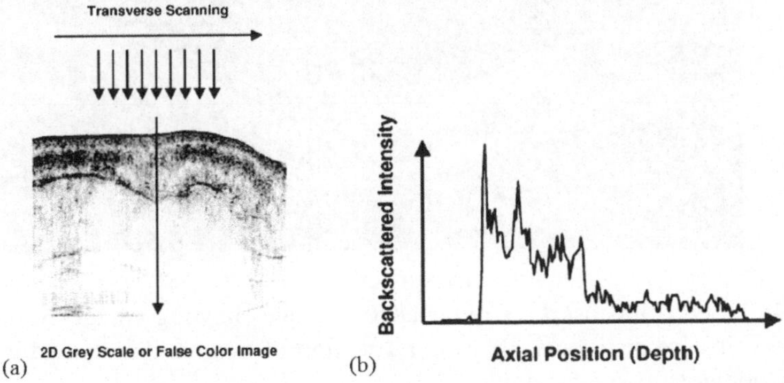

Figure 9.23: (a) 2D (and 3D) cross-sectional images are constructed by imaging at different transverse positions; (b) 1D representation of the backscattering in a cross-sectional plane of the tissue as indicated by the line through tissue in (a) [301].

partial waves for all sample beam backscatterers along a single A-scan simultaneously. It accomplishes this by dispersing the recombined beam into its spectral components by a spectrometer and performs an inverse Fourier transformation of the detected spectrum yielding an A-scan image in its entirety (see Fig. 9.23). Contrast in OCT images originates from the varying intensity of back-reflected light, and signal differences originate from subtle variations of refractive index.

Consequently, FdOCT yields higher frames rates and greater sensitivities. Although FdOCT methods require more complex post-processing, they have great potential in terms of speed of acquisition and sensitivity. For a given N pixel-based SdOCT with a depth scan range of $x_{\text{depth}} = \frac{N}{2} l_C$, a TdOCT system acquiring signal over the same total time duration as an SdOCT system will have an signal-to-noise (SNR) ratio of [303]:

$$\text{SNR}_{\text{TdOCT}} = 10 \log\left(4P_S\left(\frac{2}{N}\right)T\frac{\varepsilon}{h\nu}\right) = \text{SNR}_{\text{SdOCT}} - 10\log\left(\frac{N}{2}\right) \tag{9.26}$$

where P_S, total detected sample power; T, total signal collection time; ε, the quantum detector efficiency; and $h\nu$, the photon quantum energy. Therefore a SdOCT system is intrinsically more sensitive than a TdOCT by a factor of $N/2$ [304]. In addition to sensitivity and resolution considerations, the nominal axial imaging depth of an OCT system is derived by the following expression [305]:

$$z_{\max} = \frac{1}{4\eta}\frac{\lambda_0^2}{\Delta\lambda}N \tag{9.27}$$

where η is the average refractive index of the sample under study (for glass $\eta = 1.5$), N is the number of detector array elements ($N = 1024$); all other terms are as described previously. As the depth-to-resolution ratio of OCT is > 100, it qualifies as a high resolution imaging modality [238], and is capable of doing so down to millimeter scale depths.

Owing to its reliance on interferometry, OCT is more limited than confocal imaging in terms of signal detection. As light reflected from the specimen must be coherent with a reference beam, it cannot detect fluorescence (as this requires the illumination and detection beams to be of different wavelengths). As such, OCT appears unsuitable for analysis of immunohistochemistry or other standard gene expression assays [211]. Although OCT may be likened to US in its theoretical formulation, it also is victim to some of the associated consequences, for instance, conspicuous speckle artifacts [238]. The use of all photons as in photoacoustic imaging (see Section 9.3.5) is of considerable advantage over OCT techniques, reliant on (quasi-) ballistic interactions, due to the fact that a useful percentage of (diffuse) photons penetrates several cm into tissue. Additionally,

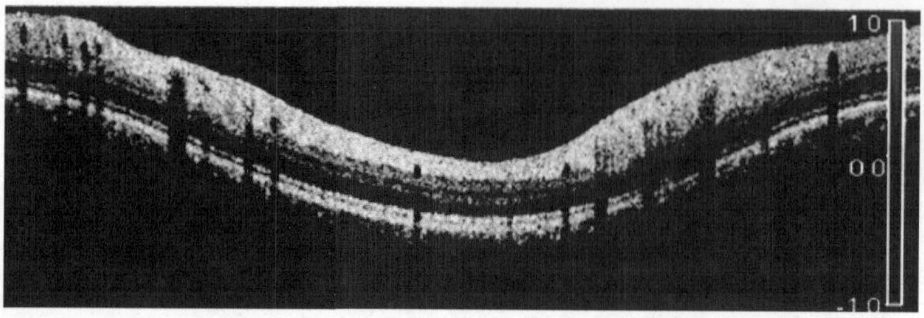

Figure 9.24: (See color insert.) Colour DOCT image showing vessels in the optic nerve head. Arteries and veins are distinguishable from direction of flow as determined by the signs (blue or red) of the Doppler shift and the angle [329].

diffuse, random, light scattering can perform uniform illumination of microvessels which may be otherwise be obscured.

Some very active research areas at present include: diagnosing dermatological diseases e.g. psoriasis [306]; assessment of arteriosclerotic plaques [307, 308]; and determining burn extent and tissue viability by defining tissue barrier layers characteristic of scarring (wound healing and graft flow) [309–311]. However, in truth, OCT has ubiquitous applications, having emerged in a variety of clinical fields: ophthalmology [312–314], intravascular imaging in cardiology [315, 316], oncology [317, 318], gastroenterology [319–321], general dermatology [322–324], dentistry [325, 326], and gynecology [327, 328], to name a few. Functional extensions of OCT have emerged: polarization-sensitive systems used, for example, in the diagnosis of neoplastic[5] processes; differential phase-sensitive methods for use in photorefractive surgery; full-field advancement of the conventional single-point OCT detection technique; and endoscopic OCT. Combining OCT with complementary techniques such as OCT with confocal microscopy (optical coherence microscopy), amalgamates the spatial sectioning and pin-hole rejection capabilities of confocal microscopy with the additional longitudinal sectioning provided by OCT coherence gating. Another asset of OCT is that it can be used to separate structure and function in 3D and to measure flow in individual microvessels. Methods which embody this ability are outlined in the following sections.

9.3.6.1 Doppler

Scanning of the reference mirror of an OCT system at a velocity v, produces a Doppler signal at a frequency $f_D = 2v/\lambda$; the dynamic constituents of the tissue (with velocity v_S) will also produce a Doppler signal. Hence, the signal of the Doppler OCT (DOCT) will be proportional to [20]:

$$A(t)\cos[2\pi(f_D - f_{Ds})t + \phi(t)] \qquad (9.28)$$

where $A(t)$ is the reflectivity and $\phi(t)$ is the phase shift defined by the scatterer position.

By simply measuring the frequency shift of moving particles in a defined vessel, it is possible to characterize blood flow and surpasses that of Laser Doppler Flowmetry (see Section 9.2.2.2) due to OCT's ability to resolve structures in depth.

Doppler ultrasound (US), the fundamental principle upon which DOCT is based, was developed as a tool for vascular disease assessment and monitoring. However, despite the advancements of DOCT techniques, a principal limitation still exists: the Doppler method is inherently 1D. The "true" velocity is extracted from this 1D information by assuming the direction of blood motion, resulting in an inaccurate determination of the flow velocity [330]. Doppler techniques are only apt for larger blood vessels with faster flow rates, in which Doppler shifts are easier to detect [331].

[5]Neoplasm: a new or uncontrolled growth of abnormal tissue, e.g., a tumor

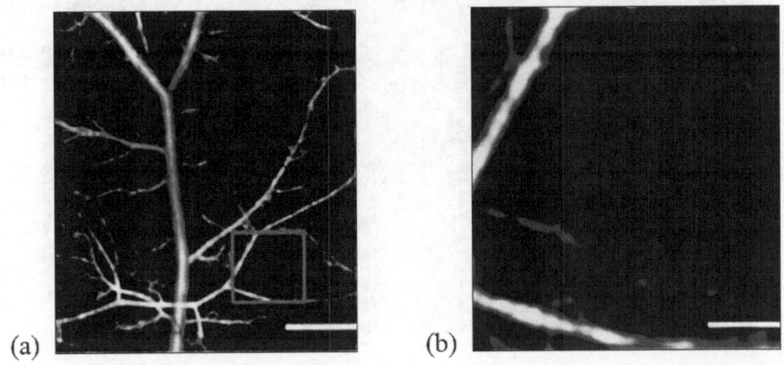

Figure 9.25: (a) SV image in dorsal window chamber of mouse (scale bar = 1 mm); (b) magnified region of interest from (a) (scale bar = 200 μm) [344].

Furthermore, as a Fourier transformation is usually preformed in sliding short-time windows, a tradeoffs between axial and velocity resolutions exist in the flow estimation [238]. DOCT is also inherently sensitive to the phase stability caused by both the system and the measurement environments [332].

The preliminary experiments regarding DOCT involved investigating picoliter blood volumes [333]. Since then, DOCT has had great success in the visualization of ocular media and related flow dynamics (see Fig. 9.24) [334–337], in addition to cerebral [338], cardiovascular [339] and urological [340] applications.

9.3.6.2 Speckle variance

Due to the extensive tortuosity of the microvasculature (especially if ailments which alter the physiology are present), the Doppler angular dependency may lead to incomplete vascular maps *in vivo*. Speckle variance (SV) techniques based on structural image intensity have been used in tumor microvascular imaging with high-frequency ultrasound [341]. The interframe speckle variance (SV_{ijk}) images of structural image of the OCT intensity (I_{ijk}) may be calculated as follows [342]:

$$SV_{ijk} = \frac{1}{N} \sum_{i=1}^{N} \left(I_{ijk} - \bar{I}\right)^2 \tag{9.29}$$

where N, the number of B-mode frames SV is calculated across; i, slice index; j and k, lateral and depth indices of the images; and $\bar{I}$, the average over the same set of pixels. SV-OCT images accentuate blood vessels as flowing portions induce localized speckle patterns and thus, are uncorrelated between frames [343].

One of the most outward advantages of SV is its independence of the Doppler angle for flow velocity computations and its simplicity, with little additional computational complexity. In addition, as it is intrinsically based on contrast, SV techniques have a potential benefit over fluorescence microscopy, especially when neovasculature exhibits increased permeability [342]. However, there are issues relating to the interpretation of the variance results obtained. The calculated variance is on the range of $\pm\infty$ and is dependent on the chosen window size. Thus, variance itself does not directly indicate flow and *a priori* structural knowledge is required to separate static and dynamic regions. In addition, SV-OCT suffers from multiple scattering induced artifacts and interframe bulk tissue motion [345]; this can lead to spurious values of artificial contrast wrongly indicating the presence of vessels beneath real blood vessels.

SV-OCT imaging has been reported in the dynamic monitoring of antivascular treatment effects (e.g., photodynamic therapy) [342]; analysis of the developing embryonic mammalian environ-

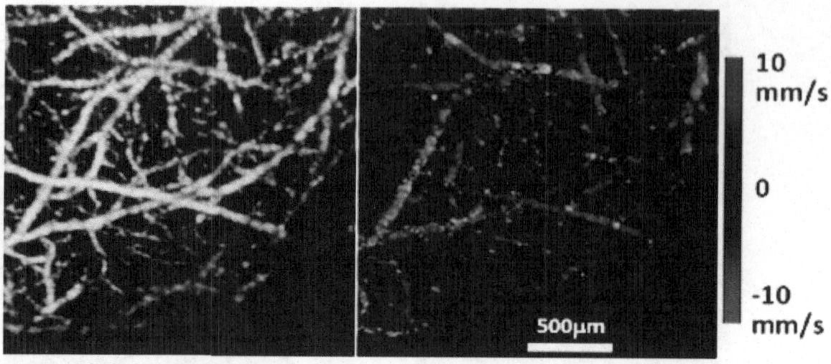

Figure 9.26: (See color insert.) Cerebral blood flow in cortical mouse brain using OMAG (left) and DOMAG (right) methods [347].

ment [346]; and with spectroscopic OCT for blood oxygen saturation analysis of the chorioallantoic membrane [343].

9.3.6.3 Optical microangiography

Optical Microangiography (OMAG) is a recently developed technique reliant on endogenous contrast, which effectively separates the moving and static scattering elements of tissue to achieve 3D high-resolution blood flow images approaching that of conventional histology, allowing for *in vivo* perfusion assessment.

In OMAG, spectral interferograms are modulated by a constant Doppler frequency (e.g., by a piezo-translation stage), thereby making separation of the moving and static scattering components within the sample feasible. The mathematical analysis involved essentially maps velocities moving into the tissue away from the surface into one image and velocities moving out of the tissue toward the surface into a second image by means of the Hilbert transform and subsequent fast Fourier transform [332]. This effectively separates the signals from moving constituents and bulk static tissue in frequency space. A further advancement of the OMAG modality came in the form of Doppler OMAG (DOMAG), a method which encompasses the advantages of both OMAG and the phase-resolved OCT methods [347]. In DOMAG, a digital frequency modulation approach is implemented to provide high-resolution 3D bi-directional flow mapping within highly scattering media. It effectively eliminates the requirement of capturing two 3D interferogram data sets, thereby reducing the computational load and thus increasing the potential temporal imaging resolution for *in vivo* imaging studies. [348].

As OMAG does not make use of OCT signal phases to assess the blood flow, it tolerates inevitable sample movement and tissue optical heterogeneity, thus limiting noise production [348]. OMAG and DOMAG have been demonstrated in the non-invasive assessment of cerebrovascular circulation in mice [332, 348, 349]; the retina [350, 351]; cutaneous skin assessments [352]; and in the diagnosis of renal pathologies using ultrahigh-sensitive optical microangiography (UHS-OMAG), with detectable velocity values ranging from $\sim 4\ \mu$m/s to ~ 30 mm/s [353].

9.3.7 Cytometric methods

Cytometry is the quantitative term for whole single cell analysis with a relatively low numerical aperture. Cells in suspension are sucked or pressed into a cytometer apparatus by overpressure or the use of mechanical pumps. Covered with sheath fluid, the cells undergo separation. Solid tissue, however, cannot be analysed by flow cytometer means without some form of initial tissue disintegration [354]. For analysis of solid tissues, slide-based cytometry is implemented by lamp

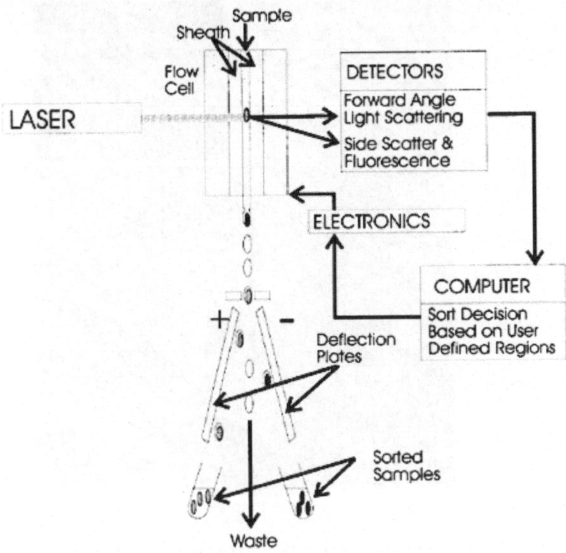

Figure 9.27: Illustration of flow cytometric cell sorting [366].

illumination [355] and camera based detection, or laser excitation and fluorescence detection [356].

In conventional flow cytometry (FCM), forward (cell size and refractive index dependent) or orthogonal (provides granularity information) light scatter is used for label-free analysis of rough leukocyte discrimination, for instance [357, 358]. Application of fluorescent dyes to label specific markers or cellular functions paved the way for gleaning additional cellular information and the characterization of biomarkers [359]. The feasibility of simultaneous analysis of many parameters lies in the multicolor approach of fluorescent dyes. Lasers or modern LEDs excite cells impregnated with fluorescent dye and the emitted fluorescence is detected by photodiodes. This allows for analysis of complex cellular structures, cell subtypes, cell-cell interactions, biological processes and identification of rare cell types. The use of fluorescence is particularly useful in cytomics, which characterizes single cells to unravel their interactions within cell systems and so to get a better insight into biological processes in organisms [354]. Polychromatic cytometry produces a complicated pattern of fluorescence to examine many parameters simultaneously in order to find cell interactions and causal connections; this reduces costs as it prevents repetitive use of markers for identifying populations. For example, cytometric systems utilizing 17 dyes simultaneously have been reported, for immunological analysis of disease patterns [360].

Cytometric procedures have enabled the separation and sorting of targeted cells by employing laser tweezers [361, 362] and lab-on-a-chip concepts [363–365]. Cells may be isolated from the larger cell collective by applications of single laser pulses or deflection in a continuous laser beam (see Fig. 9.27), and stored in a reservoir for further analysis, e.g., in the determination of relative concentration and purification.

As previously mentioned in Section 9.3.4, the use of fluorescent sources induces photobleaching with prolonged exposure therefore affecting analytical results [367]. However, this bleaching effect has itself been used as a tool for single-cell fluorescence spectroscopy [368, 369] in the discrimination of DNA information at the single-molecular level [370].

Flow cytometry may be incorporated in a wealth of different studies, notably: cell cycle analysis [373, 374]; apoptosis[6] [375–377] and stem cell investigations [378, 379]; and drug effect trials

[6]Apoptosis: cell death

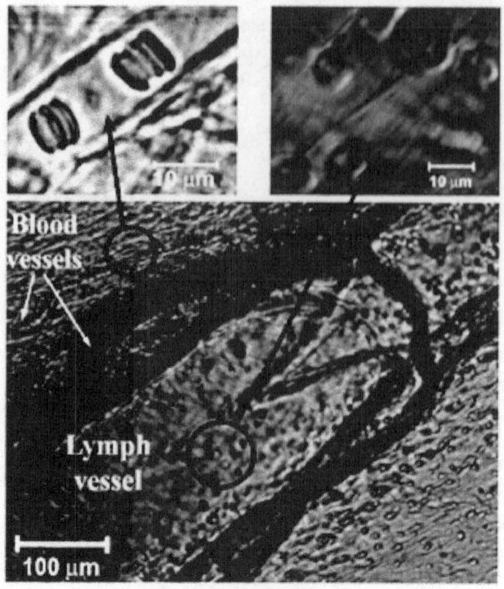

Figure 9.28: Cytometric photothermal microscopic image of rat mesentery with blood and lymph microvessels (bottom); (top left) RBCs in a capillary; (top right) cells in lymph flow [371, 372].

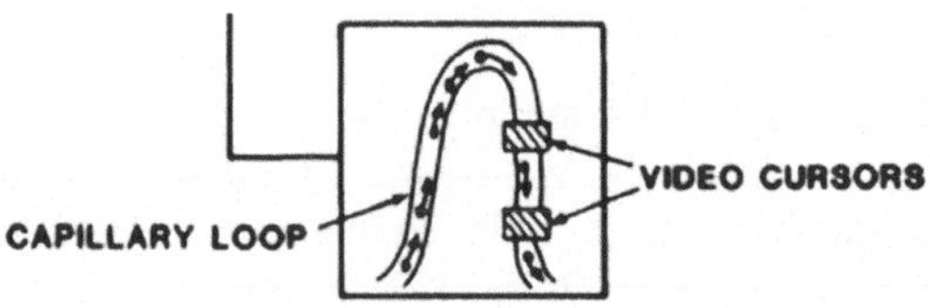

Figure 9.29: Illustration of television microscopy methods of capillary velocity estimation [397].

[380, 381]. Furthermore, flow cytometry has been used in conjunction with other complementary modalities such as: photothermal and photoacoustic applications for the study of blood and lymph flows (see Fig. 9.28) [371, 372, 382]; applications in tumor analysis and fluorescence based breast cancer imaging [383–386]; functional brain imaging [387]; and utilized with contrast enhancing fluorescence nanoparticles for HIV screening [388, 389]. Flow cytometry has also been used in a number of clinical studies for example sickle cell anaemia, with the potential for discriminating between sickled and non-sickled cells, as the sickled variety have reduced oxygen-carrying ability and more slowly through the microcirculation [390].

The temporal variations in light intensity subjected to cross-correlation computations yield transit times for photometric events moving from one cursor to another, thereby allowing the computation of red blood cell velocity (RBC_V) values. Currently, videocapillaroscopy is the clinical "gold standard" for capillary imaging and analysis. However, the depth of tissue penetration is a limiting factor and restricts capillaroscopic techniques to the nutritive portions of the skin [398].

Particle image velocimetry (PIV) is a non-intrusive measurement technique, used to measure full-field velocity data within a 2D plane of a particle-seeded flow field [399]. The fluid velocity is inferred from the motion of tracer particles which constitute a random pattern that is "tied" to the fluid, whose motion is visible through tracer pattern changes. In PIV, two sequential images are subsampled at one particular area via an interrogation window. Within these samples, an average spatial shift of particles may be observed from one sample to its counterpart in the other image [400], provided flow is present. The displacement of a tracer particle (d) in a finite time interval

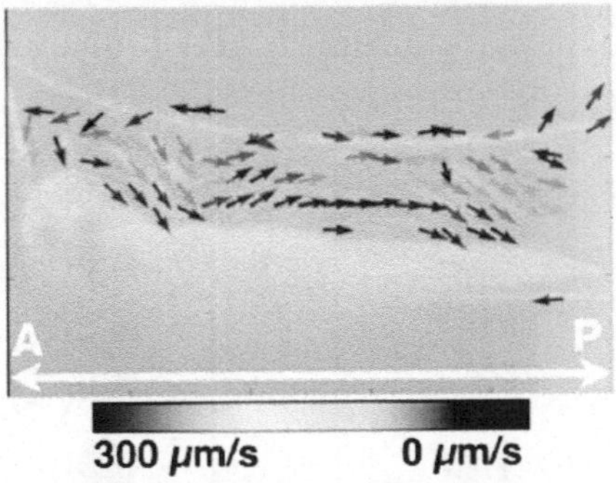

Figure 9.30: 2D, two-component flow velocity field of OCT-based particle tracking velocimetry of non-recirculatory cilia-driven fluid flow [405].

($\Delta t = t'' - t'$) may be given by [401]:

$$d(x;t',t'') = \int_{t'}^{t''} v[x(t),t]dt \tag{9.30}$$

where $v[x(t),t]$ is the tracer particle velocity. The tracer pattern does not necessarily have to be composed of discrete tracer particles; the above interpretation is likewise applicable to continuous tracers such as dyes. PIV tracer velocity values are deduced by calculation of the expectation value of the auto-correlation function for a double-exposure continuous image [401]. The temporal auto-correlation function of the scattered light intensity yields measurements of velocity gradients in a steady flow [402], thus providing a way of determining shear gradients quantitatively.

Performance of PIV methods in measuring instantaneous velocity fields were improved upon by the introduction of direct cross-correlation of image fields in place of multiple-exposure auto-correlation methods [403]. Cross-correlation methods of interrogation of successive single-exposure frames can be used to measure the separation of pairs of particle images, resulting in improvements in spatial resolution, detection rate, accuracy and reliability. A high cross-correlation value near unity is observed when many particle images in the initial image match their corresponding spatially equivalent shifted partners in the subsequent image, i.e. the higher the correlation coefficient, the greater the accuracy of the velocity data obtained [399]. PIV has been associated with certain limitations, such as directional ambiguity [401], and its use of microbeads for contrast have resulted in severe obstructions and distortion of the flow profiles [404], thus limiting its clinical application.

The clinical applicability of the PIV technique has been reported in small animal models and noteworthy in the analysis of arterioles with both bifurcation and confluence in the rat mesentery [406]. The most successful approach for employing advanced velocimetry for measurements in microfluidics (see Section 9.3.7) is microparticle image velocimetry (μPIV) using fluorescently tagged polystyrene particles [230, 407, 408]. PIV has been used as a complementary technique to a wide variety of modalities. Recently, it was coupled with OCT (see Fig. 9.30) for quantitatively characterizing the microfluidic-scale flow generated by epithelial motile cilia of *Xenopus tropicalis* embryos [405]. PIV is not restricted to optically acquired images only; US imaging has been used to measure the velocity distribution in the porcine left ventricle [4], with reported spatial and temporal resolutions of 0.4 mm and 0.5 ms, respectively [409]. In addition, x-ray velocimetry has been suggested as a means of *in vivo* wall shear stress measurement, as it is a highly influential factor for the progression of arterial disease [410].

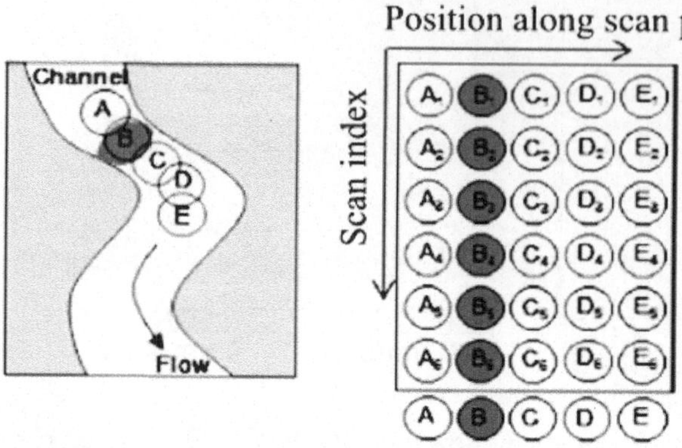

Figure 9.31: Illustration of the SLIC method for flow measurement. A laser scans many small regions, the reflected intensity is detected and pair-correlation provides a flow measurement. Image adapted from [412].

9.3.8 Correlation spectroscopy

Scanning laser image correlation (SLIC) is an optical correlation technique which traces a laser beam rapidly with respect to the motion of particles. It applies the use of pair-correlation [411] to analyse reflected fluctuations from moving particles, thus yielding temporal information between sequential images. SLIC is capable of discriminating among multiple populations of particles travelling simultaneously through the same channel at different velocities [412, 413].

In SLIC, a laser follows a trajectory across a channel, illuminating a series of (many) small regions (see Fig. 9.31). The reflected intensity for each region is measured with an optical detector. In order to perform velocity measurements, temporal comparisons need to be made of a particle initially and at a later time via cross-correlation. For SLIC computation, normalised cross-correlation is used [412] and is defined as:

$$G_{ab}(\tau) = \frac{\langle \delta I_b(t) \cdot \delta I_a(t+\tau) \rangle_t}{(\langle \delta I_a(t) \rangle_t \langle \delta I_b(t) \rangle_t)} \tag{9.31}$$

where a and b refer to the columns in Fig. 9.31; I, intensity; τ, temporal correlation shift; $\langle\rangle_t$, temporal average; and $\delta I(t) = I(t) - \langle I(t) \rangle$. 2D plots may be deduced via multidistance pair-correlation [414].

STICS is fundamentally different from other optical correlation techniques, e.g., speckle, as it does not require the use of a model and is a purely statistical method [331]. However, it is limited in the range of velocities it can measure, the maximum velocity being limited by the acquisition speed of detection [412]. SLIC has been widely implemented in assessments of vascular dynamics in, for example, zebra fish embryos [17, 415].

9.3.9 Advancements in flow assessment in OCT

Recently, techniques have been proposed for flow velocity investigations that are distinct from those which utilize phase information, frequency shifts or Doppler broadening of bandwidth. Time-varying speckle is manifested as a change in OCT (see Section 9.3.6) image spatial speckle frequencies; methods have utilized this fact to provide quantitative flow information *in vitro* [416].

Autocorrelation methods for quantitative mapping of transverse particle-flow velocity have been proposed [417], which employ the statistical nature of the intensity fluctuation of backscattered light modulated by (stochastically) flowing particles. These methods are derived from the theoretical

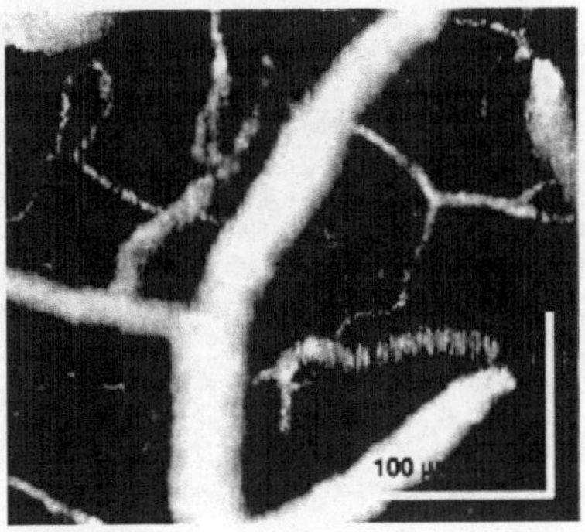

Figure 9.32: OCT maximum intensity projection angiogram of the rat somatosensory cortex with 3.6 μm transverse resolution [421].

analysis of fluorescence correlation spectroscopy [418]. Such methods are clearly advantageous, e.g., with regard to phase-resolved Doppler OCT which has a limited dynamic range of velocity caused by phase wrapping [417, 419]. Such methods have been further applied as a means of non-invasive measurement of concentration in non-flowing particle suspensions governed by Poissonian distributions [420].

Means of calculating absolute flow velocities without explicit knowledge of vessel angles have recently been reported by employing the use of surface integrals along the $x-y$ plane [421] (see Fig. 9.32) and by maximum intensity projection correlation of coincident pixels in multiple OCT B-scans [422].

OCT techniques which encompass cross-correlation have recently been introduced [423]. A 2D cross-correlation between two spatially distinct images was performed. However, in practical application, the measured velocity range was smaller than predicted; this error was attributed to the quasi-synchronous manner of image acquisition. This may be improved upon by continuously analysing the specimen using multiple, spatially disparate imaging points [424]. By performing cross-correlation analysis of the flow induced fluctuations of the OCT signal, transit times may be yielded and ergo velocity values for particle flow computed. Methods which utilize the time scale of random fluctuations in the dynamic scattering component related to RBC_V have recently been reported in quantitative studies of capillary hemodynamics [425]. The application of cross-correlation methods of velocity estimation to complex situations, e.g. turbulence, is the focus of current research. Imaging at multiple positions has been the topic of recent discussion in the imaging community; current developments are outlined in the next section.

9.3.10 Dual-beam techniques

Several investigations have reported the use of a dual-beam imaging modality [426, 427]. The classic interferometric setup of partial coherence interferometry (PCI) and OCT has the drawback of being sensitive to longitudinal object positions [428]. Efforts to overcome such limitations in ocular media have been reported, in which the cornea was used as a reference surface in a common path dual-beam interferometric set-up [429]. A dual-beam Doppler spectral domain OCT (SdOCT) system which eliminated the ambiguity associated with unknown orientation of local velocity vectors in the blood vessels of zebrafish has been reported [430].

Recent work has been proposed [431, 432], which outlines a dual-beam scan Doppler optical coherence angiography (see Fig. 9.33). A similar technique has also been reported [433], in which two laterally displaced sample beams make it possible to apply phase-resolved Doppler analysis. However, these methods are sensitive to involuntary sample motion. Regardless, dual-beam methods

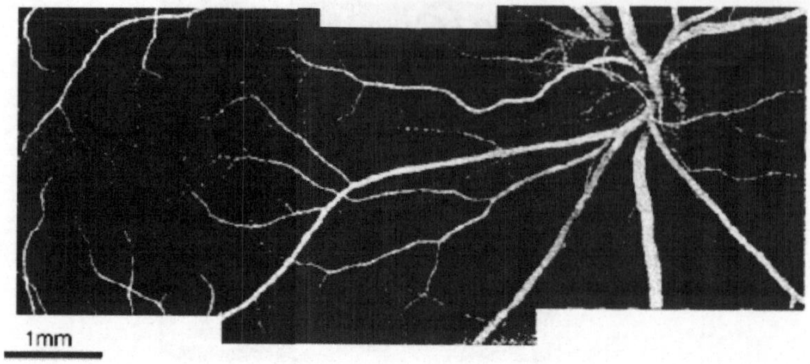

Figure 9.33: Mosaic of *en-face* images of the retinal vasculature captured using dual-velocity optical coherence angiography [431]; two different scanning beams with spatial and temporal separation provide two measurable velocity ranges enabling higher sensitivity to very low velocity flows.

have been reported to yield an increased dynamic range for detectable velocities [90] and capable of providing useful microstructural information, in addition to providing high spatial resolution velocity measurements [434].

9.4 Conclusion

This chapter has provided an extensive overview and discussion of the advancement of optical sectioning techniques applied to blood flow imaging from their initial inception to modern day, all of which are capable of relaying clinically relevant and diagnostically important morphological and functional information. The implication of these methods in the clinical realm has been outlined, in addition to an in-depth discussion of their *modus operandi*, associated advantages and limitations. Although the techniques discussed may differ inherently in their construction, operation, resolution, etc., they are yet intrinsically linked. The prevalence of complementary modalities is rife at present, utilizing supplementary information to yield multifaceted information with affirming, real-world applications.

9.5 Acknowledgment

The authors are grateful to the Irish Council for Science Engineering and Technology (IRCSET) and the National Biophotonics and Imaging Platform Ireland funded under the Higher Education Authority PRTLI Cycle 4 for supporting this research.

References

[1] G. J. Tearney, M. E. Brezinski, B. E. Bouma, S. A. Boppart, C. Pitris, J. F. Southern, and J. G. Fujimoto, "*In vivo* endoscopic optical biopsy with optical coherence tomography," *Science* **276**, 2037–2039 (1997).

[2] J.-L. Chen, L. Wei, V. Acuff, D. Bereczki, F.-J. Hans, T. Otsuka, W. Finnegan, C. Patlak, and J. Fenstermacher, "Slightly altered permeability-surface area products imply some cerebral capillary recruitment during hypercapnia," *Microvas. Res.* **48**, 190–211 (1994).

[3] A. G. Hudetz, B. B. Biswal, G. Feher, and J. P. Kampine, "Effects of hypoxia and hypercapnia on capillary flow velocity in the rat cerebral cortex," *Microvas. Res.* **54**, 35–42 (1997).

[4] P. Vennemann, R. Lindken, and J. Westerweel, "In vivo whole-field blood velocity measurement techniques," *Exp. Fluids* **42**, 495–511 (2007).

[5] D. M. McDonald, and P. L. Choyke, "Imaging of angiogenesis: from microscope to clinic," *Nat. Med.* **9**, 713–725 (2003).

[6] R. Weissleder, "Scaling down imaging: Molecular mapping of cancer in mice," *Nature Reviews Cancer* **2**, 11–18 (2002).

[7] J. D. Pearlman, R. J. Laham, M. Post, T. Leiner, and M. Simons, "Medical imaging techniques in the evaluation of strategies for therapeutic angiogenesis," *Curr. Pharma. Des.* **8**, 1467–1496 (2002).

[8] M. Neeman, "Functional and molecular MR imaging of angiogenesis: Seeing the target, seeing it work," *J. Cell. Biochem. Suppl.* **39**, 11–17 (2002).

[9] N. G. Costouros, F. E. Diehn, and S. K. Libutti, "Molecular imaging of tumor angiogenesis," *J. Cell. Biochem.* **87**, 72–78 (2002).

[10] R. Weissleder and V. Ntziachristos, "Shedding light onto live molecular targets," *Nature Medicine* **9**, 123–128 (2003).

[11] M. J. Leahy, J. O'Doherty, P. Mc Namara, and J. G. Enfield, "Biophotonic methods in microcirculation imaging," *Med. Laser App.* **22**, 105–126 (2007).

[12] J. Lighthill, *Mathematical Biofluid Dynamics*, Society for Industrial and Applied Mathematics, Philadelphia (1975).

[13] J. E. Moore Jr., A. Delfino, P.-A. Doriot, P.-A. Dorsaz, and W. Rutishauser, "Arterial fluid dynamics: the relationship to artherosclerosis and application in diagnostics," in *Biofluid methods in vascular and pulmonary systems*, CRC Press (2001).

[14] D. D. Backer and J.-L. Vincent, "Clinical applications of SDF videomicroscopy," in *Microcirculation Imaging*, Martin J. Leahy (ed.), Wiley–VCH, Weinheim (2012).

[15] L. Devgan, S. Bhat, S. Aylward, and R. J. Spence, "Modalities for the assessment of burn wound depth," *J. Burns Wounds* **5**, 7–15 (2006).

[16] V. Singh, L. Devgan, S. Bhat, and S. M. Milner, "The pathogenesis of burn wound conversion," *Annals of Plastic Surgery* **59**, 109–115 (2007).

[17] X. T. Pan, H. Yu, X. K. Shi, V. Korzh, and T. Wohland, "Characterization of flow direction in microchannels and zebrafish blood vessels by scanning fluorescence correlation spectroscopy," *J. Biomed. Opt.* **12**, 014034 (2007).

[18] J. B. West, "Ibn al-Nafis, the pulmonary circulation, and the Islamic Golden Age," *J. Appl. Physiol.* **105**, 1877–1880 (2008).

[19] P. E. Pormann and E. Savage-Smith, *Medieval Islamic Medicine*, Edinburgh University Press, Edinburgh (2007).

[20] V. Tuchin, *Tissue Optics: Light Scattering Methods and Instruments for Medical Diagnosis*, SPIE Press, Bellingham, Washington (2007).

[21] J. Ward, R. Clarke, and R. Linden, *Physiology at a Glance*, Blackwell Publishing Ltd (2005).

[22] G. J. Tortora, *Introduction to the Human Body: The Essentials of Anatomy and Physiology*, Addison Wesley Longman, New York (1997).

[23] C. I. Wright, C. I. Kroner, and R. Draijer, "Non-invasive methods and stimuli for evaluating the skin's microcirculation," *Journal of Pharmacological and Toxicological Methods* **54**, 1–25 (2006).

[24] A. I. Vinik, T. Erbas, T. S. Park, K. K. Pierce, and K. B. Stansberry, "Methods for evaluation of peripheral neurovascular dysfunction," *Diabetes Technology & Therapeutics* **3**, 29–50 (2001). (2011).

[25] B. Fagrell and M. Intaglietta, "Microcirculation: Its significance in clinical and molecular medicine," *J. Int. Med.* **241**, 349–362 (1997).

[26] T. Matsumoto and F. Kajiya, "Coronary microcirculation: Physiology and mechanics," *Fluid Dynamics Research* **37**, 6081 (2005).

[27] I. D. Swain and L. J. Grant, "Methods of measuring skin blood-flow," *Phys. Med. Bio.* **34**, 151–175 (1989).

[28] S. E. Charm and G. S. Kurland, *Blood Flow and Microcirculation*, Wiley, New York (1974).

[29] American Vein and Aesthetics Institute, *http://www.medrehab.com/Skincare.php*.

[30] E. Berardesca, J. L. Leveque, and P. Masson, "EEMCO guidance for the measurement of skin microcirculation," *Skin Pharmacology and Applied Skin Physiology* **15**, 442–456 (2002).

[31] H. A. M. Daanen, "Finger cold-induced vasodilation: a review," *European J. Appl. Physiol.* **89**, 411–426 (2003).

[32] M. J. Leahy and G. E. Nilsson, "Biophotonic functional imaging of skin microcirculation," in *Handbook of Photonics for Biomedical Science*, Valery V. Tuchin (ed.), CRC Press, Boca Raton, FL (2010).

[33] A. I. Vinik, T. Erbas, T. S. Park, K. B. Stansberry, J. A. Scanelli, and G. L. Pittenger, "Dermal neurovascular dysfunction in type 2 diabetes," *Diabetes Care* **24**, 1468–1475 (2001).

[34] R. R. Anderson and J. A. Parrish, "Optical properties of human skin," in *The Science of Photomedicine*, J. D. Regan and J. A. Parrish (eds.), Plenum Press, New York, 147–194 (1982).

[35] T. Vo-Dinh, *Biomedical Photonics Handbook*, CRC Press, Boca Raton, FL (2003).

[36] V. V. Tuchin, *Handbook of Optical Biomedical Diagnostics*, SPIE Press, Bellingham, WA (2002).

[37] M. van Gemert, S. Jacques, H. Sterenborg, and W. Star, "Skin optics," *IEEE Transactions in Biomedical Engineering* **36**, 1146–1154 (1989).

[38] J. Lee and N. Smith, "Theoretical modeling in hemodynamics of microcirculation," *Microcirculation* **15**, 699–714 (2008).

[39] J. M. Schmitt and G. Kumar, "Optical scattering properties of soft tissue: a discrete particle model," *Appl. Opt.* **37**, 2788–2797 (1998).

[40] J. Cobb and D. Claremont, "Noninvasive measurement techniques for monitoring of microvascular function in the diabetic foot," *The International Journal of Lower Extremity Wounds* **1**, 161–169 (2002).

[41] R. F. Abarquez and J. E. L. Cinco, "Microcirculation: target therapy in cardiovascular diseases – A clinical perspective," *Clinical Hemorheology and Microcirculation* **29**, 157–165 (2003).[42]

[42] M. Cutolo, C. Pizzorni, and A. Sulli, "Capillaroscopy," *Best Practice & Research Clinical Rheumatology* **19**, 437–452 (2005).

[43] S. Guiducci, R. Giacomelli, and M. M. Cerinic, "Vascular complications of scleroderma," *Autoimmunity Reviews* **6**, 520–523 (2007).

[44] M. Hahn, C. Hahn, M. Junger, A. Steins, D. Zuder, T. Klyscz, A. Buchtemann, G. Rassner, and V. Blazek, "Local cold exposure test with a new arterial photoplethysmographic sensor in healthy controls and patients with secondary Raynaud's phenomenon," *Microvas. Res.* **57**, 187–198 (1999).

[45] J. L. P. Vaz, M. A. A. Dancour, D. A. Bottino, and E. Bouskela, "Nailfold videocapillaroscopy in primary antiphospholipid syndrome (PAPS)," *Rheumatology* **43**, 1025–1027 (2004).

[46] M. Aschwanden, T. Daikeler, K. A. Jaeger, C. Thalhammer, A. Gratwohl, M. Matucci-Cerinic, and A. Tyndall, "Rapid improvement of nailfold capillaroscopy after intense immunosuppression for systemic sclerosis and mixed connective tissue disease," *Annals of the Rheumatic Diseases* **67**, 1057–1059 (2008).

[47] M. I. Perez and S. R. Kohn, "Cutaneous manifestations of diabetes-mellitus," *Journal of the American Academy of Dermatology* **30**, 519–531 (1994).

[48] G. A. Scardina and P. Messina, "Microvascular abnormalities in patients with rheumatoid arthritis," *Annals of Anatomy* **188**, 425–429 (2006).

[49] W. Grassi, P. Core, G. Carlino, and C. Cervini, "Nailfold capillary-permeability in psoriatic-arthritis," *Scandinavian Journal of Rheumatology* **21**, 226–230 (1992).

[50] J. P. Vuchetich, S. K. Miranowski, B. A. Mueller and K. O. Lim, "High nailfold plexus visibility in schizophrenia is associated with a distinct neuropsychological profile and less ventriculomegaly," *Schizophrenia Bulletin* **35**, (2009).

[51] A. L. Herrick and C. Hutchinson, "Vascular imaging," *Best Practice & Research Clinical Rheumatology* **18**, 957–979 (2004).

[52] K. Borysewicz, "Nailfold capillaroscopy (NC) evaluation in patients with hand fingers pain in inflammatory rheumatic diseases," *European Journal of Pain* **13**, 55–285 (2009).

[53] F. Ingegnoli, R. Gualtierotti, C. Lubatti, L. Zahalkova, L. Meani, P. Boracchi, S. Zeni, and F. Fantini, "Feasibility of different capillaroscopic measures for identifying nailfold microvascular alterations," *Seminars in Arthritis and Rheumatism* **38**, 289–295 (2009).

[54] P. T. Goedhart, "Sidestream Dark Field (SDF) imaging: a novel stroboscopic LED ring-based imaging modality for clinical assessment of the microcirculation," *Opt. Exp.* **15**, (2007).

[55] M. Rossi and A. Carpi, "Skin microcirculation in peripheral arterial obliterative disease," *Biomedicine & Pharmacotherapy* **58**, 427–431 (2004).

[56] K. C. Vollebregt, K. Boer, K. R. Mathura, J. C. de Graaff, D. T. Ubbink, and C. Ince, "Impaired vascular function in women with pre-eclampsia observed with orthogonal polarisation spectral imaging," *British Journal of Obstetrics and Gynaecology* **108**, 1148–1153 (2001).

[57] F. Schiavon, P. Maffei, C. Martini, E. De Carlo, C. Fais, S. Todesco, and N. Sicolo, "Morphologic study of microcirculation in acromegaly by capillaroscopy," *The Journal of Clinical Endocrinology & Metabolism* **84**, (2000).

[58] W. Haenggi, H. R. Linder, M. H. Birkhaeuser, and H. Schneider, "Microscopic findings of the nail-fold capillaries — dependence on menopausal status and hormone replacement therapy," *Maturitas* **22**, 37–46 (1994).

[59] H. Kurvers, M. Jacobs, R. J. Beuk, F. Vandenwildenberg, P. Kitslaar, D. W. Slaaf, and R. S. Reneman, "Reflex sympathetic dystrophy — evolution of microcirculatory disturbances in time," *Pain* **60**, 333–340 (1995).

[60] M. Cutolo, W. Grassi, and M. M. Cerinic, "Raynaud's phenomenon and the role of capillaroscopy," *Arthritis & Rheumatism* **48**, 3023–3030 (2003).

[61] O. Bongard, A. Boccara, B. Cense, C. Dainty, D. Malonek, and E. Beaurepaire, "Effects of oxygen inhalation on skin microcirculation in patients with peripheral arterial occlusive disease," *Circulation* **86**, 878–886 (1992).

[62] P. Gasser and O. Meienberg, "Finger microcirculation in classical migraine. A video-microscopic study of nailfold capillaries," *European Neurology* **31**, 168–171. (1991).

[63] P. Gasser and F. R. Bühler, "Nailfold microcirculation in normotensive and essential hypertensive subjects, as assessed by video–microscopy," *Journal of Hypertension* **10**, 83–86 (1992).

[64] C. S. Danzer and D. R. Hooker, "Determination of the capillary blood pressure in man with the micro-capillary tonometer," *American Journal of Physiology* **52**, (1920).

[65] P. Baumbach, *Understanding transcutaneous PO_2 and PCO_2 measurements*, Radiometer Publications, Copenhagen, 14–18 (1985).

[66] K. H. Tonnesen and P. Sejrsen, "Muscle blood flow calculated from desaturation curve of Xenon-133 and by direct recording," *Acta Physiologica Scandinavica* **68**, 202 (1966).

[67] P. Sejrsen, "Cutaneous blood flow in man studied by freely diffusible radioactive indicators," *Scandinavian Journal of Clinical & Laboratory Investigation* **19**, 52 (1967).

[68] P. Sejrsen, "Blood flow in cutaneous tissue in man studied by washout of radioactive Xenon," *Circulation Research* **25**, 215 (1969).

[69] S. G. Sakka, K. Reinhart, and A. Meier-Hellmann, "Comparison of pulmonary artery and arterial thermodilution cardiac output in critically ill patients," *Intensive Care Medicine* **25**, 843–846 (1999).

[70] W. Ganz, K. Tamura, H. S. Marcus, R. Donoso, S. Yoshida, and H. J. C. Swan, "Measurement of coronary sinus blood flow by continuous thermodilution in man," *Circulation* **44**, 181 (1971).

[71] T. Nishikawa and S. Dohi, "Errors in the measurement of cardiac-output by thermodilution," *Canadian Journal of Anaesthesia* **40**, 142–153 (1993).

[72] T. Nishikawa and S. Dohi, "Hemodynamic-changes associated with thermodilution cardiac-output determination during metabolic-acidosis or hypoxic hypoxia in dogs," *European Journal of Anaesthesiology* **10**, 321–329 (1993).

[73] A. van Grondelle, R. V. Ditchey, B. M. Groves, W. W. Wagner Jr, and J. T. Reeves, "Thermodilution method overestimates low cardiac output in humans," *American Journal of Physiology* **245**, H690–H692 (1983).

[74] F. Y. Ozbebit, F. Esen, S. Gulec, and H. Esen, "Evaluation of forearm microvascular blood flow regulation by laser Doppler flowmetry, iontophoresis, and curve analysis: contribution of axon reflex," *Microvas. Res.* **67**, 207–214 (2004).

[75] J. E. Francis, R. Roggli, T. J. Love, and C. P. Robinson, "Thermography as a means of blood perfusion measurement," *J. Biomech. Eng.* **101**, 246–249 (1979).

[76] H. P. Henderson and M. E. J. Hackett, "Value of thermography in peripheral vascular-disease," *Angiology* **29**, 65–75 (1978).

[77] J. R. T. Manson, M. M. Abd-Alrazzal, J. Ausobsky, P. A. Matthews, and R. C. Kester, *The Use of Microwave Emission Thermography in Peripheral Vascular Disease — A Preliminary Study*, Biological Engineering Society, London (1985).

[78] G. E. Nilsson, T. Tenland, and P. A. Oberg, "Laser Doppler Flowmetry — a non-invasive method for micro-vascular studies," *Phys. Med. Bio.* **25**, 987–988 (1980).

[79] G. E. Nilsson, T. Tenland, and P. A. Oberg, "Evaluation of a laser Doppler flowmeter for measurement of tissue blood-flow," *IEEE Trans. Biomed. Eng.* **27**, 597–604 (1980).

[80] C. Riva, G. B. Benedek, and B. Ross, "Laser Doppler measurements of blood-flow in capillary tubes and retinal arteries," *Investigative Ophthalmology* **11**, 936 (1972).

[81] M. D. Stern, "*In vivo* evaluation of microcirculation by coherent light scattering," *Nature* **254**, 56–58 (1975).

[82] M. J. Leahy, F. F. de Mul, G. E. Nilsson, and R. Maniewski, "Principles and practice of the laser-Doppler perfusion technique," *Technol. Health Care* **7**, 143–162 (1999).

[83] J. D. Briers, "Laser Doppler, speckle and related techniques for blood perfusion mapping and imaging," *Physiological Measurement* **22**, 35–66 (2001).

[84] A. Serov, W. Steenbergen, and F. de Mul, "Laser Doppler perfusion imaging with a complimentary metal oxide semiconductor image sensor," *Opt. Lett.* **27**, 300–302 (2002).

[85] A. Serov, B. Steinacher, and T. Lasser, "Full-field laser Doppler perfusion imaging and monitoring with an intelligent CMOS camera," *Opt. Exp.* **13**, 3681–3689 (2005).

[86] D. Watkins and G. A. Holloway, "Instrument to measure cutaneous blood-flow using Doppler-shift of laser-light," *IEEE Trans. Biomed. Eng.* **25**, 28–33 (1978).

[87] M. E. Anderson, T. L. Moore, M. Lunt, and A. L. Herrick, "Digital iontophoresis of vasoactive substances as measured by laser Doppler imaging — a non-invasive technique by which to measure microvascular dysfunction in Raynaud's phenomenon," *Rheumatology* **43**, 986–991 (2004).

[88] D. P. Dave and T. E. Milner, "Doppler-angle measurement in highly scattering media," *Opt. Lett.* **25**, 1523–1525 (2000).

[89] M. D. Kulkarni, T. G. van Leeuwen, S. Yazdanfar, and J. A. Izatt, "Velocity-estimation accuracy and frame-rate limitations in color Doppler optical coherence tomography," *Opt. Lett.* **23**, 1057–1059 (1998).

[90] H. C. Hendargo, R. P. McNabb, A.-H. Dhalla, N. Shepherd, and J. A. Izatt, "Doppler velocity detection limitations in spectrometer-based versus swept-source optical coherence tomography," *Biomed. Opt. Exp.* **2**, (2011).

[91] A. H. Bachman, R. A. Leitgeb, and T. Lasser, "Heterodyne Fourier domain optical coherence tomography for full range probing with high axial resolution," *Opt. Express* **14**, (2006).

[92] S. Monstrey, H. Hoeksema, J. Verbelen, A. Pirayesh, and P. Blondeel, "Assessment of burn depth and burn wound healing potential," *Burns* **34**, 761–769 (2008).

[93] Z. B. M. Niazi, T. J. H. Essex, R. Papini, D. Scott, N. R. McLean, and M. J. M. Black, "New laser-Doppler scanner, a valuable adjunct in burn depth assessment," *Burns* **19**, 485–489 (1993).

[94] I. Wang, S. Andersson-Engels, G. E. Nilsson, K. Wardell, and K. Svanberg, "Superficial blood flow following photodynamic therapy of malignant non-melanoma skin tumours measured by laser Doppler perfusion imaging," *British Journal of Dermatology* **136**, 184–189 (1997).

[95] W. R. Ferrell, P. V. Balint, and R. D. Sturrock, "Novel use of laser Doppler imaging for investigating epicondylitis," *Rheumatology* **39**, 1214–1217 (2000).

[96] G. Royl, C. Leithner, H. Sellien, J. P. Muller, D. Megow, N. Offenhauser, J. Steinbrink, M. Kohl-Bareis, U. Dirnagl, and U. Lindauer, "Functional imaging with laser speckle contrast analysis: Vascular compartment analysis and correlation with laser Doppler flowmetry and somatosensory evoked potentials," *Brain Research* **1121**, 95–103 (2006).

[97] N. A. Fomin, *Speckle Photography for Fluid Mechanics Measurements*, Springer, Berlin Heidelberg (1998).

[98] J. W. Goodman, *Speckle Phenomena in Optics: Theory and Applications*, Roberts & Co., Berlin (2006).

[99] M. Draijer, E. Hondebrink, T. v. Leeuwen, and W. Steenbergen, "Review of laser speckle contrast techniques for visualizing tissue perfusion," *Lasers in Medical Science* **24**, 639–651 (2009).

[100] K. R. Forrester, C. Stewart, J. Tulip, C. Leonard, and R. C. Bray, "Comparison of laser speckle and laser Doppler perfusion imaging: measurement in human skin and rabbit articular tissue," *Medical & Biological Engineering & Computing* **40**, 687–697 (2002).

[101] D. A. Boas and A. K. Dunn, "Laser speckle contrast imaging in biomedical optics," *J. Biomed. Opt.* **15**, (2010).

[102] J. D. Briers and S. Webster, "Laser speckle contrast analysis (LASCA): a non-scanning, full-field technique for monitoring capillary blood flow," *J. Biomed. Opt.* **1**, 174–179 (1996).

[103] D. D. Duncan and S. J. Kirkpatrick, "Can laser speckle flowmetry be made a quantitative tool?" *Journal of the Optical Society of America* **A 25**, 2088–2094 (2008).

[104] K. R. Forrester, C. Stewart, C. Leonard, J. Tulip, and R. C. Bray, "Endoscopic laser imaging of tissue perfusion: New instrumentation and technique," *Lasers in Surgery and Medicine* **33**, 151–157 (2003).

[105] C. J. Stewart, C. L. Gallant-Behm, K. Forrester, J. Tulip, D. A. Hart, and R. C. Bray, "Kinetics of blood flow during healing of excisional full-thickness skin wounds in pigs as monitored by laser speckle perfusion imaging," *Skin Research and Technology* **12**, 247–253 (2006).

[106] P. Zakharov, A. Volker, A. Buck, B. Weber, and F. Scheffold, "Quantitative modeling of laser speckle imaging," *Opt. Lett.* **31**, 3465–3467 (2006).

[107] D. D. Duncan, P. Lemaillet, M. Ibrahim, Q. D. Nguyen, M. Hiller, and J. Ramella-Roman, "Absolute blood velocity measured with a modified fundus camera," *J. Biomed Opt.* **15**, 056014 (2010).

[108] A. B. Parthasarathy, W. J. Tom, A. Gopal, X. J. Zhang, and A. K. Dunn, "Robust flow measurement with multi-exposure speckle imaging," *Opt. Exp.* **16**, 1975–1989 (2008).

[109] B. Choi, N. M. Kang, and J. S. Nelson, "Laser speckle imaging for monitoring blood flow dynamics in the *in vivo* rodent dorsal skin fold model," *Microvas. Res.* **68**, 143–146 (2004).

[110] Z. J. Du, T. Zan, H. Li, and Q. F. Li, "A study of blood flow dynamics in flap delay using the full-field laser perfusion imager," *Microvas. Res.* **82**, 284–290 (2011).

[111] H. Y. Cheng, Q. M. Luo, Q. Liu, Q. A. Lu, H. Gong, and S. Q. Zeng, "Laser speckle imaging of blood flow in microcirculation," *Phys. Med.Bio.* **49**, 1347–1357 (2004).

[112] A. Kharlamov, B. R. Brown, K. A. Easley, and S. C. Jones, "Heterogeneous response of cerebral blood flow to hypotension demonstrated by laser speckle imaging flowmetry in rats," *Neuroscience Letters* **368**, 151–156 (2004).

[113] P. Zakharov, A. C. Voelker, M. T. Wyss, F. Haiss, N. Calcinaghi, C. Zunzunegui, A. Buck, F. Scheffold, and B. Weber, "Dynamic laser speckle imaging of cerebral blood flow," *Opt. Exp.* **17**, 13904–13917 (2009).

[114] S. G. Demos and R. R. Alfano, "Optical polarization imaging," Appl. Opt. 36, 150–155 (1997).

[115] A. Ishimaru, "Diffusion of light in turbid material," *Appl. Opt.* **28**, 2210–2215 (1989).

[116] D. F. T. Silva, B. C. Vidal, D. M. Zezell, T. M. Zorn, S. C. Nunez, and M. S. Ribeiro, "Collagen birefringence in skin repair in response to red polarized-laser therapy," *J. Biomed Opt.* **11**, (2006).

[117] J. M. Schmitt, A. H. Gandjbakhche, and R. F. Bonner, "Use of polarized-light to discriminate short-path photons in a multiply scattering medium," *Appl. Opt.* **31**, 6535–6546 (1992).

[118] F. C. Mackintosh, J. X. Zhu, D. J. Pine, and D. A. Weitz, "Polarization memory of multiply-scattered light," *Physical Review* **B 40**, 9342–9345 (1989).

[119] J. O'Doherty, J. Henricson, C. Anderson, M. J. Leahy, G. E. Nilsson, and F. Sjberg, "Sub-epidermal imaging using polarized light spectroscopy for assessment of skin microcirculation," *Skin Research and Technology* **13**, 472–484 (2007).

[120] S. L. Jacques, J. C. Ramella-Roman, and K. Lee, "Imaging skin pathology with polarized light," *J. Biomed Opt.* **7**, 329–340 (2002).

[121] W. Groner, J. W. Winkelman, A. G. Harris, C. Ince, G. J. Bouma, K. Messmer, and R. G. Nadeau, "Orthogonal polarization spectral imaging: A new method for study of the microcirculation," *Nat. Med.* **5**, 1209–1213 (1999).

[122] J. O'Doherty, *Assessment of Tissue Viability by Polarised Light Spectroscopy*, Prof. Martin J. Leahy, University of Limerick, Doctoral Thesis (2007).

[123] M. G. D. Karlsson and K. Wardell, "Polarized laser Doppler perfusion imaging — reduction of movement-induced artifacts," *J. Biomed Opt.* **10**, (2005).

[124] Z. J. Smith and A. J. Berger, "Surface–sensitive polarized Raman spectroscopy of biological tissue," *Opt. Lett.* **30**, 1363–1365 (2005).

[125] S. M. Milner, S. Bhat, S. Gulati, G. Gherardini, C. E. Smith, and R. J. Bick, "Observations on the microcirculation of the human burn wound using orthogonal polarization spectral imaging," *Burns* **31**, 316–319 (2005).

[126] S. Langer, A. G. Harris, P. Biberthaler, E. von Dobschuetz, and K. Messmer, "Orthogonal polarization spectral imaging as a tool for the assessment of hepatic microcirculations — A validation study," *Transplantation* **71**, 1249–1256 (2001).

[127] C. A. den Uil, E. Klijn, W. K. Lagrand, J. J. Brugts, C. Ince, P. E. Spronk, and M. L. Simoons, "The microcirculation in health and critical disease," *Progress in Cardiovascular Diseases* **51**, 161–170 (2008).

[128] V. Cerny, Z. Turek, and R. Parizkova, "Orthogonal polarization spectral imaging," *Physiological Research* **56**, 141–147 (2007).

[129] J. Lindert, J. Werner, M. Redlin, H. Kuppe, H. Habazettl, and A. R. Pries, "OPS Imaging of human microcirculation: A short technical report," *Journal of Vascular Research* **39**, 368–372 (2002).

[130] M. Heger, J. F. Beek, K. Stenback, D. J. Faber, M. J. C. van Gemert, and C. Ince, "Darkfield orthogonal polarized spectral imaging for studying endovascular laser-tissue interactions *in vivo* — a preliminary study," *Opt. Exp.* **13**, 702–715 (2005).

[131] C. Ince, "The microcirculation is the motor of sepsis," *Critical Care* **9**, 13–19 (2005).

[132] P. E. Spronk, C. Ince, M. J. Gardien, K. R. Mathura, H. M. Oudemans-van Straaten, and D. F. Zandstra, "Nitroglycerin in septic shock after intravascular volume resuscitation," *Lancet* **360**, 1395–1396 (2002).

[133] Y. Sakr, M. J. Dubois, D. De Backer, J. Creteur, and J. L. Vincent, "Persistent microcirculatory alterations are associated with organ failure and death in patients with septic shock," *Critical Care Medicine* **32**, 1825–1831 (2004).

[134] H. A. Lehr, F. Bittinger, and C. J. Kirkpatrick, "Microcirculatory dysfunction in sepsis: a pathogenetic basis for therapy?" *Journal of Pathology* **190**, 373–386 (2000).

[135] A. G. Harris, I. Sinitsina, and K. Messmer, "The Cytoscan (TM) model E-II, a new reflectance microscope for intravital microscopy: Comparison with the standard fluorescence method," *Journal of Vascular Research* **37**, 469–476 (2000).

[136] K. R. Mathura, K. C. Vollebregt, K. Boer, J. C. De Graaff, D. T. Ubbink, and C. Ince, "Comparison of OPS imaging and conventional capillary microscopy to study the human microcirculation," *J. Appl. Physiol.* **91**, 74–78 (2001).

[137] P. A. Payne, R. Y. Faddoul, and S. M. Jawad, "A single channel pulsed Doppler ultrasound instrument for measurement of skin blood flow," in *Practical Aspects of Skin Blood Flow Measurement*, Biological Engineering Society, London (1985).

[138] P. Atkinson and J. P. Woodcock, *Doppler Ultrasound and its Use in Clinical Measurement*, Academic, London (1982).

[139] F. S. Foster, P. N. Burns, D. H. Simpson, S. R. Wilson, D. A. Christopher, and D. E. Goertz, "Ultrasound for the visualization and quantification of tumor microcirculation," *Cancer and Metastasis Reviews* **19**, 131–138 (2000).

[140] F. S. Foster, C. J. Pavlin, K. A. Harasiewicz, D. A. Christopher, and D. H. Turnbull, "Advances in ultrasound biomicroscopy," *Journal of Ultrasound in Medicine and Biology* **26**, 1–27 (2000).

[141] S. D. Bos and H. J. A. Mensink, "Can duplex Doppler ultrasound replace computerized tomography in staging patients with renal cell carcinoma?" *Scandinavian Journal of Urology and Nephrology* **32**, 87–91 (1998).

[142] M. I. Novis, R. H. Baroni, L. M. D. Cerri, R. L. Mattedi, and C. A. Buchpiguel, "Clinically low-risk prostate cancer: evaluation with transrectal doppler ultrasound and functional magnetic resonance imaging," *Clinics* **66**, 27–34 (2011).

[143] E. Epstein, C. Van Holsbeke, F. Mascilini, A. Masback, P. Kannisto, L. Ameye, D. Fischerova, G. Zannoni, V. Vellone, D. Timmerman, and A. C. Testa, "Gray-scale and color Doppler ultrasound characteristics of endometrial cancer in relation to stage, grade and tumor size," *Ultrasound in Obstetrics & Gynecology* **38**, 586–593 (2011).

[144] A. M. Y. Cheung, A. S. Brown, V. Cucevic, M. Roy, A. Needles, V. Yang, D. J. Hicklin, R. S. Kerbel, and F. S. Foster, "Detecting vascular changes in tumour xenografts using micro-ultrasound and micro-CT following treatment with vegfr-2 blocking antibodies," *Ultrasound in Medicine and Biology* **33**, 1259–1268 (2007).

[145] F. S. Foster, J. Mehi, M. Lukacs, D. Hirson, C. White, C. Chaggares, and A. Needles, "A new 15–50 MHz array-based micro-ultrasound scanner for precinical imaging," *Ultrasound in Medicine and Biology* **35**, 1700–1708 (2009).

[146] H. Becher and P. N. Burns, *Handbook of Contrast Echocardiography*, Springer, Berlin (2000).

[147] P. N. Burns, J. E. Powers, and T. Fritzsch, "Harmonic imaging: a new imaging and Doppler method for contrast enhanced ultrasound," *Radiology* **185**, 142 (1992).

[148] K. K. Hodge, J. E. McNeal, M. K. Terris, and T. A. Stamey, "Random systematic versus directed ultrasound guided trans-rectal core biopsies of the prostate," *Journal of Urology* **142**, 71–75 (1989).

[149] B. G. Ewigman, J. P. Crane, F. D. Frigoletto, M. L. Lefevre, R. P. Bain, and D. McNellis, "Effect of prenatal ultrasound screening on perinatal outcome," *New England Journal of Medicine* **329**, 821–827 (1993).

[150] J. Flammer, S. Orgul, V. P. Costa, N. Orzalesi, G. K. Krieglstein, L. M. Serra, J. P. Renard, and E. Stefansson, "The impact of ocular blood flow in glaucoma," *Progress in Retinal and Eye Research* **21**, 359–393 (2002).

[151] N. G. Pandian, A. Kreis, B. Brockway, J. M. Isner, A. Sacharoff, E. Boleza, R. Caro, and D. Muller, "Ultrasound angioscopy — Real-time, two-dimensional, intraluminal ultrasound imaging of blood-vessels," *American Journal of Cardiology* **62**, 493–494 (1988).

[152] G. Heiss, A. R. Sharrett, R. Barnes, L. E. Chambless, M. Szklo, and C. Alzola, "Carotid atherosclerosis measured by B-mode ultrasound in populations — Associations with cardiovascular risk-factors in the aric study," *American Journal of Epidemiology* **134**, 250–256 (1991).

[153] F. S. Foster, C. J. Pavlin, K. A. Harasiewicz, D. A. Christopher, and D. H. Turnbull, "Advances in ultrasound biomicroscopy," *Ultrasound in Medicine and Biology* **26**, 1–27 (2000).

[154] R. J. Wakefield, P. V. Balint, M. Szkudlarek, E. Filippucci, M. Backhaus, M. A. D'Agostino, E. N. Sanchez, A. Iagnocco, W. A. Schmidt, G. Bruyn, D. Kane, P. J. O'Connor, B. Manger,

F. Joshua, J. Koski, W. Grassi, M. N. D. Lassere, N. Swen, F. Kainberger, A. Klauser, M. Ostergaard, A. K. Brown, K. P. Machold, and P. G. Conaghan, "Musculoskeletal ultrasound including definitions for ultrasonographic pathology," *Journal of Rheumatology* **32**, 2485–2487 (2005).

[155] P. C. Lauterbur, "Image formation by induced local interactions: Examples employing nuclear magnetic resonance," *Nature* **242**, 190–191 (1973).

[156] P. G. Mansfield, P.K., "NMR 'diffraction' in solids?" *Journal of Physics C* **6**, L422–L426 (1973).

[157] A. Berger, "How does it work? Magnetic resonance imaging," *British Medical Journal* **324**, 35–35 (2002).

[158] F. Mirrashed and J. C. Sharp, "*In vivo* morphological characterisation of skin by MRI micro-imaging methods," *Skin Research and Technology* **10**, 149–160 (2004).

[159] C. M. Kerskens, R. M. Piech, and J. F. M. Meaney, "Imaging blood circulation using Nuclear Magnetic Resonance," in *Microcirculation Imaging*, Wiley-VCH, Weinheim (2012).

[160] R. J. Kim, E. Wu, A. Rafael, E. L. Chen, M. A. Parker, O. Simonetti, F. J. Klocke, R. O. Bonow, and R. M. Judd, "The use of contrast-enhanced magnetic resonance imaging to identify reversible myocardial dysfunction," *New England Journal of Medicine* **343**, 1445–1453 (2000).

[161] P. Caravan, J. J. Ellison, T. J. McMurry, and R. B. Lauffer, "Gadolinium(III) chelates as MRI contrast agents: Structure, dynamics, and applications," *Chemical Reviews* **99**, 2293–2352 (1999).

[162] J. K. T. Lee, S. S. Sagel, R. J. Stanley, and J. P. Heiken, *Computed Body Tomography with MRI Correlation*, Lippincott, Williams and Wilkins, Philadelphia, PA (2005).

[163] G. J. Wilson, R. M. Hoogeveen, W. A. Willinek, R. Muthupillai, and J. H. Maki, "Parallel imaging in MR angiography," *Topics in Magnetic Resonance Imaging* **15**, 169–185 (2004).

[164] E. K. Yucel, C. M. Anderson, R. R. Edelman, T. M. Grist, R. A. Baum, W. J. Manning, A. Culebras, and W. Pearce, "Magnetic resonance angiography — Update on applications for extracranial arteries," *Circulation* 100, 2284–2301 (1999).

[165] D. L. Parker, C. Yuan, and D. D. Blatter, "MR angiography by multiple thin slab 3D acquisition," *Magnetic Resonance in Medicine* **17**, 434–451 (1991).

[166] L. Faggioni, V. Zampa, S. Ortori, E. Picano, R. De Lucia, E. Soldati, M. G. Bongiorni, E. Neri, and C. Bartolozzi, "Time-resolved contrast-enhanced magnetic resonance angiography (CEMRA) of the left atrium-pulmonary veins complex with half dose of intravenous gadolinium-based contrast agent. Technical feasibility and comparison with a conventional CEMRA, full contrast dose protocol," *European Journal of Radiology* **81**, 250–256 (2012).

[167] M. Neeman and H. Dafni, "Structural, functional, and molecular MR imaging of the microvasculature," *Annual Review of Biomedical Engineering* **5**, 29–56 (2003).

[168] J. J. Oliver and D. J. Webb, "Noninvasive assessment of arterial stiffness and risk of atherosclerotic events," *Arteriosclerosis Thrombosis and Vascular Biology* **23**, 554–566 (2003).

[169] D. J. Loeffelbein, M. Souvatzoglou, V. Wankerl, A. Martinez-Moller, J. Dinges, M. Schwaiger, and A. J. Beer, "PET-MRI fusion in head-and-neck oncology: Current status and implications for hybrid PET/MRI," *Journal of Oral and Maxillofacial Surgery* **70**, 473–483 (2012).

[170] C. de Bazelaire, M. Chapellier, A. Pluvinage, A. Scemama, F. Pilehvari, P. Bourrier, J. Frija, and E. de Kerviler, "New developments in oncology MRI," *Oncologie* **12**, 187–196 (2010).

[171] A. Cuocolo, W. Acampa, M. Imbriaco, N. De Luca, G. L. Iovino, and M. Salvatore, "The many ways to myocardial perfusion imaging," *Quarterly Journal of Nuclear Medicine and Molecular Imaging* **49**, 4–18 (2005).

[172] K. Nassenstein, S. Orzada, L. Haering, A. Czylwik, M. Zenge, H. Eberle, T. Schlosser, O. Bruder, E. Muller, M. E. Ladd, and S. Maderwald, "Cardiac MRI: evaluation of phonocardiogram-gated cine imaging for the assessment of global und regional left ventricular function in clinical routine," *European Radiology* **22**, 559–568 (2012).

[173] J. W. Belliveau, D. N. Kennedy, Jr., R. C. McKinstry, B. R. Buchbinder, R. M. Weisskoff, M. S. Cohen, J. M. Vevea, T. J. Brady, and B. R. Rosen, "Functional mapping of the human visual cortex by magnetic resonance imaging," *Science* **254**, 716–719 (1991).

[174] E. R. Freilich and W. D. Gaillard, "Utility of functional MRI in pediatric neurology," *Current Neurology and Neuroscience Reports* **10**, 40–46 (2010).

[175] P. E. Valk, D. Delbeke, and D. L. Bailey, *Positron Emission Tomography: Clinical Practice*, Springer-Verlag, Berlin (2006).

[176] U. S. National Research Council, *Mathematics and Physics of Emerging Biomedical Imaging*, Committee on the Mathematics and Physics of Emerging Dynamic Biomedical Imaging (eds.), National Academy Press, Washington D.C. (1996).

[177] D. W. Townsend, "Physical principles and technology of clinical PET imaging," *Annals Academy of Medicine Singapore* **33**, 133–145 (2004).

[178] R. L. Buckner, J. R. Andrews-Hanna, and D. L. Schacter, "The brain's default network — Anatomy, function, and relevance to disease," in *Year in Cognitive Neuroscience 2008*, Wiley-Blackwell, Malden, 1–38 (2008).

[179] S. Minoshima, B. Giordani, S. Berent, K. A. Frey, N. L. Foster, and D. E. Kuhl, "Metabolic reduction in the posterior cingulate cortex in very early Alzheimer's disease," *Annals of Neurology* **42**, 85–94 (1997).

[180] C. Wilson, A. A. Lammertsma, C. G. McKenzie, K. Sikora, and T. Jones, "Measurements of blood-flow and exchanging water space in breast-tumors using positron emission tomography — a rapid and noninvasive dynamic method," *Cancer Research* **52**, 1592–1597 (1992).

[181] S. Minoshima, N. L. Foster, K. A. Frey, R. L. Wahl, J. H. Burdette, and D. E. Kuhl, "Can FDG PET distinguish dementia patients with cortical Lewy bodies from pure Alzheimer's disease?" *Journal of Nuclear Medicine* **38**, 257–257 (1997).

[182] A. M. Owen, J. Doyon, A. Dagher, A. Sadikot, and A. C. Evans, "Abnormal basal ganglia outflow in Parkinson's disease identified with PET — Implications for higher cortical functions," *Brain* **121**, 949–965 (1998).

[183] J. S. Rakshi, T. Uema, K. Ito, D. L. Bailey, P. K. Morrish, J. Ashburner, A. Dagher, I. H. Jenkins, K. J. Friston, and D. J. Brooks, "Frontal, midbrain and striatal dopaminergic function in early and advanced Parkinson's disease — A 3D [F-18]dopa-PET study," *Brain* **122**, 1637–1650 (1999).

[184] H. Stefan, G. Pawlik, H. G. Bocherschwarz, H. J. Biersack, W. Burr, H. Penin, and W. D. Heiss, "Functional and morphological abnormalities in temporal-lobe epilepsy — a comparison of interictal and ictal EEG, CT, MRI, SPECT and PET," *Journal of Neurology* **234**, 377–384 (1987).

[185] S. S. Spencer, "The relative contributions of MRI, SPECT, and PET imaging in epilepsy," *Epilepsia* **35**, 72–89 (1994).

[186] O. Muzik, E. A. da Silva, C. Juhasz, D. C. Chugani, J. Shah, F. Nagy, A. Canady, H. M. von Stockhausen, K. Herholz, J. Gates, M. Frost, F. Ritter, C. Watson, and H. T. Chugani, "Intracranial EEG versus flumazenil and glucose PET in children with extratemporal lobe epilepsy," *Neurology* **54**, 171–179 (2000).

[187] G. D. Hutchins, M. Schwaiger, K. C. Rosenspire, J. Krivokapich, H. Schelbert, and D. E. Kuhl, "Noninvasive quantification of regional blood-flow in the human heart using N-13 ammonia and dynamic positron emission tomographic imaging," *Journal of the American College of Cardiology* **15**, 1032–1042 (1990).

[188] R. O. Bonow, V. Dilsizian, A. Cuocolo, and S. L. Bacharach, "Identification of viable myocardium in patients with chronic coronary-artery disease and left-ventricular dysfunction — Comparison of Thallium scintigraphy with reinjection and PET imaging with F-18 fluorodeoxyglucose," *Circulation* **83**, 26–37 (1991).

[189] B. A. Dwamena, S. S. Sonnad, J. O. Angobaldo, and R. L. Wahl, "Metastases from non-small cell lung cancer: Mediastinal staging in the 1990s – Meta–analytic comparison of PET and CT," Radiology 213, 530–536 (1999).

[190] K. Kinkel, Y. Lu, M. Both, R. S. Warren, and R. F. Thoeni, "Detection of hepatic metastases from cancers of the gastrointestinal tract by using noninvasive imaging methods (US, CT, MR imaging, PET): A meta-analysis," *Radiology* **224**, 748–756 (2002).

[191] M. Karam, S. Roberts-Klein, N. Shet, J. Chang, and P. Feustel, "Bilateral hilar foci on F-18-FDG PET scan in patients without lung cancer: Variables associated with benign and malignant etiology," *Journal of Nuclear Medicine* **49**, 1429–1436 (2008).

[192] R. Vikram, H. D. W. Yeung, H. A. Macapinlac, and R. B. Iyer, "Utility of PET/CT in differentiating benign from malignant adrenal nodules in patients with cancer," *American Journal of Roentgenology* **191**, 1545–1551 (2008).

[193] M. L. Jan, K. S. Chuang, G. W. Chen, Y. C. Ni, S. Chen, C. H. Chang, J. Wu, T. W. Lee, and Y. K. Fu, "A three-dimensional registration method for automated fusion of micro PET-CT-SPECT whole-body images," *IEEE Transactions on Medical Imaging* **24**, 886–893 (2005).

[194] H. Corrodi and G. Jonsson, "Formaldehyde fluorescence method for histochemical demonstration of biogenic monoamines — a review on methodology," *Journal of Histochemistry & Cytochemistry* **15**, 65 (1967).

[195] K. Takano, J. Sato, H. Shirasaki, N. Yamazaki, K. Hoki, and T. Himi, "Melanin pigmented oncocytic metaplasia of the nasopharynx," *Auris Nasus Larynx* **31**, 161–163 (2004).

[196] I. C. MacDonald, A. C. Groom, and A. F. Chambers, "Cancer spread and micrometastasis development: quantitative approaches for *in vivo* models," *Bioessays* **24**, 885–893 (2002).

[197] R. J. Motzer, J. Bacik, T. Mariani, P. Russo, M. Mazumdar, and V. Reuter, "Treatment outcome and survival associated with metastatic renal cell carcinoma of non-clear-cell histology," *Journal of Clinical Oncology* **20**, 2376–2381 (2002).

[198] M. L. Woods, C. J. Koch, and E. M. Lord, "Detection of individual hypoxic cells in multicellular spheroids by flow cytometry using the 2-nitroimldazole, EF5, and monoclonal antibodies," *International Journal of Radiation Oncology Biology Physics* **34**, 93–101 (1996).

[199] A. K. H. Kwok, W. W. Y. Li, C. P. Pang, T. Y. Y. Lai, G. H. F. Yam, N. R. Chan, and D. S. C. Lam, "Indocyanine green staining and removal of internal limiting membrane in macular

hole surgery: Histology and outcome," *American Journal of Ophthalmology* **132**, 178–183 (2001).

[200] M. Mori, Y. Adachi, T. Matsushima, H. Matsuda, H. Kuwano, and K. Sugimachi, "Lugol Staining Pattern and Histology of Esophageal Lesions," *American Journal of Gastroenterology* **88**, 701–705 (1993).

[201] E. P. Walker, P. H. Butler, J. W. Pickering, W. A. Day, R. Fraser, and C. N. Vanhalewyn, "Histology of port wine stains after copper vapor laser treatment," *British Journal of Dermatology* **121**, 217–223 (1989).

[202] D. B. Apfelberg, J. Kosek, M. R. Maser, and H. Lash, "Histology of port wine stains following argon-laser treatment," *British Journal of Plastic Surgery* **32**, 232–237 (1979).

[203] J. W. Buecker, J. L. Ratz, and D. F. Richfield, "Histology of port-wine stain treated with carbon-dioxide laser," *Journal of the American Academy of Dermatology* **10**, 1014–1019 (1984).

[204] B. Sung, M. S. Kim, B. C. Lee, J. S. Yoo, S. H. Lee, Y. J. Kim, K. W. Kim, and K. S. Soh, "Measurement of flow speed in the channels of novel threadlike structures on the surfaces of mammalian organs," *Naturwissenschaften* **95**, 117–124 (2008).

[205] A. Sarasa-Renedo, A. Darrell, and J. Ripoli, "Applications of optical tomography in biomedical research," in *Handbook of Photonics for Biomedical Science*, Valery V. Tuchin (ed.), CRC Press, Boca Raton, FL (2010).

[206] J. R. Walls, J. G. Sled, J. Sharpe, and R. M. Henkelman, "Resolution improvement in emission optical projection tomography," *Phys. Med. Bio.* **52**, 2775–2790 (2007).

[207] V. V. Tuchin, "Optical clearing of tissues and blood using the immersion method," *Journal of Physics D-Applied Physics* **38**, 2497–2518 (2005).

[208] J. Sharpe, U. Ahlgren, P. Perry, B. Hill, A. Ross, J. Hecksher-Sorensen, R. Baldock, and D. Davidson, "Optical projection tomography as a tool for 3D microscopy and gene expression studies," *Science* **296**, 541–545 (2002).

[209] A. C. Kak and M. Slaney, *Principles of Computerized Tomographic Imaging*, IEEE Press (1988).

[210] J. Sharpe, "Optical projection tomography as a new tool for studying embryo anatomy," *Journal of Anatomy* **202**, 175–181 (2003).

[211] J. Sharpe, "Optical projection tomography," *Annual Review of Biomedical Engineering* **6**, 209–228 (2004).

[212] T. Alanentalo, A. Asayesh, H. Morrison, C. E. Loren, D. Holmberg, J. Sharpe, and U. Ahlgren, "Tomographic molecular imaging and 3D quantification within adult mouse organs," *Nature Methods* **4**, 31–33 (2007).

[213] M. Oldham, H. Sakhalkar, Y. M. Wang, P. Y. Guo, T. Oliver, R. Bentley, Z. Vujaskovic, and M. Dewhirst, "Three-dimensional imaging of whole rodent organs using optical computed and emission tomography," *J. Biomed Opt.* **12**, 1–10 (2007).

[214] J. Kerwin, M. Scott, J. Sharpe, L. Puelles, S. C. Robson, M. Martinez-de-la-Torre, J. L. Ferran, G. J. Feng, R. Baldock, T. Strachan, D. Davidson, and S. Lindsay, "3-dimensional modelling of early human brain development using optical projection tomography," *BMC Neuroscience* **5**, 27 (2004).

[215] M. Fauver, E. J. Seibel, J. R. Rahn, M. G. Meyer, F. W. Patten, T. Neumann, and A. C. Nelson, "Three-dimensional imaging of single isolated cell nuclei using optical projection tomography," *Opt. Exp.* **13**, 4210–4223 (2005).

[216] R. A. Rahim, M. H. F. Rahiman, C. L. Goh, S. Z. M. Muji, H. A. Rahim, and Y. M. Yunos, "Modeling orthogonal and rectilinear mixed-modality projection of optical tomography for solid-particles concentration measurement," *Sensors and Actuators A* **161**, 53–61 (2010).

[217] R. A. Rahim, P. J. Fea, C. K. San, and L. L. Chean, "Real-time image reconstruction for various flow regimes using an optical tomography sensor in a gravity flow conveyor," *Advanced Powder Technology* **16**, 399–411 (2005).

[218] R. A. Rahim, K. T. Chiam, M. H. F. Rahiman, and P. Jayasuman, "Velocity profile measurement using digital signal processor-based optical tomography system," *IEEE Sensors Journal* **9**, 1076–1083 (2009).

[219] C. G. Arques, R. Doohan, J. Sharpe, and M. Torres, "Cell tracing reveals a dorsoventral lineage restriction plane in the mouse limb bud mesenchyme," *Development* **134**, 3713–3722 (2007).

[220] R. J. Bryson-Richardson and P. D. Currie, "Optical projection tomography for spatio-temporal analysis in the zebrafish," *Cellular and Developmental Biology* **76**, 37–50 (2004).

[221] R. Kopelman and W. H. Tan, "Near-field optics — Imaging single molecules," *Science* **262**, 1382–1384 (1993).

[222] S. W. Hell and J. Wichmann, "Breaking the diffraction resolution limit by stimulated-emission — Stimulated-emission-depletion fluorescence microscopy," *Opt. Lett.* **19**, 780–782 (1994).

[223] V. Westphal, J. Seeger, T. Salditt, and S. W. Hell, "Stimulated emission depletion microscopy on lithographic nanostructures," *Journal of Physics B* **38**, 695–705 (2005).

[224] G. Donnert, J. Keller, R. Medda, M. A. Andrei, S. O. Rizzoli, R. Lurmann, R. Jahn, C. Eggeling, and S. W. Hell, "Macromolecular-scale resolution in biological fluorescence microscopy," *Proc. National Academy of Sciences* **103**, 11440–11445 (2006).

[225] E. Rittweger, K. Y. Han, S. E. Irvine, C. Eggeling, and S. W. Hell, "STED microscopy reveals crystal colour centres with nanometric resolution," *Nature Photonics* **3**, 144–147 (2009).

[226] W. L. Chao, B. D. Harteneck, J. A. Liddle, E. H. Anderson, and D. T. Attwood, "Soft X-ray microscopy at a spatial resolution better than 15 nm," *Nature* **435**, 1210–1213 (2005).

[227] T. Wilson and C. J. R. Sheppard, *Theory and Practice of Optical Scanning Microscopy*, Academic, London (1984).

[228] W. Min, S. J. Lu, S. S. Chong, R. Roy, G. R. Holtom, and X. S. Xie, "Imaging chromophores with undetectable fluorescence by stimulated emission microscopy," *Nature* **461**, 1105–1109 (2009).

[229] T. A. Klar and S. W. Hell, "Subdiffraction resolution in far-field fluorescence microscopy," *Opt. Lett.* **24**, 954–956 (1999).

[230] C. F. Kuang and G. R. Wang, "A novel far-field nanoscopic velocimetry for nanofluidics," *Lab on a Chip* **10**, 240–245 (2010).

[231] Y. Kazoe, K. Mawatari, Y. Sugii, and T. Kitamori, "Development of a measurement technique for ion distribution in an extended nanochannel by super-resolution-laser-induced fluorescence," *Analytical Chemistry* **83**, 8152–8157 (2011).

[232] K. S. Morozova, K. D. Piatkevich, T. J. Gould, J. H. Zhang, J. Bewersdorf, and V. V. Verkhusha, "Far-red fluorescent protein excitable with red lasers for flow cytometry and superresolution STED nanoscopy," *Biophysical Journal* **99**, 13–15 (2010).

[233] C. Sensen and B. Hallgremsson, *Micro-Computed Tomography*, Springer-Verlag, Berlin, (2009).

[234] L. A. Feldkamp, L. C. Davis, and J. W. Kress, "Practical cone–beam algorithm," *Journal of the Optical Society of America A—Optics Image Science and Vision* **1**, 612–619 (1984).

[235] L. Zagorchev, P. Oses, Z. W. Zhuang, K. Moodie, M. J. Mulligan-Kehoe, M. Simons, and T. Couffinhal, "Micro computed tomography for vascular exploration," *Journal of Angiogenesis Research* **2**, (2010).

[236] E. L. Ritman, "Molecular imaging in small animals — Roles for micro-CT," *J. Cell. Biochem.* Suppl. **39**, 116–124 (2002).

[237] T. L. Kline and E. L. Ritman, "Studying microcirculation with micro–CT," in *Microcirculation Imaging*, Martin J. Leahy (ed.), Wiley–VCH, Weinheim (2012).

[238] L. V. Wang and H.-I. Wu, *Biomedical Optics: Principles and Imaging*, Wiley, Hoboken, NJ (2007).

[239] R. Savai, A. C. Langheinrich, R. T. Schermuly, S. S. Pullamsetti, R. Dumitrascu, H. Traupe, W. S. Rau, W. Seeger, F. Grimminger, and A. Banat, "Evaluation of angiogenesis using micro-computed tomography in a xenograft mouse model of lung cancer," *Neoplasia* **11**, 48–56 (2009).

[240] L. Zagorchev and M. J. Mulligan-Kehoe, "Molecular imaging of vessels in mouse models of disease," *European Journal of Radiology* **70**, 305–311 (2009).

[241] M. S. Morrison, S. A. Ricketts, J. Barnett, A. Cuthbertson, J. Tessier, and S. R. Wedge, "Use of a novel Arg-Gly-Asp radioligand, (18)FAH111585, to determine changes in tumor vascularity after antitumor therapy," *Journal of Nuclear Medicine* **50**, 116–122 (2009).

[242] T. Miclau, C. Lu, Z. Thompson, P. Choi, C. Puttlitz, R. Marcucio, and J. A. Helms, "Effects of delayed stabilization on fracture healing," *Journal of Orthopaedic Research* **25**, 1552–1558 (2007).

[243] A. Garcia-Sanz, A. Rodriguez-Barbero, M. D. Bentley, E. L. Ritman, and J. C. Romero, "Three-dimensional microcomputed tomography of renal vasculature in rats," *Hypertension* **31**, 440–444 (1998).

[244] R. Iliescu, S. R. Fernandez, S. Kelsen, C. Marie, and A. R. Chade, "Role of renal microcirculation in experimental renovascular disease," *Nephrology Dialysis Transplantation* **25**, 1079–1087 (2010).

[245] V. Goh, S. Halligan, D. M. Wellsted, and C. I. Bartram, "Can perfusion CT assessment of primary colorectal adenocarcinoma blood flow at staging predict for subsequent metastatic disease? A pilot study," *European Radiology* **19**, 79–89 (2009).

[246] D. A. Steinman, "Image-based computational fluid dynamics modeling in realistic arterial geometries," *Annals of Biomedical Engineering* **30**, 483–497 (2002).

[247] J. Suo, D. E. Ferrara, D. Sorescu, R. E. Guldberg, W. R. Taylor, and D. P. Giddens, "Hemodynamic shear stresses in mouse aortas — Implications for atherogenesis," *Arteriosclerosis Thrombosis and Vascular Biology* **27**, 346–351 (2007).

[248] A. Lerman and E. L. Ritman, "Evaluation of microvascular anatomy by micro–CT," *Herz* **24**, 531–533 (1999).

[249] J. G. White, W. B. Amos, and M. Fordham, "An evaluation of confocal versus conventional imaging of biological structures by fluorescence light-microscopy," *Journal of Cell Biology* **105**, 41–48 (1987).

[250] P. J. Tadrous, "Methods for imaging the structure and function of living tissues and cells: 3. Confocal microscopy and micro-radiology," *Journal of Pathology* **191**, 345–354 (2000).

[251] J. Hueve, R. Wesselmann, M. Kahms, and R. Peters, "4Pi microscopy of the nuclear pore complex," *Biophysical Journal* **95**, 877–885 (2008).

[252] F. Helmchen and W. Denk, "Deep tissue two-photon microscopy," *Nature Methods* **2**, 932–940 (2005).

[253] C. Xu, W. Zipfel, J. B. Shear, R. M. Williams, and W. W. Webb, "Multiphoton fluorescence excitation: New spectral windows for biological nonlinear microscopy," *Proc. National Academy of Sciences* **93**, 10763–10768 (1996).

[254] W. Denk, J. H. Strickler, and W. W. Webb, "2-photon laser scanning fluorescence microscopy," *Science* **248**, 73–76 (1990).

[255] P. Theer, M. T. Hasan, and W. Denk, "Two-photon imaging to a depth of 1000 μm in living brains by use of a Ti : Al2O3 regenerative amplifier," *Opt. Lett.* **28**, 1022–1024 (2003).

[256] S. Inoué, "Foundations of confocal scanned imaging in light microscopy," in *Handbook of Biological Confocal Microscopy*, James B. Pawley (ed.), Springer, New York (2006).

[257] K. Konig, "Multiphoton microscopy in life sciences," *Journal of Microscopy-Oxford* **200**, 83–104 (2000).

[258] S. M. Potter, S. E. Fraser, and J. Pine, "The greatly reduced photodamage of 2–photon microscopy enables extended 3–dimensional time–lapse imaging of living neurons," Scanning 18, (1996).

[259] S. A. Boppart, B. E. Bouma, M. E. Brezinski, G. J. Tearney, and J. G. Fujimoto, "Imaging developing neural morphology using optical coherence tomography," *Journal of Neuroscience Methods* **70**, 65–72 (1996).

[260] D. M. Shotton, "Electronic light-microscopy — Present capabilities and future-prospects," *Histochemistry and Cell Biology* **104**, 97–137 (1995).

[261] J. M. Schmitt, M. J. Yadlowsky, and R. F. Bonner, "Subsurface imaging of living skin with optical coherence microscopy," *Dermatology* **191**, 93–98 (1995).

[262] M. Garcia–Alloza and B. J. Bacskai, "Techniques for brain imaging *in vivo*," *Neuromolecular Medicine* **6**, 65–78 (2004).

[263] Y. Tomita, N. Kubis, Y. Calando, A. T. Dinh, P. Meric, J. Seylaz, and E. Pinard, "Long-term *in vivo* investigation of mouse cerebral microcirculation by fluorescence confocal microscopy in the area of focal ischemia," *Journal of Cerebral Blood Flow and Metabolism* **25**, 858–867 (2005).

[264] Z. G. Zhang, K. Davies, J. Prostak, J. Fenstermacher, and M. Chopp, "Quantitation of microvascular plasma perfusion and neuronal microtubule-associated protein in ischemic mouse brain by laser-scanning confocal microscopy," *Journal of Cerebral Blood Flow and Metabolism* **19**, 68–78 (1999).

[265] D. C. Morris, Z. G. Zhang, K. Davies, J. Fenstermacher, and M. Chopp, "High resolution quantitation of microvascular plasma perfusion in non-ischemic and ischemic rat brain by laser-scanning confocal microscopy," *Brain Research Protocols* **4**, 185–191 (1999).

[266] M. J. Levene, D. A. Dombeck, K. A. Kasischke, R. P. Molloy, and W. W. Webb, "*In vivo* multiphoton microscopy of deep brain tissue," *Journal of Neurophysiology* **91**, 1908–1912 (2004).

[267] W. H. Kim, C. I. Kim, S. W. Lee, S. H. Lim, C. W. Park, H. Lee, and M. K. Park, "Particle image velocimetry of the blood flow in a micro-channel using the confocal laser scanning microscope," *Journal of the Optical Society of Korea* **14**, 42–48 (2010).

[268] E. A. V. Jones, M. H. Baron, S. E. Fraser, and M. E. Dickinson, "Measuring hemodynamic changes during mammalian development," *American Journal of Physiology—Heart and Circulatory Physiology* **287**, 1561–1569 (2004).

[269] N. D. Lawson and B. M. Weinstein, "In vivo imaging of embryonic vascular development using transgenic zebrafish," *Developmental Biology* **248**, 307–318 (2002).

[270] D. G. Buschke, J. M. Squirrell, H. Ansari, M. A. Smith, C. T. Rueden, J. C. Williams, G. E. Lyons, T. J. Kamp, K. W. Eliceiri, and B. M. Ogle, "Multiphoton flow cytometry to assess intrinsic and extrinsic fluorescence in cellular aggregates: Applications to stem cells," *Microscopy and Microanalysis* **17**, 540–554 (2011).

[271] W. He, H. F. Wang, L. C. Hartmann, J. X. Cheng, and P. S. Low, "*In vivo* quantitation of rare circulating tumor cells by multiphoton intravital flow cytometry," *Proc. National Academy of Sciences* **104**, 11760–11765 (2007).

[272] K. H. Kim, T. Ragan, M. J. R. Previte, K. Bahlmann, B. A. Harley, D. A. Wiktor-Brown, M. S. Stitt, C. A. Hendricks, K. H. Almeida, B. P. Engelward, and P. T. C. So, "Three-dimensional tissue cytometer based on high-speed multiphoton microscopy," *Cytometry Part A* **71**, 991–1002 (2007).

[273] E. R. Tkaczyk and A. H. Tkaczyk, "Multiphoton flow cytometry strategies and applications," *Cytometry Part A* **79**, 775–788 (2011).

[274] T. Khokhlova, I. Pelivanov, and A. Karabutov, "Advances in optoacoustic imaging," in *Handbook of Photonics for Biomedical Science*, Valery V. Tuchin (ed.), CRC Press, Boca Raton, FL (2010).

[275] R. A. Kruger, P. Y. Liu, Y. R. Fang, and C. R. Appledorn, "Photoacoustic ultrasound (PAUS) — Reconstruction tomography," *Medical Physics* **22**, 1605–1609 (1995).

[276] G. Paltauf, J. A. Viator, S. A. Prahl, and S. L. Jacques, "Iterative reconstruction algorithm for optoacoustic imaging," *Journal of the Acoustical Society of America* **112**, 1536–1544 (2002).

[277] Y. Wang, D. Xing, Y. G. Zeng, and Q. Chen, "Photoacoustic imaging with deconvolution algorithm," *Phys. Med. Bio.* **49**, 3117–3124 (2004).

[278] J. Laufer, D. Delpy, C. Elwell, and P. Beard, "Quantitative spatially resolved measurement of tissue chromophore concentrations using photoacoustic spectroscopy: application to the measurement of blood oxygenation and haemoglobin concentration," *Phys. Med. Bio.* **52**, 141–168 (2007).

[279] A. Tabuchi, M. Mertens, H. Kuppe, A. R. Pries, and W. M. Kuebler, "Intravital microscopy of the murine pulmonary microcirculation," *J. Appl. Physiol.* **104**, 338–346 (2008).

[280] X. D. Wang, Y. J. Pang, G. Ku, X. Y. Xie, G. Stoica, and L. H. V. Wang, "Noninvasive laser-induced photoacoustic tomography for structural and functional *in vivo* imaging of the brain," *Nature Biotechnology* **21**, 803–806 (2003).

[281] H. F. Zhang, K. Maslov, G. Stoica, and L. V. Wang, "Functional photoacoustic microscopy for high-resolution and noninvasive *in vivo* imaging," *Nature Biotechnology* **24**, 848–851 (2006).

[282] K. Maslov, G. Stoica, and L. H. V. Wang, "*In vivo* dark-field reflection-mode photoacoustic microscopy," *Opt. Lett.* **30**, 625–627 (2005).

[283] Z. Xie, L. V. Wang, and H. F. Zhang, "Optical fluence distribution study in tissue in dark-field confocal photoacoustic microscopy using a modified Monte Carlo convolution method," *Appl. Opt.* **48**, 3204–3211 (2009).

[284] S. Hu, K. Maslov, and L. V. Wang, "Optical-resolution photoacoustic microscopy for *in vivo* volumetric microvascular imaging in intact tissues," in *Handbook of Photonics for Biomedical Science*, Valery V. Tuchin (ed.), CRC Press, Boca Raton, FL (2010).

[285] S. Hu, K. Maslov, and L. V. Wang, "Three-dimensional optical-resolution photoacoustic microscopy," *JoVE* (2011).

[286] S. Hu, K. Maslov, and L. V. Wang, "Noninvasive label-free imaging of microhemodynamics by optical-resolution photoacoustic microscopy," *Opt. Exp.* **17**, 7688–7693 (2009).

[287] H. Fang, K. Maslov, and L. V. Wang, "Photoacoustic Doppler effect from flowing small light-absorbing particles," *Phys. Rev. Letts.* **99**, (2007).

[288] H. Fang, K. Maslov, and L. V. Wang, "Photoacoustic Doppler flow measurement in optically scattering media," *Appl. Phys. Letts.* **91**, (2007).

[289] H. Fang and L. V. Wang, "Photoacoustic Doppler effect and flow sensing," in *Photoacoustic Imaging and Spectroscopy*, Lihong V. Wang (ed.), CRC Press, Boca Raton, FL (2009).

[290] E. I. Galanzha, E. V. Shashkov, T. Kelly, J.-W. Kim, L. Yang, and V. P. Zharov, "*In vivo* magnetic enrichment and multiplex photoacoustic detection of circulating tumour cells," *Nature Nanotechnology* **4**, 855–860 (2009).

[291] S.-H. Yang, G.-Z. Yin, and D. Xing, "Pharmacokinetic monitoring of indocyanine green for tumor detection using photoacoustic imaging," *Chinese Physics Letters* **27**, (2010).

[292] M. H. Xu and L. H. V. Wang, "Universal back-projection algorithm for photoacoustic computed tomography," *Phys. Rev.* **E 71**, (2005).

[293] M. H. Xu and L. H. V. Wang, "Photoacoustic imaging in biomedicine," *Review of Scientific Instruments* **77**, (2006).

[294] L. Wang, X. Xie, J.-T. Oh, M.-L. Li, G. Ku, S. Ke, S. Similache, C. Li, and G. Stoica, "Combined photoacoustic and molecular fluorescence imaging *in vivo*," *IEEE Engineering in Medicine and Biology Society* **1**, 190–192 (2005).

[295] P. P. Joshi, Y.-S. Chen, S. Kim, J. Shah, K. Sokolov, and S. Emelianov, "Molecular therapeutic agents for noninvasive photoacoustic image-guided photothermal therapy," *IEEE Engineering in Medicine and Biology Society* **2009**, 4106–4109 (2009).

[296] D. Huang, E. A. Swanson, C. P. Lin, J. S. Schuman, W. G. Stinson, W. Chang, M. R. Hee, T. Flotte, K. Gregory, C. A. Puliafito, and J. G. Fujimoto, "Optical coherence tomography," *Science* **254**, 1178–1181 (1991).

[297] W. Drexler and J. G. Fujimoto, *Optical Coherence Tomography: Technology and Applications*, Springer–Verlag, Berlin (2008).

[298] M. R. Hee, E. A. Swanson, D. Huang, J. A. Izatt, C. P. Lin, J. S. Schuman, C. A. Puliafito, and J. G. Fujimoto, "Optical coherence tomography," *Invest. Ophthal. Vis. Sci.* **33**, 722–722 (1992).

[299] J. M. Schmitt, "Optical coherence tomography (OCT): A review," *IEEE J. Select. Top. Quant. Electr.* **5**, 1205–1215 (1999).

[300] A. F. Fercher, K. Mengedoht, and W. Werner, "Eye-length measurement by interferometry with partially-coherent light," *Opt. Lett.* **13**, 186–188 (1988).

[301] J. G. Fujimoto, "Optical coherence tomography," *Comptes Rendus De L Academie Des Sciences Serie Iv Physique Astrophysique* **2**, 1099–1111 (2001).

[302] H. C. Hendargo, R. P. McNabb, A. H. Dhalla, N. Shepherd, and J. A. Izatt, "Doppler velocity detection limitations in spectrometer-based versus swept-source optical coherence tomography," *Biomed. Opt. Exp.* **2**, 2175–2188 (2011).

[303] Z. Yaqoob, J. Wu, and C. Yang, "Spectral domain optical coherence tomography: a better OCT imaging strategy," *Bio.Techniq.* **39**, 6–13 (2005).

[304] B. Liu and M. E. Brezinski, "Theoretical and practical considerations on detection performance of time domain, Fourier domain, and swept source optical coherence tomography," *J. Biomed Opt.* **12**, (2007).

[305] P. H. Tomlins and R. K. Wang, "Theory, developments and applications of optical coherence tomography," *Journal of Physics D* **38**, 2519–2535 (2005).

[306] J. Welzel, M. Bruhns, and H. H. Wolff, "Optical coherence tomography in contact dermatitis and psoriasis," *Arch. Dermatol. Res.* **295**, 50–55 (2003).

[307] J. G. Fujimoto, "Optical coherence tomography for ultrahigh resolution *in vivo* imaging," *Nature Biotechnology* **21**, 1361–1367 (2003).

[308] H. Yabushita, B. E. Bourna, S. L. Houser, T. Aretz, I. K. Jang, K. H. Schlendorf, C. R. Kauffman, M. Shishkov, D. H. Kang, E. F. Halpern, and G. J. Tearney, "Characterization of human atherosclerosis by optical coherence tomography," *Circulation* **106**, 1640–1645 (2002).

[309] B. H. Park, C. Saxer, S. M. Srinivas, J. S. Nelson, and J. F. de Boer, "*In vivo* burn depth determination by high-speed fiber-based polarization sensitive optical coherence tomography," *J. Biomed. Opt.* **6**, 474–479 (2001).

[310] J. F. de Boer, S. M. Srinivas, A. Malekafzali, Z. P. Chen, and J. S. Nelson, "Imaging thermally damaged tissue by polarization sensitive optical coherence tomography," *Opt. Exp.* **3**, 212–218 (1998).

[311] B. S. Atiyeh, S. W. Gunn, and S. N. Hayek, "State of the art in burn treatment," *World Journal of Surgery* **29**, 131–148 (2005).

[312] J. F. Arevalo, C. F. Fernandez, and R. A. Garcia, "Optical coherence tomography characteristics of choroidal metastasis," *Ophthalmology* **112**, 1612–1619 (2005).

[313] I. Svorenova, P. Strmen, and Z. Olah, "Optical coherence tomography — a new imaging method in ophthalmology," *Bratislava Medical Journal* **111**, 306–307 (2010).

[314] C. L. Shields, M. A. Materin, and J. A. Shields, "Review of optical coherence tomography for intraocular tumors," *Current Opinion in Ophthalmology* **16**, 141–154 (2005).

[315] G. Guagliumi, G. Musumeci, V. Sirbu, H. G. Bezerra, N. Suzuki, L. Fiocca, A. Matiashvili, N. Lortkipanidze, A. Trivisonno, O. Valsecchi, G. Biondi-Zoccai, and M. A. Costa, "Optical coherence tomography assessment of *in vivo* vascular response after implantation of overlapping bare-metal and drug-eluting stents," *Cardiovascular Interventions* **3**, 531–539 (2010).

[316] A. F. Fercher, W. Drexler, C. K. Hitzenberger, and T. Lasser, "Optical coherence tomography — principles and applications," *Reports on Progress in Physics* **66**, 239–303 (2003).

[317] L. P. Hariri, G. T. Bonnema, K. Schmidt, A. M. Winkler, V. Korde, K. D. Hatch, J. R. Davis, M. A. Brewer, and J. K. Barton, "Laparoscopic optical coherence tomography imaging of human ovarian cancer," *Gynecologic Oncology* **114**, 188–194 (2009).

[318] H. J. Boehringer, E. Lankenau, F. Stellmacher, E. Reusche, G. Huettmann, and A. Giese, "Imaging of human brain tumor tissue by near-infrared laser coherence tomography," *Acta Neurochirurgica* **151**, 507–517 (2009).

[319] E. V. Zagaynova, O. S. Streltsova, N. D. Gladkova, L. B. Snopova, G. V. Gelikonov, F. I. Feldchtein, and A. N. Morozov, "*In vivo* optical coherence tomography feasibility for bladder disease," *J. Urology* **167**, 1492–1496 (2002).

[320] S. A. Boppart, "Optical coherence tomography — Principles applications and advances," *Minerva Biotecnologica* **16**, 211–237 (2004).

[321] S. Mordon, V. Maunoury, P. Bulois, P. Desreumaux, and J. F. Colombel, "Optical coherence computed tomography in gastroenterology," *Gastroenterol. Cliniq. Biol.* **29**, 618–620 (2005).

[322] T. Gambichler, V. Jaedicke, and S. Terras, "Optical coherence tomography in dermatology: technical and clinical aspects," *Arch. Dermatol. Res.* **303**, 457–473 (2011).

[323] J. Welzel, "Optical coherence tomography in dermatology: a review," *Skin Res. Technol.* **7**, 1–9 (2001).

[324] J. Welzel, E. Lankenau, R. Birngruber, and R. Engelhardt, "Optical coherence tomography of the skin," in *Current Problems in Dermatology*, 27–37 (1998).

[325] C. Gimbel, "Optical coherence tomography diagnostic imaging for dentistry," *Laser Surg. Med.* 55–55 (2009).

[326] L. L. Otis, M. J. Everett, U. S. Sathyam, and B. W. Colston, "Optical coherence tomography: A new imaging technology for dentistry," *J. Am. Dental Assoc.* **131**, 511 (2000).

[327] C. Pitris, A. Goodman, S. A. Boppart, J. J. Libus, J. G. Fujimoto, and M. E. Brezinski, "High-resolution imaging of gynecologic neoplasms using optical coherence tomography," *Obstetr. Gynecol.* **93**, 135–139 (1999).

[328] M. Ascencio, P. Collinet, M. Cosson, and S. Mordon, "The role and value of optical coherence tomography in gynecology," *J. Gynecol., Obstetriq. Biol. Reprod.* **36**, 749–755 (2007).

[329] Y. Wang, A. A. Fawzi, R. Varma, A. A. Sadun, X. Zhang, O. Tan, J. A. Izatt, and D. Huang, "Pilot study of optical coherence tomography measurement of retinal blood flow in retinal and optic nerve diseases," *Invest. Ophthal. Vis. Sci.* **52**, 840–845 (2011).

[330] B. Dunmire, K. W. Beach, K. H. Labs, M. Plett, and D. E. Strandness, "Cross-beam vector Doppler ultrasound for angle-independent velocity measurements," *Ultrasound Med. Biol.* **26**, 1213–1235 (2000).

[331] M. Rossow, W. W. Mantulin, and E. Gratton, "Spatiotemporal image correlation spectroscopy measurements of flow demonstrated in microfluidic channels," *J. Biomed Opt.* **14**, (2009).

[332] R. K. Wang, S. L. Jacques, Z. Ma, S. Hurst, S. R. Hanson, and A. Gruber, "Three dimensional optical angiography," *Opt. Exp.* **15**, 4083–4097 (2007).

[333] J. A. Izatt, M. D. Kulkami, S. Yazdanfar, J. K. Barton, and A. J. Welch, "*In vivo* bidirectional color Doppler flow imaging of picoliter blood volumes using optical coherence tomograghy," *Opt. Lett.* **22**, 1439–1441 (1997).

[334] V. Guedes, J. S. Schuman, E. Hertzmark, G. Wollstein, A. Correnti, R. Mancini, D. Lederer, S. Voskanian, L. Velazquez, H. M. Pakter, T. Pedut-Kloizman, J. G. Fujimoto, and C. Mattox, "Optical coherence tomography measurement of macular and nerve fiber layer thickness in normal and glaucomatous human eyes," *Ophthalmology* **110**, 177–189 (2003).

[335] S. Yazdanfar, A. M. Rollins, and J. A. Izatt, "*In vivo* imaging of human retinal flow dynamics by color Doppler optical coherence tomography," *Arch. Ophthal.* **121**, 235–239 (2003).

[336] J. A. Izatt, M. R. Hee, E. A. Swanson, C. P. Lin, D. Huang, J. S. Schuman, C. A. Puliafito, and J. G. Fujimoto, "Micrometer-scale resolution imaging of the anterior eye *in vivo* with optical coherence tomography," *Arch. Ophthalmol.* **112**, 1584–1589 (1994).

[337] M. Wojtkowski, A. Kowalczyk, R. Leitgeb, and A. F. Fercher, "Full range complex spectral optical coherence tomography technique in eye imaging," *Opt. Lett.* **27**, 1415–1417 (2002).

[338] C. Wang, Y. Yang, Z. Ding, J. Meng, K. Wang, W. Yang, and Y. Xu, "Monitoring of drug and stimulation induced cerebral blood flow velocity changes in rat sensory cortex using spectral domain Doppler optical coherence tomography," *J. Biomed. Opt.* **16**, (2011).

[339] P. Li, A. Liu, L. Shi, X. Yin, S. Rugonyi, and R. K. Wang, "Assessment of strain and strain rate in embryonic chick heart *in vivo* using tissue Doppler optical coherence tomography," *Phys. Med. Biol.* **56**, 7081–7092 (2011).

[340] J. Wierwille, P. M. Andrews, M. L. Onozato, J. Jiang, A. Cable, and Y. Chen, "*In vivo*, label-free, three-dimensional quantitative imaging of kidney microcirculation using Doppler optical coherence tomography," *Lab. Invest.* **91**, 1596–1604 (2011).

[341] A. Needles, D. E. Goertz, A. M. Cheung, and F. S. Foster, "Interframe clutter filtering for high frequency flow imaging," *Ultrasound Med. Biol.* **33**, 591–600 (2007).

[342] A. Mariampillai, B. A. Standish, E. H. Moriyama, M. Khurana, N. R. Munce, M. K. K. Leung, J. Jiang, A. Cable, B. C. Wilson, I. A. Vitkin, and V. X. D. Yang, "Speckle variance detection of microvasculature using swept-source optical coherence tomography," *Opt. Lett.* **33**, 1530–1532 (2008).

[343] X. Liu, K. Zhang, Y. Huang, and J. U. Kang, "Spectroscopic-speckle variance OCT for microvasculature detection and analysis," *Biomed. Opt. Exp.* **2**, 2995–3009 (2011).

[344] A. Mariampillai, M. K. K. Leung, M. Jarvi, B. A. Standish, K. Lee, B. C. Wilson, A. Vitkin, and V. X. D. Yang, "Optimized speckle variance OCT imaging of microvasculature," *Opt. Lett.* **35**, 1257–1259 (2010).

[345] J. Fingler, D. Schwartz, C. Yang, and S. E. Fraser, "Mobility and transverse flow visualization using phase variance contrast with spectral domain optical coherence tomography," *Opt. Exp.* **15**, 12636–12653 (2007).

[346] N. Sudheendran, S. H. Syed, M. E. Dickinson, I. V. Larina, and K. V. Larin, "Speckle variance OCT imaging of the vasculature in live mammalian embryos," *Laser Phys. Letts.* **8**, 247–252 (2011).

[347] R. K. Wang and L. An, "Doppler optical micro-angiography for volumetric imaging of vascular perfusion *in vivo*," *Opt. Exp.* **17**, 8926–8940 (2009).

[348] R. K. Wang, "Directional blood flow imaging in volumetric optical micro angiography achieved by digital frequency modulation," *Opt. Lett.* **33**, 1878–1880 (2008).

[349] Y. Jia, P. Li, and R. K. Wang, "Optical microangiography provides an ability to monitor responses of cerebral microcirculation to hypoxia and hyperoxia in mice," *J. Biomed. Opt.* **16**, (2011).

[350] Z. Zhi, W. Cepurna, E. Johnson, T. Shen, J. Morrison, and R. K. Wang, "Volumetric and quantitative imaging of retinal blood flow in rats with optical microangiography," *Biomed. Opt. Exp.* **2**, 579–591 (2011).

[351] R. K. Wang, L. An, P. Francis, and D. J. Wilson, "Depth-resolved imaging of capillary networks in retina and choroid using ultrahigh sensitive optical microangiography," *Opt. Lett.* **35**, 1467–1469 (2010).

[352] L. An, J. Qin, and R. K. Wang, "Ultrahigh sensitive optical microangiography for *in vivo* imaging of microcirculations within human skin tissue beds," *Opt. Exp.* **18**, 8220–8228 (2010).

[353] Z. Zhi, Y. Jung, Y. Jia, L. An, and R. K. Wang, "Highly sensitive imaging of renal microcirculation in vivo using ultrahigh sensitive optical microangiography," *Biomed. Opt. Exp.* **2**, 1059–1068 (2011).

[354] A. Mittag and A. Trnok, "Perspectives in Cytometry," in *Advanced Optical Flow Cytometry*, Valery V. Tuchin (ed.), Wiley–VCH, Weinheim, Germany (2011).

[355] V. S. Varga, L. Ficsor, V. Kamaras, V. Jonas, T. Virag, Z. Tulassay, and B. Molnar, "Automated multichannel fluorescent whole slide imaging and its application for cytometry," *Cytometry A* **75**, 1020–1030 (2009).

[356] L. A. Kamentsky, D. E. Burger, R. J. Gershman, L. D. Kamentsky, and E. Luther, "Slide-based laser scanning cytometry," *Acta Cytologica* **41**, 123–143 (1997).

[357] J. M. Hatfield and W. C. Hymer, "Flow cytometric analysis and sorting of live male-rat anterior-pituitary cell-types by forward angle and perpendicular light scatter," *Endocrinology* **119**, 2670–2682 (1986).

[358] S. Suzuki and N. Eguchi, "Leukocyte differential analysis in multiple laboratory species by a laser multi-angle polarized light scattering separation method," *Exper. Animals* **48**, 107–114 (1999).

[359] B. Rotman, "Measurement of activity of single molecules of Beta-D-Galactosidase," *Proc. Nat. Acad. Sci.* **47**, 1981 (1961).

[360] S. P. Perfetto, P. K. Chattopadhyay, and M. Roederer, "Innovation — Seventeen-colour flow cytometry: unravelling the immune system," *Nature Rev. Immunology* **4**, 648–645 (2004).

[361] X. Wang, S. Chen, M. Kong, Z. Wang, K. D. Costa, R. A. Li, and D. Sun, "Enhanced cell sorting and manipulation with combined optical tweezer and microfluidic chip technologies," *Lab on a Chip* **11**, 3656–3662 (2011).

[362] J. Enger, M. Goksor, K. Ramser, P. Hagberg, and D. Hanstorp, "Optical tweezers applied to a microfluidic system," *Lab on a Chip* **4**, 196–200 (2004).

[363] M. M. Wang, E. Tu, D. E. Raymond, J. M. Yang, H. C. Zhang, N. Hagen, B. Dees, E. M. Mercer, A. H. Forster, I. Kariv, P. J. Marchand, and W. F. Butler, "Microfluidic sorting of mammalian cells by optical force switching," *Nature Biotechnology* **23**, 83–87 (2005).

[364] C. Q. Yi, C. W. Li, S. L. Ji, and M. S. Yang, "Microfluidics technology for manipulation and analysis of biological cells," *Analytica Chimica Acta* **560**, 1–23 (2006).

[365] D. Wlodkowic and Z. Darzynkiewicz, "Rise of the Micromachines: Microfluidics and the Future of Cytometry," in *Methods in Cell Biology* **102**, 105–125 (2011).

[366] H. M. Davey and D. B. Kell, "Flow cytometry and cell sorting of heterogeneous microbial populations: The importance of single-cell analyses," *Microbiol. Rev.* **60**, 641 (1996).

[367] J. P. Rigaut and J. Vassy, "High-resolution three-dimensional images from confocal scanning laser microscopy quantitative study and mathematical correction of the effects from bleaching and fluorescence attenuation in depth," *Analyt. Quantit. Cytol. Histol.* **13**, 223–232 (1991).

[368] E. Bedner, L. T. Du, F. Traganos, and Z. Darzynkiewicz, "Caffeine dissociates complexes between DNA and intercalating dyes: Application for bleaching fluorochrome-stained cells for their subsequent restaining and analysis by laser scanning cytometry," *Cytometry* **43**, 38–45 (2001).

[369] R. M. P. Doornbos, B. G. deGrooth, and J. Greve, "Experimental and model investigations of bleaching and saturation of fluorescence in flow cytometry," *Cytometry* **29**, 204–214 (1997).

[370] T. Takada, M. Fujitsuka, and T. Majima, "Single-molecule observation of DNA charge transfer," *Proc. Nat. Acad. Sci.* **104**, 11179–11183 (2007).

[371] V. P. Zharov, E. I. Galanzha, and V. V. Tuchin, "Photothermal image flow cytometry *in vivo*," *Opt. Lett.* **30**, 628–630 (2005).

[372] V. P. Zharov, E. I. Galanzha, and V. V. Tuchin, "*In vivo* photothermal flow cytometry: Imaging and detection of individual cells in blood and lymph flow," *J. Cell. Biochem.* **97**, 916–932 (2006).

[373] G. Sitton and F. Srienc, "Growth dynamics of mammalian cells monitored with automated cell cycle staining and flow cytometry," *Cytometry A* **73**, 538–545 (2008).

[374] M. E. K. Calvert, J. A. Lannigan, and L. F. Pemberton, "Optimization of yeast cell cycle analysis and morphological characterization by multispectral imaging flow cytometry," *Cytometry A* **73**, 825–833 (2008).

[375] H. Lecoeur, "Nuclear apoptosis detection by flow cytometry: Influence of endogenous endonucleases," *Exper. Cell Res.* **277**, 1–14 (2002).

[376] N. Yasuda, S. Matzno, C. Iwano, M. Nishikata, and K. Matsuyama, "Evaluation of apoptosis and necrosis induced by statins using fluorescence-enhanced flow cytometry," *J. Pharm. Biomed. Analysis* **39**, 712–717 (2005).

[377] S. Yasuhara, Y. Zhu, T. Matsui, N. Tipirneni, Y. Yasuhara, M. Kaneki, A. Rosenzweig, and J. A. J. Martyn, "Comparison of comet assay, electron microscopy, and flow cytometry for detection of apoptosis," *J. Histochem. Cytochem.* **51**, 873–885 (2003).

[378] J. P. Nolan and L. Yang, "The flow of cytometry into systems biology," *Brief. Funct. Genom. Proteom.* **6**, 81–90 (2007).

[379] A. Castagnola, S. Eda, and J. L. Jurat-Fuentes, "Monitoring stem cell proliferation and differentiation in primary midgut cell cultures from Heliothis virescens larvae using flow cytometry," *Differentiation **81**, 192–198 (2011).*

[380] S. K. Koester, J. U. Maenpaa, V. J. Wiebe, W. J. Baker, G. T. Wurz, R. C. Seymour, R. E. Koehler, and M. W. Degregorio, "Flow-cytometry — Potential utility in monitoring drug effects in breast-cancer," *Breast Cancer Res. Treat.* **32**, 57–65 (1994).

[381] S. A. Morgan, J. V. Watson, P. R. Twentyman, and P. J. Smith, "Flow cytometric analysis of Hoechst-33342 uptake as an indicator of multi-drug resistance in human–lung cancer," *British J. Cancer* **60**, 282–287 (1989).

[382] V. P. Zharov, E. I. Galanzha, E. V. Shashkov, J.-W. Kim, N. G. Khlebtsov, and V. V. Tuchin, "Photoacoustic flow cytometry: principle and application for real-time detection of circulating single nanoparticles, pathogens, and contrast dyes *in vivo*," *J. Biomed. Opt.* **12**, (2007).

[383] K. Wang, K. Wang, W. Li, T. Huang, R. Li, D. Wang, B. Shen, and X. Chen, "Characterizing breast cancer xenograft epidermal growth factor receptor expression by using near-infrared optical imaging," *Acta Radiologica* **50**, 1095–1103 (2009).

[384] S. J. Simpson, M. Vachula, M. J. Kennedy, H. Kaizer, J. S. Coon, R. Ghalie, S. Williams, and D. Vanepps, "Detection of tumor-cells in the bone-marrow, peripheral-blood, and apheresis products of breast-cancer patients using flow-cytometry," *Exper. Hematol.* **23**, 1062–1068 (1995).

[385] E. Bergers, P. J. vanDiest, and J. P. A. Baak, "Tumour heterogeneity of DNA cell cycle variables in breast cancer measured by flow cytometry," *J. Clinic. Pathol.* **49**, 931–937 (1996).

[386] I. Brotherick, B. K. Shenton, M. Egan, W. E. Cunliffe, D. A. Browell, L. G. Lunt, J. R. Young, and M. J. Higgs, "Examination of multidrug resistance in cell lines and primary breast tumours by flow cytometry," *Europ. J. Cancer* **32**, 2334–2341 (1996).

[387] F. Villalobos-Chavez, E. Carrillo-Garcia, R. Morales-Camacho, E. Franco-Macias, J. Millan-Pascual, and J. J. Rodriguez-Uranga, "Infiltration of the meninges or brain by a non-Hodgkin's lymphoma, diagnosed by flow cytometry in cerebrospinal fluid," *Revista De Neurologia* **40**, 661–664 (2005).

[388] E. H. Park, "Small flow cytometry with a single optical system using fluorescence nanoparticles for HIV screening," *Abstr. Papers Am. Chem. Soc.* **239**, (2010).

[389] B. Gao, W.-g. Fu, Z.-h. Dong, Z.-d. Fang, Z.-j. Liu, Y. Si, X.-m. Zhang, and Y.-q. Wang, "Functional endothelial cells derived from embryonic stem cells labeled with HIV transactivator peptide-conjugated superparamagnetic nanoparticles," *Chinese Med. J.* **124**, 298–303 (2011).

[390] S. P. Morgan and I. M. Stockford, "Instrumentation for *in vivo* flow cytometry — a sickle cell anaemia case study," in *Advanced Optical Flow Cytometry*, Valery V. Tuchin (ed.), Wiley-VCH, Weinheim, Germany (2011).

[391] M. J. Rossow, W. W. Mantulin, and E. Gratton, "Scanning laser image correlation for measurement of flow," *J. Biomed. Opt.* **15**, (2010).

[392] J. D. Briers and A. F. Fercher, "Retinal blood-flow visualization by means of laser speckle photography," *Invest. Ophthal. Vis. Sci.* **22**, 255–259 (1982).

[393] B. Hebert, S. Costantino, and P. W. Wiseman, "Spatiotemporal image correlation spectroscopy (STICS) theory, verification, and application to protein velocity mapping in living CHO cells," *Biophys. J.* **88**, 3601–3614 (2005).

[394] B. Fagrell, A. Fronek, and M. Intaglietta, "Microscope-television system for studying flow velocity in human-skin capillaries," *Am. J. Physiol.* **233**, 318–321 (1977).

[395] A. Bollinger, P. Butti, J. P. Barras, H. Trachsle, and W. Siegenth, "Red blood-cell velocity in nailfold capillaries of man measured by a television microscopy technique," *Microvas. Res.* **7**, 61–72 (1974).

[396] J. D. Briers and A. F. Fercher, "Retinal blood-flow visualization by means of laser speckle photography," *Invest. Ophthal. Vis. Sci.* **22**, 255–259 (1982).

[397] H. H. Lipowsky, N. U. Sheikh, and D. M. Katz, "Intravital microscopy of capillary hemodynamics in sickle cell disease," *J. Clinic. Invest.* **80**, 117–127 (1987).

[398] B. Fagrell, "Advances in microcirculation network evaluation: An update," *Intern. J. Microcirc.* **15**, 34–40 (1995).

[399] K. Jambunathan, X. Y. Ju, B. N. Dobbins, and S. Ashforthfrost, "An improved cross-correlation technique for particle image velocimetry," *Measur. Sci. Technol.* **6**, 507–514 (1995).

[400] C. E. Willert and M. Gharib, "Digital particle image velocimetry," *Exp. Fluids* **10**, 181–193 (1991).

[401] J. Westerweel, "Fundamentals of digital particle image velocimetry," *Measur. Sci. Technol.* **8**, 1379–1392 (1997).

[402] C. Keveloh and W. Staude, "Determination of velocity-gradients with scattered-light cross-correlation measurements," *Appl. Opt.* **22**, 333–338 (1983).

[403] R. D. Keane and R. J. Adrian, "Theory of cross-correlation analysis of PIV images," *Appl. Sci. Res.* **49**, 191–215 (1992).

[404] X. T. Pan, H. Yu, X. K. Shi, V. Korzh, and T. Wohland, "Characterization of flow direction in microchannels and zebrafish blood vessels by scanning fluorescence correlation spectroscopy," *J. Biomed. Opt.* **12**, (2007).

[405] S. Jonas, D. Bhattacharya, M. K. Khokha, and M. A. Choma, "Microfluidic characterization of cilia-driven fluid flow using optical coherence tomography-based particle tracking velocimetry," *Biomed. Opt. Exp.* **2**, 2022–2034 (2011).

[406] A. Nakano, Y. Sugii, M. Minamiyama, J. Seki, and H. Niimi, "Velocity profiles of pulsatile blood flow in arterioles with bifurcation and confluence in rat mesentery measured by particle image velocimetry," *JSME Intern. J. Ser. C* **48**, 444–452 (2005).

[407] J. G. Santiago, S. T. Wereley, C. D. Meinhart, D. J. Beebe, and R. J. Adrian, "A particle image velocimetry system for microfluidics," *Exp. Fluids* **25**, 316–319 (1998).

[408] R. Lima, S. Wada, K. Tsubota, and T. Yamaguchi, "Confocal micro-PIV measurements of three-dimensional profiles of cell suspension flow in a square microchannel," *Measur. Sci. Technol.* **17**, 797–808 (2006).

[409] H. R. Zheng, L. L. Liu, L. Williams, J. R. Hertzberg, C. Lanning, and R. Shandas, "Real time multicomponent echo particle image velocimetry technique for opaque flow imaging," *Appl. Phys. Letts.* **88**, (2006).

[410] R. A. Jamison, S. Dubsky, K. K. W. Siu, K. Hourigan, and A. Fouras, "X-ray velocimetry and haemodynamic forces within a stenosed femoral model at physiological flow rates," *Ann. Biomed. Eng.* **39**, 1643–1653 (2011).

[411] M. A. Digman and E. Gratton, "Imaging barriers to diffusion by pair correlation functions," *Biophys. J.* **97**, 665–673 (2009).

[412] M. J. Rossow, W. W. Mantulin, and E. Gratton, "Scanning laser image correlation for measurement of flow," *J. Biomed. Opt.* **15**, (2010).

[413] B. Hebert, S. Costantino, and P. W. Wiseman, "Spatiotemporal image correlation spectroscopy (STICS) theory, verification, and application to protein velocity mapping in living CHO cells," *Biophys. J.* **88**, 3601–3614 (2005).

[414] S. A. Hall, D. M. Wood, E. Ibraim, and G. Viggiani, "Localised deformation patterning in 2D granular materials revealed by digital image correlation," *Granular Matter* **12**, 1–14 (2010).

[415] A. S. Forouhar, M. Liebling, A. Hickerson, A. Nasiraei-Moghaddam, H. J. Tsai, J. R. Hove, S. E. Fraser, M. E. Dickinson, and M. Gharib, "The embryonic vertebrate heart tube is a dynamic suction pump," *Science* **312**, 751–753 (2006).

[416] J. K. Barton and S. Stromski, "Flow measurement without phase information in optical coherence tomography images," *Opt. Exp.* **13**, 5234–5239 (2005).

[417] Y. Wang and R. K. Wang, "Autocorrelation optical coherence tomography for mapping transverse particle-flow velocity," *Opt. Lett.* **35**, 3538–3540 (2010).

[418] H. Asai, "Proposal of a simple method of fluorescence correlation spectroscopy for measuring the direction and magnitude of a flow of fluorophores," *Japan. J. Appl. Phys.* **19**, 2279–2282 (1980).

[419] Z. P. Chen, Y. H. Zhao, S. M. Srinivas, J. S. Nelson, N. Prakash, and R. D. Frostig, "Optical Doppler tomography," *IEEE J. Select. Top. Quant. Electr.* **5**, 1134–1142 (1999).

[420] Y. Wang and R. K. K. Wang, "Measurement of particle concentration in flow by statistical analyses of optical coherence tomography signals," *Opt. Lett.* **36**, 2143–2145 (2011).

[421] V. J. Srinivasan, S. Sakadzic, I. Gorczynska, S. Ruvinskaya, W. Wu, J. G. Fujimoto, and D. A. Boas, "Quantitative cerebral blood flow with optical coherence tomography," *Opt. Exp.* **18**, 2477–2494 (2010).

[422] J. Enfield, E. Jonathan, and M. J. Leahy, "*In vivo* imaging of the microcirculation of the volar forearm using correlation mapping optical coherence tomography (cmOCT)," *Biomed. Opt. Exp.* **2**, 1184–1193 (2011).

[423] Z. Y. Shen, M. Wang, Y. H. Ji, Y. H. He, X. S. Dai, P. Li, and H. Ma, "Transverse flow velocity quantification using optical coherence tomography with correlation," *Laser Phys. Lett.* **8**, 318–323 (2011).

[424] S. M. Daly, C. Silien, and M. J. Leahy, "Dual-beam optical coherence tomography system for quantification of flow velocity in capillary phantoms," *Proc. SPIE* **8222** (2012).

[425] V. J. Srinivasan, H. Radhakrishnan, E. H. Lo, E. T. Mandeville, J. Y. Jiang, S. Barry, and A. E. Cable, "OCT methods for capillary velocimetry," *Biomed. Opt. Exp.* **3**, 612–629 (2012).

[426] W. D. Bachalo, "Method for measuring the size and velocity of spheres by dual-beam light-scatter interferometry," *Appl. Opt.* **19**, 363–370 (1980).

[427] K. Q. Xia, Y. B. Xin, and P. Tong, "Dual-beam incoherent cross-correlation spectroscopy," *J.Opt. Soc. Am. A* **12**, 1571–1578 (1995).

[428] A. Baumgartner, C. K. Hitzenberger, E. Ergun, M. Stur, H. Sattmann, W. Drexler, and A. F. Fercher, "Resolution-improved dual-beam and standard optical coherence tomography: a comparison," *Graefes Arch. Clin. Exp. Ophthal.* **238**, 385–392 (2000).

[429] A. H. Bachmann, R. Michaely, T. Lasser, and R. A. Leitgeb, "Dual beam heterodyne Fourier domain optical coherence tomography," *Opt. Exp.* **15**, 9254–9266 (2007).

[430] N. V. Iftimia, D. X. Hammer, R. D. Ferguson, M. Mujat, D. Vu, and A. A. Ferrante, "Dual-beam fourier domain optical Doppler tomography of zebrafish," *Opt. Exp.* **16**, 13624–13636 (2008).

[431] F. Jaillon, S. Makita, E.-J. Min, B. H. Lee, and Y. Yasuno, "Enhanced imaging of choroidal vasculature by high-penetration and dual-velocity optical coherence angiography," *Biomed. Opt. Exp.* **2**, 1147–1158 (2011).

[432] S. Makita, M. Yamanari, M. Miura, and Y. Yasuno, "High-sensitive blood flow imaging of the retina and choroid by using double-beam optical coherence angiography," *Proc. SPIE* **7550** (2010).

[433] S. Zotter, M. Pircher, T. Torzicky, M. Bonesi, E. Götzinger, R. A. Leitgeb, and C. K. Hitzenberger, "Visualization of microvasculature by dual-beam phase-resolved Doppler optical coherence tomography," *Opt. Exp.* **19**, 1217–1227 (2011).

[434] Y. Imai and K. Iimura, "Velocity vector measurement based on correlation process between low coherence interference outputs," *Opt. Commun.* **271**, 219–223 (2006).

10

Optical Microangiography

Hrebesh M. Subhash

Division of Biomedical Engineering, School of Medicine, Oregon Health and Science University, 3303 SW Bond Ave, Portland, OR

Ruikang K. Wang

Biophotonics and Imaging Laboratory, Department of Bioengineering, University of Washington, Seattle, WA

Optical microangiography (OMAG) is a recently developed volumetric imaging technique based on coherence domain imaging modality, which is capable of producing 3-D images of dynamic blood perfusion within microcirculatory tissue beds *in vivo*. In this chapter, we will discuss its basic principle of operation, theoretical overview, extended functionalities, and its applications in various clinical and fundamental research fields. In addition, we will also review the principle of operation, latest technological developments and applications of ultra high sensitive OMAG, an extended version of OMAG for high sensitive imaging of very slow flow in capillary beds.

Key words: optical coherence tomography, Doppler effect, perfusion imaging, spectral domain interferometry

10.1 Introduction

The microcirculation plays a vital role in the pathophysiology of several disorders in many clinical areas including cardiology, dermatology, neurology, ophthalmology, etc. [1]. The primary function of microcirculation is referred to the process involved in the nutritive blood delivery to the tissue's capillary bed, which is vital for the homeostasis, and thereby the survival of an organ. Recent advances have highlighted the crucial involvement of the microcirculation in many basic research and clinical circumstances including cancer diagnosis and therapy, arteriosclerosis, therapeutic angiogenesis, vasopastic conditions, reconstructive surgery and also for the development and implementation of anti-vascular strategies. In clinical research, non-invasive imaging of microcirculation could be of great significance in assessing the efficacy of medical or surgical intervention in clinical trials, and in clinical practice it could be helpful to assist in the diagnosis and monitoring of disease progression or the result of therapy in individual patients. Numerous imaging techniques have been proposed in the last few decades to image microcirculation in medical research area, which vary widely according to the type of microcirculatory information that they can provide, including positron emission tomography (PET) [2], magnetic resonance imaging (MRI) [3], plethysmography [4,5] thermal [6] and radioisotope [7,8] clearance, orthogonal polarization spectral imaging [9,10], video-photometric capillaroscopy [11, 12] and Doppler ultrasound [13]. Some of these methods are limited with their imaging parameters such as spatial and temporal resolution, the ability to quantify blood flow and to obtain depth resolved information, and requirement of the injection of the contrast tracers; while others have practical limitations in clinical and basic research applications.

There has been a great deal of interests in developing non/minimally-invasive high resolution label free depth resolved imaging modality based on optical techniques for both clinical and fundamental studies. Because, in general, microvasculature imaging is a challenging task due to the requirement of relatively high spatiotemporal resolution and sensitivity to image small diameter of the blood vessels. Most of the available methods that fulfill these conditions are based on optical measurement technologies such as intravital confocal microscopy, laser Doppler technique, infrared thermography, optical intrinsic signal imaging, photo acoustic imaging and phase-resolved Doppler optical coherence tomography etc. Intravital confocal microscopy uses a fluorescence microscope to image various molecular and cellular processes *in vivo* with high resolution. However, intravital microscopy is a time consuming, invasive procedure, and the imaging depth is limited to a few hundred microns in highly scattering specimens [14, 15]. The laser Doppler technique uses the frequency shift produced by the Doppler effect to measure blood flow. This technique is capable of noninvasive and continuous recording of blood perfusion in tissue. A major limitation of laser Doppler technique is its inability to image tissue deeper than 1 mm [16, 17]. Moreover, laser Doppler is not able to measure flow in absolute units (i.e., ml/min), thus it often uses arbitrary unit of flux. Infrared thermography graphically depicts temperature gradients over a given body surface area. Generally, an increase in the blood flow can be related to a rise in temperature due to increased metabolic activity in the highly vascular region [18, 19]. This approach has lower sensitivity because a number of physiological changes involved with increased blood flow do not necessarily indicate pathology [18]. Infrared thermography is generally used in conjunction with other imaging techniques like laser Doppler technique and mammography [18]. Optical intrinsic signal imaging is another imaging modality with very high spatial and temporal resolution, but is limited to superficial two dimensional mapping and is invasive in nature [20]. Photoacoustic imaging (PAI), based on thermal-acoustic phenomena resulting from the strong light absorption of blood and the subsequent thermo-elastic expansion, has been reported to map vascular structures deep within the brain of small animals [21, 22]. However, the spatial ($\sim 100\ \mu$m) resolution of this approach is limited by the viscoelastic filtering of higher acoustic frequencies by the tissue.

Optical coherence tomography (OCT) [23–25] is a novel, non-invasive, optical imaging modality based on low coherence interferometry. OCT enables the non-invasive, non-contact imaging of cross-sectional structures in biological tissues and materials with high resolution. The technology has already made revolutionary impact in many clinical and fundamental research areas. In principle, OCT is an optical analogue to clinical ultrasound. In OCT, the temporally gated optical pulse remitted from scattering sites within the sample is localized by low-coherence interferometry (LCI) [26–28]. This is typically achieved with a Michelson interferometer, the coherence-gated information about the elementary volume of the scatters within the obscuring scattering specimen can be obtained from either the time domain measurement (TD-OCT) or the frequency domain (FD-OCT) [29, 30] measurement. As a variant coherence domain variant, FD-OCT has been widely attracted in the biomedical imaging fields due to its higher sensitivity and imaging speed compared to the conventional TD-OCT.

Soon after the invention of OCT, there was a great interest in the development of various hardware and software modules for extending the functionality of OCT for measuring functional and physical parameters such as polarization sensitive [31], spectroscopy [32], elastography [33] etc. Of these, one of the most significant and physiologically relevant functionality is to measure and quantify the blood flow within tissue microstructures. This functional extension of OCT is widely known as Doppler OCT (D-OCT) [34–37]. Since its first demonstrations in the mid-1990s, several research groups have worked intensely on extending the capabilities of D-OCT for various clinical and fundamental research applications. Most of these developments have utilized the time-domain OCT methods; very recently, both spectral and frequency domain OCT approaches have been adopted for D-OCT imaging as well [38–42]. Among them optical micronagiography (OMAG) is a very promising method for high-resolution imaging of microvascular flow within tissue beds with high flow sensitivity [43–45]. The basic principle behind OMAG is based on FDOCT. In OMAG, the imaging contrast of blood perfusion is based on the endogenous light scattering from the moving blood erythrocytes in the blood vessels; thus no exogenous contrasting agents are necessary. This is achieved by efficient separation of the moving scattering elements from the static scattering ones within tissue through the OMAG hardware associated with mathematical analysis of the optical scattering signals emerged from an illuminated tissue sample.

In the following sections, we will describe the basic principles and different configurations of OMAG in detail. We will also describe several clinical applications of OMAG, which have been demonstrated in our laboratory, such as mapping cortical microvascular perfusion for brain research, ocular flow imaging for ophthalmic applications, microcirculation within the human skin for dermatological application, and microcirculation imaging of cochlea in a mouse model,

10.2 Optical Microangiography (OMAG)

As described in the earlier section, optical micro-angiography (OMAG) is a functional extension to the FD-OCT imaging modality, which uses the spectral domain configuration capable of resolving 3D distribution of dynamic blood perfusion at the capillary level within microcirculatory beds *in vivo*. The key difference between OMAG and FD-OCT is that in OMAG the interferogram in the lateral direction (B-scan) is spatially modulated with a carrier frequency, which can separate the moving and static scattering components within a sample. This carrier modulation frequency can be introduced either by mounting the reference mirror in the reference arm onto a linear piezo-translation stage, that moves the mirror at a constant velocity across the B scan (i.e. x-direction scan) or an off-pivot scanning beam. In the earlier version of OMAG system [43–44], this is achieved by mounting the reference mirror in the reference arm onto a linear piezo-translation stage that moved the mirror at a constant velocity across the B scan (i.e. x direction scan). However, the latest version of OMAG utilizes the spatial modulation frequency provided by the inherent blood flow modulation rather than reference arm modulation [45].

10.2.1 Theoretical aspect of OMAG

The OMAG algorithm is based on rigorous mathematical analysis of the optical spectral domain interferograms, which were captured by the well-defined scanning protocol of OMAG hardware implemented with an FD-OCT system. In the earlier generation of OMAG, in order to extract microvascular imaging, the moving and static scatters were separated by introducing a carrier frequency to the captured interferogram. This carrier frequency is generated by adding a phase delay to each A-scan using a moving reference arm or an off-pivot scanning beam. However, these techniques rely on precise synchronization of reference arm modulation and B-scan acquisition, which require expensive or cumbersome modulators, and are unable to detect bidirectional flow in a single B-scan. In order to overcome this drawback, a modified Hilbert transform without the use of spatial frequency modulation is introduced in the OMAG. No frequency modulations are required and a novel OMAG signal processing algorithm based on a modified Hilbert transform is applied to the spatial frequency content across a single B-scan to obtain volumetric perfusion map with directional information. The latest version of OMAG is applicable for both spectrometer-based and swept-source OCT systems. Unlike the earlier version of OMAG [44, 46], which require two separate B-scans to detect positive and negative flow, each with modulations tuned to the desired flow direction, the second generation of OMAG is able to resolve bidirectional flow in a single B-scan pass across the sample. As described in the earlier section, in the first generation of OMAG the static and moving scatters were separated by modulating the reference arm with a modulation frequency. The following section explains the theory behind the working principle of OMAG and its theoretical aspect.

If we consider the spectral domain interferogram which is formed between the light backscattered from the sample and reflected from the mirror at each lateral (x-direction) positions captured by a spectrometer at each wavelength λ can be expressed as a function of two time variables t_1 and t_2 as shown below [47]:

$$B(t_1,t_2) = \cos(2\pi f_0 t_1 + 2\pi(f_M - f_D)t_2 + \varphi) \tag{10.1}$$

where f_0, f_M, and f_D are the frequency components, respectively and ϕ is a random phase term. In connection with the discussion below, we here assume that f_0 and f_M are two modulation frequency components whereas f_D is the Doppler frequency component. We also assume that there is no correlation between t_1 and t_2, and when t_1 varies t_2 is constant and vice versa.

In practice, at each scanning position, the interference spectrum is discretized by N segments, corresponding to the number of pixels in the camera of the SD-OCT system. For each one B-scan, the object is sampled by M times in the x direction, which will produce a data matrix with a size of (N,M). If we consider the OMAG imaging of blood flow within the microcirculation tissue beds, under a B-scanning condition, the static scatters and the moving scatters are illustrated in Fig. 10.1 (a). The depth-encoded spectral interferogram captured by the linear detector is a real function, $B(z,t)$ and can be written as:

$$B(z,t) = A(z)\cos(k_0 z) \tag{10.2}$$

where $A(z)$ is the reflective coefficient of the scatter; k_0 is the wave vector of the detected light; z relates to the detecting depth. In order to simplify the problem, we do not consider the random phase arising from the refractive index float and assume the reflective coefficient $A(z)$ of the scatter is a constant along the B-scan direction, t is the B-scan time, corresponding to the different lateral position.

According to Eq. (10.2), if we consider the non-moving scatters at a depth z, as shown in Figs. 10.1 (a) and (b), the signal $B(z,t)$ do not vary with the B-scan time t. So the corresponding signal can be viewed as a rectangular function, i.e., $\mathrm{rect}(t/\tau_0) = F(t-\tau_0/2) - F(t+\tau_0/2)$, as shown in Fig. 10.2(a). On the other hand, for the moving scatter, the signal is a rectangular enveloped cosine signal i.e. $\mathrm{rect}(t/\tau_0)_{\cos} = \cos(2\pi u_0 t)F(t-\tau_0/2) - F(t+\tau_0/2)$ which is illustrated in Fig. 10.2(c), where u_0 is the modulation frequency generated by the flow speed.

If we consider the above assumption, according to Figs. 10.1(b) and (c), the total time required for a single B-scan is T_0, and which corresponds to a total of N_0 A-lines in a B-scan frame. The scanning time for the scatter (moving or static), τ_0, depends upon the number of A-lines in the B-frame, n_0, to image the structure, and which corresponds to the physical dimension of the imaged structure within a B-scan frame, and t_0 is the B-scan time required at the center of the scattering structure as illustrated in Fig. 10.1(c). According to the above parameters, the Fourier transform $R(z,u)$ of the lateral dimension (i.e., B-scan at time t) can be expressed as:

$$R(z,u) = \frac{A(z)\cos(k_0 z)}{T_0}\int_{t_0-\frac{\tau_0}{2}}^{t_0-\frac{\tau_0}{2}} e^{-i2\pi u t}\,dt \tag{10.3}$$

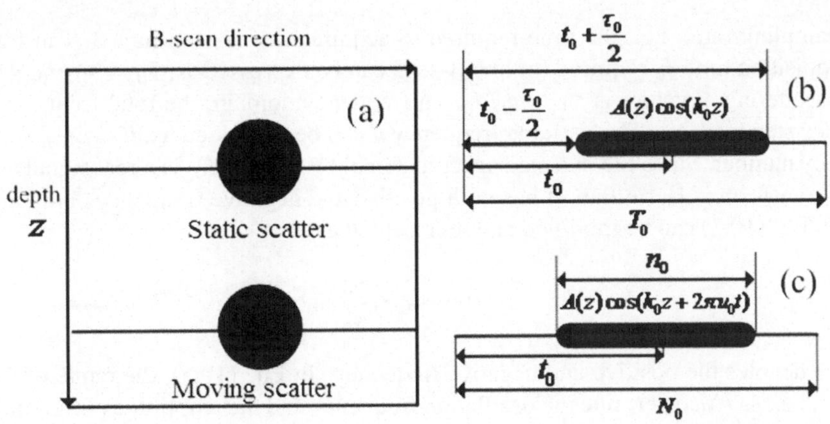

Figure 10.1: Schematic of moving and no-moving scattering structure under B-scan condition in SD-OCT.

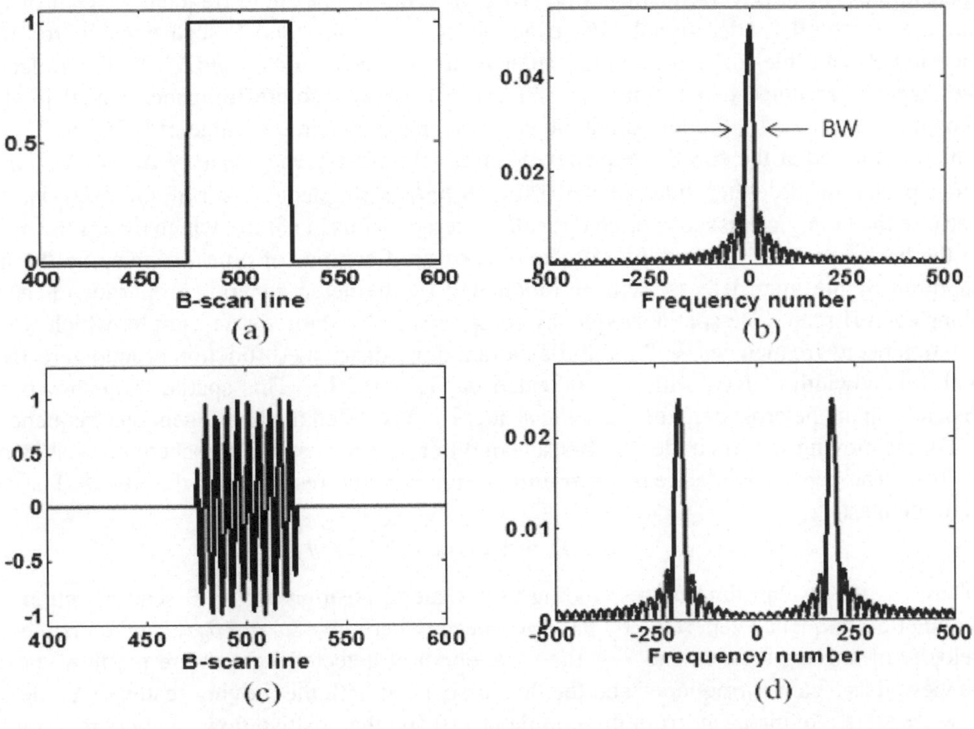

Figure 10.2: Comparison of structural signal and flow signal (a) the structural signal; (b) the absolute FFT of the structural signal; (c) the flow signal; (d) the absolute FFT of the flow signal.

where u is the Fourier transform frequency of B-scan at time t. This corresponds to the spatial frequency along the B-scan direction. After simplification, the result of Eq. (10.3) can be presented as:

$$R(z,u) = A(z)\cos(k_0 z)\frac{\sin(\pi u \tau_0)}{\pi u T_0}e^{-i2\pi u t_0} \tag{10.4}$$

If we consider the OMAG spectral detection section, the acquisition time of the linear detector is

$1/f_0$ (sampling rate), i.e., the time required to acquire each A-scan in a B-scan frame. Then the total acquisition time T_0 required for one B-scan can be expressed as: $T_0 = N_0/f_0$. The B-scan time for the scattering structure is $\tau_0 = n_0/f_0$. In frequency domain, the total frequency is f_0 and the frequency step isf_0/N_0. The variable frequency u can be expressed as, $u = nf_0/N_0$, where n is the frequency number. Since the detected spectral signal by the camera is a real signal and therefore its Fourier transform is Hermitian, it has both positive and negative frequency components. Then the equation Eq. (10.3) can be modified and represented as:

$$R_{\pm}(z,n) = A(z)\cos(k_0 z)\frac{n_0}{N_0}\text{sinc}(\frac{n_0 n}{N_0})e^{-i2\pi n t_0 \frac{f_0}{N_0}} \tag{10.5}$$

where $\pm$ denotes the positive and negative frequency. In Eq. (10.5), the range of the non-moving scatterer, i.e., n_0/N_0 determine the oscillation frequency and the amplitude of the sinc function. The depth encoded information is retained in $\cos(k_0 z)$, which is independent of the Fourier transform along the B-scan direction. Due to the Hermitian symmetry of Fourier transform, the frequency ranges from $-f_0/2$ to$f_0/2$, accordingly the frequency number n ranges from $-N_0/2$ to $N_0/2$, with the max value of sinc function $\text{sinc}(x)$ centered at $n = 0$, this means that the main signal energy concentrates at the zero frequency. Fig. 10.2(a) shows the absolute frequency signal of the non-moving structural (static) signal. For example, if we set the total B-scan lines N_0 to 1000, and the total B-scan lines of non-moving scatter n_0 to 50 (between 475 and 525). The reflectivity of the signal is assumed to be unity, i.e. $B(z,t) = 1$. The absolute frequency signal $|R_{\pm}(z,n)|$ is shown in Fig. 10.2(b), the amplitude of $|R_{\pm}(z,n)|$ has a maximum value of 0.05 ($n_0/N_0 = 0.05$), which is located at the zeroth frequency position with a frequency span of $\Delta n = 2N_0/n_0$ and the other peaks on the either sides of the 0th peak have a frequency span of $\Delta n = N_0/n_0$. This is because the biological tissue is often optically heterogeneous in nature, which means the magnitude of the backscattered light and the refractive index are functions of time variable. So the intensity captured by the liner detector will be modulated by the heterogeneous properties of the sample along each B-scan. The spatial frequency components of a static tissue sample, which we call the heterogeneous frequencies, will exhibit as a randomly distributed function around zero frequency with a bandwidth of BW, which is indicated in Fig. 10.2(b). This spatial frequency bandwidth depends on the heterogeneity of the static scatters and is called the heterogeneous frequency.

For the moving scatters under the B-scan condition, the corresponding schematic is shown in Fig. 10.1(c). The depth-encoded real spectral interference signal recorded by the SD-OCT system can be written as:

$$B(z,t) = A(z)\cos(k_0 z + 2\pi ut) \tag{10.6}$$

where t is the B-scan time corresponding to the lateral position across B-scan direction, u is the modulation frequency generated by the flow speed, where $u = 2u_0\cos\theta_d/\lambda$ and u_0 is the absolute velocity of moving scatters and λ is the wavelength of detected light. Here the flow speed u can be viewed as a carrier frequency and the flow associated with the moving scatters include negative flow (scatters moving away from the sample beam) and the positive flow (scatters moving forward to the sample beam). Then the Fourier transform of the spectral signal $B(z,t)$ can be expressed as:

$$H(z,u) = \frac{A(z)}{T_0}\int_{t_0-\frac{\tau_0}{2}}^{t_0+\frac{\tau_0}{2}} \cos(k_0 z + 2\pi ut)e^{-i2\pi u_0 t}dt$$

$$= \frac{A(z)e^{ik_0 z}}{2T_0}\int_{t_0-\frac{\tau_0}{2}}^{t_0+\frac{\tau_0}{2}} e^{-i2\pi(u-u_0)t}dt + \frac{A(z)e^{-ik_0 z}}{2T_0}\int_{t_0-\frac{\tau_0}{2}}^{t_0+\frac{\tau_0}{2}} e^{-i2\pi(u+u_0)t}dt \tag{10.7}$$

This equation includes positive and negative frequency components:

$$H(z,u) = H_{+}(z,u) + H_{-}(z,u) \tag{10.8}$$

where $H_+(z,u)$ is the positive frequency and $H_-(z,u)$ is the negative frequency. Then Eq. (10.7) can be split up as:

$$H_+(z,u) = \frac{A(z)e^{ik_0z}}{2T_0}\frac{\sin[\pi\tau_0(u-u_0)]}{\pi(u-u_0)}e^{-i2\pi(u-u_0)t_0} \tag{10.9}$$

$$H_-(z,u) = \frac{A(z)e^{-ik_0z}}{2T_0}\frac{\sin[\pi\tau_0(u+u_0)]}{\pi(u+u_0)}e^{-i2\pi(u+u_0)t_0} \tag{10.10}$$

According to the assumption described in section 10.2.1, Eq. (10.8) can also be expressed as:

$$H_+(z,n) = A(z)e^{ik_0z}\frac{n_0}{2N_0}\mathrm{sinc}(\frac{n_0}{N_0}(n-\frac{u_0N_0}{f_0}))e^{-i2\pi(\frac{nf_0}{N_0}-u_0)t_0} \tag{10.11}$$

$$H_-(z,n) = A(z)e^{-ik_0z}\frac{n_0}{2N_0}\mathrm{sinc}(\frac{n_0}{N_0}(n+\frac{u_0N_0}{f_0}))e^{-i2\pi(\frac{nf_0}{N_0}+u_0)t_0} \tag{10.12}$$

If we consider Eq. (10.9), (10.10), (10.11), and (10.12) with Eq. (10.4) and Eq. (10.5), the non-moving scatters are centered around the 0th frequency (DC) region (heterogeneous frequency) and the moving scatters are shifted away from the 0th frequency $n = 0$ to $n = \pm u_0N_0/f_0$. This shifting distance in the frequency domain can be directly related to the velocity u_0 of the moving scatters, total B-scan lines, N_0, and the acquisition rate of CCD, f_0. Since the max frequency number is $n_{\max} = \pm N_0/2$, the maximum detectable velocity with OMAG is $v_{\max} = \pm\lambda f_0/4$, which is the same with that of the Doppler OCT. Figs. 10.2(c) and (d) illustrate a simulated signal for the moving scatter and corresponding frequency shift for the signal in the frequency domain, respectively. The two shifted sinc function peaks in Fig. 10.2(d) corresponds to Eq. (10.9) and (10.10). The simulated illustrations, shown in Figs. 10.2(c) and (d), clearly show how the OMAG separates the moving scatters from non-moving scatters by flow speed modulation.

A schematic of the OMAG signal processing flow chart is illustrated in Fig. 10.3. Fig. 10.3(a) shows a B-scan frame, which includes the static and moving scatters. According to Eqs. (10.2) and (10.6), if we consider the non-moving scatters at a depth z, the signal $B(z,t)$ does not vary with the B-scan time t. Therefore, the corresponding signal can be viewed as a rectangular function. Whereas, for the moving scatters, the signal under B-scan condition is a rectangular envelope cosine signal, which is shown in Fig. 10.3(a). By applying a Fourier transformation along the B-scan direction, the spatial frequency components of a static tissue sample, which we call the heterogeneous frequencies, will exhibit as a randomly distributed function around zero frequency with a bandwidth of BW, which is indicated in Fig. 10.3(b). On the other hand, the moving scatters produce a frequency shift, which is caused by the Doppler effect of the moving particles and shifts it away from the heterogeneous frequencies due to static scatters. Next, for extracting the flow information the structural signal is filtered out in the frequency domain. This was accomplished by introducing the modified Hilbert transform algorithm. To achieve this, one of the conjugate terms was windowed out and the heterogeneous frequency centered around the 0th frequency region (DC) using a frequency shifted Heaviside function. The cut-off frequency shift of the Heaviside function depends upon the heterogeneity of the static scatters. Then, an inverse Fourier transform is applied, the inverse Fourier transform has positive and negative frequency. After inverse transforming from frequency domain, and then applying the conventional spectral Fourier transform along the depth direction, the strength of the flow signal will be retrieved. This is illustrated in Figs. 10.3(c) and (d). For the flow signal, the inverse Fourier transform (iFFT) has positive and negative frequency, which retrieves the directional flow information and can be expressed as:

$$\mathrm{iFFT}(H_+(z,n)) = \frac{A(z)e^{i(k_0z+2\pi u_0t)}}{2} \tag{10.13}$$

$$\mathrm{iFFT}(H_-(z,n)) = \frac{A(z)e^{-i(k_0z+2\pi u_0t)}}{2} \tag{10.14}$$

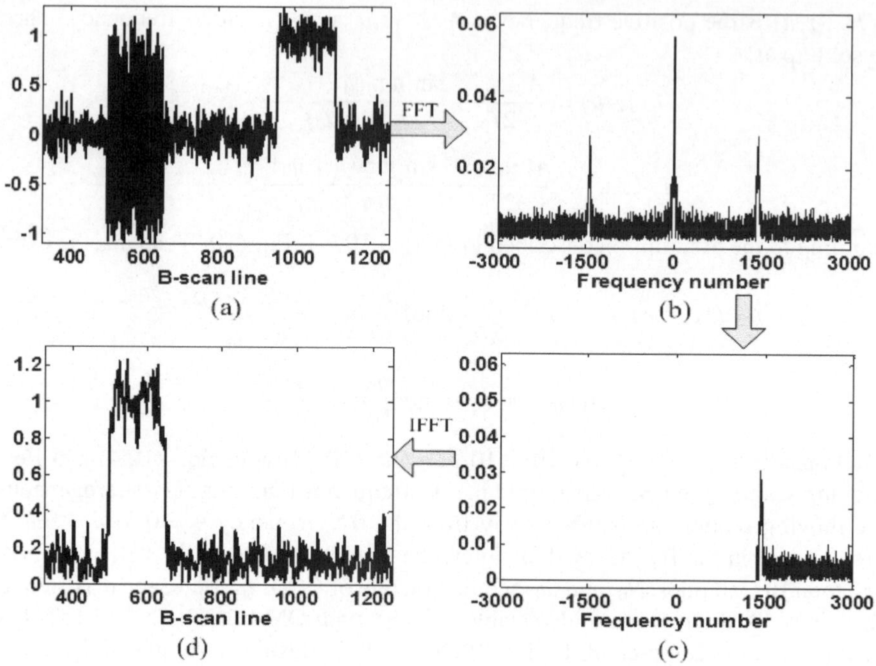

Figure 10.3: The flow chart of signal processing steps in OMAG (a) the flow signal and structural signal; (b) the flow signal and structural signal in the frequency domain; (c) filter the structural signal and negative frequency of the flow signal; (d) the flow signal inverting from the frequency domain.

Figure 10.3(d) shows the inverse Fourier transformed signal. The absolute amplitude of the flow signal obtained by taking the Fourier transform can be expressed as:

$$A(z) = 2\left|\text{iFFT}[H(z,n)]\right| \tag{10.15}$$

From Eq. (10.15) it is evident that the imaging contrast is a result that represents the optical reflectance scattered from the flow particles, and it does not relate to the flow velocity. The amplitude of the flow signal $A(z)$ can be used to reconstruct the flow, just like that in the conventional OCT.

10.2.2 Extended imaging capabilities of OMAG

In this section we explain the extended imaging features such as directional flow imaging, Doppler flow imaging and motion compensation implemented with OMAG.

10.2.2.1 Directional flow imaging

Based on the above signal processing, the real flow signal is transformed to an analytical signal by Hilbert transform, which enables the bidirectional flow configuration, i.e., the positive flow and the negative flow to be separated in different imaging plane. Fig. 10.4 shows the Hilbert transformed analytical flow signal, which is obtained by filtering out the negative frequency components and the structural signals, and then taking the inverse Fourier transform as shown below [46]:

$$\text{iFFT}[H(z,n)] = \frac{A(z)e^{ik_0 z}}{2}(\cos(2\pi|u_0|t) \pm i\sin(2\pi|u_0|t) \tag{10.16}$$

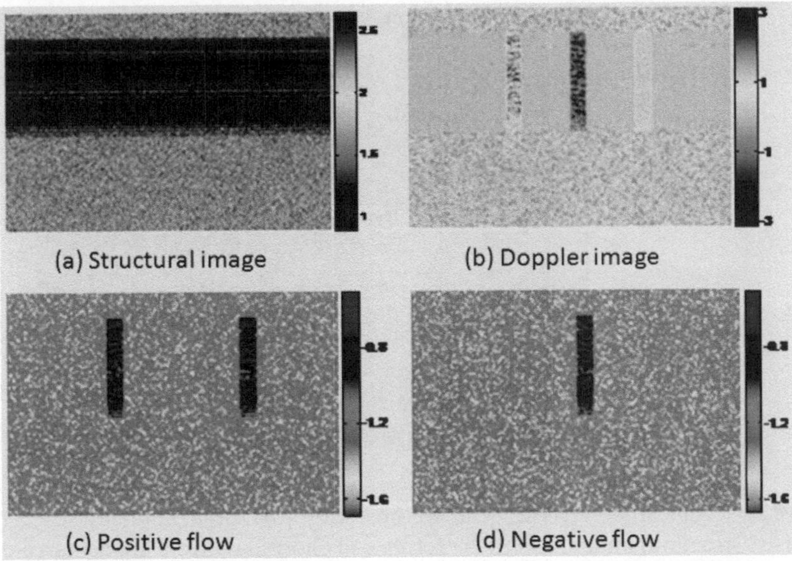

Figure 10.4: (See color insert.) Bidirectional image with OMAG: (a) the structure image, (b) the Doppler image, the left $v_0 = 7.5$ mm/s (red color), the middle $v_1 = -7.5$ mm/s (blue color); the right $v_2 = 4.5$ mm/s (orange color); (c) the positive flow image; (d) the negative flow image.

where u_0 is the modulation frequency, and which relates to the flow direction. If $u_0 > 0$, the Fourier transformation along the depth direction resolves the positive flow components in the positive image plane and if $u_0 < 0$, the negative flow components in the negative imaging plane.

The sample movement during *in vivo* imaging conditions is an inevitable artifact in OMAG (in OCT in general), and is particularly dominant for imaging of the human eye or skin. The relative sample motion represents as a Doppler shift in the light frequency between the light it emits and that it receives. This shift is imparted when the light strikes an object which is moving, relative to the probe. For the OMAG system, the Doppler frequency due to the sample motion is depicted as an additional modulation frequency, f_0, in the interferogram.

As an example to illustrate the effect of subject motion on the OMAG results, Fig. 10.5 shows a typical *in vivo* B scan of the posterior part of the human eye from a volunteer. Fig. 10.5(A) is the conventional OCT image, where the important physiological layers, such as the retina and choroids, can be delineated. Fig. 10.5(B) is the corresponding OMAG flow image where it can be seen that although the blood flow signals from retinal and choroidal layers are evident, the subject movement deteriorates the blood flow image, particularly in the right part of the image. Further analysis from Fig. 10.5(B) implies that the motion is not uniform, even during one single B-scan (within 50 milliseconds). This non-uniform subject movement can also be seen in the phase-resolved DOCT (PRDOCT) image as shown in Figs. 10.5(C) and 10.6(D).

A casual inspection of Fig. 10.5 shows that the blood flow imaging is better delivered by OMAG than that by PRDOCT, because the blood flow signals as seen in the choroidal layer in Fig. 10.5(B) are not seen in PRDOCT images (Figs. 10.5 (C) and (D)), as illustrated by the arrows. However, still, the subject movement artifacts are present. Thus, for *in vivo* OMAG imaging of human eye, a solution to the bulk motion artifacts is required so that the quality of OMAG blood flow image is improved. Because OMAG imaging has its origin in FD-OCT, the OCT signals can be directly calculated from the captured interferograms for sequential A-scans using conventional FD-OCT algorithms. It is known that the OCT signal so computed is a complex function, $\tilde{B}_{OCT}(t,z)$, which

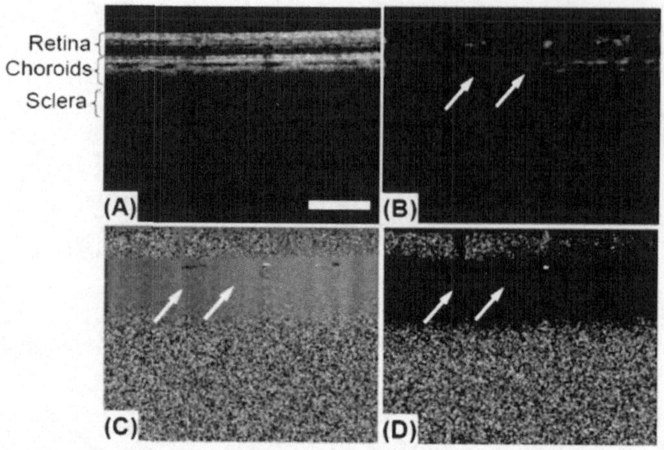

Figure 10.5: Typical in vivo B scan of posterior part of a human eye. (A) Conventional OCT/OMAG structural image, where the retina and choroidal layers are demarcated; and the corresponding (B) OMAG flow image, (C) PRDOCT image with gray levels coded from $-\pi$ (black) to π (white) and (D) Power Doppler OCT image. Scale bar = 500 μm. Images are reproduced from [67].

can be written as:

$$\tilde{B}_{\mathrm{OCT}}(t,z) = A(t,z)\exp[i\phi(t,z)] \tag{10.17}$$

where $A(t,z)$ and $\varphi(t,z)$ are the amplitude and the phase of $\tilde{B}_{OCT}(t,z)$, respectively. t is the timing when the probe beam proceeds in the B scan, and z represents the coordinate along the imaging depth. In our OMAG system, the phase term $\varphi(t,z)$ can be expressed by the following equation:

$$\phi(t,z) = \phi_P(t,z) + \phi_B(t,z) + \phi_M(t,z) \tag{10.18}$$

where $\phi_P(t,z)$ is the phase term caused by the moving red blood cells; $\phi_B(t,z)$ is the phase term caused by the subject movement; $\phi_M(t,z)$ is the phase term caused by the modulation frequency, f_M. Following PRDOCT [48, 49], the phase differences between the i-th and $(i-1)$-th A-lines can be written as:

$$\phi^i(t,z) = \Delta\phi_P^i(t,z) + \Delta\phi_B^i(t,z) + \Delta\phi_M^i(t,z) \tag{10.19}$$

where $\Delta\phi_P^i(t,z)$ and $\Delta\phi_B^i(t,z)$ are the phase changes caused by the moving particle and the subject movement between the i-th and $(i-1)$-th A-lines, respectively. Because in OMAG system the introduced modulation frequency, f_M, is constant during imaging, $\Delta\phi_M^i(t,z)$ is a constant value which is known *a priori*, i.e.:

$$\Delta\phi_M^i(t,z) = 2\pi f_M T \tag{10.20}$$

where T is the time interval between adjacent A-lines. This phase term can be directly subtracted from Eq. (10.18). Thus, the phase term directly related to the movement, $\Delta\phi_m^i(t,z)$ is:

$$\Delta\phi_m^i(t,z) = \Delta\phi_P^i(t,z) + \Delta\phi_B^i(t,z). \tag{10.21}$$

In Eq. (10.21), the variable t is the timing of the probe beam proceeding in a B scan, that corresponds to the position of the probe beam, x. Thus Eq. (10.19) can be replaced by:

$$\Delta\phi_m^i(x,z) = \Delta\phi_P^i(x,z) + \Delta\phi_B^i(x,z) \tag{10.22}$$

Because the OMAG system usually has an imaging speed of more than 20,000 A scans per second, it is reasonable to assume that the subject is static within a single A scan. Under this condition, Eq.

(10.22) represents the bulk motion of subject between adjacent A scans, plus the phase changes due to the blood flow if presented. Usually, within a single B scan, the regions occupied by the blood vessels are much smaller than the areas occupied by the surrounding tissue. Thus, the phase change between i-th and $(i-1)$-th A-scans caused by the bulk motion could be approximated by averaging all the phase differences along the A-scan to minimize the errors brought by the system noise and flow signals [50,51].

$$\mathrm{D}f_m^i(x) = \frac{1}{z}\sum f_m^i(x,z)dz \tag{10.23}$$

Here $\Delta\phi_m^i(x)$ is the bulk motion corresponding to the phase difference between i-th and $(i-1)$-th A-scans. Therefore, with reference to the first A scan in the B scan, the phases at the i-th A-line caused by the bulk subject motion, $\phi_m^i(x)$, can be obtained by a recursive function:

$$\phi_m^1(0) = 0, \quad \phi_m^i(x) = \phi_m^{i-1}(x) + \Delta\phi_m^i(x), \quad i = 2,3,......N \tag{10.24}$$

where N is the number of A scans that consists of the B scan. Thus far, the phase changes along the B scan due to the bulk tissue motion, $\phi_B^i(x,z)$, have been computed. Subtract Eq. (10.24) from Eq. (10.18), and then insert into Eq. (10.17), we have:

$$\tilde{B}'_{\mathrm{OCT}}(x,z) = A(x,z)\exp[i(\phi_P(x,z) + \phi_M(x,z))] \tag{10.25}$$

where the frequency modulation term due to the bulk tissue motion is eliminated. Subsequently, the spectral interferograms without the tissue motion effect can be obtained via an inverse FFT to Eq. (10.25):

$$b(x,\lambda) = \mathrm{FFT}^{-1}\left[\tilde{B}'(x,z)\right] \tag{10.26}$$

Finally, the conventional OMAG algorithm as detailed in the last section is applied to Eq. (10.26) to obtain the OMAG flow image that would be ideally free of motion artifacts. In Eq. (10.23), the phase due to the bulk tissue motion is estimated by the averaged value of phase changes along the A scan. However, the phases are random for the OCT signals that fall below the system noise floor. This will have a dramatic effect on the estimation of bulk tissue motion. To reduce this effect, we often use the OCT structural image to segment the regions of interest, $R(x,z)$, within which the OCT signals are 15 dB above the system noise level. Only the phases within the region of interest are calculated. Below, we detail the steps to perform the segmentation to find $R(x,z)$.

First, the SD-OCT structural image is used to segment the regions of interest that represent retina and choroids. Two boundaries are determined. One corresponds to the vitreo-retinal interface, i.e., anterior boundary, and the other to the deepest penetration points, posterior boundary. The anterior boundary is obtained by using an algorithm which is similar to that described by Mujat et al. [53]. A Gaussian filter with a standard deviation of 4×4 pixels is used to blur the cross-sectional image (B scan) obtained previously. Then the edge of the image is obtained by calculating the gradient of the blurred structural image. It is then converted to a binary image by setting a threshold. The first nonzero points of the binary image, represented by a curve, are detected, and the speckle noises are eliminated. The anterior boundary is then obtained by fitting and smoothing this curve.

The posterior boundary is obtained by setting a threshold to the blurred retina structural image, which is equal to the noise floor of the image obtained. The intensity is treated as the signal if it is larger than the threshold and set it to unity; on the other hand, it is treated as noise if it is smaller than the threshold and is set to zero. Using this method, the structure image is converted to a binary image. The posterior boundary is obtained by the last nonzero points after the isolated speckle noises are eliminated. The final posterior boundary is then obtained by a fitting and smoothing procedure. Finally, the region of region $R(x,z)$ is obtained by bounding the anterior and posterior boundaries as described above. The phase estimation in Eq. (10.23) is therefore performed within this region of interest:

$$\Delta\phi_m^i(x) \approx \frac{1}{z}\int \Delta\phi_m^i(x,z)dz; \quad z \in R(x,z). \tag{10.27}$$

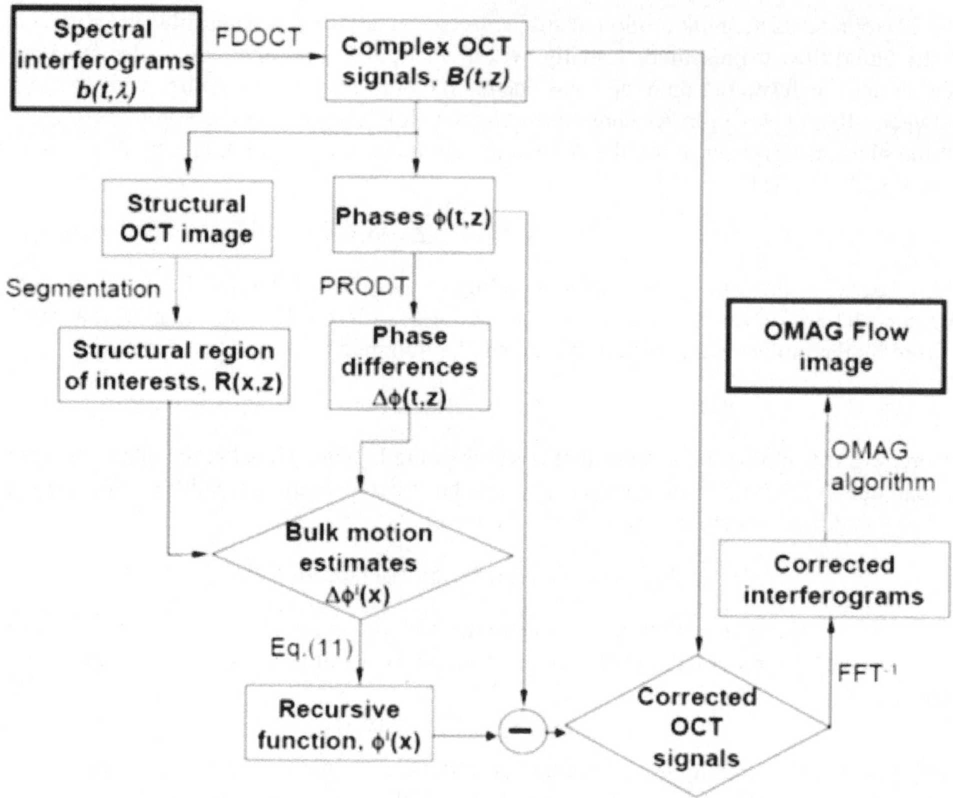

Figure 10.6: Flow chart detailing the steps to computationally compensate the bulk tissue motion artifacts in OMAG imaging of blood perfusion in retina and choroids. Image is reproduced from [52].

To further improve the accuracy of the phase estimation, the phases in Eq. (10.27) are only calculated for the OCT signals that are stronger than a preset threshold, which is 15 dB above the system noise floor. Figure 10.6 illustrates the flow chart of the operations that are used to calculate the final OMAG flow images with the subject motion artifacts minimized.

This motion compensation algorithm is described by using retinal imaging as an example. The algorithm is however applicable to other cases where the biological tissues other than retina are concerned. However, the steps for treating the motion compensation would need to be considered according to the specific tissue types and the motion characteristics.

10.2.2.2 Doppler OMAG

The key advantage of OMAG is that only the signals backscattered by the moving blood appear in the OMAG flow output plane, this makes the blood flow imaging almost free of artifact induced noise. However, the OMAG is incapable of providing flow velocity information. This is because in the OMAG flow image, the regions that are occupied by the microstructural signals are rejected by OMAG, thus the required correlation between the adjacent A-scans within the static tissue regions are totally lost, leading to a rather noisy appearance in the output plane of flow velocity. To overcome this problem, a useful method is recently proposed to digitally reconstruct an ideal static background tissue that is totally optically homogeneous to replace the real heterogeneous tissue

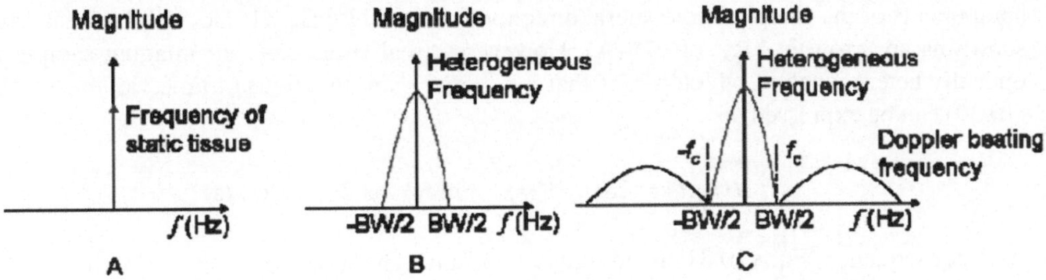

Figure 10.7: Diagram of frequency components for different tissue samples: (A) an ideal tissue sample (optically homogeneous sample) with no moving particles; (B) a real tissue sample (optically heterogeneous sample) with no moving particles; (C) a real tissue sample (optically heterogeneous sample) with moving particles. Images are reproduced from [54].

sample in OMAG [54]. This ideal background tissue provides a constant background signal that makes the adjacent A-scans totally correlated, leading to a dramatic increase of the phase signal to noise ratio (SNR) for the phase-resolved signals that represent flow velocities. This method inherits the advantages of both OMAG and PRDOCT.

The spectral interference signal captured by each pixel of the CCD camera in OMAG/SD-OCT is essentially the same except the wavelength, λ. We assume the wavenumbers of the broad band light source are from k_0 to k_0+, where $k_0 = 2\pi/\lambda_0$, and these wavenumbers cover 1024 pixels of the line scan camera respectively. Consequently, the camera records the spectral interference fringe signal formed between the reference light and the light backscattered from within sample, which can be written as a function of k_j:

$$I(k_j) = S(k_j)\left\langle \left| E_R \exp(i2k_j r) + \int_{-\infty}^{\infty} a(z)\exp\{i2k_j[r+nz]\}dz \right|^2 \right\rangle \quad j = 1,2,3,\ldots,1024 \qquad (10.28)$$

where $i = -1$, $\langle\rangle$ is the time average, k_j is the wavenumber of the light captured by the j-th detector (pixel) of the CCD camera, $I(k_j)$ is the light intensity captured by the j-th detector, $S(k_j)$ is the spectral density of the light source at k_j, r is the optical path length for the light travelled in the reference arm, n is the refractive index of the sample, $a(z)$ is the magnitude of the light backscattered at depth z. In our system, each B-scan contains 1500 A-lines and covers about 2.5 mm in the lateral direction. Thus the signal captured by the j-th pixel in each B scan can be written as a function of time variable t that relates to the position of focus beam spot on the sample, steered by the x scanning mirror thus:

$$I(k_j,t) = S(k_j)\left\langle \left| E_R \exp(i2k_j r) + \int_{-\infty}^{\infty} a(z)\exp\{i2k_j[r+nz]\}dz \right|^2 \right\rangle \quad j = 1,2,3\ldots1024 \qquad (10.29)$$

Because the light backscattered from the sample is quite weak compared to the light reflected from the reference mirror, we do not consider the self cross-correlation between the light backscattered from different positions within the sample. We also do not consider the DC signals because they do not contribute to useful OMAG signals. Therefore, Eq. (10.29) can be written as:

$$I(k_j,t) = 2S(k_j)E_R \int_{-\infty}^{\infty} a(z,t)\cos(2k_j nz)dz \qquad (10.30)$$

It is clear that Eq. (10.29) is constant if the sample is totally optically homogeneous, which means that $a(z,t)$ and n do not vary within the entire sample. If this is the case, then the spatial frequency components of the sample in the lateral direction presented by Eq. (10.30) will be a delta function, shown as an arrow in Fig. (10.7) (A). However in real situations, our imaging sample is often optically heterogeneous, which means that $a(z,t)$ and n are functions of time variable t. Thus, Eq. (10.30) can be expressed as:

$$I(k_j,t) = 2S(k_j)E_R \int_{-\infty}^{+\infty} a(z_1)\cos[2k_j n(z,t)zdz] \tag{10.31}$$

As a consequence, Eq. (10.31) is no longer constant. The intensity captured by the CCD camera will be modulated by the heterogeneous properties of the sample along each B-scan. The spatial frequency components of a static tissue sample, which we call the heterogeneous frequencies, will exhibit as a randomly distributed function around zero frequency with a bandwidth of BW, as shown in Fig. 10.7(B) [54].

When there is a patent blood vessel buried within motionless tissue at position (z_1,t_1), we assume the blood cells (scattering particles) within the vessel move towards the incident beam at a velocity v. The frequency of the light backscattered from these blood cells will be modulated by its velocity. Then, Eq. (10.31) can be expressed as:

$$I(k_j,t) = 2S(k_j)E_R \left[\int_{-\infty}^{\infty} a(z,t)\cos(2k_j n(t)z)dz + a(z_1,t_1)\cos[2k_j n(t)(z_1 - vt)]\right] \tag{10.32}$$

Here we also do not consider the self cross-correlation signal from within the sample. The first term on the right side of Eq. (10.31) represents backscattering signals from a static sample with reflectivity of $a(z,t)$, while the second term represents backscattering from the moving particles with reflectivity of $a(z_1,t_1)$ with a velocity of v at position (z_1,t_1). Moving particles produce a frequency shift caused by the Doppler effect of the moving particles. This is illustrated in Fig. 10.7(C), the blue curve is the Doppler beat frequency part. Recall that the phase-resolved technique requires a correlation between adjacent A scans to determine v of the moving particles [48], and the correlation, in conventional PRDOCT, provided by the first term on the right-side of Eq. (10.32) is also required to suppress the noise signals in the non-flow regions in order to increase the flow imaging contrast. Because of the optical heterogeneity $n(z,t)$ of a tissue, $n(z,t)$ imposes a noise background onto the blood flow signals, making it difficult for PR-DOCT to measure precisely the blood flow velocity, particularly in capillaries [60, 65, 67]. In contrast, OMAG eliminates the first term on the right side of Eq. (10.32) in order to image blood flow. This elimination renders the noise production due to $n(z,t)$ to a minimum, but unfortunately, results in OMAG losing its correlation condition between adjacent A scans for the heterogeneous tissue regions. Consequently, the phase-resolved technique cannot be directly applied to OMAG blood flow signals. To solve this problem, our proposed strategy is to digitally re-construct an ideal sample background with a constant backscattering coefficient a_0 and a refractive index n_0 throughout the sample, thus creating a totally homogeneous sample which reinforces a complete correlation among OMAG A scan signals.

$$I_0(k_j,t) = 2S(k_j)E_R \left[\int_{-\infty}^{\infty} a_0(z,t)\cos\left(2k_j n_0(z,t)z\right)dz\right] \tag{10.33}$$

where $a_0(z,t) \equiv a_0$ and $n_0(z,t) \equiv n_0$ throughout the scanned tissue sample. In condition, $a_0 = 10^{-6}$ and $n_0 = 1.35$ when we construct the homogenous tissue background using Eq. (10.33). These values were taken according to the typical optical properties of biological tissues, i.e. the average reflectivity is between 10^{-4} and 10^{-7} and the average refractive index is 1.35 [55]. The digitally reconstructed homogenous tissue sample subsequently replaces the first term on the right side of Eq. (10.32). In doing so, OMAG blood flow signal now becomes:

$$I'(k_j,t) = 2S(k_j)E_R \left[\int_{-\infty}^{\infty} a_0(z,t)\cos(2k_j n_0 z)dz + E_R a(z_1,t_1)\cos[2k_j n(z_1,t_1)(z_1 - vt)]\right] \tag{10.34}$$

The construction of the ideal tissue sample does not affect OMAG signals of blood flow because it only replaces the tissue background signals with a homogeneous background without affecting the blood flow signals within the B scan. If we treat time variable t as a constant and apply a Fourier transform upon wavelength k, then we can obtain:

$$\tilde{I}(z,t) = \mathrm{FT}^{-1}\left\{I(k_j,t)\right\}|k = A(z,t)\exp[i\phi(z,t)] \tag{10.35}$$

where $\phi(z,t)$ is the phase of the analytic signal. The phase difference between adjacent A scans, n and $n-1$, is then evaluated:

$$\Delta\phi(z,t) = \tan^{-1}\left[\frac{\mathrm{Im}[\tilde{I}(z,t_n)\cdot\tilde{I}(z,t_{n-1})]}{\mathrm{Re}[\tilde{I}(z,t_n)\cdot\tilde{I}(z,t_{n-1})]}\right] \tag{10.36}$$

Based on the linear relationship between phase difference between adjacent A-lines and velocity [35, 48], the velocity of flow signal imaged by OMAG can be directly written as:

$$v(z,t) = \frac{\lambda\Delta\phi(z,t)}{4\pi\Delta t} \tag{10.37}$$

where $v(z,t)$ is the flow velocity at depth z, Δt is the time interval between adjacent A-lines. Note that there is a small constant offset induced by a_0 in Eq. (10.34), which may perturb the evaluated $\Delta\phi(z,t)$. However, the small offset is usually at least 2 orders of magnitude smaller than the OMAG flow signals, leading to a negligible effect on the final evaluated $\Delta\phi(z,t)$.

The flow chart of the processing procedure is illustrated in Fig. 10.8. It is because the image data was achieved by scanning of the scanner, the variable t present in the theory section could be directly replaced by the position of the x direction. In this case, we use x to replace t for better illustration of the cross section image. The raw spectral interference signal, $I(k,x)$, is first separated into two parts based on the heterodyne technique by a carefully selected frequency, f_c along lateral direction, which depends on the characteristic of the sample and system setup. The static signal, $I_s(k,x)$, the low frequency part, is reconstructed following the theory described above. An ideal simulation sample, $I_{\text{ideal}}(k,x)$, with no optical heterogeneity could be achieved by Eq. (10.30). Using a frequency synthesizing method, the flow signal, $I_f(k,x)$, extracted from the original interference data by applying a high pass filter at each wavelength, and the static signal, extracted from the ideal simulation sample by applying a low pass filter at each wavelength, are recombined to a new synthesizing signal, $I_{\text{syn}}(k,x)$. After applying the PRDOCT algorithm, we could obtain the Doppler OMAG phase difference image. Base on the following linear relationship between phase difference and velocity [34, 49], we could directly obtain the velocity information of the sample.

Because the background tissue signal is rejected previously, the Doppler OMAG image provides two great improvements on two aspects. Firstly, based on phase resolved technology, the flow velocity is directly provided by Doppler OMAG, compared to traditional OMAG. Secondly, the texture pattern artifacts caused by the optical heterogeneity which could greatly reduce the performance of the PRDOCT is successfully rejected. In consequence, the phase stocktickerSNR of the Doppler OMAG is greatly improved compared to PRDOCT.

10.3 Applications of OMAG

Because of its exceptionally high spatial resolution and velocity sensitivity, several basic research and clinical applications of OMAG have been demonstrated, which includes monitoring cortical hemodynamics and cerebral vascular perfusion mapping in rodent models for brain research,

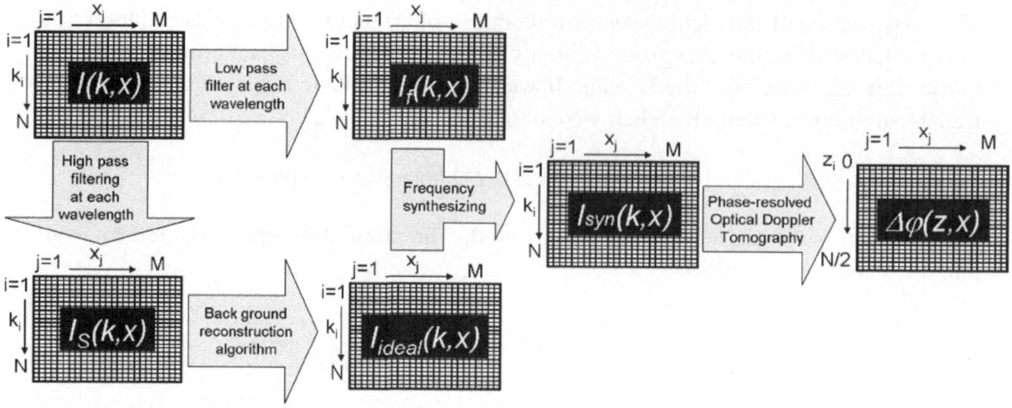

Figure 10.8: Flow chart showing the steps for DOMAG to evaluate the velocities of blood flow from a B scan data set, $I(k,t)$. The data coordinates are indicated in the lower right corner of each data block, where t is the time variable of probe beam scanning over a sample, k is the wavenumber, f is the spatial frequency, and z is the imaging depth. FT$|t$ represents the Fourier transform (FT) against the time variable t in the B scan, FT$-1|f$ indicates the inverse FT against the spatial frequency, f, and FT$|k$ is FT against the wavenumber k.

cerebral blood perfusion and vascular plasticity following traumatic brain injury in rodent models, screening vasoactive drugs, monitoring changes in tissue morphology and hemodynamics following pharmacological intervention and mapping, and imaging ocular blood flow.

10.3.1 *In vivo* imaging of mouse cerebral blood perfusion and vascular plasticity following traumatic brain injury using OMAG

Traumatic brain injury (TBI) often causes alterations in cerebral blood flow (CBF) that are thought to influence secondary pathophysiology and neurologic outcome in human brain. Inadequate CBF is an important contributor to mortality and morbidity after TBI [56]. Despite the importance of cerebral vascular dysfunction in TBI pathophysiology, the effect of trauma on CBF has been less well studied than the effect of trauma on the brain [57]. Similarly, our understanding of the rehabilitation and autoregulation of cerebrovascular blood circulation after TBI also remains incomplete. In this regard, a non-invasive technique for imaging *in vivo* blood flow, down to capillary level resolution, would be of great value.

Due to its non-invasiveness and its capillary-level imaging resolution, OMAG has been reported to longitudinally image cerebral blood perfusion and vascular plasticity in animal models following traumatic brain injury [58]. A typical series of OMAG CBF images of a mouse following TBI are shown in Fig. 10.9 and the cross-sectional structure and perfusion images corresponding to the dashed line positions are shown in Fig. 10.10. Fig. 10.9(A) is the OMAG image from baseline, i.e., the control, where it shows the capability of OMAG to delineate the dynamic CBF, down to capillary level resolution, within the cortex while the skull was left intact. At 30 minutes after TBI, a reduction of CBF (cerebral ischemia) over the entire cortex was seen in OMAG image (Fig. 10.9(B)). The reduction of CBF might be due to the post-traumatic hemorrhage caused by the external injury that leaves the blood in the space between the meninges and cortex, near the TBI site (pointed by the green arrow). However, the CBF reduction was not even across the cortex as seen in Fig. 10.9(B), with the ipsilateral reduction more severe than the contralateral region. Another possible reason for the reduction of CBF seen in the OMAG image might be the possible bleeding that partially

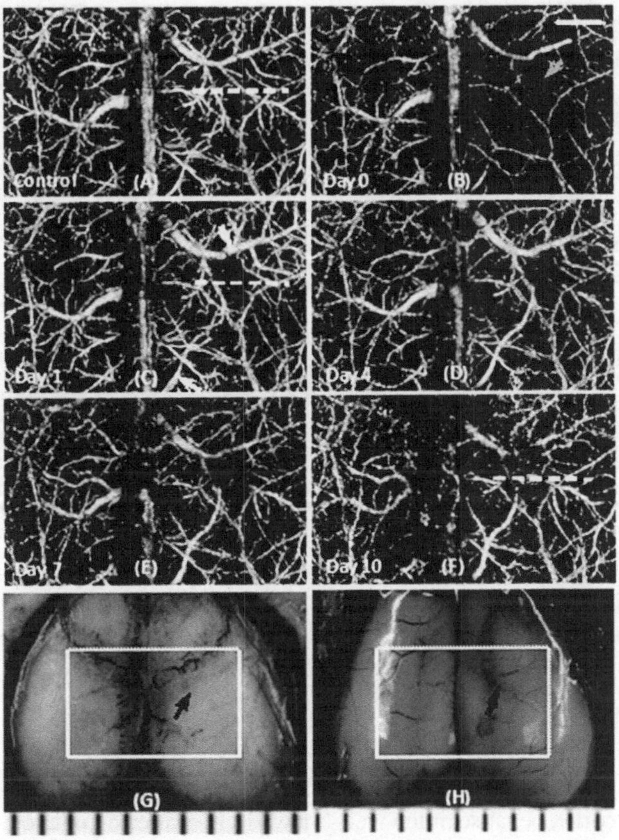

Figure 10.9: (See color insert.) 3D OMAG imaging of the cortex during TBI in mice. Compared to baseline (A), progressive vessel regulation (vessels are pointed by white arrows) and neovascularization at traumatic area develop during TBI rehabilitation. The site of injury is pointed by green arrow. (G) and (H) are the photographs of the brain cortex with and without skull on the same mouse. The area in (A)-(F) corresponds to the area marked with dashed white box in (G) and (H). The scale bar represents 1.0 mm. Images are reproduced from [58].

blocks the light penetration into the deeper tissues (i.e. light absorption due to the clotted blood), however, the clotted blood will be most likely localised near the TBI site. At the TBI site, the blood flow was totally ceased, due to hemostasis. Furthermore, the vessel constriction was apparent in the ipsilateral region that might be caused by acute cerebrovascular regulation to prevent the occurrence of hypoxic-ischemic reaction [59].

During the progress of rehabilitation, OMAG is able to visualize the changes of CBF on the same injured animal over time. At Day 1, vasoconstriction disappeared and the blood perfusion almost returned to the baseline, apart from the site at injury (Fig. 10.9 (C)). However, the vessel dilation seemed occurred near the TBI site, particularly for the vessels pointed by the white arrows and their associated branches. The needle-induced lesion area is still absent from the blood circulation (Fig. 10.9(C) and Fig. 10.10(B)). From Day 4 to Day 7, the new blood vessels started to appear in the traumatic region, indicating the neovascularization was happening (Fig. 10.9(D) and 10.9(E). The neovascularization was more evident at Day 10 (Fig. 10.9(F) and Fig. 10.10(C)), however the blood flows over the cortex seen in the previous OMAG images was increasingly difficult to detect by the OMAG system at Day 10. The reason for this difficulty is that the thickness of cranium doubled

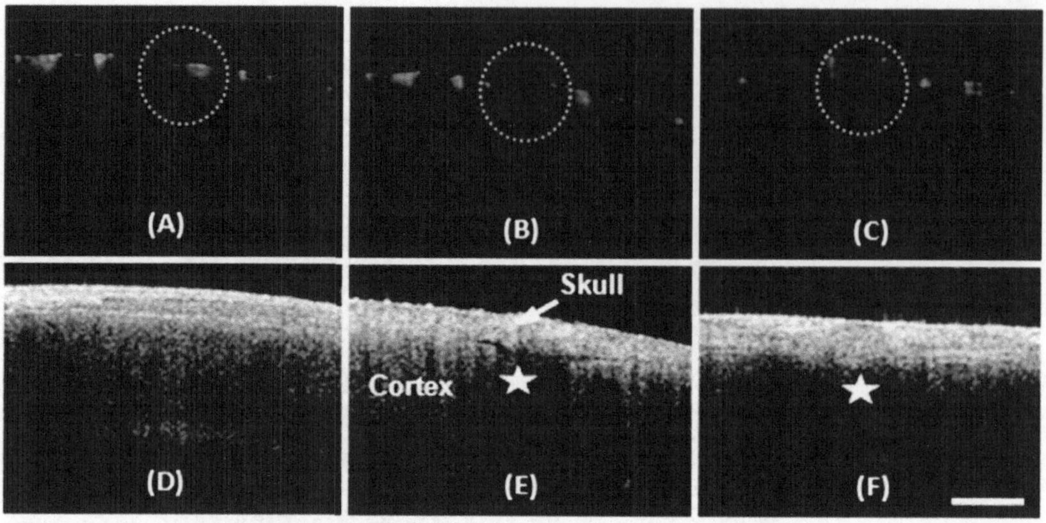

Figure 10.10: Cross-sections (slices) of microstructure (A–C) and blood perfusion (D–F) of the mouse brain during pre- (A&D) and post- (B&E, C&F) traumatic phases. They correspond to the dashed line position in Fig. 10.9. The areas in dashed circle show the evolution of neovascularization and the trauma zone in the cortex is pointed by a white star. Images are reproduced from [93].

(Fig. 10.10(F)) when compared with the control (Fig. 10.10(D)) and that reduced the amount of light to reach the cortex because of the well-known light scattering phenomenon [55]. The increased thickness of cranium was most probably due to the infection caused by the experimental procedures, although the antibiotics were applied daily to the animal. This can be eliminated for future systematic studies on TBI through careful and skilled surgical procedures. Despite this infection in the current study that doubled the cranium thickness, OMAG still offers the opportunity to visualize the changes of global CBF that may aid our understanding of the cerebral vascular plasticity upon TBI.

For comparison, the direct photographs of the brain cortex with and without skull just after the OMAG imaging at day 10 are shown in Fig. 10.9(G) and Fig. 10.9(H), respectively, where the TBI site is identified by the black arrow. Seeing the blood vessels through the cranium is almost impossible (Fig. 10.9(G)). Comparing between Fig. 10.9(H) and OMAG images, the agreement on the major vascular network over the brain cortex is achieved. More importantly, the microvessels unobserved in the photograph of Fig. 10.9(H) are seen in OMAG images, suggesting the OMAG capability to monitor the cerebral vascular circulation after TBI at capillary level resolution.

The ability to non-invasively record and map the variations of cerebral blood flow would greatly contribute to our understanding of the complex nature involved following TBI. Because the moving red blood cells in patent vessels, including capillaries can be precisely localized in OMAG, any functional vessel up to the depth of 2.00 mm is able to be imaged under OMAG. The experimental results reported so far have shown the capability of OMAG to monitor the response of the cerebral circulation to TBI and to visualize the neovascularization following TBI. The noted increases in newly formed vessels after TBI may serve to alleviate secondary neuronal damage by improving local blood flow and metabolite delivery to the nutrient deprived neurons. Our understanding of the mechanism of new vessel formation still remains incomplete. Based on the volumetric imaging of OMAG with improved resolution, OMAG may provide a powerful tool to investigate and visualize neovascularization following TBI on the same animal over a long period of time. Specifically, if combined with immunocytochemistry, OMAG may aid the investigations on elucidating whether both angiogenesis and vasculogenesis or either of them participates in promoting neovascularization [60]. However, due to the coagulation of red blood cells from broken vessels on the site of injury in the current study, observation of the generation of precursor microvessels will possibly be inhibited, if this beginning event happens before the blood clot is partially absorbed. Currently, research groups are continuing to develop algorithms to quantitatively assess the CBF from the OMAG measurements so that the accurate angiodynamics following TBI can be provided.

10.3.2 Mapping retinal and choroidal microvascular perfusion

Accurate 3D imaging of microvascular blood perfusion has great significance in ophthalmology. There is a growing body of evidence suggests that vascular abnormalities and dysregulation may contribute to the development of several major ocular diseases as different as glaucoma, diabetic retinopathy, or age related macular degeneration etc. Much effort has been made to investigate the ocular microvascular perfusion in detail. However, direct 3D visualization and investigation of the ocular microcirculation is complicated by the fact that the posterior pole of the eye is nourished mainly by two different vascular beds, the retina and the choroid, in which the retina have several layers and sub layers. In terms of physiological and pathological conditions, the retinal and choroidal microvascular systems exhibit significant differences, which are reviewed elsewhere [61]. High-resolution noninvasive techniques for depth resolved *in vivo* imaging of ocular microvascular perfusion are not currently available as a diagnostic tool in ophthalmology. Such a technique could have a significant impact on better understanding of retinal pathogenesis and early diagnosis and facilitating preventive retinal treatment.

Research groups have reported the use of OMAG to image the ocular blood perfusion within the posterior segment of the eye *in vivo*. Figure 10.11 shows the *in vivo* imaging results produced by one volume data set captured at a position near the optic disk. Figure 10.11(A) gives the OCT fundus projection image obtained by integrating signals along the depth direction from the volumetric OCT structural images using the method proposed by Jiao et al. [62], where the major blood vessels over the retina can be seen, but not in the choroid. Figure 10.11(B) represents one cross-sectional image within the volumetric OCT image at the position marked by the yellow line in Fig. 10.11(A). Figure 10.11(C) shows 2D OMAG flow image of the cross sections after the bulk motion was corrected as described in the above section, where it can be seen that the blood flows within the retina and choroidal layers are clearly delineated. In the retinal region, not only some big vessels, but also the capillary vessels are presented. Although the blood flows in the vessels in the choroid region are slow, which are difficult to be detected by PRDOCT, they can be captured by OMAG imaging method. Because OMAG gives the volumetric structural and flow images simultaneously, the 3D vasculatures can be merged into the 3D structural image. Such merged volumetric image is illustrated in Fig. 10.11(D), where a cut-through view in the center of volumetric structural image is used to better appreciate how the blood vessels innervate the tissue. To render the volumetric flow image, the blood flow signals are coded with green color (retina) and red color (choroid). The result is shown in Fig. 10.11(E), where the flow image shows us two vessel networks with good connection between vessels.

Currently, the OMAG imaging system has a limited field of view. One typical 3D image covers a volume of $2\times2\times2$ mm^3 in the posterior segment of the eye. Figure 10.12 shows one example of 3D perfusion maps from a healthy volunteer. Figs. 10.12(A) and 10.12(B) demonstrate the 3-D volumetric blood vessel networks in the retina and choroid. In Fig. 10.12(C), the retinal blood vessels (coded with green) and choroidal blood vessels (coded in red) are merged together to present their relative positions. Together with a cross section B-scan structure image, Fig. 10.12(C) also demonstrates the positions of blood vessels relative to the structure.

To achieve wide field imaging of fundus vasculature (7.4 mm$\times$7.4 mm) with this technique, different areas of the posterior part of human eye can be sequentially scanned to obtain multiple 3D datasets, which are then stitched together to form a wide field of view. The images in Fig. 10.13 were created from sixteen 3D datasets captured using a predesigned scan pattern. Figs. 10.13

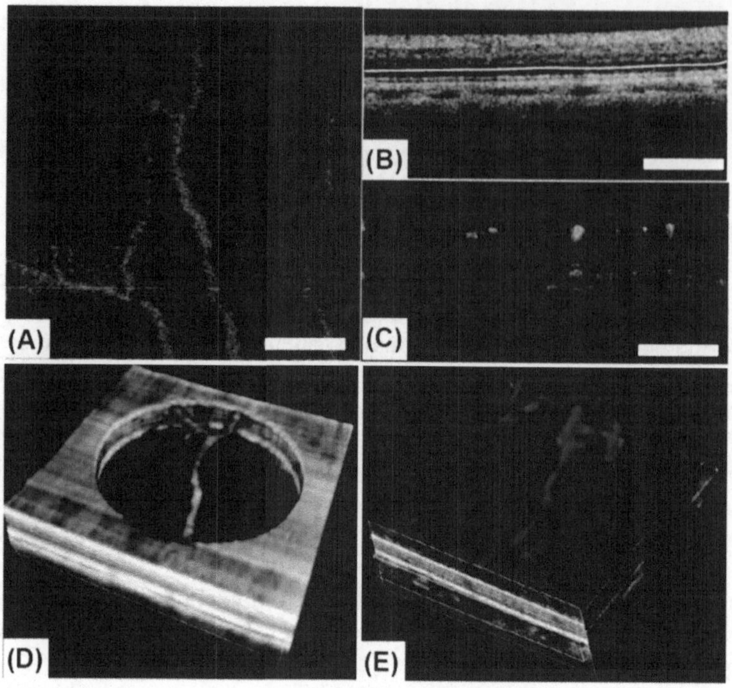

Figure 10.11: (See color insert.) *In vivo* volumetric imaging of the posterior chamber of an eye from a volunteer. (A) OCT fundus image of the scanned volume as described in [33]. (B) OCT cross-sectional image at the position marked yellow in (A), in which four lines as shown result from the segmentation method that is used to separate the blood flows in retina and choroids. (C) Fly through movie that represents the 2D OMAG flow images within the scanned volume. (D) Volumetric rendering of the merged structural and flow images with a cut through in the center of structural image. (E) Volumetric rending of the blood flow image where flows in retina are coded with green and those in choroids with red. Scale bar = 500 μm. Images are reproduced from [52].

(A) and (B) are blood-flow maps from the retina and choroid using OMAG. These results compare favorably with clinical fluorescein angiography (FA)—see Figure 10.13(C)—and indocyanine green angiography (ICGA) — see Figure 10.13(D)—from the same volunteer. Furthermore, OMAG sees more micro-blood vessels in the foveal region than FA (marked by the white ellipse).

By comparison, the OMAG results demonstrated very good agreement with the clinical FA and ICGA results. Through scrutinizing the appearances of the blood vessels, almost all noticeable vessels presented by FA and ICGA images are demonstrated by OMAG imaging. Furthermore, in the retinal perfusion map Fig. 10.13(A), the OMAG results demonstrated more microcirculation information in the fovea region than that of the FA image. The main advantages of OMAG compared to FA and ICGA are that the images are obtained without injected contrast agents and the vessels can be correlated with the depth of location in the retina or choroid. These two advantages of OMAG wide field of view perfusion maps indicate this imaging modality will potentially be a very powerful tool for *in vivo* clinical application in the future.

10.3.3 Volumetric imaging of cochlear blood perfusion in rodent

The motivation behind the study of cochlear microcirculation is the hypothesis that it plays an important role in maintaining the normal homoeostatic environment in the inner ear and also by the

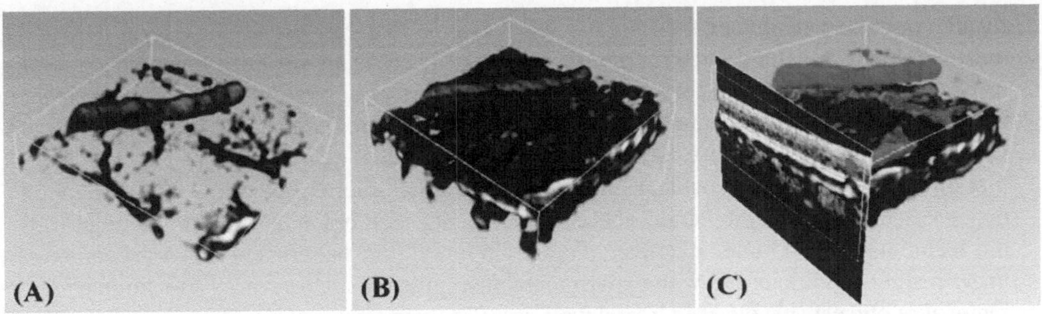

Figure 10.12: (See color insert.) Volumetric image of blood vessel networks in (a) retina and (b) choroid. (c) Combined volumetric image, together with a cross section structure image. Images are reproduced from [63].

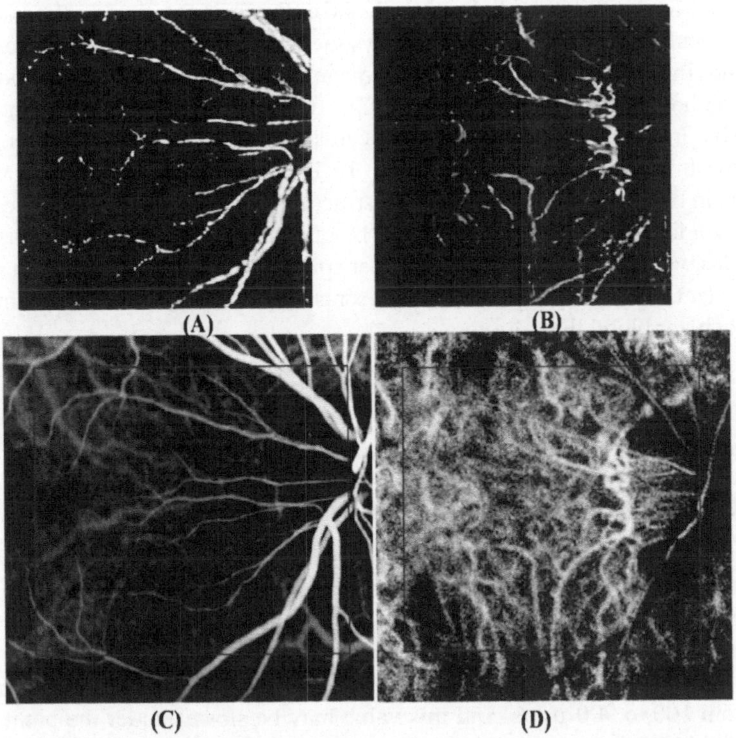

Figure 10.13: Wide field of view blood perfusion maps for (A) retina and (B) choroids, compared with (C) fluorescein angiography and (D) indocyanine green angiography. Images are reproduced from [63].

assumption that some cochlear diseases are vascular in nature. It is hypothesized that these disorders can be treated by increasing blood flow to the inner ear. It is known that there is high metabolic demand of cochlear tissues such as stria vascularis [64, 65], and that ischemia may have potential role in cochlear injury following noxious insults such as sound [66–68] or ototoxic drugs [69]. It is also possible that vascular change scan be part of etiology of sudden deafness syndrome [70, 71] and Meniere's disease [72, 73]. Imaging to measure cochlear blood flow could be accomplished for the vascular network of the osseous spiral lamina that can be visualized via the round window membrane, a natural opening into the cochlea. There is a clear need for understanding of the mechanisms controlling the cochlear blood flow. The study of blood flow in cochlea has interested auditory investigators for centuries. There have been many research activities, with applications of various techniques to measure cochlear blood flow. Intravital microscopy [74, 75] was used for the first direct observation of cochlear blood flow. Intravital microscopy allowed visualization of the major vascular beds of the lateral wall and the basilar membrane in the living animal [69]. With this technique, vessel lumen diameter, changes in blood flow pattern, and flow rate can be assessed under resting conditions and with experimental manipulations. However, the technique requires the removal of otic capsule over the lateral wall vessels to permit direct visualization. Under the best of conditions, it is a very invasive procedure.

Recently, OMAG has been demonstrated to have potential for studying *in vivo* cochlear blood flow and imaging the cochlear microstructures for small animal models. In one study, the investigators selected gerbil as the animal model because of its relatively thin bony otic capsule [76]. Fig. 10.14 (A) shows *in vivo* 3D OMAG image of gerbil cochlea. The imaging volume was $2 \times 2 \times 2$ mm^3. The final images were scaled to the physical dimensions using a refractive index of 1.35 for typical biological tissues. Fig. 10.14(A) shows the image of the microstructures within the imaged tissue volume. In Fig. 10.14(B), 3D OMAG image of the blood vessels in the bone and in the tissue just inside the bony otic capsule is shown. Fig. 10.14(C) is the 2D projection of the 3D image in Fig. 10.14(B). In the projection image, one can see the blood vessel network, including the capillaries, in the first turn of the cochlea. Fig. 10.14(D) illustrates the visualization of the osseous spiral lamina in the base of the cochlea. This structure can easily be seen via the thin round window membrane avoiding attenuation of the signal by otic capsule bone. The osseous spiral lamina contains arterioles, venules and capillaries. Deeper spiral modiolar artery and vein might be accessible for measurement. This lamina possibly represents the easiest location to obtain an estimate of the quality of cochlear blood flow.

10.4 Ultra High Sensitive OMAG (UHS-OMAG)

The minimal flow sensitivity which could be achieved with OMAG methods was 160 μm/s [54] within the reach for imaging microcirculations within the tissue beds. The minimal flow sensitivity of OMAG *in vivo* studies is limited mainly by the phase noise introduced by the motion artifact and the scanning protocol, which requires relatively long scanning time for acquiring volumetric data set for 3D reconstruction. Since the flow velocity of microcirculation within the capillary is in the range from 100 to 900 μm/s, and this value may be slower under the pathological conditions, conventional OMAG is incapable of imaging capillary microcirculation with high sensitivity. In order to overcome this limitation, the sensitivity of OMAG must be improved, and its imaging acquisition time needs to be reduced. Moreover, in OMAG the flow contrast is based on the Doppler flow which is essentially determined by the axial flow component parallel to the imaging direction of the OMAG system. This component is designated by $v(\cos\theta)$, where v is the velocity of the flow and θ is the angle of the flow direction relative to the imaging direction. For cases such as in the retina, the primary direction of the blood flow is nearly perpendicular to the imaging direction such that $\theta \sim 90°$. In such cases, to visualize the blood vessels with the OMAG technique, the velocity, v, of the flow must be large enough to have a sufficient axial component to surpass the phase noise at that point, which is determined by the local signal-to-noise ratio. In order to overcome these limitations of OMAG, new and exciting approach has been proposed to image very slow capillary microcirculation in tissue beds. In the following section, we describe the implementations of UHS-

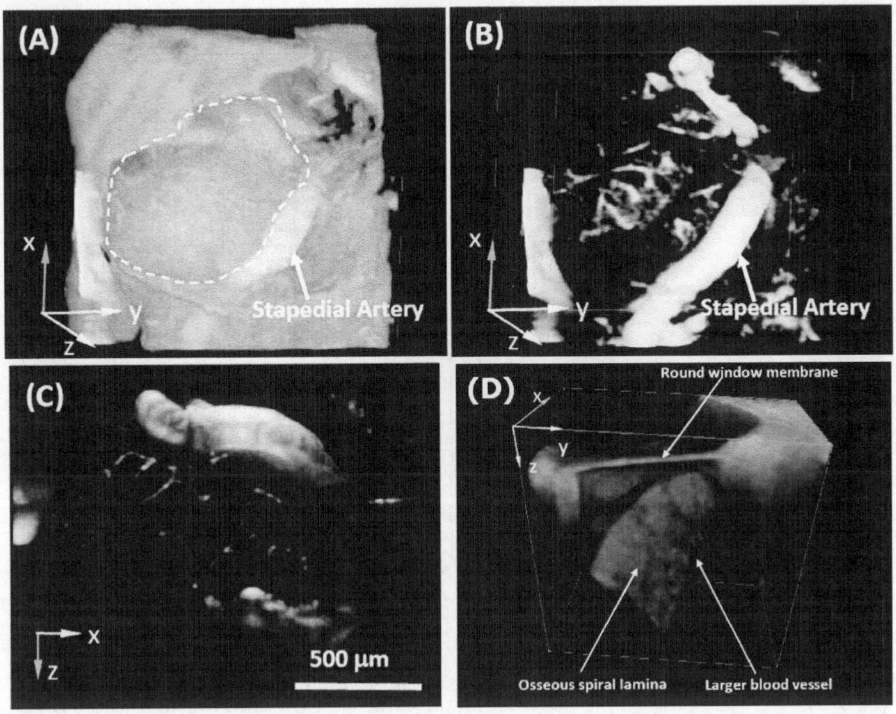

Figure 10.14: (See color insert.) OMAG image of the gerbil cochlea in 3-D. Image volume is $2.0 \times 2.0 \times 2.0\ \text{mm}^3$. (A) Image of microstructures within the scanned tissue, where the location of the cochlea is indicated by the dashed outline. (B) Corresponding volumetric image of the blood perfusion within the cochlea. (C) 2-D projection view ($x - z$ view) of blood flow in the cochlea; the image shows the blood vessel network, including capillaries, in the first turn of the cochlea. (D) OMAG imaging of cochlea in gerbils through the round window *in vivo*. The imaged tissue volume $= 2.0 \times 2.0 \times 2.0\ \text{mm}^3$ $(x - y - z)$. The OMAG probe beam was directed from the top. Images are reproduced from [76].

OMAG and image processing algorithm for volumetric capillary flow imaging. We also describe extended features such as full range imaging and ultra-high resolution imaging with supercontinnum source in the following section.

10.4.1 Scanning protocol and algorithm

Unlike conventional OMAG, to achieve ultrahigh sensitive imaging of slow microcirculation, UHS-OMAG employs a new scanning protocol and novel flow reconstruction algorithm. UHS-OMAG acquires low density B-scan frame (i.e. fast scan), therefore for a given imaging speed of the system, the frame rate can be dramatically improved [77]. However, in the elevation scanning direction (i.e. slow scan), high density scans is used.

The 3D spectral interference signals captured by the UHS-OMAG system can be written as:

$$I(t,k_j) = S(t,k_j)\left\{E_R^2 + 2E_R\int_{-\infty}^{\infty} a(z,t)\cos[2k_j n(t)z]dz + 2E_R a(z_l)\cos[2k_j n(t)(z_l - \nu t)]\right\} \tag{10.38}$$

where $j = 1,2,\ldots,N$ is the pixel number of the line scan CCD camera, k_j is the wave number of

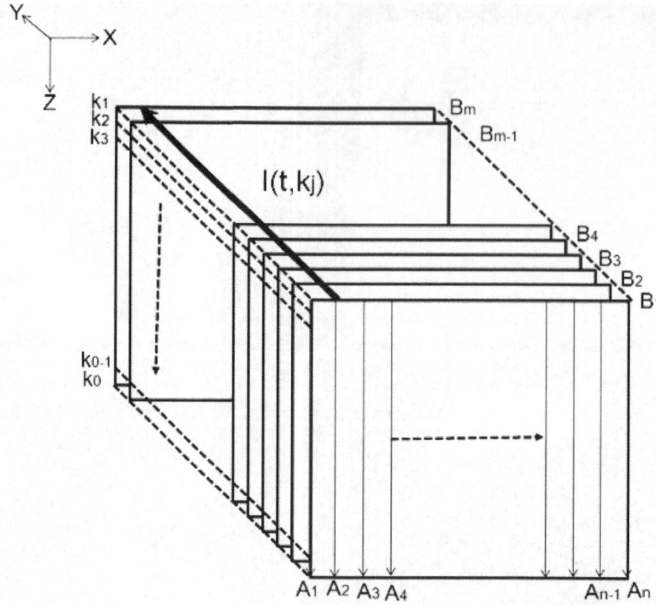

Figure 10.15: Schematic of scanning protocol and signal processing method employed in UHS-OMAG. B_1 to B_m are the B-scans in the 3D data cube, A_1 to A_n are the A-scan in B frame. k_j is the wavenumber of the light captured by the j-th pixel, where $j = 1,2,\ldots,N$ is the pixel number of the line scan CCD camera. The solid black arrow shows the high pass filtering direction in UHS-OMAG signal processing.

the light captured by the j-th pixel; $I(k_j)$ is the light intensity detected by the j-th detector; t is the time variable when one A-line, $I(k)$, was captured in the Y-direction (C scan direction), as shown in Fig. 10.15; $S(k_j)$ is the spectral density of the light source at k_j; n is the refractive index; $a(z)$ is the amplitude of the back scattered light and z is the depth from which the light back scattered from; v is the velocity of a moving particle, for example blood cells, which are buried in the tissue at depth z_1. In Eq. (10.38), we ignore the self cross-correlation term that occurred between the light backscattered within the sample, because it is relatively weak compared to that reflected from the reference mirror. Then the first term in Eq. (10.38) is the DC signal produced by the light reflected from the reference mirror. The second term is the spatial frequency component of the static tissue sample, which we call the heterogeneous frequency component, which can provide the static structural information of the sample. The third term is the Doppler beating signal, which is introduced by the moving particles in the tissue sample. Depending upon the magnitude of the moving particles velocity, the Doppler beating signal shifts away from the static interference signals caused by the microstructures of the sample.

For obtaining slow the microcirculation within capillary vessels, UHS-OMAG algorithm uses the high pass filtering along the slow scan direction as shown in Fig. 10.15, rather than in the B-scan direction in conventional OMAG, in order to remove the DC signal and the static signals due to the microstructures of the sample. The high pass filtering in signal processing is implemented by applying a differential operation on the captured B-scan spectral interferograms along the slow-scan direction. The differential operation is equivalent to high pass filtering, which suppresses the DC and scattering signals from the static elements within the scanned volume, i. e.,

$$I_{\text{FLOW}}(t_i, k_j) = I(t_i, k_j) - I(t_{i-1}, k_j),\ i = 1,2,3,\ldots,N \tag{10.39}$$

where i represents the index of the B-scans in the slow-scan direction. Then, by applying the fast Fourier transform (FFT) upon every wavenumber k (keeping t constant) the depth resolved blood flow signals are obtained, where $\lambda - k$ is obtained by using cubic spline interpolation on the captured interferogram. The movement artifact is one of the most distracting issues for *in vivo* imaging of slow microcirculations, which is caused by the involuntary movement of sample and can seriously deteriorate the image quality. We implemented the motion compensation algorithm described in the above section to effectively resolve the movement artifact issues.

In UHS-OMAG, the maximum detectable velocity that is not wrapped is determined by the adjacent time spacing, Δt_B, between adjacent B-scans in the Y-direction, i.e., $V = \lambda/2n\Delta t_B$, where λ is the central wave length of the light source. If the system imaging system has a B-scan frame rate of 300 fps, then $\Delta t_B \sim 3.3$ ms. Therefore, considering that the slow-scan direction is densely sampled with an oversampling factor of ~ 12, the maximum unambiguous detectable velocity would be 141 μm/s. It must be emphasized that the maximum velocity that can be detected by the system is determined by the system imaging speed. If the imaging speed is of an A-scan rate of 47,000 per second, the maximum detectable velocity is ~ 30 mm/s. However, if flow velocity is > 141 μm/s, the UHS-OMAG will not be able to provide the actual velocity values because of the well-known phase wrapping effect in the interference signals, unless a specific phase-unwrapping algorithm is used to un-wrap the phases. The minimum velocity that the system can detect is determined by the system phase noise floor, which can be expressed by the intensity signal to noise ratio, S, of the OMAG/OCT system by $\sigma^2_{\Delta\varphi} = 1/S$ [78, 79]. At an imaging speed of 47,000 A-scan per second, a minimum detectable velocity of ~ 4 μm/s has been reported [80].

By the use of the scanning protocol and algorithm described above, Fig. 10.16 shows the UHS-OMAG imaging results obtained from human skin located at the palm (the area marked as square box in Fig. 10.16(B). Fig. 10.16(A) shows a schematic drawing of the blood vessel system of the human skin, in which an interconnected network of vessels is characterized by regular structures on all levels. The human skin is composed of the cutis and the subcutis (hypodermis [HD]). The cutis is further divided into the epidermis (EP) and the dermis (DR). The dermis and subcutis are pervaded with a complex system of blood vessels, while the epidermis is free of vessels. A superficial network comprises the interface between papillary (PD) and reticular dermis (RD), while a lower network is located on the border between dermis and subcutis. Vertical vessels connect both networks and thus make it complete. Because the UHS-OMAG sensitivity is as low as ~ 4 μm/s, even the dynamics of sweat glands are imaged. Fig 10.16(C) gives the projection view at the depths from 400 to 450 μm, which depth corresponds to the papillary dermis where the capillary vessels are dense (e.g., pointed by the arrows). At the depths from 450 to 650 μm, the vessels are almost vertical that connects vessel networks between papillary dermis and reticular dermis, seen as the bright spots in Fig. 10.16(D). The blood vessel network in reticular dermis is given in Fig. 10.16(E) where the vessel diameter is seen to be smaller than those situated in the hypodermis in Fig. 10.16(F). These observations from ultrahigh sensitive OMAG are almost identical to that described in the standard reference, for example given in Fig. 16(A), demonstrating the power of the ultrahigh sensitive OMAG in the investigations of pathological conditions in dermatology.

10.4.2 Ultra-high resolution imaging using Supercontinuum source

High axial resolution is a critical parameter for imaging capillary level microcirculation with UHS-OMAG, and which scales with the bandwidth and center wavelength of the source, where higher resolution is achieved with a light source having larger spectral bandwidth and lower center wavelength. In biological applications, scattering and water absorption, which are highly wavelength dependent, become important factors in the selection of an appropriate light source. Water absorption increases with increasing wavelength and scattering increases with decreasing wavelength. Broadband light sources having wavelengths of $\sim$1300 nm are especially attractive as they offer an excellent compromise between depth penetration, water absorption, and axial resolution. A

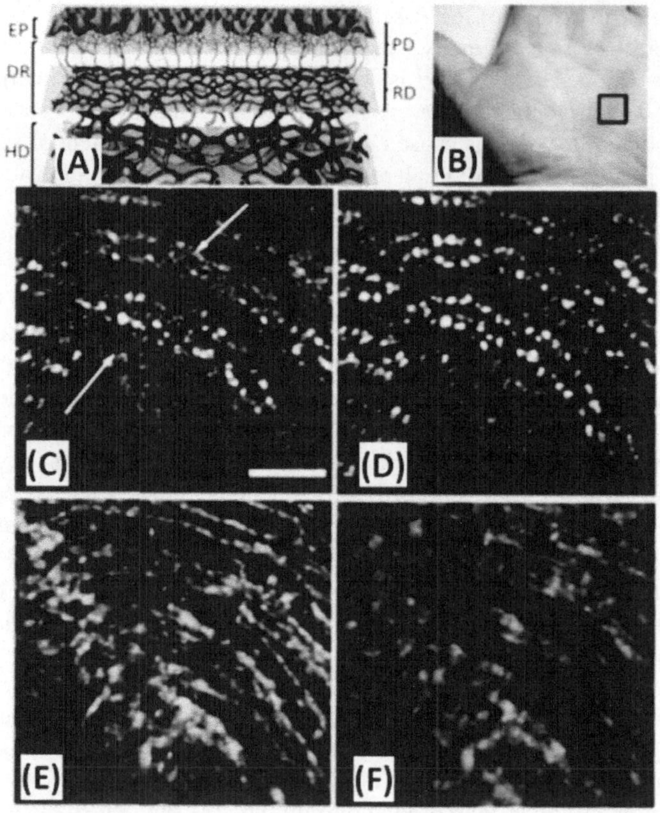

Figure 10.16: (See color insert.) Schematic diagram of the blood vessel system of the human skin; (B) photograph of palm showing the scanning area ($2 \times 2\text{mm}^2$). UHS-OMAG provides detailed projection views of microcirculation network at different depths of skin obtained from: (C) 400–450 μm (closely representing papillary dermis), (D) 450–650 μm, (E) 650–780 μm (closely representing reticular dermis) and (F) 780–1100 μm (part of hypodermis), respectively. The strength of reflectance signals in the images is displayed within a range between 20 dB (dark) and 50 dB (bright). [80]

number of reports (e.g., [81, 82]) have demonstrated the use of state-of the-art femtosecond lasers to achieve a 2–3 μm axial resolution, but with the disadvantage of being expensive and bulky, limiting their use to a few research laboratories. Being spectrally very broad and visually very bright, supercontinuum (SC) light sources have become attractive recently as excellent alternatives for OCT imaging to achieve subcellular axial resolution [83]. The feasibility of the Fianium SC source for time-domain and spectral-domain OCT (SD-OCT) was demonstrated by several groups [84, 85].

To achieve ultrahigh resolution and ultrahigh-sensitive imaging of tissue microcirculations, a UHS-OMAG system based on SC source has been reported [86]. The schematic of the system is shown in Fig. 10.17, but with the design consideration and the use of components that can handle the high intensity and broad bandwidth of an SC light source. In this system, the light source applied was a Super K Versa Supercontinuum Source (Koheras A/S, Denmark) pumped by an Nd:YAG laser, which provides an output spectrum from 460 to 2400 nm and a total output power of 1.5 W. The output light from the SC source then was passed through an optical filter that was specially designed to filter and reshape the incoming SC light into the light that centers at 800 nm with a bandwidth of 120 nm. The filtered light was then collimated and coupled into an optical fiber

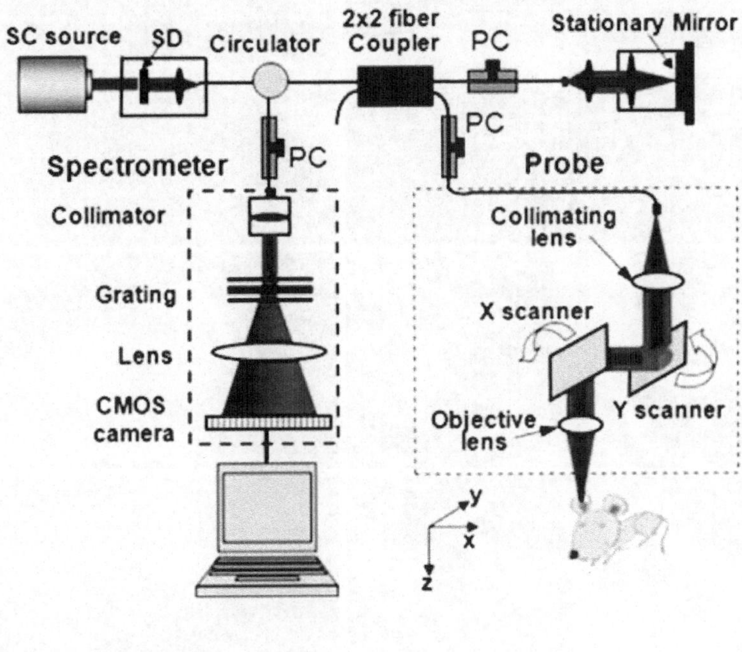

Figure 10.17: Schematics of the system and setup; SD - spectral filter.

(single-mode)-based SD-OCT system via an optical circulator (AC Photonics, USA). All the optic-fiber components used were specified at 800 nm with a spectral bandwidth of at least 120 nm. The output power from the single-mode fiber in the sample arm was measured at ∼12 mW. It is known that the capillary vessels have an average diameter of 6–8 μm. Therefore, to resolve the capillary vessels within microcirculatory tissue beds, the system had the measured spatial resolutions of 3.2 μm (axial) and 5.8 μm (lateral) over a depth range from 0 to 2 mm [86].

Figure 10.18 gives typical UHS-OMAG results of a mouse ear skin, scanned using an UHS-OMNAG system that used supercontinuum light source. The system not only offers the ability that a typical ultrahigh resolution OCT system offers because the typical, layered micro-structural features of the mouse pinna, e.g., epidermis, dermis, and auricular cartilage, can be can be delineated (Fig. 10.18(a)), but also visualizes the abundant capillary blood vessels perfused through the micro-circulation tissue beds (Fig. 10.18(b)). Fig. 10.18(c) gives the 2D maximum-intensity projection view of a 3D OMAG image of microcirculation obtained from a field of view of 0.5 mm × 0.5 mm, that provides a clearer demonstration of the system capability to resolve single capillary vessels within tissue beds, where the looped structures of the capillary network, a common feature in skin microcirculation can be seen due to the system's ultrahigh spatial resolution. The capillaries indicated by the thick arrows (Fig. 10.18(c)) have the measured diameter of ∼6 μm, close to the lateral resolution of the system. Even the individual red blood cells (thin arrows) moving in the capillaries can be identified in the OMAG flow image. Figure 10.18(d) illustrates a 3D view rendered by merging the microstructural image with the blood vessel image, where the capillary vessels (white arrows) on top of the big vessel could be seen more clearly.

The UHS-OMAG system has a broad detectable velocity range, from ∼4 μm/s to ∼15mm/s [86], which enables us to image not only the big arteries and veins but also the detailed capillary bed within tissue. By scanning multiple small regions and combining them together afterward, Fig. 10.19 shows the detailed and impressive vascular perfusion map of the whole ear, where the insert is a photograph of the mouse ear imaged. Since the densely patterned capillary beds and plexus

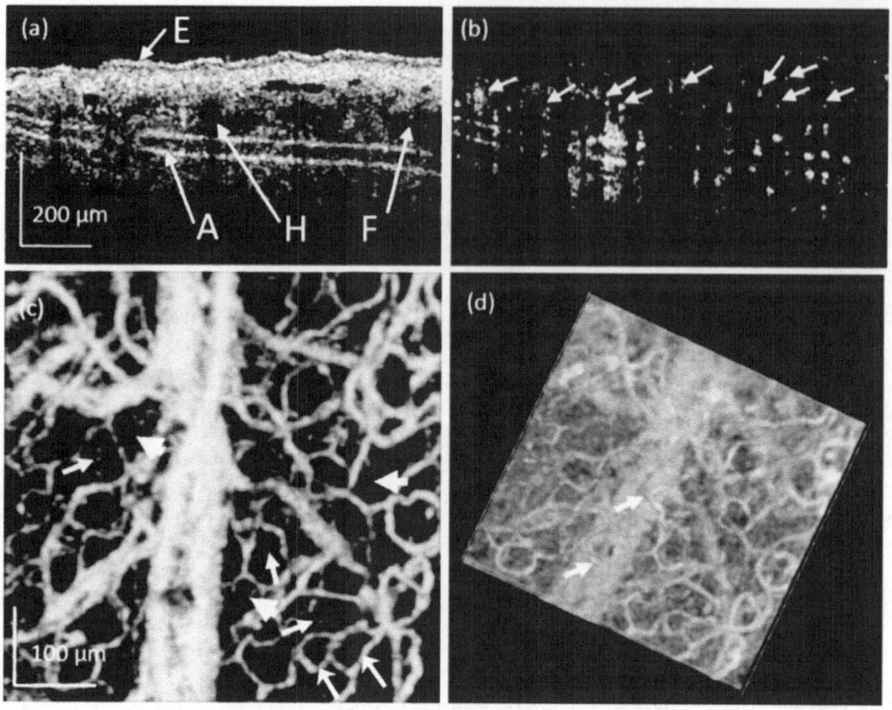

Figure 10.18: (a) Cross-sectional structural image of mouse pinna *in vivo*: A, auricular cartilage; E, epidermis; H, hair follicle; F, fatty subcutaneous tissue; and (b) corresponding blood flow image. (c) 2D projection view of a 3D OMAG image of blood vessels within a $\sim$500 μm$\times$500 μm area and (d) a 3D view rendered by merging the structure with the blood vessels. [86]

(circles) can be imaged and resolved clearly, this image demonstrates the power of OMAG imaging of microcirculations within tissue beds *in vivo*.

10.5 Summary

OMAG and UHS-OMAG are emerging imaging modalities with clear potential in many basic research and medical imaging applications. Because of their exceptionally high spatial resolution and velocity sensitivity, they may provide useful information regarding microcirculation in a number of applications, both in clinical and basic research. For example, OMAG/UHS-OMAG may one day be used to screen for vasoactive drugs, monitor changes in tissue morphology and hemodynamics following pharmacological intervention and photodynamic therapy, evaluate the efficacy of laser treatment in patients with a vascular birthmark (port wine stain), assess the depth of burn wounds, map cortical hemodynamics for brain research, and image blood flow around the eye. Quantification of the local metabolic rate of oxygen consumption would be an exciting extension for OMAG/UHS-OMAG. Another interesting direction would be to combine OMAG with other high-resolution imaging tools, such as laser speckle imaging, confocal microscopy and two-photon microscopy. The fruitful cellular and molecular information provided by these modalities, based on scattering or fluorescence contrast, will be highly complementary.

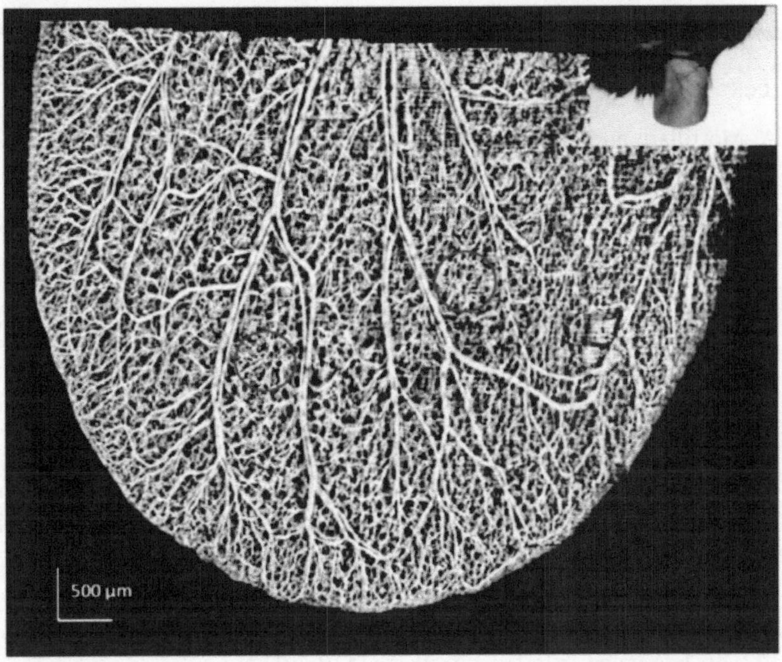

Figure 10.19: Whole-ear vascular network of a living mouse imaged by an SC light source coupled UHS-OMAG system. Insert is a picture of the mouse ear [86].

Acknowledgments

We thank many of our colleagues who have contributed to the OMAG project at the Wang laboratory, particularly the graduate students and postdoctoral fellows. Dr. Wang also acknowledges grant supports from the National Heart, Lung, and Blood Institute (R01 HL093140, R01HL093140S), National Institute of Biomedical Imaging and Bioengineering (R01EB009682), National Institute on Deafness and Other Communication Disorders (R01DC010201, R01DC010201S) and the American Heart Association Grant-in-Aid (0855733G).

References

[1] N.A. Mortillaro and A.E. Taylor, *The Pathophysiology of the Microcirculation*, CRC Press (1994).

[2] P.G. Camici, "Positron emission tomography and myocardial imaging," *Heart* **83**, 75–80 (2000).

[3] P.R. Schvartzman and R.D. White, "Magnetic resonance imaging," in *Textbook of Cardiovascular Medicine*, E.J. Topol (ed.), 2nd ed. Philadelphia: Lippincott Williams & Wilkins, 213–1256 (2002).

[4] A.B. Hertzman and C.R. Spealman, "Observation on the finger volume pulse recorded photoelectrically," *Am. J. Physiol.* **119**, 334 (1937).

[5] A.V.J. Challoner, "Photoelectric plethysmography for estimating cutaneous blood flow," in *Non- Invasive Physiological Measurements*, P. Rolfe (ed.), Vol. 1, Academic Press, London, p. 125 (1979).

[6] G. Holti and K.W. Mitchell, "Estimation of the nutrient skin blood flow using a non-invasivesegmented thermal probe," in *Non-Invasive Physiological Measurements*, P. Rolfe (ed.), Vol. 1, Academic Press, London, p. 113 (1979).

[7] S.S. Kety, "Measurement of regional circulation by the local clearance of radioactive sodium," *Am. Heart J.* **38**, 321 (1949).

[8] P. Sejrsen, "Measurement of cutaneous blood flow by freely diffusable radioactive isotopes. Methodological studies on the washout of krypton-85 and xenon-13 from the cutaneous tissue in man," *Dan. Med. Bull.* **18**, (Suppl. 3), 9 (1971).

[9] W. Groner, J.W. Winkelman, A.G. Harris, C. Ince, G.J. Bouma, K. Messmer, and R.G. Nadeau, "Orthogonal polarization spectral imaging: a new method for study of the microcirculation," *Nat. Med.* **5** (10), 1209 (1999).

[10] R.G. Nadeau and W. Groner,"The role of a new noninvasive imaging technology in the diagnosis of anemia," *J. Nutr.* **131** (5), 1610S (2001).

[11] H. Wayland and P.C. Johnson, "Erythrocyte velocity measurements in microvessels by a two-slit photometric method," *Am. J. Physiol.* **22**, 333 (1967).

[12] A. Bollinger, P. Butti, J.P. Barras, H. Trachsler, and W. Siegenthaler, "Red blood cell velocity in nailfold capillaries of man measured by a television microscopy technique," *Microvasc. Res.* **7**, 61 (1974).

[13] J.G. Stevenson, M.A. Brandestini, T. Weiler, E.A.Howard, M. Eyer, "Digital multigate Doppler with color echo and Doppler display - Diagnosis of atrial and ventricular septal defects," *Circulation* **60**, 205 (1979).

[14] A.M. Iga, S. Sarkar, K M. Sales, M C. Winslet, and A M. Seifalian, "Quantitating therapeutic disruption of tumor blood flow with intravital video microscopy," *Cancer Res.* **66**, 11517-11519 (2006).

[15] R.K. Jain, L.L. Munn, and D. Fukumura, "Dissecting tumour pathophysiology using intravital microscopy," *Nat. Rev. Cancer* **2**, 266–276 (2002).

[16] J.D. Briers, "Laser Doppler, speckle and related techniques for blood perfusion mapping and imaging," *Physiol. Meas.* **22**, 35–66 (2001).

[17] A. Caselli, D.S. Bedi, C. O'Connor, C. Shah, and A. Veves, "Assessment of laser Doppler perfusion imager's *in vivo* reliability: Can it be used for a prospective analysis," *J. Laser Appl.* **14**, 198–202 (2002).

[18] M. Hassan, R.F. Little, A. Vogel, K. Aleman, K. Wyvill, R. Yarchoan, and A.H. Gandjbakhche, "Quantitative assessment of tumor vasculature and response to therapy in Kaposi's sarcoma using functional noninvasive imaging," *Technol. Cancer Res. Treat.* **3**, 451–457 (2004).

[19] J. Sorensen, M. Bengtsson, E.L. Malmqvist, G. Nilsson, and F. Sjoberg, "Laser Doppler perfusion imager (LDPI)–for the assessment of skin blood flow changes following sympathetic blocks," *Acta Anaesthesiol. Scand.* **40**, 1145-1148 (1996).

[20] A. Grinvald, E. Lieke, R.D. Frostig, C.D. Gilbert, and T.N. Wiesel, "Functional architecture of cortex revealed by optical imaging of intrinsic signals," *Nature* **324**, 361–364 (1986).

[21] X.D. Wang, Y. Pang, G. Ku, X. Xie, G. Stoica, and L.-H. Wang, "Non-invasive laser-induced photoacoustic tomography for structural and functional imaging of the brain *in vivo*," *Nat. Biotechnol.* **21**, 803–806 (2003).

[22] H.F. Zhang, K. Maslov, G. Stoica, and L.H.V. Wang, "Functional photoacoustic microscopy for high resolution and noninvasive in vivo imaging," *Nat. Biotechnol.* **24**, 848–851 (2006).

[23] D. Huang, E.A. Swanson, C.P. Lin, J.S. Shuman, W.G. Stinson, W. Chang, M.R. Hee, T. Flotte, K. Gregory, C.A. Puliafito, and J.G. Fujimoto. "Optical coherence tomography," *Science* **254**, 1178–1181, (1991).

[24] A.F. Fercher, W. Drexler, C.K. Hitzenberger, and T. Lasser, "Optical coherence tomography principles and applications," *Rep. Progr. Phys.* **66**, 239–303 (2003).

[25] W. Drexler and J.G. Fujimoto (eds.), *Optical Coherence Tomography: Technology and Applications*, Springer, Berlin (2008).

[26] B.L. Danielson and C.D. Whittenberg, "Guided-wave reflectometry with micrometer resolution," *Appl. Opt.* **26**, 2836–2842 (1987).

[27] K. Takada, I. Yokohama, K. Chida, and J. Noda, "New measurement system for fault location in optical waveguide devices based on an interferometric technique," *Appl. Opt.* **26**, 1603–1606 (1987).

[28] A.F. Fercher, K. Mengedoht, and W. Werner, "Eye-length measurement by interferometry with partially coherent light," *Opt. Lett.* **13**, 1867–1869 (1988).

[29] G. Hausler and M.W. Lindner, "Coherence radar and Spectral radar- new tools for dermatological diagnosis," *J. Biomed. Opt.* **3**, 21–31 (1998).

[30] E.A. Swanson, J.A. Izatt, M.R. Hee, D. Huang, C.P. Lin, J.S. Schuman, C A. Puliafito, and J.G. Fujimoto, "*In vivo* retinal imaging by optical coherence tomography," *Opt. Lett.* **18**, 1864–1866 (1993).

[31] M.R. Hee, D. Huang, E.A. Swanson, J.G. Fujimoto, "Polarization sensitive low-coherence reflectometer for birefringence characterization and ranging," *JOSA* B **9**, 903–908 (1992).

[32] S.J. Matcher, M. Cope, and D.T. Delpy, "*In vivo* measurements of the wavelength dependence of tissue-scattering coefficients between 760 and 900 nm measured with time-resolved spectroscopy," *Appl. Opt. 36*, 386–396 (1997).

[33] J.M. Schmitt, "OCT elastography: Imaging microscopic deformation and strain of tissue," *Opt. Express* **3**, 199–211 (1998).

[34] Z.P. Chen, T.E. Milner, D. Dave, and J.S. Nelson, "Optical Doppler tomographic imaging of fluid flow velocity in highly scattering media," *Opt. Lett.* **22**, 64–66 (1997).

[35] Z.P. Chen, T.E. Milner, S. Srinivas, X.J. Wang, A. Malekafzali, M.J.C. van Gemert, and J.S. Nelson, "Noninvasive imaging of in vivo blood flow velocity using optical Doppler tomography," *Opt. Lett.* **22**, 1–3, (1997).

[36] J.A. Izatt, M.D. Kulkarni, S. Yazdanfar, J.K. Barton, and A.J. Welsh, "*In vivo* color Doppler imaging of picoliter blood volumes using optical coherence tomography," *Opt. Lett.* **22**, 1439–1441 (1997).

[37] Z. Chen, Y. Zhao, S.M. Srinivas, J.S. Nelson, N. Prakash, and R.D. Frostig, "Optical Doppler tomography," *IEEE J. Sel. Top. Quantum Electron.* **5**, 1134–1141 (1999).

[38] B.R. White, M.C. Pierce, N. Nassif, B. Cense, B.H. Park, G.J. Tearney, B.E. Bouma, T.C. Chen, and J.F. de Boer, "*In vivo* dynamic human retinal blood flow imaging using ultra-high-speed spectral domain optical Doppler tomography," *Opt. Express* **11**, 3490–3497 (2003).

[39] R.A. Leitgeb, L. Schmetterer, W. Drexler, A.F. Fercher, R.J. Zawadzki, and T. Bajraszewski, "Real-time assessment of retinal blood flow with ultrafast acquisition by color Doppler Fourier domain optical coherence tomography," *Opt. Express* **11**, 3116–3121 (2003).

[40] R.A. Leitgeb, L. Schmetterer, C.K. Hitzenberger, A.F. Fercher, F. Berisha, M. Wojtkowski, and T. Bajraszewski, "Real-time measurement of *in vitro* flow by Fourier-domain color Doppler optical coherence tomography," *Opt. Lett.* **29**, 171–173 (2004).

[41] S. Makita, Y. Hong, M. Yamanari, T. Yatagai, and Y. Yasuno, "Optical coherence angiography," *Opt. Express* **14**, 7821–7840 (2006).

[42] R.K. Wang, "High resolution visualization of fluid dynamics with Doppler Optical Coherence Tomography," *Measurement Science and Technology* **15**, 725–733 (2004).

[43] R.K. Wang, S.L. Jacques, Z. Ma, S. Hurst, S. Hanson, and A. Gruber, "Three dimensional optical angiography," *Opt. Express* **15**, 4083–4097 (2007).

[44] R.K. Wang and S. Hurst, "Mapping of cerebro-vascular blood perfusion in mice with skin and skull intact by Optical Micro-AngioGraphy at 1.3 μm wavelength," *Opt. Express* **15**, 11402 (2007).

[45] R. K. Wang and H.M. Subhash, "Optical microangiography: high-resolution 3-D imaging of blood flow," *Optics & Photonics News* **20**, 40–46 (2009).

[46] R.K. Wang, "Directional blood flow imaging in volumetric optical microangiography achieved by digital frequency modulation," *Opt. Lett.* **33**, 1878–1880 (2008).

[47] R.K. Wang, "*In vivo* full range complex Fourier domain optical coherence tomography," *Appl. Phys. Lett.* **90**, 054103 (2007).

[48] Y.H. Zhao, Z.P. Chen, Z.H. Ding, H. Ren, and J.S. Nelson, "Real-time phase-resolved functional optical coherence tomography by use of optical Hilbert transformation," *Opt. Lett.* **25**, 98–100 (2002).

[49] H.W. Ren, Z.H. Ding, Y.H. Zhao, J. Miao, J.S. Nelson, and Z.P. Chen, "Phase-resolved functional optical coherence tomography: simultaneous imaging of *in situ* tissue structure, blood flow velocity, standard deviation, birefringence, and Stokes vectors in human skin," *Opt. Lett.* **27**, 1702 (2002).

[50] B.R. White, M.C. Pierce, N. Nassif, B. Cense, B. Park, G. Tearney, B. Bouma, T. Chen, and J. de Boer, "*In vivo* dynamic human retinal blood flow imaging using ultra-high-speed spectral domain optical Dopplertomography," *Opt. Express* **11**, 3490–3497 (2003).

[51] V.X.D. Yang, M.L. Gordon, A. Mok, Y. Zhao, Z. Chen, R.S.C. Cobbold, B.C. Wilson, and I.A. Vitkin, "Improved phase-resolved optical Doppler tomography using the Kasai velocity estimator and histogramsegmentation," *Opt. Commun.* **208**, 209–222 (2002).

[52] L. An and R.K. Wang, "*In vivo* volumetric imaging of vascular perfusion within human retina and choroids with optical micro-angiography," *Opt. Express* **16**, 11438–11452 (2008).

[53] M. Mujat, R.C. Chan, B. Cense, B.H. Park, C. Joo, T. Akkin, T. C. Chen, and J.F. de Boer, "Retinal nerve fiber layer thickness map determined from optical coherence tomography images," *Opt. Express* **13**, 9480–9491(2005).

[54] R.K. Wang and Lin An, "Doppler optical micro-angiography for volumetric imaging of vascular perfusion *in vivo*," *Opt. Express* **17**, 8926–8940 (2009).

[55] V. Tuchin, *Tissue Optics: Light Scattering Methods and Instruments for Medical Diagnosis*. ISBN number: 0819464333. SPIE (2007).

[56] C. Werner and K. Engelhard, "Pathophysiology of traumatic brain injury," *Br. J. Anaesth.* **99** (1), 4–9 (2007).

[57] G.J. Bouma and J.P. Muizelaar, "Cerebral blood flow, cerebral blood volume, and cerebrovascular reactivity after severe head injury," *J. Neurotrauma* **9**, S333–S348 (1992).

[58] Y. Jia, N. Alkayed and R.K. Wang, "Potential of optical microangiography to monitor cerebral blood perfusion and vascular plasticity following traumatic brain injury in mice *in vivo*," *J. Biomed. Opt.* **14**, 040505 (2009).

[59] C.A. Guyton, "Local and humoral control of blood flow by the tissue," in *Textbook of Medical Physiology*, Philadelphia: W.B. Saunders, 195–202 (2006).

[60] R. Morgan, C.W. Kreipke, G. Roberts, M. Bagchi, J.A. Rafols, "Neovascularization following traumatic brain injury: possible evidence for both angiogenesis and vasculogenesis," *Neurological Research* **29** (4), 375–381 (2007).

[61] A. Bill and G.O. Sperber, "Control of retinal and choroidal blood flow," *Eye* **4**, 319–325 (1990).

[62] S. Jiao, R. Knighton, X. Huang, G. Gregori, and C.A. Puliafito, "Simultaneous acquisition of sectional and fundus ophthalmic images with spectral-domain optical coherence tomography," *Opt. Express* **13**, 444–452 (2005).

[63] Lin An, Hrebesh M. Subhush, David J. Wilson, and Ruikang K. Wang, "High-resolution wide-field imaging of retinal and choroidal blood perfusion with optical microangiography," *J. Biomed. Opt.* **15**, 026011 (2010).

[64] J.T.Y. Chou and K. Rodgers, "Respiration of tissues lining the mammalian membranous labyrinth," *J. Laryngol. Otol.* **76**, 341–351 (1962).

[65] R. Thalmann, T. Miyoshi, and I. Thalmann, "The influence of ischemia upon the energy reserves of inner ear tissues," *Laryngoscope* **82**, 2249–2272 (1972).

[66] A. Axelsson, D. Vertes, and J. Miller, "Immediate noise effects on cochlear vasculature in the guinea pig," *Acta Otolaryngol.* **91**, 237–246 (1981).

[67] J. Hawkins, Jr., "The role of vasoconstriction in noise-induced hearing loss," *Ann. Otol. Rhinol. Laryngol.* **80**, 903–913 (1971).

[68] W.S. Quirk and M.D. Seidman, "Cochlear vascular changes in response to loud noise," *Otol. Neurotol.* **16**, 322–325 (1995).

[69] M. Lawrence, "Circulation in the capillaries of the basilar membrane," *Laryngoscope* **80**, 1364–1375 (1970).

[70] S. Millen, R. Toohill, and R. Lehman, "Sudden sensorineural hearing loss: Operative complication in non-otologic surgery," *Laryngoscope* **92**, 613–617 (1982).

[71] H. Plasse, F. Spencer, M. Mittleman, and J. Frost, "Unilateral sudden loss of hearing: An unusual complication of cardiac operation," *J. Thorac. Cardiovasc. Surg.* **79**, 822–826 (1980).

[72] J. Prazma, G. K. Rodgers, and H.C. Pillsbury, "Cochlear blood flow: Effect of noise," *Arch. Otolaryngol.* **109**, 611–615 (1983).

[73] Z. Selmani, I. Pyykkö, H. Ishizaki, and T.I. Marttila, "Cochlear blood flow measurement in patients with Meniere's disease and other inner ear disorders," *Acta Otolaryngol.* **121**, 10–13 (2001).

[74] F.L. Weille, S.R. Gargano, R. Pfister, D. Martinez, and J.W. Irwin, "Circulation of the spiral ligament and stria vascularis of living guinea pig: Experimental study," *AMA Arch. Otolaryngol.* **59**, 731–738 (1954).

[75] H.B. Perlman and R.S. Kimura, "Observations of the living blood vessels of the cochlea," *Ann. Otol. Rhinol. Laryngol.* **64**, 1176–1192 (1955).

[76] N. Choudhury, F. Chen, X. Shi, A.L. Nuttall, and R.K. Wang, "Volumetric imaging of blood flow within cochlea in gerbil *in vivo*," *IEEE J. Sel. Top. Quantum Electron.* **16**, 524–529 (2009).

[77] R.K. Wang, L. An, P. Francis, and D.J. Wilson, "Depth-resolved imaging of capillary networks in retina and choroid using ultrahigh sensitive optical microangiography," *Optics letters* **35**(9), 1467–1469 (2010).

[78] B.J. Vakoc, S.H. Yun, J.F. de Boer, G.J. Tearney, and B.E. Bouma, "Phase-resolved optical frequency domain imaging," *Opt. Express* **13**, 5483–5492 (2005).

[79] B.H. Park, M.C. Pierce, B. Cense, S.H. Yun, M. Mujat, G.J. Tearney, B.E. Bouma and J.F. de Boer, "Real-time fiber-based multi-functional spectral-domain optical coherence tomography at 1.3 μm," *Opt.Express* **13**, 3931–3944 (2005).

[80] Lin An, Jia Qin, and Ruikang K Wang, "Ultrahigh sensitive optical microangiography for *in vivo* imaging of microcirculations within human skin tissue beds," *Opt. Express* **18**, 8220–8228 (2010).

[81] W. Drexler, U. Morgner, F.X. Krtner, C. Pitris, S.A. Boppart, X. D. Li, E.P. Ippen, and J.G. Fujimoto, "*In vivo* ultrahigh-resolution optical coherence tomography," *Opt. Lett.* **24**, 1221–1223 (1999).

[82] R. Leitgeb, W. Drexler, A. Unterhuber, B. Hermann, T. Bajraszewski, T. Le, A. Stingl, and A. Fercher, "Ultrahigh resolution Fourier domain optical coherence tomography," *Opt. Express* **12**, 2156–2165 (2004).

[83] B. Povazay, K. Bizheva, A. Unterhuber, B. Hermann, H. Sattmann, A.F. Fercher, W. Drexler, A. Apolonski, W.J. Wadsworth, J.C. Knight, P.St.J. Russell, M. Vetterlein, and E. Scherzer, "Submicrometer axial resolution optical coherence tomography," *Opt. Lett.* **27**, 1800–1802 (2002).

[84] Stefan Kray, Felix Spöler, Michael Först, and Heinrich Kurz, "High-resolution simultaneous dual-band spectral domain optical coherence tomography," *Opt. Lett.* **34**, 1970–1972 (2009).

[85] Felix Spöler, Stefan Kray, Patrik Grychtol, Barbara Hermes, Jörg Bornemann, Michael Först, and Heinrich Kurz, "Simultaneous dual-band ultra-high resolution optical coherence tomography," *Opt. Express* **15**, 10832–10841 (2007).

[86] Zhongwei Zhi, Jia Qin, Lin An, and Ruikang K. Wang, "Supercontinuum light source enables *in vivo* optical microangiography of capillary vessels within tissue beds," *Opt. Lett.* **36**, 3169–3171 (2011).

11

High-Speed Photoacoustic Tomography

Liang Song

Institute of Biomedical and Health Engineering, Shenzhen Institutes of Advanced Technology, Chinese Academy of Sciences, Shenzhen, China, LIANG.SONG@SIAT.AC.CN

Zijian Guo and Lihong V. Wang*

Optical Imaging Laboratory, Department of Biomedical Engineering, Washington University in St. Louis, St. Louis, Missouri

**Corresponding author: LHWANG@WUSTL.EDU*

11.1 Introduction

Traditional diagnostic imaging technologies—including ultrasound, x-ray computed tomography, and magnetic resonance imaging—have dramatically improved patient care in the clinic. However, these technologies still have limited ability to detect small lesions. In most cases, the detectable lesions are ~ 1 cm in diameter, corresponding to $\sim 10^9$ cells (including circulating and microscopic metastatic deposits) and representing $\sim 2/3$ of the natural history of a cancer [1]. Consequently, the window of opportunity for treatment before a tumor reaches its lethal stage is narrow. Hence, it is imperative to develop novel technologies capable of detecting neoplasia early.

Nonionizing biomedical optical imaging is highly desirable because of its rich contrast. In particular, optical absorption—to which photoacoustic tomography is sensitive—can be used to obtain physiological parameters such as the total concentration and oxygenation of hemoglobin. While the total concentration of hemoglobin is related to angiogenesis, the oxygenation of hemoglobin is related to hyper-metabolism. Since both angiogenesis and hypermetabolism are hallmarks of cancer, photoacoustic tomography can potentially provide early-cancer detection.

11.1.1 Fundamentals of photoacoustic tomography

Photoacoustic (or optoacoustic) tomography (PAT) is a novel hybrid imaging modality based on the photoacoustic effect, which describes the generation of acoustic waves upon absorption of photons [2, 3]. Although Alexander Graham Bell discovered this effect as far back as 1880 [4], it was not until the early 1990s—after the technological advances of lasers, computers, and computed tomography—that its medical applications started to become apparent [5, 6]. When a short laser pulse is absorbed by structures (such as microvessels) in biological tissue, wideband ultrasonic (photoacoustic) waves are produced from a thermal- and stress-confined thermoelastic expansion [7]. Photoacoustic signals are then detected and reconstructed to form an image, whose amplitude reflects, essentially, the optical absorption properties and the Grueneisen parameter of issue. In PAT, both ballistic and diffuse photons are utilized to generate photoacoustic signals, and the spatial resolution is determined primarily by ultrasonic rather than optical detection. Since ultrasonic scattering in biological tissue is two to three orders of magnitude weaker than optical scattering per unit path-length, high spatial resolution can be achieved at depths beyond the optical transport mean free path.

In general, if the laser excitation conforms with both the thermal and the stress confinements, the initial local acoustic pressure rise p_0 can be described by [8]:

$$p_0 = \Gamma \eta_{th} \mu_a F, \tag{11.1}$$

where Γ is the dimensionless Grueneisen parameter, η_{th} is the percentage of the deposited optical energy ($\mu_a \times F$) converted into heat, μ_a is the optical absorption coefficient (cm^{-1}), and F is the optical fluence (J/cm^2). It can be seen that p_0 depends on the optical energy deposition as well as the thermal and mechanical properties of the tissue. In conventional photoacoustic soft tissue imaging, Γ and η_{th} are usually treated as constants, and the initial pressure rise reflects, essentially, the optical energy deposition.

In biological tissue, the primary endogenous chromophores in the visible spectral region are oxy- and deoxy-hemoglobin (HbO_2 and HbR) and melanin. The strong intrinsic absorption of HbO_2 and HbR enables blood vessels to be readily imaged photoacoustically, with high contrast and without using ionizing radiation. With multi-wavelength measurements, changes in both the concentration and the oxygen saturation of hemoglobin can be quantified. Hence, photoacoustic functional imaging of endogenous hemoglobin contrast is feasible with both high sensitivity and high resolution at great depths.

Existing high-resolution, purely optical imaging technologies—including confocal microscopy [9], two-photon microscopy [10], and optical coherence tomography (OCT) [11]—have had a profound impact on biomedicine. However, they rely on the detection of ballistic photons, and thus cannot image beyond the optical transport mean free path ($\sim$ 1 mm in human skin) [8]. Furthermore, since none of them sense optical absorption directly, label-free functional imaging is not easily available with these modalities.

PAT overcomes the limitations of existing high-resolution optical imaging technologies; it combines excellent optical contrast with high ultrasonic resolution at depths beyond the quasi-ballistic regime or the optical diffusion limit, defined by the optical transport mean free path [2, 3]. In addition, the maximum imaging depth and the spatial resolution of PAT are scalable with ultrasonic and optical parameters [12]. PAT is emerging as a viable technology for both clinical and preclinical imaging. It has demonstrated many biomedical applications, including the imaging of tumor angiogenesis [13-16], tumor hypoxia [17], gene expression [18], hemoglobin oxygenation [19, 20], breast cancer [21], and sentinel lymph nodes [22–25].

Figure 11.1 shows the principles of a representative PAT system and two *in vivo* functional images acquired with the system. In the system, a Q-switched Nd:YAG laser was adopted to provide 532-nm laser pulses with a pulse width of 6.5 ns. A single-element, unfocused 3.5-MHz ultrasonic transducer (V383, Panametrics) with an 88% −6-dB bandwidth was used to detect the photoacoustic waves. To produce a tomographic image, the transducer was scanned around the object to detect, with laser illumination, the photoacoustic signals at each scanning position. Then, a photoacoustic back-projection algorithm was used for image reconstruction [26].

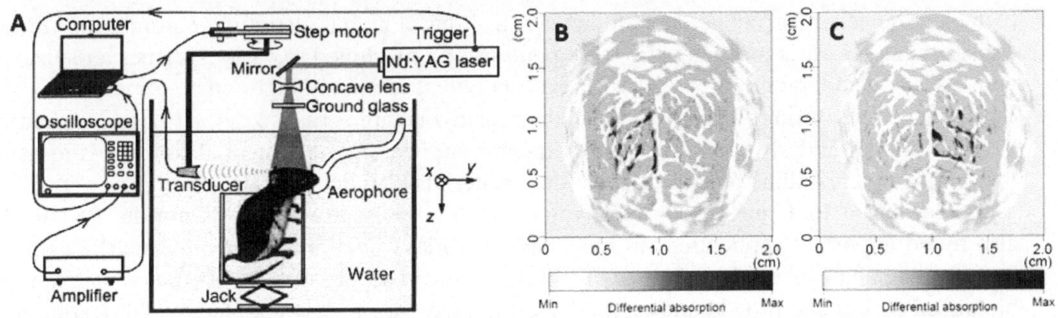

Figure 11.1: (See color insert.) Representative PAT system and functional photoacoustic images. (A) Schematic of the PAT system for noninvasive *in vivo* transdermal and transcranial imaging; (B,C) *In vivo* functional PAT images corresponding to the left- and right-side whisker stimulations, respectively, acquired in a rat with the skin and skull intact. The two PAT images of functional representations of whiskers (red) are superimposed on a PAT image of the vasculature (gray) in the cerebral cortex. Reprinted with permission from reference [26].

11.1.2 Motivations for high-speed photoacoustic tomography

High imaging speed is valuable to both clinical practice and preclinical research. In the clinic, time is critical; to make decisions promptly, clinicians increasingly require real-time imaging. High-speed imaging is highly desirable in preclinical research as well, such as small animal imaging for drug discovery, where high-throughput is important. In addition, a high imaging speed enables PAT (i) to reduce motion artifacts that are due to, for instance, the breathing of subjects, (ii) to reduce cost and patient discomfort, and (iii) to potentially reduce risks associated with minimally invasive clinical procedures, such as intravascular imaging.

From a historical perspective, ultrasonic array technology has revolutionized ultrasonography by enabling real-time imaging; it is now the standard technology for clinical ultrasonic imaging systems. The recent use of ultrasonic arrays for PAT has also led to high-speed and even real-time photoacoustic imaging. In addition, PAT based on ultrasonic arrays can make full use of commercial diagnostic ultrasonic instruments. If we can leverage existing commercial ultrasonic platforms for developing novel PAT technologies, we will not only enable high imaging speed but also provide a technology that can be easily accepted by physicians. Since ultrasonic transducer arrays represent such an important enabling technology for high-speed PAT, we have dedicated the section below to introducing the basic principles and technology development of modern ultrasonic transducer arrays.

11.2 Ultrasonic Transducer Arrays and Image Formation

11.2.1 Materials for ultrasonic transducers

The heart of an ultrasonic transducer is a piezoelectric element that can convert acoustic energy to electrical signals and vice versa. Although a number of natural materials, including quartz and tourmaline, are piezoelectric, their piezoelectric properties are not strong enough to make efficient medical ultrasonic transducers. Presently, lead-zirconate-titanate (PZT), a ferroelectric ceramic of strong piezoelectric properties, is the most popular material for conventional diagnostic ultrasonic transducers. PZT has many advantages for fabricating ultrasonic transducers [27, 28]: (i) it has a high electromechanical conversion efficiency; (ii) it has a high transmitting constant for ultrasonic transmission; (iii) it is mechanically strong and can be machined to various shapes and sizes; (iv) with a Curie temperature of $\sim$ 190°C, it can operate at relatively high temperatures and is stable over long periods of time. However, due to their relatively large grain sizes (5–10 μm), conventional PZT are not particularly suited for high-frequency applications. A potential solution is to develop fine-grain polycrystalline ferroelectric ceramic materials [29].

In addition to PZT, piezoelectric polymers, such as polyvinylidence difluoride (PVDF), have also found important applications in medical ultrasonics. Such materials are usually flexible and inexpensive, and possess both low acoustic impedance (which allows impedance matching with biological tissue) and broad bandwidth. Therefore, they are widely adopted for fabricating miniature hydrophones, which are useful for probing and measuring the beam characteristics of medical ultrasonic transducers. However, due to their low transmitting constant and low electromechanical conversion efficiency (sensitivity), they are seldom used for making transmit-receive ultrasonic transducers, and are not widely used for PAT as well.

Recently, a new type of material, composite piezoelectric ceramic, has emerged as one of the most promising candidates for fabricating high-performance, high-frequency ultrasonic transducers [30]. These composites are usually mixed with a piezoelectric ceramic and a low-density polymer. In general, they have both a lower acoustic impedance and a higher electromechanical coupling coefficient than ordinary ceramic. Compared with conventional PZT, composites often provide higher sensitivity and wider bandwidth: both are important for high-frequency applications. Recent progress in fabrication technology has enabled the preparation of PZT-polymer 1-3 composites for applications in the 1–80 MHz range [31, 32].

Relaxor-based ferroelectric single crystals—such as lead magnesium niobate-lead titanate (PMN-PT) and lead zinc niobate-lead titanate (PZN-PT)—can also be used to fabricate medical ultrasonic transducers. In particular, single crystals show great promise for high-frequency ultrasonic transducer applications. They possess superior piezoelectric properties, including a high electromechanical coupling coefficient ($k_{33} > 0.9$), a dielectric constant of 1000–5000 with low dielectric loss, and an exceptional piezoelectric coefficient of $d_{33} > 2000pC/N$. However, for single crystals to be effectively used for high-frequency applications, further investigations in crystal growth, micromachining techniques, and testing are still needed [30].

11.2.2 Ultrasonic array construction and image formation

A simple single-element ultrasonic transducer primarily consists of a piezoelectric element, a front matching layer, and a backing layer. The piezoelectric element resonates at a vibrational frequency given by (with the lowest resonant frequency being $n = 1$):

$$f_0 = n\frac{c}{2L}, \tag{11.2}$$

where c is the speed of sound, L is the thickness of the piezoelectric element, and n is an odd integer. In other words, the thickness is an odd-integer multiple of the half-wavelength (with an even-integer multiple, the signal would vanish). When an ultrasonic transducer is excited by an electrical source, it rings at its natural resonance frequency. For continuous wave (CW) application, the transducers are air-backed to direct as much energy in the forward direction (i.e., the direction toward the transducer front surface or biological tissue) as possible, which also generates reverberation (i.e., multiple reflections). However, for most medical applications, a short ultrasonic pulse is desirable for high axial resolution. Thus, an absorbing backing layer is employed to damp out reverberation. In addition, to overcome the acoustic impedance mismatch between the active layer and the medium for efficient energy transmission, a front matching layer is adopted.

In most of today's clinical ultrasonic imaging settings—in which relatively low ultrasonic frequencies of 1–15 MHz are used—ultrasonic transducer arrays, rather than single-element transduc-

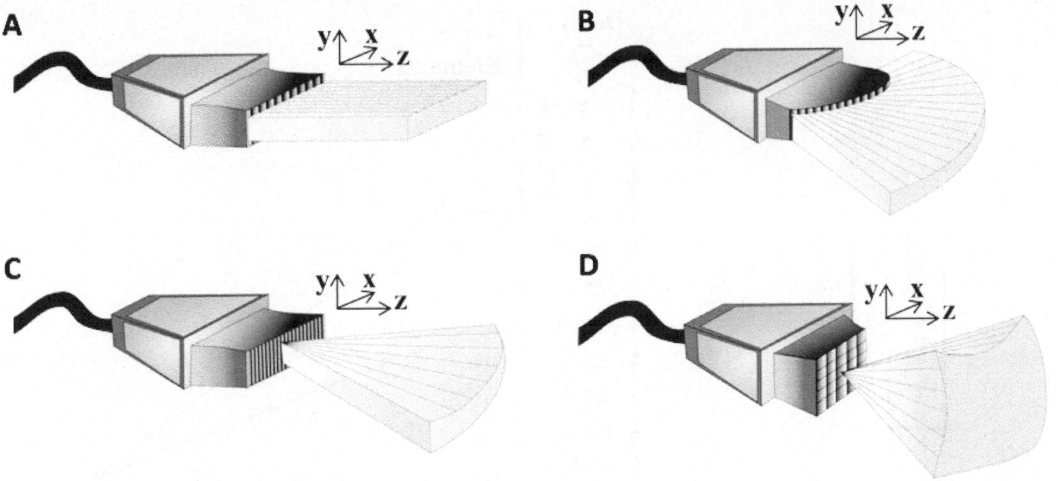

Figure 11.2: Constructions of various ultrasonic arrays and their respective imaging fields. (A) Linear array; (B) curvilinear array; (C) phased array; (D) 2D array. Coordinates x, y, and z represent the azimuthal, elevational, and axial directions, respectively. In D, x and y become symmetric.

ers, are employed. A transducer array consists of a group of closely spaced piezoelectric elements; each element has its own electrical connections. This allows elements to be activated individually or in groups to emit and/or to receive ultrasonic waves, enabling image formation by electronically sweeping an ultrasonic beam.

The active elements of ultrasonic transducer arrays can be arranged into various forms, resulting in different types of arrays. In this section, we will review the basics of the following types of arrays (Fig. 11.2): (i) linear array; (ii) curvilinear array; (iii) phased array; (iv) 2D array.

Linear and curvilinear arrays consist of groups of rectangular piezoelectric elements arranged side by side (Fig. 11.2(A,B)). They are usually ~ 1 cm wide and 10–15 cm long, with 128–512 active elements. Individual ultrasonic beams are emitted or received by activating groups of elements in succession. As a result, to produce a 2D image, instead of mechanically scanning a single-element transducer, an ultrasonic beam is electronically scanned across the face of the transducer array. If the electronic sequencing is sufficiently fast, high-frame-rate (>30 Hz) imaging can be achieved. Since the ultrasonic beams travel essentially perpendicular to the surface of the array, the linear array has a rectangular image field, while the curvilinear array has a fan-shaped image field. The size of a pitch—the distance between the centers of two neighboring elements—in a linear or curvilinear array ranges from $\lambda/2$ to $3\lambda/2$, where λ is the center ultrasonic wavelength.

Phased arrays are similar to linear arrays in construction, but are operated quite differently. Compared with a linear array, a phased array (Fig. 11.2(C)) is usually smaller (1–3 cm long) and possesses fewer active elements (64–256 elements), with a pitch of $\lambda/2$ or smaller. Individual ultrasonic beams are produced or received by activating all elements in the array, with appropriate delays applied to the stimuli applied to or signals received by each element. As a result, the generated or received ultrasonic beams can be both steered and focused.

Taking reception as an example, Fig. 11.3 shows the basic principles of the delay-and-sum beamformation, which is used to form B-scan images in most clinical ultrasonic imaging systems. With respect to an image point $P(R, \theta)$, where R and θ are the radius and polar angle, respectively, in a polar coordinate system with the pole zero set at the center of the ultrasonic array (Figure 11.3), the

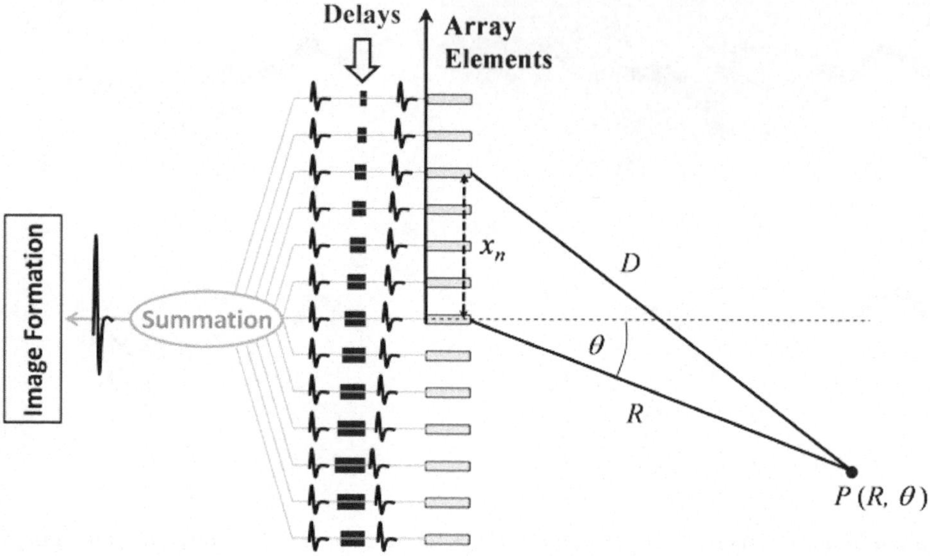

Figure 11.3: Schematic of the delay-and-sum beam formation. x_n, distance between element n and the center element; θ, steering angle ($-90° \leq \theta \leq 90°$); $P(R,\theta)$, image point.

time difference for acoustic waves to reach the center element and element n is given by:

$$\tau_n(R,\theta) = \frac{\sqrt{(x_n - R\sin\theta)^2 + R^2\cos^2\theta}}{c} - \frac{R}{c}, \tag{11.3}$$

where x_n is the distance between element n and the center element, c is the speed of sound in the medium, and θ satisfies $-90° \leq \theta \leq 90°$. As a result, for the signals received by each element n, by first applying a delay τ_n relative to the center element, and then adding the delayed signals together, we approximately recover the signals from the image point P. To enhance the image quality, similar delays can be applied during ultrasonic transmission, so that the emitted ultrasonic waves can also be steered toward a specific direction and/or focused at a specific point (transmit focus).

In reality, additional off-axis radiations resulting from grating lobes and side lobes may exist. If they are not handled properly, the lateral resolution will deteriorate. The grating lobes originate from the division of the transducer into regularly spaced individual elements. They are similar to the diffraction pattern from an optical grating. The angles at which the diffraction peaks emerge can be computed by the following equation:

$$\alpha_g = \sin^{-1}(\frac{n\lambda}{d}), \tag{11.4}$$

where $n = \pm 1, \pm 2, \ldots, \lambda$ is the acoustic wavelength, and d is the pitch of the array. For grating lobes to occur at angles greater than 90°, d needs to be smaller than $\lambda/2$, under which the ultrasonic array is said to be fully sampled. In addition, randomizing the pitches between elements is another way to suppress grating lobes. To reduce the side lobes, apodization can be used. Apodization means gradually decreasing the vibrational amplitudes across the transducer elements with an increasing distance from the center of the transducer. It is usually accomplished by using more power to excite the innermost elements.

Linear arrays—including curvilinear and phased linear arrays—can be focused and/or steered in only one plane: the azimuthal plane. In the elevational plane, focusing is usually achieved with a cylindrical acoustic lens or a cylindrically curved transducer surface. At present, the elevational resolution is the worst measure among all resolutions for linear-array ultrasonic imaging systems.

A 2D ultrasonic array provides not only high-speed 3D imaging but also improved elevational resolution. A 2D ultrasonic array (Fig. 11.2(D)) consists of a 2D matrix of active elements, and thus is also termed as the matrix array. With a 2D array, electronic focusing can then be performed in both of the transverse directions, resulting in a more uniform lateral resolution. However, due to the huge number of elements required for 2D array construction, the fabrication—the handling of electrical interconnections, electrical impedance mismatching, and the processing of small elements—of 2D arrays is still quite challenging [28, 33]. At present, only a very limited choice of commercial 2D arrays (e.g., the Philips xMATRIX array) is available [34].

Other types of ultrasonic arrays, not discussed above, include, for example, annular arrays that can achieve dynamic and isotropic lateral focusing but require mechanical sector scanning for 2D imaging. In addition, some types of ultrasonic arrays (such as circular arrays) uncommon in today's clinical ultrasonic imaging settings are nonetheless particularly useful for building PAT systems (For details, please refer to Section 11.3).

11.3 Photoacoustic Tomography Using Low-Frequency Ultrasonic Arrays

Among the numerous advantages of PAT, imaging scalability and penetration depth are highly beneficial for many preclinical and clinical applications [7, 35], such as small animal imaging [26, 36], breast cancer imaging [37–39], and sentinel lymph node image guided biopsy [40–42]. Properly designed photoacoustic imaging systems have demonstrated imaging depths of several centimeters in tissue [38, 40, 43–51]. On the detection side, PAT resembles ultrasonography (US) [52], where acoustic attenuation limits the detectable penetration of sound waves in the biological tissue. Since ultrasonic wave attenuation in biological tissue has a power law dependence on the frequency, most of the clinical ultrasonic scanners operate between 1–15 MHz to allow centimeters penetration depth. In this section, we review the recent development of high-speed low-frequency PAT which can image several centimeters deep in biological tissues with optical absorption contrast and ultrasonic resolution. Three representative systems with cylindrical (circular), spherical (arc), and planar (linear) detection geometries are discussed in detail.

11.3.1 Systems based on cylindrical or circular detection geometry

Figure 11.4(A) shows the schematic of a PAT system for small animal imaging based on a ring array [36, 48]. The irradiation source was a tunable Ti-Sapphire laser with a 12-ns pulse duration and a 10-Hz pulse repetition rate. The laser beam passed through a conical lens to form a ring-shaped cross-section, which was projected around the object. The fluence of each laser pulse on the tissue was well below 20 mJ/cm^2, the American National Standards Institute (ANSI) safety standard. The detection side of the PA imaging system is a 512-element full-ring array. The diameter of the ring is 5 cm, and the center frequency of each element is 5 MHz with 80% bandwidth. Each array element is cylindrically focused, forming an imaging slice of about 1 mm thickness within a central imaging region of a diameter of 20 mm. The system provides uniform radial and tangential resolutions of around 0.1 mm. With 64 data acquisition (DAQ) channels, a complete 2D scan requires eight laser shots. The system provides an imaging frame rate of 0.625 Hz without averaging. By vertically scanning samples, the system resembles the cylindrical detection geometry and 3D PAT images are obtained.

The unique full-ring design enables high quality cross-sectional imaging of small animals. Fig-

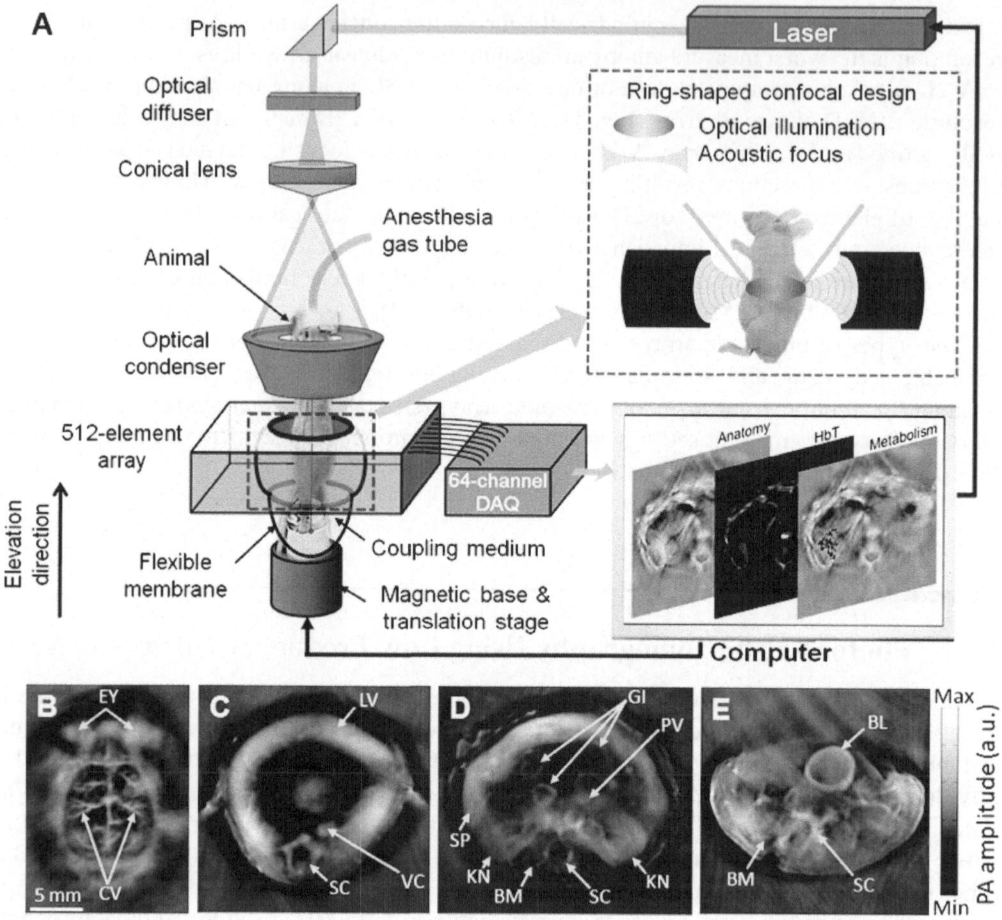

Figure 11.4: (See color insert.) (A) System configurations of the full-ring photoacoustic computed tomography system. (B)—(E) *In vivo* PAT images of nude mice at different anatomical locations. BL, bladder; BM, backbone muscle; CV, cortical vessels; EY, eyes; GI, GI tract; KN, kidney; LV, liver; PV, portal vein; SC, spinal cord; SP, spleen; VC, vena cava. Reprinted with permission from reference [53].

ures 11.4(B)—(E) show serial cross-sectional images of $\sim$ 6-week-old healthy athymic mice in axial views. Figure 11.4(B) is an *in vivo* cortical vessel image acquired through the intact scalp and skull. Figures 11.4(C)—(E) showing the endogenous hemoglobin contrast were acquired at 760 nm. The liver, spleen, and kidneys are clearly visible. Additionally, detailed vascular structures within these organs are also visible, demonstrating that the system can be used for whole-body angiographic imaging without injecting exogenous contrasts. The spinal cord, stomach, and gastrointestinal tracts are shown in the image due to their surrounding microvasculature. Major blood vessels, such as *vena cava*, are also clearly visible. Figure 11.4(E) is an *in vivo* image of a mouse bladder acquired 30 minutes after tail vein administration of IRDye800-2DG. Using exogenous optical contrast (e.g., near-infrared dyes), the system can also image organs with little blood. The urinary bladder showed strong contrast as it was filled with the dye excreted by the kidneys.

The ring-array based PAT system provides high quality cross-sectional images in real time. In principle, it can obtain cross-sectional images in real-time at a frame rate equal to the laser pulse repetition rate. However, it also suffers from non-uniform spatial resolution in three dimensions.

The elevational resolution (∼1 mm), which relies on fixed acoustic foci, is usually worse than the in-plane resolution (radial and tangential resolutions, ∼ 0.1 mm) due to the cylindrical detection geometry. A novel reconstruction algorithm was developed to partially mitigate this issue [36].

11.3.2 Systems based on spherical or arc detection geometry

As shown in Fig. 11.5(A), a spherical detection geometry was developed [54] to obtain 3D PAT images with relatively uniform spatial resolutions. The imaging system consists of four main components: fiber-optic light delivery, a mouse holder, an ultrasonic array, and DAQ electronics. Two laser sources were employed: (i) an Alexandrite laser (Ta-2, Light Age, Inc., Somerset, New Jersey), operating at a 755-nm wavelength, a 10-Hz pulse repetition rate, energy of ∼100 mJ per pulse, and a pulse duration of ∼75 ns; and (ii) Nd:YAG laser (Brilliant, Quantel, Bozeman, Montana), operating at a 1064-nm wavelength, a 10-Hz pulse repetition rate, ∼100 mJ of energy per pulse, and a pulse duration of ∼15 ns. Light delivery was performed orthogonally to the array of acoustic transducers by a bifurcated, randomized fiber bundle (Schott AG, Germany) of 48 inches in length. After leaving the fiber, the two light beams were respectively expanded to a diameter of 8 cm at the target.

The PA signals were acquired with a 64-element arc-shaped piezocomposite array custom-built by Imasonic, SAS (France). The center frequency of the ultrasonic transducers was 3.1 MHz with a −6 dB bandwidth of 80%. Each element, spaced 0.7 mm apart, had a square dimension of 2 mm. The focal length of the arc array in the lateral direction was 65 mm and the overall angular aperture between elements 1 and 64 was 152 degree, which gave an angle of 2.4 degree between elements. The step size for the rotation was set to 2.4 deg to ensure even detector spacing in the lateral and elevational directions. The DAQ system consists of three custom-designed 48 channel analog amplifiers. Data digitalization was performed with two 32-channel boards containing analog-to-digital (AD) converters with a sampling rate of up to 40 MHz. By rotating the mouse around the central axis, the system resembles a spherical detection geometry with 9600 virtual transducers placed on the reconstruction sphere with an animal enclosed in its center. Three-dimensional tomographic reconstruction was performed using a 3-D reconstruction-algorithm-based radial back projection of filtered and simultaneously integrated PA signals.

PAT volume image acquired from a male mouse scan is shown in Fig. 11.5(B). The mouse was illuminated with the alexandrite laser (755 nm). The spinal region as well as other internal organs is clearly shown in the image. A PAT volume image of another mouse (Fig. 11.5(C)) was acquired using the Nd:YAG laser at 1064 nm. It shows the descending aorta, the abdominal aorta, three tail veins, and the kidneys.

The time required to acquire a 3-D image dataset averaged over 32 laser pulses is 8 min. The time for 3-D image reconstruction using standard computer processing units (CPUs) is several hours, which can be reduced to a few minutes by using multiple graphical processing units (GPU).

In comparison to the ring-array system, the arc-array system with spherical detection geometry provides uniform spatial resolutions in all directions. However, it cannot provide any cross-sectional image in real-time and require simultaneous light illumination of the 3D volume, which limits the fluence when the total laser pulse energy is limited.

11.3.3 Systems based on planar or linear detection geometry

PAT array systems based on linear detection geometry were also developed. Figure 11.6(A) shows a PAT system built on a clinical ultrasound imaging system (iU22; Philips Healthcare, Andover, MA). The modified system allowed access to raw per-channel photoacoustic data, while all imaging capabilities of the commercial ultrasonic scanner were retained. Raw photoacoustic and US data were transferred to a custom-built data acquisition system for image display and postprocessing, providing dual-modality imaging. Photoacoustic images were reconstructed using a Fourier beam-

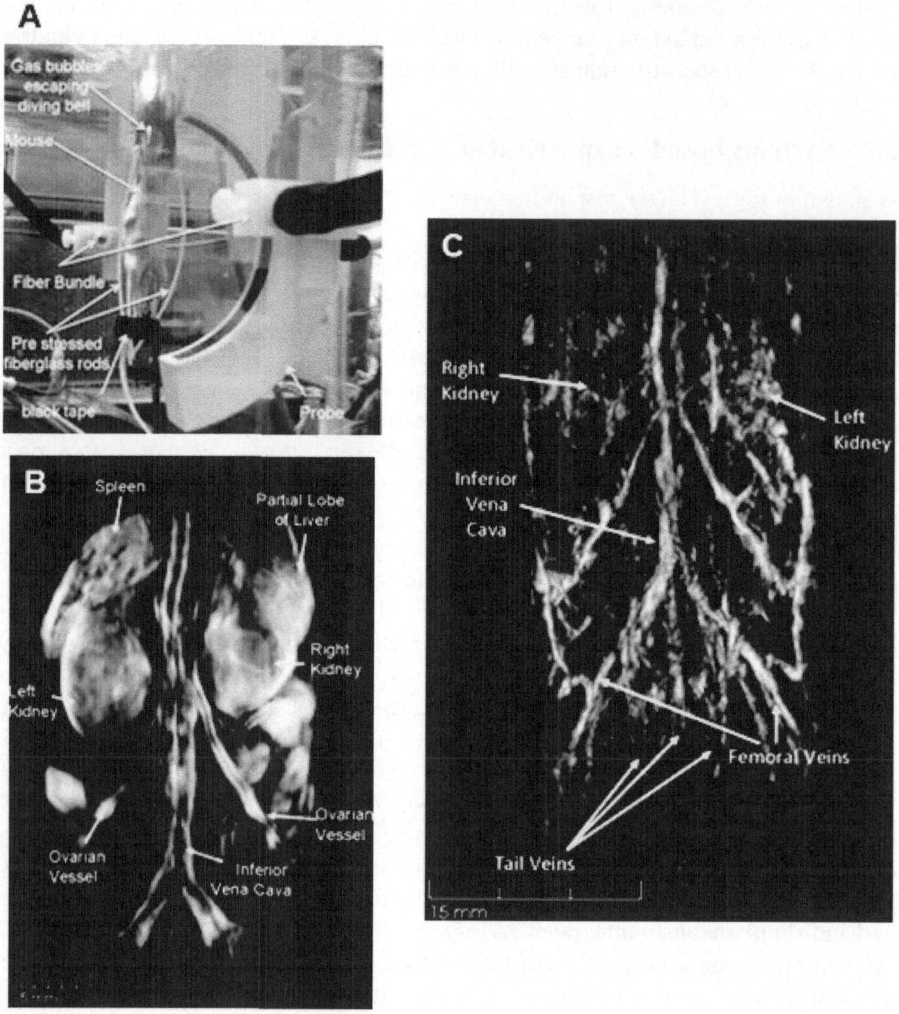

Figure 11.5: (A) Picture showing the placement of a mouse and light illumination with respect to the arc array of wideband ultrasonic transducers. (B) Three-dimensional PAT image of a nude mouse illuminated at 755 nm with optical fluence of 1 mJ/cm^2, showing an area of the mouse with the bifurcation of the inferior *vena cava* extended into the gonadal (ovarian) veins. Both kidneys are visualized as well as the spleen and a partial lobe of the liver. (C) Three-dimensional PAT image of a nude mouse illuminated at 1064 nm, with optical fluence of 1 mJ/cm^2, showing the mouse body vasculature including descending inferior vena cava and its bifurcation into the external and internal femoral veins and the three tail veins. Additionally, there is a partial view of the left and right kidney vasculature. Reprinted with permission from reference [54].

forming algorithm [55] implemented in software (MATLAB; MathWorks, Natick, MA), generating a photoacoustic B-mode image from one laser shot. A FPGA-based electronic board synchronized data acquisition with the laser firing. Photoacoustic data capture at a frame rate of 10 frames per second was limited by the current laser repetition rate. Light from a tunable dye laser (ND6000; Continuum, Santa Clara, CA), pumped by a Q-switched Nd:YAG laser (Brilliant B; Quantel, Les Ulis, France) with a 6.5-nanosecond pulse duration and a 10-Hz pulse repetition rate, was delivered

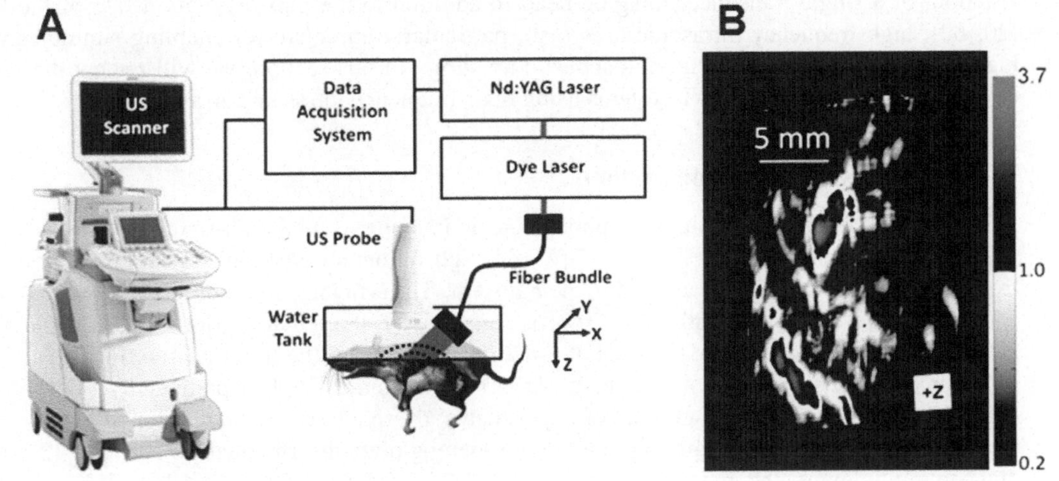

Figure 11.6: (See color insert.) *In vivo* PAT MAP images of rat axillary region. (A) Experimental setup of photoacoustic imaging system adapted from a US imaging system. x = x-axis, y = y-axis, z = z-axis. (B) Volumetric photoacoustic image of rat axilla acquired 20 minutes following methylene blue injection. Reprinted with permission from reference [24].

through a high-temperature epoxy, multimode fiber bundle (Schott Fiber Optics, Southbridge, MA). The optical wavelength was tunable between 606 and 678 nm. The light fluence on the skin was less than 5 mJ/cm^2, well within the ANSI safety limits.

The system was used clinically for noninvasive imaging of sentinel lymph nodes (SLNs) for axillary lymph node staging in breast cancer patients. The feasibility was demonstrated with animal studies. As shown in Fig. 11.6(A), the photoacoustic probe was partially immersed in a water tank, which had an opening at the bottom sealed with a thin, disposable, clear membrane. Rats were placed below the water tank, in contact with the membrane by means of ultrasonic coupling gel. Baseline PAT images acquired prior to methylene blue injection showed the network of blood vessels in rat axillae. After methylene blue injection, photoacoustic signals from the lymph vessel and SLN increased, while signal amplitudes from blood vessels remained largely unchanged after injection. Figure 11.6(B) shows PAT maximum amplitude projection (MAP) images of rat SLNs and blood vessels. A composite color map consisting of gray-scale and blue portions was chosen to visualize the blood vessels, the lymph vessels, and the lymph node in the same image.

11.4 Photoacoustic Tomography Using High-Frequency Ultrasonic Arrays

Recently, high-frequency (>20 MHz) ultrasound that is capable of imaging fine details with high spatial resolution has attracted wide attention. In particular, the emerging high-frequency ultrasonic array technology has excited researchers in both clinical and preclinical imaging areas [56–58]. Compared with a single-element high-frequency ultrasonic transducer, a high-frequency ultrasonic array is able to image with an extended depth of focus and a much higher frame rate, enabling not only high-resolution structural imaging, but also functional blood flow imaging in real time [59].

The development of high-frequency ultrasonic array technology has also stimulated a great interest in applying it for PAT. Since the imaging speed of PAT is limited largely by the mechanical scanning of a single-transducer imaging head in addition to the pulse repetition rate of the laser [20, 60], high-frequency ultrasonic arrays are particularly attractive for enabling simultaneously high-speed and high-resolution photoacoustic imaging. In this section, we will review the recent development of high-speed PAT systems using high-frequency ultrasonic arrays.

11.4.1 Acoustic-resolution systems

The first proof-of-concept study on photoacoustic imaging using a high-frequency ultrasonic array was conducted by Zemp et al. in 2007 [61]. A high-frequency ultrasonic linear array, fabricated from a 2-2 piezo-composite, was used in their system. The array had a center frequency of 30 MHz and a reception-only bandwidth of $\sim$ 70%; it consisted of 48 elements with a 100-μm pitch; its 2-mm elevational aperture was focused at $\sim$8.2 mm away from the transducer surface. The laser source used in the system was a tunable dye laser (Continuum, ND6000), pumped by a Q-switched Nd:YAG laser (Quantel, Brilliant B). For experiments, the dye laser output was tuned to 584 nm—an isosbestic point at which the oxy- and deoxy-hemoglobin absorb equally. Through 12:1 time division multiplexing, the image data were acquired using a four-channel digital oscilloscope (Tektronix, TDS5034). A 6-μm-diameter carbon fiber was imaged to characterize the system's spatial resolution, which showed an axial and a lateral resolution of $\sim$25 μm and $\sim$100 μm, respectively, much higher than those offered by clinical-frequency ultrasound. In addition, it was demonstrated that images were focused across the entire 4-mm depth of imaging—a significant improvement over single-element-transducer PAT. Due to a low laser repetition rate (10 Hz) and the 12:1 multiplexing in data acquisition (DAQ), the system did not really achieve a significant improvement in imaging speed over a single-element-transducer PAT system. Nonetheless, it had demonstrated the feasibility of developing high-performance PAT using a high-frequency ultrasonic array.

Using the same 30-MHz ultrasonic array described above, Zemp et al. further developed their PAT system and significantly improved its performance [62]. This new system (Fig. 11.7) was able to perform real-time photoacoustic imaging and display at 50 Hz. As the light source, a tunable dye laser (Cobra, Sirah GmbH, Germany) pumped by a Q-switched Nd:YLF laser (INNOSLAB, Edgewave GmbH, Germany) was employed. This laser system was capable of operating at an $\sim$1-kHz repetition rate, with a 40-nm wavelength tunable range (560–600 nm). Photoacoustic signals from the 48 ultrasonic transducer array elements were amplified, 6:1 time-division down-multiplexed, and streamed into an eight-channel high-speed DAQ card (Octopus 8389, GaGe Applied Systems, USA). With a quad-core dual-processor PC, the photoacoustic image was reconstructed with a receive-only delay-and-sum beamformation (Eq. (11.2)), which was implemented using parallel programming in C++. To offload the computation burden of CPU, the scan conversion and image display after beamformation were allocated to the GPUs of the graphics card (128 MB PCIe x16 nVidia Quadro NVS 285). For the first time, this system achieved real-time photoacoustic imaging and display at 50 Hz (fps). Using this system, the first *in vivo* photoacoustic cardiovascular dynamic imaging in a murine model was performed [63].

However, one important feature lacking in this real-time B-scan PAT system was robust 3D imaging. To overcome this issue, L. Song et al. further developed a robust light delivery and linear translation scheme for the system, enabling high-speed 3D photoacoustic imaging consisting of 166 B-scan frames at 1 Hz [64, 65]. Figure 11.8 shows several representative *in vivo* microvascular images acquired using this high-speed 3D PAT system [65].

The realization of high-speed 3D imaging has greatly expanded the application spectrum of high-frequency linear-array PAT. For example, using this 3D linear-array PAT system and a murine model, the feasibility of noninvasive photoacoustic sentinel lymph node mapping was demonstrated [23]. In particular, the 3D dynamic imaging capability was found quite helpful for differentiating the sentinel lymph node from other lymphatic structures, such as the lymphatic valves. Recently, the system has also been utilized to study human pulsatile dynamics *in vivo*, in which both the hemoglobin concentration dynamics and the arterial pulsatile motions were imaged and measured quantitatively

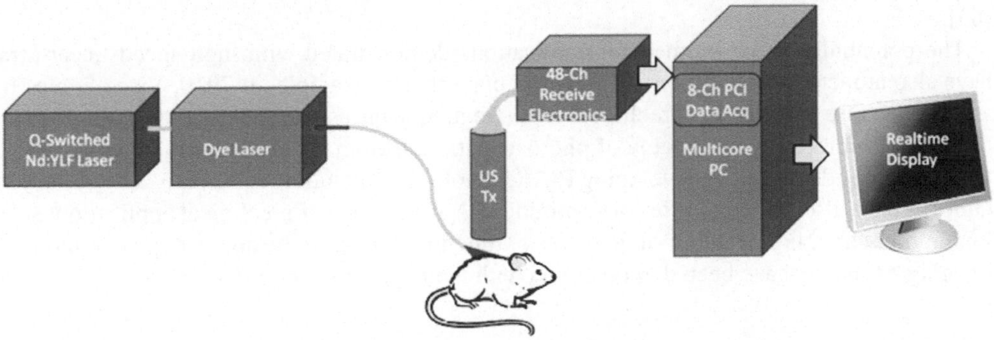

Figure 11.7: Architecture of the real-time PAT system using a high-frequency ultrasonic array. Key components shown include a KHz-repetition rate Q-switched laser, a dye laser, a fiber optic cable, an ultrasound transducer (US TX), receive electronics, an 8-core PC with an 8-Channel DAQ card, and a monitor for real-time display. Reprinted with permission from reference [62].

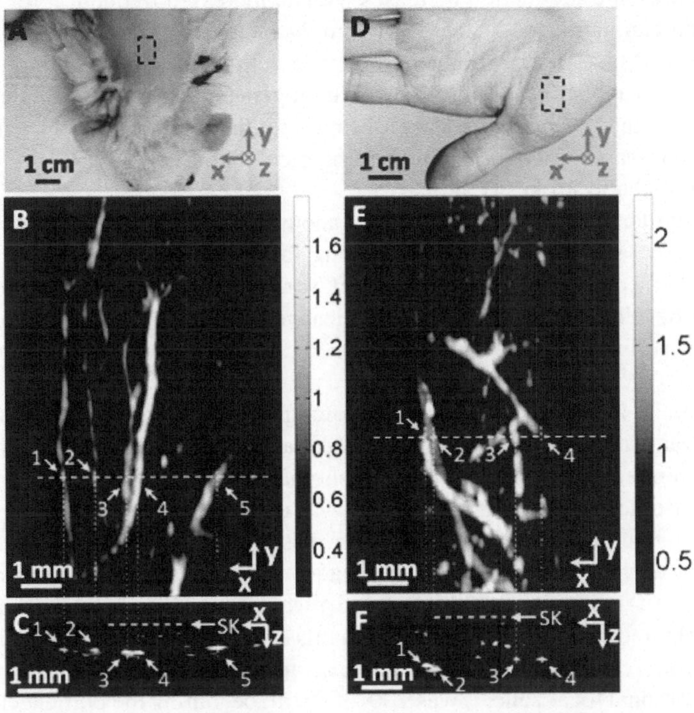

Figure 11.8: Noninvasive *in vivo* photoacoustic images acquired with the 3D linear-array PAT system. (A) Photograph of a Sprague Dawley rat with hair removed before imaging. Coordinates x, y, and z represent the lateral, elevational, and axial (depth) directions, respectively. The dashed rectangle indicates the imaged area. (B) Photoacoustic maximum amplitude projection (MAP) image of the rat. The grayscale represents relative optical absorption. (C) Photoacoustic B-scan image corresponding to the dashed horizontal line in (B), showing the depths of the blood vessels. SK, skin surface. Numbers 1–5 indicate corresponding blood vessels in (B) and (C). (D) Photograph of a human hand. The dashed rectangle indicates the imaged area. (E) Photoacoustic MAP image of the hand. (F) Photoacoustic B-scan image corresponding to the dashed horizontal line in (E). Numbers 1–4 indicate corresponding blood vessels in (E) and (F). Reprinted with permission from reference [65].

[65].

The potentially broad biomedical applications demonstrated with high-speed linear-array PAT have also attracted the attention of industrial players. For example, in 2010, VisualSonics Inc., the world's leading supplier for preclinical high-frequency ultrasonic imaging systems, has started to offer commercial systems capable of photoacoustic-ultrasonic dual-modality imaging [66]. Meanwhile, startups dedicated in developing PAT technologies (including Endra Inc. and i-Thera Medical GmbH.) have also started to offer their products. A wide range of preclinical applications, including longitudinal imaging of tumor angiogenesis, functional imaging of tumor hypoxia, and molecular imaging of cancer, have been demonstrated with their systems [66–68].

11.4.2 Optical-resolution systems

The development of optical-resolution photoacoustic microscopy (OR-PAM) has stimulated great interests in the biomedical research community [60]. By focusing a pulsed illumination laser beam into a diffraction-limited spot, OR-PAM can provide micrometer or even sub-micrometer spatial resolution, enabling *in vivo* imaging of individual capillaries or even individual red blood cells (RBCs). Because the ultrasonic attenuation increases with an increased frequency, for *in vivo* imaging, such high resolution can hardly be achieved by simply increasing the ultrasonic frequency. In only a few years, OR-PAM has demonstrated numerous preclinical and clinical applications. For instance, OR-PAM has been applied to: (i) the study of angiogenesis and the oxygen metabolic rate of tumors [69–71]; (ii) the study of ocular diseases through retina and microvascular imaging [72–74]; (iii) the study of neurovascular coupling and neurological diseases [75, 76]; and (iv) the study of brain functions and ischemic strokes [77].

However, similar to mechanical-scanning acoustic-resolution photoacoustic microscopy (AR-PAM), mechanical scanning is a major limiting factor for the improvement in imaging speed of OR-PAM. In this section, we will review recent work exploring the use of high-frequency ultrasonic arrays for the development of high-speed optical-resolution photoacoustic tomography. Although this research is still in its infancy, it has produced promising results that indicate a bright future for this technology.

The first optical-resolution photoacoustic tomography system developed with a high-frequency ultrasonic linear array employed cylindrical optical focusing. As a result, the system (Fig. 11.9 (A)) was also termed as section-illumination photoacoustic microscopy or SI-PAM [78]. The high-frequency ultrasonic array used in this system was the same as the one described in Section 11.1.

The motivation for using section illumination was two-fold: (i) to overcome the bottleneck spatial resolution—the elevational resolution—associated with a linear ultrasonic array (for details, refer to Section 11.2.2); (ii) to maintain the high-speed advantage that can be offered by an ultrasonic array. For the 30-MHz linear ultrasonic array used in this study, the lateral and axial resolutions were $\sim$80 μm and $\sim$25 μm, respectively. In contrast, the acoustic elevational resolution was rather poor; even within the elevational focal zone, it was 200–300 μm, becoming the bottleneck of the overall image quality. With section illumination, the elevational resolution was then defined by optical diffraction-limited cylindrical focusing, which was one to two orders of magnitude higher than that defined acoustically. As shown in the study, the section illumination enabled an elevational resolution of $\sim$28 μm, $\sim$10-fold better than the original acoustical elevational resolution (Fig. 11.9(B)–(G)). In addition, because section illumination can photoacoustically excite the entire B-scan imaging region with each laser pulse, it makes full use of the ultrasonic array for high-speed imaging. Indeed, the system has achieved an impressive 249-Hz B-scan imaging rate and a 0.5-Hz 3D imaging rate (each 3D image consists of 498 B-scan frames) [78].

Using the developed SI-PAM system and Evans blue dye, microvascular perfusion dynamics in mice were studied *in vivo* in real time. In experiments, the Evans blue dye was injected through the mouse tail vein; meanwhile, the mouse ear was continuously imaged in 3D by SI-PAM for several minutes, with a temporal resolution of $\sim$2 s. The results showed details of the perfusion process of

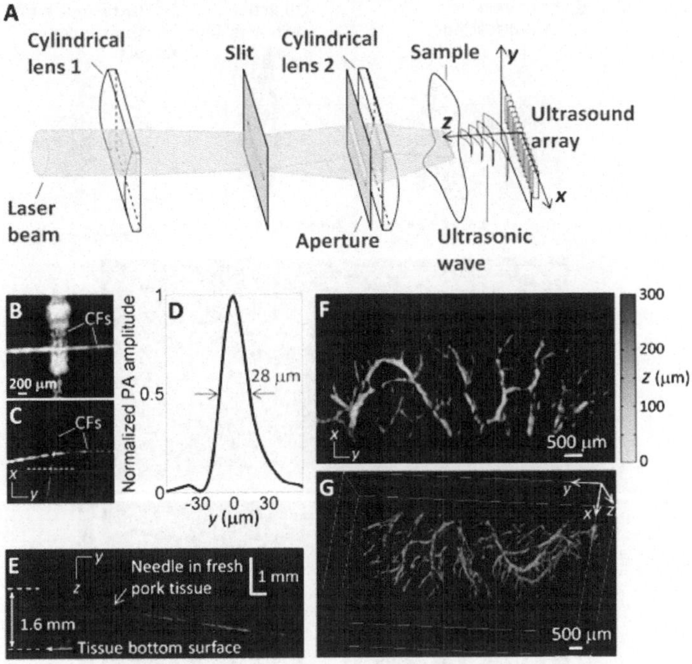

Figure 11.9: (See color insert.) (A) Schematic of SI-PAM. The widths of the slit and the aperture along the y axis are 50 μm and 5 mm, respectively. Coordinates x, y, and z represent the lateral, elevational, and axial directions of the ultrasonic array, respectively. (B,C) MAP images of two crossed 6-μm diameter carbon fibers (CFs) acquired without and with section illumination, respectively. (D) Distribution of photoacoustic (PA) amplitude from the vertical carbon fiber along the dashed line in (C). (E) MAP (along x) image of a 250-μm diameter black needle inserted in a fresh pork specimen. (F) MAP image of a mouse ear microvasculature. Depth (z) is encoded by color. (G) 3D image showing the microvasculature in (F). Reprinted with permission from reference [78].

the Evans blue dye, including Evans blue's perfusion into the arterial networks, exchange within the capillary beds, and returning from the venous networks [78]. The combined high spatial and temporal resolutions demonstrated through these *in vivo* experiments may have profound implications for future preclinical and clinical applications, in particular, for the study of tumor angiogenesis and the assessment of microvascular complications in diabetic patients.

However, to enable optical diffraction-limited resolution in both the elevational and lateral directions, spherical (rather than cylindrical) focusing is required. To achieve this goal, L. Song et al. developed a novel multi-focal approach for this high-frequency linear-array PAT [79]. It is worth noting that, although ultrasonic arrays were employed to improve the imaging speed of PAT since 2005, this was the first demonstration of truly optical-resolution PAT using an ultrasonic array.

For photoacoustic excitation, the system used a micro-lens array to provide 20 focused illumination laser beams, spreading uniformly in the lateral direction (Fig. 11.10(A)). Compared with a single focus, this multiple foci reduced the scanning load and increased the imaging speed significantly. The system achieved a 10-μm uniform lateral resolution and was capable of acquiring $1000\times500\times200$ voxels within only 4 min, $\sim$four times faster than conventional mechanical-scanning single-element OR-PAM. Through engineering improvements, for example, by reducing the data multiplexing and using more focusing beams, the imaging speed can potentially be further increased by more than 10-fold. In addition to the improvements in spatial resolution and imaging speed, the system also achieved a high signal-to-noise ratio (SNR), enabling not only high-quality

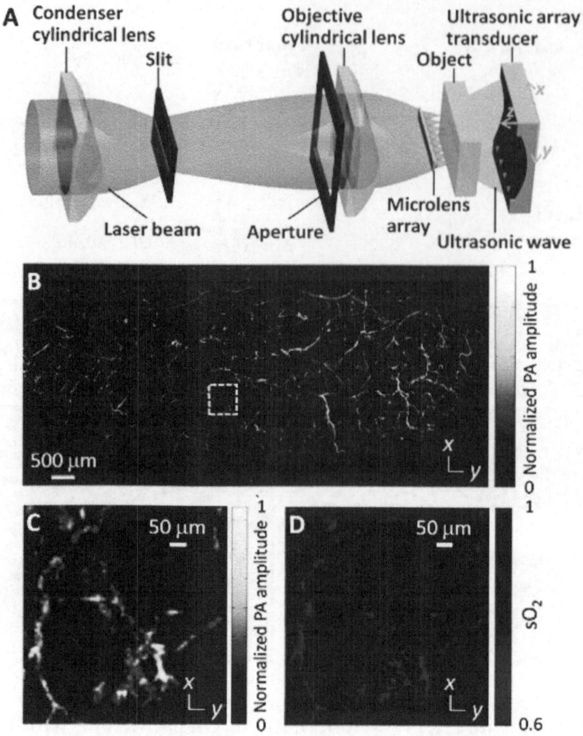

Figure 11.10: (See color insert.) (A) Schematic of the multi-focal optical-resolution photoacoustic tomography system. The widths of the slit and the aperture along y are 50 μm and 5 mm, respectively. (B) MAP image acquired at 570 nm. (C) Close-up of the vasculature in the dashed box in (B). (D) Oxygen saturation (sO_2) mapping for vessels in (C). Reprinted with permission from reference [79].

structural imaging of microvasculature, but also *in vivo* quantification of oxygenation in individual vessels (Fig. 11.10 (B)-(D)).

11.5 Other Variations of High-Speed Photoacoustic Tomography

Although ultrasonic arrays have played a critical role in the development of high-speed PAT, a variety of other approaches have also been explored to improve the imaging speed of PAT. In this final section, we will review the development of high-speed PAT based on optical-scanning, hybrid-scanning, and voice-coil scanning schemes, respectively.

11.5.1 Optical-scanning systems

It is well known that optical scanning using an oscillating mirror can be orders of magnitude faster than mechanical scanning. Based on this idea, Z. Xie et al. developed the first *in vivo* laser-scanning optical-resolution photoacoustic microscopy (LSOR-PAM) [80]. In their system, an unfocused single-element ultrasonic transducer was kept stationary; during data acquisition, the laser beam was raster scanned within the transducer's field of view (FOV). This design, together with a kHz-repetition-rate laser, enabled their system to acquire an image of 256×256 pixels in ∼2 min, with a lateral resolution of 7.8 μm. Compared with conventional mechanical-scanning OR-PAM, this imaging speed was an obvious progress (2 min vs. 20 min). Using this system, *in vivo* imaging of the microvasculature of a mouse ear was demonstrated.

Nevertheless, there are a few shortcomings with this system. Most significantly, the FOV of LSOR-PAM relied essentially on the FOV of the stationary ultrasonic transducer, which could be quite limited. In clear media, a maximum FOV of ∼6 mm in diameter was presented. Because of the degradation of detection sensitivity toward the edges of the FOV, the maximum effective FOV for *in vivo* imaging was even smaller. In addition, the oblique detection used in the system can potentially deteriorate the SNR of the system.

However, the great potential of optical-scanning photoacoustic imaging demonstrated in this work should not be dwarfed by these shortcomings. In fact, most of them can potentially be resolved or improved with engineering advancements. The recent development of PAT systems based on similar optical-scanning schemes has shown further improvements in both imaging speed and spatial resolution [81, 82].

11.5.2 Hybrid-scanning systems

The main motivation for developing hybrid-scanning optical-resolution photoacoustic microscopy (HSOR-PAM) was to provide both high speed and high SNR for optical-resolution photoacoustic imaging [83]. Unlike LSOR-PAM, which employed raster laser scanning for 3D imaging, a combination of fast 1D laser scanning and linear mechanical scanning was used for 3D imaging in HSOR-PAM. Furthermore, instead of using an unfocused ultrasonic transducer, as in LSOR-PAM, a cylindrically focused ultrasonic transducer was utilized to improve the photoacoustic detection sensitivity in HSOR-PAM. With a pulsed laser capable of operating at a 5-kHz repetition rate, the HSOR-PAM system achieved a B-scan imaging rate of 6.25 Hz (consisting of 800 A-scans), with a lateral resolution of 3.5 μm. More importantly, the HSOR-PAM system demonstrated a higher SNR compared with that in LSOR-PAM. The high imaging speed and high SNR of HSOR-PAM were demonstrated through *in vivo* microvascular imaging of both the iris and the ear in mice [83].

11.5.3 Voice-coil-based systems

Because laser beams need to be scanned—either in 1D or 2D—within the FOV of an ultrasonic transducer, neither LSOR-PAM nor HSOR-PAM can employ a spherically focused ultrasonic transducer for detection, resulting in an inevitable loss of detection sensitivity. To address this issue, an alternative approach was developed, in which a voice-coil fast scanner together with a focused ultrasonic transducer was employed. The first prototype system using this scheme emerged in 2009 [84]. Figure 11.11(A) shows the architecture of the system's imaging head, which consists of a voice-coil-based fast scanner (VCS-10-023-BS-01, H2W Technologies Inc.), a spherically focused 25-MHz single-element ultrasonic transducer (V324-SM, Panametrics), and a custom-built light delivery system. In this work, the scanning range and frequency of the voice-coil scanner was ∼9 mm and 10 Hz, respectively. Therefore, the system was capable of performing ultrasonic B-scan imaging at 20 Hz in real time. However, due to the use of a low-repetition-rate (20-Hz) laser, it took 10 s to acquire a photoacoustic B-scan image consisting of 200 A-scan lines. Using acoustic focusing, the system achieved a photoacoustic lateral and axial resolution of ∼180 μm and ∼40 μm, respectively. The photoacoustic imaging depth of the system was estimated to be ∼2 mm. Figure 11.11(B) shows a co-registered photoacoustic-ultrasonic *in vivo* image of a human finger acquired with the system.

Later on, also using a voice-coil stage, L. Wang et al. independently developed another high-speed optical-resolution photoacoustic imaging system, which was capable of real-time photoacoustic B-scan imaging at 20 Hz over a 9-mm scanning range and up to 40 Hz over a 1-mm scanning

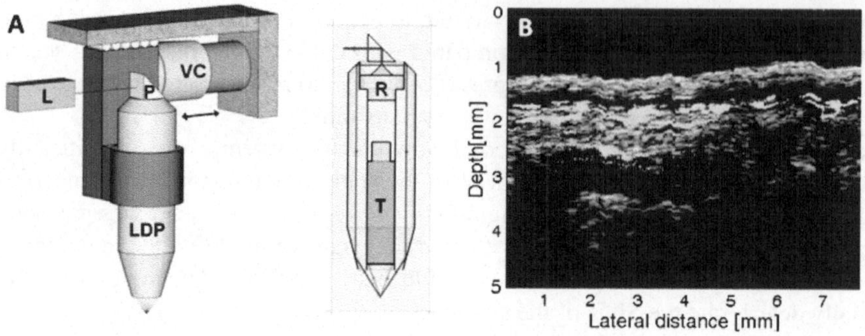

Figure 11.11: (See color insert.) (A) Voice-coil photoacoustic-ultrasonic scanning system and cross section of light delivery probe (LDP). Incident light from laser (L) is diverted towards the reflective cone (R) by the prism (P). Ultrasound transducer (T) is mounted inside the LDP. (B) Representative *in vivo* image acquired by the system. Gray scale, ultrasonic image; color scale, photoacoustic image. Reprinted with permission from reference [84].

range [85]. With an imaging depth of $\sim$1.4 mm, the system provided a fine optical lateral resolution of $\sim$3.4 μm, capable of imaging a single red blood cell *in vivo*. As shown in Fig. 11.12(A), the key enabling components of the system include a pulsed laser capable of operating at 4 kHz, a voice-coil scanning stage (VCS-1010, Equipment Solutions), a high-precision linear actuator with a stepper motor (for 3D imaging), a 75-MHz single-element ultrasonic transducer (V2022 BC, Olympus NDT), and a custom-developed light delivery system. *In vivo* imaging of individual capillaries and RBCs were demonstrated with the system (Fig. 11.12(B, C)). In addition, with a B-scan imaging rate of 40 Hz, highly dynamic processes can be continuously imaged in real time. For example, travelling RBCs in individual capillaries of a nude mouse ear were imaged *in vivo*. Furthermore, using auto-correlation analysis, the average flow speed of these RBCs was computed ($\sim$0.13 mm/s). To our knowledge, this is the first time that OR-PAM has demonstrated a B-scan frame rate of up to 40 Hz, representing a promising direction for future studies.

11.6 Conclusions

Photoacoustic tomography (PAT) is a rapidly growing emerging biomedical imaging technology with applications already being explored in many medical branches, including vascular biology, oncology, neurology, ophthalmology, dermatology, gastroenterology, and cardiology [3]. As a breakthrough hybrid imaging modality, PAT combines the advantages of optical absorption contrast and ultrasonic resolution, which enables functional and molecular imaging at depths well beyond the optical ballistic and quasi-ballistic regimes. To fully exert the potential of PAT for both clinical and preclinical applications, a high imaging speed is important. In the clinic, clinicians increasingly require real-time imaging to make decisions promptly. In preclinical research, such as small animal imaging for drug discovery, high throughput is usually crucial. In addition, a high imaging speed enables PAT (i) to reduce motion artifacts, (ii) to reduce cost and patient discomfort, and (iii) to potentially reduce risks associated with minimally invasive clinical procedures. To achieve high-speed imaging, ultrasonic arrays have been employed for both low-frequency and high-frequency PAT. In low-frequency ultrasonic array PAT, systems based on various detection geometries, including cylindrical, spherical, and planar geometries, have been constructed. Properly designed low-frequency

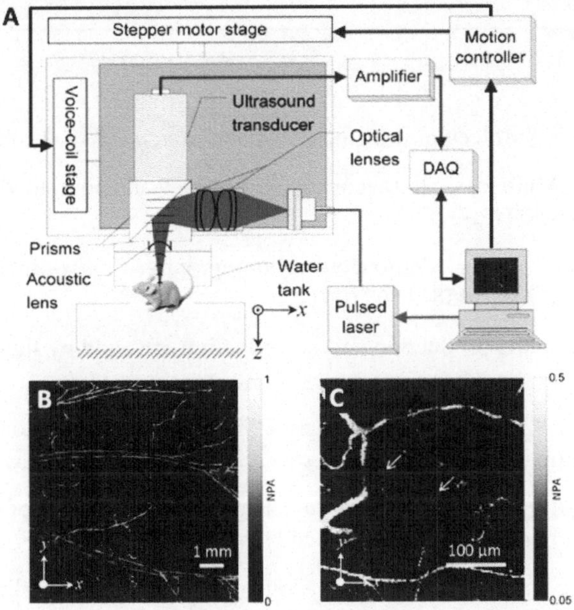

Figure 11.12: (A) Schematic of the voice-coil OR-PAM system. (B) *In vivo* image of mouse ear vasculature. (C) Close-up of the region enclosed by the dashed box in (B); arrows denote capillaries. NPA, normalized photoacoustic amplitude. Reprinted with permission from reference [85].

PAT systems using ultrasonic arrays have demonstrated imaging depths of several centimeters in biological tissue, and have been explored for both preclinical and clinical applications, including clinical detection and diagnosis of breast cancer, whole-body small animal imaging, and noninvasive clinical imaging of sentinel lymph nodes. In high-frequency ultrasonic array PAT, systems capable of offering both real-time imaging and high spatial resolution have been developed. In particular, using a 30-MHz linear ultrasonic array together with section illumination and/or multi-focal illumination, PAT systems offering optical diffraction-limited spatial resolution and high imaging speed have been developed. Furthermore, for high-frequency, high-speed PAT, besides the use of ultrasonic arrays, alternative approaches—with the use of laser scanning, hybrid scanning, and voice-coil scanning schemes—have also been explored. The continuously rapid development of high-speed PAT is expected to accelerate both the clinical translation of PAT and important new scientific discoveries in preclinical PAT studies.

Acknowledgments

This work was sponsored in part by National Institutes of Health grants R01 EB000712, R01 EB008085, R01 CA134539, U54 CA136398, R01 EB010049, and 5P60 DK02057933 to L.W., and the Shenzhen Development and Reform Commission Fund [2010] 1599, the Guangdong Innovation Research Team Fund for Low-Cost Healthcare Technologies (GIRTF-LCHT), the Low-Cost Health Engineering Research Program of the Chinese Academy of Sciences [2011] to L.S.. L.W. has a financial interest in Microphotoacoustics, Inc. and Endra, Inc., which, however, did not support this work.

References

[1] R. Weissleder, "Molecular imaging in cancer," *Science* **312**, 1168–1171 (2006).

[2] L.V. Wang, "Multiscale photoacoustic microscopy and computed tomography," *Nature Photonics* **3**, 503–509 (2009).

[3] L.V. Wang and S. Hu, "Photoacoustic tomography: *in vivo* imaging from organelles to organs," *Science* **335**, 1458–1462 (2012).

[4] A.G. Bell, "On the production and reproduction of sound by light," *Am. J. Sci.* **20**, 305–324 (1880).

[5] R.A. Kruger, P.Y. Liu, Y.R. Fang, and C.R. Appledorn, "Photoacoustic Ultrasound (Paus)-Reconstruction Tomography," *Med. Phys.* **22**, 1605–1609 (1995).

[6] A.A. Oraevsky, S.L. Jacques, and F.K. Tittel, "Determination of tissue optical properties by piezoelectric detection of laser-induced stress waves," *Proc. SPIE* **1882**, 86–101 (1993).

[7] M.H. Xu and L.H.V. Wang, "Photoacoustic imaging in biomedicine," *Rev. Sci. Instruments* **77**, 041101 (2006).

[8] L.V. Wang and H.-I. Wu, *Biomedical Optics: Principles and Imaging* (John Wiley & Sons, Inc., Hoboken, NJ, 2007).

[9] R.H. Webb, "Confocal optical microscopy," *Rep. Progr. Phys.* **59**, 427–471 (1996).

[10] W. Denk, J.H. Strickler, and W.W. Webb, "Two-photon laser scanning fluorescence microscopy," *Science* **248**, 73–76 (1990).

[11] D. Huang, E.A. Swanson, C.P. Lin, J.S. Schuman, W.G. Stinson, W. Chang, M.R. Hee, T. Flotte, K. Gregory, C.A. Puliafito, et al., "Optical coherence tomography," *Science* **254**, 1178–1181 (1991).

[12] L.V. Wang, "Prospects of photoacoustic tomography," *Med. Phys.* **35**, 5758–5767 (2008).

[13] G. Ku, X. D. Wang, X. Y. Xie, G. Stoica, and L. H. V. Wang, "Imaging of tumor angiogenesis in rat brains *in vivo* by photoacoustic tomography," *Appl. Opt.* **44**, 770–775 (2005).

[14] S. Hu and L. V. Wang, "Photoacoustic imaging and characterization of the microvasculature," *J. Biomed. Opt.* **15**, 011101 (2010).

[15] J. Jose, S. Manohar, R.G.M. Kolkman, W. Steenbergen, and T.G. van Leeuwen, "Imaging of tumor vasculature using Twente photoacoustic systems," *J. Biophotonics* **2**, 701–717 (2009).

[16] Y.Q. Lao, D. Xing, S.H. Yang, and L.Z. Xiang, "Noninvasive photoacoustic imaging of the developing vasculature during early tumor growth," *Phys. Med. Biol.* **53**, 4203–4212 (2008).

[17] M.L. Li, J.T. Oh, X.Y. Xie, G. Ku, W. Wang, C. Li, G. Lungu, G. Stoica, and L. V. Wang, "Simultaneous molecular and hypoxia imaging of brain tumors *in vivo* using spectroscopic photoacoustic tomography," *Proc. IEEE* **96**, 481–489 (2008).

[18] L. Li, R.J. Zemp, G. Lungu, G. Stoica, and L.H.V. Wang, "Photoacoustic imaging of lacZ gene expression *in vivo*," *J. Biomed. Opt.* **12**, 020504 (2007).

[19] H.F. Zhang, K. Maslov, M. Sivaramakrishnan, G. Stoica, and L.H.V. Wang, "Imaging of hemoglobin oxygen saturation variations in single vessels *in vivo* using photoacoustic microscopy," *Appl. Phys. Lett.* **90**, 053901 (2007).

[20] H.F. Zhang, K. Maslov, G. Stoica, and L.H.V. Wang, "Functional photoacoustic microscopy for high-resolution and noninvasive *in vivo* imaging," *Nat. Biotechnol.* **24**, 848–851 (2006).

[21] S.A. Ermilov, T. Khamapirad, A. Conjusteau, M.H. Leonard, R. Lacewell, K. Mehta, T. Miller, and A.A. Oraevsky, "Laser optoacoustic imaging system for detection of breast cancer," *J. Biomed. Opt.* **14**, 024007 (2009).

[22] K.H. Song, E.W. Stein, J.A. Margenthaler, and L.V. Wang, "Noninvasive photoacoustic identification of sentinel lymph nodes containing methylene blue *in vivo* in a rat model," *J. Biomed. Opt.* **13**, 054033 (2008).

[23] L. Song, C. Kim, K. Maslov, K.K. Shung, and L.H.V. Wang, "High-speed dynamic 3D photoacoustic imaging of sentinel lymph node in a murine model using an ultrasound array," *Med. Phys.* **36**, 3724–3729 (2009).

[24] T.N. Erpelding, C. Kim, M. Pramanik, L. Jankovic, K. Maslov, Z. Guo, J.A. Margenthaler, M.D. Pashley, and L.V. Wang, "Sentinel lymph nodes in the rat: noninvasive photoacoustic and US imaging with a clinical US system," *Radiology* **256**, 102–110 (2010).

[25] C. Kim, T.N. Erpelding, K. Maslov, L. Jankovic, W.J. Akers, L. Song, S. Achilefu, J.A. Margenthaler, M.D. Pashley, and L.V. Wang, "Handheld array-based photoacoustic probe for guiding needle biopsy of sentinel lymph nodes," *J. Biomed. Opt.* **15**, 046010 (2010).

[26] X.D. Wang, Y.J. Pang, G. Ku, X.Y. Xie, G. Stoica, and L.H.V. Wang, "Noninvasive laser-induced photoacoustic tomography for structural and functional *in vivo* imaging of the brain," *Nat. Biotechnol.* **21**, 803–806 (2003).

[27] R.L. Goldberg, S.W. Smith, J.G. Mottley, and K.W. Ferrara, "Ultrasound," in *The Biomedical Engineering Handbook,* 2nd ed., J. D. Bronzino, ed. (CRC Press, Boca Raton, FL, 2000).

[28] K.K. Shung and M. Zipparo, "Ultrasonic transducers and arrays," *IEEE Eng. Med. Biol. Mag.* **15**, 20–30 (1996).

[29] H. F. Wang, B. Jiang, T. R. Shrout, and W. W. Cao, "Electromechanical properties of fine-grain, 0.7 Pb(Mg1/3Nb2/3)O-3-0.3PbTiO(9.3) ceramics," *IEEE Trans. Ultrasonics Ferroelectrics and Frequency Control* **51**, 908–912 (2004).

[30] K.K. Shung, J.M. Cannata, and Q.F. Zhou, "Piezoelectric materials for high frequency medical imaging applications: A review," *J. Electroceramics* **19**, 141–147 (2007).

[31] Q.F. Zhou, S.T. Lau, D.W. Wu, and K. Shung, "Piezoelectric films for high frequency ultrasonic transducers in biomedical applications," *Progr. Mater. Sci.* **56**, 139–174 (2011).

[32] R.B. Liu, K.A. Harasiewicz, and F.S. Foster, "Interdigital pair bonding for high frequency (20–50 MHz) ultrasonic composite transducers," *IEEE Trans. Ultrasonics Ferroelectrics and Frequency Control* **48**, 299–306 (2001).

[33] J.R. Noble, M.P. Fronheiser, and S.W. Smith, "Real-time stereo 3D ultrasound," *Ultrasonic Imaging* **28**, 245–254 (2006).

[34] Y. Wang, T. Erpelding, L. Jankovic, Z. Guo, J.-L. Robert, G. David, and L.V. Wang, "*In vivo* three-dimensional photoacoustic imaging based on a clinical matrix array ultrasound probe," *J. Biomed. Opt.* (2012, in press).

[35] C. Li and L.H.V. Wang, "Photoacoustic tomography and sensing in biomedicine," *Phys. Med. Biol.* **54**, R59–R97 (2009).

[36] J. Xia, Z.J. Guo, K. Maslov, A. Aguirre, Q. Zhu, C. Percival, and L.H.V. Wang, "Three-dimensional photoacoustic tomography based on the focal-line concept," *J. Biomed. Opt.* **16**, 090505 (2011).

[37] G. Ku, B.D. Fornage, X. Jin, M. Xu, K.K. Hunt, and L.V. Wang, "Thermoacoustic and photoacoustic tomography of thick biological tissues toward breast imaging," *Tech. Cancer Res. Treatment* **4**, 559–566 (2005).

[38] A.A. Oraevsky, E. V. Savateeva, S.V. Solomatin, A.A. Karabutov, V. G. Andreev, Z. Gatalica, T. Khamapirad, and P.M. Henrichs, "Optoacoustic imaging of blood for visualization and diagnostics of breast cancer," in *Proc. SPIE* (2002), pp. 81–94.

[39] R.A. Kruger, H.E. Reynolds, W.Kiser, D.R. Reinecke, and G.A. Kruger, "Thermoacoustic computed tomography for breast imaging," *Radiology* **210**, 587–587 (1999).

[40] T.N. Erpelding, C. Kim, M. Pramanik, L. Jankovic, K. Maslov, Z.J. Guo, J.A. Margenthaler, M.D. Pashley, and L.H.V. Wang, "Sentinel lymph nodes in the rat: Noninvasive photoacoustic and US imaging with a clinical US system," *Radiology* **256**, 102–110 (2010).

[41] C. Kim, T.N. Erpelding, K. Maslov, L. Jankovic, W.J. Akers, L.A. Song, S. Achilefu, J.A. Margenthaler, M.D. Pashley, and L.H.V. Wang, "Handheld array-based photoacoustic probe for guiding needle biopsy of sentinel lymph nodes," *J. Biomed. Opt.* **15**, 046010 (2010).

[42] C. Kim, C. Favazza, and L.H.V. Wang, "*In vivo* photoacoustic tomography of chemicals: High-resolution functional and molecular optical imaging at new depths," *Chem. Rev.* **110**, 2756–2782 (2010).

[43] B. Yin, D. Xing, Y. Wang, Y. Zeng, Y. Tan, and Q. Chen, "Fast photoacoustic imaging system based on 320-element linear transducer array," *Phys. Med. Biol.* **49**, 1339–1346 (2004).

[44] J. Gamelin, A. Aguirre, A. Maurudis, F. Huang, D. Castillo, L.V. Wang, and Q. Zhu, "Curved array photoacoustic tomographic system for small animal imaging," *J. Biomed. Opt.* **13**, 024007 (2008).

[45] R.G. Kolkman, P.J. Brands, W. Steenbergen, and T.G. van Leeuwen, "Real-time *in vivo* photoacoustic and ultrasound imaging," *J. Biomed. Opt.* **13**, 050510 (2008).

[46] P. Ephrat, L. Keenliside, A. Seabrook, F.S. Prato, and J.J. Carson, "Three-dimensional photoacoustic imaging by sparse-array detection and iterative image reconstruction," *J. Biomed. Opt.* **13**, 054052 (2008).

[47] S. Vaithilingam, T.J. Ma, Y. Furukawa, I.O. Wygant, X. Zhuang, A. De La Zerda, O. Oralkan, A. Kamaya, S.S. Gambhir, R.B. Jeffrey, Jr., and B.T. Khuri-Yakub, "Three-dimensional photoacoustic imaging using a two-dimensional CMUT array," *IEEE Transactions on Ultrasonics, Ferroelectrics, and Frequency Control* **56**, 2411–2419 (2009).

[48] C.H. Li, A. Aguirre, J. Gamelin, A. Maurudis, Q. Zhu, and L.V. Wang, "Real-time photoacoustic tomography of cortical hemodynamics in small animals," *J. Biomed. Opt.* **15**, 010509 (2010).

[49] X. Wang, J.B. Fowlkes, J.M. Cannata, C. Hu, and P.L. Carson, "Photoacoustic imaging with a commercial ultrasound system and a custom probe," *Ultrasound Med. Biol.* **37**, 484–492 (2011).

[50] H. Park, J. Yang, S. Seo, K. Kim, J. Suh, D. Kim, S. Haam, and K. H. Yoo, "Multifunctional nanoparticles for photothermally controlled drug delivery and magnetic resonance imaging enhancement," *Small* **4**, 192–196 (2008).

[51] R. Olafsson, D. R. Bauer, L. G. Montilla, and R. S. Witte, "Real-time, contrast enhanced photoacoustic imaging of cancer in a mouse window chamber," *Opt. Express* **18**, 18625–18632 (2010).

[52] L. V. Wang, "Tutorial on photoacoustic microscopy and computed tomography," *IEEE J. Sel. Top. Quantum Electron.* **14**, 171–179 (2008).

[53] J. Xia, M. Chatni, K. Maslov, Z. Guo, K. Wang, M.A. Anastasio, and L.V. Wang, "Whole-body ring-shaped confocal photoacoustic computed tomography of small animals *in vivo*," *J. Biomed. Opt.* **17**, 050506 (2012).

[54] H.P. Brecht, R. Su, M. Fronheiser, S.A. Ermilov, A. Conjusteau, and A. A. Oraevsky, "Whole-body three-dimensional optoacoustic tomography system for small animals," *J. Biomed. Opt.* **14**, 064007 (2009).

[55] K.P. Kostli and P.C. Beard, "Two-dimensional photoacoustic imaging by use of Fourier-transform image reconstruction and a detector with an anisotropic response," *Appl. Opt.* **42**, 1899–1908 (2003).

[56] J.W. Xuan, M. Bygrave, H.Y. Jiang, F. Valiyeva, J. Dunmore-Buyze, D. W. Holdsworth, J.I. Izawa, G. Bauman, M. Moussa, S.F. Winter, N.M. Greenberg, J. L. Chin, M. Drangova, A. Fenster, and J.C. Lacefield, "Functional neoangiogenesis imaging of genetically engineered mouse prostate cancer using three-dimensional power Doppler ultrasound," *Cancer Res.* **67**, 2830–2839 (2007).

[57] C.M. Trivedi, Y. Luo, Z. Yin, M.Z. Zhang, W.T. Zhu, T. Wang, T. Floss, M. Goettlicher, P.R. Noppinger, W. Wurst, V.A. Ferrari, C.S. Abrams, P.J. Gruber, and J.A. Epstein, "Hdac2 regulates the cardiac hypertrophic response by modulating Gsk3 beta activity," *Nature Medicine* **13**, 324–331 (2007).

[58] F.S. Foster, M.Y. Zhang, Y.Q. Zhou, G. Liu, J. Mehi, E. Cherin, K. A. Harasiewicz, B.G. Starkoski, L. Zan, D.A. Knapik, and S.L. Adamson, "A new ultrasound instrument for *in vivo* microimaging of mice," *Ultrasound Med. Biol.* **28**, 1165–1172 (2002).

[59] F.S. Foster, J. Mehi, M. Lukacs, D. Hirson, C. White, C. Chaggares, and A. Needles, "A new 15–50 MHz array-based micro-ultrasound scanner for preclinical imaging," *Ultrasound Med. Biol.* **35**, 1700–1708 (2009).

[60] K. Maslov, H.F. Zhang, S. Hu, and L.V. Wang, "Optical-resolution photoacoustic microscopy for *in vivo* imaging of single capillaries," *Opt. Lett.* **33**, 929–931 (2008).

[61] R.J. Zemp, R. Bitton, M.L.Li, K.K. Shung, G. Stoica, and L.V. Wang, "Photoacoustic imaging of the microvasculature with a high-frequency ultrasound array transducer," *J. Biomed. Opt.* **12**, 010501 (2007).

[62] R.J. Zemp, L. Song, R. Bitton, K.K. Shung, and L.V. Wang, "Realtime photoacoustic microscopy *in vivo* with a 30-MHz ultrasound array transducer," *Opt. Express* **16**, 7915–7928 (2008).

[63] R.J. Zemp, L. Song, R. Bitton, K.K. Shung, and L.V. Wang, "Realtime photoacoustic microscopy of murine cardiovascular dynamics," *Opt. Express* **16**, 18551–18556 (2008).

[64] L. Song, K. Maslov, R. Bitton, K.K. Shung, and L.V. Wang, "Fast 3-D dark-field reflection-mode photoacoustic microscopy *in vivo* with a 30-MHz ultrasound linear array," *J. Biomed. Opt.* **13**, 054028 (2008).

[65] L. Song, K. Maslov, K.K. Shung, and L.H.V. Wang, "Ultrasound-array-based real-time photoacoustic microscopy of human pulsatile dynamics *in vivo*," *J. Biomed. Opt.* **15**, 021303 (2010).

[66] P. Ephrat, A. Needles, C. Bilan, A. Trujillo, C. Theodoropoulos, D. Hirson, and S. Foster, *Photoacoustic Imaging of Murine Tumors Using the Vevo 2100 Micro-Ultrasound System* (Visualsonics White Paper, 2010).

[67] i-Thera Medical GmbH., retrieved http://www.ithera-medical.com/index.php?id=12.

[68] Endra Inc., retrieved http://www.endrainc.com/content/products/.

[69] S. Oladipupo, S. Hu, J. Kovalski, J. J. Yao, A. Santeford, R. E. Sohn, R. Shohet, K. Maslov, L. H. V. Wang, and J. M. Arbeit, "VEGF is essential for hypoxia-inducible factor-mediated neovascularization but dispensable for endothelial sprouting," *Proc. Nat. Acad. Sci. U.S.A.* **108**, 13264–13269 (2011).

[70] S. S. Oladipupo, S. Hu, A. C. Santeford, J. J. Yao, J. R. Kovalski, R. V. Shohet, K. Maslov, L. V. Wang, and J. M. Arbeit, "Conditional HIF-1 induction produces multistage neovascularization with stage-specific sensitivity to VEGFR inhibitors and myeloid cell independence," *Blood* **117**, 4142–4153 (2011).

[71] J. J. Yao, K. I. Maslov, Y. Zhang, Y. N. Xia, and L. V. Wang, "Label-free oxygen-metabolic photoacoustic microscopy *in vivo*," *J. Biomed. Opt.* **16**(2011).

[72] S. L. Jiao, M. S. Jiang, J. M. Hu, A. Fawzi, Q. F. Zhou, K. K. Shung, C. A. Puliafito, and H. F. Zhang, "Photoacoustic ophthalmoscopy for *in vivo* retinal imaging," *Opt. Express* **18**, 3967–3972 (2010).

[73] S. Hu, B. Rao, K. Maslov, and L. V. Wang, "Label-free photoacoustic ophthalmic angiography," *Opt. Lett.* **35**, 1–3 (2010).

[74] A. de la Zerda, Y. M. Paulus, R. Teed, S. Bodapati, Y. Dollberg, B. T. Khuri-Yakub, M. S. Blumenkranz, D. M. Moshfeghi, and S. S. Gambhir, "Photoacoustic ocular imaging," *Opt. Lett.* **35**, 270–272 (2010).

[75] S. Hu, P. Yan, K. Maslov, J. M. Lee, and L. H. V. Wang, "Intravital imaging of amyloid plaques in a transgenic mouse model using optical-resolution photoacoustic microscopy," *Opt. Lett.* **34**, 3899–3901 (2009).

[76] S. Hu and L. V. Wang, "Neurovascular photoacoustic tomography," *Front Neuroenergetics* **2**, 10 (2011).

[77] S. Hu, K. Maslov, V. Tsytsarev, and L. V. Wang, "Functional transcranial brain imaging by optical-resolution photoacoustic microscopy," *J. Biomed. Opt.* **14**, 040503 (2009).

[78] L. Song, K. Maslov, and L. V. Wang, "Section-illumination photoacoustic microscopy for dynamic 3D imaging of microcirculation *in vivo*," *Opt. Lett.* **35**, 1482–1484 (2010).

[79] L. Song, K. Maslov, and L. V. Wang, "Multifocal optical-resolution photoacoustic microscopy *in vivo*," *Opt. Lett.* **36**, 1236–1238 (2011).

[80] Z. X. Xie, S. L. Jiao, H. F. Zhang, and C. A. Puliafito, "Laser-scanning optical-resolution photoacoustic microscopy," *Opt. Lett.* **34**, 1771–1773 (2009).

[81] B. Rao, K. Maslov, A. Danielli, R. M. Chen, K. K. Shung, Q. F. Zhou, and L. V. Wang, "Real-time four-dimensional optical-resolution photoacoustic microscopy with Au nanoparticle-assisted subdiffraction-limit resolution," *Opt. Lett.* **36**, 1137–1139 (2011).

[82] W. Shi, P. Hajireza, P. Shao, A. Forbrich, and R. J. Zemp, "*In vivo* near-realtime volumetric optical-resolution photoacoustic microscopy using a high-repetition-rate nanosecond fiber-laser," *Opt.Express* **19**, 17143–17150 (2011).

[83] B. Rao, L. Li, K. Maslov, and L. H. Wang, "Hybrid-scanning optical-resolution photoacoustic microscopy for *in vivo* vasculature imaging," *Opt. Lett.* **35**, 1521–1523 (2010).

[84] T. Harrison, J. C. Ranasinghesagara, H. H. Lu, K. Mathewson, A. Walsh, and R. J. Zemp, "Combined photoacoustic and ultrasound biomicroscopy," *Opt.Express* **17**, 22041–22046 (2009).

[85] L. D. Wang, K. Maslov, J. J. Yao, B. Rao, and L. H. V. Wang, "Fast voice-coil scanning optical-resolution photoacoustic microscopy," *Opt. Lett.* **36**, 139–141 (2011).

12

Optoacoustic Molecular Imaging: Methods and Applications

Adrian Taruttis and Vasilis Ntziachristos
Institute for Biological and Medical Imaging and Chair for Biological Imaging, Helmholtz Zentrum München and Technische Unversität München, Ingolstädter Landstr. 1, Neuherberg, Germany

Key words: molecular imaging, optical imaging, optoacoustic imaging, photoacoustic imaging

12.1 Introduction

Optical imaging at tissue depths of several millimeters to centimeters becomes feasible by operating in the far-red and near-infrared (NIR) wavelength range, i.e., 630 nm–900 nm. In the NIR, light absorption by tissue is much lower than in the visible spectrum, as evident by the red appearance of light seen penetrating tissue after illumination with a white light source [1]. While simple tissue epi-illumination and transillumination results in an image blurred in appearance due to strong photon scattering in tissue, optical tomography methods have demonstrated the abilility to quantitatively resolve fluorescent molecules delivered *in vivo* in tissues [2, 3] or intrinsic tissue chromophores, such as hemoglobin concentration [4]. However, optical imaging, even in tomographic mode, is limited by the scattering of light by tissue cellular interfaces and organelles, resulting in reduced scattering coefficients of tissue in the range of $\mu_s \sim 10\ \text{cm}^{-1}$ in the NIR [5]. As a result of photon scattering, light coming from a collimated laser beam incident on tissue becomes completely diffusive within 1 mm of photon propagation. Tomographic methods only partially resolve the loss in imaging resolution that derives as a result of photon diffusion in tissue. For example, fluorescence molecular tomography (FMT), a modality based on detection at several projections of diffuse light that has propagated several millimeters to centimeters in tissues, achieves spatial resolutions in the order of 1 mm at depths of approximately 1–2 cm.

Resolution in optical imaging can however significantly improve via the use of optoacoustics, a technique that is insensitive to photon scattering and instead obeys the resolution limitations of ultrasound imaging, even though it resolves optical contrast. The method operates by capitalizing on the photoacoustic effect, i.e., the generation of sound waves resulting from the absorption of light of transient intensity in materials. The light energy absorbed causes local heating and the resulting thermal expansion gives rise to pressure differentials. This results in pressure waves (sound), which propagate outwards. Optoacoustic imaging has been considered for several decades in imaging applications of biological tissues [6–8]. In tissues, contrast can be generated by several intrinsic or extrinsically administered photo-absorbing molecules and nanoparticles. Both forms of hemoglobin, i.e., oxygenated and deoxygenated, absorb light over a broad wavelength spectrum, providing an important contrast to optoacoustic imaging. Melanin is also a strong absorber of light and therefore an optoacoustic contrast source. Introducing exogenous optical agents to the tissue provides further sources of contrast. In a single optoacoustic image, the contrast resulting from each applied excitation wavelength could be coming from a number of different photo-absorbing sources. Differentiating between sources of contrast in the context of functional and molecular imaging applications requires further information. One approach is the collection of baseline measurements, i.e., images obtained before the administration of an exogenous contrast agent. Then images obtained after the agent administration can be subtracted from the baseline measurement to derive contrast coming only from the agent biodistribution. This strategy is generally limited in scope as it is only available within short time frames after agent injection so that new images collected can relate to the baseline image. Successful examples of this approach have been documented, a salient one being lymphatic mapping, because of the short times over with the contrast enhancement takes place [9]. However, over an extended period of time, obtaining the same image from a subject that moves and changes shape is highly challenging. An example could be imaging a subcutaneous tumor in a mouse over a period of days. The tumor is soft, possibly changing in size and structure: obtaining exactly the same image for comparison of different time points is impractical. Therefore, an alternative and more potent strategy in differentiating photo-absorbing agents in tissues is the use of multi-wavelength illumination to spectroscopically image a number of different photo-absorbing agents present in an image virtually simultaneously. Correspondingly, multispectral optoacoustic tomography (MSOT) was developed for functional and molecular optoacoustic imaging of tissues. MSOT obtains images at multiple excitation wavelengths and after spectral processing delivers images of the biodistribution of different chromophores of distinct spectral signatures [10, 11]. MSOT therefore offers a high resolution optical imaging approach that can resolve specific contrast from several millimeters to centimeters deep within tissues, without the need for baseline measurements, and could be applicable not only to biological research but also clinical imaging.

This chapter presents an overview of the physical principles that relate to optoacoustic signal generation and propagation, and then describes the instrumentation and optoacoustic imaging implementations reported in the literature. An overview of corresponding image reconstruction and spectral processing methods pertaining to MSOT is also presented. Finally, the chapter offers a discussion on sources of contrast for optoacoustic imaging, including related imaging applications.

12.2 Optoacoustic Signal Generation

The photoacoustic effect can be understood as follows: incident photons from a pulse of light are absorbed by some matter. At least part of this absorbed energy causes a local rise in temperature, that is, the matter is heated by the pulse. This local temperature increase gives rise to a local volume expansion (thermoelastic expansion), which causes a pressure differential, thus giving rise to acoustic waves propagating through the medium. The following equations are adapted from Li et al. [12] and Diebold et al. [13]. The energy $h(\mathbf{r})$ absorbed per unit volume during a pulse of length

τ can be defined as:

$$h(\mathbf{r}) = \int_0^\tau \mu_a(\mathbf{r})\Phi(\mathbf{r},t)dt = \mu_a(\mathbf{r})\phi(\mathbf{r}), \tag{12.1}$$

where $\Phi(\mathbf{r},t)$ is the fluence rate (J $s^{-1}m^{-2}$) and ϕ(r) is the fluence (J m^{-2}), at a point $\mathbf{r}$ in space. Assuming that the pulse duration is short enough that changes during the pulse can be neglected, then the local temperature rise is given by:

$$\Delta T = \frac{h}{\rho c_V}, \tag{12.2}$$

where ρ is the density and c_V is the specific heat capacity at constant volume. The change in pressure due to this temperature change is given by:

$$\Delta p = \frac{\beta \Delta T}{K_T}, \tag{12.3}$$

where β is the volume thermal expansivity (K^{-1}) and K_T is the isothermal compressibility (m^2/N). By substituting Eq. (12.2), we obtain:

$$\Delta p = \frac{\beta h}{K_T \rho c_V}. \tag{12.4}$$

Using $v_s^2 = c_p/(K_T \rho c_V)$, where v_s is the speed of sound in the medium and c_p ($JK^{-1}g^{-1}$) is the specific heat at constant pressure, and defining $\Gamma = \beta v_s^2/c_p$, we have:

$$\Delta p = \Gamma h, \tag{12.5}$$

with Γ a dimensionless constant representing the relevant thermodynamic properties of the absorber, referred to as the Grüneisen coefficient. By substitution of Eq. (12.1):

$$\Delta p = \Gamma \mu_a \phi, \tag{12.6}$$

which relates the change in pressure to the local optical absorption properties and local fluence. This pressure change is the initial condition that gives rise to (opto)acoustic waves propagating through the medium, and is the quantity that optoacoustic images visualize. To obtain an estimate of realistic values for pressure and temperature increases in typical optoacoustic imaging scenarios, consider the excitation of oxygenated whole blood at 900 nm. Assume a fluence of 50 mJ/cm^2: this represents the maximum permissible skin exposure (American National Standard for safe use of lasers, ANSI Z136.1-2007), so the calculation is relevant for a very superficial blood vessel. $\mu_a \approx 6.4$ cm^{-1}, from known values for blood absorption. Using a value of $\Gamma = 0.25$ [12], we obtain Δp= 80 kPa. Now, using K_T= 4.6 $\times$ 10^{-10} m^2/N (value for water) and β = 4$\times 10^{-4}K^{-1}$, we have a temperature increase of ΔT = 92 mK.

12.3 Optoacoustic Wave Propagation

By considering the change in pressure Δp as the initial condition $p_0(\mathbf{r})$ from which acoustic waves propagate, we can write the wave equation [13]:

$$\left(\nabla^2 - \frac{1}{v_s^2}\frac{\partial^2}{\partial t^2}\right) p(\mathbf{r},t) = \frac{p_0(\mathbf{r})}{v_s^2}\frac{d\delta(t)}{dt}, \tag{12.7}$$

where $p(\mathbf{r},t)$ is the acoustic pressure wave at point $\mathbf{r}$, which is the quantity that can be measured using ultrasound detectors. Solutions for the pressure can be found using Green's functions, yielding [12]:

$$p(\mathbf{r},t) = \frac{1}{4\pi v_s^2}\frac{\partial}{\partial t}\left[\frac{1}{v_s t}\int d\mathbf{r}' p_0(\mathbf{r}')\delta\left(t - \frac{|\mathbf{r}-\mathbf{r}'|}{v_s}\right)\right]. \tag{12.8}$$

Therefore, if we place a detector at a certain position $\mathbf{r}$, then the pressure signal received will originate from a sphere with radius $v_s t$, which is intuitive since the acoustic wave propagates out from the sources to the detector at the speed of sound. We can examine the expected pressure signals by simulation, in this case by applying an analytical solution to the governing wave equation. The simulation is performed on a plane (2D) for a circular absorber with a diameter of 2 mm and a paraboloid absorption profile (Fig. 12.1a). The detector position is at a distance of 10 mm away from the center of the absorber. Note the bipolar nature of the signal (Fig. 12.1b). By changing the time axis to a distance axis (multiplying by the speed of sound), we can visualize this signal as a distance-resolved profile (Fig. 12.1c). From this plot, we observe that the bipolar signal starts 9mm from the detector and ends 11mm from the detector, as expected from the size of the absorber and the distance from the detector, that is, information about the spatial characteristics of the absorber is contained in the signal. Correspondingly, an absorber with a larger diameter would result in a wider bipolar signal, and a narrower absorber in a narrower signal. In frequency terms, we therefore expect larger features to produce lower signal frequencies and smaller features to produce higher frequencies.

12.4 Instrumentation and Implementations

What is the simplest conceivable MSOT imaging system? For excitation, nanosecond pulsed lasers, commonly Q-switched Nd:YAG systems, are suitable. In the case of multispectral imaging, the wavelength should be tunable, so an optical parametric oscillator (OPO) or some other mechanism for varying the wavelength is essential. To detect the ultrasound signals generated by the photoacoustic effect, an ultrasound detector is necessary. Signals from the detector are collected by an analog-to-digital converter and stored in a computer. For tomography, the ultrasound waves should be sampled at multiple angles (projections) around the object imaged. This can be achieved by moving the detector around the object, or alternatively, by using a detector array. Figure 12.2 shows an example schematic for such a system. Once the optoacoustic signals have been recorded, they are fed into an image reconstruction algorithm to produce the image. To summarize, there are three main technical tasks in optoacoustic imaging: illumination, ultrasound detection and image reconstruction.

Correspondingly, tomographic optoacoustic imaging systems generally rely on sampling the acoustic field in space and then applying an inversion scheme to reconstruct volumetric images. Although implementations scanning single detectors have been reported [14, 15], systems of improved performance employ fixed, multi-element detection arrays [16–18], or a combination of scanning and multi-element detection [19, 20]. Such systems, depending on geometry, either scan one 2D slice at a time using cylindrically focused detection (see Fig. 12.3), or produce 3D volumes, which requires sufficient sampling in all spatial dimensions and therefore either a greater amount of detectors or a longer mechanical scanning time. While the vast majority of reported results from such imaging systems are of small animals, preliminary examples of studies on human subjects have also been reported [21–23].

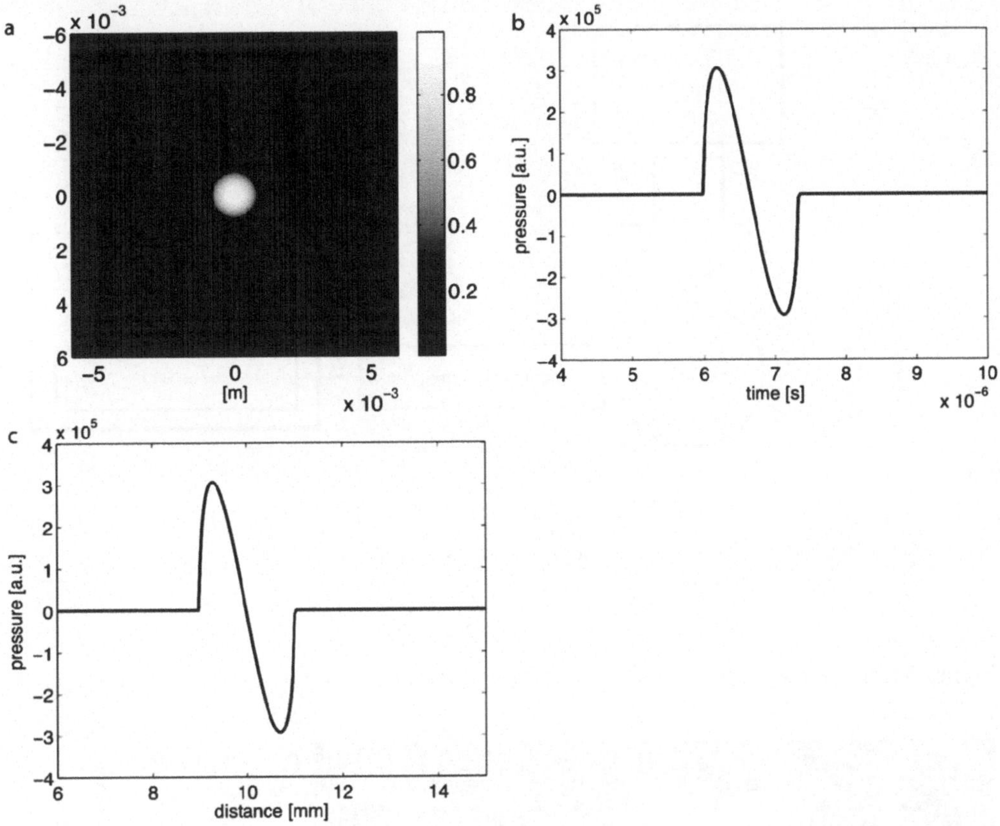

Figure 12.1: Simulation of an optoacoustic signal. (a) Originating absorption profile with paraboloid intensity inside a 2 mm diameter circle. (b) Resulting simulated optoacoustic signal detected at a point 10 mm from the absorber's center. (c) The same signal plotted against distance.

12.4.1 Optical backward-mode detection

While detection in optoacoustic systems is typically performed using technology developed for ultrasound imaging, i.e., piezoelectric technology, potent alternatives to optoacoustic detection utilize interferometric methods. In particular, a Fabry-Perot interferometer film transparent to excitation light pulses has been demonstrated for enabling illumination and detection to conveniently come from the same angle [25]. High quality 3D images result from a broad detection bandwidth and dense spatial sampling. However, the need to scan a laser beam over the film to obtain signals from individual sample points reduces the acquisition speed and may result in disadvantageous acquisition times, reported at 15 minutes for single wavelength images.

12.4.2 Optoacoustic microscopy

Optoacoustic microscopy systems produce high resolution images close to the skin surface. There are two major approaches. Optical resolution optoacoustic microscopy, where focused excitation light governs the lateral resolution, has been reported with diffraction limited optical resolutions of less than 1 μm [26]. Since the resolution obtained depends on the focusing of light, the imaging depth is comparable to laser scanning microscopy (generally less than 1 mm [5]). In this case the commonly cited advantage of optoacoustic imaging, i.e., the insensitivity of the method to tissue

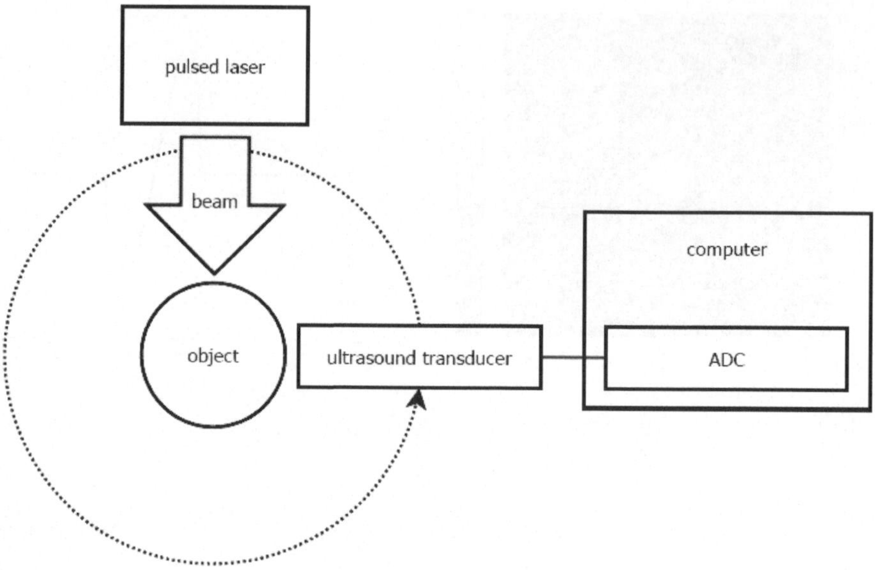

Figure 12.2: A basic optoacoustic tomography system.

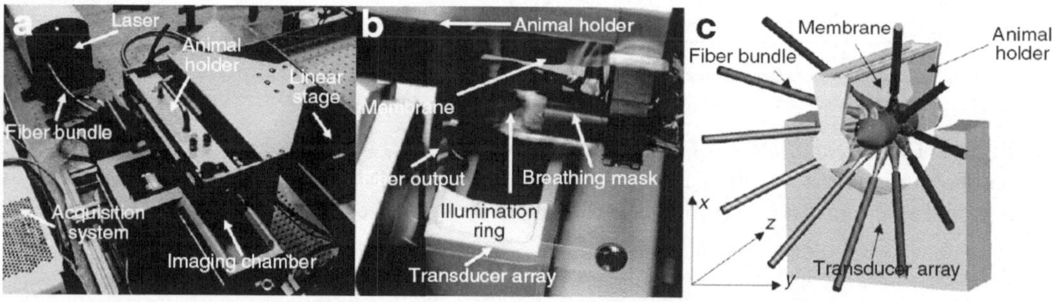

Figure 12.3: Real-time small-animal imager. Produces two-dimensional slice images at 10 frames/s. Adapted from [24].

scattering no longer applies. However, the natural sensitivity of optoacoustic imaging to hemoglobin is still considered sufficiently advantageous to render optical resolution optoacoustic microscopy an interesting alternative to conventional tissue sectioning optical microscopy, such as confocal or multi-photon microscopy or optical coherence tomography. The second approach to optoacoustic microscopy is the use of strongly focused ultrasound detectors to produce images with acoustically governed resolution, that is, resolution obeying the ultrasonic diffraction limit. In this case there is no requirement for using tightly focused light and therefore the penetration depth achieved can be greater than with optical focusing, defined by the attenuation of the high-frequency ultrasound components. An example of such a system has been reported capable of imaging at depths greater than 1mm and resolutions measured in tens of microns [27]. The chromophores typically visualized by optoacoustic microscopy are oxy- and deoxyhemoglobin as well as melanin, pointing to applications in imaging of functional parameters of melanoma and other skin tumors. Ophthalmic angiography is a further potential application area: contrast-rich images from small animals were reported in 2010 by Hu et al. [28] and Jiao et al. [29].

12.4.3 Intravascular catheters and endoscopes

Early detection and accurate characterization of atherosclerotic plaques remains one of the primary challenges in biomedical imaging [30]. Since optoacoustic signals can reveal the composition of tissues by spectral analysis, a significant effort has been invested in the development of intravascular optoacoustic catheter systems to probe atherosclerotic plaques. The most common approach is to add an optical fiber for excitation to an intravascular ultrasound (IVUS) system, which represents an established modality for plaque visualization. This allows IVUS and optoacoustic imaging with the same catheter [31]. One notable development demonstrated the detection of lipid deposits in human coronary artery specimens *ex vivo* by multispectral excitation around 1200 nm, where lipids display an absorption peak [32]. Currently, reported acquisition times in tens of seconds in the absence of blood highlight the need for further technical improvements before this technology can be used in patients. Similarly, optoacoustic endoscopic imaging is possible and can benefit from the increased resolution of optoacoustic imaging at greater depths. Systems in early stages of development employing spinning illumination and ultrasound detection [33] or ring illumination and multi-element detection [34] have been reported.

12.4.4 Flow cytometry

Although *in vivo* optoacoustic flow cytometry is not, strictly speaking, imaging, it is a highly promising method that equally relies on optoacoustic signal generation and detection. In this technique, a superficial blood vessel is illuminated and cells labelled with a targeted optical agent cause optoacoustic signal spikes as they flow past the excitation/detection point. This has been demonstrated, for example, on circulating cancer cells by Galanzha et al. in 2009 [35] and can be employed in a theranostic process for monitoring photothermal cell eradication [36].

12.5 Image Reconstruction and Processing

12.5.1 Image reconstruction for optoacoustic tomography

We refer to image reconstruction as the procedure to obtain an image from optoacoustic signals measured at multiple positions. The discussion is restricted to 2D tomography. The methods can generally be extended to the third dimension if necessary. For image reconstruction, two approaches are considered: delay-and-sum type methods and a linear model-based inversion.

12.5.2 Delay-and-sum

Whether based on simple beamforming equations [37] or more rigorously derived analytical formulas [38, 39], a common approach to reconstructing optoacoustic images boils down to summing signals onto a grid which maps the time-resolved signals to distances away from the detectors. This is accompanied by frequency filtering to more accurately approximate the originating image as well as model the detector frequency response. While some weighting factors to account for detection geometry have been proposed [37, 39], there is limited scope for taking complicated, non-uniform detector geometries into account in a holistic way. Moreover, despite efforts to derive exact analytical reconstruction algorithms, results show inaccuracies due to idealized assumptions in their derivations [40]. The primary advantage of delay-and-sum type formulas is their relative simplicity and fast computation times.

12.5.3 Model-based inversion

A model-based optoacoustic image reconstruction method for 2D slice imaging was described by Rosenthal et al. in 2010 [40]. A semi-analytical model of optoacoustic signal propagation is built on a grid. This model can then be inverted and multiplied with the measured signals to give the optoacoustic image. More formally:

$$\mathbf{p} = \mathbf{M}\mathbf{z} \tag{12.9}$$

where $\mathbf{p}$ is a vector containing the measured optoacoustic signals, $\mathbf{M}$ is the model matrix that describes the imaging system and optoacoustic generation and propagation, and $\mathbf{z}$ is a vector containing the pixels of the originating image, which is the unknown to solve for. $\mathbf{M}$ is calculated for a specific geometry by interpolating analytical solutions of integrals over arcs, which represent the time domain of the optoacoustic signals on the image grid. As with many simple problems in experimental linear algebra, the solution (image) is found by least squares:

$$\mathbf{z}_s = \text{argmin}_{\mathbf{z}} \|\mathbf{p} - \mathbf{M}\mathbf{z}\| \tag{12.10}$$

where $\mathbf{z}_s$ is the solution image that minimizes the square error. Commonly, iterative algorithms are employed to compute the image. The advantage of the model-based approach is that the model can be adapted to account for non-ideal or non-uniform characteristics in the measurement system. A salient example of the necessity of such modeling is given in scenarios where the spatial sampling of the acoustic field is not uniform: Buehler et al. [41] applied a model-based approach to reconstruct images from such geometries. Since light needs to be delivered to the tissue from somewhere, such non-uniform detection geometries are likely simply for mechanical reasons, as gaps in detectors are needed to let light through. Another assumption in analytical formula-driven reconstructions is that the acoustic field is sampled at points. However, a realistic detector has a finite size, and to obtain adequate SNR, these diameters are often significantly wide. This has a negative effect on lateral resolution [42]. Rosenthal et al. [43] showed how a model incorporating finite-sized detectors could be used to recover lateral resolution (see Fig. 12.4). In time, it is highly likely that additional system characteristics will be included in models used for inversion, resulting in increasingly accurate images. A drawback of model-based approaches is, however, an increased computation time over simple analytical formulas. Modeling additional system characteristics further increases this time in many cases. The computation time should be considered to have two distinct parts: first, the model matrix is computed, then image reconstruction is performed by feeding the model matrix and the measurement data into an iterative algorithm. Since the model matrix depends on fixed system characteristics, it can be computed once and used repeatedly after that for reconstructions. The only caveat is that the speed of sound, a parameter of the model, varies with temperature, but this is advisable to keep to a controlled constant value in *in vivo* experiments in any case. Therefore, the reconstruction time for each image does not include the time taken for computing the model matrix.

12.5.4 Spectral unmixing

Spectral unmixing is the process of converting the images, which each correspond to a specific excitation wavelength, into a new set of images where each one corresponds to the distribution of a specific absorber. Two approaches will be described in the following: linear spectral unmixing where the source absorption spectra are known a priori, and blind source separation where the source spectra are determined from the measurement data.

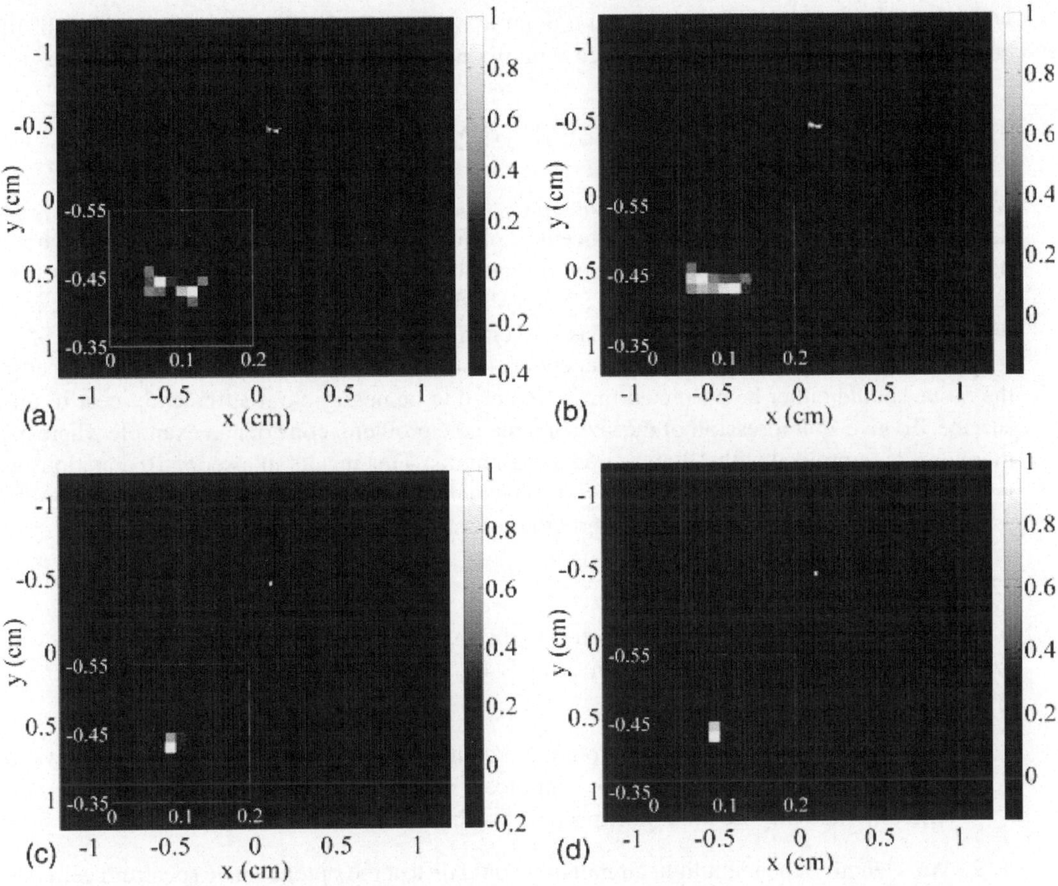

Figure 12.4: Experimental reconstructions of an optoacoustic point source detected by a flat detector with a width of 1.3 cm obtained using a delay-and-sum algorithm (a), a model-based inversion modeled with a point detector (b) a model-based inversion modeled with a 1.3-mm flat detector using spatial convolution (c) and a model-based inversion modeled with a 1.3-mm flat detector using temporal convolution (d). The point source was obtained by applying plane-selective illuminating on a black hair embedded in a clear agar phantom. Adapted from [43].

12.5.4.1 Linear spectral unmixing with known source spectra

This method works as follows: for each pixel in the image, the total measured optoacoustic spectrum is fitted to the known absorption spectra of the absorption sources expected to be present in the tissue. If a particular absorber makes significant signal contributions, its spectrum should be included, otherwise those contributions may be erroneously attributed to a different absorber. In a typical case, the included source spectra would be that of an exogenous contrast agent, and those of oxy- and deoxyhemoglobin, plus a flat (constant) spectrum to account for measurement offsets or spectrally flat absorbers. The fitting is performed using least-squares on the set of linear equations resulting from the multispectral measurements (1 equation per excitation wavelength). The initial pressure distribution that underlies optoacoustic images is proportional to local light fluence in addition to the absorption properties, that is:

$$p_0 \propto \phi \mu_a, \tag{12.11}$$

where p_0 denotes the initial pressure at a point in space, ϕ is the fluence and μ_a is the absorption coefficient. The equations used for spectral unmixing, for each pixel, are then of the form:

$$\phi\mu_a(\lambda_i) = \phi \sum_{j=1}^{N} \varepsilon_j(\lambda_i)c_j, \tag{12.12}$$

where λ_i is the wavelength, $\phi\mu_a(\lambda_i)$ is the optoacoustic response for that pixel, ε_j is the wavelength-dependent absorption coefficient per concentration for the absorber represented by the spectral component j, and c_j is the local concentration of that absorber. The unknown quantities solved for by least-squares are then ϕc_j for $j = 1,...,N$. Note that the images must be corrected for possible wavelength-dependent fluctuations in laser excitation energy, so that ϕ is independent of wavelength. Additionally, the wavelength-dependence of the fluence due to the absorption spectrum of the tissue should either be corrected for or assumed to be negligible if sufficiently near to the skin surface. To give an impression of the size of a realistic problem, consider an example where 5 chromophores are unmixed with 10 measured wavelengths. This results in a set of 10 equations with 5 unknowns each, that is, a 10×5 matrix. Since the matrix is comparatively small, the Moore-Penrose pseudoinverse can easily be applied to find the solution giving the least square error.

12.5.4.2 Blind source separation

Blind source separation, that is, spectral unmixing where the source spectra are unknown, was proposed for MSOT by Glatz et al. in 2011 [44]. There are two motivating factors behind this approach:

1. While we often consider hemoglobin, in its different oxygenation states, and whatever agent we may have injected, as the only significant absorbers in tissue in the wavelength range of interest, there may be other unexpected absorbers contributing to image contrast.

2. Wavelength-dependent light attenuation could distort the optoacoustic spectrum generated by absorbers, since the initial pressure is proportional to the local absorption coefficient and the local fluence.

Both cases are a problem in linear spectral unmixing with known source spectra because the unexpected or distorted signals would be fitted to combinations of the known input spectra. Blind unmixing approaches attempt to find the significant spectral contributions from the measurement data itself. From Glatz et al., the two proposed methods for blind spectral unmixing are principle component analysis (PCA) and independent component analysis (ICA). Unmixing by PCA is based on the assumption that the spectral components are statistically uncorrelated. The result of PCA is a linear orthogonal transformation where components are in the order of largest variance. The method can be used for dimension reduction: when the number of excitation wavelengths exceeds the number of source spectra, the remainder of the components may represent noise that can be discarded. ICA, on the other hand, seeks a transformation into source spectra based on components having a maximum statistical independence. While blind source separation has been reported to resolve unique absorber distributions with a superior SNR to linear spectral unmixing with known sources [44], there are situations where these methods cannot be robustly applied. For example, if the objective is to resolve oxy- and deoxyhemoglobin distribution or hemoglobin oxygen saturation, it is unlikely that either PCA or ICA will identify purely oxygenated or deoxygenated hemoglobin as the source spectra, but rather some combination of the two, since such combinations are likely to be present in the measurement data in higher amounts than the pure states. In general, depending on the imaging data, these approaches might combine or split spectra in unexpected ways.

12.6 Sources of Contrast

This section discusses sources of image contrast in MSOT. We have seen that optoacoustic image intensity (initial pressure distribution) is given by:

$$p_0 = \Gamma \phi \mu_a, \tag{12.13}$$

where Γ, the Grüneisen coefficient, describes the thermodynamic properties of the material being heated, ϕ is the light fluence, and μ_a is the absorption coefficient. We see that the initial pressure is proportional to the product of the local light fluence and absorption coefficient, that is, the optoacoustic image represents the amount of optical energy absorbed at each point in space. The fluence at each point depends on the illumination, as well as the optical properties of the tissue. Spatial variations in fluence are relatively smooth due to the high scattering of light in tissue. As a result, the factor providing by far the most defined (high frequency) image contrast is μ_a, the local absorption coefficient. Contrast sources are therefore materials that absorb light.

12.6.1 Endogenous tissue absorption

12.6.1.1 Hemoglobin contrast

To appreciate why optoacoustic imaging is capable of producing high contrast images of blood vessels, consider the difference in absorption coefficients between blood and surrounding tissue. As an example, at a wavelength of 800 nm, hemoglobin, whether oxygenated or not, has a molar extinction coefficient of approximately 800 $cm^{-1}M^{-1}$. A typical value of hemoglobin concentration in whole blood is 150 g/l, resulting in an absorption coefficient of $\mu_a = 2.3$ cm^{-1}. Assume the tissue surrounding the blood vessel has an absorption coefficient in the region of 0.2 cm^{-1} [45]. Taking into account the fact that the optoacoustic signal amplitude is directly proportional to the absorption coefficient, we have an order of magnitude higher signal from blood than from the surrounding tissue. As a result, vascular imaging is a natural application of optoacoustic imaging. To illustrate this point, Fig. 12.5 shows an optoacoustic image through the liver of a mouse *in vivo* taken at an excitation wavelength of 850 nm without any signal averaging, that is, produced from a single laser pulse (system described in Fig. 12.2). Several blood vessels of various sizes are clearly visible, even though the liver tissue surrounding the blood vessels is quite absorbing compared to other tissue types.

In addition to simply producing images of vasculature at single wavelengths, we can gain further information by multispectral imaging: hemoglobin displays a change in absorption spectrum based on its oxygenation state. The corresponding extinction spectra are plotted in Fig. 12.6.

By MSOT, it is thus possible to resolve the concentrations of the two oxygenation states and therefore related measures, such as blood oxygen saturation. The relevant formula is as follows:

$$S_{O_2} = \frac{HbO_2}{HbO_2 + Hb}, \tag{12.14}$$

where S_{O_2} is the oxygen saturation to be calculated, HbO_2 is the concentration of oxygenated hemoglobin and Hb is the concentration of deoxygenated hemoglobin. This functional imaging capability has been demonstrated in different variations over the past years, including the use of two visible wavelengths in microscopic imaging of superficial vasculature [46] and deep tissue sensing [47].

Figure 12.7 shows blood oxygen saturation in blood vessels in the tail of a mouse as an example of functional imaging of hemoglobin oxygenation by MSOT. The experimental and processing steps used that example were as follows:

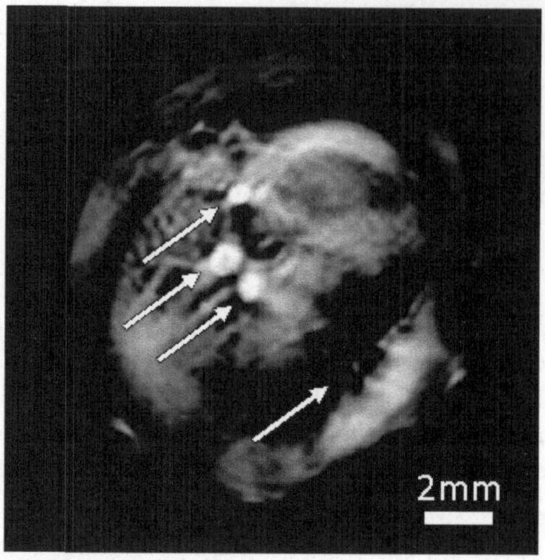

Figure 12.5: Blood vessels visible in an optoacoustic image taken at 850 nm through the liver of a mouse.

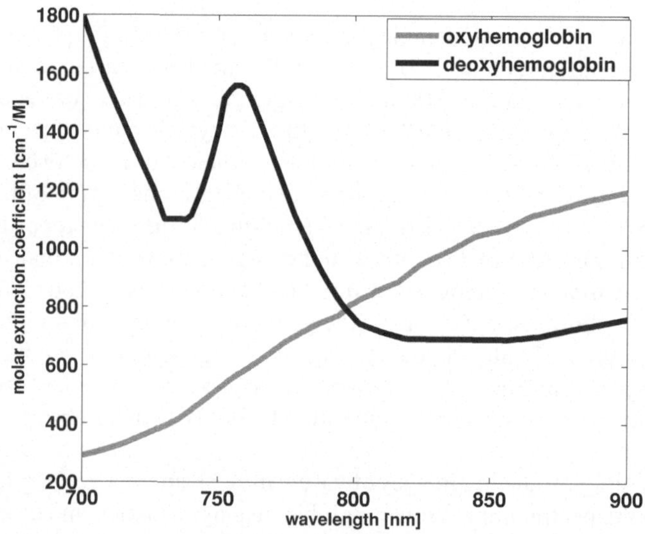

Figure 12.6: Extinction spectra of deoxyhemoglobin (black) and oxygenated hemoglobin (grey). Data compiled by Scott Prahl, Oregon Medical Laser Center (http://omlc.ogi.edu/spectra), from multiple sources.

1. MSOT imaging was performed at multiple wavelengths: 700 nm, 730 nm, 760 nm, 790 nm, 810 nm, and 850 nm.

2. The spectral contributions of oxy- and deoxyhemoglobin were computed per pixel by linear spectral unmixing.

The image is composed of two layers. In the background, using a grayscale to represent intensity, is a single wavelength optoacoustic image taken at 850 nm. This image provides anatomical

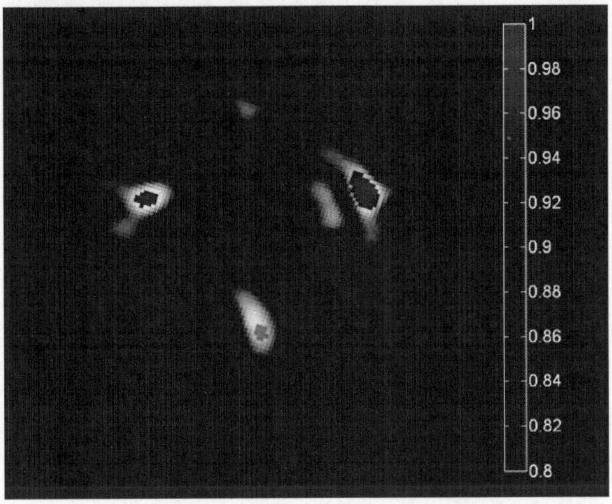

Figure 12.7: (See color insert.) Blood oxygenation in veins and artery of a mouse tail. The scale bar indicates blood oxygen saturation (S_{O_2}) as a fraction.

structures of the tail. The overlay, in a color scale from blue (less oxygenation) to red (maximum oxygenation) shows the functional information, in this case oxygen saturation. Potential applications of such measurements are numerous: for one, blood oxygen saturation in arteries is a measure of hypoxemia.

12.6.1.2 Further tissue-intrinsic sources of contrast

Melanin is a biological pigment found in the skin and hair, and represents a strong absorber of light, which has been exploited in optoacoustic imaging. For example, Oh et al. used the absorption of melanin to produce microscopic optoacoustic images of melanoma [48]. An absorption spectrum taken from the literature of eumelanin, a common form of melanin, is shown in Fig. 12.8. Note that melanin is present in large enough concentrations in pigmented skin for strong optoacoustic signals to be generated, even in the near infrared (see Fig. 12.9).

Water concentration in tissue is of much interest as a pathophysiological biomarker, displaying elevated levels in tumors, and has been reported to be distinguishable by MSOT in initial studies by Xu et al. [49]. Water has an absorption spectrum as shown in figure 5.10, with a local peak around 975 nm. A challenge in imaging water is its relatively high normal tissue concentration, which could serve to attenuate the excitation light on its way to the target. However, water does represent a promising additional intrinsic tissue parameter that can potentially be extracted by MSOT.

Lipids display an optical absorption peak at around 1200 nm, which has values an order of magnitude lower in NIR wavelengths up to 1100 nm [50]. Since lipids form an important component of atherosclerotic plaques, some efforts at their detection by intravascular optoacoustic imaging have been reported [32, 51]. The high absorption of water in this wavelength range, however, makes it challenging to perform lipid detection noninvasively at macroscopic scales.

12.6.2 Exogenous contrast agents

Table 12.1 provides several examples of light absorbing contrast agents that have been reported in the literature for optoacoustic imaging applications. The selection of contrast agents for MSOT is generally application driven. However, some essential properties are universal. Obviously, in order to generate an optoacoustic signal, the agent must absorb light. Typically, for imaging at depth, this

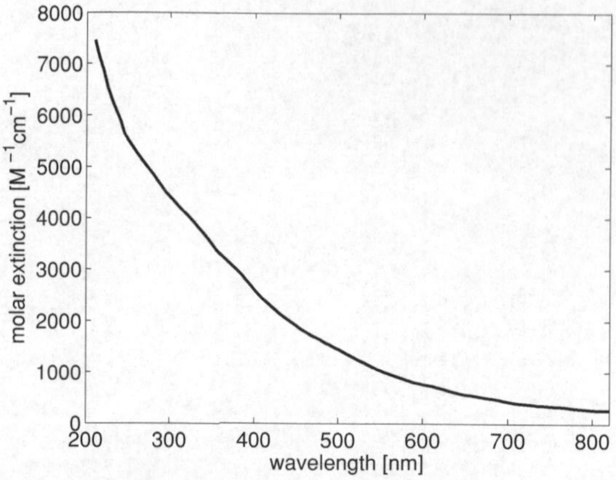

Figure 12.8: Extinction spectrum of eumelanin. Data compiled by Steven Jacques, Oregon Medical Laser Center (http://omlc.ogi.edu/spectra).

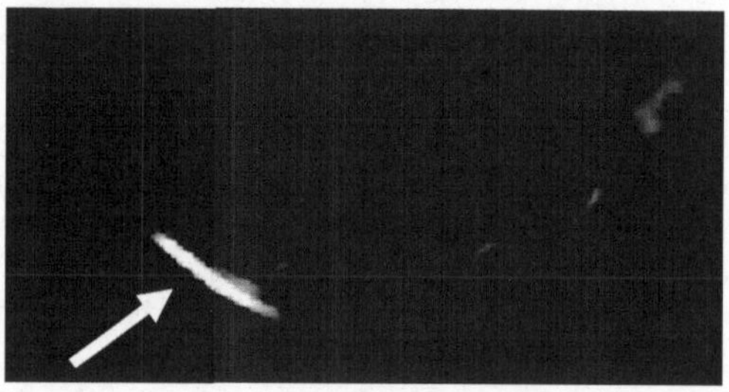

Figure 12.9: Strong optoacoustic contrast produced by melanin, indicated by arrow, in the skin of a mouse (black 6). Excitation at 900 nm.

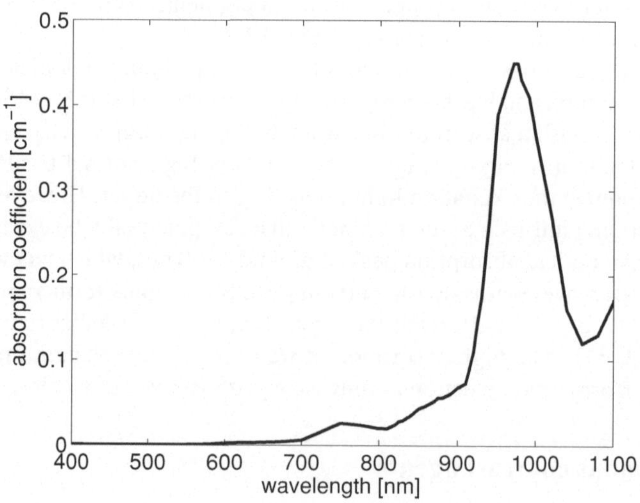

Figure 12.10: Water absorption spectrum. Data compiled by Scott Prahl, Oregon Medical Laser Center (http://omlc.ogi.edu/spectra).

absorption should occur in the NIR, so that light can reach the agent. Absorption in the NIR would be sufficient if the imaging was performed in a time series where an increase (or decrease) in contrast over time is measured in an unchanging background. A number of examples of such imaging, which can be performed at a single wavelength, have been documented. Salient examples include the use of gold nanocages for imaging of the sentinel lymph node in rats [9] and imaging of tumors in mice using targeted carbon nanotubes [52]. However, an unchanging background (or unmoving tissue) is not always realistic. In *in vivo* experiments where imaging agents should be visualized over the course of several hours or days, it is impractical to position the tissue in exactly the same way during each imaging session. As soon as the tissue background changes, there is a problem distinguishing the imaging agent from the intrinsic background tissue absorption. Therefore, to detect signal specific to the contrast agent in question, that is, to suppress the background signal, it is essential to image at multiple wavelengths and unmix the resulting images to obtain the various spectral signatures, including that of the agent. This adds another requirement for suitable MSOT contrast agents: they should have an absorption spectrum that uniquely distinguishes them from intrinsic tissue absorbers. In the ideal case, an MSOT contrast agent would have a very thin peak in its absorption spectrum: when imaging at the applicable wavelength, the agent would absorb a lot of light and generate a high optoacoustic signal; when slightly changing the wavelength, so that the background absorption does not significantly change, the agent would not absorb any light or generate any signal at all. The two images could be subtracted from one another to obtain a spatial map of the contrast agent, without significant background. In reality, the absorption peaks of potential contrast agents are generally too wide to allow such an approach: in the wavelength range from peak to off-peak absorption there is usually a significant change in the spectra of tissue intrinsic absorbers, therefore making more sophisticated spectral unmixing approaches mandatory. However, it still holds that the narrower the absorption peak, the easier it is to uniquely identify to agent. So we have, from a technical view, a set of requirements for MSOT contrast agents: they should display high absorption in the NIR with a narrow absorption peak. Note that not all of the agents listed in Table 12.1 display very sharp absorption peaks: for example, carbon nanotubes have a relatively flat characteristic spectrum. Generally, many of the reported imaging results in the table employed single wavelength imaging with some sort of reference threshold to detect contrast enhancement after agent injection or accumulation. Since the concept of MSOT is based on separation of specific absorbers based on their spectra, agents that have been used in this manner are not necessarily ideal for MSOT imaging. Ntziachristos et al. introduced a measure of absorption, corrected for quantum (fluorescence) yield, per unit of mass concentration, in an attempt to compare the optoacoustic efficiency of different contrast agents [53]. The results show that near infrared fluorescent dyes display higher values than a range of other agents, such as gold nanorods. However, it is difficult to compare such a range of vastly different agents when characteristics like weight and pharmacokinetic profiles may vary by orders of magnitude. The selection of agents for real-world imaging applications depends on many other factors than signal efficiency, such as whether the agent is approved for use in patients (ICG is, gold nanoparticles are not), whether the dimensions of the molecules or particles are suitable for certain physiological effects (gold nanoparticles can be made in the right size range to accumulate by enhanced tumor vascular permeability, for example), whether the agent can be conjugated to targeting ligands (ICG has no available reactive group for this purpose) et cetera. Other characteristics should also be considered in the context of efficient generation of optoacoustic signals. For example, plasmonic nanoparticles can undergo coupling when brought close together, a fact which was exploited by Mallidi et al. by targeting gold nanospheres to closely packed receptors [54]. However, this could be a major disadvantage: gold nanorods can also be coupled *in vivo*, for example when taken up by inflammatory cells, causing their absorption spectrum to change unpredictably. Additionally, gold nanorods are known to change shape (and therefore absorption spectrum) due to melting from the heating energy of pulsed lasers [55, 56], which could limit the fluence and number of pulses used for quantitative optoacoustic imaging, an issue that requires further investigation. On the other hand, organic dyes are well known to undergo photobleaching

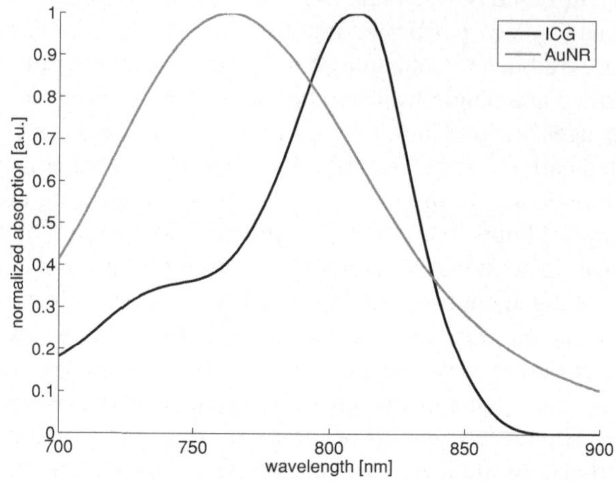

Figure 12.11: Normalized absorption spectra of indocyanine green (ICG) and gold nanorods (AuNR).

under intense illumination, also resulting in alterations to their absorption spectra. All these factors need to be taken into account when selecting MSOT contrast agents. We discuss two different types of contrast agents in the following: organic dyes and gold nanorods. Organic dyes are in very widespread use in biomedicine, in particular for use as fluorescent agents in imaging ranging from microscopy using immunofluorescence to deep-tissue diffuse optical techniques [5]. They are available in various wavelength regions, including the NIR. Additionally, they have been incorporated into a multitude of molecular imaging agents, by adding targeting ligands or by dequenching mechanisms upon specific enzymatic action (activatable probes). Many of these molecular imaging agents are commercially available. A further advantage of organic dyes is their clinical potential, for example, indocyanine green (ICG), is clinically (FDA) approved. In fact, ICG has been established as a tool to investigate a variety of different clinical endpoints such as hepatic function [57]. As for gold nanorods, they are an example of nanostructures with high absorption in the NIR region and tunable longitudinal plasmon resonances dependent on their aspect ratio. Due to their well established surface conjugation chemistry, gold nanorods can be easily linked to specific ligands in order to target molecular entities such as cell receptors [58]. In addition, the intense photothermal properties due to the conversion of optical energy into heat via non-radiative electron relaxation dynamics, can be used for therapeutic purposes [59] and allow light-mediated drug release [60]. The absorption spectra of ICG (in water) and selected gold nanorods (AuNR, nominal absorption peak around 780 nm, Ntracker 30-PM-780, Nanopartz Inc.), normalized to their maxima, are plotted in Fig. 12.11. From the plot we can see that both agents display an absorption peak in the NIR and can be considered as suitable MSOT contrast agents.

Correspondingly, Fig. 12.12 shows results from phantom imaging experiments, where both ICG and AuNR were detected by MSOT. Tissue-mimicking cylindrical phantoms of 2 cm diameter were prepared by molding 1.3% weight of Agar powder (Sigma-Aldrich) black India ink (Higgins) and 6% of Intralipid 20% emulsion (Sigma-Aldrich) to obtain a background with an optical absorption coefficient of $\mu_a \approx 0.2$ cm^{-1} and a reduced scattering coefficient of $\mu_s' \approx 10$ cm^{-1}. A cylindrical inclusion with a diameter of approximately 3 mm in the center of the background cylinder additionally contained 0.8 μM ICG or 1.4 μg/ml AuNR, corresponding to an additional absorption of $\mu_a \approx 0.2$ cm^{-1} as determined using a spectrometer. MSOT data sets of the phantoms were recorded between 720 nm and 850 nm with 10 nm steps using 100 signal averages. The results in Fig. 12.12 show that

TABLE 12.1: A selection of contrast agents reported in the literature for optoacoustic imaging.

Contrast medium	Absorption features	Reported applications
Methylene blue	677 nm peak	Lymphatic mapping in 2008 by Song et al. [61].
indocyanine green (ICG)	810 nm peak (in plasma)	Brain angiography in 2004 by Wang et al. [62] and numerous other applications.
IRDye 800CW (Licor)	774 nm peak	Conjugated with RGD peptide to target brain tumors in 2008 by Li et al. [11].
Gold nanorods	Tunable NIR	Multispectral identification in the circulation in 2010 [17].
Gold nanospheres	Increase in NIR absorption when closely coupled	Tumor targeting and subsequent resonance coupling by antibody conjugation in 2009 by Mallidi et al. [54].
Hollow gold nanospheres	Tunable peak in NIR	Contrast enhanced imaging of the brain vasculature in 2010 by Lu et al. [63].
Gold nanocages	Tunable peak in NIR	Bioconjugated to target melanoma in 2010 by Kim et al. [64].
Gold-enhanced carbon nanotubes	Increased NIR absorption	Optoacoustic and photothermal flow cytometry in 2009 by Kim et al. [65].
Silver nanoplates	Absorption in 1000 nm region	Demonstrated as contrast agent for imaging at 1064 nm in 2010 by Homan et al. [66].
Single-walled carbon nanotubes (SW-CNT)	Relatively flat spectrum	Conjugated with RGD peptide for tumor targeting in 2008 by de le Zerda et al. [52].
ICG-enhanced single-walled carbon nanotubes	Spectrum defined by ICG	Conjugated with RGD peptide for tumor targeting in 2010 by de le Zerda et al. [67].

images acquired at 790 nm and 780 nm, near the peak absorption wavelengths of ICG and AuNR respectively display no clear contrast from the inclusions because of strong light attenuation inside the phantoms and low concentrations of the agents. However, by imaging at multiple wavelengths and employing spectral unmixing, the ICG and AuNR could be resolved: the target-to-background ratios (TBR) of the inclusions increased from approximately 1 to 2.6 and 3.0 respectively. The location of the inclusions was at approximately 1 cm depth from the phantom surface, representing a challenging imaging scenario and indicating the feasibility of spatially resolved detection of these agents by MSOT.

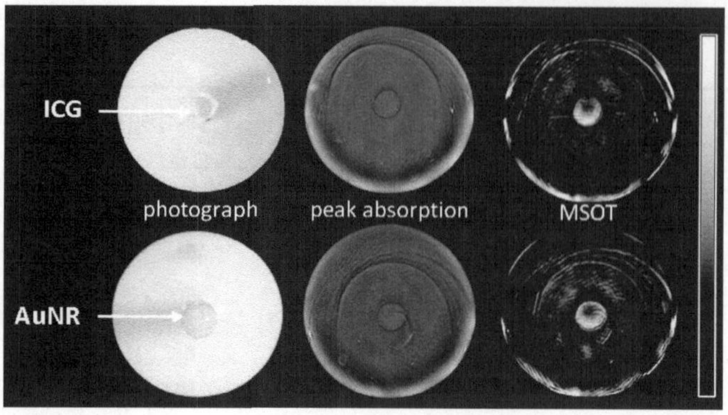

Figure 12.12: Multispectral optoacoustic tomography of phantoms containing Indocyanine green (ICG) and gold nanorods (AuNR).

In vivo, MSOT reveals exogenous contrast agents simultaneously to tissue-intrinsic absorption. In the example shown in Fig. 12.13, MSOT was applied to visualize ICG entering the kidneys of a mouse [16]. Because of hemoglobin contrast, the kidneys are clearly visible even in optoacoustic images taken at single wavelengths (Fig. 12.13 a and b). High-rate dynamic imaging (10 frames/s) enabled by the parallel read-out from multi-element ultrasound detector arrays allows the inflow of ICG to be detected simply by the increase in absorption it provides over time (Fig. 12.13 c and d). Multispectral imaging with subsequent spectral unmixing provides the specific ICG distribution at a single time point (Fig. 12.13 e).

12.6.2.1 Activatable agents

Activatable fluorescent agents, which are initially optically silent but become fluorescent when cleaved by enzymes, have proven to be a uniquely powerful tool for imaging specific protease activity [68, 69]. These probes work by positioning multiple fluorochromes close enough together that their fluorescence is quenched; cleaving by proteases then separates the fluorochromes which can then be seen by fluorescence imaging. Since the dequenching is also associated with a change is the absorption spectrum of the probe in question, detection by MSOT could be feasible. This ability to detect an activatable fluorescent probe by MSOT based on the change in its absorption spectrum on activation was exploited in imaging of matrix metalloproteinase (MMP) activity in human carotid plaque specimens by Razansky et al. in 2011 [70]. In vitro activation of the agent confirmed a change in the absorption spectrum (Fig. 12.14 a). MSOT imaging in phantoms also detected this change: in the image at 635 nm excitation, the inactive probe inclusion produces more signal than the active agent (Fig. 12.14 b); at 675 nm the active inclusion increases in intensity (Fig. 12.14 c). By subtracting the two images (Fig. 12.14 d) it is possible to enhance the active inclusion and suppress the inactive inclusion and background absorption because of the presence of the absorption peak at 675 nm.

12.6.3 Reporter genes

Fluorescent proteins find daily application in biological research, and efforts are continuing to shift their excitation and emission wavelengths into the NIR to enable imaging in deeper tissues [71]. In the meantime, Razansky et al. demonstrated MSOT detection of fluorescent proteins, largely in the red wavelength range, in model organisms such as Zebrafish in 2009 (see Fig. 12.15) [72]. Additionally, recent work has led to reporter gene imaging specifically conceived for optoacoustic

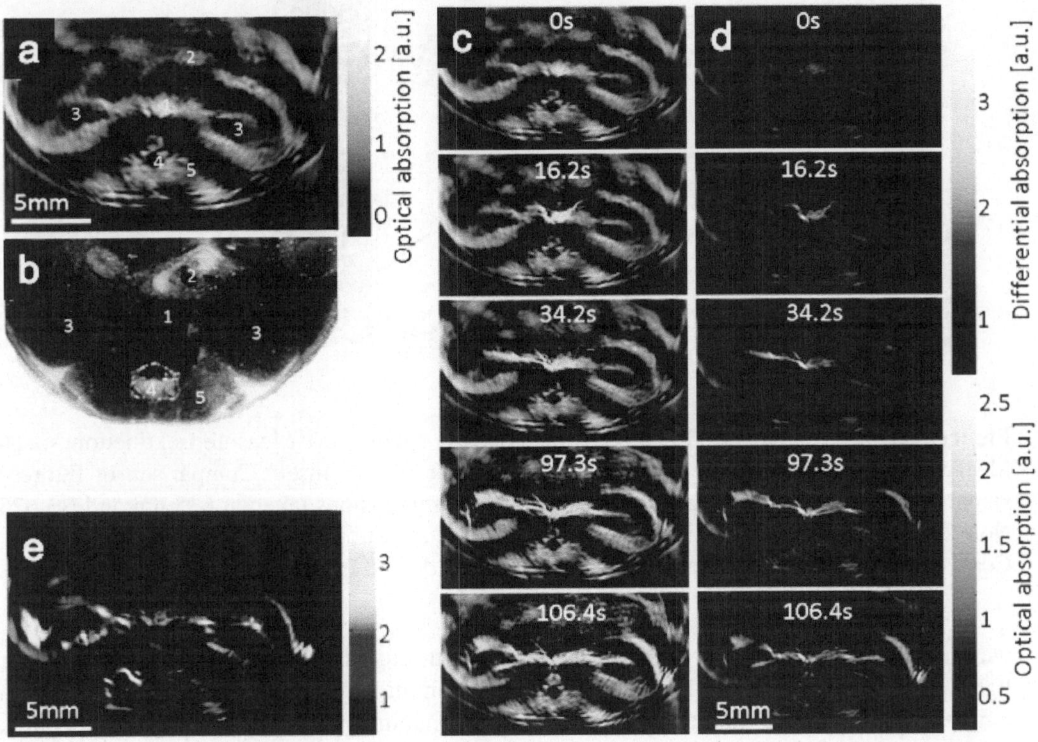

Figure 12.13: (See color insert.) Indocyanine green (ICG) entering the kidneys of a mouse. (a) Optoacoustic slice image through the kidneys. 1 - vena cava, 2 - portal vein, 3 - kidneys, 4 - spine. (b) Corresponding cryosection photograph showing the same structures. (c) Selected images from single laser pulses at 800 nm during ICG injection showing increased contrast from the agent. (d) Overlay of differential contrast highlighting the ICG enhancement. (e) Overlay showing the distribution of ICG in the same animal by spectral unmixing after imaging at multiple wavelengths (750, 770, 790, 810, 830, 850, 870, 890, and 910 nm). Note the agreement with areas of increased contrast in (d). Adapted from [16].

imaging: by introducing the gene encoding tyrosinase, which is responsible for producing melanin, cells have been reported to produce an order of magnitude more optoacoustic signal [73]. These advances suggest a role for MSOT imaging of reporter genes in basic biological research, allowing a higher resolution in deep tissue than the fluorescence approaches employed thus far.

12.7 Conclusion

The purpose of this chapter was to provide an overview of the physical principles, implementation considerations, reconstruction approaches and potential sources of contrast for molecular optoacoustic imaging. Multispectral optoacoustic tomography (MSOT), based on the ultrasound detection of optical absorption via the optoacoustic effect, can provide images that probe the underlying biological processes involved in disease. The technique combines rich optical contrast, provided by intrinsic tissue absorbers like hemoglobin and a multitude of optical imaging agents,

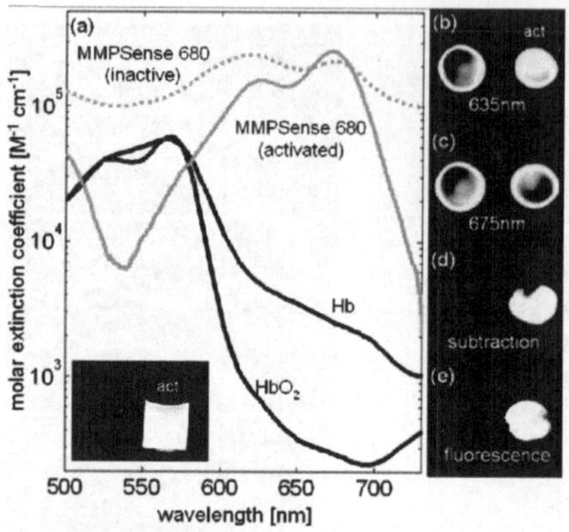

Figure 12.14: Imaging of MMP-activated optical agent. (a) Measured extinction spectra of MMPSense 680 (PerkinElmer) in active and inactive states. Inset: Comparison of fluorescence signal. (b) Optoacoustic image of inactive and active inclusions taken at 635 nm and (c) 675 nm. Note the change in intensity in the active inclusion. (d) Subtraction of the two wavelengths. (e) Corresponding fluorescence image of the phantom. Adapted from [70].

with ultrasound resolution in deep tissues, breaking through the barrier that the high scattering of light raises after the first millimeter. By employing multi-wavelength illumination, MSOT distinguishes absorbers based on their spectral signatures, enabling multichannel images of specific chromophores of interest, including the different hemoglobin oxygenation states and exogenous optical contrast agents. There is a wide range of potential application areas for MSOT, ranging from small animal imaging, where the ability to visualize reporter genes at high resolutions could be a valuable addition to the biologists toolset, to clinical diagnostics and treatment monitoring, including fields as diverse as dermatological examinations, breast cancer screening, noninvasive lymphatic mapping, and functional vascular assessment.

Acknowledgments

VN acknowledges support from the ERC Advanced Investigator Award and the German Ministry of Education and Research (BMBF) Innovation in Medicine Award.

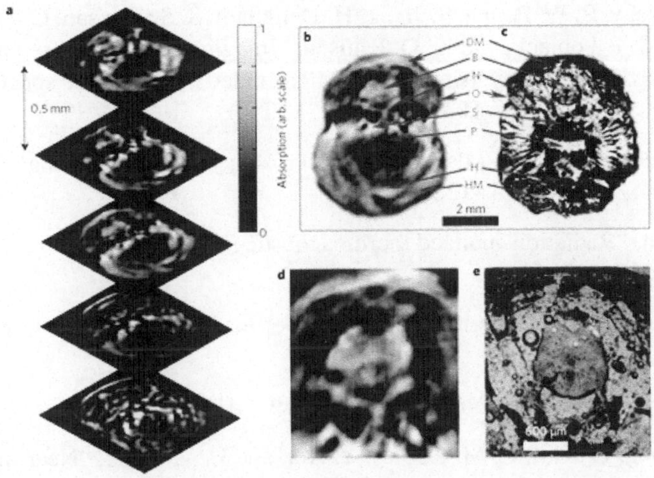

Figure 12.15: (See color insert.) *In vivo* imaging through the brain of an adult (six-month-old) mCherry-expressing transgenic zebrafish. (a) Five transverse optoacoustic imaging slices through the hindbrain area at the level of crista cerebellaris of a living zebrafish taken at 585 nm. (b) Example of an imaged slice and (c) its corresponding histological section in inverted colors. DM, dorsal fin musculature; B, hindbrain; N, lateral line nerve; O, operculum; S, skull bones; P, pharynx; H, heart; HM, hypobranchial musculature. (d) MSOT image of the brain (enlarged) with mCherry expression shown in color. (e) Corresponding fluorescent histology of a dissected fish at the hindbrain level. Adapted from [72].

References

[1] R. Weissleder and V. Ntziachristos, "Shedding light onto live molecular targets," *Nat. Med.* **9**, 123–128 (2003).

[2] V. Ntziachristos, A. G. Yodh, M. Schnall, and B. Chance, "Concurrent MRI and diffuse optical tomography of breast after indocyanine green enhancement," *Proc. Natl. Acad. Sci. U. S. A.* **97**, 2767–2772 (2000).

[3] A. Ale, R. B. Schulz, A. Sarantopoulos, and V. Ntziachristos, "Imaging performance of a hybrid x-ray computed tomography-fluorescence molecular tomography system using priors," *Med. Phys.* **37**, 1976–1986 (2010).

[4] B. Brooksby, B. W. Pogue, S. Jiang, H. Dehghani, S. Srinivasan, C. Kogel, T. D. Tosteson, J. Weaver, S. P. Poplack, and K. D. Paulsen, "Imaging breast adipose and fibroglandular tissue molecular signatures by using hybrid MRI-guided near-infrared spectral tomography," *Proc. Natl. Acad. Sci. U. S. A.* **103**, 8828–8833 (2006).

[5] V. Ntziachristos, "Going deeper than microscopy: the optical imaging frontier in biology," *Nat. Methods* **7**, 603–614 (2010).

[6] T. Bowen, "Radiation-induced thermoacoustic soft tissue imaging," *IEEE Ultrasonics Symposium*, 817–822 (1981).

[7] G. Busse, "Imaging with the optoacoustic effect," *Optics & Laser Technology* **12**, 149–154 (1980).

[8] A. Rosencwaig, "Photoacoustic spectroscopy," *Annu. Rev. Biophys. Bioeng.* **9**, 31–54 (1980).

[9] K. H. Song, C. Kim, C. M. Cobley, Y. Xia, and L. V. Wang, "Near-infrared gold nanocages as a new class of tracers for photoacoustic sentinel lymph node mapping on a rat model," *Nano Lett.* **9**, 183–188 (2009).

[10] D. Razansky, C. Vinegoni, and V. Ntziachristos, "Multispectral photoacoustic imaging of fluorochromes in small animals," *Opt. Lett.* **32**, 2891–2893 (2007).

[11] M. L. Li, J. T. Oh, X. Xie, G. Ku, W. Wang, C. Li, G. Lungu, G. Stoica, and L. V. Wang, "Simultaneous molecular and hypoxia imaging of brain tumors in vivo using spectroscopic photoacoustic tomography," *Proc. IEEE* **96**, 481–489 (2008).

[12] C. Li and L. V. Wang, "Photoacoustic tomography and sensing in biomedicine," *Phys. Med. Biol.* **54**, R59–97 (2009).

[13] G. J. Diebold, T. Sun, and M. I. Khan, "Photoacoustic monopole radiation in one, two, and three dimensions," *Phys. Rev. Lett.* **67**, 3384–3387 (1991).

[14] X. Wang, Y. Pang, G. Ku, X. Xie, G. Stoica, and L. V. Wang, "Noninvasive laser-induced photoacoustic tomography for structural and functional in vivo imaging of the brain," *Nat. Biotechnol.* **21**, 803–806 (2003).

[15] R. Ma, A. Taruttis, V. Ntziachristos, and D. Razansky, "Multispectral optoacoustic tomography (MSOT) scanner for whole-body small animal imaging," *Opt. Express* **17**, 21414–21426 (2009).

[16] A. Buehler, E. Herzog, D. Razansky, and V. Ntziachristos, "Video rate optoacoustic tomography of mouse kidney perfusion," *Opt. Lett.* **35**, 2475–2477 (2010).

[17] A. Taruttis, E. Herzog, D. Razansky, and V. Ntziachristos, "Real-time imaging of cardiovascular dynamics and circulating gold nanorods with multispectral optoacoustic tomography," *Opt. Express* **18**, 19592–19602 (2010).

[18] J. Gamelin, A. Maurudis, A. Aguirre, F. Huang, P. Guo, L. V. Wang, and Q. Zhu, "A real-time photoacoustic tomography system for small animals," *Opt. Express* **17**, 10489–10498 (2009).

[19] R. A. Kruger, W. L. Kiser, D. R. Reinecke, G. A. Kruger, and K. D. Miller, "Thermoacoustic molecular imaging of small animals," *Mol. Imaging* **2**, 113–123 (2003).

[20] H. P. Brecht, R. Su, M. Fronheiser, S. A. Ermilov, A. Conjusteau, and A. A. Oraevsky, "Whole-body three-dimensional optoacoustic tomography system for small animals," *J. Biomed. Opt.* **14**, 064007 (2009).

[21] R. A. Kruger, R. B. Lam, D. R. Reinecke, S. P. Del Rio, and R. P. Doyle, "Photoacoustic angiography of the breast," *Med. Phys.* **37**, 6096–6100 (2010).

[22] S. Manohar, S. E. Vaartjes, J. C. G. van Hespen, J. M. Klaase, F. M. van den Engh, W. Steenbergen, and T. G. van Leeuwen, "Initial results of in vivo non-invasive cancer imaging in the human breast using near-infrared photoacoustics," *Opt. Express* **15**, 12277–12285 (2007).

[23] S. A. Ermilov, T. Khamapirad, A. Conjusteau, M. H. Leonard, R. Lacewell, K. Mehta, T. Miller, and A. A. Oraevsky, "Laser optoacoustic imaging system for detection of breast cancer," *J. Biomed. Opt.* **14**, 024007 (2009).

[24] D. Razansky, A. Buehler, and V. Ntziachristos, "Volumetric real-time multispectral optoacoustic tomography of biomarkers," *Nat. Protoc.* **6**, 1121–1129 (2011).

[25] J. Laufer, E. Zhang, G. Raivich, and P. Beard, "Three-dimensional noninvasive imaging of the vasculature in the mouse brain using a high resolution photoacoustic scanner," *Appl. Opt.* **48**, D299–D306 (2009).

[26] C. Zhang, K. Maslov, and L. V. Wang, "Subwavelength-resolution label-free photoacoustic microscopy of optical absorption in vivo," *Opt. Lett.* **35**, 3195–3197 (2010).

[27] H. F. Zhang, K. Maslov, G. Stoica, and L. V. Wang, "Functional photoacoustic microscopy for high-resolution and noninvasive in vivo imaging," *Nat. Biotechnol.* **24**, 848–851 (2006).

[28] S. Hu, B. Rao, K. Maslov, and L. V. Wang, "Label-free photoacoustic ophthalmic angiography," *Opt. Lett.* **35**, 1–3 (2010).

[29] S. Jiao, M. Jiang, J. Hu, A. Fawzi, Q. Zhou, K. K. Shung, C. A. Puliafito, and H. F. Zhang, "Photoacoustic ophthalmoscopy for in vivo retinal imaging," *Opt. Express* **18**, 3967–3972 (2010).

[30] J. Sanz and Z. A. Fayad, "Imaging of atherosclerotic cardiovascular disease," *Nature* **451**, 953–957 (2008).

[31] S. Sethuraman, S. R. Aglyamov, J. H. Amirian, R. W. Smalling, and S. Y. Emelianov, "Intravascular photoacoustic imaging using an IVUS imaging catheter," *IEEE Trans. Ultrason. Ferroelectr. Freq. Control* **54**, 978–986 (2007).

[32] K. Jansen, A. F. W. Van der Steen, H. M. M. van Beusekom, J. W. Oosterhuis, and G. van Soest, "Intravascular photoacoustic imaging of human coronary atherosclerosis," *Opt. Lett.* **36**, 597–599 (2011).

[33] J. M. Yang, K. Maslov, H. C. Yang, Q. Zhou, K. K. Shung, and L. V. Wang, "Photoacoustic endoscopy," *Opt. Lett.* **34**, 1591–1593 (2009).

[34] Y. Yuan, S. Yang, and D. Xing, "Preclinical photoacoustic imaging endoscope based on acousto-optic coaxial system using ring transducer array," *Opt. Lett.* **35**, 2266–2268.

[35] E. I. Galanzha, E. V. Shashkov, T. Kelly, J. W. Kim, L. Yang, and V. P. Zharov, "In vivo magnetic enrichment and multiplex photoacoustic detection of circulating tumour cells," *Nat. Nanotechnol.* **4**, 855–860 (2009).

[36] E. I. Galanzha, E. V. Shashkov, P. M. Spring, J. Y. Suen, and V. P. Zharov, "In vivo, noninvasive, label-free detection and eradication of circulating metastatic melanoma cells using two-color photoacoustic flow cytometry with a diode laser," *Cancer Res.* **69**, 7926–7934 (2009).

[37] C. G. A. Hoelen, and F. F. M. de Mul, "Image reconstruction for photoacoustic scanning of tissue structures," *Appl. Opt.* **39**, 5872–5883 (2000).

[38] R. A. Kruger, P. Liu, and C. R. Appledorn, "Photoacoustic ultrasound (PAUS)–reconstruction tomography," *Med. Phys.* **22**, 1605–1609 (1995).

[39] M. Xu and L. V. Wang, "Universal back-projection algorithm for photoacoustic computed tomography," *Phys. Rev. E* **71**, 016706 (2005).

[40] A. Rosenthal, D. Razansky, and V. Ntziachristos, "Fast semi-analytical model-based acoustic inversion for quantitative optoacoustic tomography," *IEEE Trans. Med. Imaging* 29, 1275–1285 (2010).

[41] A. Buehler, A. Rosenthal, T. Jetzfellner, A. Dima, D. Razansky, and V. Ntziachristos, "Model-based optoacoustic inversions with incomplete projection data," *Med. Phys.* **38**, 1694–1704 (2011).

[42] M. Xu and L. V. Wang, "Analytic explanation of spatial resolution related to bandwidth and detector aperture size in thermoacoustic or photoacoustic reconstruction," *Phys. Rev. E* **67**, 056605 (2003).

[43] A. Rosenthal, V. Ntziachristos, and D. Razansky, "Model-based optoacoustic inversion with arbitrary-shape detectors," *Med. Phys.* **38**, 4285–4295 (2011).

[44] J. Glatz, N. C. Deliolanis, A. Buehler, D. Razansky, and V. Ntziachristos, "Blind source unmixing in multi-spectral optoacoustic tomography," *Opt. Express* **19**, 3175–3184 (2011).

[45] M. J. Niedre, G. M. Turner, and V. Ntziachristos, "Time-resolved imaging of optical coefficients through murine chest cavities," *J. Biomed. Opt.* **11**, 064017 (2006).

[46] Z. Guo, S. Hu, and L. V. Wang, "Calibration-free absolute quantification of optical absorption coefficients using acoustic spectra in 3D photoacoustic microscopy of biological tissue," *Opt. Lett.* **35**, 2067–2069 (2010).

[47] Y. Y. Petrov, I. Y. Petrova, I. A. Patrikeev, R. O. Esenaliev, and D. S. Prough, "Multiwavelength optoacoustic system for noninvasive monitoring of cerebral venous oxygenation: a pilot clinical test in the internal jugular vein," *Opt. Lett.* **31**, 1827–1829 (2006).

[48] J. T. Oh, M. L. Li, H. F. Zhang, K. Maslov, G. Stoica, and L. V. Wang, "Three-dimensional imaging of skin melanoma in vivo by dual-wavelength photoacoustic microscopy," *J. Biomed. Opt.* **11**, 034032 (2006).

[49] Z. Xu, C. Li, and L. V. Wang, "Photoacoustic tomography of water in phantoms and tissue," *J. Biomed. Opt.* **15**, 036019 (2010).

[50] C. L. Tsai, J. C. Chen, and W. J. Wang, "Near-infrared absorption property of biological soft tissue constituents," *J. Med. Biol. Eng.* **21**, 7–14 (2001).

[51] S. Sethuraman, J. H. Amirian, S. H. Litovsky, R. W. Smalling, and S. Y. Emelianov, "Spectroscopic intravascular photoacoustic imaging to differentiate atherosclerotic plaques," *Opt. Express* **16**, 3362–3367 (2008).

[52] A. De La Zerda, C. Zavaleta, S. Keren, S. Vaithilingam, S. Bodapati, Z. Liu, J. Levi, B. R. Smith, T. J. Ma, and O. Oralkan, "Carbon nanotubes as photoacoustic molecular imaging agents in living mice," *Nat. Nanotechnol.* **3**, 557–562 (2008).

[53] V. Ntziachristos and D. Razansky, "Molecular Imaging by Means of Multispectral Optoacoustic Tomography (MSOT)," *Chem. Rev.* **110**, 2783–2794 (2010).

[54] S. Mallidi, T. Larson, J. Tam, P. P. Joshi, A. Karpiouk, K. Sokolov, and S. Emelianov, "Multiwavelength photoacoustic imaging and plasmon resonance coupling of gold nanoparticles for selective detection of cancer," *Nano Lett.* **9**, 2825–2831 (2009).

[55] S. S. Chang, C. W. Shih, C. D. Chen, W. C. Lai, and C. R. C. Wang, "The shape transition of gold nanorods," *Langmuir* **15**, 701–709 (1999).

[56] C. L. Didychuk, P. Ephrat, A. Chamson-Reig, S. L. Jacques, and J. J. L. Carson, "Depth of photothermal conversion of gold nanorods embedded in a tissue-like phantom," *Nanotechnology* **20**, 195102 (2009).

[57] D. B. Hunton, J. L. Bollman, and H. N. Hoffman, "Studies of hepatic function with indocyanine green," *Gastroenterology* **39**, 713–724 (1960).

[58] Z. Li, P. Huang, X. Zhang, J. Lin, S. Yang, B. Liu, F. Gao, P. Xi, Q. Ren, and D. Cui, "RGD-conjugated dendrimer-modified gold nanorods for in vivo tumor targeting and photothermal therapy," *Mol. Pharmacol.* **7**, 94–104 (2010).

[59] E. B. Dickerson, E. C. Dreaden, X. Huang, I. H. El-Sayed, H. Chu, S. Pushpanketh, J. F. McDonald, and M. A. El-Sayed, "Gold nanorod assisted near-infrared plasmonic photothermal therapy (PPTT) of squamous cell carcinoma in mice," *Cancer Lett.* **269**, 57–66 (2008).

[60] A. G. Skirtach, C. Dejugnat, D. Braun, A. S. Susha, A. L. Rogach, W. J. Parak, H. Mohwald, and G. B. Sukhorukov, "The role of metal nanoparticles in remote release of encapsulated materials," *Nano Lett.* **5**, 1371–1377 (2005).

[61] K. H. Song, E. W. Stein, J. A. Margenthaler, and L. V. Wang, "Noninvasive photoacoustic identification of sentinel lymph nodes containing methylene blue in vivo in a rat model," *J. Biomed. Opt.* **13**, 054033 (2008).

[62] X. Wang, G. Ku, M. A. Wegiel, D. J. Bornhop, G. Stoica, and L. V. Wang, "Noninvasive photoacoustic angiography of animal brains in vivo with near-infrared light and an optical contrast agent," *Opt. Lett.* **29**, 730–732 (2004).

[63] W. Lu, Q. Huang, G. Ku, X. Wen, M. Zhou, D. Guzatov, P. Brecht, R. Su, A. Oraevsky, and L. V. Wang, "Photoacoustic imaging of living mouse brain vasculature using hollow gold nanospheres," *Biomaterials* **31**, 2617–2626 (2010).

[64] C. Kim, E. C. Cho, J. Chen, K. H. Song, L. Au, C. Favazza, Q. Zhang, C. M. Cobley, F. Gao, Y. Xia, and L. V. Wang, "In vivo molecular photoacoustic tomography of melanomas targeted by bioconjugated gold nanocages," *ACS Nano* **4**, 4559–4564 (2010).

[65] J. W. Kim, E. I. Galanzha, E. V. Shashkov, H. M. Moon, and V. P. Zharov, "Golden carbon nanotubes as multimodal photoacoustic and photothermal high-contrast molecular agents," *Nat. Nanotechnol.* **4**, 688–694 (2009).

[66] K. Homan, S. Kim, Y. S. Chen, B. Wang, S. Mallidi, and S. Emelianov, "Prospects of molecular photoacoustic imaging at 1064 nm wavelength," *Opt. Lett.* **35**, 2663–2665 (2010).

[67] A. Zerda, Z. Liu, S. Bodapati, R. Teed, S. Vaithilingam, B. T. Khuri-Yakub, X. Chen, H. Dai, and S. S. Gambhir, "Ultrahigh sensitivity carbon nanotube agents for photoacoustic molecular imaging in living mice," *Nano Lett.* **10**, 2168–2172 (2010).

[68] J. Deguchi, M. Aikawa, C. H. Tung, E. Aikawa, D. E. Kim, V. Ntziachristos, R. Weissleder, and P. Libby, "Inflammation in Atherosclerosis," *Circulation* **114**, 55–62 (2006).

[69] V. Ntziachristos, C. H. Tung, C. Bremer, and R. Weissleder, "Fluorescence molecular tomography resolves protease activity in vivo," *Nat. Med.* **8**, 757–761 (2002).

[70] D. Razansky, N. J. Harlaar, J. L. Hillebrands, A. Taruttis, E. Herzog, C. J. Zeebregts, G. M. van Dam, and V. Ntziachristos, "Multispectral optoacoustic tomography of matrix metalloproteinase activity in vulnerable human carotid plaques," *Mol. Imaging Biol.* **14**, 277–285 (2012).

[71] X. Shu, A. Royant, M. Z. Lin, T. A. Aguilera, V. Lev-Ram, P. A. Steinbach, and R. Y. Tsien, "Mammalian expression of infrared fluorescent proteins engineered from a bacterial phytochrome," *Science* **324**, 804–807 (2009).

[72] D. Razansky, M. Distel, C. Vinegoni, R. Ma, N. Perrimon, R. W. Koster, and V. Ntziachristos, "Multispectral opto-acoustic tomography of deep-seated fluorescent proteins in vivo," *Nature Photon.* **3**, 412–417 (2009).

[73] A. Krumholz, S. J. VanVickle-Chavez, J. Yao, T. P. Fleming, W. E. Gillanders, and L. V. Wang, "Photoacoustic microscopy of tyrosinase reporter gene in vivo," *J. Biomed. Opt.* **16**, 080503 (2011).

13

Multimodal Microscopy for Comprehensive Tissue Characterizations

Shuliang Jiao

Department of Ophthalmology, University of Southern California

Hao F. Zhang

Department of Biomedical Engineering, Northwestern University

This chapter describes the integration of photoacoustic microscopy (PAM) with other optical microscopic imaging modalities to achieve simultaneous multimodal imaging. We first discuss solving the compatibility issue among PAM and other imaging modalities by introducing the laser-scanning optical-resolution PAM. We then discuss the integration of PAM with optical coherence tomography (OCT) and confocal microscopy for providing both optical absorption and optical scattering contrasts. We also discuss improving the lateral resolution of PAM with adaptive optics. Finally, as an important application, we discuss multimodal imaging of the retina.

Key words: photoacoustic imaging, photoacoustic microscopy, multimodal imaging, absorption contrast, optical coherence tomography, ophthalmic imaging, retinal imaging, adaptive optics, autofluorescence imaging, retinal blood vessels, retinal pigment epithelium, melanin, lipofuscin

13.1 Introduction

Developing multimodal microscopic imaging technology covering different contrast mechanisms to achieve comprehensive physiological information of biological tissues is becoming increasingly important in biomedical research [1–3]. As an example of multimodal imaging, we can combine two imaging modalities one of which is sensitive to optical scattering while the other is sensitive to optical absorption, we can then simultaneously image the scattering and absorption properties of biological tissues. Usually, the scattering properties of biological tissues can provide anatomical information, e.g. the organization of the cellular layers of the retina, and the absorption properties can provide molecular information, e.g. the concentration of hemoglobin.

Almost all optical imaging modalities are based on the detection of either the illuminating light reflected from the sample or fluorescent light stimulated in the sample. The challenge in measuring optical absorption in scattering media such as biological tissues is that once the photons are absorbed, they cannot be directly quantified by imaging technologies that rely on back-travelling photons. Photoacoustic (PA) imaging is currently the only optical absorption based imaging modality. Its contrasts can be provided by both endogenous and exogenous contrast agent. As a result, integrating PA imaging with other optical imaging modalities can provide complementary contrasts.

PA is a scalable imaging technology that detects laser-induced ultrasonic waves to image the three-dimensional distribution of the optical energy deposition. PA imaging has been investigated intensively during the past decade owing to its ability to achieve both physiologically specific optical absorption contrast and good spatial resolution in deep tissue. Several different designs were reported, and potential applications in a wide spectrum of both biomedical research and clinical diagnostics also were demonstrated [4, 5].

Among all the PA imaging technologies, only photoacoustic microscopy (PAM) [6–8] has demonstrated capabilities to image biological tissue at a microscopic scale. PAM usually employs a focused single-element high-frequency ultrasonic transducer and a spatially overlapped optical illumination. Depending on the relative sizes of the optical and ultrasonic focuses in PAM, the spatial (lateral) resolution can be provided either ultrasonically or optically.

To image biological tissue beyond one optical transport mean free path, where photons are randomly scattered, ultrasonic resolution is required owing to the much weaker ultrasonic scattering in tissue. By using a 50 MHz focused ultrasonic transducer, a lateral resolution of 45 μm was achieved at a maximum depth of 3 mm [7]. When the object is optically thin (within one transport mean free path) or optically transparent, optical resolution can be employed to further improve the spatial resolution of PAM. An optical-resolution PAM (OR-PAM) was recently reported, where a lateral resolution of 5 μm was achieved [8].

This chapter discusses the integration of PAM with other optical microscopic imaging modalities to achieve simultaneous multimodal imaging. It is organized as follows. In Section 13.2, we discuss solving the compatibility issues of PAM with other optical imaging modalities. We then discuss the integration of PAM with optical coherence tomography (OCT), the integration of PAM with confocal microscopy, and multimodal imaging of the retina. The last section summarizes the conclusions.

13.2 Laser-Scanning Optical-Resolution Photoacoustic Microscopy

When integrating into a multimodal imaging system compatibility among different imaging modalities is an essential requirement. When compatible, the different imaging modalities can potentially provide registered images of different contrast mechanisms.

The integration of PAM with existing optical microscopic imaging modalities such as confocal microscopy, two-photon microscopy, and optical coherence tomography has been hampered, because existing PAMs require mechanical scanning of the ultrasonic optical assembly, which is not compatible with other optical microscopic imaging modalities. Since PAM uses ultrasonic detection whereas other methods use optical detection, the only possible solution for compatibility is to use the same optical scanning mechanism as other optical microscopic imaging modalities.

Laser-scanning OR-PAM (LSOR-PAM) [9] was first reported in 2009 to demonstrate the feasibility of employing optical scanning in PAM. In LSOR-PAM (Fig. 13.1), the ultrasonic detector is kept stationary, and only the laser light is raster scanned within the field of view (FOV) during data acquisition. A tunable dye laser pumped by an Nd:YLF laser system (pulse duration: 6 ns) was

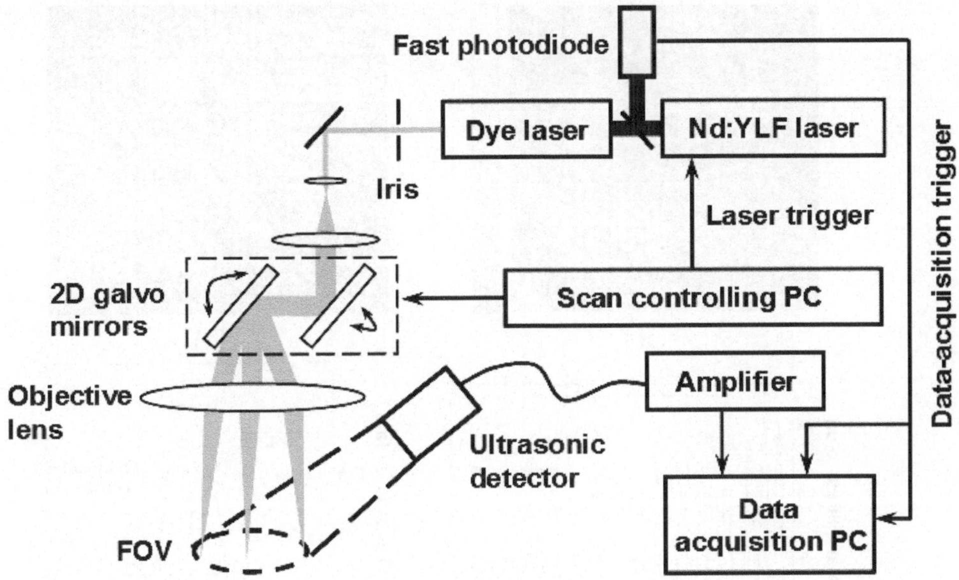

Figure 13.1: Schematic of the LSOR-PAM experimental setup.

used as the irradiation source. The laser system can operate with a pulse repetition rate (PRR) of up to 5 kHz in an optical wavelength tuning range between 540 nm to 900 nm. The output laser light from the dye laser was spatially filtered by an iris and expanded to reach a beam diameter of 8 mm. After attenuated by a neutral density filter, the expanded laser beam then passed through an x–y galvanometer scanner and a 60 mm focal length objective lens.

A PC-controlled (scan-controlling PC) analog output board synchronized the laser triggering and the optical scanner. The induced PA waves were detected by a commercial, unfocused ultrasonic transducer (V312, Olympus NDT; center frequency: 10 MHz; bandwidth: 80%; active element diameter: 6 mm). The ultrasonic transducer was placed 30 mm away from the sample and tilted about 15°. The detected PA signals were first amplified by a wideband amplifier and then digitized and stored by a data acquisition board controlled by the data acquisition PC for further processing. A fast photodiode detected the laser pulses and triggered the data acquisition to avoid the impact of laser jittering. The energy of each laser pulse was also recorded from the photodiode to compensate for the pulse energy instability. The sampling rate of the data acquisition board was 200 MS/s, and the PA signals were recorded for 3 s. No signal averaging was employed during data acquisition.
The FOV and spatial resolution of the LSOR-PAM were quantified through phantom imaging. The FOV of LSOR-PAM is determined by the ultrasonic beam size of the unfocused ultrasonic detector, since only the optical focus was raster scanned. According to our simulation on the ultrasonic beam profile the beam diameter (−6 dB) of the unfocused ultrasonic detector is comparable to its active element size (6 mm in diameter) within at least 30 mm away from its transducer surface. Fig. 13.2a gives the experimental measurement of the FOV in LSOR-PAM. The sample was a black mesh grid printed on a transparency using a commercial laser printer. The measured grid size was 865 m by using an optical microscope. During the experiments, the grid and the ultrasonic detector were immersed in deionized water inside a water tank. The scanning area was 8 mm × 8 mm. The laser pulse energy was 0.04 J. After the volumetric data were acquired, the maximum-amplitude-projection (MAP) image was calculated. As Fig. 13.2a shows, a maximum contrast-to-noise ratio (CNR) of 26 dB was achieved without any image processing except that high frequency noise above 100 MHz was digitally removed. Based on the size of the grid, a circular FOV with a diameter of >6 mm was achieved (at least seven grids can be clearly observed with a local CNR >6 dB).

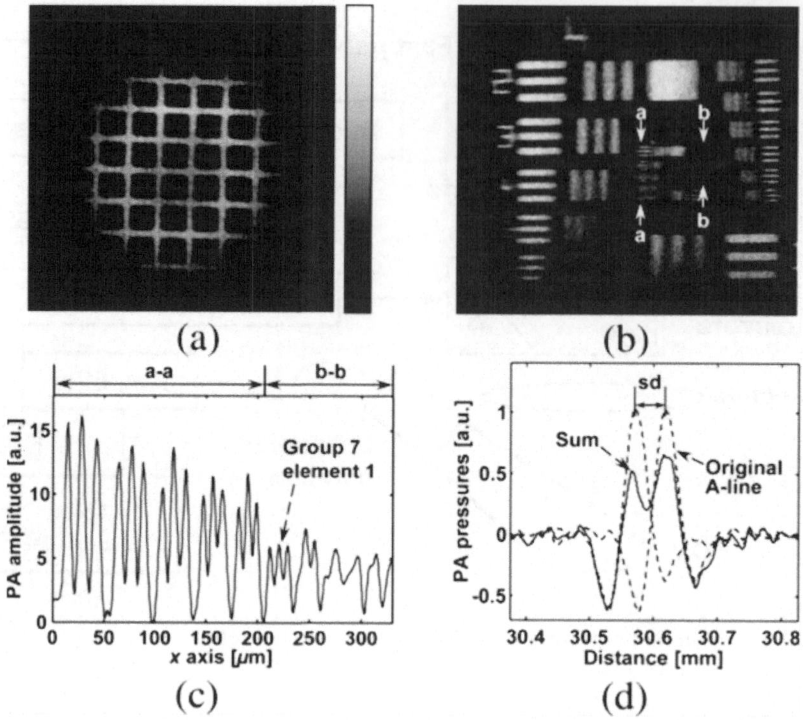

Figure 13.2: Quantification of the FOV and the spatial resolutions. (a) LSOR-PAM image of the printed mesh grid. (b) LSOR-PAM image of the USAF resolution target. (c) PA values at the cross sections highlighted by a-a and b-b in (b). (d) Estimate of axial resolution from a typical A-line acquired from blood vessel. sd: shift distance.

The lateral resolution of the LSOR-PAM was quantified by imaging an USAF 1951 resolution test target (IT-20-P-TM, Applied Image). Fig. 13.2b shows the MAP image of the resolution target. Fig. 13.2c shows the magnitude of the PA signals measured at the two locations as marked in Fig. 13.2 (b), where the smallest resolvable bar spacing is 7.82 m (group 7, element 1). Hence, the lateral resolution is better than 7.8 m. Considering the influence of the refraction at the water surface, we estimated the theoretical optical focal diameter to be 7 m. This experimental result shows 11% degradation. In tissue imaging, optical scattering reduces the spatial resolution; however, when the sample is optically thin, the deterioration of the lateral resolution is insignificant [8]. The lateral resolutions along the x and y axes shown here are not identical, which is possibly due to optical misalignment. It can be solved by a better alignment of the objective lens and the two galvanometer mirrors. To quantify the axial resolution, a typical A-line [Fig. 13.2d] was used as an approximation of the 1D axial point-spread-function (PSF). We first shifted the 1D PSF by a distance and added it to the original PSF. Then the Rayleigh criterion was applied to the sum. The smallest shifted distance that still allows resolving the two peaks (by 10% amplitude difference) was considered as the resolution along that direction. Hence, the estimated axial resolution is around 50 m, which is primarily determined by the ultrasonic center frequency and bandwidth [6].

In vivo imaging of microvasculature in the ear of a Swiss Webster mouse (Charles River Labs; body weight: 20 g) was acquired. Before experiments, the hairs on the right ear were gently removed using commercial human hair-removing lotion. During experiments, the animal was placed on a homemade animal holder, and a mixture of 1% isoflurane with medical grade oxygen was ventilated to the animal through a commercial non-rebreathing anesthesia system (M3000, LEI Medical) at a

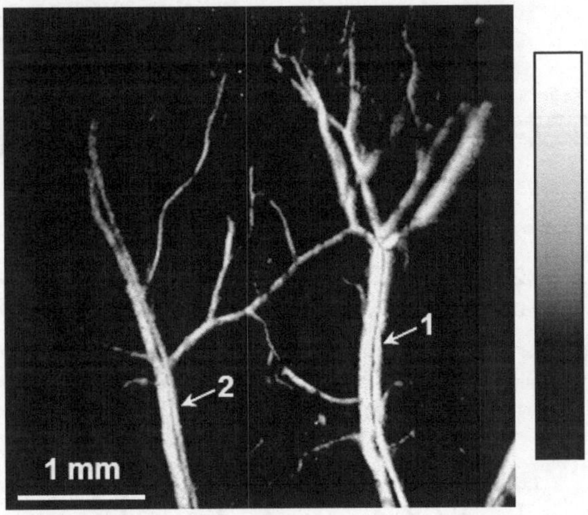

Figure 13.3: LSOR-PAM image of vasculature in a Swiss Webster mouse ear *in vivo*. Two pairs of parallel veins and arteries are highlighted by 1 and 2.

flow rate of 1 l /min to keep the animal motionless. Unlike other work [10] no optical clearing agent was applied to the skin here. The LSOR-PAM image of the microvasculature is shown in Fig. 13.3. As previously demonstrated [8], OR-PAM is able to resolve capillary network with high quality and offers the potential to study associated physiological changes in the capillaries. Although LSOR-PAM has lower spatial resolution comparable with OR-PAM, it shows comparable image quality in imaging microvascular structures. Up to seven orders of vessel branching can be observed, and the smallest vessel is imaged by a single pixel in the image.

The average CNR in Fig. 13.3 is 30 dB, which is lower than that from the OR-PAM image. Two reasons contribute to the reduced CNR: (i) A flat ultrasonic transducer was used in LSOR-PAM, while the previous OR-PAM used a strongly focused ultrasonic transducer. Since geometrical focusing increases ultrasonic detecting sensitivity and rejects unwanted signals from the out-of-focus regions, the confocal design in OR-PAM greatly improves CNR. A focused ultrasonic transducer can be employed in LSOR-PAM to increase the CNR, as well; however, a trade-off between the CNR and the FOV needs to be reached, because the focused transducer has a reduced beam diameter. (ii) The distance between the ultrasonic detector and the sample in LSOR-PAM (30 mm) is much longer than that in OR-PAM (5 mm), which leads to lower detected PA signal amplitude owing to the decay of a propagating spherical PA wave.

The advantages of LSOR-PAM stem from several aspects. First, removing the bulky load (all the optical and ultrasonic components) that used to be translated together in OR-PAM can potentially achieve higher scanning speed. For imaging systems with low-laser PRR where the data acquisition speed is primarily limited by the PRR, the use of optical scanning is not critical; however, when the PRR is higher than 10 kHz, the bottleneck for increasing the data acquisition speed is the scanning system. Hence, optical scanning presents an opportunity to further speed up the data acquisition. Second, optical scanning allows sophisticated scanning patterns to be performed, such as a complete raster scanning followed by localized measurements on a single vessel. Lastly, the optical delivery and scanning mechanism in LSOR-PAM are similar to most existing optical microscopic modalities, which lay the foundation for future integration of LSOR-PAM to other modalities.

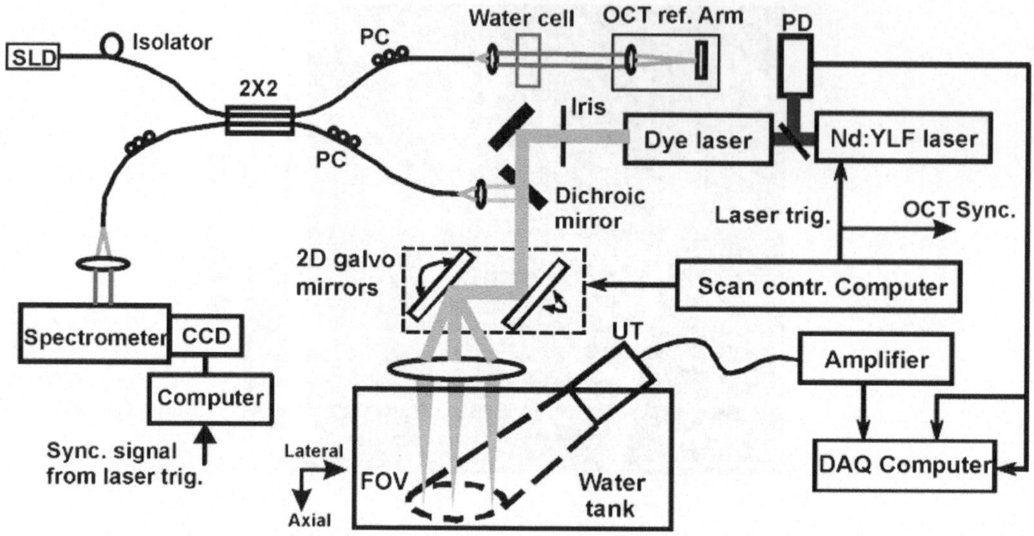

Figure 13.4: Schematic of the integrated PAM and OCT experimental system. SLD: superluminescent diode; PC: polarization controller; PD: photodiode; FOV: field of view; UT: ultrasonic transducer.

13.3 Fused PAM and Spectral-Domain OCT

PAM and OCT [11, 12] are two imaging modalities that can provide complementary contrasts for imaging biological tissues and are good candidates for an integrated multimodal system [13]. OCT is a low coherence interferometer based imaging modality that can provide 3D microscopic imaging of biological tissues. OCT detects the interference in the interferometer in either time domain or spectral domain between the back-reflected light from the sample and reference arms. By using a broadband light source OCT resolves the depth of a scatterer through coherence gating. Various optical properties of biological tissues can provide contrasts for OCT while light scattering property predominates. Although optical Doppler tomography (ODT), a branch of OCT, can provide functional information of blood flow by measuring the Doppler shift impinged on the backscattered sample light, imaging hemoglobin oxygen saturation (sO_2) is still beyond the reach of conventional OCT. As a result, combining OCT with PAM can potentially provide comprehensive information of biological tissues including the tissue anatomy, blood flow, and sO_2 from a single instrument.

The development of LSOR-PAM solved the incompatibility issue and cleared the way for integrating PAM with OCT. Figure 13.4 shows a schematic of an integrated PAM and OCT system. The configuration of the PAM subsystem including ultrasonic detection and data acquisition is the same as that described in Section 13.2. The output laser light from the dye laser was merged with the OCT probing light by a dichroic mirror. The combined light beams were scanned by an x–y galvanometer and were focused on the sample by an achromatic lens.

The fiber-based spectral-domain OCT (SD-OCT) subsystem is similar to that reported in our previous publications [14]. The SD-OCT consists of a superluminescent diode light source (SLD-371, Superlum Diodes, Russia), a 3-dB fiber coupler, a reference arm, a sample arm coupled with the PAM, and a spectrometer for detecting the interference signals in the spectral domain. The light source has a center wavelength of 840 nm and a FWHM bandwidth of 50 nm. The exposure time of the line scan CCD camera (Aviiva, e2V, Chelmsford) in the spectrometer was set to 36 μs, which can acquire OCT images with a line rate of 24 kHz. The measured sensitivity was better than 95

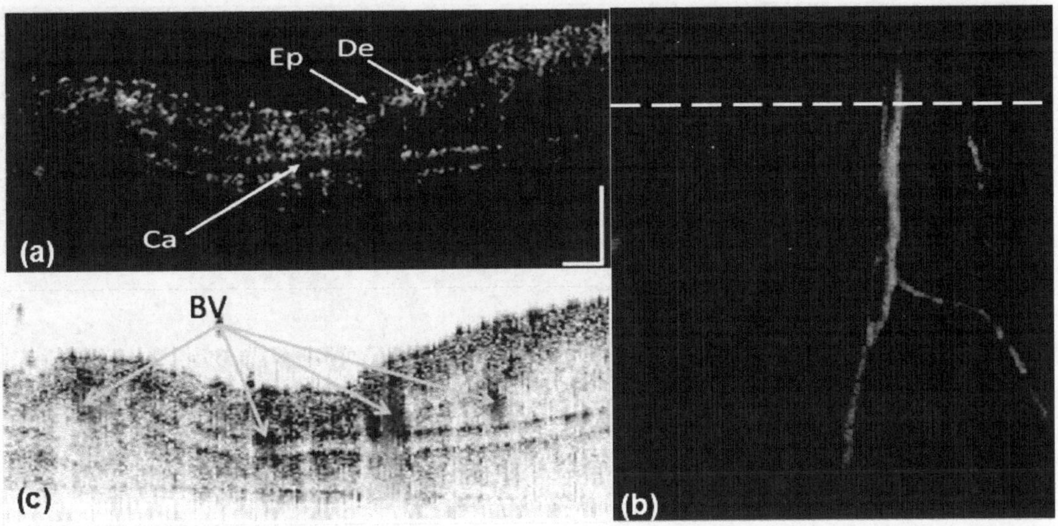

Figure 13.5: (See color insert.) Simultaneously acquired OCT and PAM images of a mouse ear. (a) OCT B-scan at the location marked in panel b by the dashed line; (b) PAM image; (c) fused OCT and PAM B-scan images at the same location. Ep: epidermis; De: dermis; Ca: cartilaginous backbone; BV: blood vessels; bar: 200 μm.

dB. The calibrated depth resolution is 6 μm in tissue and the lateral resolution is estimated to be 20 μm.

To ensure automatic registration of the two imaging modalities under all circumstances the timing of the PAM laser triggering and data acquisition, the scanning of the galvanometer scanner, and the OCT data acquisition need to be controlled on the same time base. We employed an analog output board to trigger both the image acquisition board for the CCD camera in the OCT spectrometer, the PAM laser, and the galvanometer scanner. The PAM data acquisition was triggered by the photodiode to avoid laser jittering. As a result, the two imaging systems are synchronized despite the difference in their achievable imaging speed.

The *in vivo* images of the ears of a Swiss Webster mouse are shown in Fig. 13.5. Figure 13.5a shows one typical cross-sectional OCT image consisting of 400 $\times$ 220 (depth $\times$ lateral) pixels at the location marked in Fig. 13.5b. The image clearly depicts the microscopic structures of the mouse ear. Different anatomical layers including epidermis, dermis, and the cartilaginous backbone can be clearly seen [15, 16]. There are also shadows on the images casted by either blood vessels or clusters of scatterers, presumably from various glands that blocked the light from probing tissues below them. Unlike OCT images of the retina, where shadows casted by blood vessels can be clearly recognized [8], we cannot tell the exact locations of the blood vessels.

Figure 13.5b shows MAP of the simultaneously acquired PAM image in the same area in the mouse ear. Since PAM image visualizes the distribution of optical energy deposition, only the blood vessels appear clearly in the image whereas no information about skin anatomy can be observed. Figures 13.5 a and b demonstrate the complementary nature of the contrasts contributing to OCT and PAM.

When PAM and OCT images are fused, both the skin anatomy and microvasculature can be visualized in a single volumetric image. Figure 13.5c shows the fused B-scan images at the location marked in Fig. 13.5b. The registration of the two images along the lateral directions was automatic and was guaranteed by the system design. To register the two B-scan images along the axial direction we first determined the depth relationship (pixel shift) between the two modalities by imaging

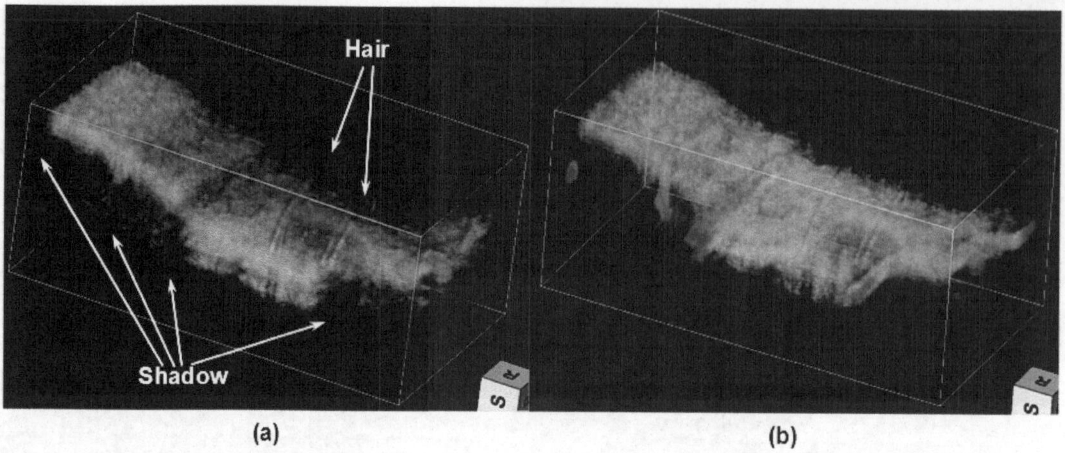

Figure 13.6: (See color insert.) Volume renderings of (a) the OCT data and (b) the final fused image. In the fused image, the blood vessels are pseudo-colored red and the opacity of the OCT voxels was set to 0.8.

the top surface of a printed mesh grid [9]. Then the PAM volumetric image was shifted accordingly along the axial direction to register with the OCT volumetric image. The OCT color map in Fig. 13.5c was inverted to highlight the blood vessels revealed by PAM. The blood vessels are pseudo-colored red in the PAM B-scan image.

The volume rendering of the OCT image and the final fused image are shown in Fig 13.6. Fig. 13.6a shows the volume rendering of the OCT data using a commercial software (Volview, Kitware), where we can distinguish blood vessels except the shadows created by them. Figure 13.6b shows the volume rendering of the fused OCT and PAM data, where the vessels imaged by PAM agree with the shadows in the OCT image very well. The fused image shows clearly the spatial distributions of the tissue properties of scattering and absorption at wavelengths of the OCT and PAM, respectively, which are not available in either of the modalities alone. In addition to the image shown here, the integrated system has the potential to image the blood velocity using ODT and sO_2 using multiple wavelength PAM imaging [7].

The experimental results demonstrated the feasibility of integrating OCT and PAM in the most suitable configuration for high speed simultaneous multimodal imaging. The imaging speed of the integrated system (60 second per volume acquisition) is determined by the PAM subsystem, which is currently limited by the PRR of the tunable laser. By using a laser with a PRR of 24 kHz the PAM can match the maximal imaging speed of the current OCT subsystem.

Again, the contrast-to-noise ratio (CNR) in the current PAM configuration is lower than that of existing optical resolution PAM (OR-PAM) due to the unfocused transducer used and the longer distance from the sample to the transducer. The longer distance is necessary for potential applications in ophthalmic imaging, the most popular application for OCT. However, the CNR can be improved by optimizing the ultrasonic transducer.

13.4 Fused PAM and Confocal Microscopy

When short pulsed laser light interacts with biological tissues some of the photons may be absorbed and their energy is converted to heat. These photons contribute to the signals for PAM. In

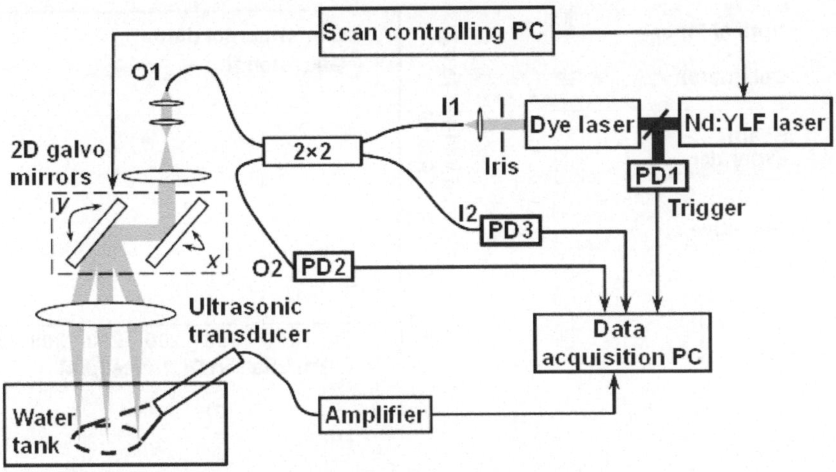

Figure 13.7: Schematic of the fused laser-scanning confocal microscopy and photoacoustic microscopy. PD: photodiode; 2×2: fiber coupler.

the mean time some of the photons are scattered back. When these photons are collected with a confocal arrangement, the function of confocal microscopy can be achieved simultaneously.

In this section we describe the integration of LSOR-PAM with a fiber-optic confocal microscope (FOCON) [17, 18] to achieve multimodal imaging of both optical absorption and optical scattering contrasts. The axial resolution of the confocal microscopy was quantified both theoretically and experimentally. The complementary contrast was demonstrated in both phantoms and small animals *in vivo*.

Figure 13.7 shows a schematic of the experimental system. The same laser was used as in Section 13.2 and 13.3. Different from that in Fig. 13.1 the laser light from the dye laser was coupled into a 2×2 single-mode optical fiber coupler. The output light from arm O1 was collimated and expanded to 10 mm in diameter and then scanned by a 2D galvanometer scanner. An achromatic lens with a focal length of 40 was used as the objective lens. The output light from the second output arm O2 was detected by a photodiode (PD2) to record the energy of each laser pulse to compensate for the energy instability. The laser pulse energy out of the output arm O1 was 0.04 μJ.

The reflected light from the sample was detected by a 10-MHz Si photodiode (PD3) to form an FOCON image. A custom-built, high-frequency, unfocused ultrasonic transducer (center frequency: 40 MHz, active element size: 1 mm) detected the induced PA signals to form a PAM image. The data acquisition was triggered by laser pulses detected by PD1 to avoid laser jittering.

13.4.1 Spatial resolution of LSOR-PAM

The lateral resolution of LSOR-PAM is determined by the size of the optical focus. As detailed in [9], the lateral resolution approaches the diffraction limit of the objective lens at the illuminating wavelength, which was 2.8 μm (a detailed description of the numerical aperture is provided in the next section). The axial resolution is determined by the center frequency and bandwidth of the ultrasonic detector; this was quantified to be 23 μm using the "shift-and-sum" method as shown in [9].

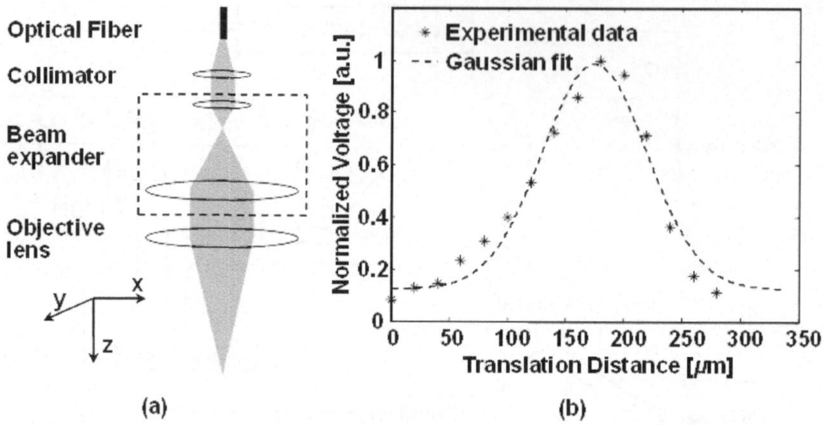

Figure 13.8: Axial resolution of the confocal microscopy. (a) schematic of the optical illumination and detection for theoretical estimation; (b) experimental measurement of axial resolution.

13.4.2 Spatial resolution of FOCON

Figure 13.8a gives a detailed schematic of the optical illumination and detection in the FOCON. The optical fiber (SM600, Thorlabs) has a numerical aperture (NA) of 0.12 and a mode field diameter of 4.6 μm. The fiber collimator has a NA of 0.29 and an output beam waist diameter of 1.2 mm. The beam was further expanded to 10 mm in diameter before it was focused by the objective lens, which yields an objective NA of 0.125.

Because the optical fiber acts as the pinhole, the lateral resolution of FOCON improves from the lateral resolution of the LSOR-PAM and can be calculated as $k\lambda/NA$, where λ is the optical wavelength, NA is the numerical aperture of objective lens, k is a coefficient from 0.37 to 0.51 depending on the mode field radius of the optical fiber [17]. Taking $\lambda = 0.578$ μm, $NA = 0.125$, and the mode field radius of 2.3 μm, the lateral resolution of the confocal microscope is around 2 μm in air.

The axial resolution of FOCON was first estimated theoretically. The axial resolution r can be expressed as $r = \lambda A/(\pi n NA_1^2)$ [19], where λ is the optical wavelength, n is the refractive index of the medium, NA_1 is the NA of the objective lens, A is the normalized fiber spot size and is expressed as $(2\pi r_0 NA_2)^2$, where r_0 is the mode field radius of the optical fiber and NA_2 is the minimum of the NA of the optical fibers and the collimating lens. Taking $\lambda = 0.578$ μm, $NA_1 = 0.125$, $r_0 = 2.3$ μm, and $NA_2 = 0.12$, we have $r = 106$ μm in air.

The axial resolution of FOCON in air was also quantified experimentally. A silver mirror was used as the sample and was translated along the z axis. A total distance of 300 μm was translated at a step size of 20 m. The normalized reading from PD3 at each step is shown in Figure 13.8b. The experimental data were then fit by a Gaussian function $a\exp(-((x-b)/c)^2)+d$, where a, b, c, and d are unknown constants and d counts for the light reflection directly from the fiber tip of arm O1. The full-width-half-max (FWHM) value of the fitted Gaussian function gives the experimental measurement of axial resolution at 108 μm, which agrees with the theoretical estimation very well.

13.4.3 Phantom imaging

To demonstrate the complementary contrast of multimodal imaging, we imaged a printed mesh grid (grid size: 865 μm) as used in [9]. The grid has carbon lines on a printing transparency, where the dark lines have strong optical absorption. Figure 13.9 shows the imaging results. As can be observed, FOCON and PAM imaged opposite contrasts: the black printed lines induced strong PA

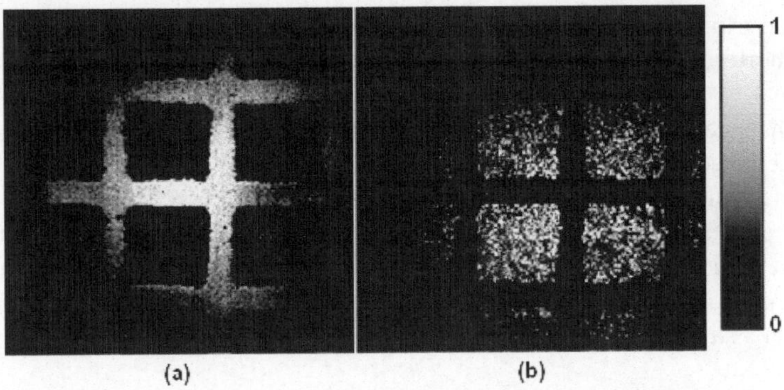

Figure 13.9: Images of a printed mesh grid using the fused PAM and FOCON. (a) FOCON image; (b) LSOR-PAM image

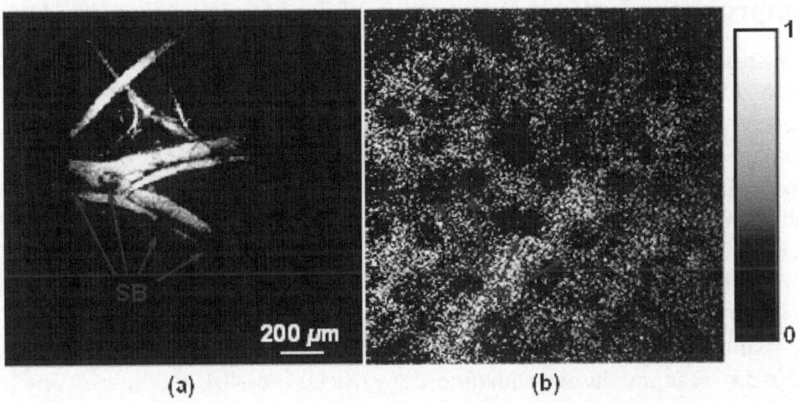

Figure 13.10: *In vivo* multimodal imaging of mouse ears. (a) LSOR-PAM image showing microvasculature; (b) FOCON image showing skin structure. SB: sebaceous gland

signal (Fig. 13.9a) but very weak back-scattered photons for confocal microscopy (Fig. 13.9b) due to stronger optical absorption compared with the transparency. Since the LSOR-PAM and confocal microscopy share the same optical focus, the two images are intrinsically registered.

13.4.4 *In vivo* animal imaging

The *in vivo* images of a mouse ear are shown in Fig. 13.10. Because the source of optical absorption is mainly hemoglobin and the Swiss Webster mouse has low skin melanin concentration, LSOR-PAM revealed the anatomy of microvessels (Fig. 13.10a) well. Sebaceous glands are embedded in the dermis and have higher optical absorption compared with the dermis; hence, they create shadows in the LSOR-PAM image, as highlighted by arrows.

Completely different anatomical features are observed in the FOCON image (Fig. 13.10b). The detected photons are primarily reflected from epidermis and dermis. Since the sebaceous gland is more optically absorptive compared with dermal tissues, fewer photons were back-reflected and the glands appeared to be dark regions in the image. As highlighted in Fig. 13.10, the spatial locations of the glands correspond well in the two images. We noticed that blood vessels do not manifest themselves as dark regions in the FOCON image. It is, presumably, because that LSOR-PAM relies on only single-trip photon propagation while FOCON requires round-trip photons propagation and thus has a shorter penetration depth and less sensitivity in order to image blood vessels without contrast agents.

The significance of this work is that it exhibits the feasibility of integrating LSOR-PAM with the well-established confocal scanning laser ophthalmoscope (cSLO) [20] for potential multimodal ophthalmic imaging based on a single light source. The 0.15 NA of the objective lens used in this study was specifically chosen to be comparable with the optical parameters of human eyes [21]. Although not demonstrated experimentally, this system is readily expandable to conduct confocal fluorescence microscopy [22] by adding the appropriate band-pass filter and high-sensitivity optical detector (such as a photon multiplication tube), yet still sharing the same light source with LSOR-PAM.

13.5 Improve the Lateral Resolution of PAM with Adaptive Optics

The axial resolution of PAOM is determined by the bandwidth and center frequency of the ultrasonic transducer. The lateral resolution of PAOM is determined by the smallest achievable spot size of the illuminating light on the sample. In imaging the eye *in vivo*, for large pupil diameters, monochromatic aberrations of the eye are the major factors that limit the achievable resolution of retinal images [23]. Although the depth resolution of PAOM could be improved by increasing the bandwidth of the ultrasonic detecting system, the lateral resolution of PAOM is still limited by the optics. One possible approach for correcting the ocular aberrations to decrease the spot size of the illuminating light on the retina, and therefore improve the lateral resolution of PAOM, is to use adaptive optics (AO) [24, 25]. AO has been applied to ophthalmic imaging with great success, which makes it possible to image single photo-receptors [26–29]. AO has also been successfully integrated in OCT [30–35], scanning laser ophthalmoscopy (SLO) [36–40], and microscopy [41–45].

This section presents a feasibility study on the integration of AO with PAM for *ex vivo* imaging of ocular tissues, which is a technical preparation for the ultimate AO-PAOM for *in vivo* retinal imaging. The goal of the current study is to correct the aberrations of the optical system for delivering the illuminating light to the sample.

Figure 13.11 shows a schematic of the AO-PAM experimental system. A compact close-loop AO system was integrated into a LSOR-PAM. The AO system consists of a real-time Shack-Hartmann wavefront sensor (SH sensor, 39x31 maximum active lenslets, Thorlabs, USA) operating at 15Hz and a 141-element MEMS-based deformable mirror (DM, Thorlabs, USA).

The illumination light source of the PAM was a frequency-doubled Q-switched Nd:YAG laser with the following parameters: wavelength = 532 nm, pulse energy = 10 J/pulse, pulse duration = 2 ns, and maximal pulse repetition rate = 30 kHz. The output laser light was attenuated with a neutral density (ND) filter before coupled into a single mode optical fiber (SMF). The light reflected from the surface of the ND filter is detected by a photodiode, which provided trigger for PAM signal acquisition. The output laser light from the SMF was first collimated into a beam diameter of 4.4 mm, passed through a two-f system (L1 and L2, f = 75mm), and was then projected onto the DM (Clear aperture: 4.4mm$\times$4.4mm). Another two-f system (L3 and L4, f = 100 mm and f = 225 mm, respectively) expanded the beam reflected from the DM into 10 mm in diameter and projected the beam onto an X-Y galvanometer scanner. The X-Y galvanometer, DM, and SH were conjugated with each other. The light beam was finally focused on the sample by an objective lens (f = 30 mm, Φ = 25.4 mm, Achromatic Lens, VIS-NIR coated). The galvanometer scanner was controlled by an analogue-output board, whose sample clock was used to trigger the laser.

To avoid speckles formed by the interference of the reflected light from the sample, a superlu-

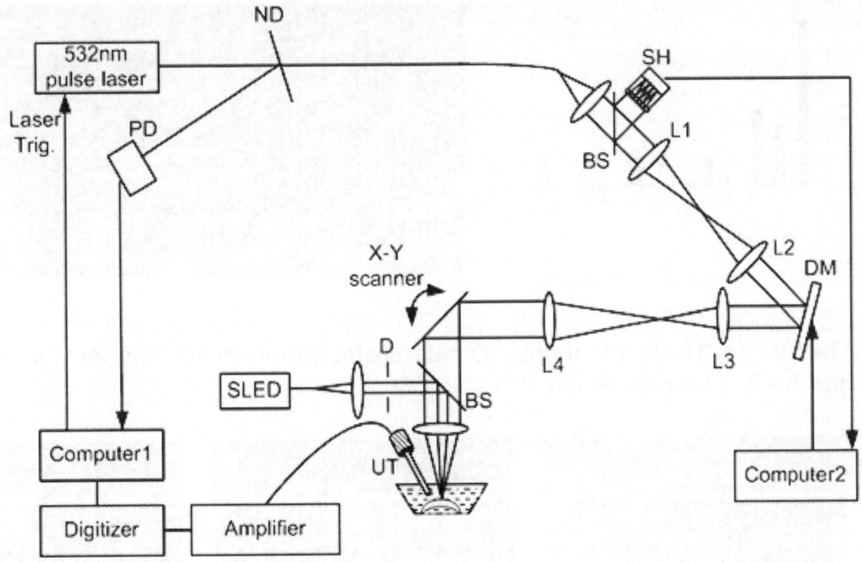

Figure 13.11: Schematic of the experimental AO-PAM system. ND: neutral density filter; PD: photodiode; D: diaphragm; L1-L4: achromatic lenses; DM: deformable mirror; SH: Shack-Hartmann wavefront sensor; BS: pellicle beamsplitter (reflection: 8%, transmission 92%); UT: ultrasonic transducer.

minescent diode (SLD, power = 10 mW, bandwidth = 50 nm, central wavelength = 840 nm) was used as the AO light source. The AO beam was first collimated (beam diameter < 1 mm) and then coupled into the center line of the PAM illuminating light path by a pellicle beam-splitter (BP-108, Uncoated, Throlabs, USA), which reflects 8% of the AO light onto the objective lens while transmitting 92% of the back-scattered light from the sample. The diffusely reflected light from the sample could be considered to have a spherical wavefront emitted from a point light source. This wavefront passed through the DM and was delivered into the SH by another pellicle beam-splitter. Therefore, the AO beam travelled through the same path as the PA laser beam illuminating the samples. The DM consists of a continuous mirror membrane that is deformed by electrostatic actuators ensuring deformation without hysteresis. Each actuator provides a stroke of 3.5 μm over a compact area with low influence on neighboring actuators. The control software AOkit (Thorlabs, USA) [46] minimized the wavefront errors by analyzing the signals from the SH and determined the appropriate drive signals for the DM actuators to compensate for the wavefront aberrations. After successfully correcting the wavefront errors for the reflected AO beam, the surface profile of the DM was recorded and used to compensate for the PAM light.

The induced PA waves from the sample were detected by a custom-built needle ultrasonic transducer (30 MHz; bandwidth: 50%; active element diameter: 1 mm). The detected PA signals were first amplified by 80 dB and then digitized by a high-speed digitizer at a sampling rate of 200 MS/s. The laser pulse energy was measured to be 40 nJ at the sample surface, which is within the ANSI laser safety limit for eye imaging [7]. As described in Section 13.2, the depth resolution is 23 μm. In the experiments the laser was triggered at a pulse repetition rate of 24 kHz. The acquisition of one three-dimensional PAM dataset consisting of 256$\times$256 A-lines took 2.7 seconds. During imaging, the samples were immersed in a water tank and the transducer was positioned about 4 mm away from them.

A white paper was first used as a sample for the measurement and correction of the wavefront errors. Figure 13.12a shows the first four order Zernike coefficients before and after wavefront

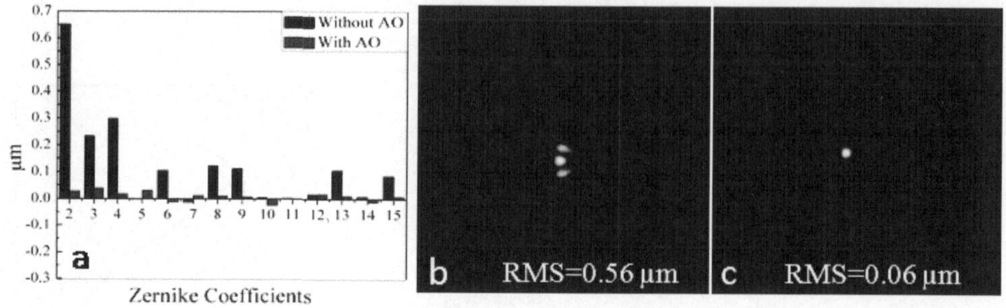

Figure 13.12: (a) The first four order Zernike coefficients without/within AO, (b) corresponding PSF without AO, (c) corresponding PSF with AO.

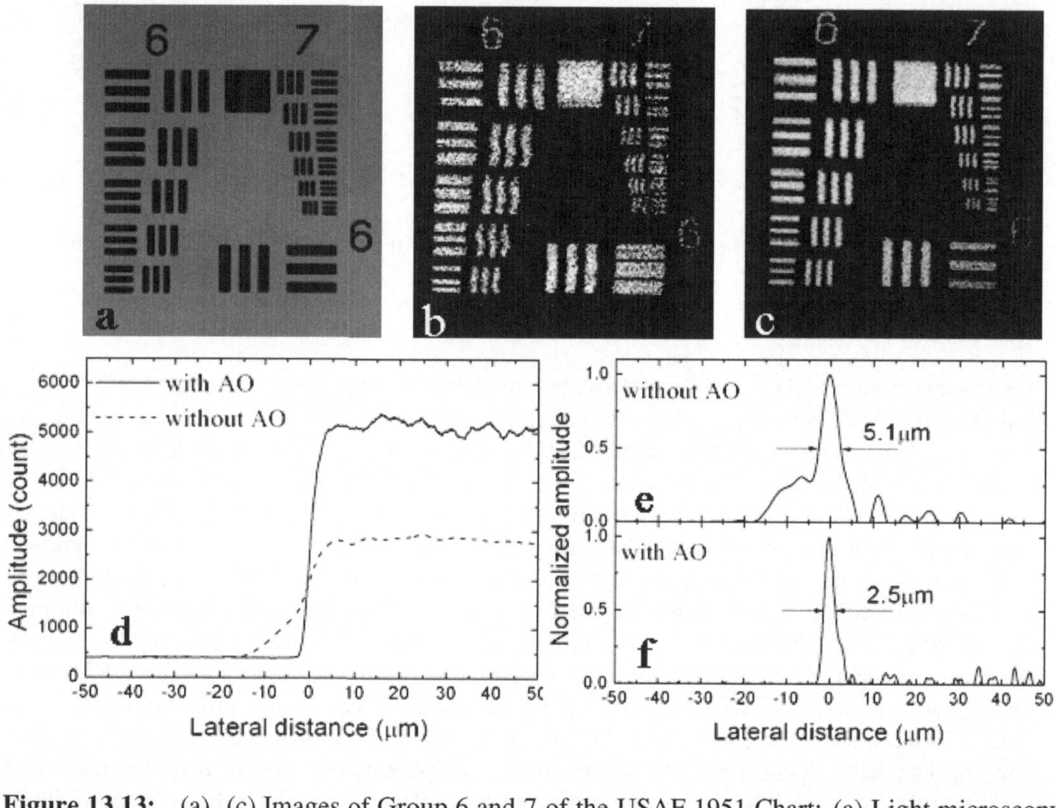

Figure 13.13: (a) (c) Images of Group 6 and 7 of the USAF 1951 Chart: (a) Light microscopy image, (b) MAP of the PAM image without AO, (c) MAP of the PAM image of the same target with AO. d: measured edge response; e: PSF calculated from the data in (d) without AO; f: PSF calculated from the data in (d) with AO.

correction. The Zernike coefficients, especially the lower-order Zernike coefficients (the first and second orders) decreased significantly after AO correction. Figures 13.12b and c show the corresponding point-spread-functions (PSFs) and RMS wavefront errors with and without AO calculated from the measured wavefronts, respectively. The results demonstrated the effective measurement and correction of the lower and higher order aberrations using the AO light. After the correction capability of the system was demonstrated, the surface profile of the DM was saved for the next experiments.

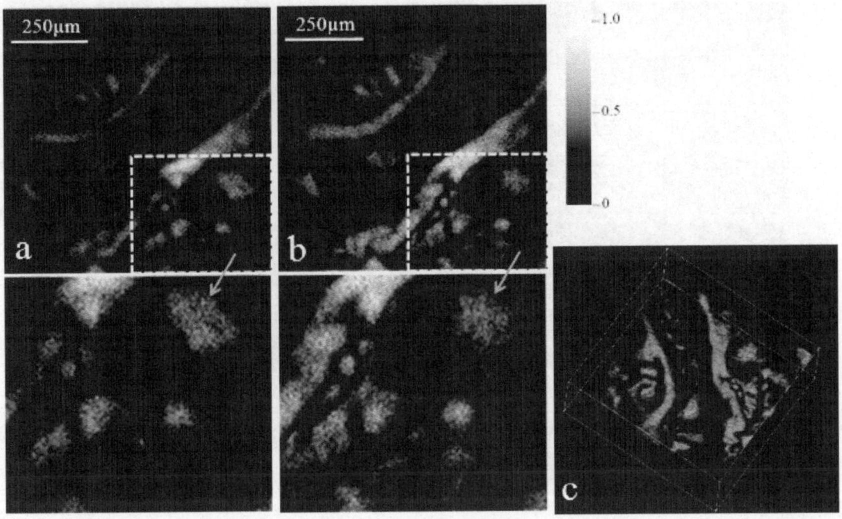

Figure 13.14: MAP of the PAM images of the ciliary body of a pig eye: (a) without AO, (b) with AO, (c) 3D rendering of the PAM dataset. The area outlined in each image was enlarged and shown as pointed by the arrows.

The lateral resolution of the AO-PAM was first evaluated by imaging a United States Air Force resolution target (USAF 1951 Chart, Edmund Optics, Inc.), which reached element 6 of Group 7, corresponding to a resolution of 2.19 μm (228.07 cycles/mm). The measured images of Group 6 and 7 of the target are shown in Fig. 13.13: (a) light microscopy image, (b) maximum amplitude projection (MAP) of the PAM image without AO, and (c) MAP of the PAM image with AO. The bars within the 6th element of Group 7 were clearly resolved in Fig. 13.13c. The edge response was also measured by imaging the edge of the black square on the same resolution target (Fig. 13.13d). The PSFs (Fig. 13.13c and d) were calculated from the measured edge response by differentiation. The calculation showed that the lateral resolution was improved from 5.1 μm without AO to 2.5 μm with AO. From the images we can also see that our system has uniform lateral resolutions in the X and Y directions.

The system was then tested on imaging excised biological samples *ex vivo*. The ciliary body of a pig eye was first imaged. The eye was acquired from a local slaughter house and was fixed in 10% formalin. The eyeball was cut in half to expose the ciliary body. Figure 13.14 shows the experimental results. Figure 13.14a and b show the MAP of the PAM images without and with AO corrections, respectively. Each image consists of 256×256 pixels covering an area of about 1mm×1mm. Figure 13.14c is a 3D rendering of the PAM dataset. The images showed interesting melanin distributions in the ciliary body. Compared with the image without AO correction, the PAM image with AO correction resolved many more details of the sample (see the enlarged areas pointed by the arrows). Due to better light energy concentration within the focus with AO correction, the PA signals are also stronger in Fig. 13.14b than in Fig. 13.14a. As a result, the images with AO correction also have a better signal-to-noise ratio (SNR).

The PAM images of the RPE of the same pig eye without and with AO correction are shown in Fig. 13.15a and b, respectively. The MAP images consist of 256×256 pixels covering an area of 0.4 mm×0.4 mm. From the images we can see significant resolution improvement of the image with AO compared with the image without AO. In the image with AO single RPE cells are well resolved while in the image without AO the RPE cells are barely recognizable.

Since PAM images the absorption contrast, Fig. 13.15b shows the concentration of absorbers at

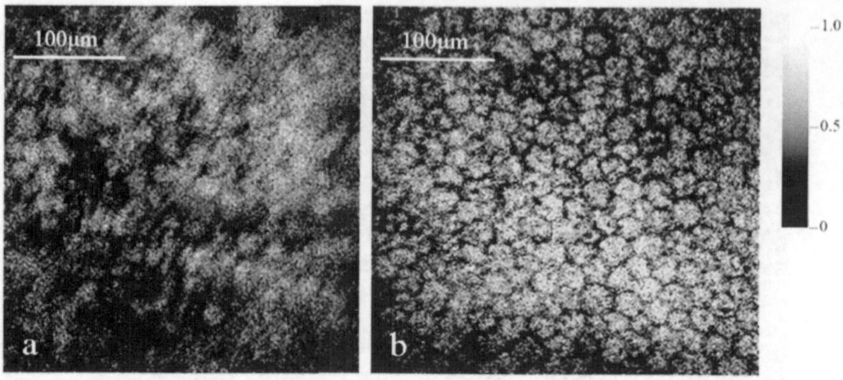

Figure 13.15: MAP of the PAM images of the RPE of the pig eye: (a) without AO, (b) with AO.

the wavelength of the laser light (532 nm). The main light-absorbing substances in RPE at 532 nm are melanin and lipofusin. It has been verified in previous experiments with lipofusin control slides that lipofusin does not generate detectable PA signals at the same experimental conditions, i.e., the same illuminating wavelength, pulse energy, and ultrasonic detecting system. As a result, it can be concluded that Fig. 13.15b shows the melanin distribution in and outside the RPE cells. From the image it can be seen that the boundaries among the RPE cells have no or weak PA signals, which means that RPE melanin concentrates inside the cells. Dark spot inside each RPE cell can also be observed. It was hypothesized that the dark spot represents the location of the nucleus.

13.6 Multimodal *In Vivo* Retinal Imaging

13.6.1 *In vivo* LSOR-PAM and auto-fluorescence imaging of the retina

Melanin and lipofuscin are two major pigments in the retinal pigment epithelium (RPE). RPE is a monolayer of pigmented cells located between the choriocapillaris and light-sensitive outer segments of the photoreceptors. Melanin protects RPE cells from oxidative damage by acting as an antioxidant [47]. Unfortunately, melanin may lose its protective function with aging and also can be photobleached irreversibly as a result of longtime light exposure [48]. On the other hand, lipofuscin is a byproduct of phagocytosis of the photoreceptor outer segments, which accumulates with aging of the retina. Excessive levels of lipofuscin accumulation could compromise essential RPE functions and contribute to the pathogenesis of age-related macular degeneration (AMD) [49]. AMD is one of the major blinding diseases affecting millions of people in the developed countries. Hence, *in vivo* imaging of melanin and lipofuscin can provide important aging information of the retina, which is important for AMD research and clinical diagnosis [50].

To specifically image melanin and lipofuscin with optical imaging modalities their most distinctive optical signatures should be captured. The most distinctive optical property of melanin is its high optical absorption coefficient in a wide optical spectral range. For lipofuscin the optical signature is its fluorescent spectrum in 580–700 nm when excited by light of 364–633 nm [51, 52]. The distinctive optical properties of melanin and lipofuscin can thus be sensed by photoacoustic ophthalmoscopy (PAOM) [53, 54] and autofluorecence (AF) imaging when illuminated with laser pulses at 532 nm. The integration of PAM with AF for simultaneously imaging melanin and lipofuscin in *ex vivo* ocular samples was first demonstrated in [30]. Combining PAOM with AF imaging for *in vivo*

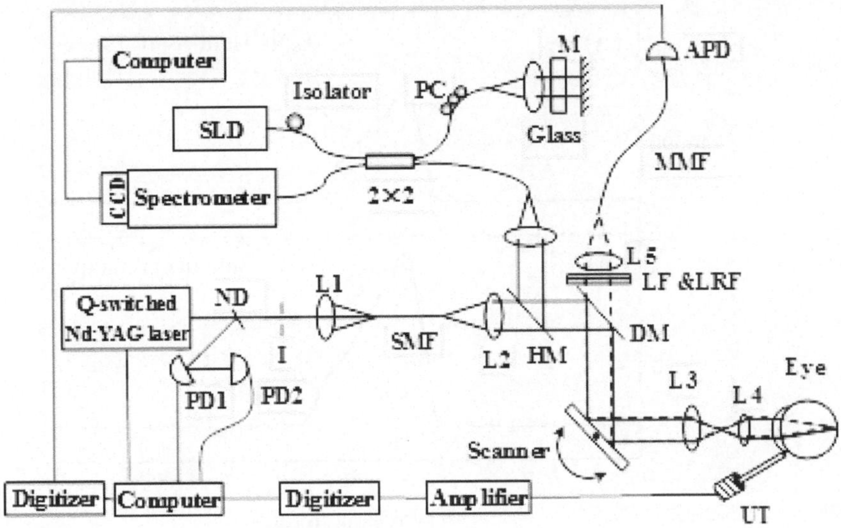

Figure 13.16: Schematic of the fused laser-scanning confocal microscopy and photoacoustic microscopy. PD: photodiode; 2×2: fiber coupler.

imaging of RPE melanin and lipofuscin was demonstrated in [55].

Figure 13.16 shows a schematic of the experimental system. The illuminating light source for both PAOM and AF is a frequency-doubled Q-switched Nd:YAG laser (SPOT-10-100-532, Elforlight Ltd, UK: 532 nm; 10 μJ/pulse; 2 ns pulse duration; maximal pulse repetition rate: 30 kHz). The output laser light was first attenuated with a neutral density (ND) filter before coupled into a single mode optical fiber. The output laser light from the fiber was collimated into a beam diameter of 6 mm, combined with the probing light of a SD-OCT by a hot mirror, reflected by a dichroic mirror, scanned by a X-Y galvanometer, and finally delivered to the eye through a lens system consisting of an achromatic relay lens ($f = 60$ mm) and an objective lens ($f = 19$ mm). The galvanometer scanner was controlled by an analogue-output board, whose sample clock was used to trigger the laser.

The back-travelling AF light emitted from the sample passed through the objective lens, the relay lens, the dichroic mirror, a long-pass filter (FEL0550, cut on wavelength: 550nm, Thorlabs, Inc), a 532 nm laser rejection filter (532-D2C, Omega Optical), and then was coupled into a multimode optical fiber (MMF) with a core diameter of 50 μm. The light exiting the MMF was detected by an avalanche photodetector (APD110A, Thorlabs, Inc). The combination of the long-pass filter and the laser rejection filter provides an attenuation of 10^8 (OD = 8) to the reflected excitation light. The AF signal was digitized and stored by a high speed digitizer (CompuScope 22G8, Gage Applied Technologies) at a sampling rate of 2 GS/s.

The induced PA waves from the sample were detected by a custom-built needle ultrasonic transducer (30 MHz; bandwidth: 50%; active element diameter: 1 mm), which was placed in contact with the eyelid coupled by ultrasound gel. The detected PA signals were first amplified by 80 dB and then digitized by another high-speed digitizer (CompuScope14200, Gage Applied Technologies) at a sampling rate of 200 MS/s.

The laser pulse energy was measured to be 40 nJ after the objective lens, which is lower than the ANSI safety limit. The OCT imaging system was used mainly for imaging guidance to reduce visible light exposure to the eye. During alignment only the OCT light was on. After the retinal region of interest was identified and the OCT image was optimized, the OCT light was turned off and the PAOM imaging mode was activated.

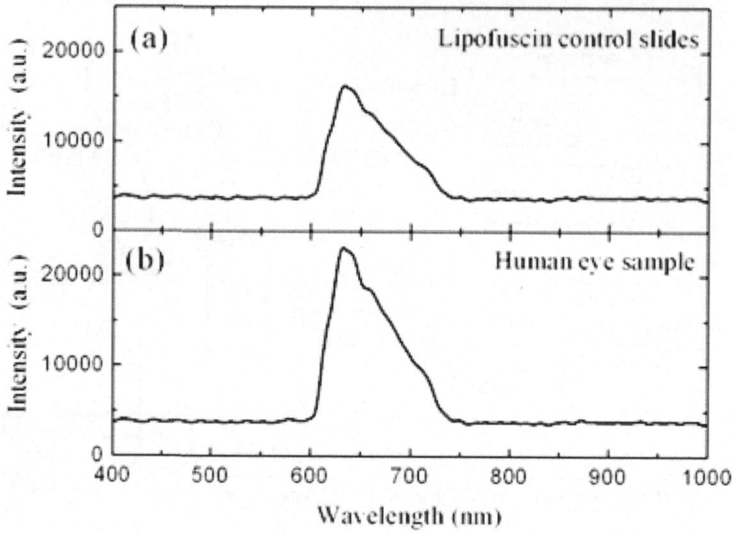

Figure 13.17: (a) and (b): autofluorescent spectra of the lipofuscin and the human RPE sample with excitation wavelength of 532 nm

The AF spectra of a human RPE sample and a lipofuscin control slides (American MasterTech Scientific Inc) were first measured with a commercial spectrometer (USB4000, Ocean Optics Inc). The similarity of the AF spectra (Fig. 13.17) verified the molecular contrast of the AF imaging. In the meantime, no phtoacoustic signal was detected for the lipofuscin control slides. The results demonstrated that lipofuscin had no contribution to the PAM image. Furthermore, it has been previously proved that RPE melanin has no contribution to the AF image [30].

The eyes of Long Evans and Sprague Dawley rats with normal retina were imaged to assess the imaging capability for pigmented and albino rats. Figure 13.18 shows the AF (Figs. 13.18a1 and a2) and PAOM (Figs. 13.18b1 and b2) images of the retina of pigmented rats at 10 and 18 weeks old, respectively. Figure 13.19 shows the AF and PAOM images of the albino rats with the same ages as in Figure 13.18.

The images demonstrated that the AF and PAM imaging modes are perfectly registered. The AF retinal images represent the lipofuscin distribution in the RPE: the stronger the AF signals the higher the lipofiscin concentration. In both the pigmented and albino rats we can see that lipofuscin concentration increased with age, which is in agreement with the literature [56]. From the images we can also see that for the same age the lipofusin concentration is higher in the albino rats than that in the pigmented rats. There are significant differences in the appearance of the PAOM images between the pigmented and albino rats. Since there is no melanin in the RPE of the albino rats, the RPE layer did not show up in the PAM images. Instead, the laser light penetrated the RPE and generated PA signals in the choroidal blood vessels. In contrast, in the pigmented rats the RPE layer appears as the brightest layer in the PAM images. Due to that the laser light was totally blocked by the RPE layer no signal from the choroidal vessels can be observed.

To further demonstrate the accumulation of lipofuscin with age the histogram of AF intensity in Fig. 13.18 and Fig. 13.19 was calculated. The results are shown in Fig. 13.20. From the histogram we can see clearly that the distribution of the AF intensity increased significantly with aging. For the same age the AF intensity of albino rats is stronger than that of the pigmented rats. When the rats became older the increase of the AF intensity is obvious especially in the albino rats. The experiments showed the evidence of increased lipofuscin concentration with aging. Possibly

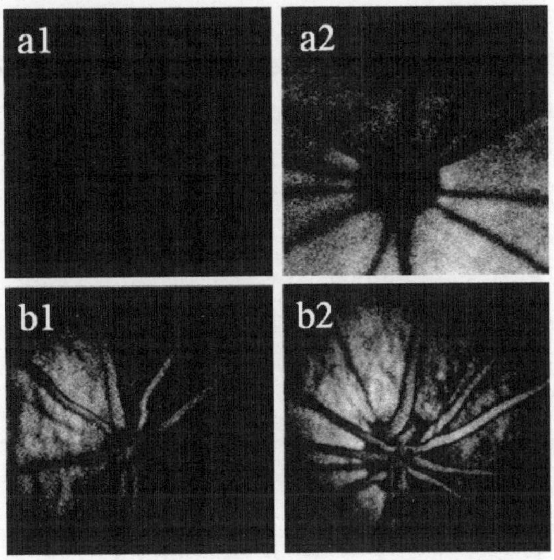

Figure 13.18: AF (a1 and a2) and PAOM (b1 and b2) images of pigmented rats. a1 and b1: 10 weeks-old; a2 and b2: 18 weeks-old.

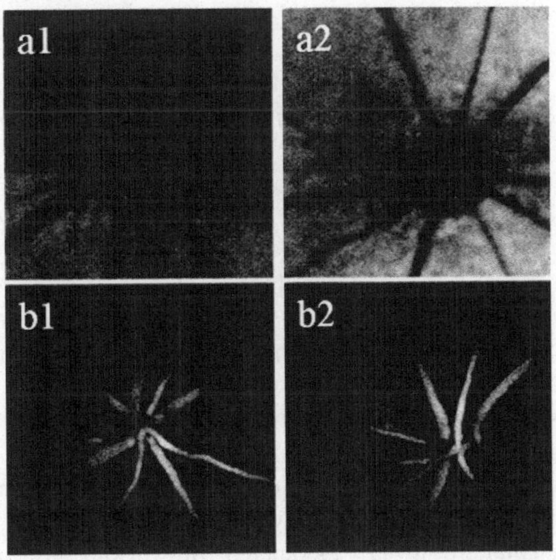

Figure 13.19: AF (a1 and a2) and PAOM (b1 and b2) images of albino rats. a1 and b1: 10 weeks-old; a2 and b2: 18 weeks-old.

due to the protective functions of RPE melanin in the pigmented rats the increase of lipofuscin concentration is not as significant as in the albino rats.

13.6.2 Integrated LSOR-PAM, OCT, and SLO for *in vivo* retinal imaging

In the previous sections we introduced the integration of LSOR-PAM with SD-OCT for multimodal imaging of both optical absorption and scattering properties of biological tissues. We also introduced the integration of PAM for non-ophthalmic applications with confocal scanning laser mi-

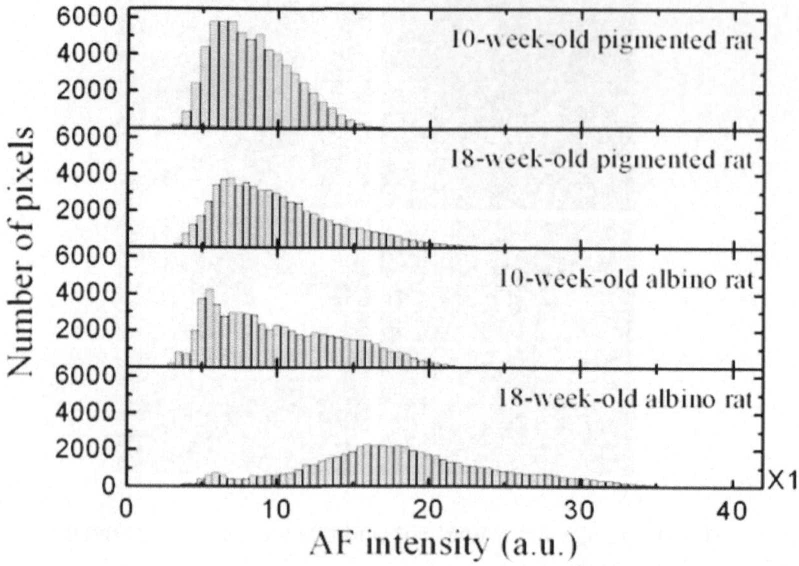

Figure 13.20: Calculated AF intensity distributions of the different rats.

croscopy with the same illuminating light source by simultaneously collecting the reflected photons. When adapted to retinal imaging, by collecting the reflected portion of the PAOM illumination light, a SLO can be added to the system without increasing retinal light exposure. These integration capabilities further demonstrate the compatibility advantages of PAOM with current major ophthalmic imaging techniques.

SLO is an optical scattering-based ophthalmic imaging technology and is widely used in screening, diagnosis, and assessing treatments in patients. Also, SLO is extensively combined with contrast agents, such as fluorescein and indocyanine green (ICG) [57] to improve imaging contrast and develop functional imaging capability.

SD-OCT provides cross-sectional retinal imaging at less than 10 μm axial resolution and is invaluable for the diagnosis and management of several severe blinding diseases [58]. Moreover, SD-OCT can measure the retinal blood flow by detecting the Doppler shift impinged on the reflected photons [59]. The limitation of SD-OCT, however, is that it is not sensitive to the optical absorption properties of the retina that are strongly associated with various physiological parameters, including oxygen saturation (sO_2) and melanin concentration in RPE.

PAOM is an optical absorption-based ophthalmic imaging modality, which demonstrates the capability of imaging retinal and choroidal vessels and melanin in RPE at high contrast by detecting photoacoustic (PA) signals as a result of strong laser absorption of hemoglobin in blood vessels and melanin in RPE [4, 60, 61]. Also, PAOM has the potential to map the sO_2 in retinal vessels based on spectroscopic measurements [62–64]. Although PAOM and SD-OCT have comparable lateral resolutions, the axial resolution of PAOM is not as good as that of SD-OCT [4], which makes PAOM not suitable for visualizing the fine layer structures in the retina.

Therefore, a multimodal system has the potential to combine the merits of SLO, SD-OCT and PAOM for a more comprehensive evaluation of the retina based on their complementary contrast mechanisms. By combining SD-OCT with PAOM, a high-resolution cross-sectional anatomic retinal layer structure could be obtained together with the high-contrast vascular image from PAOM. More importantly, the future combination of Doppler SD-OCT, which shows retinal blood flow, with spectroscopic PAOM, which provides retinal sO_2, can eventually evaluate the oxygen metabolism [14, 15] in the retina. By combining SLO with PAOM, the PAOM light source will be shared with SLO without increasing retinal light exposure. While PAOM detects PA signals from the absorbed portion of the illumination photons, the SLO will generate a scattering-based image by collecting the reflected portion of the illumination photons, which would otherwise be discarded. By adding a 488-nm laser excitation and detecting the corresponding fluorescence emissions, the integration of PAOM, SD-OCT and FA-SLO can be further achieved.

A schematic of the experimental system is shown in Fig. 13.21. A frequency-doubled Nd:YAG laser was used as the illumination source for reflection-SLO and PAOM. The laser output was coupled into a single-mode optical fiber and was further collimated to 2 mm in diameter. A galvanometer scanned the laser beam and delivered the light onto the retina with a telescope configuration (L1 and L2). In PAOM, the induced PA signals from the retina were detected by an unfocused needle ultrasonic transducer (40-MHz central frequency, 15-MHz bandwidth, 0.5×0.5 mm^2 active element size), which was placed in contact with the eyelid coupled by ultrasound gel. The detected PA signals were amplified by 60 dB and were digitized by a data acquisition board (CS14200, Gage Applied) at a sampling rate of 200 MS/s. The reflection-SLO shared the same illumination laser with PAOM and the reflected light from the retina was detected by an amplified photodiode (PD2). A high-speed data acquisition board (CS Cobra, Gage Applied) digitized the SLO signals at a sampling rate of 2 GS/s. The laser pulse energy was 40 nJ, which was reported to be eye safe by different groups [4, 65]. Because reflection-SLO and PAOM shared the same optical illumination, pulse energy was the same as that for PAOM only.

For FA-SLO, a continuous 488-nm argon-ion laser (161C-410-21, Spectra Physics) was added as the excitation source. A dichroic mirror (T495lpxr, Chroma Technology) was used to combine the 532-nm and 488-nm light. After further combined with the SD-OCT sample arm by a hot mirror (FM02, Thorlabs), the three beams shared the same scanning and delivery mechanisms as described above. The emitted fluorescence light passed through a long-pass filter (FEL0500, Thorlabs; cut-off wavelength: 500 nm; labeled by the dotted-line since it was not used in reflection-SLO), and was detected by an avalanche photodetector (APD, APD110A2, Thorlabs). Due to laser safety concerns, we perform FA-SLO and PAOM sequentially rather than simultaneously.

A fiber-based SD-OCT was integrated with PAOM and SLO as previously detailed [66]. Briefly, the SD-OCT consists of a broadband light source (IPSDD0804, InPhenix; center wavelength: 840 nm; 6-dB bandwidth: 50 nm), a 50×50 single-mode fiber coupler, a reference arm, a sample arm coupled with the PAOM by a hot mirror, and a home-built spectrometer. The exposure time of the line scan CCD camera (Aviiva SM2, e2v) in the spectrometer was 36 μs, which gave an OCT A-line rate of 24 kHz.

The axial resolution of PAOM and SD-OCT was previously quantified to be 23 μm and 6 μm, respectively [4]. The reflection-SLO and FA-SLO only provided poor axial resolution because no pin-hole was used to eliminate the out-of-focus signals and the effective numerical aperture of a rat eye is very low. Both SD-OCT and PAOM were shown to have comparable lateral resolution when imaging the retina *in vivo* [4], and both reflection-SLO and FA-SLO were expected to have comparable lateral resolution with SD-OCT and PAOM with a minor difference caused by the differences in optical wavelengths [67].

The retinas of both of albino (Sprague Dawley rat, 500 g, Harlan Laboratories) and pigmented rats (Long Evans rat, 500 g, Harlan Laboratories) were imaged *in vivo*. During the experiment, the animal was anesthetized by a mixture of 1.5% isoflurane and regular air, and the pupils were dilated with 1% Tropicamide ophthalmic solution. Anesthetized animals were restrained in a home-built holder, which was then placed on an adjustable platform with five degree of freedom. For FA-SLO, the fluorescein solution (10%, 0.1 mL/kg, Fluka, Sigma-Aldrich) was administered through tail veins.

To acquire multimodal images, SD-OCT was always used initially to identify the region of interest in the retina and to align the optical focus. When the reflection-SLO was conducted, images

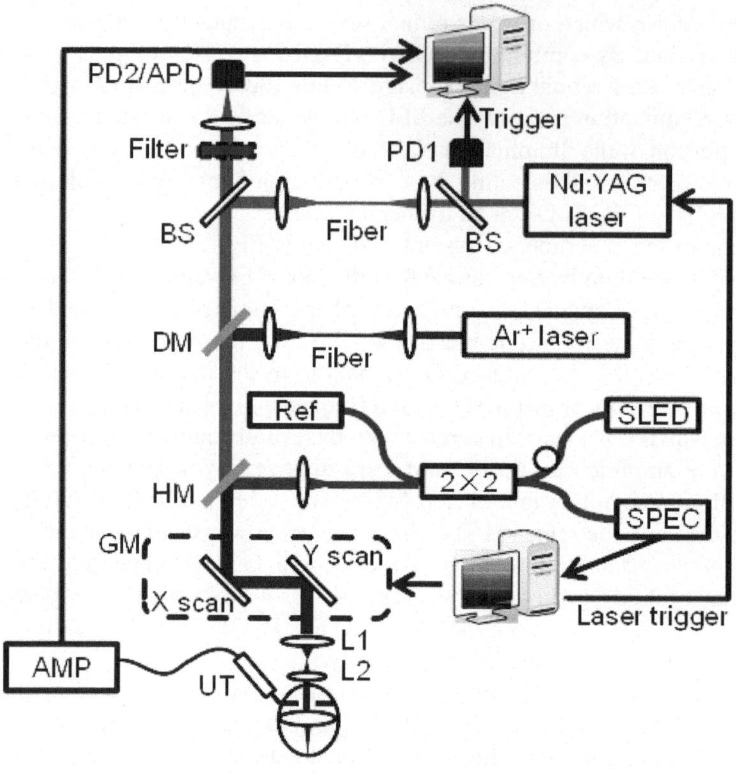

Figure 13.21: Schematic of the integrated PAOM, SD-OCT, and SLO system. SLD: super luminescent diode; SPEC: spectrometer; Ref: OCT reference arm; PD: photodiode; APD: avalanche photodetector; DM: dichroic mirror; HM: hot mirror; GM: 2D galvanometer; BS: beam splitter; UT: ultrasonic transducer; AMP: amplifier. A long-pass filter (labeled by dotted line) and an APD were introduced to acquire the fluorescence emission in the fluorescein angiography SLO. The PD2 replaced the APD and the filter was removed in the reflection SLO.

of SD-OCT, PAOM, and reflection SLO were acquired simultaneously with an image acquisition time of 2.7 s. When the FA-SLO was conducted, only SD-OCT and PAOM images were acquired simultaneously, and the FA-SLO image was acquired afterwards.

In the reflection-SLO experiments, the *in vivo* fundus images are shown in Fig. 13.22, where the images on the left column are acquired from an albino rat and the images on the right column are from a pigmented rat. In PAOM (Fig. 13.22a), the PA signals generated from retinal vessels are high (bright) due to the strong optical absorption of hemoglobin; in comparison, the retinal vessels appear to be dark in the SLO image (Fig. 13.22b) because fewer photons were reflected. Since PAOM and SLO shared the same optical illumination but detected different groups of photons (absorbed photons vs. reflected photons), the two modalities show a naturally registered image of retinal vessels with opposite contrasts. Additionally, PAOM demonstrates the capability of visualizing choroidal vasculatures (CV in Fig. 13.22a) at high contrast due to the minimal melanin concentration in RPE of albino eyes. In the *en face* SD-OCT fundus image (Fig. 13.22c), similar back-scattering contrast with SLO is revealed and the image difference between Fig. 13.22b and Fig. 13.22c is primarily caused by the different illumination wavelengths (532 nm in SLO and 840 nm in SD-OCT). Because SD-OCT and PAOM/SLO illumination light were well aligned before *in vivo* imaging, the SD-OCT image is registered with both the PAOM and SLO images.

Figure 13.22d-f show the images acquired simultaneously in a pigmented rat eye, where the

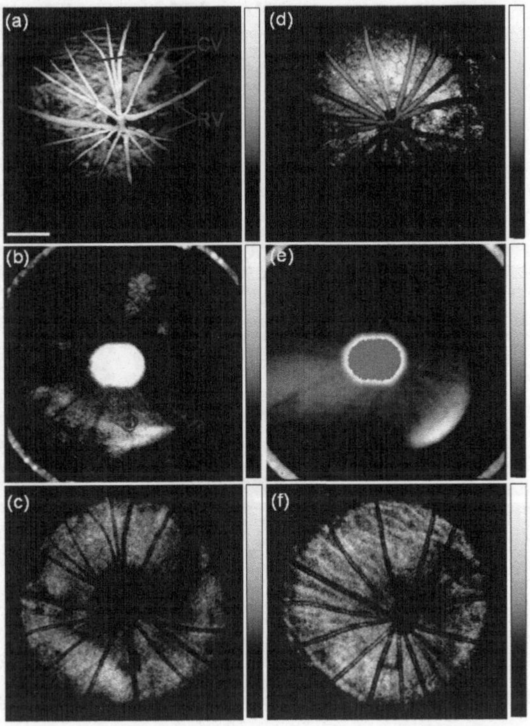

Figure 13.22: *In vivo* multimodal imaging of an albino rat (left column) and a pigmented rat (right column) when the SLO worked in reflection mode. Panels (a) and (d) are PAOM fundus images; panels (b) and (e) are reflection SLO images; and panels (c) and (f) are *en face* SD-OCT images. RV: retinal vessels; CV: choroidal vessels. Bar: 500 μm

differences among the three modalities are similar to those seen in the albino eye. When we compare results between albino and pigmented eyes, the differences are in the visualization of the RPE and choroid. In PAOM images of the albino eye, vessels in both the retina and choroid can be observed although the choroidal vessels are not clearly resolved. In the pigmented eye, the high melanin concentration in the RPE strongly absorbs the illumination light of PAOM, which creates high amplitude PA signals and, consequently, permits the visualization of melanin in RPE. On the other hand, the PAOM laser cannot penetrate through the RPE due to its strong optical absorption and, as a result, the vessels in the choroid cannot be imaged. For a similar reason, SLO shows worse contrast in the pigmented eye than in the albino eye because the RPE is highly absorptive in the pigmented eye. The bright spots at the center of both reflection-SLO images are caused by the specular reflection from the L2 (Fig. 13.21) and can be removed by optimizing the optical setup.

Figure 13.23 shows the imaging results with FA-SLO. In both albino eye (left column) and pigmented eye (right column), the image quality from PAOM and SD-OCT are comparable to those in Fig. 13.22. However, when we compare the FA-SLO images (Fig. 13.23b and Fig. 13.23e) and the reflection-SLO images (Fig. 13.22b and Fig. 13.22e), the image quality was markedly improved as a result of fluorescence detection. Additionally, the FA-SLO image of the pigmented eye (Fig. 13.23e) shows a much better contrast than that of the albino eye (Fig. 13.23b) because the background fluorescence emission from the choroid is absent due to the strong optical absorption by the melanin in the RPE in the pigmented eye.

To further demonstrate the complementary nature among these three modalities, PAOM B-scan, 1D FA-SLO profile, and SD-OCT B-scan are compared in Fig. 13.24. The dashed-line in Fig.

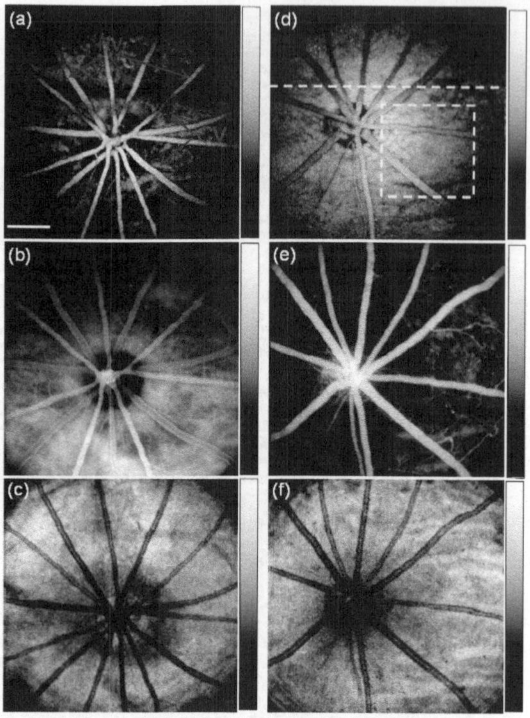

Figure 13.23: *In vivo* multimodal retinal imaging of an albino rat (left column) and a pigmented rat (right column) when the SLO worked in FA mode. Panels (a) and (d) are PAOM fundus images, panels (b) and (e) are FA SLO images; and panels (c) and (f) are *en face* SD-OCT images. RV: retinal vessels; CV: choroidal vessels. Bar: 500 μm.

13.23d indicates the locations of the 1D profile and B-scan images in their corresponding original images. The PAOM B-scan (Fig. 13.24a) specifically imaged five individual retinal vessels and the RPE with high contrast due to strong optical absorption of hemoglobin and melanin. Unlike highly resolved multiple retinal layers in the SD-OCT B-scan, other anatomic layers except for vasculature and RPE were invisible in the PAOM B-scan due to their low optical absorption coefficients [68] and worse axial resolution in the PAOM [29]. The 1D profile in FA-SLO (Fig. 13.24b) is an integration of all the fluorescence emissions along the depth of each illumination position in the retina, where the fluorescence intensity peaks correspond to retinal vessels, where the local concentration of the fluorescein is the highest. The SD-OCT B-scan (Fig. 13.24c) resolved the anatomic layers well based on the different optical scattering properties in each retinal layer, but demonstrated low contrast in visualizing the retinal vessels as a result of the back scattering determined contrast mechanism. The vertical lines in Fig. 13.24 highlight the locations of the retinal vessels in each modality and further demonstrate the spatial registration among the three modalities.

When we compare the PAOM and FA-SLO images, much finer details of the retinal capillaries can be observed in the FA-SLO image than in the PAOM image. Figure 13.25 shows the magnified views of the regions highlighted by the dashed-box in Fig. 13.22d. In both PAOM (Fig.13.25a) and FA-SLO (Fig. 13.25b) images, the major retinal vessels with a diameter of about 100 μm can be observed with high contrast; however, only the FA-SLO visualized the single capillary network as highlighted by the group 1 arrows in Fig. 13.25b. Although the capillary network itself was not imaged by PAOM, the shadows created by the capillaries are observed in the RPE and correspond well with the imaged capillaries by the FA-SLO as pointed out by the group 2 arrows.

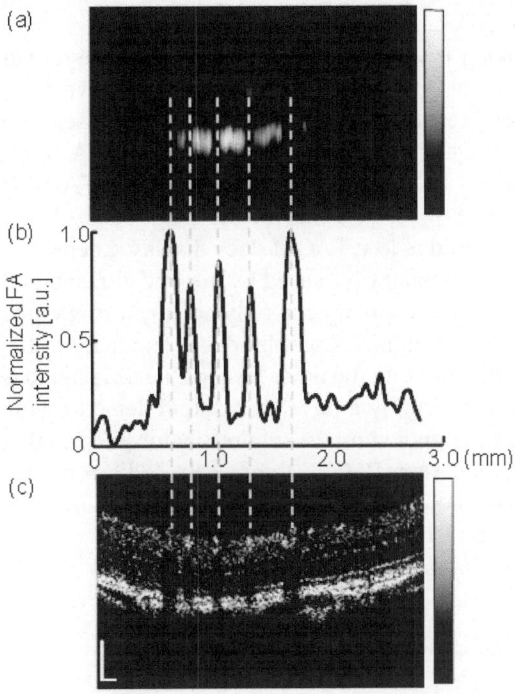

Figure 13.24: Comparison of (a) PAOM B-scan, (b) 1D FA profile, and (c) SD-OCT B-scan acquired from the same spatial location (as highlighted by dashed line in Fig. 13.23d) in a pigmented eye. Bar: 100 μm.

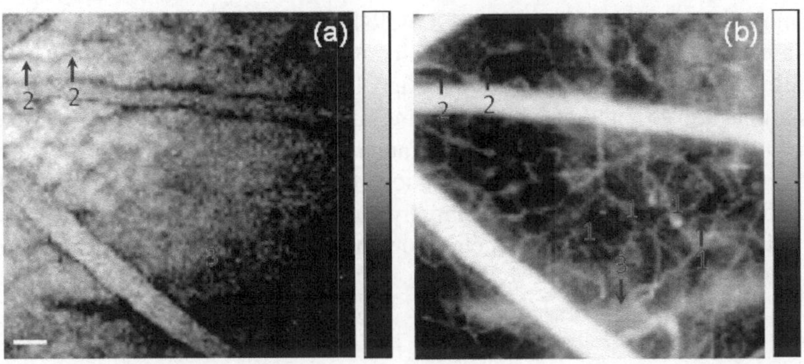

Figure 13.25: Comparison of (a) PAOM and (b) FA-SLO images within the regions highlighted by the dashed square in Fig. 13.23d. Bar: 100 μm.

A more interesting finding in comparing PAOM with FA-SLO is highlighted by the group 3 arrows. The dark region imaged by PAOM in the RPE can potentially be attributed to a lower melanin concentration in the RPE. This hypothesis is supported by the FA-SLO, where the dark region of the PAOM image becomes bright. The reason is that when the melanin concentration is high in the RPE, the fluorescence excitation light is significantly attenuated and the fluorescence emission from the choroid is blocked and cannot be detected; however, in RPE regions with low melanin concentration, more fluorescence emission can be detected and lead to high signal amplitude in the

FA-SLO as shown in Fig. 13.25b.

A question worth asking is why PAOM cannot visualize the retinal capillary at the same level as the FA-SLO does. In retinal imaging, PAOM and FA-SLO have comparable lateral resolution as in both modalities the lateral resolutions are determined by the effective numerical aperture of the subject eye and the optical wavelengths of PAOM (532 nm) and FA-SLO (488 nm) are not dramatically different. One possible reason is that in the pigmented eye, FA-SLO has much lower background signal than PAOM because of the presence of the RPE melanin; however, even in the albino eye, where the PAOM background is low, PAOM does display a densely-packed capillary network. We hypothesize that such a discrepancy is caused by the low ultrasound detection sensitivity in PAOM. With a finite lateral resolution, capillary can only occupy a single pixel in PAOM and its PA amplitude is usually much lower than the PA amplitudes of the major retinal vessels. As a result, the PA signal from capillaries may fall into the noise level of the ultrasound detector and cannot be imaged. The potential solution is to employ a novel ultrasound detector with much lower noise equivalent pressure values, such as the optical micro-ring resonator [69]. Although FA-SLO delineated more detailed retinal vasculatures than PAOM, fluorescein sodium may cause side effects in some patients [70] and FA-SLO is not capable of measuring sO_2 and melanin concentration in RPE due to its fluorescence based contrast mechanism.

13.7 Conclusion

Multimodal microscopy can provide more comprehensive characterization of biological tissues by providing complementary contrast mechanisms. By integrating PAM with other optical imaging modalities it is promising to provide both anatomical and functional information based on optical absorption and optical scattering contrasts. One important issue of integrating multiple microscopic imaging modalities is their compatibility. LSOR-PAM solved the incompatibility issue of classical PAM with other optical imaging modalities like OCT by employing a stationary unfocused ultrasonic transducer and scanning the illuminating light with a galvanometer scanner. LSOR-PAM provides a platform to integrate other imaging modalities like OCT, SLO, and auto-fluorescence imaging. One important application of the integrated multimodal imaging system is to image the retina. By providing high resolution information of the retinal vasculature and the RPE pigmentation the multimodal imaging system can potentially play an important role in the research and diagnosis of major blinding diseases like diabetic retinopathy and age-related macular degeneration.

References

[1] D.A. Sipkins, X. Wei, J. W. Wu, J.M. Runnels, D. Côtè, T.K. Means, A.D. Luster, D.T. Scadden, and C.P. Lin, "*In vivo* imaging of specialized bone marrow endothelial microdomains for tumour engraftment," *Nature* (London) **435**, 969–973 (2005).

[2] C.A. Patil, N. Bosschaart, M.D. Keller, T.G. van Leeuwen, and A. Mahadevan-Jansen, "Combined Raman spectroscopy and optical coherence tomography device for tissue characterization," *Optics Letters*, **33** 1135–1137 (2008).

[3] S. Tang, T.B. Krasieva, Z. Chen, G. Tempea, and B.J. Tromberg, "Effect of pulse duration on two-photon excited fluorescence and second harmonic generation in nonlinear optical microscopy," *J. Biomed. Opt.*, **22** 020501 (2006).

[4] A.A. Oraevsky and A.A. Karabutov, "Optoacoustic tomography," Chap. 34 in *Biomedical Photonics Handbook*, T. Vo-Dinh, Ed., Vol. PM125, pp. 34/1–34/34, CRC Press, Boca Raton, FL (2003).

[5] X. Wang, Y. Pang, G. Ku, X. Xie, G. Stoica, and L.V. Wang, "Noninvasive laser-induced photoacoustic tomography for structural and functional in vivo imaging of the brain," *Nat. Biotechnol.* **25**, 114–116 (2003).

[6] H.F. Zhang, K. Maslov, and L.V. Wang, "*In vivo* imaging of subcutaneous structures using functional photoacoustic microscopy," *Nat. Protocols* **4**, 797–804 (2007).

[7] H. F. Zhang, K. Maslov, G. Stoica, and L. V. Wang, "Functional photoacoustic microscopy for high-resolution and noninvasive in vivo imaging," *Nat. Biotechnol.* **24**, 848–851 (2006).

[8] K. Maslov, H. F. Zhang, S. Hu, and L.V. Wang, "Optical-resolution photoacoustic microscopy for in vivo imaging of single capillaries," *Opt. Lett.* **33**, 929–931 (2008).

[9] Zhixing Xie, Shuliang Jiao, Hao Zhang, and Carmen A. Puliafito, "Laser-scanning optical resolution photoacoustic microscopy," *Opt. Lett.* 34, 1771– 1773 (2009).

[10] V.P. Zharov, E.I. Galanzha, E.V. Shashkov, N.G. Khlebtsov, and V.V. Tuchin, "*In vivo* photoacoustic flow cytometry for monitoring of circulating single cancer cells and contrast agents," *Opt. Lett.* **31**, 3623–3625 (2006).

[11] D. Huang, E.A. Swanson, C.P. Lin, J.S. Schuman, W.G. Stinson, W. Chang, M.R. Hee, T. Flotte, K. Gregory, C.A. Puliafito, and J.G. Fujimoto, "Optical coherence tomography," *Science* **254**, 1178–1181 (1991).

[12] M. Wojtkowski, V. Srinivasan, T. Ko, J. Fujimoto, A. Kowalczyk, and J. Duker, "Ultrahigh-resolution, high-speed, Fourier domain optical coherence tomography and methods for dispersion compensation," *Opt. Express* **12**, 2404–2422 (2004).

[13] L. Li, K.I. Maslov, G. Ku, and L.V. Wang, "*In vivo* imaging of microcirculation using integrated photoacoustic and optical coherence microscopy," *Proc. SPIE* **7177**, 71770I (2009).

[14] S. Jiao, R. Knighton, X. Huang, G. Gregori, and C. Puliafito, "Simultaneous acquisition of sectional and fundus ophthalmic images with spectral-domain optical coherence tomography," *Opt. Express* **13**, 444–452 (2005).
http://www.opticsinfobase.org/abstract.cfm?URI=oe-13-2-444

[15] J.H. Barker, F. Hammersen, I. Bondàr, E. Uhl, T.J. Galla, M.D. Menger, and K. Messmer, "The hairless mouse ear for *in vivo* studies of skin microcirculation," *Plast. Reconstr. Surg.* **83**, 948–959 (1989).

[16] P.T. C. So, H. Kim, and I.E. Kochevar, "Two-photon deep tissue *ex vivo* imaging of mouse dermal and subcutaneous structures," *Opt. Express* **3**, 339–350 (1998).

[17] T. Dabbs and M. Glass, "Fiber-optic confocal microscope: FOCON," *Appl. Opt.* **31**, 3030–3035 (1992).

[18] H.F. Zhang, J. Wang, Q. Wei, T. Liu, S. Jiao, and C.A. Puliafito, "Collecting back-reflected photons in photoacoustic microscopy," *Opt. Express* **18**, 1278–1282 (2010).

[19] M. Gu, *Principles of Three-Dimensional Imaging in Confocal Microscopes*, World Scientific, Singapore (1996).

[20] R.H. Webb, G.W. Hughes, and F.C. Delori, "Confocal scanning laser ophthalmoscope," *Appl. Opt.* **26**, 1492–1499 (1987).

[21] D.A. Atchison and G. Smith, *Optics of Human Eye*, Butterworth-Heinemann, Oxford, (2000).

[22] S. Schmitz-Valckenberg, M. Fleckenstein, A.P. Gbel, K. Sehmi, F.W. Fitzke, F.G. Holz and A. Tufail "Evaluation of autofluorescence imaging with the scanning laser ophthalmoscope and the fundus camera in age-related geographic atrophy," *Am. J. Ophthalmol.* **146**, 183–192 (2008)

[23] P. Artal, A. Guirao, E. Berrio, and D. Williams, "Compensation of corneal aberrations by the internal optics in the human eye," *J. Vision* **1**, 1– 8 (2001).

[24] J. Liang, D. Williams, and D. Miller, "Supernormal vision and high-resolution retinal imaging through adaptive optics," *J. Opt. Soc. Am.* A **14**, 2884–2892 (1997).

[25] E. Fernandez, I. Iglesias, and P. Artal, "Closed-loop adaptive optics in the human eye," *Opt. Lett.* **26**, 746–748 (2001).

[26] K. Li, and A. Roorda, "Automated identification of cone photoreceptors in adaptive optics retinal images," *J. Opt. Soc. Am.* A **24**, 1358–1363 (2007).

[27] M. Pircher, R. Zawadzki, J. Evans, J. Werner, and C. Hitzenberger, "Simultaneous imaging of human cone mosaic with adaptive optics enhanced scanning laser ophthalmoscopy and high-speed transversal scanning optical coherence tomography," *Opt. Lett.* **33**, 22–24 (2008).

[28] J. Liang, D. Williams, and D. Miller, "Supernormal vision and high-resolution retinal imaging through adaptive optics," *J. Opt. Soc. Am.* A **14**, 2884–2892 (1997).

[29] T. Chui, H. Song, and S. Burns, "Adaptive-optics imaging of human cone photoreceptor distribution," *J. Opt. Soc. Am.* A **25**, 3021–3029 (2008).

[30] B. Hermann, E. Fernandez, A. Unterhuber, H. Sattmann, A. Fercher, W. Drexler, P. Prieto, and P. Artal, "Adaptive-optics ultrahigh-resolution optical coherence tomography," *Opt. Lett.* **29**, 2142–2144 (2004).

[31] R. Zawadzki, S. Jones, S. Olivier, M. Zhao, B. Bower, J. Izatt, S. Choi, S. Laut, and J. Werner, "Adaptive-optics optical coherence tomography for high-resolution and high-speed 3D retinal in vivo imaging," *Opt. Express* **13**, 8532–8546 (2005).
http://www.opticsinfobase.org/abstract.cfm?id=85806.

[32] Y. Zhang, B. Cense, J. Rha, R. Jonnal, W. Gao, R. Zawadzki, J. Werner, S. Jones, S. Olivier, and D. Miller, "High-speed volumetric imaging of cone photoreceptors with adaptive optics spectral-domain optical coherence tomography," *Opt. Express* **14**, 4380–4394 (2006).
http://www.opticsinfobase.org/abstract.cfm?id=89918&CFID=113107704
&CFTOKEN=11132256

[33] Y. Zhang, J. Rha, R. Jonnal, and D. Miller, "Adaptive optics parallel spectral domain optical coherence tomography for imaging the living retina," *Opt. Express* **13**, 4792–4811 (2005). http://www.opticsinfobase.org/abstract.cfm?URI=oe-13-12-4792

[34] R. Zawadzki, S. Choi, S. Jones, S. Oliver, and J. Werner, "Adaptive optics-optical coherence tomography: optimizing visualization of microscopic retinal structures in three dimensions," *J. Opt. Soc. Am.* A **24**, 1373–1383 (2007).

[35] K. Kurokawa, K. Sasaki, S. Makita, M. Yamanari, B. Cense, and Y. Yasuno, "Simultaneous high-resolution retinal imaging and high-penetration choroidal imaging by one-micrometer adaptive optics optical coherence tomography," *Opt. Express* **18**, 8515–8527 (2010). http://www.opticsinfobase.org/abstract.cfm?URI=oe-18-8-8515

[36] A. Roorda, F. Romero-Borja, W. Donnelly, H. Queener, T. Hebert, and M. Campbell, "Adaptive optics scanning laser ophthalmoscopy," *Opt. Express* **10**, 405–412 (2002), http://www.opticsinfobase.org/abstract.cfm?URI=OE-10-9-405

[37] D. Merino, C. Dainty, A. Bradu, and A. Podoleanu, "Adaptive optics enhanced simultaneous en-face optical coherence tomography and scanning laser ophthalmoscopy," *Opt. Express* **14**, 3345–3353 (2006),
http://www.opticsinfobase.org/oe/abstract.cfm?URI=oe-14-8-3345

[38] Y. Zhang, S. Poonja, and A. Roorda, "MEMS-based adaptive optics scanning laser ophthalmoscopy," *Opt. Lett.* **31**, 1268–1270 (2006).

[39] D. Hammer, R. Ferguson, C. Bigelow, N. Iftimia, T. Ustun, and S. Burns, "Adaptive optics scanning laser ophthalmoscope for stabilized retinal imaging," *Opt. Express* **14**, 3354–3367 (2006).
http://www.opticsinfobase.org/abstract.cfm?id=89323
&CFID=113107704&CFTOKEN=11132256

[40] S. Burns, R. Tumbar, A. Elsner, D. Ferguson, and D. Hammer, "Large-field-of-view, modular, stabilized, adaptive-optics-based scanning laser ophthalmoscope," *J. Opt. Soc. Am.* A **24**, 1313–1326 (2007).

[41] L. Sherman, J. Ye, O. Albert, and T. Norris, "Adaptive correction of depth-induced aberrations in multiphoton scanning microscopy using a deformable mirror," *J. Microscopy* **206**, 65–71 (2002).

[42] M. Booth, M. Neil, R. Juskaitis, and T. Wilson, "Adaptive aberration correction in a confocal microscope," *PNAS* **99**, 5788–5792 (2002).

[43] P. Marsh, D. Burns, and J. Girkin, "Practical implementation of adaptive optics in multiphoton microscopy," *Opt. Express* **11**, 1123–1130 (2003).
http://www.opticsinfobase.org/abstract.cfm?&id=72382

[44] J. Girkin, S. Poland, and A. Wright, "Adaptive optics for deeper imaging of biological samples," *Current Opinion in Biotech.* **20**, 106–110 (2009).

[45] J. W. Cha, J. Ballesta, and P. T. C. So, "Shack-Hartmann wavefront-sensor-based adaptive optics system for multiphoton microscopy," *J. Biomed. Opt.* **15**, 046022 (2010).

[46] Thorlabs, "Operation Manual of AOkit."
http://www.thorlabs.com/NewGroupPage9.cfm?ObjectGroup_ID=3208

[47] M.A. Ostrovsky, N.L. Sakina, and A.E. Dontsov, "An antioxidative role of ocular screening pigments," *Vis. Res.* **27**, 893–899 (1987).

[48] T. Sarna, J. M. Burke, W. Korytowski, M. Rozanowska, C.M.B. Skumatz, A. Zareba, M. Zareba, "Loss of melanin from human RPE with aging: possible role of melanin photooxidation," *Exp. Eye Res.* **76**, 89–98 (2003).

[49] F.C. Delori, D.G. Goger, and C.K. Dorey, "Age-related accumulation and spatial distribution of lipofuscin in RPE of normal subjects," *Invest. Ophthalmol. Vis. Sci.* **42**, 1855–1866 (2001).

[50] J.J. Weiter, F.C. Delori, G.L. Wing, and K.A. Fitch, "Retinal pigment epithelial lipofuscin and melanin and choroidal melanin in human eyes," *Invest. Ophthalmol. Vis. Sci.* **27**, 145–152(1986).

[51] A.D. Marmorstein, L.Y. Marmorstein, H. Sakaguchi, and J.G. Hollyfield, "Spectral profiling of autofluorescence associated with lipofuscin, Bruch's membrane, and sub-RPE deposits in normal and AMD eyes," *Invest. Ophthalmol. Vis. Sci.* **43**, 2435–2441 (2002).

[52] F.C. Delori, C.K. Dorey, G. Staurenghi, O. Arend, D.G. Goger, and J.J. Weiter, "*In Vivo* fluorescence of the ocular fundus exhibits retinal pigment epithelium lipofuscin characteristics," *Invest. Ophthalmol. Vis Sci.* **36**, 718-729 (1995).

[53] S. Jiao, M. Jiang, J. Hu, A. Fawzi, Q. Zhou, K. K. Shung, C.A. Puliafito, and H.F. Zhang, "Photoacoustic ophthalmoscopy for *in vivo* retinal imaging," *Opt. Express* **18**, 3967–3972 (2010).

[54] X. Zhang, M. Jiang, A. A. Fawzi, X. Li, K.K. Shung, C.A. Puliafito, H.F. Zhang, and S. Jiao "Simultaneous dual molecular contrasts provided by the absorbed photons in photoacoustic microscopy," *Opt. Lett.* **35**, 4018–4020 (2010).

[55] X.Y. Zhang, H.F. Zhang, C.A. Puliafito, and S. Jiao, "Simultaneous in vivo imaging of melanin and lipofuscin in the retina with multimodal photoacoustic ophthalmoscopy," *J. Biomed. Opt.* **16**, 080504 (2011).

[56] P. Mukherjee, S. Bose, A. A. Hurd, R. Adhikary, H. Schonenbrucher, A.N. Hamir, J. A. Richt, T.A. Casey, M.A. Rasmussen, and J.W. Petrich, "Monitoring the accumulation of lipofuscin in aging murine eyes by fluorescence spectroscopy," *Photochemistry and Photobiology* **85**, 234–238 (2009).

[57] W.R. Freeman, D. Bartsch, A.J. Mueller, A.S. Banker, and R.N. Weinreb, "Simultaneous indocyanine green and fluorescein angiography using a confocal scanning laser ophthalmoscope," *Arch. Ophthalmol.* **116**, 455–463 (1998).

[58] G.J. Jaffe, J. Caprioli, "Optical coherence tomography to detect and manage retinal disease and glaucoma," *Am. J. Ophthalmol.* **137**, 156–169 (2004).

[59] H. Wehbe, M. Ruggeri,S. Jiao, G. Gregori, C.A. Puliafito, and W. Zhao, "Automatic retinal blood flow calculation using spectral domain optical coherence tomography," *Opt. Express* **15**, 15193–15206 (2007).

[60] Q. Wei, T. Liu, S. Jiao, and H.F. Zhang, "Image chorioretinal vasculature in albino rats using photoacoustic ophthalmoscopy," *J. Mod. Opt.* **58**, 1997–2001(2011).

[61] X. Zhang, H. Zhang, C. Puliafito, and S. Jiao, "Simultaneous *in vivo* imaging of melanin and lipofuscin in the retina with photoacoustic ophthalmoscopy and autofuorescence imaging," *J. Biomed. Opt.* **16**, 080504 (2011).

[62] S. Hu, L. V. Wang, "Photoacoustic imaging and characterization of the microvasculature," *J. Biomed. Opt.* **15**, 011101 (2010).

[63] J. Yao, K. I. Maslov, Y. Zhang, Y. Xia, and L. V. Wang, "Label-free oxygen-metabolic photoacoustic microscopy *in vivo*," *J. Biomed. Opt.* **16**, 076002 (2011).

[64] T. Liu, Q. Wei, J. Wang, S. Jiao, and H.F. Zhang, "Combined photoacoustic microscopy and optical coherence tomography can measure metabolic rate of oxygen," *Biomed. Opt. Express* **2**, 1359–1365 (2011).

[65] S. Hu, B. Rao, K. Maslov, and L.V. Wang, "Label-free photoacoustic ophthalmic angiography," *Opt. Lett.* **35**, 1–3 (2010).

[66] S. Jiao, Z. Xie, H. Zhang, and C. Puliafito, "Simultaneous multimodal imaging with integrated photoacoustic microscopy and optical coherence tomography," *Opt. Lett.* **34**, 2961–2963 (2009).

[67] H. Zhang, J. Wang, Q. Wei, T. Liu, S. Jiao, and C.A. Puliafito, "Collecting back-reflected photons in photoacoustic microscopy," *Opt. Express* **18**, 1278–1282 (2010).

[68] M. Hammer, A. Roggan, D. Schweitzer, and G. Muller, "Optical properties of ocular fundus tissues-an in-vitro study using the double-integrating-sphere technique and inverse Monte-Carlo simulation," *Phys. Med. Biol.* **40**, 963–978 (1995).

[69] T. Ling, S. L. Chen, and L.J. Guo, "High-sensitivity and wide-directivity ultrasound detection using high Q polymer microring resonators," *Appl. Phys. Lett.* **98**, 204103 (2011).

[70] H.F. Fine, J.L. Prenner, and D. Roth, "Fluorescein angiography," Chapter 3 in *Medical Retina Focus on Retinal Imaging*, F.G. Holz and R.F. Speide, Eds., pp.19–25, Springer, Berlin (2010).

14

Adaptive Optics Scanning Laser Ophthalmoscopy (AOSLO)

Yuhua Zhang, Christopher A. Girkin

Department of Ophthalmology, University of Alabama at Birmingham, Birmingham, AL

Jacque L. Duncan

Department of Ophthalmology, University of California, San Francisco, CA

Austin Roorda

School of Optometry, University of California, Berkeley, CA

14.1 Introduction

The AOSLO [1] is an advanced imaging modality for the living eye. In most applications the imaging target of the AOSLO is the retina, a thin, transparent, multi-layered neural tissue lining the inner surface of the eye that initiates and processes visual signals at the earliest stage [2–4]. The retina is actually a piece of brain tissue, and one of a few parts of the central nervous system (CNS) that can be visualized non-invasively [5]. Direct assessment of the retinal structure and function at the single cell level in the living eye is important for both basic science research and clinical research on the retina; this task may be facilitated by advanced retinal imaging technology. The scanning laser ophthalmoscopy (SLO) [6, 7] is a retinal imaging modality that was developed in the early 1980s. Like most ophthalmic imaging instruments, the SLO works essentially with the principle of the ophthalmoscope that was invented by Charles Babbage in 1847 and Hermann von Helmholtz in 1851 [8, 9], i.e., shining the light into the eye to illuminate the retina and (simultaneously) recording the light scattering back to form the image. The SLO is a confocal imaging system; thus it has the potential for enhanced spatial resolution, improved image contrast, and fine optical sectioning ability, which are the fundamental merits of the confocal imaging mechanism [10, 11]. However, the SLO must use the optical system of the human eye, including the cornea, lens, and vitreous; hence, the human eye is an essential component of the SLO and plays the role of the objective lens in a microscope. Unfortunately, the optics of the human eye, although exquisitely designed, are not perfect. Theoretically, when the pupil of the human eye measures 6 mm in diameter, the cone photoreceptors in the central region of the retina should be resolved; but this was not achieved until Liang et al. introduced adaptive optics (AO) to compensate for the optical defects of the human eye in a flood illuminated ophthalmoscope [12]. In 2002, Roorda et al. reported the first AO assisted SLO [1], which provided video rate retinal images with unprecedented resolution and contrast. The invention of the AOSLO represented an important advance in high-resolution ophthalmoscopy. In the decade since the first AOSLO was reported, AOSLO has gained significant progress in engineering, in basic science, and in clinical application. Many fundamental advantages of the confocal imaging nature of the SLO have been realized or capitalized, but the AOSLO is still at an early stage. This chapter will be dedicated to describing this emerging technology. First, we will briefly review the structural and optical properties of the human eye and the retina to describe the major challenges to *in vivo* high-resolution retinal imaging; then, we will review the SLO working principle and the spatial and temporal properties of the human eye's optical defects, which will elucidate the requirements of the ophthalmic AO system. Next, we will discuss the AOSLO including the design of the optical system, the selection of the light sources, the optimization of photon detection, and image acquisition as well as image processing. We will present specific examples of AOSLO imaging of the retinal structure and function. Finally, we will summarize and discuss the emerging trend and applications.

The adaptive optics scanning laser ophthalmoscopy is a methodology that involves the instrument, i.e., the adaptive optics scanning laser ophthalmoscope, and related techniques for image processing, analysis, and interpretation. For simplicity, we will use the term AOSLO to represent both the methodology and the instrument based upon the context we are discussing.

14.2 The Structural and Optical Properties of the Human Eye and the Retina

14.2.1 The human eye

As a major optical component, the structural and the optical properties of the human eye are important parameters in the design of an AOSLO. Fig. 14.1 illustrates the most relevant components of the eye's optical system, consisting of the cornea, the aqueous humor, the lens, and the vitreous humor. The cornea and lens are two refracting elements that form the image of an object on the retina; of those, the cornea contributes most of the total refractive power of the eye (about 2/3 of the total power of a relaxed eye), and the lens makes up the rest. Although the lens contributes less in light refraction, it can provide adjustable power that allows objects at various distances from the eye to be imaged on the retina. This function is called accommodation, and occurs when the lens shape is changed by the ciliary muscle contraction or relaxation. The iris is a thin, pigmented, contractile diaphragm with a central aperture, known as the pupil, which regulates the light entering the eye and is the ultimate optical aperture stop of the ophthalmic imaging system. The retina lines the inside wall of the globe and is supported by the choroid, a thin (about 214 μm) and pigmented vascular tissue. The choroid supplies the essential nourishment to the neuronal retina and plays many important roles, such as providing a conduit for vessels traveling to other parts of the eye and absorbing light, thereby preventing unwanted light from scattering back through the retina. Outside

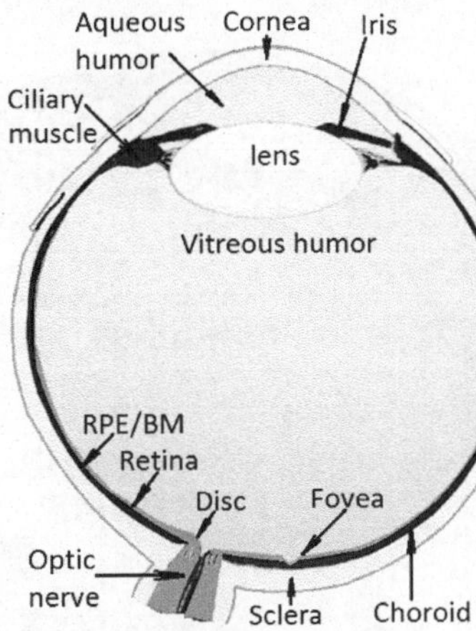

Figure 14.1: The structure of the human eye.

the choroid is the sclera, a fibrous tissue that surrounds and supports the eye [13, 14].

The pupil size may vary from 1 mm to 8 mm under different levels of illumination; the accommodation can change the optical power of the eye to bring an object of interest into focus onto the retina [13]. While accommodation is critical to vision performance, it is adverse to high-resolution retinal imaging. First, a large pupil is preferable for retinal imaging because it provides a larger numerical aperture (NA), allowing for better resolution; thus, AO-assisted retinal imaging systems are best performed with a dilated pupil. Second, the eye should maintain a constant pupil size and a stable focus during the imaging. Therefore, in the AOSLO, as well as other AO assisted retinal imaging systems, the pupil is very often dilated and the accommodation is paralyzed with mydriatic or cycloplegic drugs, e.g., one or two drops of phenylephrine (2.5%) (for mydriasis) and tropicamide (1%) combination or cyclopentolate hydrochloride (1%) (for longer-acting cycloplegia) are applied topically to the eye at the beginning of the imaging session.

14.2.2 The retina

Figure 14.2 is a typical fundus photograph of a living human eye showing the retinal structures that we have marked and will mention in later discussion. The macula is the central posterior portion of the retina, with an area 6 mm, or 21.5° of visual angle [15], in diameter. It contains the densest concentration of photoreceptors, the essential light-sensitive cells, in the retina. The macula is responsible for high-resolution visual acuity, central visual field and color vision. In the central macula resides the fovea, a small area that is about 0.8 mm (2.75°) in diameter [16] that will be described in more detail next. About 15 degrees away from the fovea nasally, the optic nerve head (ONH) is comprised of ganglion cell axons (described next) that carry the visual signal. The ONH is the exit point for ganglion cell axons, and is also the entry and exit point for major blood vessels, arteries and veins, which supply the retina [14]. This image of the retina includes only large structures such as blood vessels and the optic disc; no individual cells are visible. Furthermore, this ''en-face" image provides little information about the cross-sectional structure of the retina (however, a trained ophthalmologist may examine depth information relevant to disease through stereo images of the fundus to perceive information about the retinal thickness and structure).

Figure 14.3 shows the neuronal layers of the retina under high magnification microscopy [2]. On the outermost border of the retina, Bruch's membrane, an acellular tissue consisting of 5 layers with a total thickness of 2–4 μm [14], lies between the retina and the choroid. Tight junctions between retinal pigment epithelial cells provide the outer blood-retinal barrier. Towards the vitreous, the

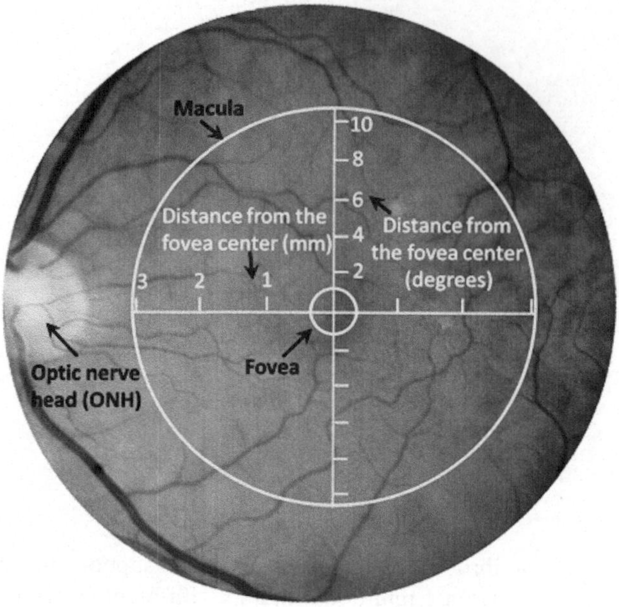

Figure 14.2: Photograph of the retina.

basement membrane of the retinal pigment epithelium (RPE) forms the innermost layer of Bruch's membrane. The RPE is a monolayer of cells that directly supports the photoreceptors, delivering nutrients to the photoreceptors, participating in the regeneration of vitamin A in the visual cycle and phagocytosing photoreceptor outer segments [14, 17]. The thickness of the RPE is about 10–14 μm. Healthy RPE cells are critical for maintaining the normal structure of the retina and for preserving normal photoreceptor function. The photoreceptors, cones and rods, which are named for their shapes, reside proximal to the RPE cells [14]. Photoreceptors are the essential light-sensitive cells that capture photons of light with their outer segments and convert the photo-signal into a neural-signal that is transmitted by the inner segments [14]. The human eye has three types of cones that are sensitive to long-wavelength (peak sensitivity at approximately 565 nm), middle-wavelength (peak at approximately 545 nm), and short-wavelength (peak at approximately 440 nm) light [3, 5]. Cone density and size vary in the retina. The cone density peaks at the foveal center and decreases with increasing eccentricity [16]. The fovea is dominated by cones. In the central fovea, there are only cone photoreceptors. Outside of the fovea, the parafovea is dominated by rods. As a whole, the macula is cone-enriched but not cone-dominated [18]. The cone size and cell-to-cell spacing increase with increasing eccentricity from the foveal center. The inner segment diameter of the cones at the foveal center is about 2 μm, whereas in the area beyond 2 degrees of eccentricity the cone size can be 5–8 μm [16]. The rod inner segment is about 2 μm (diameter) in macula, and slightly increases across the entire eccentricity range with most noticeable diameter of about 3 μm observed between 8 and 16 mm, eccentric to the fovea [16]. Rod density increases with increasing eccentricity; the highest rod densities are within in a broad, horizontally-oriented elliptical ring approximately 15 degrees from the foveal center [3–5, 16]. The photoreceptors are like optical fibers, guiding the incident light into the outer segment and the reflected light back to the inner retina [19–22]. As we will see later in this chapter, the waveguide nature of the photoreceptors significantly increases the contrast between the photoreceptors and the surrounding tissue in optical

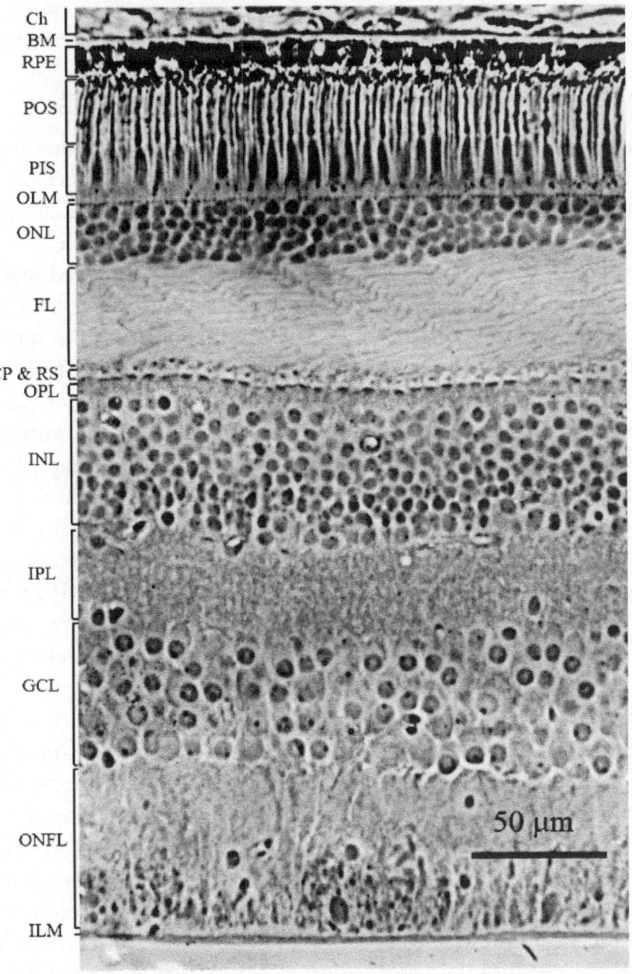

Figure 14.3: The picture was taken of a retinal section about 1.25 mm from the center of the fovea and was photographed by phase-contrast microscopy. Magnification ratio: 550X. Ch, choroid; BM, Bruch's membrane; RPE, retina pigment epithelium; POS, photoreceptor (rods and cones) outer segments; PIS, photoreceptor (rods and cones) inner segments; OLM, outer limiting membrane; ONL, outer nuclear layer; FL, fiber layer; CP & RS, cone pedicles and rod spherules (photoreceptor terminals); OPL, outer plexiform layer; INL, inner nuclear layer; IPL, inner plexiform layer; GCL, ganglion cell layer; ONFL, optic nerve fiber layer; ILM, inner limiting membrane. Modified from [2] with permission of Philosophical Transactions of the Royal Society of London.

imaging, allowing the cell mosaic to be clearly resolved by the AOSLO. The visual signal generated by the photoreceptors is transmitted to the horizontal cells and the bipolar cells, whose cell bodies reside in the inner nuclear layer, then to the ganglion cells with cell bodies in the ganglion cell layer. The axons of the retinal ganglion cells form nerve fiber bundles which exit the eye through the ONH and send the visual signal to the brain. The inner-limiting membrane separates the neuronal retina and the collagenous vitreous. This vitreo-retinal interface is a strong light reflector in the fundus and may obscure the tissues underneath it [23].

14.3 Challenges to High-Resolution Retinal Imaging

The organization of the human eye's optical system and the retina makes the eye an effective objective lens for in-vivo imaging of the retina, which enables direct observations of neural, glial and vascular tissue in a living subject. While the eye provides the unique availability for optical imaging, its unique structure also imposes serious limits to cellular level imaging.

First, it is difficult to collect adequate photons to achieve a good signal to noise ratio (SNR). The human eye has a small numerical aperture (NA); with a fully dilated pupil of 8 mm, the NA is only 0.24, inefficient for collecting the light scattered back from the retina, and the reflectivity of the retina is only about 0.08. For imaging based upon reflectance, it is estimated that, on average, only 1 out of 10,000 photons that enter the eye can reach the detector [23, 24]. For imaging based upon fluorescence, even fewer photons can be detected [25, 26]. Additionally, the amount of light that can be delivered safely into the eye is restricted, i.e., retinal imaging must be conducted under the maximum permitted exposure (MPE) level to avoid any damage to the human eye [27–29]; therefore, the SNR of the retinal image cannot be increased simply by increasing the illumination light. When the retina is imaged within a small field of view (FOV) and with high speed, under the MPE level, the photons caught by an individual image pixel are significantly less than in large FOV imaging. Therefore, a high-resolution retinal imaging system must be able to efficiently illuminate the retina and collect the reflected photons. A large pupil size is preferred, which allows not only collection of more light for imaging but also better resolution.

Second, the retina is transparent, and many cells have similar refractive indices, making it difficult to obtain images with high contrast by reflectance imaging. Non-invasive imaging of the human retina must rely on natural contrast sources, i.e., scattering from structures with different indices of refraction and the absorption of ocular pigments such as oxy-hemoglobin and deoxy-hemoglobin (in retinal and choroidal blood vessels), melanin (in the RPE and choroid), macular pigment (in the axons of the photoreceptors), and the visual pigments (in the photoreceptors) [24–26, 30–33]. When imaging diseased eyes, the image contrast can be seriously impaired by the scattering in the lens, vitreous, and retinal structures due to accumulation of extracellular material (e.g., drusen) [34–43]. Modern molecular biotechnology has developed novel, easily imaged fluorescent proteins that can be expressed in particular cells, allowing researchers to target particular cells for the expression of contrast agents (such as green fluorescent protein, or GFP) in animal models. The ability to visualize endogenous (autofluorescence) and exogenous (added novel fluorescent probes) fluorophores is highly desirable.

Third, the eye is in continual motion, even when fixating on a target [44–48]. The amplitude spectrum of retina motion spans a wide frequency range up to several hundred Hz and the power spectrum follows a reciprocal relationship to frequency ($1/f$) [49, 50]. For a 30 frame per second (fps) image acquisition, the high frequency jitters or tremors cause distortions within a single frame, while the slow frequency motion leads to misplacement of successive frames. Sophisticated methods must be developed to achieve accurate image registration [51, 52]. However, the algorithms are vulnerable to the noise in the image. This problem can be exacerbated in patient populations that have lower reflection and inferior fixation ability. Inaccurate image registration reduces the fidelity of the averaged image, making measurements of structural morphology inaccurate. To overcome motion artifacts, Riggs et al. suggested that the image acquisition rate should be at least 100 fps [47], Potsaid et al. [53] and Rha et al. [54] suggested that the ideal frame acquisition time should be less than 0.004 second. However, it will be very challenging to achieve decent image SNR with this speed.

Fourth, the optical system of the human eye is not perfect but has many defects, which are described by wavefront aberrations and will be discussed in detail later in this chapter. Optical aberrations prevent us from achieving diffraction-limited resolution. Theoretically, since the lateral

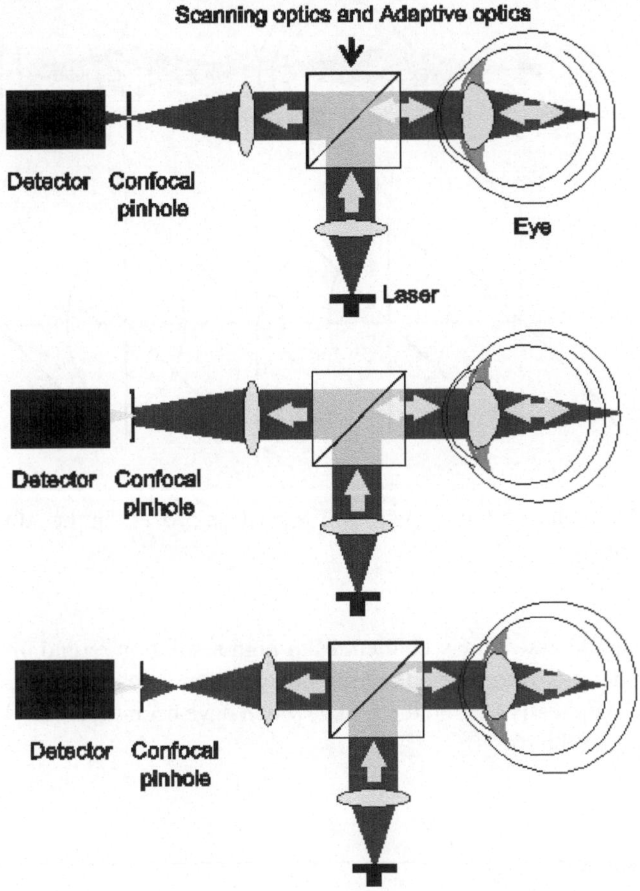

Figure 14.4: The reduced AOSLO system.

resolution is proportional to the diameter of the pupil and the axial resolution is proportional to the square of the pupil diameter, we might expect to increase 3-dimensional spatial resolution by enlarging the pupil size, e.g., by dilating the pupil. However, the optical aberration of the human eye increases with pupil size [55–58]. Further, optical aberrations of the human eye are dynamic [59, 60] and vary from person to person. With advanced design and manufacturing technology, sophisticated optical systems may be developed with minimized optical aberration; but when the human eye is incorporated, the imaging system will never be diffraction-limited. This is the major challenge that this chapter addresses. We will present how we can apply AO, a technique originally conceived for use in astronomical imaging [61] to compensate for time-varying aberrations in the atmosphere, into the SLO to correct for the imperfections in the cornea and lens of the eye, allowing *in vivo* images of unprecedented resolution and contrast [1].

Given these challenges, the retinal imaging system must be highly efficient in light illumination and collection. Confocal imaging has the potential to meet this requirement. As will be discussed in the next section, an SLO only illuminates or focuses light on the point to be imaged; further, the SLO only collects light that is exactly in focus, whereas out-of-focus scattered light is blocked by a confocal pinhole placed in front of the photo detector, thereby improving the image contrast and allowing intrinsic imaging of different layers of the retina with good axial resolution by moving the focus axially; in other words, permitting optical sectioning the retina. Thus, the SLO is an excel-

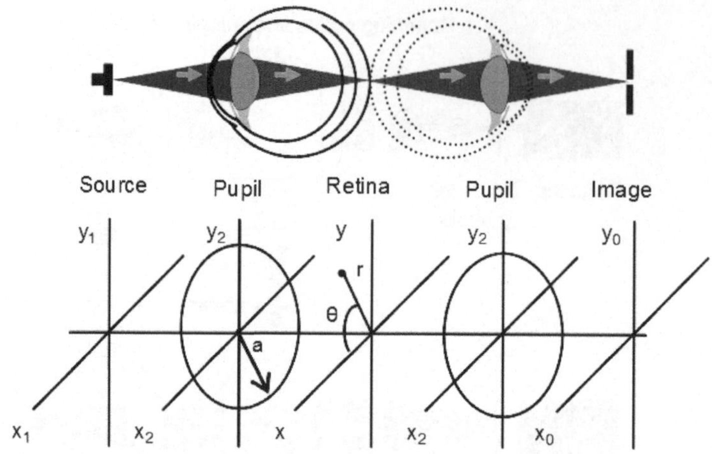

Figure 14.5: The reduced double path PSF formation process in the AOSLO. The characters are defined in the context.

lent modality that addresses many challenges to high resolution retinal imaging. The fundamental advantages include improved efficiency in light collection, enhanced resolution, improved contrast and the capacity to optically section the retina, which have been very well described by Wilson [11], Sheppard [62] and Webb [6, 7].

14.4 The Imaging Characteristics of the SLO

The SLO was invented by Webb et al. [6, 7]. Its basic principles of operation are the same as a confocal scanning laser microscope, which was designed in 1955 by Minsky [63]. The only difference is that a SLO uses the human eye as its objective lens. Basically, the SLO system can be reduced to consist of a point light source, a set of intermediate scanning optics, the human eye, a confocal pinhole, and a photo-detector, as shown in Figure 14.4. The human eye serves as both the objective lens that focuses the light onto the retina and the collection lens that focuses the light reflected from the retina to the pinhole (and the detector). Only the light from the volumetric focal region in the retina that is conjugate to the pinhole can reach the detector (the top panel), because the out-of-focus scattering is blocked by the pinhole (the middle and bottom panels). The image formation of the SLO basically follows that of the confocal optical microscopy that has been vigorously treated with scalar theory and electro-magnetic wave vector theory [11, 64–69]. However, much of the analysis for confocal microscopy was performed assuming that the sample was a plane reflector or a point reflector. Because the retina is a relatively transparent tissue with densely packed multilayer neural cells, the light scattering from the retina cannot be simply treated as reflections from a point or a plane. Therefore, the definition of the imaging performance of standard confocal optical microscopy, such as the transverse resolution and the depth resolution, may only be used for heuristic assessments or characterizations of the SLO performance.

Imaging characteristics of the SLO: Assuming the amplitude point spread function (PSF) of the eye's optics is $h(x,y)$, the retinal amplitude reflectance is $r(x,y)$, then the field of the point (x,y) at the retina is $h(x,y)r(x,y)$. Thus, the field of point x_0, y_0 at the image plane, denoted by $\Phi(x_0,y_0)$, is the convolution of field of the retina and the PSF of the eye, as depicted in Figure 14.5,

$$\Phi(x_0, y_0) = \int_{-\infty}^{\infty}\int_{-\infty}^{\infty} h(x,y)r(x,y)h(x_0/M - x, y_0/M - y)dxdy, \tag{14.1}$$

where M is the magnification ratio from the retina plane to the image plane. With **an infinitesimal pinhole**, $x_0 = y_0 = 0$, the intensity at the detector is:

$$I = \left|\int_{-\infty}^{\infty}\int_{-\infty}^{\infty} h(x,y)r(x,y)h(-x,-y)dxdy\right|^2 = |h^2 \otimes r|^2, \tag{14.2}$$

where $\otimes$ denotes the convolution operation. The amplitude PSF of the SLO is given by $h^2(x,y)$ and the image of the SLO is the convolution of $h^2(x,y)$ and the retinal amplitude reflectance; thus, the image of the SLO is linear in intensity. Here we should note the assumption of the point pinhole. When a large pinhole is used, the intensity at the detector will become $I = |h \otimes r|^2$, i.e., the amplitude PSF of the SLO becomes $h(x,y)$. Under this situation, the SLO image is no longer linear in intensity but linear in amplitude, meaning that the SLO imaging is coherent.

Following [68], we introduce v as the normalized optical coordinate,

$$v \approx 2\pi ar/\lambda f, \tag{14.3}$$

where a is the radius of the eye pupil, f is the focal length of the eye, and λ is the laser wavelength in the eye which is a quotient of the laser wavelength in air over the eye's refractive index. With a circular pupil [68],

$$I(v) = I_0\left[2J_1(v)/v\right]^4, \tag{14.4}$$

where I_0 is the peak intensity of the image of a point object and $J_1(v)$ is the first-order Bessel function of the first kind. From Eq. (14.4) we derive the **lateral two-point resolution** d, according to Rayleigh criterion [11, 68, 70],

$$d = 0.56\lambda f/a. \tag{14.5}$$

However, as proved by Sheppard and Wilson [10, 11], with increasing pinhole size, this resolution will quickly deteriorate to that of a conventional microscope.

$$d = 0.61\lambda f/a \tag{14.6}$$

Eq. (14.6) can be used as a practical estimation of the SLO resolution, as there is always a trade-off between the resolution that requires a small pinhole and the imaging signal to noise ratio that needs a large pinhole. As we analyzed in Section 14.3, the signal photons are precious in imaging of the living human eye. We have to compromise with a relatively large pinhole in order to collect enough photons for imaging. On the other hand, even with an ideal point pinhole, the benefit gained in lateral resolution is only 8% [10, 11, 70]. However, as will be discussed next, the major advantage of the SLO is not for its lateral resolution, but for its improved axial resolution and the ability to reject the out-of-focus scattering thereby improving contrast.

Depth response of the SLO [70]**:** Based upon scalar theory, the depth response of the SLO for a plane reflector can be expressed as

$$V(z) = e^{-jknz(1+\cos\theta_0)}\frac{\sin[knz(1-\cos\theta_0)]}{knz(1-\cos\theta_0)}. \tag{14.7}$$

For a point reflector

$$V(z) = e^{-jknz(1+\cos\theta_0)}\left[\frac{\sin[knz(1-\cos\theta_0)/2]}{knz(1-\cos\theta_0)/2}\right]^2, \tag{14.8}$$

where $k = 2\pi/\lambda$, $\cos\theta_0 = f/\sqrt{f^2+a^2}$, n is the refractive index of the eye, and z is the depth variable. Eq. (14.7) and Eq. (14.8) indicate that, with the change of the depth, the optical field not only varies in amplitude but also changes in phase which is described by the term $e^{-jknz(1+\cos\theta_0)}$. The presence of the phase term is of great importance, implying that there can be interference between the scatterings from different depths, which very likely occurs in the retina. This may give rise to speckle that degrades the fidelity of the retinal image, as will be demonstrated later.

The intensity on the photo-detector for a plane reflector can be expressed as

$$I(z) = \left[\frac{\sin[knz(1-\cos\theta_0)]}{knz(1-\cos\theta_0)}\right]^2, \tag{14.9}$$

and for a point reflector

$$I(z) = \left[\frac{\sin[knz(1-\cos\theta_0)/2]}{knz(1-\cos\theta_0)/2}\right]^4. \tag{14.10}$$

From these two equations, we have the axial resolution of the SLO, commonly defined as the full width at half maximum (FWHM) distance or -3 dB resolution. For a plane reflector this can be expressed as

$$d = 0.90\lambda(f/a)^2, \tag{14.11}$$

and for a point reflector,

$$d = 1.24\lambda(f/a)^2. \tag{14.12}$$

The meaning of a plane reflector or a point reflector in the retina could be obscure, thus the estimation of the resolution under these assumptions would be somewhat arbitrary. However, despite the difference between the resolution derived from the plane reflector and the point reflector, it is clear that the lateral resolution of the SLO is inversely proportional to the numerical aperture of the eye, whereas the axial resolution is inversely proportional to the square of the numerical aperture. When the confocal pinhole is optimized, the lateral and axial resolutions for a 6 mm pupil and 600 nm light are about 2 μm and 30 μm, respectively. However, the SLO must use the human eye as its objective lens, whose optical quality is unfortunately far from the diffraction-limited state, especially for large pupils, preventing us from taking full advantage of the confocal imaging nature and obtaining diffraction-limited retinal images. The typical axial resolution is limited to over 200 μm and the transverse resolution to about 10 μm [7]. To achieve diffraction-limited resolution and take advantage of the confocal imaging merits, it is critical to correct for ocular aberrations. This is why AO was introduced for the SLO.

14.5 The Aberration of the Human Eye

The optical defects in the eye are described by the wave aberration, the deviation of light waves from the ideal shape, e.g., if the eye's optics were perfect, the wavefront of a point source outside the eye would have converged with a perfect spherical wavefront inside the eye and formed a point image, i.e., Airy disk, on the retina; inversely, the wavefront of a point source on the retina would have become perfectly flat when the light exits from the eye. Such perfect wavefront conversion and image formation never happens in a real eye; a point source will form a dispersed pattern on the retina and the wavefront of the light coming out the eye from a point source is of a complex shape. Depending on the spectrum of the illumination light, the wavefront aberration can be monochromatic or chromatic. A detailed discussion of the optical aberrations of the human eye is beyond the scope of this chapter, and interested readers are referred to the available reference texts [23, 71].

14.5.1 Mathematical expression of the ocular optical aberration

The wavefront aberration of the human eye can be expressed by Zernike polynomials, which have traditionally been used to describe the wavefront in optical systems with circular pupils. A number of mathematical properties make Zernike polynomials suitable for representing the ocular aberration. First, they are a complete set of orthonormal functions over a unit circle, meaning that an arbitrarily complex **continuous** surface can be accurately described by a series of independent bases, given enough terms. Second, the first several orders of the polynomials directly correspond to traditional optical aberrations, such as defocus, astigmatism, coma, and spherical aberration, allowing for easy understanding and interpretation.

The Optical Society of America (OSA) [71] recommended a double indexing scheme and a single indexing scheme for representing the ocular aberration. With the OSA double indexing scheme, Zernike polynomials are defined as

$$Z_n^m(\rho,\theta) = \begin{cases} N_n^m R_n^m(\rho)\cos m\theta, & m \geq 0; \\ -N_n^m R_n^m(\rho)\sin m\theta, & m < 0, \end{cases} \tag{14.13}$$

where n is the radial order, $n \geq 0$; m is the azimuthal order, $m = -n, -n+2, -n+4, \ldots n$.

$$R_n^m(\rho) = \sum_{s=0}^{(n-|m|)/2} \frac{(-1)^s (n-s)!}{s!\,[0.5(n+|m|-s)]!\,[0.5(n-|m|-s)]!}\rho^{n-2s} \tag{14.14}$$

and

$$N_n^m = \sqrt{2(n+1)/(1+\delta_{m0})}, \tag{14.15}$$

where N_n^m is the normalization factor, and δ_{m0} is the Kronecker delta, $\delta_{m0} = 1$ when $m = 0$, and $\delta_{m0} = 0$ when $m \neq 0$.

The wavefront aberration can be decomposed as weighted sum of Zernike modes, in the double indexing scheme,

$$W(\rho,\theta) = \sum_n^N \sum_{m=-n}^n W_n^m Z_n^m(\rho,\theta) =$$

$$= \sum_n^N \left\{ \sum_{m=-n}^{-1} W_n^m[-N_n^m R_n^{|m|}(\rho)\sin(m\theta)] + \sum_{m=0}^n W_n^m[N_n^m R_n^{|m|}(\rho)\cos(m\theta)] \right\}, \tag{14.16}$$

whereas in the single indexing scheme,

$$W(\rho,\theta) = \sum_{j=0}^J a_j z_j(\rho,\theta) \quad , \tag{14.17}$$

where the Zernike polynomials $z_j(\rho,\theta)$ are described by a single indexing scheme, j is the index of the order and J is the highest order of the series. According to the OSA recommendation, the conversion between j and the values of n and m can be done with the following equations.

$$j = [n(n+2)+m]/2 \tag{14.18}$$

and

$$n = \text{roundup}[(-3+\sqrt{9+8j})/2] \tag{14.19}$$

$$m = 2j - n(n+2). \tag{14.20}$$

Metrics for estimating the ocular aberration:

1. **The peak-to-valley (P-V)** wavefront aberration. This is simply the maximum departure of the actual wavefront from the desired wavefront in both positive and negative directions, but it tells nothing about the area over which this error is occurring.

2. **Root-mean-square (RMS)** wavefront aberration. This is a description of the standard deviation from the ideal wavefront shape over the pupil. Expressed by the Zernike polynomials, the coefficient of each Zernike mode is essentially its standard deviation. Because the polynomials are mathematically independent, the variance of the sum of modes is equal to the sum of the variances of each individual mode, therefore,

$$\mathrm{RMS} = \sqrt{\sum_{j=3}^{J} a_j^2}, \tag{14.21}$$

where j starts at 3, because the first three terms of Zernike modes z_0^0, z_1^{-1}, z_1^1 are not considered as wavefront aberration; they represent wavefront piton and tilt along x, y direction.

Metrics for defining the image quality:

1. **The point spread function (PSF)**. It is a measure of a light intensity distribution on the retina at the image point. Assuming the pupil function is $P(r, \theta)$, and wavefront aberration is $W(r, \theta)$, the PSF can be calculated by Fourier transform

$$PSF = C\left|FT\left[P(r,\theta)e^{-i2\pi W(r,\theta)/\lambda}\right]\right|^2, \tag{14.22}$$

where C is a constant. FT denotes Fourier transform. The PSF is one of the most important factors for assessing image quality not only in the eye but also in all optical imaging systems. It is an effective estimation of the performance of an optical system. Other metrics, such as modulation transfer function (MTF) of the optical system, can be directly derived from the PSF through a Fourier transform.

2. **The Strehl ratio (SR)**. It is a measure of the light intensity at the image point in the presence of aberration over the intensity that would be obtained if no aberration were present. It is defined as the peak height of the PSF in a real optical system over the peak height for the same optical system without any aberrations (i.e., diffraction-limited). Given the wavefront aberration $W(r,\theta)$, a good approximation (for *SR* as small as 0.1) of the *SR* is given by [72],

$$SR \approx e^{-[2\pi W(r,\theta)/\lambda]^2}. \tag{14.23}$$

This implies that when the aberration is small, the *SR* is independent of the nature of the aberration and is smaller than the ideal value of unity by an amount proportional to the variance of the wavefront aberration. Generally, an optical system can be considered as diffraction-limited when the $SR \geq 0.8$, which requires the root mean square (RMS) of the wavefront aberration $W(r, \theta) \leq 0.071\lambda$. This is the Marechal criterion or Rayleigh limit.

3. **Optical transfer function (OTF)**. This is a measure of the contrast and phase change of the spatial frequency components of an object imaged by an optical system [73]. It is the normalized Fourier transform of the intensity PSF of an optical imaging system [74]. The OTF provides a complete assessment of the performance of an optical system to linearly transfer various spatial frequency components from the object to the image. The modulus of OTF is called modulation transfer function (MTF), which is the measure of the contrast reduction of the spatial frequency components of an object through an optical system; whereas

the phase of OTF is called phase transfer function, which is the measure of the phase change of each frequency component of the object at the image plane. Given the **intensity** PSF of the optical system, the OTF can be calculated by the Fourier transform.

$$OTF = FT\left[PSF\right]/FT\left[PSF\right]|_{\text{zero frequency}} \tag{14.24}$$

FT denotes Fourier transform, $FT\left[PSF\right]|_{\text{zero frequency}}$ represents the zero frequency components of the Fourier transform of the PSF. The MTF can be calculated by

$$MTF = \left|FT\left[PSF\right]/FT\left[PSF\right]_{\text{zero frequency}}\right| \tag{14.25}$$

These metrics are not only used for assessing the image quality of the human eye but also for estimating the performance of the ophthalmic imaging system. The wavefront aberration is the fundamental factor; once $W(r,\theta)$ is measured, the PSF and OTF can then be calculated. For this reason, the most commonly used metric for evaluation of the performance of the AOSLO is the RMS of the wavefront aberration.

14.5.2 The spatial property of human ocular wavefront aberrations

The optical aberrations of the eye vary greatly from person to person and are influenced by many parameters, such as pupil size, age, etc. For direct relevance to AO compensation for the ocular aberration, we summarize the results of two independent studies that were completed by the University of Rochester and Indiana University. These studies provided statistical distribution of Zernike components in the living human eye.

Porter et al. (University of Rochester) measured 109 subjects through a 5.7 mm pupil with a Shack-Hartmann wavefront sensor [75]. This study demonstrated that the majority of the power lies within the low order modes: the defocus and astigmatism, i.e., Z_2^0, Z_2^{-2}, Z_2^2, which account for over 92% of the total wavefront aberrations. For high-order ($n\ ge3$) aberrations, the means of Zernike modes, except for spherical aberration, are approximately zero and have a large inter-subject variability. The magnitudes of the higher-order aberrations reduce with increasing order. Another important result of this study is that it proved that Zernike polynomials were efficient basis functions for representing the wavefront aberration of the human eye. Further, this study predicted that a Strehl ratio greater than 0.8 could be achieved in over 91% of the subjects by correcting 17 Zernike modes. Because most of the subjects were from a clinic at Bausch & Lomb who tended to be myopic, so the magnitude of the defocus coefficient is larger than that for a purely randomly selected, normal population.

Thibos et al. (Indiana University) investigated 200 eyes from 100 subjects [76]. This population was relatively young; the age range was 22–35 years. The results of this study proved again that the majority of the power lies within the low order modes; the average amount of higher order aberrations present for a 7.5 mm pupil was equivalent to the wave-front error produced by less than 0.25 D of defocus. More importantly, this study demonstrated that the ocular wavefront aberration increases with increasing pupil size, as shown by Figure 14.6 (b).

These two population studies have important implications for AO compensation of the wavefront aberration in the living human eye. As will be discussed later, Doble et al. derived the peak to valley (P-V) wavefront aberrations against pupil size from the two studies and predicted the stroke (the maximum actuation distance of the actuator in the deformable mirror) requirement of the deformable mirror [23, 77, 78].

14.5.3 The temporal property of human ocular wavefront aberration

Due to continuous eye movement, micro-fluctuations of accommodation, and tear film thickness changes over the cornea, the optical wavefront aberration of the human eye is not static but varies

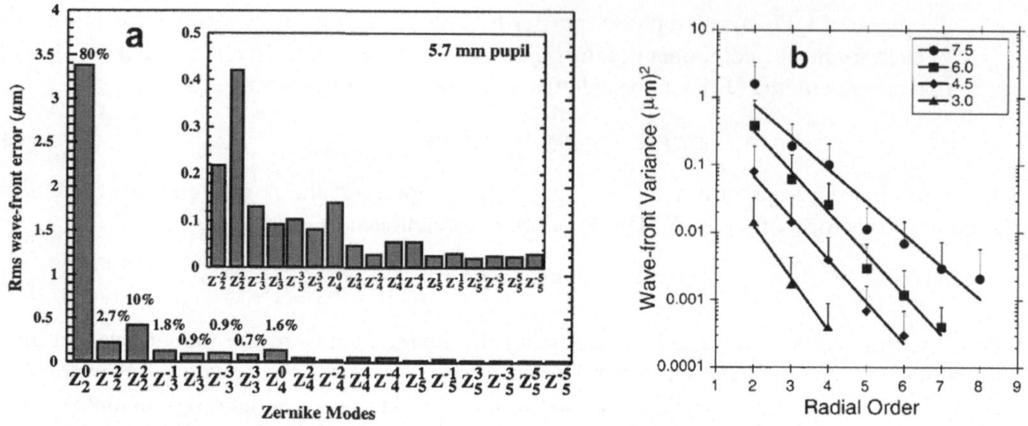

Figure 14.6: (a) The wavefront aberration decomposed into Zernike polynomials for a large human population over a 5.7-mm pupil [75]. The majority of the aberration power is found in the low order modes, i.e., defocus. The percentages above the first eight modes indicate the percentage of the total wavefront variance. (b) Variation of wavefront variance with radial order of Zernike modes for different pupil diameters [76]. Symbols indicate mean values and error bars indicate standard deviation of the population. Data sets are parameterized by pupil diameter, which was varied by applying the appropriately scaled mask to the array of centroids before computing Zernike coefficients. Data from left and right eyes are pooled ($N = 140$ for pupil diameter 7.5 mm; $N = 200$ for other pupil diameters). Regression lines on semi-log coordinates indicate exponential decline. Reproduced with permission from the Optical Society of America (OSA).

over time. With a real time Shack-Hartmann wavefront sensor, Hofer et al. measured the temporal dynamics of the human eye's aberrations [59]. They observed that all Zernike modes of the ocular wavefront aberration exhibited temporal instability and shared similar spectra and bandwidths both within and between subjects. Although the power of the wavefront aberration can be measured within a spectral range up to 5–6 Hz, beyond 1–2 Hz the power density becomes too small to significantly impact image quality. Thus, they suggested that an AO system with a closed-loop bandwidth 1–2 Hz could achieve diffraction-limited imaging in the human eye with a pupil size of 5.8 mm. Indeed, this assertion has been proved true by later research, e.g., an AO system that is operated at a closed-loop bandwidth of several hertz can reduce the RMS wavefront aberration to less than 0.1 μm (over the spectral region 500–840 nm) in most cases, which has been evidenced by later publications. However, Diaz-Santana et al. [79] later suggested that ocular aberrations could present dynamic behavior faster than 30 Hz and thus demand even faster AO correction. While the precise bandwidth of the temporal variation of the ocular wavefront aberration remains to be further determined, it is obvious that high-speed AO is desirable, particularly when it is used in clinical imaging applications. (We would prompt readers not to mistake the term "closed-loop bandwidth" with a similar term "closed-loop frequency or refreshing frequency." Practically, to achieve a closed-loop bandwidth of 1–2 Hz, the closed-loop refreshing frequency should be 3–10 times of the closed-loop bandwidth. Hence, most current ophthalmic AO systems are operated with a closed-loop refreshing frequency of 10–30 Hz.)

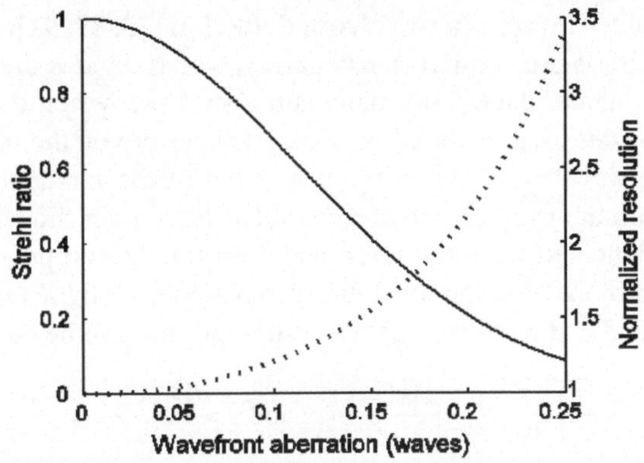

Figure 14.7: The solid curve demonstrates the Strehl ratio as a function of RMS wave aberration, while the dashed curve shows the normalized lateral resolution varying with the RMS wave aberration. Reproduced with permission from [80].

14.6 Adaptive Optics for the Human Eye

AO was originally developed to facilitate diffraction-limited astronomical imaging by compensating for time-varying wavefront aberrations induced by the atmosphere. A classical AO system consists of a wavefront sensor (WFS) and a wavefront corrector that measures and compensates for the wavefront aberration in real time. Normally, AO implies a dynamic control system, which is often operated with a closed-loop feedback scheme.

The first successful AO system for the human eye was demonstrated by Liang et al. [12], which consisted of a Shack-Hartman WFS and a deformable mirror (DM) wavefront corrector. For the first time, they demonstrated the ability to compensate for high-order aberrations in the living human eye and achieved unprecedented spatial resolution; the retinal image revealed individual foveal cone photoreceptors. In an ophthalmic AO system, the dynamic compensation has dual significance: first, AO corrects for the aberrations that vary from person to person; second, AO compensates for the time-varying wavefront aberrations in individual eye. Figure 14.7 illustrates the lateral resolution improved by AO compensation for the wavefront aberration [80]. AO has been proved to be an indispensable mechanism for high quality ophthalmic optical imaging, and has been implemented in various retinal imaging modalities, e.g., flood illumination fundoscopy [12, 54, 60], AOSLO [1, 81–83], and AO-OCT [84–88]. In this section, we will discuss the key components, namely, wavefront detection and correction, specifically for ophthalmic AO systems. Interested readers are also referred to extensive treatment on how an AO system works in general [89], or specifically for vision applications [23].

14.6.1 Wavefront detection

Although there are various techniques for measuring the wavefront [90], the most commonly employed wavefront sensor for ophthalmic AO is a Shack-Hartmann wavefront sensor (SHWS), which provides objective measurement of the wavefront aberration with high speed, making it possible for AO to correct ocular wavefront aberration in real time. The SHWS has become a standard device for diagnosing the ocular wavefront aberration in optometry and ophthalmology. Here we summarize the basic principle of Shack-Hartmann wavefront detection and provide a description of the practical procedures for building a SHWS.

The principle of Shack-Hartmann wavefront detection [23, 89, 91]. As depicted in Figure 14.8, the key element of a SHWS is a micro-lenslet array, which divides the optical aperture of the pupil plane, or a pupil conjugate plane, into many sub-apertures. When the incident light wavefront is perfectly flat, each lenslet focuses the light within its aperture on the focal plane, forming reference positions for the flat wavefront. When the wavefront of the incident light is aberrated, the local wavefront within a sub-aperture can be considered as tilted over the lenslet, thus the focus position of the light will be deflected from the reference position. Decomposing the deflection into X and Y directions, denoted by Δx, Δy, the local wavefront slopes along X and Y directions, or the partial differential along X and Y direction, within the sub-aperture can be calculated by

$$\frac{\partial W(x,y)}{\partial x} = \frac{\Delta x(x,y)}{f} \quad \text{and} \quad \frac{\partial W(x,y)}{\partial y} = \frac{\Delta y(x,y)}{f}$$

Where f is the focal length of the lenslet. Expanding the wavefront aberration into Zernike polynomials,

$$W(x,y) = \sum_{j}^{J} a_j Z_j(x,y)$$

The X and Y slopes within the sub-aperture can be expressed as

$$\frac{\partial W(x,y)}{\partial x} = \sum_{j}^{J} a_j \frac{\partial Z_j(x,y)}{\partial x} \quad \text{and} \quad \frac{\partial W(x,y)}{\partial y} = \sum_{j}^{J} a_j \frac{\partial Z_j(x,y)}{\partial y}.$$

Substituting partial derivatives with the local slopes,

$$\frac{\Delta x(x,y)}{f} = \sum_{j}^{J} a_j \frac{\partial Z_j(x,y)}{\partial x} \quad \text{and} \quad \frac{\Delta y(x,y)}{f} = \sum_{j}^{J} a_j \frac{\partial Z_j(x,y)}{\partial y}.$$

Assuming there are N sub-apertures,

$$\begin{bmatrix} \frac{\Delta x(x_1,y_1)}{f} \\ \vdots \\ \frac{\Delta x(x_N,y_N)}{f} \\ \frac{\Delta y(x_1,y_1)}{f} \\ \vdots \\ \frac{\Delta y(x_N,y_N)}{f} \end{bmatrix} = \begin{bmatrix} \frac{\partial Z_3(x_1,y_1)}{\partial x}, \cdots\cdots & \frac{\partial Z_J(x_1,y_1)}{\partial x} \\ \cdots\cdots\cdots\cdots & \cdots\cdots\cdots\cdots \\ \frac{\partial Z_3(x_N,y_N)}{\partial x}, \cdots\cdots & \frac{\partial Z_J(x_N,y_N)}{\partial x} \\ \frac{\partial Z_3(x_1,y_1)}{\partial y}, \cdots\cdots & \frac{\partial Z_J(x_1,y_1)}{\partial y} \\ \cdots\cdots\cdots\cdots & \cdots\cdots\cdots\cdots \\ \frac{\partial Z_3(x_N,y_N)}{\partial y}, \cdots\cdots & \frac{\partial Z_J(x_N,y_N)}{\partial y} \end{bmatrix} \begin{bmatrix} a_3 \\ a_4 \\ \vdots \\ \vdots \\ a_J \end{bmatrix}. \tag{14.26}$$

Hence, the coefficients of Zernike polynomials of the wavefront aberration can be solved from Eq. (14.26). Normally this equation is over-determined. An approximate solution can be obtained by singular value decomposition (SVD) or least-square fitting method. Interested readers are referred to the available references [23, 71, 89].

Practical procedure of building a Shack-Hartmann wavefront sensor

Selecting a lenslet array: A suitable lenslet array is determined by the pupil size, the desired dynamic range, and the desired sensitivity of the wavefront measurement. Yoon [23] estimated that, in general, the number of lenslets used for measuring the wavefront aberration should not be less than the number of Zernike modes to be determined; e.g., for a 6-mm pupil, with a lenslet array whose pitch size is 0.3 mm, there will be 277 lenslets across the pupil; thus, a maximum 277 Zernike modes (up to 22nd order) could be determined. However, in practice, to ensure more accurate measurement of high order aberrations, more lenslets are adopted. Detailed discussion can be found in references [23].

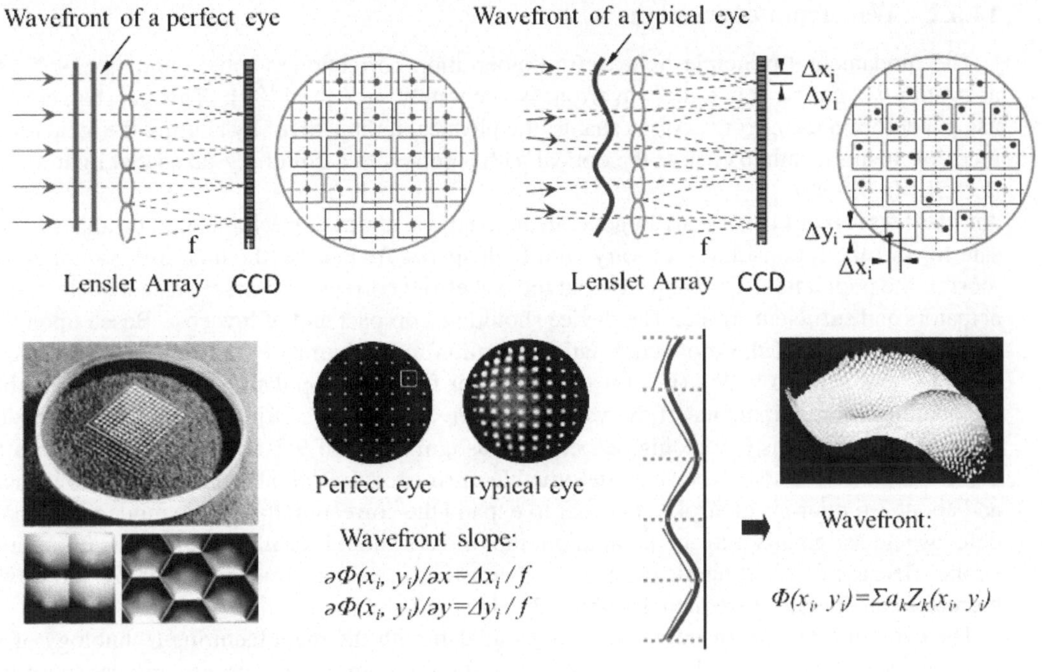

Figure 14.8: Shack-Hartmann wavefront detection.

Selecting a camera: The camera should provide good spectral response over a broad spectral range and high frame rates. In general, a CCD camera has better spectral responsivity in the visible light region (450–650 nm). Recently developed CMOS cameras have demonstrated better spectral responsivity in near infrared region. As discussed in the previous section, to compensate the dynamic variation of the ocular wavefront aberration, depending on the light budget, the wavefront sensor in the AOSLO system should be able to be operating with frame rates greater than 10 Hz.

Calibration of the SHWS: The classic method for calibrating the SHWS should be interferometry [90]. Here we describe a simple way to calibrate the wavefront sensor. First, the wavefront sensor is illuminated by a well collimated beam, the focus spots of each sub-aperture is minimized by adjusting the position of the lenslet array relative to the camera chip; then, a point source is placed at a different distance to the wavefront sensor, thereby generating a testing wavefront with various powers. Measuring the distance, thereby calculating the power and comparing this measured result with the wavefront sensor measurement, the system error can be examined. The system error can be minimized by carefully adjusting the position of the lenslet array. Because the power of the testing wavefront is inversely proportional to the distance, the measurement error is inversely proportional to the square of the distance; thus, this method is insensitive to the measurement error of the distance. For example, assuming that the distance between the point source and the wavefront sensor is 2 meters but the measurement is 2.002 meters, i.e., there is a measurement error of 2 mm, which results in a measurement error of $0.002/2^2 = 0.0005$ (diopter). Obviously this is not a rigorous calibration method, as it can only generate a testing wavefront of a single Zernike mode, and the wavefront is diverging. However, this method has proven to be very useful and fairly accurate, particularly during the development of the SHWS.

14.6.2 Wavefront correction

The fundamental principle of wavefront aberration correction is 'phase conjugation," i.e., the aberration is "nulled" once the wavefront is accurately measured [89]. This can be achieved by using a deformable mirror (DM) to change the physical light path, or by altering the local refractive index of the light path to change the optical path length with a liquid crystal spatial light modulator (LC-SLM) [92–98].

An ideal wavefront corrector. In general, an ideal wavefront corrector should be able to compensate for the aberrations that may vary with high spatial frequency (the high order aberrations) for most of the population. This requires that the wavefront corrector possesses an adequate number of actuators and sufficient stroke. The device should be compact and of low cost. Based upon the two population studies of the monochromatic aberration in the human eye, Doble and Miller derived the statistical peak to valley (P-V) wavefront error for large populations, and thereby established the quantitative requirements of the wavefront corrector [23, 77, 78]. For example, correcting the high order aberrations (excluding defocus and astigmatism) of 95% of typical eyes over a 6 mm pupil using a continuous face sheet deformable mirror requires about 100 actuators over the pupil and about 3-6 microns of stroke. In order to expand the correction to include moderate amounts of defocus and astigmatism in the population, the mirrors should ideally have at least 30 microns of stroke. Because of the dynamic changes in aberrations in the eye, it is important that the wavefront corrector can operate at frequencies above 30 Hz [77, 78].

The evolution of AO for human eyes is paralleled with the manufacturing technology of wavefront correctors. Dreher et al. used a 13-segment DM to compensate for the astigmatism of the eye [99]. Liang et al. [12] employed a mechanical DM (Xinetics, Andover, MA) which has a continuous mirror face sheet offering a 46 mm effective optical aperture that is fixed to an array of individually addressable lead zirconate-titanate (PZT) actuators with stroke up to 2 microns, to correct high order ocular aberrations. In 2001, Fernandez et al. reported a closed-loop dynamic AO retinal imaging system that was based upon a micromachined membrane deformable mirror (MMDM) with 37 actuators (OKO Technologies, Holland) [100], and Hofer et al. [60] built a closed-loop dynamic AO retinal imaging system with a 97-actuator Xinetics lead magnesium niobate (PMN) DM. The closed-loop AO effectively improved the imaging quality. The first AOSLO employed the Xinetics 37-actuator DM [1]. In order to map the human pupil to the effective aperture of the DM, relay telescopes with large magnification ratios had to be developed, thus leading to a large overall system structure. The cost of this type of DM is high, about $1500/actuator. Several inexpensive wavefront correctors such as membrane mirrors and bimorph mirrors were also employed. Fernandez et al. [100] and Hermann et al. [84] used 37-channel micromachined membrane DMs (OKO Technologies, Holland). These DM have large stroke but are limited in their ability to correct sufficiently high-order aberrations for the eye. While the great potential of AO compensation for the wavefront aberration in the living human eye was successfully demonstrated by use of early DMs, the drawbacks that limit wider applications of AO for vision science and clinical research were also revealed clearly.

In the late 1990s, advances in micro-electro-mechanical system (MEMS) technology paved the way to make compact DMs with densely packed actuators that could be operated with high speed, and potentially at lower cost through massive production. In 2002, Doble et al. [101] reported the first prototype MEMS DM (Boston Micromachines Co., Boston, MA) for AO in the human eye. This DM had 140 actuators fixed to a 4 mm optical face. Although the actuator stoke was only 1 micron, this MEMS DM demonstrated significant advantages in building a robust AO system. By 2005, Boston Micromachines (BMC) had pushed the MEMS DM from prototype to a real product [102, 103] that, to a reasonable degree, met the requirements for an effective AO system for vision applications [23, 76, 77]. Boosted by two Bioengineering Research Partnerships (BRP) that were supported by the National Institutes of Health [104], the MEMS DMs have been widely adopted in the development of the new generation AO retinal imaging systems including AOSLO [81–83,

105] and AO-OCT [86, 87]. However, to date the MEMS DM is still challenged by limited stroke, which currently is about 5.5 μm. Interestingly, mechanical DMs with discrete actuators recently re-emerged with significantly improved stroke and a more compact structure. For example, the mirao^{TM} 52-e electromagnetic DM (Imagine Eyes SA, France) has a mirror face of 15 mm driven by 52 actuators whose stroke can be up to 50 μm [106], and the high-speed DM97-15 (Alpao AS, France) has a mirror face of 13.5 mm driven by 97 actuators whose stroke can be up to 30 μm (3×3 actuators) [107–110]. These DMs demonstrate excellent ability to correct for the wide ranging aberrations found in eyes, though they don't have the ideal number of actuators.

On the other hand, the LC-SLMs have a high density of actuators, and also have been used in several applications [92–98, 111–114]. To compensate for wavefront aberrations greater than 2π (one wavelength), a technique called phase wrapping is needed. The major drawback of the LC-SLM is its inherent polarization dependence. Material dispersion and phase wrapping are two other LC properties that reduce SLM performance in polychromatic light or if there is a difference between the wave front sensing and imaging wavelengths. To date the LC-SLM can't match the performance of the discrete actuator DM.

In ophthalmic AO systems, a DM is preferred because it can provide excellent reflectance to avoid photon loss and it does not cause light dispersion, which is critical for retinal imaging systems that use broadband light.

Wavefront reconstruction and correction. Given the time-varying property of the human eye's wavefront aberration, it is clear that AO correction is a dynamic process and preferably operated with a feedback closed-loop. The wavefront measurement and compensation must be done in real time, and the system must be robust and stable. For detailed treatment of general theory and modeling of AO control, readers are referred to references [23, 89].

The key to closed-loop AO correction is wavefront reconstruction, a process to derive the commands for each actuator from the slopes of the wavefront aberration measured by the Shack-Hartmann wavefront sensor. In early AO systems, the wavefront measured by the SHWS was fitted to Zernike polynomials, from which the control commands of each actuator were calculated. This is called modal reconstruction. The advantage of this method is that the actuator commands can always be determined, even when the wavefront sensor fails to measure the wavefront slopes in some sub-apertures. The modal-based reconstruction from the wavefront slopes to the actuator commands is indirect. Boyer et al. [115] and Jiang et al. [116] proposed a direct method to obtain the actuator commands from the wavefront slopes. The rationale of this method is that the local wavefront shape (specifically, the slope) change can be considered as a linear superimposition of the actions of each actuator, i.e.,

$$S(x,y) = \sum_{m=1}^{M} h_m(x,y)c_m, \tag{14.27}$$

where $S(x,y)$ denotes wavefront slope along x, y directions over the sub-aperture x_i, y_i) measured by the SHWS, M is the number of actuators, c_m is the command (e.g., voltage or current that is applied to the actuator, m), $h_m(x,y)$ is the contribution of the actuator m to the slope over the sub-aperture (x_i,y_i).

Expressing $S = [S_{x1}, S_{x2}, ...S_{xN}, S_{y1}, S_{y2}, ...S_{yN}]^T$, S_{xi} and S_{yi} are x, y components of the wavefront slope over sub-aperture i respectively, T stands for transpose. Denoting the command vector of the actuators $C = [C_1, C_2, ...C_M]^T$, M is the number of actuators, Eq. (14.26) can be written as

$$S = HC. \tag{14.28}$$

H is the actuator-wavefront interaction (or influence) matrix, it can be tested by measuring the response of the wavefront slopes (over each sub-aperture of the SHWS) to the action of each individual actuator driven by unit command. H has a dimension of $(2N \times M)$.

Assuming S_m is column matrix of the wavefront slopes measured by the SHWS, the commands to the actuators can be obtained by $C = RS$; R is the wavefront reconstructor, which, in many cases, may be a truncated inversed interaction matrix H^{-1} obtained via the singular value decomposition (SVD) algorithm, in which small singular values of H are simply discarded to avoid saturating the actuators, or system divergence. A more elegant reconstructor may be obtained by adding a constant regularization factor α to all the singular values instead of dropping the small singular values [117], i.e.,

$$R = -(H^T H + \alpha^2 I)^{-1} H^T, \tag{14.29}$$

where I is the $M \times M$ identity matrix, α is the noise to signal ratio of the system and may be experimentally determined. More sophisticated reconstructors such as local waffle penalty, Kolmogorov penalty, and Zernike modal reconstruction have been reported to improve the AO performance in the human eye [117]. Once the reconstructor is determined, the AO loop may be closed with an integral controller,

$$C[t] = C[t-1] + GRS_m, \tag{14.30}$$

where $C[t]$ is the command to the DM at time t, and G is the loop gain, which can be theoretically estimated and experimentally optimized.

Woofer-Tweeter scheme. As described earlier, current mechanical DMs lack adequate numbers of actuators for correct for high order aberration, whereas the MEMS DMs lack the necessary stroke to compensate aberrations of large dynamic range that mainly manifest in low orders; thus, a single DM could be inefficient to achieve diffraction-limited imaging. To cope with this problem, a "woofer-tweeter" scheme consisting of two DMs was developed, in which a large stroke DM with fewer actuators provides low order correction and a small stroke DM with more actuators (usually a MEMS DM) provides high order correction [82, 87, 118–123]. The two DMs may be operated either successively or simultaneously. In the successive mode, the "woofer" DM is first applied to minimize the low order aberrations, then the "tweeter" DM takes over to compensate for the residual high-order aberrations [82, 87]; whereas in the simultaneous mode, the wavefront aberration is distributed or partitioned to the "woofer" and the "tweeter," which work simultaneously to compensate for the aberration [118–123].

14.7 AOSLO Development

14.7.1 Optical system

Raster scanning. Shown in Figure 14.9 is a basic configuration of the AOSLO. The light from a laser is usually coupled into a single mode optical fiber. The light emitted from the tip of the fiber output forms a point source, which is collimated and relayed by the telescope and the beam splitter (BS) to the DM, the horizontal scanner (HS) which is usually a resonant scanner operating at 8–16 KHz (the line rate), the vertical scanner (VS) which is usually a galvo scanner operating at 15–30 Hz (the frame rate), finally to the eye, forming a raster scan on the retina. The diffusely reflected light from the retina transmits inversely along the ingoing path to the beam splitter, where most of the light passes through and is relayed by a telescope to the collection lens. A confocal pinhole is placed at the focal point of the collection lens, and the signal is received by the photo-detector, most likely a photomultiplier tube (PMT) or an avalanche photodiode (APD), further processed, and acquired by the computer for storage and display.

Optical conjugation relationships. The DM, the lenslet array of the Shack-Hartmann wavefront sensor, the HS, VS and the collection lens are aligned so that they are all conjugate to the entrance pupil of the eye. The center of the pupil plane should be the pivot point of the scanning beam. To ensure the wavefront at the pupil plane will be precisely relayed to the DM, relay telescopes must be

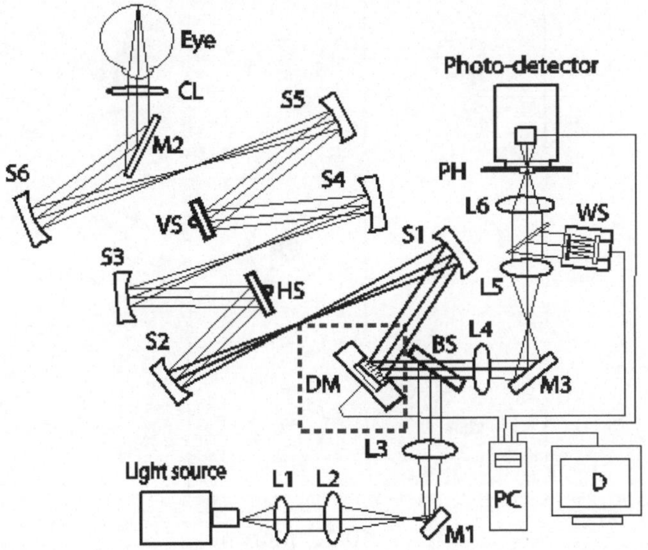

Figure 14.9: PC, computer; D: display; BS: beam splitter; HS: horizontal scanner, VS: vertical scanner. In this configuration, the DM is placed at a pupil conjugate plane that is away from the eye.

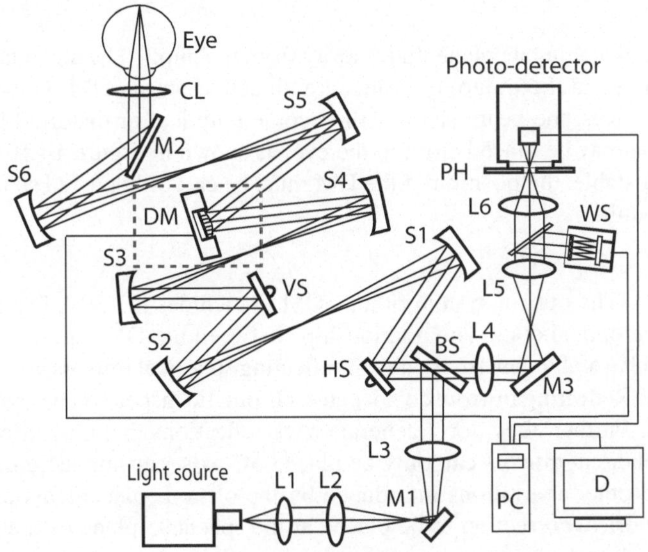

Figure 14.10: The DM is placed at a pupil conjugate plane that is close to the eye.

used between the HS, the VS, the DM, and the pupil plane. It is critical to carefully design the relay optics to ensure these conjugation relationships and to ensure the beam will enter the eye without being clipped by the pupil. This can be achieved by optimizing the positions of the HS and the VS.

DM position. An important feature of the AOSLO is that the AO corrects for the wavefront aberration in both the ingoing light path (for a sharp focus on the retina) and the outgoing light path (for a sharp image of the focused spot on the confocal pinhole). As shown in Figure 14.9, the DM may

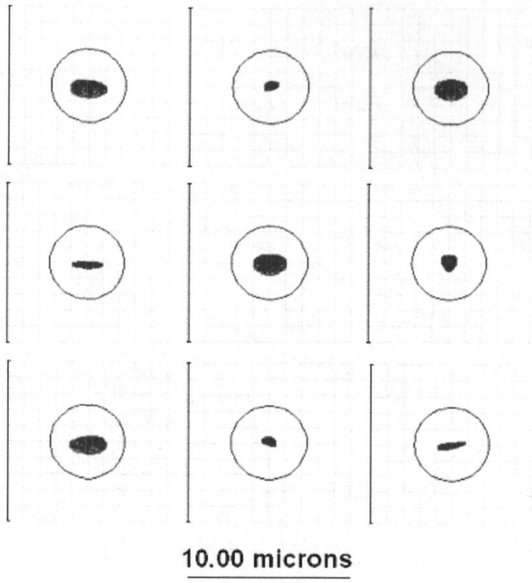

Figure 14.11: Geometric spot diagrams of the scanning optical system at 9 points over its 3 degree scanning field. The circles are Airy disks.

be placed at a pupil conjugate plane that is away from the pupil. The advantage of this configuration is that the ingoing and the outgoing beams are all stable on the DM. However, when the eye has large refractive errors, the beam shape will become elliptical or distorted [87]. To overcome this problem, the DM may be placed close to the eye, as shown in Figure 14.10. Now that beam on the DM is no longer stable, the position of the DM must be carefully placed so that the DM is precisely imaged on the pupil.

Optical layout. The optical system of an AOSLO includes the DM, fast and slow scanners, and relay optics. The optical conjugate relationships between the DM and the scanners are formed by relay optics which usually consist of pairs of reflecting spherical mirrors arranged in the format of an afocal telescope. Reflecting mirrors do not cause chromatic dispersion which allow for imaging with broadband light. Further, they don't generate back reflections that may affect wavefront detection. However, the spherical mirrors can only be placed off-axis, causing astigmatism. To eliminate the astigmatism and other aberrations introduced by the off-axis placements of the mirrors, one may allow for a cylindrical correction to be placed at the spectacle plane of the eye and then minimize the remaining high-order system aberrations by optimizing the system design [1, 81–83, 87, 105]. In this way, all components are placed in a plane. An alternative design is to fold the optical system [107, 124–126], i.e., minimizing the astigmatism and other system aberrations by tilting the mirrors within each telescope in orthogonal directions. This has become a popular configuration in recent AOSLO optical designs.

14.7.2 Optimal pinhole size

AO enables diffraction-limited confocal imaging, forming a compact light spot, i.e., Airy disk, on the focal plane of the collection lens, allowing a small pinhole to be used. However, to achieve the theoretical lateral resolution of the confocal imaging, the ideal pinhole size, in the normalized optical coordinate v, should be less than 0.5, which is much smaller than the Airy disk ($v = 3.83$)

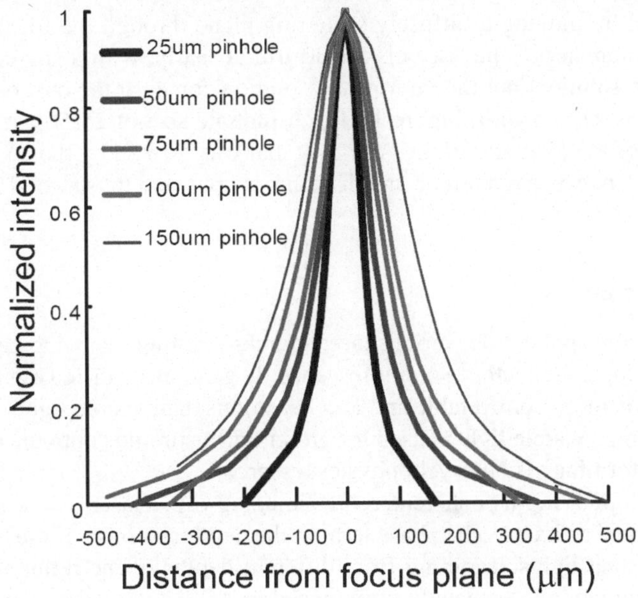

Figure 14.12: The measured axial intensity distribution through focus with pinholes of different diameters. Reproduced with permission from the SPIE.

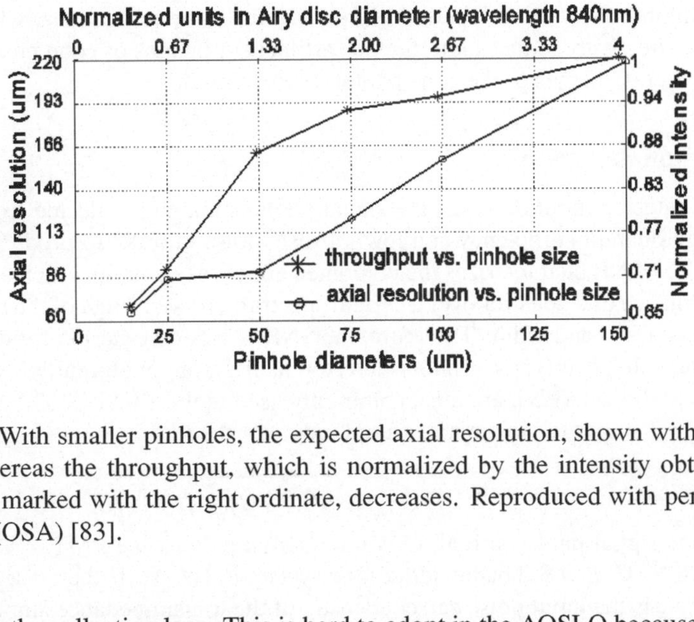

Figure 14.13: With smaller pinholes, the expected axial resolution, shown with the left ordinate, is improved, whereas the throughput, which is normalized by the intensity obtained by the 150 μm pinhole and marked with the right ordinate, decreases. Reproduced with permission from the Optical Society (OSA) [83].

that is formed by the collection lens. This is hard to adopt in the AOSLO because the signal would be too weak to produce an image with sufficient SNR. Therefore, the optimal pinhole size is always a trade-off between resolution and SNR. In practice, an optimal size of the pinhole is near the size of the Airy disk formed by the collection lens, ensuring most of the photons from the retina are collected (Fig. 14.11). With a pinhole of this size, on one hand, the AOSLO is unable to take advantage of enhanced lateral resolution of the confocal mechanism; on the other hand, the depth discrimination ability of the AOSLO is much more forgiving to the enlarged pinhole, a satisfactory axial sectioning performance is still attainable [10, 11, 62, 64, 70, 80, 127]. Figure 14.12 plots an experimental test of the improvement of the axial resolution with the decrease of the pinhole size as measured by moving a diffusely scattering plane through the focal plane of a model eye. In this test, the diameter of the Airy disk is 30 μm. Clearly, with a smaller pinhole, the AOSLO has better axial resolution, but the improved resolution comes at the cost of reduced throughout of the signal photons, as shown in Figure 14.13. A pinhole size of 25-50 μm, which corresponds to 0.74-1.48 times of the diameter of the Airy disk that was formed by the collection lens, could be a good compromise between resolution and light throughput, and thus a good imaging signal-to-noise ratio.

14.7.3 Light sources

Depending on the application, various laser sources emitting visible to near infrared light can be adopted for imaging by reflectance or fluorescence. In general, infra-red light has deeper penetration in the retina and is more comfortable and less hazardous than visible light, and thus is mostly used for clinical imaging. Visible light is used for presenting a stimulus onto the retina for testing retinal function and performing visual psychophysics research.

Because laser light is highly coherent, retinal imaging with a laser will be inevitably accompanied by light interference artifacts. The phase term in the depth response of the SLO [Eq.(14.7) and Eq. (14.8)] indicates that lights scattering from different depths of the retina will interfere with each other. This phenomenon is especially pronounced in AOSLO imaging, which produces images in a small field of view with high magnification. The interference artifact can remarkably degrade the fidelity of the retinal image, as shown in Figure 14.14. To mitigate this problem, low coherent light sources such as superluminescent laser diodes (SLD) are preferable [83, 128, 129]. Figure 14.14 shows images taken with an 840 nm infra-red highly coherent laser light (the left panel) and a SLD (Broadlighter S840-HP, Superlum, Russia) at the same retinal area. Clearly, the use of low-coherent light effectively reduces interference artifacts in images of cone photoreceptors, allowing much higher fidelity images of the cone photoreceptor mosaic.

14.7.4 Photon detection

The photo-detector should convert the signal photons that are collected from the retina to electrons with high quantum efficiency and low intrinsic noise in order to produce a video signal with a good SNR. The SNR characterizes the combined effects of quantum efficiency and noise, i.e., the overall performance of a detector over a certain spectrum, power range of the signal light and a specific imaging system bandwidth. Therefore, the SNR is a good criterion for deciding on a suitable detector. Technically, two types of photo-detector, namely, the photomultiplier tube (PMT) and the avalanche photo diode (APD), are most commonly used in the AOSLO. The SNR is defined as the ratio of the signal amplitude to the noise amplitude. For the PMT,

$$SNR = I_P G / \sqrt{2eBG^2 N_F (I_P + I_D) + i_a^2 B}, \tag{14.31}$$

where, I_P is the signal photo current, G is the internal gain of the PMT, e is the electron charge, $e = 1.602 \times 10^{-19}$ C, B is the bandwidth of the system in Hz, N_F is the noise figure, I_D is the dark photo current, i_{in} is the input noise current density of the transimpedance amplifier in A/Hz$^{1/2}$.
The APD's internal photon multiplication mechanism is different from that of the PMT. For the APD

$$SNR = I_P G / \sqrt{2eBG^2 F (I_P + I_{DG}) + 2eBI_{DS} + i_a^2 B}, \tag{14.32}$$

where I_{DS} is the surface leakage dark current, which flows through the interface between the PN junction and the Si oxide layer and does not flow through the avalanche region and thus is not multiplied. I_{DG} is the internal dark current which is generated inside the Si substrate and flows in the avalanche region so it is multiplied with the gain factor G of the APD. F is the excess noise figure, which is determined by the APD gain and the excess noise index of the detector's material.

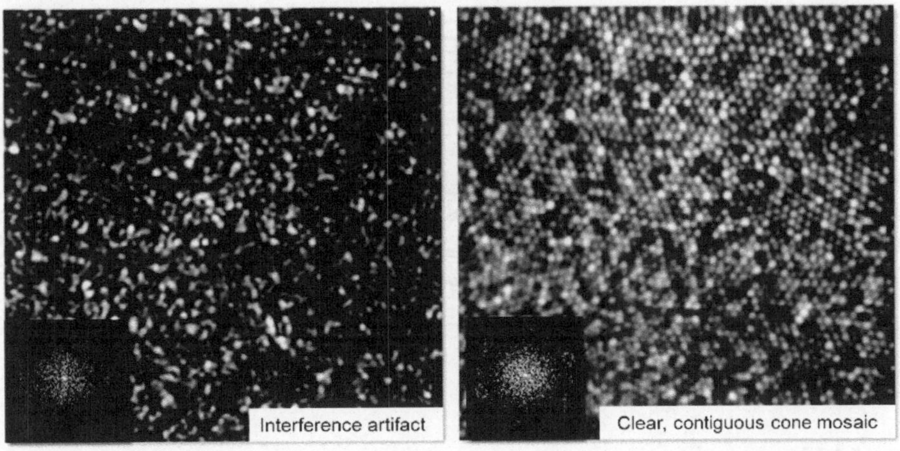

Figure 14.14: Two retinal images of the same retinal areas in a healthy eye. Images were taken from a location 0.50 degrees nasal from the fovea. The field of view subtends 0.8 degrees, or approximately 240 μm on a side. Both images are a registered sum of 20 frames from a single video. The left image is taken with a coherent 840 nm light and the right is taken with low-coherence 840 nm light. All the images were taken with the same illumination power level and the same settings of the AOSLO imaging system. The low-coherence image taken with the SLD reveals more of the contiguous closely packed cone photoreceptor array and the spatial spectrum (Fourier transform) of the image (lower left inset) reveals a better defined hexagonal pattern corresponding to foveal cone mosaic.

As a heuristic estimation, the bandwidth of the AOSLO video signal is

$$B \approx \alpha(300/r_d)f_l/t_d, \tag{14.33}$$

where α is the scanning angle in degrees, r_d is the lateral resolution in μm, f_l is the line scanning frequency in Hz, and the t_d is the duty cycle of the valid video signal, which is normally the most linear region of the sinusoidal scanning path during which time the imaging data acquisition system records the image.

The light power reaching the photo detector is estimated in a range over 0.01 to 10 nano-watts (nW). This light level was tested in a healthy human eye with an AOSLO.

Figure 14.15 gives an example of the SNRs calculated from commercially available photo detectors including 4 PMTs and 3 APDs from Hamamatsu Corporation (Hamamatsu Corporation, Japan) and PerkinElmer (PerkinElmer, Waltham, MA). A transimpedance amplifier C6438-01 (Hamamatsu Corporation, Japan) was used in the computation.

Other PMT modules such as the H7422-40 (Hamamatsu Corporation, Japan) have better quantum efficiency, but its maximum output signal current at the anodes is rated at only 2 μA, which converts to a permissible illumination on the cathode of 0.011 nW. This is far below the normal AOSLO power range. Exposures beyond this permissible level do not necessarily burn down the anode (even after long exposure times) but can damage the photocathode. Nevertheless, the H7422-40 PMT module is an attractive detector for imaging situations where the returning light is very low. Low light situations include confocal imaging of the weakest scattering layers in the inner retina, such as the ganglion cells or autofluorescence imaging.

Over the estimated signal power and spectral ranges of the AOSLO, the PMT is more forgiving to the input noise of the transimpedance amplifier than the APD, but with a delicate design of a low noise transimpedance amplifier, the APD can be comparable for the AOSLO photo signal detection.

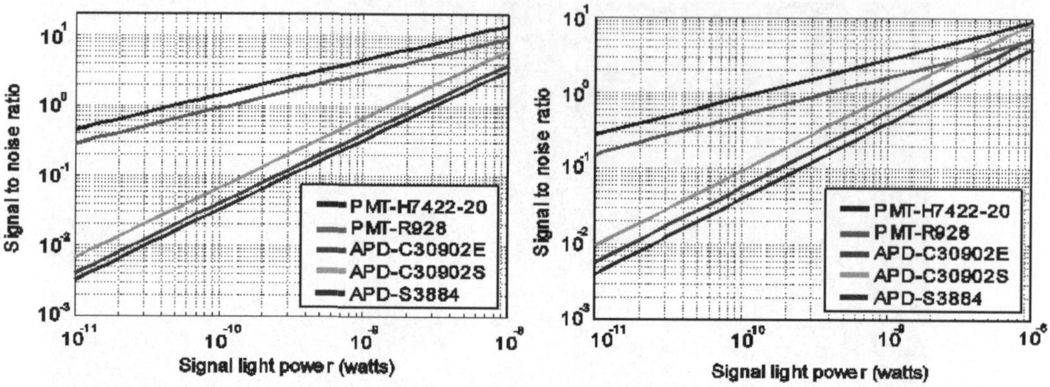

Figure 14.15: Calculated signal to noise ratio of photo-detectors. The left chart shows the SNRs that were calculated at 680 nm, whereas the right plots the SNRs that were calculated at 840 nm [130]. Reproduced with permission from the Optical Society of America.

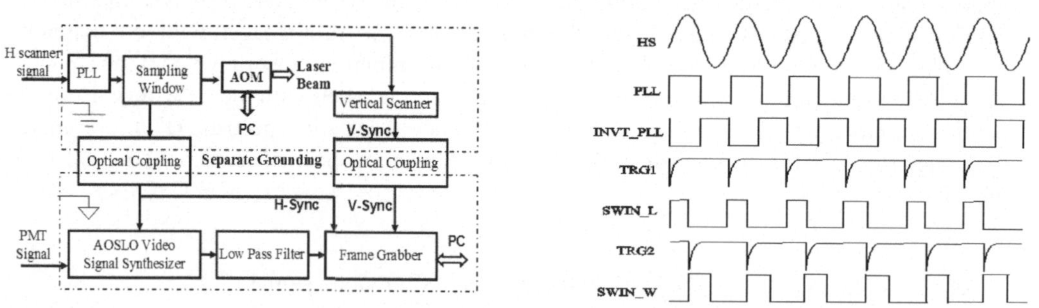

Figure 14.16: AOSLO imaging signal conditioning and timing.

14.7.5 Image signal conditioning and acquisition

Before being acquired by the computer, the analog signal generated by the photo-detector should be conditioned to a pseudo-video format so that the signal can be rendered as 2-D images. A frame grabber (imaging acquisition card) is normally used to record the video signal. The composite video signal contains the horizontal (line) and vertical (frame) synchronization signals (the Hsync and the Vsync), a DC-black level, and the active line signals. Figure 14.16 depicts a design example. A phase locked-loop (PLL) is designed to produce a square wave that is in phase with the sinusoidal line scanning signal, which generally serves as the master clock of the imaging system. A trigger signal TRG1 is derived from the falling edge of the inverted PLL output. With a proper delay from TRG1, a second trigger signal TRG2 is generated as the starting edge of the sampling window. A sampling window corresponding to the most linear part of the forward direction of the sinusoidal scanning path of the horizontal scanner, which comprises about 40% of one cycle of the horizontal scan, is formed and sent to the acousto-optical modulator (AOM) controller to modulate the laser beam such that the light is only projected on the retina within the sampling window and during the rest of the cycle there is no light on the retina. Within this window, the computer can also send a more sophisticated control signal to the AOM for phase and intensity modulation of the beam (discussed in Section 14.9). The sampling window signal is sent to the video signal synthesizer via an optical coupler. The PLL signal is also sent to the vertical scanner driver which gives the vertical (frame) synchronization signal. V-Sync is sent to the frame grabber via an optical coupler. Separate grounding is designed to prevent the video signal from being affected by the noisy PLL circuit and the AOM as well as the vertical scanner driver modules. Normally images are acquired and stored uncompressed in a digital format.

14.7.6 Laser safety

The American Standards for the Safe Use of Lasers (ANSI Z136.1-2010) specifies the maximum permissible exposure (MPE) levels to protect persons from hazardous exposures to lasers in various application fields with an emphasis on exposures of the eye. The MPE values are specified by the light wavelength, the eye condition and the scanning field as well as the exposure time.

In the AOSLO, a focused laser spot is raster-scanned across the retina. Each point on the retina is exposed to a series of repeated focused laser pulses with a frequency that is equal to the frame rate of the system. Under this light regime, The ANSI Standard applies three "rules" that define the MPEs, yielding the highest protection is used. Rule 1: "The exposure from any single pulse in a train of pulses shall not exceed the MPE for a single pulse of that pulse duration." Rule 2: "Average power MPE for thermal and photochemical hazards. The [total] exposure from any group of pulses delivered in time T shall not exceed the MPE for time T." Rule 3: "Multiple pulse MPE for thermal hazards. The exposure for any single pulse within a group of pulses ... shall not exceed the single pulse MPE multiplied by a multiple-pulse correction factor C, which is $n^{-0.25}$, where n is the total number of pulses." As a guideline, ANSI Z 136.1-2000 suggests: "... it is good practice to maintain exposure levels as far below the MPE as is possible." [25] Normally, we take a value that is at least 10 times lower than the ANSI MPE as the AOSLO MPE.

14.8 AOSLO Image Processing

Image processing is an important component of the AOSLO. Because the AOSLO imaging is limited by safe limit of light exposure, the image SNR of a single frame may not be good enough for analysis; thus, co-adding a sequence of frames is required to generate a static image with improved SNR. This could be achieved by cross-correlation analysis of frame-to-frame shifts in the video frames. However, the distortion within a frame (as described earlier) caused by the high frequency motion prevents the successive frames from being precisely registered. Removing the distortions is an important step to render high-fidelity visualization of the retina. This can be done by dividing each AOSLO frame into a series of strips that are less affected from the eye motion artifacts and then calculating the shifts of each strip relative to the corresponding zone in the reference frame, as depicted in Figure 14.17. To be completely free from distortion, the ideal frame acquisition time should be less than 0.004 second [53, 54] , which, for an AOSLO with a line scanning rate of 16 KHz, corresponds to 64 lines; therefore, for a frame consisting of 512 lines, each frame should be divided into at least 8 strips.

Let $E(x)$ denote the reflectivity of point $X(t)$ of the AOSLO image, and τ denote the frame scan period. For an individual strip of the AOSLO image, assuming the retina drifts with constant velocity v, then,

$$E(X(t_i+\tau)) = E(X(t_i)+\tau v), \tag{14.34}$$

where t_i denotes discrete pixel recording times, v can be detected by cross-correlations. For a pair of discrete rectangular images E and E', the cross-correlation is

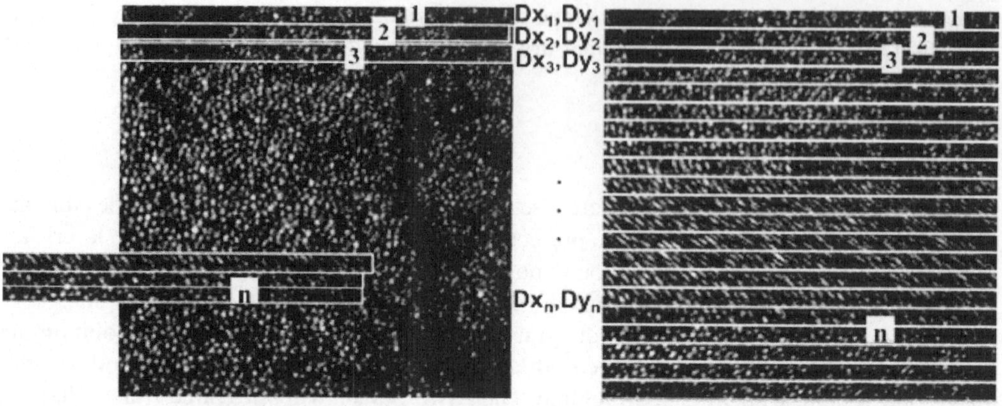

Figure 14.17: To conduct the cross-correlation, the AOSLO image are divided into stripes that are free of the distortion caused by the retinal motion.

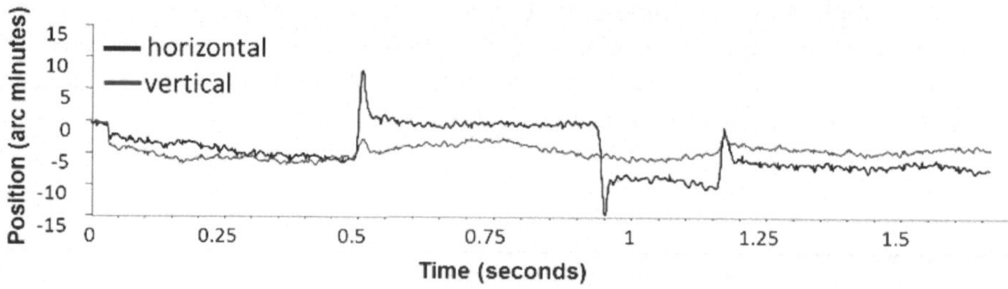

Figure 14.18: High-speed and high-precision measurement of the retinal movement.

$$\text{corr}(E,E')m,n = \sum_i \sum_j E(i+m, j+n)E'(i,j). \tag{14.35}$$

By finding the indices m, n, k, which maximize cross-correlation between consecutive pairs of discrete strips, one can obtain an estimate for the offset τv, and then extract the drift velocity v. The standard approach to cross-correlation of discrete images is the fast Fourier transform (FFT). Vogel et al. proposed a novel computational technique called the map-seeking circuit (MSC) algorithm [52], which has much lower computational complexity than Fourier approaches; hence it may allow real-time motion estimation. Once motion estimates are available, one can compensate for the motion-induced image distortions, i.e., “dewarping.” The distortion in the reference frame may be extracted by taking the average relative shift found for all other frames, assuming that the actual average shift is zero for a fixating eye, or by a weighting scheme that is based on linear interpolation.

A very useful by-product of great importance of the image registration is retinal motion traces that provide a high-speed and high-precision measurement of retinal movement, shown in Figure 14.18. Temporal measurement speed can be potentially up to 16 kHz if all scan lines in a frame are analyzed, and spatial precision can be a fraction of the size of a foveal cone photoreceptor. This ability enables important studies that require tracking the retinal motion, which will be presented later in this chapter.

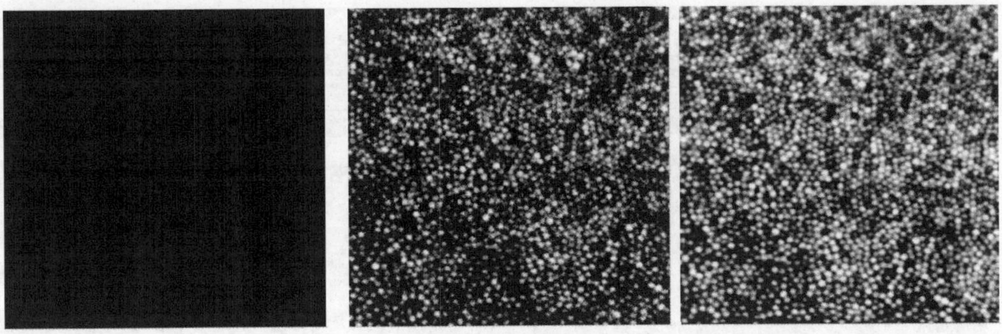

Figure 14.19: AOSLO images taken from a living human eye. The left panel is a single frame taken before AO correction but after best correction of defocus and astigmatism with trial lenses, whereas the middle panel is a single frame taken after AO correction. The right panel shows a registered set of 10 AO-corrected images. All images have been corrected for distortions due to eye movements. These images were taken from a retinal location about 1 degree from the center of the fovea. The field of view subtends 0.9 degrees, or approximately 270 μm on a side. The image was taken with a 840-nm SLD.

14.9 AOSLO Imaging Modes

14.9.1 Reflectance imaging

In this mode, the AOSLO utilizes direct reflecting light to form retinal images. Figure 14.19 demonstrates the threefold benefit brought by AO for retinal imaging: increased brightness, improved contrast, and enhanced lateral resolution. Figure 14.20 is a montage of retinal images, revealing small, tightly packed cones in the fovea; away from the foveal center, cones become larger in size, and rods appear in the peripheral retina. Both Figure 14.19 and Figure 14.20 were taken through a 5.5-mm pupil. The robustness of the AO is also demonstrated by its formation of a very compact focused spot at the confocal pinhole via the collection lens. This enables us to use smaller pinholes while maintaining a decent SNR for imaging, allowing the retina to be optically sectioned, as illustrated in Figure 14.21. Figure 14.22 shows images taken in a living macaque eye with the same AOSLO instrument. Because the macaque eye length is only about 2/3 of the length of the human eye, the numerical aperture of the macaque eye is 1.5 times greater than that of the human eye; thus, AOSLO images taken in the macaque eye show better resolution.

14.9.2 Fluorescence imaging

Fluorescence imaging may produce high contrast images of otherwise invisible cells in the retina and can be readily achieved by incorporating excitation light sources into the AOSLO. Researchers at the University of Rochester have demonstrated the fluorescence AOSLO imaging of the retinal pigment epithelial (RPE) cells and ganglion cells in the living non-human primate eye [105, 131] and living human eye [132]. To image the RPE cells, they excited the autofluorescence of the lipofuscin in the RPE cells with the light from a 568-nm Ar/Kr laser and recorded the fluorescence emission at 624 nm. Because the autofluorescence signal is extremely weak, many frames (up to 2000 frames) had to be averaged to improve the SNR of the image. However, a single autofluorescence image doesn't have enough contrast for image registration. To overcome this problem, they developed a dual simultaneous imaging and registration technique, in which they applied an

Figure 14.20: AOSLO retinal images taken in the eye of a human subject with healthy retina. All the image strips have a size of 2×0.25 degrees (width $\times$ height) in the human eye, corresponding to about $600\,\mu m \times 75\,\mu m$. From the top, (a) and (b) are images taken at the superior retina at the eccentricity of 2 degrees and 1 degree from the fovea center, respectively; (c) is an image that was taken across the fovea center, which is marked by the white cross; (d) and (e) are images taken at the inferior retina at an eccentricity of 1 degree and 2 degrees away from the fovea center, respectively. These images show well resolved and contiguous cone mosaics. These images also show photoreceptors ranging in size as a function of eccentricity from the fovea center. (f) and (g) are images that were taken along the equator of the retina temporally, the image locations (eccentricities) are marked at the edges of the images, whereas (h) is an image that was taken along the equator of the retina nasally. These images reveal that cones (the large spots) are surrounded by rods (small spots). The images were taken with the 840 nm SLD light source. All images are a registered set of 20 AO-corrected images and have been corrected for distortions due to eye movements.

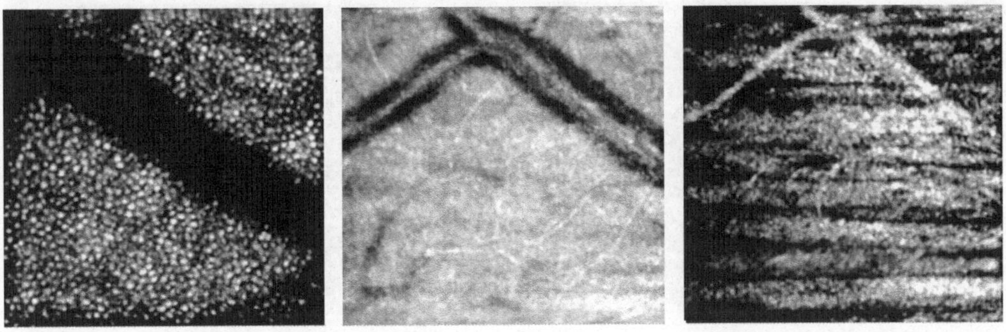

Figure 14.21: Optical sectioning of the retinal layers. In the left panel, the AOSLO was focused on the outer limiting membrane and shows the cone mosaic. The middle is an optical section of the inner retina, showing light scattered from the blood vessels. The right is an optical section with the focus on the surface of the retina, showing the striation of the nerve fiber bundles. The image is from a location about 2.7 degrees superior to the foveal center. These images were taken in a living human eye. All images have been corrected for distortions due to eye movements. The field of view subtends 0.9 degrees, or approximately 270 m on a side. The light source is a SLD whose wavelength is 840 nm.

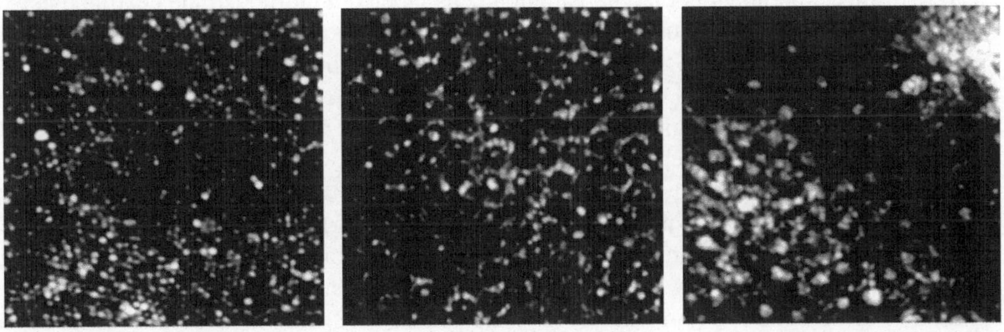

Figure 14.22: AOSLO images taken from a living macaque eye. The left image was taken at the foveal center (rod free zone), showing only the cone photoreceptor moasic; the middle image was taken at a location 6 degrees away from the foveal center nasally, revealing that cones (the large spots) are surrounded by rods (small spots); the right image was taken on the edge of the optic nerve head, approximately 12 degrees away from the foveal center; cones are further enlarged whereas the size of rods remain unchanged. All these images are a registered set of 20 AO-corrected images and have been corrected for distortions due to eye movements. The field of view subtends 0.45 degrees, or approximately 90 μm on a side. The eye was imaged with a 840 nm SLD.

830 nm superluminescent laser diode to scan the retina with the excitation light and recorded the reflectance and autofluorescence images simultaneously. They calculated the retinal motion through the reflectance images and then applied the motion correction for the simultaneously collected autofluorescence images. Figure 14.23 shows the RPE cells imaged in a living macaque eye. The RPE cell mosaic appears in a honeycomb pattern, where the cell nucleus is a dark spot surrounded by the fluorescent lipofuscin granules. With the same AOSLO system, they also imaged retinal ganglion cells in the living Macaca mulatta monkey eye. In these experiments, ganglion cell bodies and axons were labeled with retrograde transport of rhodamine dextran or Alexa 594 injected into the lateral geniculate nucleus (LGN). Rhodamine dye was excited with 530 nm light and the fluorescence was

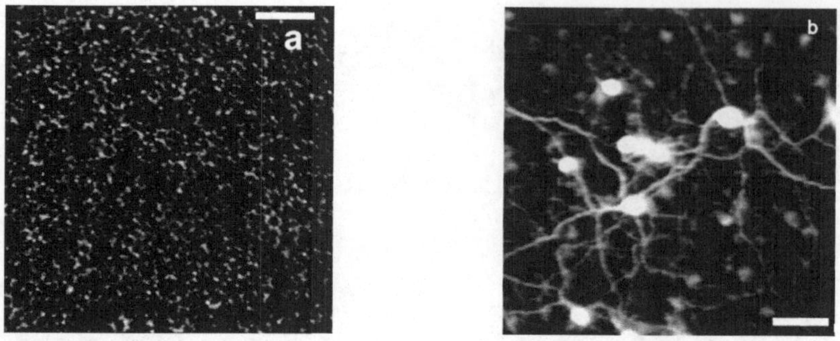

Figure 14.23: Fluorescence AOSLO imaging. The left panel shows an autofluorescence image that reveals the retinal pigment epithelium mosaic in the fovea of a macaque [105]. The right panel shows a fluorescence image of ganglion cells labeled with rhodamine dextran dye [131]. Ganglion cell bodies and their dendrites are resolved. Both images are averages of 1000 frames. For the RPE image, the scale bar is 75 μm; for the ganglion cell image, the scale bar is 50 μm. Adapted from [105, 131] with permission of OSA and IOVS.

imaged at 593 nm, while Alexa 594 dye was excited at 568 nm and imaged at 624 nm. An important feature of this experiment is that the ganglion cells labeled with rhodamine dextran dye exhibited substantially increased brightness when the retinal light exposure was increased by three times, a procedure called "photo filling," which effectively enhanced imaging of ganglion cell dendrites and axons.

Geng et al. reported imaging of the mouse eye [124, 133, 134] with a fluorescence AOSLO. In this study, an 843-nm laser diode (LD) was used as the wavefront sensing source. A 789-nm SLD with 11.5-nm bandwidth was used as the reflectance imaging light source. An air-cooled Argon laser provided multiple spectral lines between 457 and 514 nm for fluorescence imaging. The instrument provided diffraction-limited imaging of the photoreceptor mosaic, nerve fiber bundles, fine capillaries and blood flow. Ganglion cells were fluorescently labeled with yellow fluorescence protein (YFP) by one of two methods. The first was a transgenic mouse line that expresses YFP in a small subset of retinal ganglion cells (B6.Thy1-YFPH). In the second method, retinal ganglion cells in an adult C57BL/6J mouse were sparsely labeled with YFP via transduction from retrograde viral vectors. Ganglion cell bodies, dendrites and axons were clearly resolved, as shown in Figure 14.24. Imaging resolution characterized directly from *in vivo* images was sub-micron laterally, and $\sim 10\,\mu$m axially. This research demonstrated the great potential of the fluorescence AOSLO for imaging a variety of retinal structures including individual pericytes, Müller glial cells, bipolar cells and amacrine cells that are fluorescently labeled in transgenic mice, or using cell-specific adeno-associated virus (AAV) and lentiviral vectors. In addition to structural imaging, fluorescence imaging may provide measures of retinal function at a cellular and subcellular scale. The combination of the high-resolution imaging ability and advanced molecular techniques for engineering the mouse may open new opportunities for broad applications on investigating retinal development and disease mechanisms and evaluating therapeutic efficacy.

14.9.3 *In vivo* two-photon retinal imaging

Hunter et al. [125] recently demonstrated two-photon fluorescence imaging of the retina in a living macaque eye. The retina was excited by a Ti-sapphire laser at 730 nm. This source had an 80 MHz repetition rate and a pulse width less than 70 fs in air. The two-photon fluorescence was detected in a region under 550 nm. To improve the SNR of the extremely low two-photon fluorescence image, up to 16,500 individual fluorescence frames (12 minute acquisition) were recorded

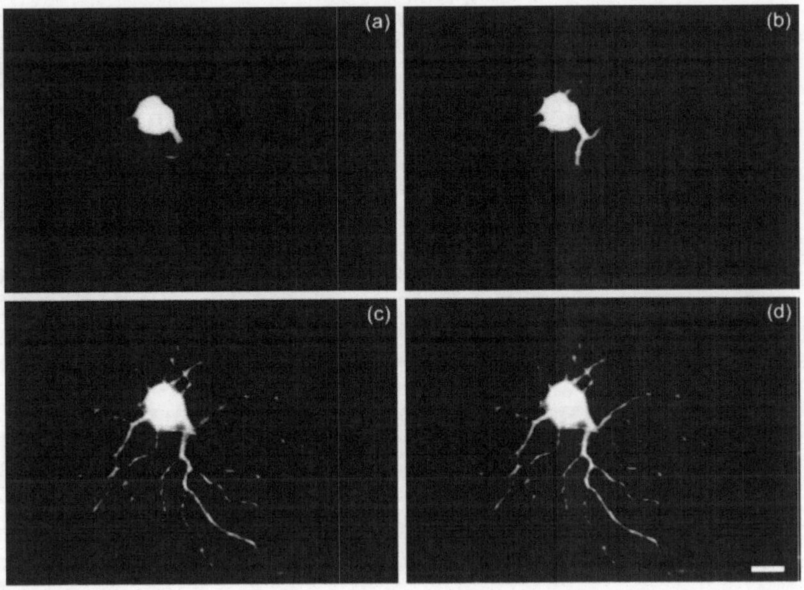

Figure 14.24: *In vivo* fluorescence images of a ganglion cell expressing YFP. (a-c) Individual images from three of the focuses, at focus steps of 11.6 μm, (a) is at the innermost focus and (c) is at the outermost focus. Each image at an individual focus step was a registered image average of 500 frames. (d) Maximum intensity projection image generated from 5 separate *in vivo* images taken at focus steps of 5.8 μm. Confocal pinhole diameter was 3.9 Airy disks. All images were contrast stretched identically to preserve their relative brightness. Scale bar: 20 μm. Reproduced with permission from the Optical Society of America (OSA).

and registered to produce the final image. As described earlier for one-photon fluorescence imaging, a simultaneous dual-frame imaging mechanism was adopted. Figure 14.25 shows the cone mosaic imaged by AOSLO two-photon fluorescence and by direct reflectance. The ability to image the retina in the living eye with two-photon excitation is important for a number of reasons. First, it allows the fluorophores whose excitation spectrum falls below 400 nm to be excited, since the wavelength of 400 nm is the spectral cut-off of the mammalian eye where the one-photon excitation can't reach. Second, two-photon imaging using near-infrared light to excite the retina can avoid intense visual stimulation. Third, two-photon fluorescence imaging possesses intrinsically better axial resolution than one-photon fluorescence imaging by preferentially exciting fluorophores near the focal plane.

The AO two-photon retinal imaging in living primates eye represented a major advance in *in vivo* high-resolution retinal imaging; it not only extended the ability of the AOSLO imaging of important retinal fluorophores that cannot be accessed in the living eye by single-photon fluorescence imaging but also opened the door to study retinal function at the cellular scale. As reported by [125], increased fluorescence emission was observed in response to photoreceptor bleaching in the living macaque eye, indicating the creation of new fluorescent molecules or an increase in the concentration of existing fluorescent molecules either directly by the two-photon excitation light or by its stimulation of a visual response. Two-photon imaging allows excitation of multiple endogenous fluorophores, such as NADH, that are functional markers of cell metabolism. Many of the transparent retinal cell-types contain two-photon excitable intrinsic fluorophores, and can be imaged with high contrast on a two-photon microscope ex-vivo, suggesting that both the structure and function of any retinal cell types may be imaged by two-photon excitation *in vivo* without the use of exogenous

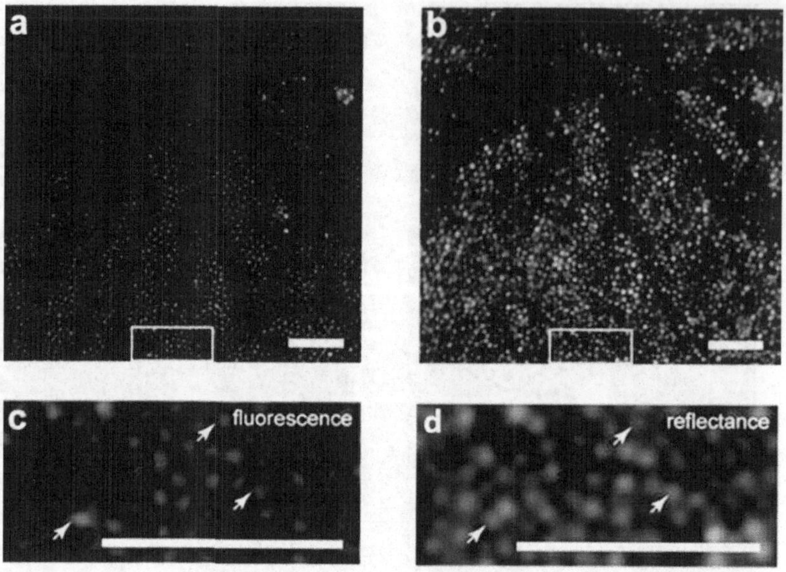

Figure 14.25: (a) Two-photon image and (b) reflectance image of the cone photoreceptor in a living macaque eye. (c) and (d) are the magnified sections in (a) and (b) respectively. White arrows indicate corresponding individual cones observed in both images, whereas black arrows mark a cone that was not reflecting light but shows a strong fluorescence signal. Reproduced with permission from the Optical Society of America (OSA).

fluorophores. Because NIR light is used, the AO two-photon retinal imaging leads to reduced photo damage and deeper penetration. Due to the quadratic dependence on the intensity, two-photon excitation is limited to the focal area only. Thus, cells out-of-focus experience only the innocuous infrared light with negligible photodamage or phototoxicity and photo-bleaching of fluorophores is minimized.

14.10 AOSLO for Visual Stimulus Presentation

Due to the scanning imaging nature of the AOSLO, visual stimuli can be directly presented onto the retina by modulating the scanning light. The light modulation may be conducted by an acousto-optic modulator (AOM). The shape, size, luminance, and the position of the stimuli can be precisely encoded directly into the scanning raster. If the modulation is applied on the imaging laser, the image will be encoded with the spatial pattern of the modulation. In Figure 14.26 a photo of one of the authors was mapped to the scanning field. In accordance with the AOSLO imaging system timing, the spatial position of each pixel of the photo was transformed to a series of time points, and the grey level of each pixel was converted to analog voltage for modulation of the beam intensity at the exact corresponding time point of the scanning field. Thus, the scanning beam projects the photo on the retina. This image is a single frame of a 1.2-degree field of view, 512×512 pixels, and the video was taken at 30 frames per second. Although the method of modulating the laser beam is not new, a distinguished feature is that the AOSLO can present an AO-corrected visual stimulus; therefore, the subject sees an ultra-sharp image. This function significantly facilitated

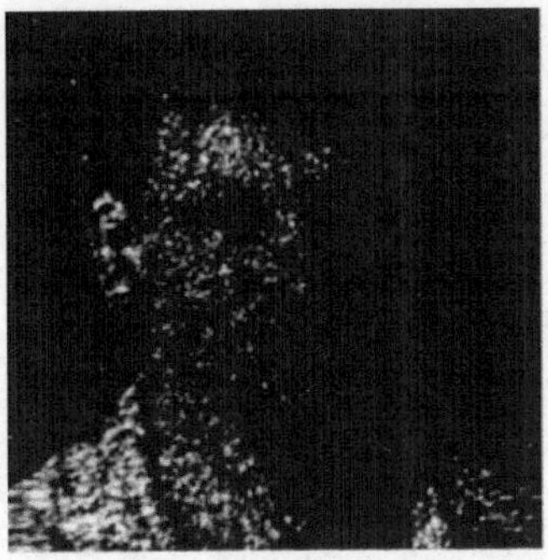

Figure 14.26: AOSLO projects a photo on the retina by modulating the imaging laser beam.

high-resolution functional imaging, psychophysics and visual neuroscience, as we will present here, the stimuli can be delivered and localized on the scale of a single cone photoreceptor. Here we describe two studies that capitalize on AOSLO visual stimulation capabilities.

14.10.1 AOSLO imaging of retinal function by measuring intrinsic signal

Retinal intrinsic signals are retinal scattering changes that occur in response to visual stimulation, e.g., when the retina is flashed by a visible light stimulus, photopigment molecules in photoreceptors will be photoisomerized, ions will be transported in and out of the photoreceptor cells and other retinal neurons, and choroidal and retinal blood flow will be redirected. Any or all of these changes may cause changes in the scattering of the light in the retina. The location, time course, and magnitude of the scattering changes in response to visible light stimulation will encode details of these changes, much like the electroretinogram records the electrical changes in the retina. Therefore, intrinsic retinal signal is a measure of the instantaneous ensemble change of the optical properties of the retina and thus it may provide a noninvasive measure of retinal function. Grieve et al. [135] measured the retinal intrinsic signals in the living human eye and non-human primate eye with an AOSLO.

In this study, the AOSLO was adapted to be a dual-wavelength mode, in which a visible light of wavelength 658 nm was used to stimulate the retina and an infrared SLD with 840 nm wavelength was used to take a high resolution image of the retina while and after the stimulus was presented onto the retina. Modulation of each laser beam using acousto-optic modulators allowed the integration of complex, patterned stimuli into the projected raster, whose exact locations on the retina were recorded into the movie in real time. The retina has very low spectral sensitivity at 840 nm, implying that the photopigment absorption of the imaging light is very low; thus, the images taken with the 840 nm light recorded essentially no changes in reflectance as a function of changes in the concentration of pigment within the cones. Therefore, the intrinsic signals observed with the 840 nm light were not confounded by changes in absorption of the photopigments caused by photobleaching with the 658-nm stimulus. Stimulus luminance was 12,000 cd/m^2. For each test, 20 to 30 second movies were recorded, with stimulation occurring at 5 seconds. The stimulus covered half the field, either in a half-field pattern, covering the top half of the square field, or in a 2×2 checkerboard pattern, covering one top and one bottom quadrant, as shown in Figure 14.27. In five human subjects, results showed a clear increase in infrared light scattering in the stimulated region with respect to its surroundings, reproduced in four subjects across multiple imaging sessions. Signal increase began immediately at the onset of the stimulus, reached a peak 2 to 3 seconds after stimulus onset, and decreased to baseline within 2 to 10 seconds. The experiment found that the magnitude of the increase over the stimulated area varied from 0% to 5% between subjects. The results suggested

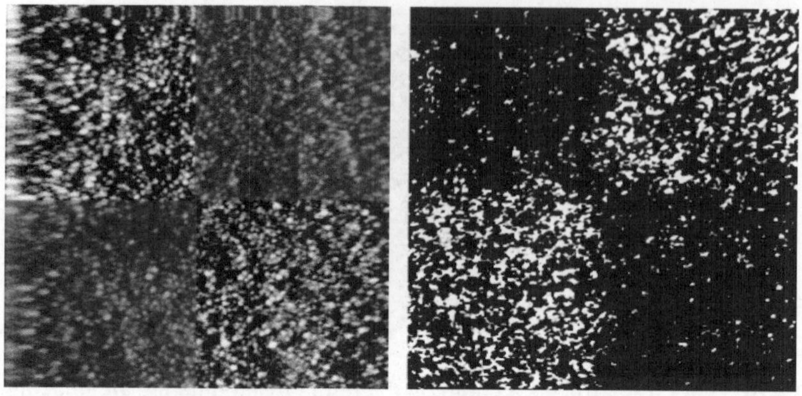

Figure 14.27: AOSLO study of the retinal intrinsic signal. The left panel illustrates the stimulus projected onto the retina through the AOSLO visual stimulus delivery channel. The semitransparent red check-board pattern indicates where the stimulation was delivered. The right panel shows a difference image of the infrared images of the retina at maximum response minus baseline. The form of the stimulus is clearly revealed as an increase in scattered infrared light following stimulation. Right panel courtesy of Kate Grieve.

that the signal originated in the cone photoreceptors, though not all cones contributed to the same extent. In individual cones, signal increases over 20% were measured.

14.10.2 Precise visual stimuli presentation

Figure 14.28 is the layout of a dual-wavelength confocal AOSLO that was developed in the University of California at Berkeley for precise visual stimulus delivery. This instrument has a dual source – retina – detector confocal configuration. The beams from two light sources whose wavelengths are 680 nm and 840 nm, respectively, share the same scanning path but are independently modulated. The 840 nm source produces real-time high resolution retinal images while the 680 nm source presents AO corrected light stimuli of various configurations. The stimulus position is guided by images taken with the 840 nm source and the stimulus intensity is controlled by the acoustic-optic-modulator. The longitudinal and transverse ocular chromatic aberrations differed between the two wavelengths and were minimized by adjusting the positions of the source, the retinal plane and the pinholes of the detectors to be exactly conjugate with each other in both light channels, ensuring that both beams accurately focus on the lateral and longitudinal position of interest in the retina. In the human eye, with a field of view of 1.2 degree, the AOSLO can deliver and maintain the stimulus on a single foveal cone with the 3-D positioning precision as high as 0.7 μm $\times$ 0.7 μm $\times$ 60 μm.

This dual-wavelength AOSLO enabled an important study of the contribution of single cone photoreceptors to the response of central visual neurons. In a collaboration with Lawrence Sincich, PhD and Jonathan Horton, MD, PhD at University of California at San Francisco, we used the AOSLO to deliver micron-scale light stimuli to the receptive field centers of neurons in the macaque lateral geniculate nucleus (LGN), i.e., we stimulated single cones in the living macaque eye, and simultaneously recorded the firings (action potentials) of the ganglion cells through proxy neurons in the LGN with an extracellular electrode [138]. This ability is of great importance for *in vivo* characterization of a neuron's response properties under stimulation. As demonstrated in this study, AOSLO can create precise maps of the cones that underlie the receptive fields of visual neurons by precisely stimulating individual cone photoreceptors. Such cone maps will be useful for answering definitively how chromatic sensitivity depends on the balance of cone ratios between receptive field centers and surrounds. Previously, a neuron's response properties are characterized by presenting

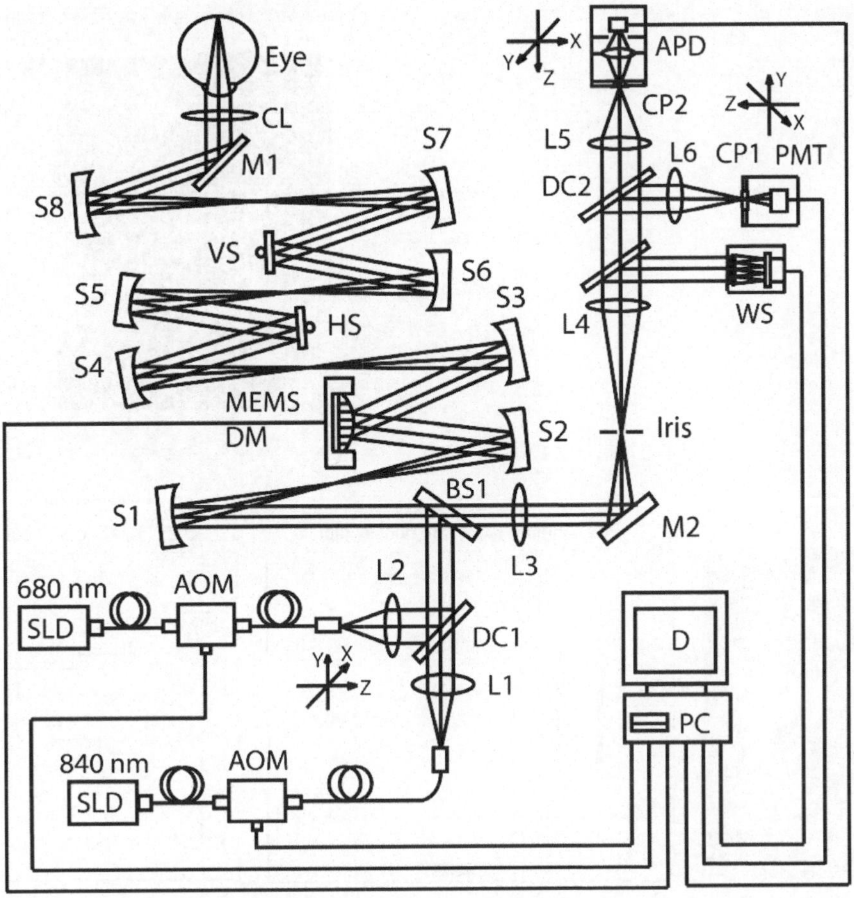

Figure 14.28: Dual wavelength confocal AOSLO for precise visual stimulation.

stimuli on an external screen while recording action potentials with an extracellular electrode. Such a method does not provide direct identification of the cones feeding the receptive field. This method is also challenged by ocular optical aberrations, scatter, and eye movement, all of which degrade visual stimuli. These limitations alter the location and spectral intensity of light impinging on the photoreceptors, making it difficult to map the cone field precisely, especially near the fovea, where cone spacing is only a few microns.

In this experiment, the real-time high-resolution retinal images taken with the 840 nm light provided high-speed, high-precision measurement of retinal motion; the AO correction for wavefront aberration ensured the light stimulus was delivered with ultra-sharp precision. By tracking retinal movement, most of the energy in the stimulus is likely to fall within a single cone. The size and geometry of the stimulus were defined and controlled by the AOM. We could record reliable responses from an isolated LGN neuron while stimulating a cone with 680 nm light. The position of the stimulus was selected manually at one point, specifying either a row or a column position centered on that location. When the stimulus sequence was started, stimuli were flashed in pseudorandom order an equal number of times at each specified position, as shown in Fig. 14.29. This study revealed that receptive field centers of LGN neurons close to the foveal center are comprised of multiple cones. Because LGN neurons respond reliably when only one of their cone inputs is stimulated, it suggests that single cone activation is sufficient for perception, even away from the fovea.

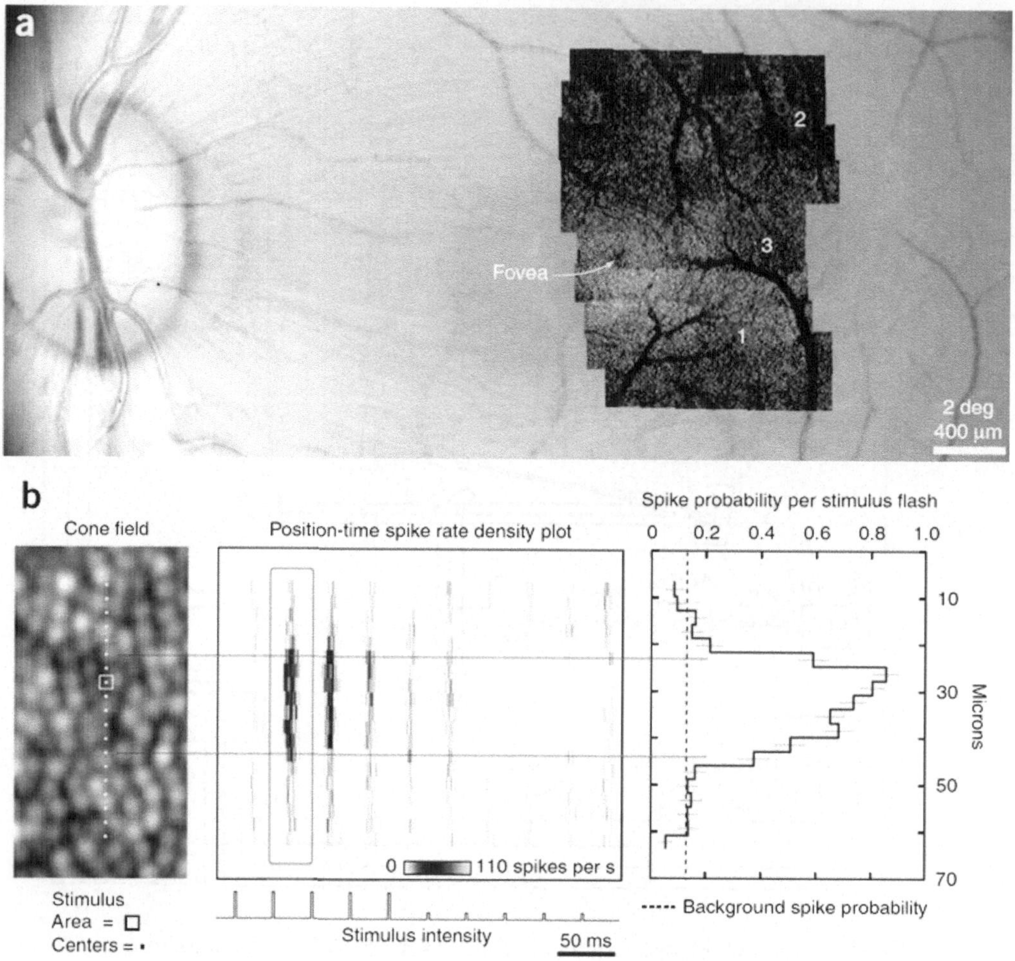

Figure 14.29: (a) color fundus photograph of macaque retina with an AOSLO montage overlay where receptive fields (red circles) were recorded. (b) Stimuli flashed at 19 contiguous locations across the cone field of neuron 1 (left) led to an adapting ON response and an inhibitory OFF response (middle, each row in the spike density plot represents the temporal response of one position in the cone field). Response latency was $\sim$ 45 ms. Residual light in the optical path generated background activity at the frame rate. Activity above the background rate occurred over a region spanning four cones, indicated by red lines. Mean spike probability (right, $\pm$ s.e.m.) was measured in the blue outlined area of the spike density plot. Reproduced with permission from [138].

14.11 AOSLO *In Vivo* Study of Retinal Degenerative Diseases

The robust AO correction for the wavefront aberration of the living human eye has enabled studies of the retinal diseases, including cone–rod dystrophy (CRD), retinitis pigmentosa (RP) [139], acute zonal occult outer retinopathy (AZOOR) [140], Stargardt disease [141], neurogenic weakness, ataxia, and retinitis pigmentosa (NARP) [142], and age-related macular degeneration (AMD). A common feature of these diseases is that they all cause progressive death of photoreceptors. For example, in RP, rod loss precedes cone loss, whereas in CRD, cone loss precedes rod loss. Eventually cones and rods are lost in patients with both conditions. The mechanisms underlying photoreceptor death in patients with these diseases are not well understood, partly because photoreceptors couldn't be easily visualized in living eyes. Conventionally, most understanding of retinal degenerations has come from histology on animal models and human donor eyes with advanced or end stages of disease. In clinical practice, the disease presence and severity are diagnosed based on funduscopic appearance during standard ophthalmoscopy which is often supplemented by fundus photography, fluorescein angiography, SLO and OCT. However, none of these methods can provide assessment on the single cell scale due to the imperfect optics of the human eye; consequently, these approaches are limited since the critical cellular elements of the disease processes are not observable. In addition, functional characteristics (e.g., visual acuity) are often poorly correlated with disease severity, further complicating interpretation of disease severity.

AOSLO images provide new insights into possible mechanisms of cone vision loss in patients with these conditions. In a study of the macular photoreceptor structure in patients with inherited retinal degenerations including CRD and RP [139], the photoreceptor structure data from RP and CRD patients were compared with data from normal subjects. Cone spacing at 1 degree from the fovea was compared to standard measures of central visual function including best-corrected visual acuity (BCVA), foveal threshold, multifocal electroretinogram amplitude and timing, and microperimetry. This study revealed that cone spacing values were significantly different from normal subjects for both RP and CRD patients, and demonstrated a statistically significant correlation

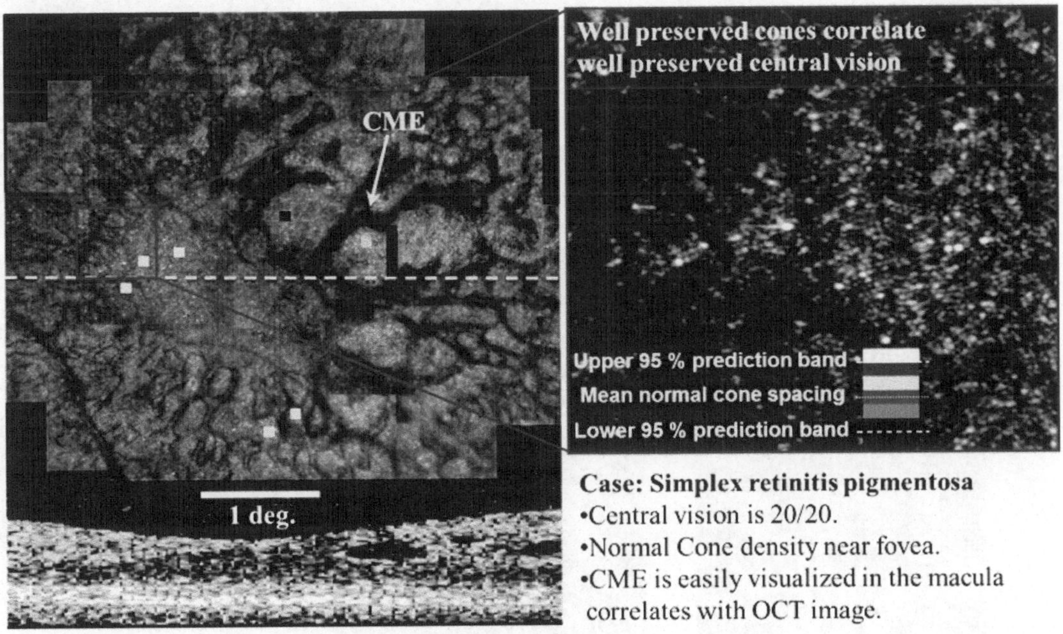

Figure 14.30: AOSLO images of patient with RP show cyst walls of cystoid macular edema (CME), a feature commonly seen in patients with RP. The CME was also detected by OCT (color image). Despite the presence of cystoid spaces, cones were readily visualized and demonstrated normal cone spacing throughout the region: cone spacing falls within 95% predictive values for subjects with healthy eyes. Although normal macular cone spacing was observed in this patient and many other patients with RP, when evaluated as a group, cone structures near the foveas of patients with RP were significantly different from subjects with healthy eyes. Modified from [139] with permission.

with foveal threshold, best-corrected visual acuity, and multifocal electroretinogram amplitude, as shown in Figure 14.30. Although many RP patients showed normal cone spacing within 1 degree of fixation, cones could not be unambiguously identified in several retinal regions. Cone spacing increased in all CRD patients, even those with early disease.

For the first time, AOSLO images also revealed mosaics of RPE cells in regions where it appeared that cones were missing [143]. RPE cell shape, size, and distribution compared well with measurements from the literature. Fundus-related microperimetry results indicated scotomas that corresponded to the locations where RPE cells were visible, shown in Figure 14.31.

AMD is the leading cause of blindness in people 60 years of age or older in the developed world. Although treatments are available for exudative AMD, an advanced form of the disease, there are no effective treatments for early to intermediate disease. High-resolution imaging of the retinas may facilitate direct assessment of the photoreceptors, but imaging in elderly patients has been challenging due to disease related changes of the eye's optical system. In a recent study, we have demonstrated that AOSLO can produce high-resolution images in elderly patients. A total of 39 subjects (24 males and 15 females) have been enrolled in this study, including 34 AMD patients and 5 age-matched normal subjects. Their ages range from 50 to 87 years old, with a mean of 72.10 years. The patients were selected from the clinic registry of the Department of Ophthalmology of

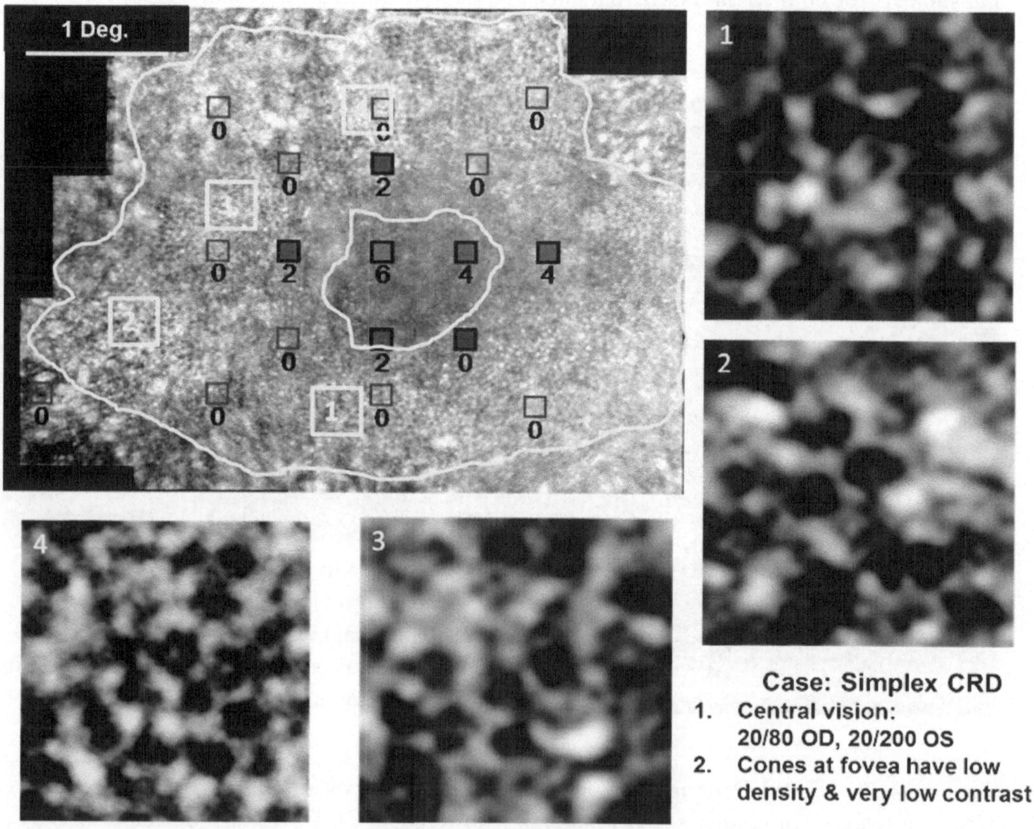

Figure 14.31: Patient with cone-rod dystrophy. RPE cells appear as a regular array surrounding the central cone-preserved region, as shown on the upper-left panel. Microperimetry data are overlayed on the AOSLO image. Numbers indicate the attenuation scale in decibels. Absolute scotomas, indicated by empty red squares and labeled '**0**', correspond with regions with absent cones and visible RPE cells. Modified from [143] with permission.

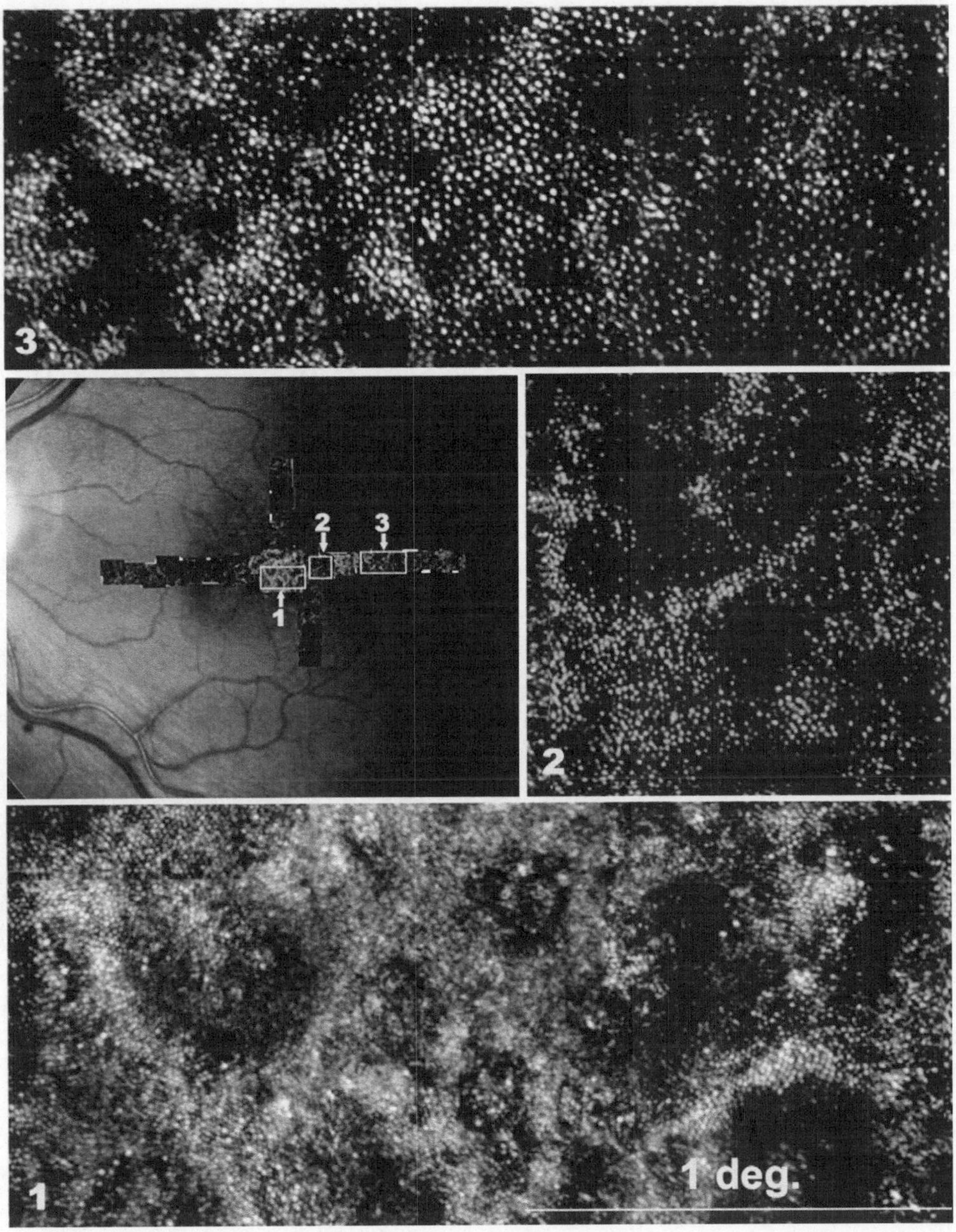

Figure 14.32: AOSLO retinal images of a patient with AMD at intermediate stage (Age-Related Eye Disease Study (AREDS) grade 6). The images reveal reduced brightness of the cones over drusen (dark areas) and reduced cone density in the fovea.

the University of Alabama at Birmingham by reviewing the clinic charts but without any further examination before they were imaged by the AOSLO. Images were successfully obtained from 38 eyes of 26 subjects. AOSLO revealed the pathological structure changes with high-resolution in patients with AMD at various stages. The cone photoreceptors that overlay drusen showed reduced reflectivity and moderately increased cell spacing, as shown in Figure 14.32 and Figure 14.33. In patients with advanced stage of disease, shown in Figure 14.34, AOSLO produced high-resolution

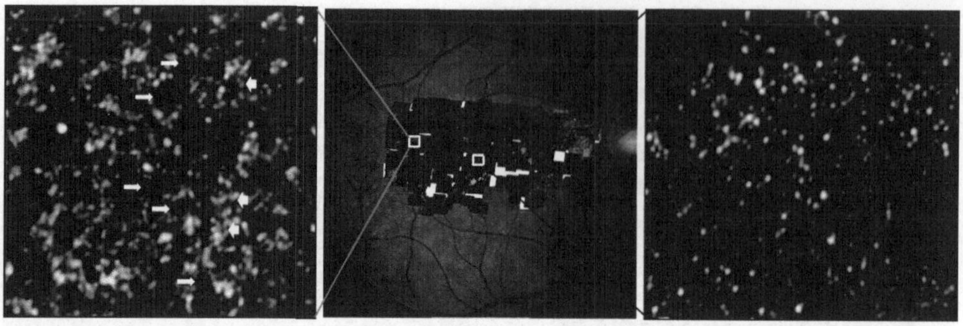

Figure 14.33: AOSLO retinal images of a patient with AMD at intermediate stage (AREDS grade 6). In the fovea, cone photoreceptors were preserved but with significantly reduced density (right panel). In the parafovea, cones showed reduced reflectivity compared with rods, as shown in the left panel, the thin arrows point to cones and the thick arrowheads point to rods. The inset images (the left and the right panels) subtend 0.5 degrees, or approximately 150 μm on a side.

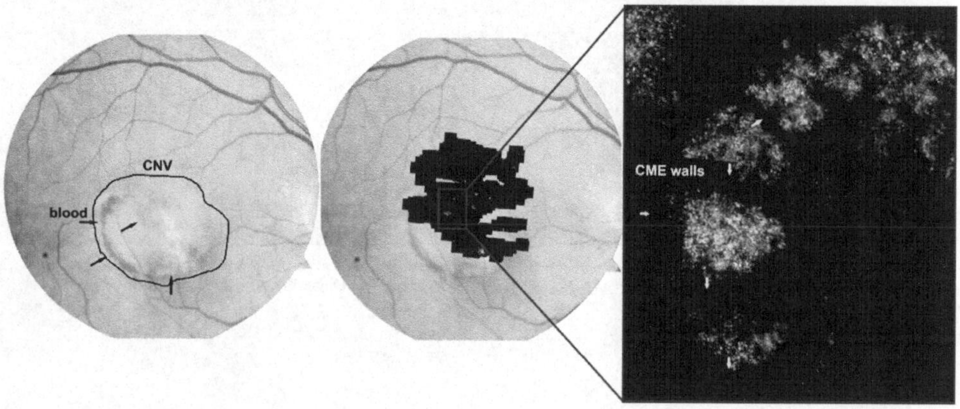

Figure 14.34: AOSLO retinal image of a patient with advanced AMD (AREDS grade 11, wet AMD with CNV). The CME walls were confirmed by OCT imaging (not shown here).

images of the area with choroidal neovascularization (CNV). On the CNV area, the cone mosaic was severely disrupted. This study demonstrates that AOSLO holds promise to provide new insight into the pathophysiology of AMD.

14.12 Summary

To date AO retinal imaging has been realized in three modalities, i.e., flood illumination funduscopy, optical coherence tomography (AO-OCT), and AOSLO. Compared with AO flood-illumination ophthalmoscopes, AOSLO is a scanning imaging system, highly efficient for illuminating the retina and collecting photons from the eye. The spatial sampling is not restricted by the available pixels of a 2D imaging chip. It is a confocal system that can reject the contrast-reducing out-of-focus scattering light, thereby improving resolution and contrast. Moreover, the AOSLO can be operated at a frame rate of 30 frames/second or higher, sufficient to record dynamic activities such as blood flow in the retinal capillaries. Compared with AO-OCT, AOSLO renders arguably the best "en-face" retinal image. This allows us to correlate the AOSLO findings with clinical "gold standard" color fundus photos and fundus autofluorescence (FAF) images easily. While the AO-OCT produces cross-sectional retinal images with superb axial resolution and fast speed, its en-face retinal images must be reconstructed from a series of cross-sectional images. A 3D volumetric OCT image may be acquired at the time scale of 1 second with the fastest OCT imaging system to date; hence, the reconstruction is vulnerable to eye movement. Further, the AO-OCT images are intrinsically accompanied by light interference artifact, i.e., speckle, reducing image fidelity.

The AOSLO is an excellent platform for multifunctional and multispectral imaging of retinal structure and function at the cellular and even the sub-cellular level in the living eye. In-vivo cellular level fluorescence retinal imaging with single-photon or multi-photon excitation can be readily realized. This has important implications. Recent advances in molecular biotechnology have made it possible to label a variety of retinal cells with fluorescent markers, such as cones, rods, ganglion cells, RPE cells, pericytes, Müller glial cells, bipolar cells and amacrine cells, promising to resolve cells and cellular details not accessible with reflectance imaging of the unlabelled retina. To date the AOSLO is the only imaging modality that has achieved *in-vivo* cellular-level retinal fluorescence images. With multi-photon excitation, further improvement of the ability to image endogenous and exogenous fluorophores is expected.

In summary, AOSLO is a promising tool for basic science research on the retina and clinical diagnosis as well as treatment of retinal diseases.

Acknowledgment

The research has been supported by National Eye Institute Grants NIH-NEI EY002162 (JLD), EY14375 (AR), and the National Science Foundation Science and Technology Center for Adaptive Optics, managed by the University of California at Santa Cruz under cooperative agreement AST-9876783 (AR). EyeSight Foundation of Alabama (YZ), International Retina Research Foundation (YZ), EY021903 (YZ), Songs for Sight (CAG), Buck Trust of Alabama (CAG), Research to Prevent Blindness (CAG, JLD) and the Foundation Fighting Blindness (JLD, AR).

The authors thank Mark Clark, BS, for providing the fundus photo of Figure 14.2 and advising on the labeling of Figure 14.34.

References

[1] A. Roorda et al., "Adaptive optics scanning laser ophthalmoscopy," *Opt. Express* **10** (9), 405–412 (2002).

[2] B.B. Boycott, J.E. Dowling, Helga Kolb, "Organization of the primate retina: light microscopy," *Phil. Trans. Roy. Soc. London. Series B, Biol. Sci.* **255** (799), 109–184 (1969).

[3] *WEBVISION. The Organization of the Retina and Visual System*, H. Kolb, R. Nelson, E. Fernandez, and B.W. Jones (eds.) http://retina.umh.es/Webvision/index.html (2012).

[4] R.W. Rodieck, *The First Step in Seeing* (Sinauer Associates, Sunderland, MA, 1998).

[5] J.E. Dowling, *The Retina: An Approachable Part of the Brain* (Belknap Press of Harvard University Press, Cambridge, MA, 1987).

[6] R.H. Webb and G.W. Hughes, "Scanning laser ophthalmoscope," *IEEE Trans. Biomed. Eng.* **28**(7), 488–492 (1981).

[7] R.H. Webb, G.W. Hughes, and F.C. Delori, "Confocal scanning laser ophthalmoscope," *Appl. Opt.* **26**(8), 1492–1429 (1987).

[8] H. Friedenwald, "The history of the invention and of the development of the ophthalmoscope," *J. Am. Med. Assoc.* **38**, 549-552 (1902).

[9] C.R. Keeler, "The ophthalmoscope in the lifetime of Hermann von Helmholtz," *Arch. Ophthalmol.* **120**(2), 194–201 (2002).

[10] T. Wilson, "The role of the pinhole in confocal imaging systems," Chap. 11 in *The Handbook of Biological Confocal Microscopy*. 2nd Edition, J. B. Pawley, Ed. (Plenum, New York, 1995, pp. 167-182).

[11] T. Wilson and C. Sheppard, *Theory and practice of scanning optical microscopy* (Academic Press, London, Orlando, 1984).

[12] J. Liang, D.R. Williams, and D.T. Miller, "Supernormal vision and high-resolution retinal imaging through adaptive optics," *J. Opt. Soc. Am. A. Opt. Image Sci. Vis.* **14**(11), 2884–2892 (1997).

[13] D.A. Atchison G. Smith, *Optics of the Human Eye* (Butterworth-Heinemann, Oxford, Boston, 2000).

[14] J.V. Forrester, *The Eye: Basic Sciences in Practice,* 3rd ed. (Saunders, Edinburgh, New York, 2007).

[15] R. Klein et al., "The Wisconsin age-related maculopathy grading system," *Ophthalmology* **98**(7), 1128–1134 (1991).

[16] C.A. Curcio et al., "Human photoreceptor topography," *J. Comp. Neurol.* **292**(4), 497–523 (1990).

[17] O. Strauss, "The retinal pigment epithelium in visual function," *Physiol. Rev.* **85**(3) 845–881 (2005).

[18] C.A. Curcio, C. Owsley, and G.R. Jackson, "Spare the rods, save the cones in aging and age-related maculopathy," *Invest. Ophthalmol. Vis. Sci.* **41**(8), 2015–2018 (2000).

[19] W.S.C. Stiles, B.H. Crawford, "The luminous efficiency of rays entering the eye pupil at different points," *Proc. Roy. Soc. London* **112**, 428–450 (1932).

[20] S.A. Burns et al., "Variations in photoreceptor directionally across the central retina," *J. Opt. Soc. Am. A Opt. Image Sci. Vis.* **14**(9), 2033–2040 (1997).

[21] J.M.Gorrand and F.C. Delori, "Reflectance and curvature of the inner limiting membrane at the foveola," *J. Opt. Soc. Am. A Opt. Image Sci. Vis.* **16**(6), 1229–1237 (1999).

[22] A. Roorda and D.R. Williams, "Optical fiber properties of individual human cones," *J. Vis.* **2**(5), 404–412 (2002).

[23] J. Porter, *Adaptive Optics for Vision Sscience: Principles, Practices, Design, and Applications* (Wiley-Interscience, Hoboken, NJ, 2006).

[24] F.C. Delori and K.P. Pflibsen, "Spectral reflectance of the human ocular fundus," *Appl. Opt.* **28**(6), 1061–1077 (1989).

[25] F.C. Delori, "Spectrophotometer for noninvasive measurement of intrinsic fluorescence and reflectance of the ocular fundus," *Appl. Opt.* **33**(31) 7439–7452 (1994).

[26] F.C. Delori et al., "*In vivo* fluorescence of the ocular fundus exhibits retinal pigment epithelium lipofuscin characteristics," *Invest. Ophthalmol. Vis. Sci.* **36**(3) 718–729 (1995).

[27] Z136.4, A., American National Standard Recommended Practice for Laser Safety Measurements for Hazard Evaluation, 2010.

[28] F.C. Delori et al., "Maximum permissible exposures for ocular safety (ANSI 2000), with emphasis on ophthalmic devices," *J. Opt. Soc. Am. A Opt. Image Sci. Vis.* **24**(5), 1250–1265 (2007).

[29] J.J. Hunter et al., "The susceptibility of the retina to photochemical damage from visible light," *Prog. Retin. Eye Res.* **31**(1), 28-42 (2012).

[30] F.C. Delori, "Autofluorescence method to measure macular pigment optical densities fluorometry and autofluorescence imaging," *Arch. Biochem. Biophys.* **430**(2), 156-162 (2004).

[31] F.C. Delori and E.S. Gragoudas, "Light source for monochromatic ophthalmoscopy and fluorescein angiography," *Arch. Ophthalmol.* **97**(7), 1349–1350 (1979).

[32] F.C. Delori et al., "Monochromatic ophthalmoscopy and fundus photography. The normal fundus," *Arch. Ophthalmol.* **95**(5), 861–868 (1977).

[33] A.E. Elsner et al., "Infrared imaging of sub-retinal structures in the human ocular fundus," *Vision Res.* **36**(1), 191–205 (1996).

[34] S.R. Freeman et al., "Optical coherence tomography-raster scanning and manual segmentation in determining drusen volume in age-related macular degeneration," *Retina* **30**(3), 431–435 (2010).

[35] T.R. Friberg, R.A. Bilonick, and P.M. Brennen, "Analysis of the relationship between drusen size and drusen area in eyes with age-related macular degeneration," *Ophthalmic Surg. Lasers Imaging* **42**(5), 369–375 (2011).

[36] A.A. Khanifar et al., "Drusen ultrastructure imaging with spectral domain optical coherence tomography in age-related macular degeneration," *Ophthalmology* **115**(11), 1883–1890 (2008).

[37] G. Landa et al., "Drusen characteristics revealed by spectral-domain optical coherence tomography and their corresponding fundus autofluorescence appearance in dry age-related macular degeneration," *Ophthalmic Res.* **47**(2), 81–86 (2012).

[38] D. Pauleikhoff et al., "Drusen and their significance in age related macular degeneration," *Fortschr. Ophthalmol.* **87**(5), 429–432 (1990).

[39] J.P. Sarks, S.H. Sarks, and M.C. Killingsworth, "Evolution of soft drusen in age-related macular degeneration," *Eye (Lond.)* **8**, 269–283 (1994).

[40] S. Schmitz-Valckenberg et al., "Reticular drusen associated with geographic atrophy in age-related macular degeneration," *Invest. Ophthalmol. Vis. Sci.* **52**(9), 5009–5015 (2011).

[41] S.G. Schuman et al., "Photoreceptor layer thinning over drusen in eyes with age-related macular degeneration imaged *in vivo* with spectral-domain optical coherence tomography," *Ophthalmology* **116**(3), 488–496 (2009).

[42] K. Yi et al., "Spectral domain optical coherence tomography for quantitative evaluation of drusen and associated structural changes in non-neovascular age-related macular degeneration," *Br. J. Ophthalmol.* **93**(2), 176–181 (2009).

[43] C. Cavallotti and L. Cerulli, *Age-related changes of the human eye. Aging medicine*, Humana Press, Totowa, N.J., 2008.

[44] H.B. Barlow, "Eye movements during fixation," *J. Physiol.* **116**(3), 290–306 (1952).

[45] M. Eizenman, P.E. Hallett, and R.C. Frecker, "Power spectra for ocular drift and tremor," *Vision Res.* **25**(11), 1635–1640 (1985).

[46] S. Martinez-Conde, S.L. Macknik, and D.H. Hubel, "The role of fixational eye movements in visual perception," *Nat. Rev. Neurosci.* **5**(3), 229–240 (2004).

[47] L.A. Riggs, J.C. Armington, and F. Ratliff, "Motions of the retinal image during fixation," *J. Opt. Soc. Am.* **44**(4), 315–321 (1954).

[48] T.N. Cornsweet, "Determination of the stimuli for involuntary drifts and saccadic eye movements," *J. Opt. Soc. Am.* **46**(11), 987–993 (1956).

[49] J.M. Findlay, "Frequency analysis of human involuntary eye movement," *Kybernetik*, **8**(6), 207–214 (1971).

[50] S.B. Stevenson, A. Roorda, and G. Kumar, "Eye tracking with the adaptive optics scanning laser ophthalmoscope," in *Proceedings of the 2010 Symposium on Eye-Tracking Research & Applications*. Austin, TX: ACM, NY (2010).

[51] S.B. Stevenson, A. Roorda, "Correcting for miniature eye movements in high resolution scanning laser ophthalmoscopy," in *Ophthalmic Technologies XI*, SPIE, San Jose, 2005.

[52] C.R. Vogel et al., "Retinal motion estimation in adaptive optics scanning laser ophthalmoscopy," *Opt. Express* **14**(2), 487–497 (2006).

[53] B. Potsaid et al., "Ultrahigh speed spectral / Fourier domain OCT ophthalmic imaging at 70,000 to 312,500 axial scans per second," *Opt. Express* **16**(19), 15149–1569 (2008).

[54] J. Rha et al., "Adaptive optics flood-illumination camera for high speed retinal imaging," *Opt. Express* **14**(10), 552–569 (2006).

[55] F.W. Campbell and D.G. Green, "Optical and retinal factors affecting visual resolution," *J. Physiol.* **181**(3), 576–593 (1965).

[56] F.W. Campbell and R.W. Gubisch, "Optical quality of the human eye," *J. Physiol.* **186**(3), 558–578 (1966).

[57] H.C. Howland and B. Howland, "A subjective method for the measurement of monochromatic aberrations of the eye," *J. Opt. Soc. Am.* **67**(11), 1508–1518 (1977).

[58] J. Liang and D.R. Williams, "Aberrations and retinal image quality of the normal human eye," *J. Opt. Soc. Am. A Opt. Image Sci. Vis.* **14**(11), 2873–2883 (1997).

[59] H. Hofer et al., "Dynamics of the eye's wave aberration," *J. Opt. Soc. Am. A Opt. Image Sci. Vis.* **18**(3), 497–506 (2001).

[60] H. Hofer et al., "Improvement in retinal image quality with dynamic correction of the eye's aberrations," *Opt. Express* **8**(11), 631–643 (2001).

[61] H.W. Babcock, "The possibility of compensating astronomical seeing," in *Publications of the Astronomical Society of the Pacific* **65**(386), 229–236 (1953).

[62] C.J.R. Sheppard, D.M. Shotton, *Confocal microscopy*, Springer-Verlag Inc., New York, 1997.

[63] M. Minsky, "Memoir on inventing the confocal microscope," *Scanning* **10**, 128–138 (1988).

[64] T.R. Corle, C.H. Chou, and G.S. Kino, "Depth response of confocal optical microscopes," *Opt. Lett.* **11**(12), 770–772 (1986).

[65] I.J. Cox, D.K. Hamilton, C.J.R.Sheppard, "Observation of optical signatures of materials," *Appl. Phys. Lett.* **41**, 604–606 (1982).

[66] B. Richards, E. Wolf, "Electromagnetic diffraction in optical systems. II. Structure of the image field in an aplanatic system," *Proc. Roy. Soc. London A* **253**(1274), 358–379 (1959).

[67] G.S. Kino, G.G. Xiao, "Real-time scanning optical microscope," in *Confocal Microscopy*, ed. T. Wilson, Academic Press, 1990.

[68] M. Born and E. Wolf, *Principles of optics: electromagnetic theory of propagation, interference and diffraction of light.* 7th expanded ed. (Cambridge University Press, Cambridge, New York, 1999).

[69] J.B. Pawley, "The role of the pinhole in confocal imaging systems," Chap. 11 in *Handbook of biological confocal microscopy* (Springer, New York, 2006).

[70] T.R. Corle and G.S. Kino, "Depth and transverse resolution," Chap. 3 in *Confocal scanning optical microscopy and related imaging systems* (Academic Press, San Diego, 1996).

[71] R.R. Krueger, R.A. Applegate, and S. MacRae, *Wavefront customized visual correction: the quest for super vision II* (Thorofare, NJ, 2004).

[72] J.C. Wyant and K. Creath, "Basic wavefront aberration theory for optical metrology," Chap. 1 in *Applied Optics and Optical Engineering*, Vol. XI, Ed. R. R. Shannon and J. C. Wyant (Academic Press, San Diego, CA, 1992).

[73] G. Smith and D.A. Atchison, *The eye and visual optical instruments* (Cambridge University Press, Cambridge, UK, New York, NY, 1997).

[74] J.W. Goodman, *Introduction to Fourier optics*, 3rd ed. (Roberts & Company Publishers, Englewood, CO, 2005).

[75] J. Porter et al., "Monochromatic aberrations of the human eye in a large population," *J. Opt. Soc. Am. A Opt. Image Sci. Vis.* **18**(8), 1793–1803 (2001).

[76] L.N. Thibos et al., "Statistical variation of aberration structure and image quality in a normal population of healthy eyes," *J. Opt. Soc. Am. A Opt. Image Sci. Vis.* **19**(12), 2329–2348 (2002).

[77] N. Doble et al., "Requirements for discrete actuator and segmented wavefront correctors for aberration compensation in two large populations of human eyes," *Appl. Opt.* **46**(20, 4501–4514 (2007).

[78] D. Miller, L. Thibos, and X. Hong, "Requirements for segmented correctors for diffraction-limited performance in the human eye," *Opt. Express* **13**(1), 275–289 (2005).

[79] L. Diaz-Santana, C. Torti, I. Munro, P. Gasson, and C. Dainty, "Benefit of higher closed loop bandwidths in ocular adaptive optics," *Opt. Express* **11**(20), 2597–2605 (2003).

[80] Y. Zhang and A. Roorda, "Evaluating the lateral resolution of the adaptive optics scanning laser ophthalmoscope," *J. Biomed. Opt.* **11**(1), 014002 (2006).

[81] S.A. Burns et al., "Large-field-of-view, modular, stabilized, adaptive-optics-based scanning laser ophthalmoscope," *J. Opt. Soc. Am. A Opt. Image Sci. Vis.* **24**(5), 1313–1326 (2007).

[82] D.C. Chen et al., "High-resolution adaptive optics scanning laser ophthalmoscope with dual deformable mirrors," *J. Opt. Soc. Am. A Opt. Image. Sci. Vis.* **24**(5), 1305–1312 (2007).

[83] Y. Zhang, S. Poonja, and A. Roorda, "MEMS-based adaptive optics scanning laser ophthalmoscopy," *Opt. Lett.* **31**(9), 268–270 (2006).

[84] B. Hermann et al., "Adaptive-optics ultrahigh-resolution optical coherence tomography," *Opt. Lett.* **29**(18), 2142–2144 (2004).

[85] R.J. Zawadzki et al., "Adaptive optics-optical coherence tomography: optimizing visualization of microscopic retinal structures in three dimensions," *J. Op.t Soc. Am. A Opt. Image Sci. Vis.* **24**(5), 1373–1383 (2007).

[86] R.J. Zawadzki et al., "Adaptive-optics optical coherence tomography for high-resolution and high-speed 3D retinal *in vivo* imaging," *Opt. Express* **13**(21), 8532–8546 (2005).

[87] Y. Zhang et al., "High-speed volumetric imaging of cone photoreceptors with adaptive optics spectral-domain optical coherence tomography," *Opt. Express* **14**(10), 4380–4394 (2006).

[88] Y. Zhang et al., "Adaptive optics parallel spectral domain optical coherence tomography for imaging the living retina," *Opt. Express* **13**(12), 4792-4811 (2005).

[89] R.K. Tyson, *Principles of adaptive optics*, 3rd ed. Series in optics and optoelectronics, CRC Press, Boca Raton, FL, 2011.

[90] D. Malacara, *Optical shop testing*, 3rd ed. Wiley series in pure and applied optics, Wiley-Interscience, Hoboken, N.J., 2007.

[91] J. Liang et al., "Objective measurement of wave aberrations of the human eye with the use of a Hartmann-Shack wave-front sensor," *J. Opt. Soc. Am. A Opt. Image Sci. Vis.* **11**(7), 1949–1957 (1994).

[92] E.J. Fernandez, P.M. Prieto, and P. Artal, "Wave-aberration control with a liquid crystal on silicon (LCOS) spatial phase modulator," *Opt. Express* **17**(13), 11013–11025 (2009).

[93] H. Huang, T. Inoue, and H. Tanaka, "Stabilized high-accuracy correction of ocular aberrations with liquid crystal on silicon spatial light modulator in adaptive optics retinal imaging system," *Opt. Express* **19**(16), 15026–15040 (2011).

[94] G.D. Love, "Wave-front correction and production of Zernike modes with a liquid-crystal spatial light modulator," *Appl. Opt.* **36**(7), 1517–1520 (1997).

[95] S. Manzanera et al., "Liquid crystal Adaptive Optics Visual Simulator: Application to testing and design of ophthalmic optical elements," *Opt. Express* **15**(24), 16177–16188 (2007).

[96] T. Shirai, "Liquid-crystal adaptive optics based on feedback interferometry for high-resolution retinal imaging," *Appl. Opt.* **41**(19), 4013–4023 (2002).

[97] F. Vargas-Martin, P.M. Prieto, and P. Artal, "Correction of the aberrations in the human eye with a liquid-crystal spatial light modulator: limits to performance," *J. Opt. Soc. Am. A Opt. Image Sci. Vis.* **15**(9), 2552–2562 (1998).

[98] S. Ooto et al, "High-resolution imaging of the photoreceptor layer in epiretinal membrane using adaptive optics scanning laser ophthalmoscopy," *Ophthalmology* **118**(5), 873–881 (2011).

[99] A.W. Dreher, J.F. Bille, and R.N. Weinreb, "Active optical depth resolution improvement of the laser tomographic scanner," *Appl. Opt.* **28**(4), 804-808 (1989).

[100] E.J. Fernandez, I. Iglesias, and P. Artal, "Closed-loop adaptive optics in the human eye," *Opt. Lett.* **26**(10), 746–748 (2001).

[101] N. Doble et al., "Use of a microelectromechanical mirror for adaptive optics in the human eye," *Opt. Lett.* **27**(17), 1537–1539 (2002).

[102] T.G. Bifano, J.A. Perreault, P.A. Bierden, and C.E. Dimas, "Micromachined deformable mirrors for adaptive optics," in *Proc. SPIE: High Resolution Wavefront Control: Methods, Devices, and Applications IV*, J.D. Gonglewski, M.A. Vorontsov, M.T. Gruneisen, S.R. Restaino, and R.K. Tyson, Eds., **4825**, 10–13, Bellingham, WA (2002).

[103] J.A. Perreault, T.G. Bifano, B.M. Levine, and M. Horenstein, "Adaptive optic correction using microelectromechanical deformable mirrors," *Optical Engineering* **41**, 561–566 (2002).

[104] Center for Visual Science, University of Rochester, Bioengineering Research Partnership, http://www.cvs.rochester.edu/brp/index.html. 2007-04-12.

[105] D.C. Gray et al., "*In vivo* fluorescence imaging of primate retinal ganglion cells and retinal pigment epithelial cells," *Opt. Express* **14**(16), 144–158 (2006).

[106] E.J. Fernandez et al., "Adaptive optics with a magnetic deformable mirror: applications in the human eye," *Opt. Express* **14**(20), 8900–8917 (2006).

[107] A. Dubra and Y. Sulai, "Reflective afocal broadband adaptive optics scanning ophthalmoscope," *Biomed. Opt. Express* **2**(6), 1757–1768 (2011).

[108] A. Dubra et al., "Noninvasive imaging of the human rod photoreceptor mosaic using a confocal adaptive optics scanning ophthalmoscope," *Biomed. Opt. Express* **2**(7), 1864–1876 (2011).

[109] Y. Zhang, X. Wang, R.A. Myers, J.J. Alexander, T. Ye, A. Roorda, P.D. Gamlin, "Broad-spectrum adaptive optics scanning laser ophthalmoscopy," *Invest. Ophthalmol. Vis. Sci.* **52**, ARVO E-Abstract(5869) (2011).

[110] Y. Zhang, X. Wang, J. Wang, "High-speed adaptive optics scanning laser ophthalmoscope (AOSLO)," *Invest. Ophthalmol. Vis. Sci.* **52**, ARVO E-Abstract(2311) (2010).

[111] S. Ooto et al., "High-resolution imaging of resolved central serous chorioretinopathy using adaptive optics scanning laser ophthalmoscopy," *Ophthalmology* **117** (9), 1800–1809 (2010).

[112] S. Ooto et al., "High-resolution photoreceptor imaging in idiopathic macular telangiectasia type 2 using adaptive optics scanning laser ophthalmoscopy," *Invest. Ophthalmol. Vis. Sci.* **52** (8), 5541–5550 (2011).

[113] S. Ooto et al., "Photoreceptor damage and foveal sensitivity in surgically closed macular holes: an adaptive optics scanning laser ophthalmoscopy study," *Am. J. Ophthalmol.* (2012).

[114] S.Ooto, M. Hangai, and N. Yoshimura, "Photoreceptor restoration in unilateral acute idiopathic maculopathy on adaptive optics scanning laser ophthalmoscopy," *Arch. Ophthalmol.* **129**(12), 1633-1635 (2011).

[115] C. Boyer, V. Michau, and G. Rousset, "Adaptive optics: Interaction matrix measurements and real time control algorithms for the COME-ON project," *Proc. SPIE* **1271**, 63–81 (1990).

[116] W. Jiang, H. Li, "Hartmann-Shack wavefront sensing and wavefront control algorithm," in *Adaptive Optics and Optical Structures. Proc. SPIE* **1271**, 82–93 (1990).

[117] K.Y. Li et al., "Comparison of control algorithms for a MEMS-based adaptive optics scanning laser ophthalmoscope," *Proc. Am. Control. Conf.* **2009**, 3848–3853 (2009).

[118] C. Li et al., "A correction algorithm to simultaneously control dual deformable mirrors in a woofer-tweeter adaptive optics system," *Opt. Express* **18**(16), 16671–1684 (2010).

[119] W. Zou and S.A. Burns, "High-accuracy wavefront control for retinal imaging with adaptive-influence-matrix adaptive optics," *Opt. Express* **17**(22), 20167–20177 (2009).

[120] W. Zou, and S.A. Burns, "Testing of Lagrange multiplier damped least-squares control algorithm for woofer-tweeter adaptive optics," *Appl. Opt.* **51**(9), 1198–1208 (2012).

[121] W. Zou, X. Qi, and S.A. Burns, "Wavefront-aberration sorting and correction for a dual-deformable-mirror adaptive-optics system," *Opt. Lett.* **33**(22), 2602–2604 (2008).

[122] W. Zou, X. Qi, and S.A. Burns, "Woofer-tweeter adaptive optics scanning laser ophthalmoscopic imaging based on Lagrange-multiplier damped least-squares algorithm," *Biomed. Opt. Express* **2**(7), 1986–2004 (2011).

[123] W. Zou et al., "Improving wavefront boundary condition for *in vivo* high resolution adaptive optics ophthalmic imaging," *Biomed. Opt. Express* **2**(12), 3309–3320 (2011).

[124] Y. Geng et al., "Adaptive optics retinal imaging in the living mouse eye," *Biomed. Op. Express* **3**(4), 715–734 (2012).

[125] J.J. Hunter et al., "Images of photoreceptors in living primate eyes using adaptive optics two-photon ophthalmoscopy," *Biomed. Opt. Express* **2**(1), 139–148 (2010).

[126] D. Merino et al., "Observation of cone and rod photoreceptors in normal subjects and patients using a new generation adaptive optics scanning laser ophthalmoscope," *Biomed. Opt. Express* **2**(8), 2189–2201 (2011).

[127] F. Romero-Borja et al., "Optical slicing of human retinal tissue *in vivo* with the adaptive optics scanning laser ophthalmoscope," *Appl. Opt.* **44**(19),4032–4040 (2005).

[128] Y. Zhang, S. Poonja, and A. Roorda, "AOSLO: from benchtop to clinic," *Proc. SPIE*, **6306**, 63060V (2006).

[129] N.M. Putnam et al., "Modeling the foveal cone mosaic imaged with adaptive optics scanning laser ophthalmoscopy," *Opt. Express* **18**(24), 24902–24916 (2010).

[130] Y. Zhang and A. Roorda, "Photon signal detection and evaluation in the adaptive optics scanning laser ophthalmoscope," *J. Opt. Soc. Am. A Opt. Image Sci. Vis.* **24**(5), 1276–1283 (2007).

[131] D.C. Gray et al., "*In vivo* imaging of the fine structure of rhodamine-labeled macaque retinal ganglion cells," *Invest. Ophthalmol. Vis. Sci.* **49**(1), 467–473 (2008).

[132] J.I. Morgan et al., "*In vivo* autofluorescence imaging of the human and macaque retinal pigment epithelial cell mosaic," *Invest. Ophthalmol. Vis. Sci.* **50**(3), 1350–1359 (2009).

[133] Y. Geng et al., "*In vivo* imaging of microscopic structures in the rat retina," *Invest. Ophthalmol. Vis. Sci.* **50**(12), 5872–5879 (2009).

[134] Y. Geng et al., "Optical properties of the mouse eye," *Biomed. Opt. Express* **2**(4), 717–738 (2011).

[135] K. Grieve and A. Roorda, "Intrinsic signals from human cone photoreceptors," *Invest. Ophthalmol. Vis. Sci.* **49**(2), 713–719 (2008).

[136] K. Grieve, P. Tiruveedhula, Y. Zhang, and A. Roorda, "Functional imaging with the multi-wavelength adaptive optics scanning laser ophthalmoscope," *Proc. SPIE* **6426**, 64261M, (2007)

[137] Y. Zhang, P. Tiruveedhula, L. Sincich, J. Horton, and A. Roorda, "Adaptive optics scanning laser ophthalmoscope (AOSLO) for precise visual stimulus presentation," *Journal of Vision* **15**, article 116 (2007).

[138] L.C. Sincich et al., "Resolving single cone inputs to visual receptive fields," *Nat. Neurosci.* **12**(8), 967–969 (2009).

[139] J.L. Duncan et al., "High-resolution imaging with adaptive optics in patients with inherited retinal degeneration," *Invest. Ophthalmol. Vis. Sci.* **48**(7), 3283–3291 (2007).

[140] M. Mkrtchyan et al., "Outer retinal structure in patients with acute zonal occult outer retinopathy," *Am. J. Ophthalmol.* **153**(4), 757–768 (2012).

[141] Y. Chen et al., "Cone photoreceptor abnormalities correlate with vision loss in patients with Stargardt disease," *Invest. Ophthalmol. Vis. Sci.* **52**(6), 3281–3292 (2011).

[142] M.K. Yoon et al., "Adaptive optics scanning laser ophthalmoscopy images in a family with the mitochondrial DNA T8993C mutation," *Invest. Ophthalmol. Vis. Sci.* **50**(4), 1838–1847 (2009).

[143] A. Roorda, Y. Zhang, and J.L. Duncan, "High-resolution in vivo imaging of the RPE mosaic in eyes with retinal disease," *Invest. Ophthalmol. Vis. Sci.* **48**(5), 2297-2303 (2007).

15

Intrinsic Optical Signal Imaging of Retinal Function at Cellular Resolution

Xin-Cheng Yao

Department of Biomedical Engineering, Vision Sciences Research Center, University of Alabama at Birmingham, Birmingham, AL

This chapter discusses intrinsic optical signal (IOS) monitoring of functional activities in the retina. Basic principles of IOS imaging instruments and data processing algorithms are described. Stimulus-evoked IOS responses in retinal photoreceptors and inner neurons are reviewed. Both *ex-vivo* and *in-vivo* IOS experiments are presented. Potential applications of the IOS imaging technology for retinal study and disease diagnosis are discussed.

Key words: intrinsic optical signal (IOS), near infrared (NIR), retina, photoreceptor, ganglion cell, inner neuron, electrophysiology, electroretinogram (ERG), confocal microscopy, optical coherence tomography (OCT)

15.1 Introduction

In the retina, multiple types of photoreceptors and inner neurons function together as a complex neural network to provide sensitive detection of light energy and preliminary processing of visual information. Different eye diseases, such as glaucoma [1–3], age-related macular degeneration (AMD) [4–7], diabetic retinopathy [8, 9], retinitis pigmentosa (RP) [10], etc., are known to target different types of retinal cells, causing localized lesions or cell loss at early stage of the disease. Early detection of eye diseases and reliable evaluation of treatment outcomes require high resolution examination of retinal function.

Morphological evaluation of the retina, such as conventional fundus examination, can provide valuable information for disease diagnosis and treatment evaluation. Recently emerging adaptive optics and optical coherence tomography (OCT) provide improved imaging resolution for morphological evaluation, and even allow quantitative assessment of individual retinal cells and/or functional layers. However, morphological and functional changes in the retina are not always directly correlated [6, 11, 12], in terms of time course and spatial location. Electroretinogram (ERG) [13], focal ERG [26], multifocal ERG [14, 15], perimetry [16, 17], etc., have been established for functional examination of the retina. However, spatial resolution and signal selectivity of ERG and perimetry may not be high enough to provide precise separation of outer and inner retinal cell dysfunctions. Given the delicate structures and complicated functional interactions of the retina, detection of localized dysfunction of different cell populations requires a method that can examine stimulus-evoked retinal activities at high spatial and temporal resolutions. While it is possible to combine morphological (e.g., high resolution OCT) with functional (e.g., ERG) evaluation [18] to improve retinal study and disease diagnosis, conducting these separate measurements is time-consuming and cost-inefficient.

Intrinsic optical signal (IOS) imaging promises a method for concurrent morphological and functional evaluation of the retina at high spatial resolution. Stimulus-evoked transient IOSs have been used for spatiotemporal mapping of dynamic brain activities [19–27]. Without the requirement of exogenous biomarkers, IOS imaging is label-free and totally noninvasive. Recently, several imaging techniques have been demonstrated for IOS imaging of stimulus-evoked retinal activation. Conventional fundus cameras were modified to detect IOSs in anesthetized animals, such as cats [28], macaques [29, 30], as well as awake humans [31]. Functional optical coherence tomography (OCT) [32–35], confocal microscopy [36–38], and adaptive optics [39–41] systems were used to improve spatial resolution of IOS imaging in isolated animal retinas [32, 33, 37, 38], intact animals [34, 36] and living humans [35].

Although IOS recordings have been successfully demonstrated [31, 34, 39, 40, 42], practical applications of IOS imaging for retinal study and diagnosis is presently challenged by its complexity and inconsistency, in terms of time courses and signal polarities, of reported IOSs. In principle, both stimulus-evoked retinal neural activity and corresponding hemodynamic and metabolic changes can produce transient IOSs associated with retinal stimulation. While hemodynamic and metabolic changes [31, 42] associated IOSs can provide important information in healthy assessment of the visual system, they are relatively slow and cannot directly track fast neural activities in the retina. Fast IOSs, which have time courses comparable to electrophysiological kinetics, are desirable for direct evaluation of the physiological health of photoreceptors and inner neurons. Fast IOSs closely associated with action potentials and postsynaptic potentials have been observed in stimulus-activated neural tissue [43, 44]. Signal sources and mechanisms of fast IOSs in neural tissues have been discussed by Rector [45] and others [43, 44, 46–48]. Briefly, several processes, e.g. neurotransmitter secretion [49], reorientation of membrane proteins and phospholipids [43, 44, 50], and refractive index change of neural tissues [51] associated with neural activity, have been proposed as possible mechanisms of fast IOSs observed in neural tissues. Water influx in response to ionic currents through gated channels during depolarization causes cellular swelling that can also produce light scattering [46, 47, 52, 53] and polarization changes [48] in stimulus activated neurons.

It was generally believed previously that fast IOSs correlated with stimulus-evoked neural activity were inherently tiny signals only obtainable at high background light intensity and difficult for practical applications. However, using optimized near infrared (NIR) light illumination, improved imaging resolution, sophisticated retinal stimulation and data processing, we recently demonstrated fast IOS imaging of stimulus-evoked activities in the retina. Both *ex vivo* [32, 37, 38, 54–60] and *in vivo* [36] preparations were used to characterize the correlation between IOS responses and electrophysiological kinetics.

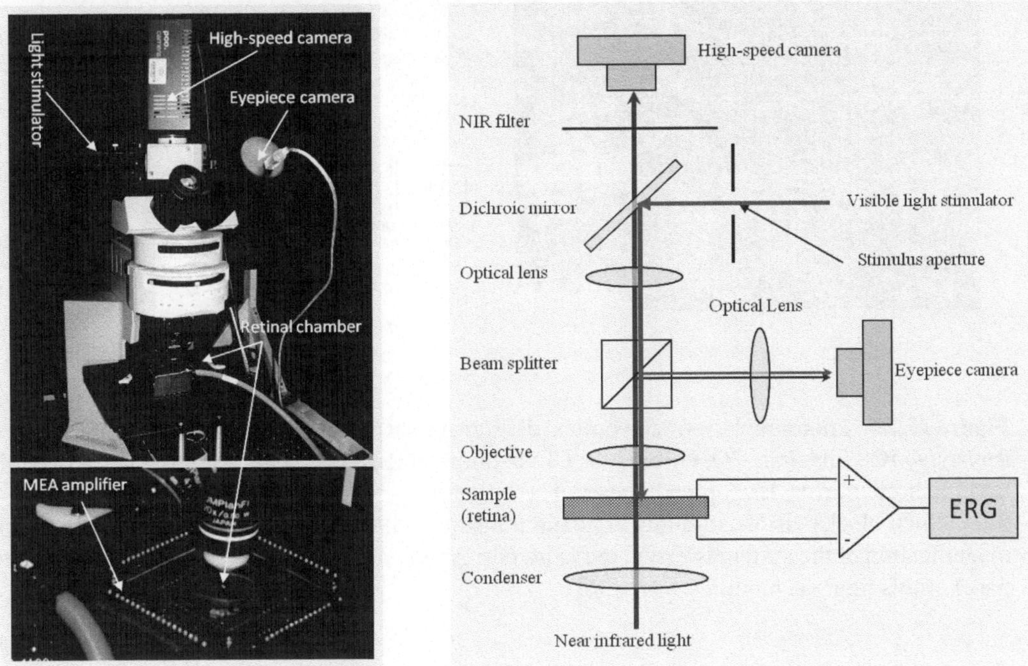

Figure 15.1: Photograph (left) and optical diagram (right) of a NIR light microscope for *ex vivo* IOS imaging. During measurements, isolated frog retina is illuminated continuously by the NIR light. The visible light stimulator is used to produce visible light flashes for retinal stimulation. A 60 channel multiple electrode array (MEA) system is used for concurrent ERG measurement of retinal activation. The dichroic mirror reflects visible stimulus light and passes the NIR recording light. The high-speed camera is used for IOS imaging, and the eyepiece camera is used to adjust visible light stimulus aperture at the retina. In order to ensure light efficiency for intrinsic optical signal imaging, the beam splitter is removed from the optical path after the visible light stimulator is adjusted. The NIR filter before the high-speed camera is used to block visible stimulus light, and allow the NIR probe light to reach the detector for recording stimulus-evoked IOSs. (This figure is modified from [58]).

15.2 IOS Imaging Setups

Several imaging modalities, including conventional light microscope [54–57], confocal microscope [36–38] and OCT [32] has been validated for fast IOS imaging of retinal activation. Representative *ex vivo* and *in vivo* IOS imaging systems are discussed as follows.

15.2.1 *Ex vivo* imaging system

Figure 15.1 shows representative system for *ex vivo* IOS imaging of retinal tissues. As shown in Fig. 15.1, a conventional microscope can be modified for transmitted light microscopy of dynamic IOSs in stimulus activated isolated retinas. The IOS imaging system consists of two (i.e., NIR and visible) light sources. The NIR light is used for IOS recording, and the visible light is used for retinal stimulation. The NIR light is produced by a 12-V 100-W halogen lamp (PHILIPS7724) with a band-pass filter (wavelength band: 800–1000 nm) in front, and the visible light stimulator

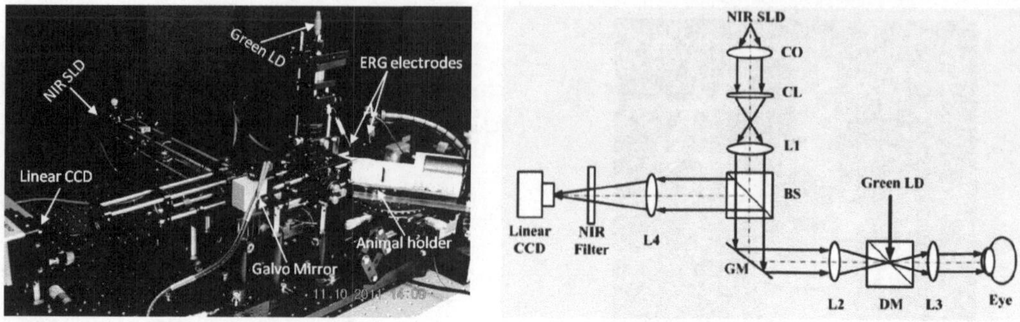

Figure 15.2: Photograph (left) and optical diagram (right) of a line-scan confocal ophthalmoscope for *in vivo* IOS imaging. CO: collimator; CL: cylindrical lens; BS: beam splitter; GM: galvo mirror; DM: dichroic mirror; Lx: optical lenses. The NIR filter, in front of the linear CCD, is a long-pass filter which blocks visible stimulus light and transmits NIR light reflected from the retina. Optical magnification of the system is estimated ∼14, corresponding to 1 μm/pixel in retinal image. (Right panel of this figure is modified from [36]).

is a fiber-coupled green light emitting diode (LED) with the central wavelength at 505 nm. The overall power of the NIR light delivered at the retina is typically ∼ 1mW. The high speed camera is used for IOS imaging, and the eyepiece camera is used to adjust visible light stimulus pattern at the retina. Both high resolution charge coupled device (CCD) 54, 55] and complementary metal-oxide-semiconductor (CMOS) [59, 60] cameras have been validated for IOS imaging at sub-cellular resolution. The CCD camera ((PCO1600, PCO AG, Kelheim, Germany) can provide 12.5 ms (80 Hz) temporal resolution (Figs. 15.4 and 15.5), while the high speed CMOS camera (PCO1200, PCO AG, Kelheim, Germany) can provide 1 ms (1000 Hz) temporal resolution (Figs. 15.6–15.11).

15.2.2 *In vivo* imaging system

Figure 15.2 shows a line-scan confocal ophthalmoscope for *in vivo* IOS imaging of intact animals [36]. In this system, a fast linear CCD camera (SG-11-01k80-00R, DALSA), with pixel size of 14 μm × 14 μm and pixel sampling rate up to 80 MHz, is employed to achieve high-speed and high-resolution imaging. A NIR (center wavelength: 830 nm; bandwidth: 60 nm) superluminescent laser diode (SLD) (SLD-35-HP, Superlum) is used for IOS imaging, and a green light-emitting diode (LED) is used for retinal stimulation. The cylindrical lens (CL) condenses the NIR recording light in one dimension to produce a focused line illumination, which is conjugated with the retina and linear CCD. Lateral and axial resolutions of the system are theoretically estimated ∼1 μm and ∼10 μm, respectively.

15.3 IOS Data Processing

The purpose of IOS data processing is to calculate dynamic optical changes relative to pre-stimulus baseline. Basic IOS images can be reconstructed through following procedures [56]:

1. The raw images (e.g., Fig. 15.4a) from the pre-stimulus baseline recording phase is averaged,

pixel by pixel, and the averaged intensity of each pixel is taken as the background intensity I of each pixel.

2. The background intensity I is subtracted from each subsequent recorded frame, pixel by pixel, to get the dynamic light change, ΔI, of each pixel.
3. The $\Delta I/I$ images (e.g., Fig. 15.4b) are reconstructed to show the dynamic optical changes correlated with retinal activation.

Dynamic differential IOS data processing can act as a high-pass filter to separate fast IOS from slow optical changes in activated tissues [60]. Dynamic differential IOS images (e.g., Fig. 15.7b) can be constructed [61]:

$$IOS_{t(x,y)} = \frac{I_{t(x,y)} - I_{ref(x,y)}}{I_{ref(x,y)}} \tag{15.1}$$

where $I_{t(x,y)}$ is the intensity value of a pixel (x,y) at a time point t; $I_{ref(x,y)}$ is the dynamic reference baseline of m consecutive frames, which can be quantified by:

$$I_{ref(x,y)} = \frac{\sum_{i=t-m}^{i=t-1} I_{i(x,y)}}{m} \tag{15.2}$$

In other words, the averaged pixel value of m consecutive frames recorded before the time point t is used as a reference baseline to calculate the differential IOS. For the dynamic differential IOSs shown in this chapter (Figs. 15.7–15.9), we selected $m = 100$ (i.e., images recorded over 100 ms) for the dynamic reference baseline. Based on the IOS image sequence, stimulus-evoked retinal dynamics can be analyzed with μm spatial resolution and ms temporal resolution.

15.4 *Ex Vivo* IOS Imaging

Freshly isolated retinas, free from the complications of hemodynamic changes and eye movements, provide a simple preparation for investigating the sources and mechanisms of fast IOSs, which is essential for optimizing the design of retinal imaging instruments. Both amphibian (frog and salamander) and mammalian (mouse) retinas have been used to characterize fast IOSs correlated with retinal activation. In order to simply the description, all IOS images shown in this article were collected from Leopard frog (*Rana Pipiens*) retinas.

15.4.1 Preparation of isolated retinas

Leopard frogs (*Rana Pipiens*) were used for IOS imaging of the retina. All experiments were performed following protocols approved by the Institutional Animal Care and Use Committee of the University of Alabama at Birmingham. 20–30 minutes dark-adaptation was typically implemented before the dissection of the retina. During the experiment, the frog was rapidly euthanized by decapitation and double pithing before the eyes were removed. The procedure was conducted in a dark room with dim red illumination. The dissection of the retina was performed in Ringer's solution containing (in mM) [62]: 110 NaCl, 2.5 KCl, 1.6 $MgCl_2$, 1.0 $CaCl_2$, 22 $NaHCO_3$, and 10 D-glucose. After removing the intact eye, we hemisected the globe below the equator with fine scissors to remove the lens and anterior structures before removing the retina without retinal pigment epithelium (RPE). Finally, the retina was transferred into the recording chamber for optical imaging. During the recording, the retina was immersed in a chamber filled with Ringer's solution.

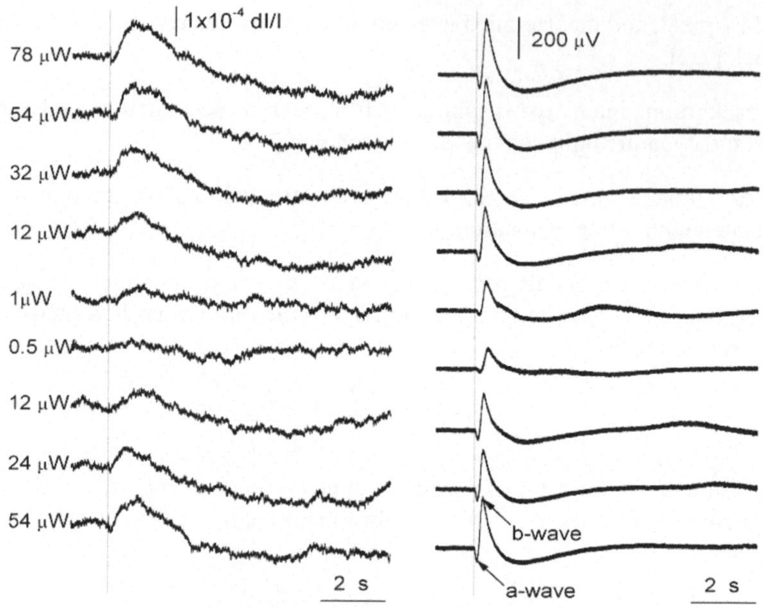

Figure 15.3: Single-channel transmission recording of integral IOS responses corresponding to stimulus intensities (0.5–78 μW). The experiment employed a custom-built microscope with optical configuration similar to the system shown in Fig. 15.1. A high sensitivity photodiode (UDT-555UV/LN, UDT Sensors, Hawthorne, CA) was used for IOS recording. Illumination source was a single high output LED at ~950 nm. Left panel illustrates optical responses, measured in a transmitted light geometry. Right panel illustrates the corresponding electrophysiological changes measured with electrodes above and below the retina. The light stimulus was a 0.1 ms flash that covered the entire retina. Each trace was from a single pass trial. (This figure is from reference [55]).

The retina was pressed to the bottom of the sample chamber with moderate pressure using a micromesh sheet [32]. Both flat mount intact retinas and retinal slices have been tested. Flat-mounted retinas provided a simple preparation for depth-resolved mapping of neural activities at individual functional layers [56]; while sliced retinas allowed parallel monitoring of visual signal propagation from the photoreceptors to inner retinal neurons [59].

15.4.2 Photodiode recording of integral IOS response in flat-mount retina

In our early experiments, a single-channel recording system, i.e., using a fast photodiode to replace the high-speed camera in Fig. 15.1, was used to demonstrate and optimize NIR light detection of retinal response. Several coherent and incoherent light sources for IOS recoding were compared. Our experiments indicated that the signal-to-noise ratio (SNR) of optical measurements using an incoherent light source, such as a NIR light-emitting diode (LED) or a halogen lamp with NIR filter as shown in Fig. 15.1, was at least 3 times better than optical measurements with coherent light sources, such as a NIR laser diode [55]. With an incoherent NIR light source, clear IOSs from single pass measurements could routinely be recorded. The magnitude peak of IOSs recorded by the fast photodiode was at the level of 10^{-4} $\Delta I/I$ (Fig. 15.3). Small magnitude of the transient optical response agreed with previous photodiode measurements of IOSs in the retina [63, 64] and other neural tissue. [43, 44, 46, 48, 65]. Both a-wave (negative peak) and b-wave (positive peak) could be clearly recorded in simultaneous electrophysiological measurements (right panel, Fig. 15.3), but

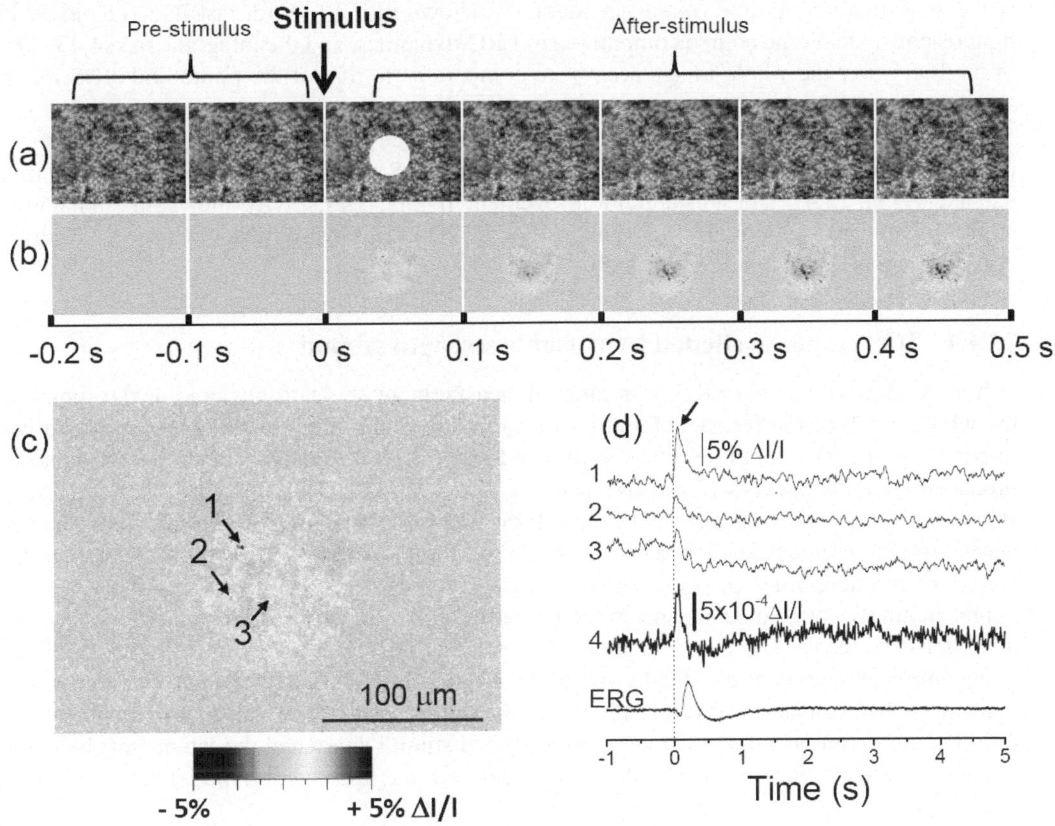

Figure 15.4: High resolution imaging of IOSs in isolated frog retina. (a) Representative raw image sequence of the retina, without differential processing. The images were recorded with a CCD camera at a speed of 80 frames/s. The white spot in the third frame shows the visible stimulus pattern. (b) IOS images. Each illustrated frame is an average over 100 ms interval (8 frames). 200 ms pre-stimulus and 500 ms post-stimulus images are shown. (c) Enlarged image of the third frame shown in (b). (d) Temporal changes of IOSs. The numbered traces 1–3 are representative IOSs of individual pixels, corresponding to arrowheads 1–3 showing retinal points in (c). Trace 4 is averaged optical responses of the whole image area. Vertical lines indicate the stimulus onset. (This figure is from reference [58]).

a positive-going (increasing) NIR transmitted light change dominated the corresponding IOSs (left panel, Fig. 15.3). Both IOS and ERG magnitudes changed corresponding to different stimulus intensities. All IOS and ERG recordings were collected from the same retina, with $\sim$ 2-minutes time interval between two traces in sequence (from top to bottom).

15.4.3 High resolution IOS imaging of flat-mount retina

Although the photodiode recording, which detected the integral optical response of the retina, was dominated by a positive IOS (Fig. 15.3), high resolution IOS imaging disclosed both negative (decreasing) and positive (increasing) signals (Fig. 15.4). In Figure 15.4, both fast and slow IOSs can be observed. While the fast optical response could reach a magnitude peak (arrowheads, Fig. 15.4d) within tens of milliseconds after the stimulus delivery; slow components of the transient IOSs lasted a relatively long time (many seconds). As shown in Fig. 15.4d, fast IOS (i.e., early-phase light response) had time course comparable to ERG dynamics, and the integral (trace 4, Fig. 15.4d) of the IOSs over the whole image area were comparable to that of the photodiode IOS recording shown in Fig. 15.3.

Given the fact that high resolution imaging could differentiate localized IOSs with opposite (positive and negative) polarities, it is noteworthy that large IOSs could often exceed 5% $\Delta I/I$ in individual pixels (Fig. 15.4). The substantial improvement in optical sensitivity allows functional imaging with sub-cellular resolution in single passes [54, 55]. Optical sensitivity could improve further with dark-filed and polarization imaging [55].

15.4.4 IOS response elicited by variable strength stimuli

It is well known that the ERG is an integral measurement of electrophysiological responses over the whole depth of the retina. Similarly, transmission microscopy of the IOSs may also consist of contributions from multiple retinal layers and cells. Stimulus-activated frog retinas consistently produced complex patterns of positive and negative IOSs [32, 54, 55]. While low light strength stimuli activated positive-going (increasing) IOSs first [57]; strengthened stimuli elicited additional negative-going (decreasing) responses (Fig. 15.5). Further strengthened stimuli shortened the latencies of the magnitude peaks of both negative-going and positive going responses. Given the nonlinear amplification mechanisms in the retina [66–68], the positive-going responses activated by low light stimulus may be partly related to second- or third-order neurons in the retina. Negative-going dominant responses elicited by strengthened stimulus may reflect increasing contributions of dynamic IOSs associated with light phototransduction procedures in activated photoreceptors [63, 69]. The observed phenomenon that a strengthened stimuli shortened the latency of the negative-going response to reach the amplitude peak agrees with the transduction model proposed by Lamb et al. [70].

15.4.5 Depth-resolved IOS imaging

By adjusting the axial (depth) location of the NIR imaging plane, IOS images could be recorded from the photoreceptor, inner nuclear (middle), and ganglion layers [56]. Using a step (1 s) visible light stimulus to activate the retina, both ON and OFF responses correlated with the stimulus onset and offset could be observed (Fig. 15.6). A rapid on-going phase of the IOSs began within 5 ms after the stimulus onset (Fig. 15.6b). Both positive (increasing) and negative (decreasing) IOSs were observed at the photoreceptor and inner layers of the retina. The distribution of IOSs with opposite polarities showed a center-surround pattern. At the photoreceptor layer, negative IOSs dominated the center area illuminated by the stimulus light spot, and positive signals dominated the surrounding area. At the inner retinal layers, on the other hand, positive IOSs dominated the center area covered by the stimulus light spot, and negative IOSs were mainly observed in the surrounding area.

Our preliminary studies [56, 57] suggest that major negative IOSs observed in the retina may relate to dynamic phototransduction procedures of photoreceptors, and that positive IOSs result primarily from the inner retinal neurons. In principle, when the NIR probe light is focused on the photoreceptor layer, the IOS image should be dominated by the IOSs produced by the photoreceptors. Although cross-talk response (defocused transmitted or scattered light) of the IOSs from other layers may also enter the CCD/CMOS imaging device, these light photons should spread (blurred) over a relatively larger area. In comparison, the IOSs directly originating in the photoreceptor layer were in focus. Whenever the NIR probe light is focused at the inner retinal layers, the intrinsic optical signal image should be dominated by the IOSs originating at the corresponding retinal depth. Thus, the positive IOSs in the surrounding area of the photoreceptor layer may result from the defocused IOSs associated with the responses of inner retinal neurons; while the negative IOSs in the

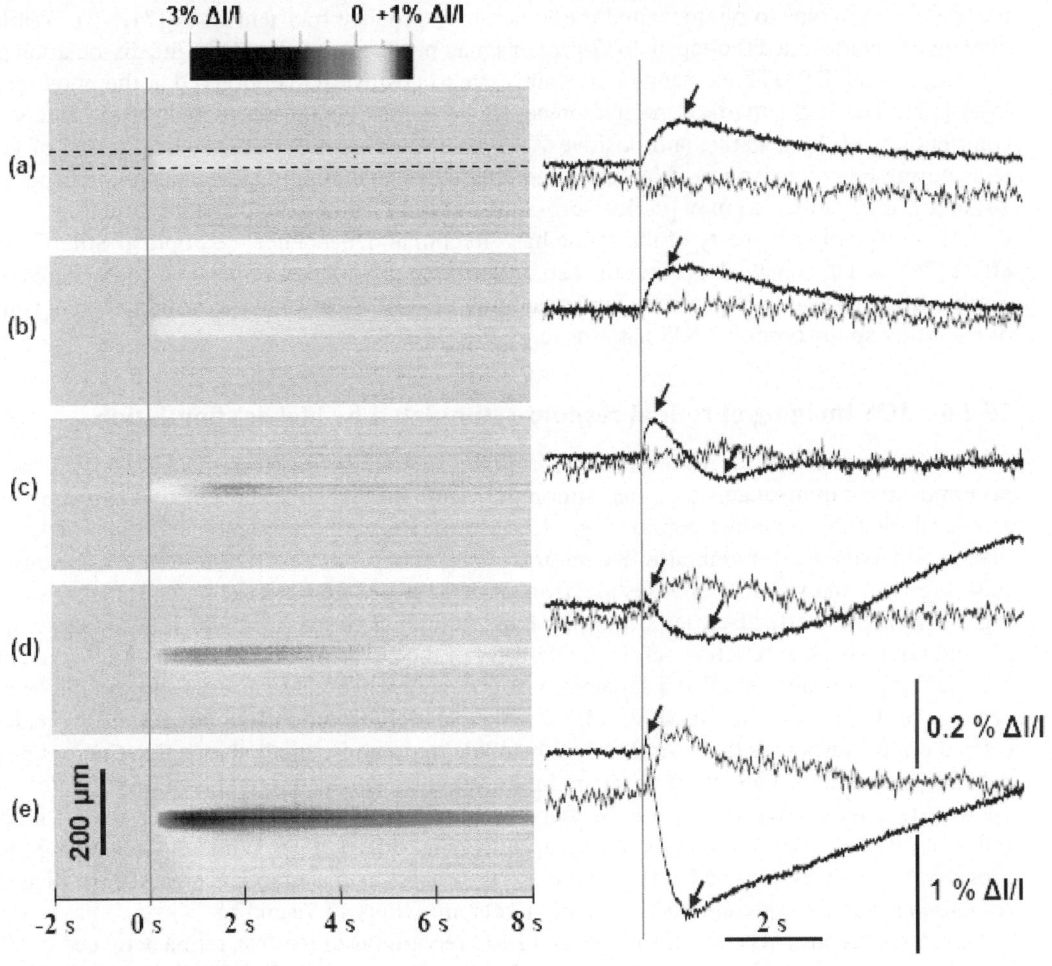

Figure 15.5: (See color insert.) IOSs elicited by variable strength stimuli. Left: M-sequence images of IOSs. Right: Black traces and red traces represent temporal changes of averaged IOSs of the stimulus covered retinal area (the area between the two dashed lines indicated in the left of panel a) and not stimulus covered area, respectively. Raw CCD images were acquired at 80 frames/s. The visible light stimuli were 8×10^{-6}(a), 8×10^{-5} (b), 8×10^{-4} (c), 8×10^{-3} (d), and 8×10^{-2} μJ (e), respectively. The top image sequence (a) was recorded first and the following sequences were recorded at 2-min intervals. The vertical lines indicate the onset of the stimuli. Green and blue arrows in the right panels indicate amplitude peaks of positive and negative IOSs, respectively. (This figure is from reference [57]).

surrounding area of the inner retinal layers may result from the defocused IOSs associated with photoreceptor response. In comparison with the inner nuclear layer, the negative IOSs at the ganglion layer spread over a relatively larger area, but with decreased signal amplitude. This agrees with the fact that the ganglion layer is at a relatively larger distance from the photoreceptor layer, and thus the light from the photoreceptor layer may be defocused (blurred) over a relatively larger area.

However, multiple other sources and mechanisms can contribute to the production and distribution of these positive and negative IOSs. Previous studies have disclosed that both binding and release of G-proteins to photoexcited rhodopsin may produce transient IOSs [71, 72]. While the binding of photoexcited rhodopsin to G-proteins may produce negative IOSs, the dissociation of the complex upon GDP/GTP exchange may contribute to positive IOSs observed at the photoreceptor layer [72]. The IOS pattern of the photoreceptor layer may also result partially from antagonistic contributions of the negative and positive IOSs associated with dynamic redistribution of G proteins during retinal activation. Moreover, the optical waveguiding property of photoreceptors [73, 74] and Muller cells [75] may produce cross-talk of the IOSs among different retinal layers. The optical waveguiding property of the retina has directional dependence, i.e., optical Stile-Crawford effect [76], and thus may also affect the center-surround distribution of positive and negative IOSs. Further investigation is required for understanding the effects of center-surround antagonism [77] of the retina on the observed IOS patterns (e.g., Fig. 15.6).

15.4.6 IOS imaging of retinal response stimulated by flicker stimulation

Both fast and slow IOSs were observed in Figs. 15.4–15.6. As shown in Fig. 15.6b, fast IOS occurred almost immediately (< 5 ms) after retinal stimulation, while some slow IOS did not totally recover during the recording period (Figs. 15.4–15.6). Recently, we combined retinal flicker stimulation and dynamic differential IOS data processing to separate fast IOS from slow IOS response [60]. Fig. 15.7 shows IOS responses in a frog retina activated by 1 Hz visible light flicker stimulus. Fig. 15.7a consistently discloses slow, high magnitude IOS component, which lasted much longer and did not go back to baseline before the delivery of the next stimulus flash (Fig. 15.7d). Dynamic differential processing revealed a separate, fast IOS component that closely followed the temporal changes of the flicker stimulus (Fig. 15.7b). High spatial resolution IOS images also revealed localized optical responses that correlated with cellular structures, and both positive (increasing) and negative (decreasing) IOSs were observed in the stimulus activated retinal area (Fig. 15.7c). Overall, the first stimulus flash evoked IOSs that were dominantly positive-going, and IOSs elicited by following flashes were dominantly negative-going (Fig. 15.7b, d–f). While the negative-going response was primarily confined to the center of the stimulus activated retinal area, the positive-going response appeared to spread into a relatively larger area (Figs.15.7a and b).

Figure 15.8 represents concurrent IOS and ERG recordings of the frog retina activated by flicker stimuli from 1.0 to 6.0 Hz. As shown in Fig. 15.8, the time courses of both IOS and ERG responses were tightly correlated with the flicker stimulus. In order to ensure the repeatability of the IOSs, two experimental trials were conducted at each stimulus frequency. The results shown in Fig. 15.8c and Fig. 15.8d indicate that both IOS and ERG responses were very repeatable. The experiments demonstrated that the dynamic differential IOSs can follow flicker stimuli up to at least 6 Hz. For higher frequency flickers (4 and 6 Hz), an additional OFF response (arrowheads in Fig. 15.8c) was detected in both IOS and ERG signals. For the 6 Hz flicker stimulus, the IOS and ERG OFF response reached their magnitude peaks at $\sim$350 ms and $\sim$325 ms after the onset of the last flash, respectively. Dynamic differential IOS imaging consistently showed positive and negative optical responses. Fig. 15.8c shows that the fast IOSs in response to the first visible light flash was positive-going, and the fast IOSs elicited by the following flashes were negative-going IOSs. The peak magnitude (4.1–4.5%) and the time-to-peak ($\sim$120 ms) of the fast IOS response evoked by the first stimulus flash are almost constant across the stimulus frequencies (1–6 Hz). However, the magnitude and time delay of the IOS responses evoked by following flashes were gradually reduced with increasing stimulus frequency (Figs. 15.9b and c).

Similar electrophysiological changes were also observed in concurrent ERG recording (Fig. 15.8c). In each retinal flicker measurement, the first visible light flash typically evoked a rapid (time-to-peak: $\sim$100 ms), but low magnitude, negative (decreasing) a-wave which was followed by a high magnitude positive (increasing) b-wave (Fig. 15.8c and Fig. 15.9d). The ERG signals elicited by the following flashes were mainly positive b-waves (Fig. 15.8c). The time-to-peak ($\sim$110 ms) of the ERG a-wave evoked by the first stimulus flash is constant across the stimulus frequencies (1–6

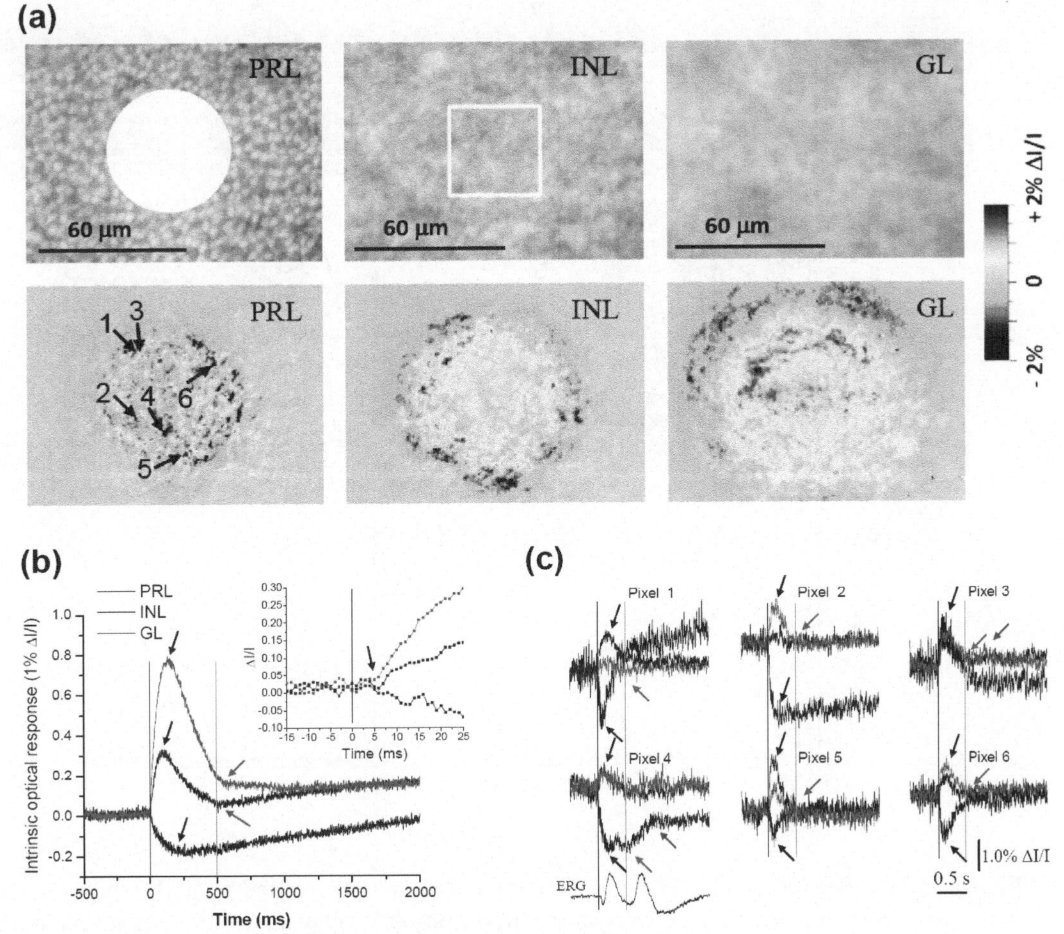

Figure 15.6: (See color insert.) (a) Top: Representative NIR light images of the photoreceptor layer (PRL), inner nuclear layer (INL), and ganglion layers (GL) of the retina before differential processing. The white spot in the PRL image shows the visible stimulus pattern. Bottom: IOS images of the PRL, INL, and GL. (b) Averaged transient IOSs of central retinal area (40×40 pixels, area marked by the white square in middle frame of (a) covered by the stimulus light. (c) Transient IOSs of individual pixels. In each subpanel, Pixels 1–6 indicates the location of each representative pixel pointed by the arrowheads 1–6 in (a). Black, blue, and red tracings correspond to the intrinsic optical signal images recorded from PRL, INL, and GL. Vertical lines indicate the stimulus onset and offset. Black arrows point to ON response of the IOSs corresponding to the stimulus onset. Green and purple arrows point to OFF response of the IOSs corresponding to the stimulus offset. (This figure is modified from [56]).

Hz). The peak magnitude (108–125 mV) and time-to-peak ($\sim$ 200 ms) of the first b-wave is also quite repeated (Fig. 15.8c). However, the magnitude and time delay of the ERG responses evoked by the following flashes were reduced with increasing stimulus frequency (Figs. 15.9e and f).

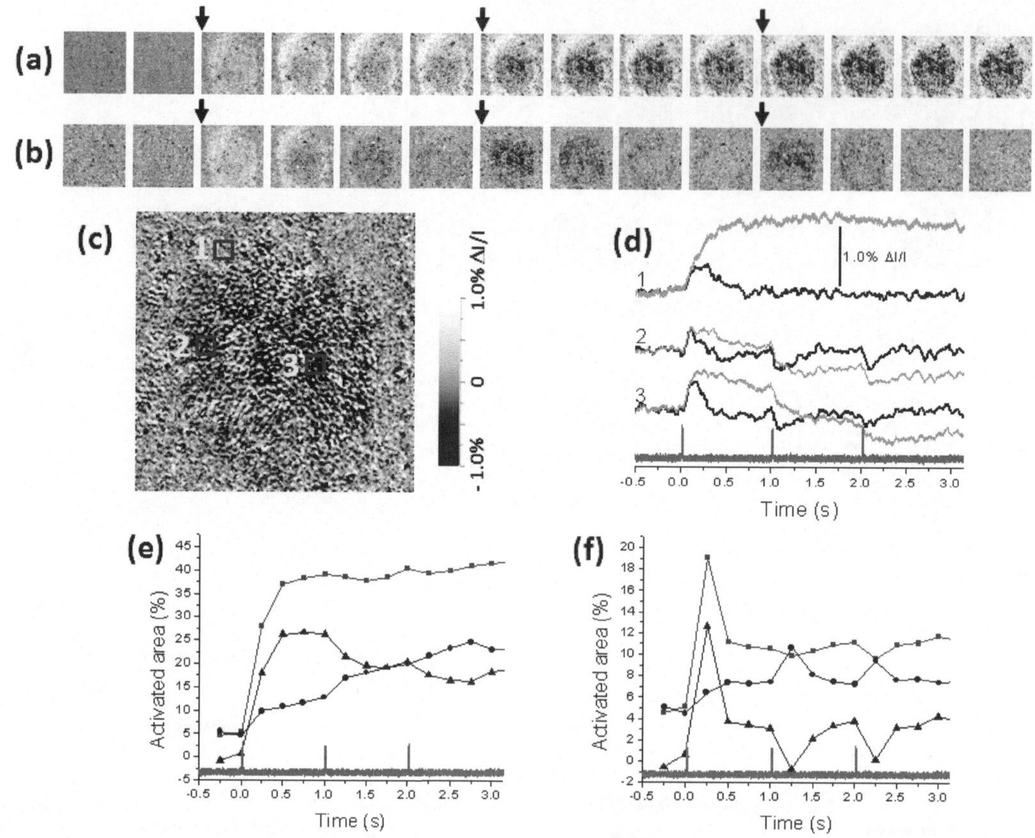

Figure 15.7: (See color insert.) (a) IOS imaging of frog retina activated by 1.0 Hz flicker stimulation. Arrowheads represent the delivery of the flicker pulses. (b) Dynamic differential IOS imaging of the same retina shown in (a). Raw images were acquired with a frame speed of 1000 frames/s. Each illustrated frame is an average of 250 frames over 250 ms interval. Each stimulus pulse lasted 10 ms (c) Enlargement of the 7th frame in (b). (d) Gray and black traces 1–3 show IOSs and dynamic differential IOSs of retinal areas marked by the red squares 1–3 in (c). Green trace depicts the flicker stimuli. (e) Statistics of IOSs in the activated retina shown in (a). (f) Statistics of dynamic differential IOSs in the activated retina shown in (b). A threshold (0.5% $\Delta I/I$) was used to reduce the effect of background noises on the statistics. In (e) and (f), the red and blue traces present the ratios of retinal areas with positive and negative IOSs, respectively. The black trace shows the difference (i.e., subtraction of the red and blue traces) of the retinal areas with positive and negative IOSs. (This figure is from reference [60]).

15.4.7 IOS imaging of retinal slice

Better understanding IOS sources and advanced study of the retinal signal processing mechanism can benefit from simultaneous measurement of different types of retinal neurons working together. Retinal slice, which opens a cross-section of the retina, allows parallel monitoring of visual signal propagation from the photoreceptors to inner retinal neurons [59]. Figure 15.10 represents IOS images of retinal slices. Rapid IOS imaging revealed a complex but consistent spatiotemporal pattern of retinal activation over multiple functional layers. Robust IOSs were consistently detected from stimulus activated photoreceptor outer segments, IPL, and ganglion cells (black arrowheads in Fig.

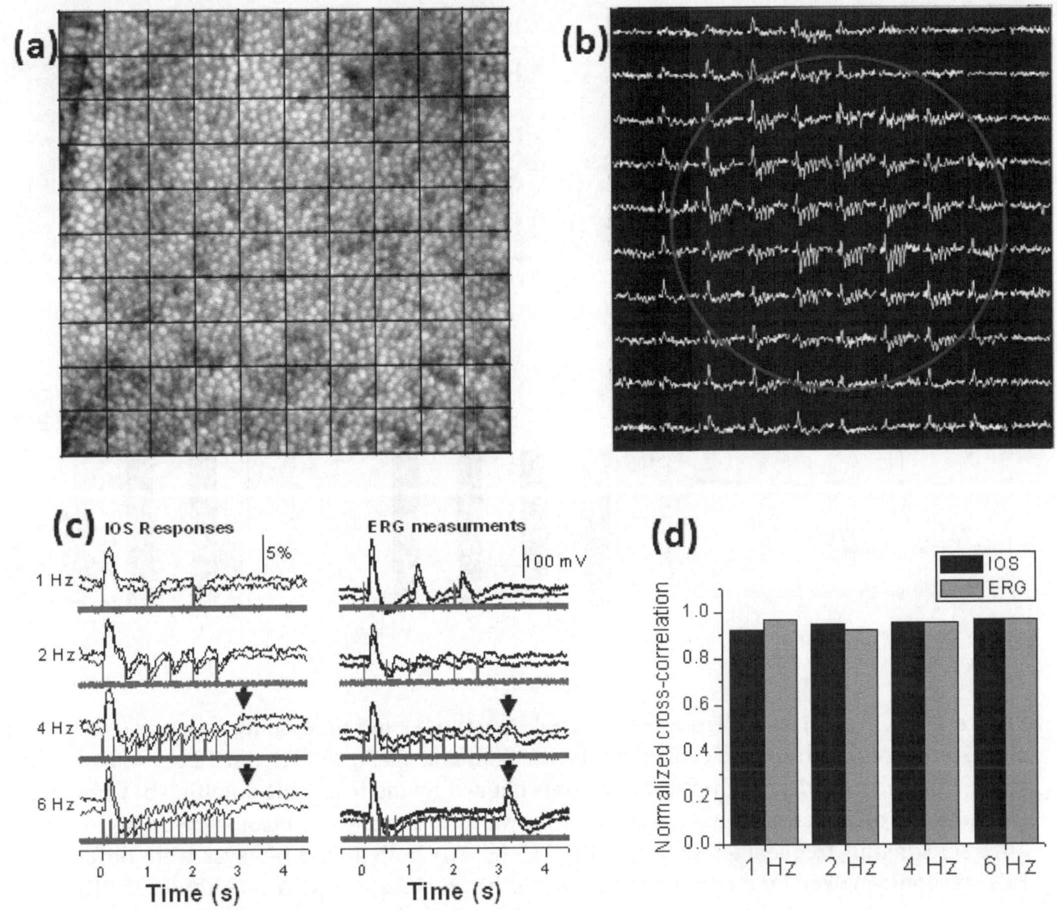

Figure 15.8: (a) Representative raw image of isolated frog retina. The retinal image (400 × 400 pixels) was split to 10 × 10 sub-images for statistics of localized dynamic differential IOSs shown in (b). (b) Optical responses activated by the localized visible light spot (circle). Each trace shows the fractional difference of positive and negative dynamic differential IOSs in each sub-image (40 × 40 pixels) shown in (a). (c) Averaged dynamic differential IOSs (left) and concurrent ERG measurements (right) activated by 1–6 Hz flicker stimuli. Two experimental trials were conducted for each stimulus frequency. (d) Normalized cross-correlation ratio of two retinal recording trails for each stimulus frequency shown in (c). Black bars show IOS responses, and gray bars show ERG measurements. (This figure is from reference [60]).

15.10d); and weak IOSs (red arrowheads in Fig. 15.10d) could be occasionally identified in the outer nuclear layer (IPL), outer plexiform layer (IPL), and inner nuclear layer (INL) between the photoreceptor and IPL. At the photoreceptor layer, high magnitude IOSs were mainly confined to the area (~120 μm) covered by the visible stimulus light (white square shown in Fig. 15.10d). In comparison, IOSs of the IPL and ganglion layer could spread beyond the whole image area (~ 400 μm). GC1 and GC2 in Fig. 15.10d show ganglion cell layer activities directly beneath the visible light stimulus and at the edge of the recording area, respectively.

Both positive and negative optical responses were observed in the retinal slice. Figure 15.11c shows the statistics of positive and negative optical signals throughout retinal depth, from the photoreceptor to ganglion layers. High resolution IOS images showed complex spatial distributions

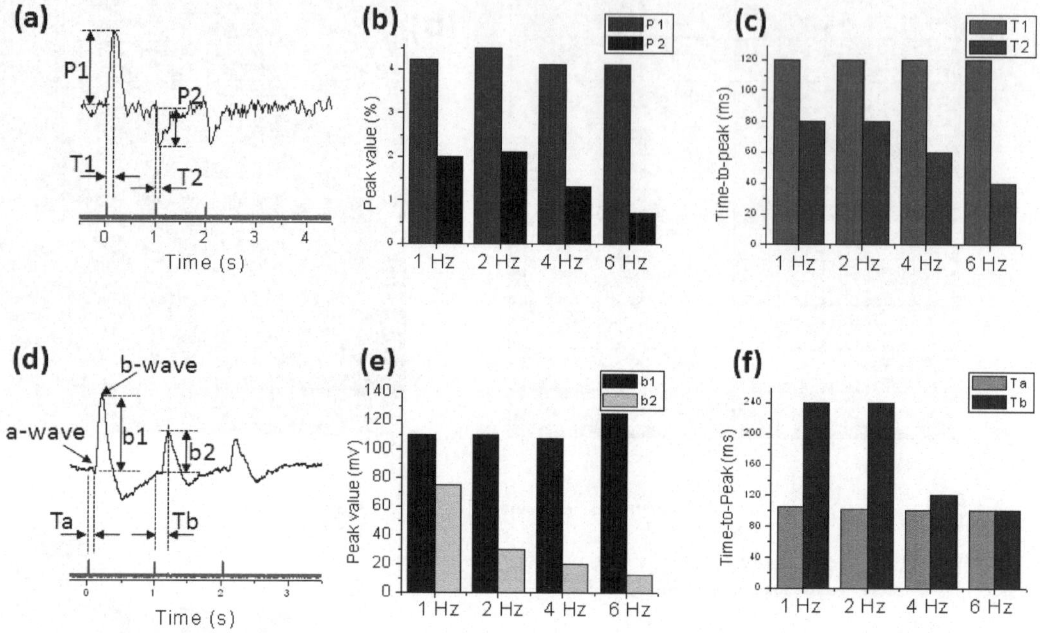

Figure 15.9: (a) P1 and T1 present the peak magnitude and time delay (relative to the stimulus onset) of the optical response evoked by the first stimulus flash, and P2 and T2 show averaged peak magnitude and time delay of optical responses elicited by the following stimuli. (b) Comparison of P1 and P2 at different stimulus frequencies shown in Fig. 15.8c. (c) Comparison of T1 and T2 at different stimulus frequencies shown in Fig. 15.8c. (d) Both a- and b-waves were observed in the ERG response evoked by the first stimulus flash. b1 and b2 show peak magnitude of ERG b-waves elicited by the first and subsequent stimulus flashes. Ta and Tb show the time delays, relative to the stimulus onset, of the a- and b-waves. (e) Comparison of b1 and b2 at different stimulus frequencies shown in Fig. 15.8c. (f) Comparison of Ta and Tb at different stimulus frequencies shown in Fig. 15.8c. (This figure is from reference [60]).

of positive and negative IOSs at different retinal layers ((Fig. 15.11b). At the photoreceptor and ganglion layers, positive and negative optical responses were mixed at a sub-cellular scale. We speculate that the positive and negative signal complexity might result from different types of localized light scattering and transmission changes that could happen on a single activated photoreceptor or ganglion cell. Previous investigations have indicated that both cellular (i.e., swelling or shrinking change of the cell body) [47, 53] and sub-cellular (e.g., nuclear infoldings)[78] changes occur during neural activation. We consistently observed that the IPL was dominated by positive-going optical responses. It is well established that the bipolar, amacrine and ganglion cells interact in the IPL through nerve terminals, and thus we hypothesize that the positive signal that dominated the IOS response in the IPL might be related to light scattering changes due to light-regulated release of synaptic vesicles at nerve terminals [49]. Figure 15.11d-f show spatiotemporal IOS images that provide simultaneous depiction of the temporal (lateral coordination) and spatial (vertical coordination) dynamics of IOSs in the retinal slice. In the photoreceptor and ganglion layers, fast optical responses occurred almost immediately, and rapidly reached their magnitude peaks within $\sim$100 ms after the onset of the visible light stimulus (Fig. 15.11d). At the IPL, IOS images consistently disclosed detectable optical signal in middle part (arrowheads in Fig. 15.11e and f) of the IPL first, and the response gradually spread into the whole layer of the IPL. Overall optical response of the

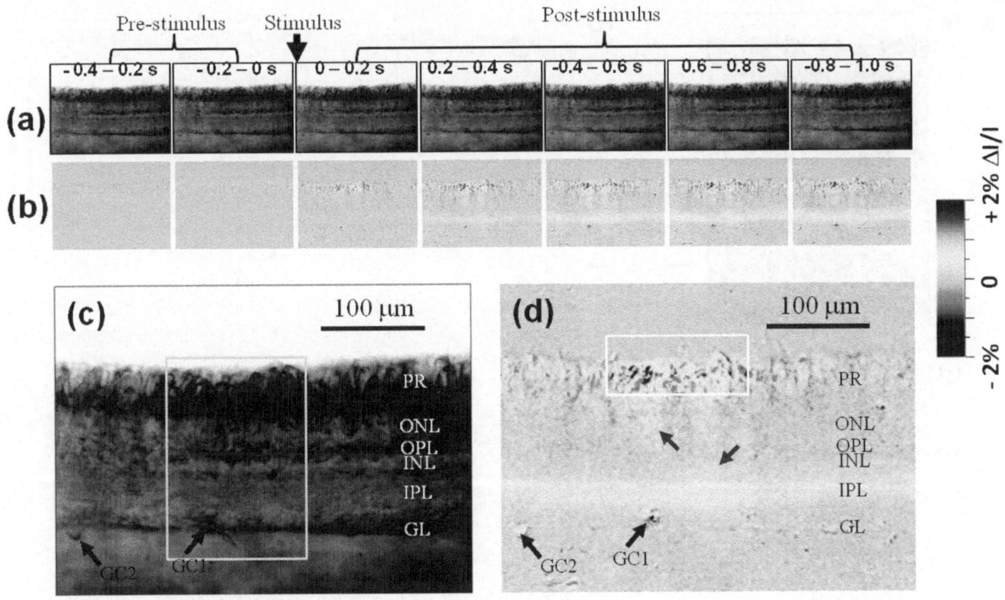

Figure 15.10: (See color insert.) (a) Raw image sequence of the retinal slice before differential processing. (b) IOS image sequence. The raw images were recorded with a speed of 500 frame/s. Each illustrated frame is an average over 200 ms interval (100 frames). (c) Enlarged image of the fifth frame in (a). (d) Enlarged image of the fifth frame in (b). The white square indicates the visible light stimulus aperture. Black arrowheads point to the somas of two ganglions cells (GC1 and GC2). (The figure is from reference [59]).

IPL reached its magnitude peak after the offset of the stimulus (Fig. 15.11f).

15.5 *In Vivo* IOS Imaging

The line-scan confocal ophthalmoscope shown in Fig. 15.2 was employed to demonstrate fast IOS imaging of retinal response *in vivo* [36]. The frog (*Rana Pipiens*) was selected for taking advantage of high (~0.4) numerical aperture [79] and large size photoreceptor (cone: ~3μm, rod: ~ 6 μm [80]), which made it possible to resolve individual photoreceptor *in vivo* without the requirement of adaptive optics. After 2 to 4 hours' dark adaptation, the frog was anesthetized by immersing into tricaine methane sulfocnate (TMS, MS-222) solution (500 mg/L) [81]. After confirmation of the anesthesia, the frog was placed in a home-built animal holder for IOS imaging. The animal holder provided five degrees of freedom to allow easy adjustment of the animal orientation and retinal area for IOS measurement. During IOS recording, the frog eye was continuously illuminated by the NIR light. With the line-scan confocal system, high resolution *in vivo* confocal imaging revealed individual photoreceptors (bright spots in left panel, Fig. 15.12). With visible light stimulation, rapid imaging disclosed fast IOSs that were tightly correlated with retinal stimulation (right panel, Fig. 15.12).

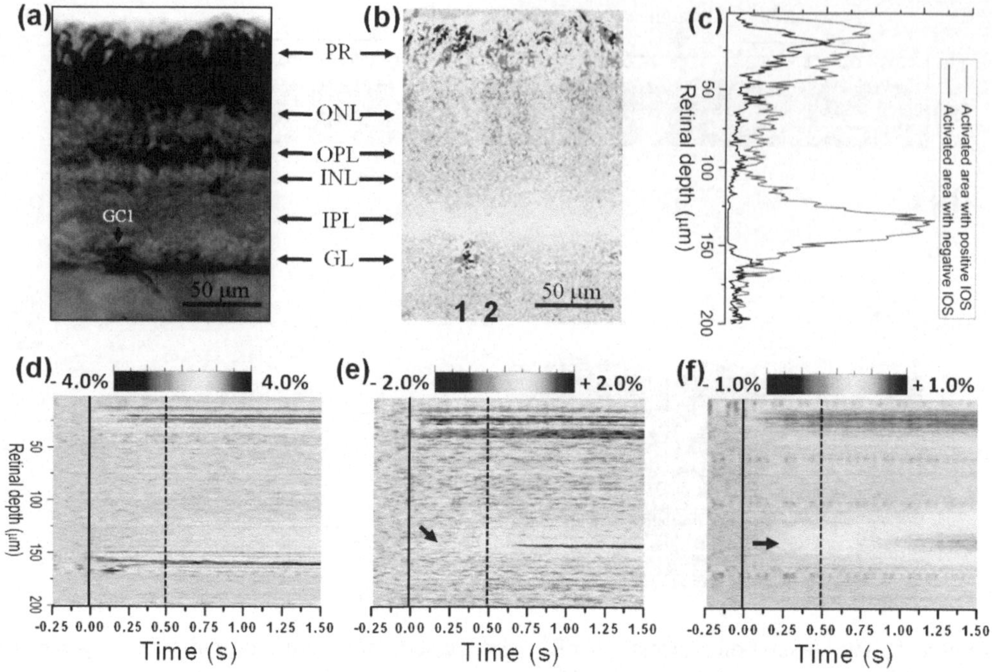

Figure 15.11: (See color insert.) (a) and (b) show enlarged raw and IOS images of the area marked by the white square in Fig. 15.10c. (c) Statistics of positive and negative signals over the retinal slice shown in Fig. 15.10b. (d) and (e) are spatiotemporal images of the line areas 1 and 2 in (b). (f) Averaged spatiotemporal image of the retinal slice shown in (b). At each time point (i.e. each frame), the IOSs were averaged in the lateral direction, and thus a two dimensional IOS image, such as (b), was condensed to a one dimensional vertical line in the spatiotemporal image (f). In d–f, the vertical solid and dash lines indicate the onset and offset of the visible light stimulus. (The figure is from reference [59]).

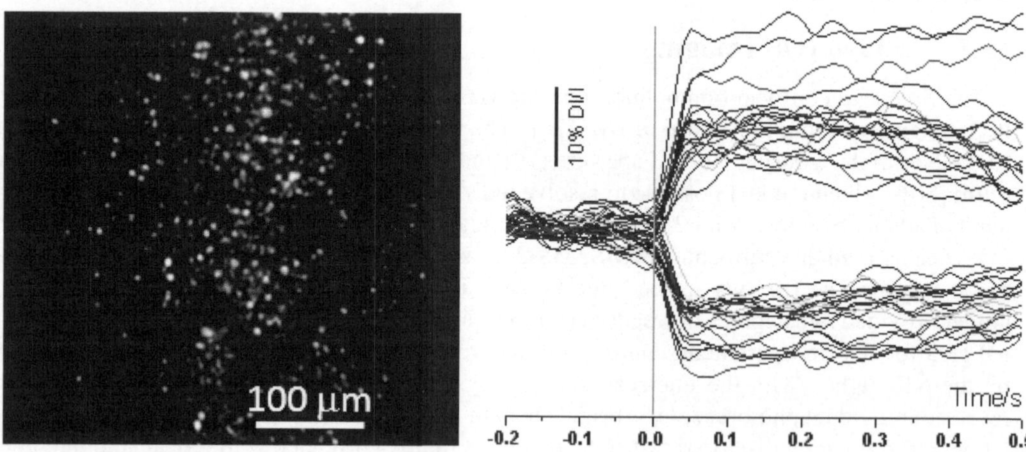

Figure 15.12: *In vivo* cellular-resolution image of frog retina (left panel). Representative IOS responses of individual pixels (right panel). Vertical line indicates the delivery of retinal stimulation.

15.6 Conclusion

In summary, fast IOS imaging of isolated retina, retinal slice and intact animal has been demonstrated. Fast IOSs, which occurred almost immediately after the stimulus delivery, were observed in photoreceptors and inner neurons (Fig. 15.6). Fast IOSs showed time course comparable to ERG response. Our experiments consistently revealed both positive and negative in adjacent retinal areas, which suggests that high spatial resolution is critical to minimize spatial pooling for robust detection of fast IOSs. Although physical sources and physiological mechanisms of fast IOSs are complicated, there is no doubt for the feasibility of imaging fast IOSs tightly coupled to electrophysiological dynamics during neural activation. So far, normal animal retinas have been used for technical validation of *ex vivo* and *in vivo* IOS imaging. Our next step is to employ diseased animal modes to test the relationship between IOS abnormalities and retinal dysfunctions; and to further instrument developments to pursue functional IOS imaging of human retinas.

Acknowledgments

This work was supported in part by Dana Foundation (Brain and Immuno-Imaging Grant program), Eyesight Foundation of Alabama, National Institutes of Health (R21RR025788 and R21EB01 2264), and National Science Foundation (CBET-1055889).

References

[1] R. W. Nickells, "Ganglion cell death in glaucoma: from mice to men," *Vet. Ophthalmol.* **10** Suppl. 1, 88–94 (2007).

[2] R. S. Harwerth, and H. A. Quigley, "Visual field defects and retinal ganglion cell losses in patients with glaucoma," *Arch. Ophthalmol.* **124**, 853–859 (2006).

[3] L. M. Ventura, N. Sorokac, R. De Los Santos, W. J. Feuer, and V. Porciatti, "The relationship between retinal ganglion cell function and retinal nerve fiber thickness in early glaucoma," *Invest. Ophthalmol. Vis. Sci.* **47**, 3904–3911 (2006).

[4] C. A. Curcio, N. E. Medeiros, and C. L. Millican, "Photoreceptor loss in age-related macular degeneration," *Invest. Ophthalmol. Vis. Sci.* **37**, 1236–1249 (1996).

[5] G. R. Jackson, C. Owsley, and C. A. Curcio, "Photoreceptor degeneration and dysfunction in aging and age-related maculopathy," *Ageing Research Reviews* **1**, 381–396 (2002).

[6] R. E. Hogg, and U. Chakravarthy, "Visual function and dysfunction in early and late age-related maculopathy," *Prog. Retin. Eye Res.* **25**, 249–276 (2006).

[7] B. Falsini, S. Serrao, A. Fadda, G. Iarossi, G. Porrello, F. Cocco, and E. Merendino, "Focal electroretinograms and fundus appearance in nonexudative age-related macular degeneration. Quantitative relationship between retinal morphology and function," *Graefes Arch. Clin. Exp. Ophthalmol.* **237**, 193–200 (1999).

[8] B. Meyer-Rusenberg, M. Pavlidis, T. Stupp, and S. Thanos, "Pathological changes in human retinal ganglion cells associated with diabetic and hypertensive retinopathy," *Graefes Arch. Clin. Exp. Ophthalmol.* **245**, 1009–1018 (2007).

[9] Y. W. Qin, G. Z. Xu, and W. J. Wang, "Dendritic abnormalities in retinal ganglion cells of three-month diabetic rats," *Curr. Eye Res.* **31**, 967–974 (2006).

[10] D. Nagy, B. Schonfisch, E. Zrenner, and H. Jagle, "Long-term follow-up of retinitis pigmentosa patients with multifocal electroretinography," *Invest. Ophthalmol. Vis. Sci.* **49**, 4664–4671 (2008).

[11] B. Falsini, D. Marangoni, T. Salgarello, G. Stifano, L. Montrone, F. Campagna, S. Aliberti, E. Balestrazzi, and A. Colotto, "Structure-function relationship in ocular hypertension and glaucoma: interindividual and interocular analysis by OCT and pattern ERG," *Graefes Arch. Clin. Exp. Ophthalmol.* (2008).

[12] A. Oishi, A. Otani, M. Sasahara, M. Kurimoto, H. Nakamura, H. Kojima, and N. Yoshimura, "Retinal nerve fiber layer thickness in patients with retinitis pigmentosa," *Eye* (2008).

[13] H. P. Scholl, and E. Zrenner, "Electrophysiology in the investigation of acquired retinal disorders," *Surv. Ophthalmol.* **45**, 29–47 (2000).

[14] D. C. Hood, J. G. Odel, C. S. Chen, and B. J. Winn, "The multifocal electroretinogram," *J. Neuroophthalmol.* **23**, 225–235 (2003).

[15] D. C. Hood, "Assessing retinal function with the multifocal technique," *Prog. Retin. Eye Res.* **19**, 607–646 (2000).

[16] H. A. Quigley, E. M. Addicks, and W. R. Green, "Optic nerve damage in human glaucoma. III. Quantitative correlation of nerve fiber loss and visual field defect in glaucoma, ischemic neuropathy, papilledema, and toxic neuropathy," *Arch. Ophthalmol.* **100**, 135–146 (1982).

[17] L. Frisen, and H. A. Quigley, "Visual acuity in optic atrophy: a quantitative clinicopathological analysis," *Graefes Arch. Clin. Exp. Ophthalmol.* **222**, 71–74 (1984).

[18] S. G. Jacobson, A. V. Cideciyan, A. Iannaccone, R. G. Weleber, G. A. Fishman, A. M. Maguire, L. M. Affatigato, J. Bennett, E. A. Pierce, M. Danciger, D. B. Farber, and E. M. Stone, "Disease expression of RP1 mutations causing autosomal dominant retinitis pigmentosa," *Invest. Ophthalmol. Vis. Sci.* **41**, 1898–1908 (2000).

[19] A. Grinvald, E. Lieke, R. D. Frostig, C. D. Gilbert, and T. N. Wiesel, "Functional architecture of cortex revealed by optical imaging of intrinsic signals," *Nature* **324**, 361–364 (1986).

[20] B. Chance, Q. Luo, S. Nioka, D. C. Alsop, and J. A. Detre, "Optical investigations of physiology: a study of intrinsic and extrinsic biomedical contrast," *Philos. Trans. Roy. Soc. Lond., B Biol. Sci.* **352**, 707–716 (1997).

[21] D. M. Rector, K. M. Carter, P. L. Volegov, and J. S. George, "Spatio-temporal mapping of rat whisker barrels with fast scattered light signals," *Neuroimage* **26**, 619–627 (2005).

[22] M. M. Haglund, G. A. Ojemann, and D. W. Hochman, "Optical imaging of epileptiform and functional-activity in human cerebral-cortex," *Nature* **358**, 668–671 (1992).

[23] Y. Hoshi, I. Oda, Y. Wada, Y. Ito, Y. Yamashita, M. Oda, K. Ohta, Y. Yamada, and M. Tamura, "Visuospatial imagery is a fruitful strategy for the digit span backward task: a study with near-infrared optical tomography," *Cognitive Brain Res.* **9**, 339–342 (2000).

[24] G. Strangman, J. P. Culver, J. H. Thompson, and D. A. Boas, "A quantitative comparison of simultaneous BOLD fMRI and NIRS recordings during functional brain activation," *Neuroimage* **17**, 719–731 (2002).

[25] N. Pouratian, S. A. Sheth, N. A. Martin, and A. W. Toga, "Shedding light on brain mapping: advances in human optical imaging," *Trends Neurosci.* **26**, 277–282 (2003).

[26] D. Rector, and R. Harper, "Imaging of hippocampal neural activity in freely behaving animals," *Behav. Brain Res.* **42**, 143–149 (1991).

[27] S. Chen, P. Li, W. Luo, H. Gong, S. Zeng, and Q. Luo, "Time-varying spreading depression waves in rat cortex revealed by optical intrinsic signal imaging," *Neurosci. Lett.* **396**, 132–136 (2006).

[28] Y. Okawa, T. Fujikado, T. Miyoshi, H. Sawai, S. Kusaka, T. Mihashi, Y. Hirohara, and Y. Tano, "Optical imaging to evaluate retinal activation by electrical currents using suprachoroidal-transretinal stimulation," *Invest. Ophthalmol. Vis. Sci.* **48**, 4777–4784 (2007).

[29] K. Tsunoda, Y. Oguchi, G. Hanazono, and M. Tanifuji, "Mapping cone- and rod-induced retinal responsiveness in macaque retina by optical imaging," *Invest. Ophthalmol. Vis. Sci.* **45**, 3820–3826 (2004).

[30] G. Hanazono, K. Tsunoda, Y. Kazato, K. Tsubota, and M. Tanifuji, "Evaluating neural activity of retinal ganglion cells by flash-evoked intrinsic signal imaging in macaque retina," *Invest. Ophthalmol. Vis. Sci.* **49**, 4655–4663 (2008).

[31] M. D. Abramoff, Y. H. Kwon, D. Ts'o, P. Soliz, B. Zimmerman, J. Pokorny, and R. Kardon, "Visual stimulus-induced changes in human near-infrared fundus reflectance," *Invest. Ophthalmol. Vis. Sci.* **47**, 715–721 (2006).

[32] X. C. Yao, A. Yamauchi, B. Perry, and J. S. George, "Rapid optical coherence tomography and recording functional scattering changes from activated frog retina," *Appl. Opt.* **44**, 2019–2023 (2005).

[33] K. Bizheva, R. Pflug, B. Hermann, B. Povazay, H. Sattmann, P. Qiu, E. Anger, H. Reitsamer, S. Popov, J. R. Taylor, A. Unterhuber, P. Ahnelt, and W. Drexler, "Optophysiology: depth-resolved probing of retinal physiology with functional ultrahigh-resolution optical coherence tomography," *Proc. Nat. Acad. Sci. U. S. A.* **103**, 5066–5071 (2006).

[34] V. J. Srinivasan, M. Wojtkowski, J. G. Fujimoto, and J. S. Duker, "In vivo measurement of retinal physiology with high-speed ultrahigh-resolution optical coherence tomography," *Opt. Lett.* **31**, 2308–2310 (2006).

[35] V. J. Srinivasan, Y. Chen, J. S. Duker, and J. G. Fujimoto, "In vivo functional imaging of intrinsic scattering changes in the human retina with high-speed ultrahigh resolution OCT," *Opt. Express* **17**, 3861–3877 (2009).

[36] Q. X. Zhang, R. W. Lu, Y. G. Li, and X. C. Yao, "In vivo confocal imaging of fast intrinsic optical signals correlated with frog retinal activation," *Opt. Lett.* **36**, 4692–4694 (2011).

[37] Q. X. Zhang, J. Y. Wang, L. Liu, and X. C. Yao, "Microlens array recording of localized retinal responses," *Opt. Lett.* **35**, 3838–3840 (2010).

[38] Y. G. Li, L. Liu, F. Amthor, and X. C. Yao, "High-speed line-scan confocal imaging of stimulus-evoked intrinsic optical signals in the retina," *Opt. Lett.* **35**, 426–428 (2010).

[39] R. S. Jonnal, J. Rha, Y. Zhang, B. Cense, W. H. Gao, and D. T. Miller, "In vivo functional imaging of human cone photoreceptors," *Opt. Express* **15**, 16141–16160 (2007).

[40] K. Grieve, and A. Roorda, "Intrinsic signals from human cone photoreceptors," *Invest. Ophthalmol. Vis. Sci.* **49**, 713–719 (2008).

[41] J. Rha, B. Schroeder, P. Godara, and J. Carroll, "Variable optical activation of human cone photoreceptors visualized using a short coherence light source," *Opt. Lett.* **34**, 3782–3784 (2009).

[42] D. A. Nelson, S. Krupsky, A. Pollack, E. Aloni, M. Belkin, I. Vanzetta, M. Rosner, and A. Grinvald, "Special report: Noninvasive multi-parameter functional optical imaging of the eye," *Ophthal. Surg. Las. Im.* **36**, 57–66 (2005).

[43] L. B. Cohen, R. D. Keynes, and B. Hille, "Light scattering and birefringence changes during nerve activity," *Nature* **218**, 438–441 (1968).

[44] I. Tasaki, A. Watanabe, R. Sandlin, and L. Carnay, "Changes in fluorescence, turbidity, and birefringence associated with nerve excitation," *Proc. Nat. Acad. Sci. U. S. A.* **61**, 883–888 (1968).

[45] D. M. Rector, X. C. Yao, R. M. Harper, and J. S. George, "In-vivo observations of rapid scattered light changes associated with neurophysiological activity," in *In-Vivo Optical Imaging of Brain Function*, Second Edition (Frontiers in Neuroscience). Ed. Ron Frostig, CRC Press: Boca Raton, FL, 143–170 (2009).

[46] L. B. Cohen, "Changes in neuron structure during action potential propagation and synaptic transmission," *Physiol. Rev.* **53**, 373–418 (1973).

[47] X. C. Yao, D. M. Rector, and J. S. George, "Optical lever recording of displacements from activated lobster nerve bundles and Nitella internodes," *Appl. Opt.* **42**, 2972–2978 (2003).

[48] X. C. Yao, A. Foust, D. M. Rector, B. Barrowes, and J. S. George, "Cross-polarized reflected light measurement of fast optical responses associated with neural activation," *Biophys. J.* **88**, 4170–4177 (2005).

[49] B. M. Salzberg, A. L. Obaid, and H. Gainer, "Large and rapid changes in light scattering accompany secretion by nerve terminals in the mammalian neurohypophysis," *J. Gen. Physiol.* **86**, 395–411 (1985).

[50] D. Landowne, "Measuring nerve excitation with polarized light," *Japan. J. Physiol.* **43** Suppl. 1, S7–11 (1993).

[51] R. A. Stepnoski, A. LaPorta, F. Raccuia-Behling, G. E. Blonder, R. E. Slusher, and D. Kleinfeld, "Noninvasive detection of changes in membrane potential in cultured neurons by light scattering," *Proc. Nat. Acad. Sci. U. S. A.* **88**, 9382–9386 (1991).

[52] G. H. Kim, P. Kosterin, A. L. Obaid, and B. M. Salzberg, "A mechanical spike accompanies the action potential in mammalian nerve terminals," *Biophys. J.* (2007).

[53] I. Tasaki, and P. M. Byrne, "Rapid structural changes in nerve fibers evoked by electric current pulses," *Biochem. Biophys. Res. Commun.* **188**, 559–564 (1992).

[54] X. C. Yao, and J. S. George, "Dynamic neuroimaging of retinal light responses using fast intrinsic optical signals," *Neuroimage* **33**, 898–906 (2006).

[55] X. C. Yao, and J. S. George, "Near-infrared imaging of fast intrinsic optical responses in visible light-activated amphibian retina," *J. Biomed. Opt.* **11**, 064030 (2006).

[56] X. C. Yao, and Y. B. Zhao, "Optical dissection of stimulus-evoked retinal activation," *Opt. Express* **16**, 12446–12459 (2008).

[57] Y. B. Zhao, and X. C. Yao, "Intrinsic optical imaging of stimulus-modulated physiological responses in amphibian retina," *Opt. Lett.* **33**, 342–344 (2008).

[58] X. C. Yao, "Intrinsic optical signal imaging of retinal activation," *Japan. J. Ophthalmol.* **53**, 327–333 (2009).

[59] Y. C. Li, C. Strang, F. R. Amthor, L. Liu, Y. G. Li, Q. X. Zhang, K. Keyser, and X. C. Yao, "Parallel optical monitoring of visual signal propagation from the photoreceptors to the inner retina layers," *Opt. Lett.* **35**, 1810–1812 (2010).

[60] Y. G. Li, Q. X. Zhang, L. Liu, F. R. Amthor, and X. C. Yao, "High spatiotemporal resolution imaging of fast intrinsic optical signals activated by retinal flicker stimulation," *Opt. Express* **18**, 7210–7218 (2010).

[61] X. C. Yao, L. Liu, and Y. G. Li, "Intrinsic optical signal imaging of retinal activity in frog eye " *J. Innovat. Opt. Health Sci.* **2**, 201–208 (2009).

[62] P. A. Sieving, K. Murayama, and F. Naarendorp, "Push-pull model of the primate photopic electroretinogram: a role for hyperpolarizing neurons in shaping the b-wave," *Vis. Neurosci.* **11**, 519–532 (1994).

[63] D. R. Pepperberg, M. Kahlert, A. Krause, and K. P. Hofmann, "Photic modulation of a highly sensitive, near-infrared light-scattering signal recorded from intact retinal photoreceptors," *Proc. Nat. Acad. Sci. U. S. A.* **85**, 5531–5535 (1988).

[64] S. M. Dawis, and M. Rossetto, "Light-evoked changes in near-infrared transmission by the ON and OFF channels of the anuran retina," *Visual. Neurosci.* **10**, 687–692 (1993).

[65] A. J. Foust, and D. M. Rector, "Optically teasing apart neural swelling and depolarization," *Neuroscience* **145**, 887–899 (2007).

[66] D. A. Baylor, and A. L. Hodgkin, "Changes in time scale and sensitivity in turtle photoreceptors," *J. Physiol.* **242**, 729–758 (1974).

[67] M. Mizunami, "Nonlinear signal transmission between second- and third-order neurons of cockroach ocelli," *J. Gen. Physiol.* **95**, 297–317 (1990).

[68] C. J. Dong, and W. A. Hare, "Contribution to the kinetics and amplitude of the electroretinogram b-wave by third-order retinal neurons in the rabbit retina," *Vision Res.* **40**, 579–589 (2000).

[69] H. H. Harary, J. E. Brown, and L. H. Pinto, "Rapid light-induced changes in near infrared transmission of rods in Bufo marinus," *Science* **202**, 1083–1085 (1978).

[70] T. D. Lamb, and E. N. Pugh, Jr., "A quantitative account of the activation steps involved in phototransduction in amphibian photoreceptors," *J. Physiol.* **449**, 719–758 (1992).

[71] V. Y. Arshavsky, T. D. Lamb, and E. N. Pugh, Jr., "G proteins and phototransduction," *Annu. Rev. Physiol.* **64**, 153–187 (2002).

[72] H. Kuhn, N. Bennett, M. Michel-Villaz, and M. Chabre, "Interactions between photoexcited rhodopsin and GTP-binding protein: kinetic and stoichiometric analyses from light-scattering changes," *Proc. Nat. Acad. Sci. U. S. A.* **78**, 6873–6877 (1981).

[73] W. Gao, B. Cense, Y. Zhang, R. S. Jonnal, and D. T. Miller, "Measuring retinal contributions to the optical Stiles-Crawford effect with optical coherence tomography," *Opt. Express* **16**, 6486–6501 (2008).

[74] A. Roorda, and D. R. Williams, "Optical fiber properties of individual human cones," *J. Vis.* **2**, 404–412 (2002).

[75] K. Franze, J. Grosche, S. N. Skatchkov, S. Schinkinger, C. Foja, D. Schild, O. Uckermann, K. Travis, A. Reichenbach, and J. Guck, "Muller cells are living optical fibers in the vertebrate retina," *Proc. Nat. Acad. Sci. U. S. A.* **104**, 8287–8292 (2007).

[76] W. S. Stiles, and B. H. Crawford, "The luminous efficiency of rays entering the eye pupil at different points," *Proc. Roy. Soc. Lond. B.* **112**, 428–450 (1933).

[77] S. Barnes, "Center-surround antagonism mediated by proton signaling at the cone photoreceptor synapse," *J. Gen. Physiol.* **122**, 653–656 (2003).

[78] M. Wittmann, G. Queisser, A. Eder, J. S. Wiegert, C. P. Bengtson, A. Hellwig, G. Wittum, and H. Bading, "Synaptic activity induces dramatic changes in the geometry of the cell nucleus: interplay between nuclear structure, histone H3 phosphorylation, and nuclear calcium signaling," *J. Neurosci.* **29**, 14687–14700 (2009).

[79] G. Li, H. Zwick, B. Stuck, and D. J. Lund, "On the use of schematic eye models to estimate retinal image quality," *J. Biomed. Opt.* **5**, 307–314 (2000).

[80] S. E. Nilsson, "An electron microscopic classification of the retinal receptors of the leopard frog (Rana Pipiens)," *J. Ultrastruct. Res.* **10**, 390–416 (1964).

[81] Y. Cakir, and S. M. Strauch, "Tricaine (MS-222) is a safe anesthetic compound compared to benzocaine and pentobarbital to induce anesthesia in leopard frogs (Rana pipiens)," *Pharmacological Reports: PR* **57**, 467–474 (2005).

16

Isometric 3D Imaging of Cellular Samples Using Optical Projection Tomographic Microscopy

Ryan L. Coe, Qin Miao, Kenny F. Chou
Dept. Bioengineering and Human Photonics Lab, University of Washington, Seattle, WA

Michael G. Meyer
VisionGate Inc., 445 N. Fifth St., Phoenix, AZ

Eric J. Seibel
Dept. Mechanical Engineering and Human Photonics Lab, University of Washington, Seattle, WA

This chapter describes 3D cellular imaging and analysis using the technique of optical projection tomography microscopy (OPTM). The theory, simulation, and method of image formation of OPTM is similar to x-ray computed tomography (CT), but images cells with light in the optical spectrum. Instead of rotating the scanner and detector around the object being imaged, a cellular specimen is rotated while the optical axis is fixed. By capturing a series of projection images around the specimen, a three-dimensional (3D) image can be reconstructed. Absorption-based stains are still the mainstay of clinical diagnosis, and thus 3D imaging based upon monochrome absorption is the primary focus. OPTM could play a role in bringing clinical cytopathology and histopathology into the third dimension. Advanced 3D visualization techniques and multimodal capabilities are demonstrated, such as 3D fluorescence imaging in epi-illumination that co-registers with nuclear chromatin morphology stained with common absorptive stains.

Key words: optical projection tomography (OPT), optical projection tomographic microscopy (OPTM), Cell-CT^{TM}, three dimensional (3D) imaging, bright field absorption, epi-illumination fluorescence, cytometry, Mie scattering, lung cancer

16.1 Introduction

Over the last hundred years, optical microscopy of biopsy and cellular specimens has become the gold standard for disease diagnosis [1]. Microscopic images of cells and tissue are correlated to clinical outcomes forming the basis of clinical pathology. For cancer diagnosis based on tissue specimens, pathologists routinely image at low magnification to determine tissue architecture [2]. Higher magnification is typically required for isolated cells, as cytological analysis relies on viewing the morphology, densitometry, and texture of the chromatin within the nucleus [3, 4]. Image contrast from light transmittance is provided by absorptive stains and counter stains to the chemically fixed cells. These stains reveal certain morphological signatures with the cells that enable various clinical objectives. For example, the Pap test is based on a stain, developed by George Papanicolaou, which has helped to reduce the cervical cancer mortality rate from the leading cause to now the eighth most common cause of cancer death for women [1]. Hematoxylin is the most widely used stain where with its counter stain, eosin (H&E), continues to be the standard contrast agents for diagnostic surgical pathology [5, 6].

The practice of cytopathology is slow to change. For example, immunohistochemical (antibody), cytogenetic, and molecular genetic assays provides molecular-specific detection capabilities that augment conventional cytology and pathology [5, 7]. These molecular probes are routinely imaged and quantified using fluorescence microscopy in research labs around the world [8]. However, the detection of these molecular probes using high-contrast fluorescence imaging is not common practice in hospital and clinical settings. In a second example, confocal microscopy has been available for over fifty years [9] and well established as the conventional form of 3D optical microscopy in research. However, clinical practice has not moved into the third dimension for disease diagnosis, possibly because of the expense involved with confocal equipment, technical difficulties associated with use, and because transmission confocal microscopes have not yet been developed that can image absorptive stains [10, 11]. Within the last decade there have been tremendous advances in 3D optical microscopy bringing unprecedented spatial resolution [12]. Due to the high cost, low throughput, and reliance on fluorescence, these advances [13–15] present significant barriers to entry into the clinical fields of pathology and cytology. These limitations could be overcome by an optical imaging technology that bridges the gap between clinical diagnoses based on absorptive stains and research that is reliant on 3D microscopy with fluorescence and other contrast modalities.

Techniques have been proposed for generating 3D images based on the method of computed tomography (CT). Three important criteria make this technology feasible including: first, the ability to image absorptive stains as well as fluorescence from fixed cells; second, to provide high throughput for imaging thousands of cells to make a diagnosis for an entire specimen; third, to be cost effective in dollars per sample analyzed. Furthermore, the 3D imaging technique should overcome the anisotropy in spatial resolution of all single-perspective optical microscopes (limited NA objective lens), such as confocal microscopy [12]. Unlike confocal microscopy, which provides a single perspective through the specimen, there are advanced optical 3D imaging techniques that provide isometric resolution by imaging from multiple perspectives. One technique involves scanning a beam of light through a stationary specimen from different angles of incidence [16–20]. This method allows for rapid image acquisition times due to fast optical scanning which is ideal for live cells and tissues [21, 22]. However, the use of a single objective lens to deliver all the scanned beams requires *a priori* assumptions about the specimen for performing the 3D reconstruction, and there remains some degradation in the axial resolution versus the lateral resolution. Alternatively, multiple objective lenses can surround the specimen to compensate for the reduction in axial resolution in any single lens [23, 24]. This method increases signal collection for weak fluorescence imaging with a significant increase in cost and complexity. Another technique rotates the specimen within a transmission optical imaging system that remains stationary [25–27]. The necessity of rotating the specimen makes this technique less attractive for imaging live cellular organisms, but it also eliminates the risk of biohazard where disease diagnosis is made after the cellular specimen is fixed. High resolution imaging can be achieved by scanning the focal plane through the specimen from a high NA-objective lens to form a projection image, which is repeated at angle increments as the specimen is rotated. The series of projections across 360 degrees provides input to a filtered back-projection reconstruction algorithm [28]. The resulting 3D image of a single cell provides a volumetric image at isometric submicron resolution for advanced cytological analysis.

At the University of Washington, the Human Photonics Laboratory and VisionGate, Inc., (Phoenix, AZ) have collaborated towards the development of the Optical Projection Tomographic Microscopy (OPTM) technique for 3D cellular imaging. The OPTM technique is being developed for the purpose of performing fast automated specimen analysis to detect cancer or pre-neoplastic cells (dysplasia). Since the OPTM methodology produces 3D cellular images that are produced in the same way as x-ray CT images, this technique is being commercialized and further developed by VisionGate as the Cell-CT^{TM} 3D imaging platform. Innovations have been implemented to achieve high throughput and detection of a variety of diagnostic features in 3D cellular images. The OPTM 3D images are reconstructed from 2D bright field microscope images using the filtered back-projection technique. These images are collected by rotating a micro-capillary containing the cells around its central axis while at the same time continually sweeping the focal plane through the cell and integrating the result onto the CCD camera. A simplified diagram of the OPTM components necessary for screening cellular specimens in absorptive mode is shown in Fig. 16.1. Cells are fixed, stained (i.e., with Hematoxylin), and embedded into optical gel. The optical gel is index matched to the micro-capillary which contains the cells. The capillary is contained by coverslips which is index matched to the capillary by an optical oil. Thus, near refraction-free imaging is achieved [29]. Pressure applied to the gel in the capillary advances cells into position for imaging between a condenser and objective. Once a cell is within the field of view (FOV), the focal position of the cell is tracked as it is rotated so that projections can be acquired. At each step in rotation, the focal plane is scanned through the cell, leaving the camera (CCD) shutter open to obtain an optical projection image by optically integrating through the entire cell. The micro-capillary (and cell) is rotated to the next position and another projection is acquired. After projections are acquired from all desired angles, the cell images must be corrected to account for cell drift that takes place as the cell images are captured. The corrected images are reconstructed into the 3D image using the filtered back-projection method [28] and visualized on a computer monitor. While theoretically possible to image cells over 180 degrees, our practical experience shows that residual refraction and scattering produce images at 0 and 180 degrees that depart from the mirror image ideal. To average out these differences, cells are imaged through 360 degrees. Various commercial applications of the Cell-CT device require different resolutions in the 3D image. For research, cells are typically oversampled by collecting 500 projection images around 360 degrees with pixel sizes of 0.75 microns on the side. The focal plane scanning is determined *a priori* in accordance with the size of the cells being imaged. For example, lung epithelial cells are approximately 10 μm in diameter, so the scan distance is set to 12 μm.

16.2 Theory Underlying Optical Projection Tomography Microscopy (OPTM)

In x-ray CT, there are two important approximations: the line approximation and Lambert-Beer's attenuation approximation. These two approximations work well in X-ray where the X-ray wavelength is much smaller than the features inside the human body. However, these two approximations may not be suitable for visible light wavelengths necessary to image cells.

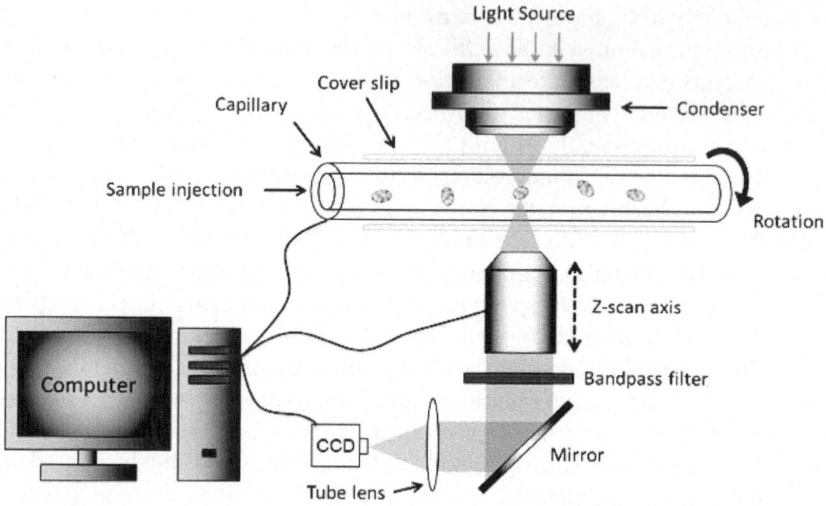

Figure 16.1: Diagram of the image formation process utilized in OPTM where projection images are produced by scanning the focal plane of the objective to optically integrate through the cell. Scanning the focal plane is accomplished by scanning the objective lens or a focal plane conjugate. Projections are acquired from desired angles by rotating the micro-capillary between the condenser and objective. The projections are reconstructed using the filtered back-projection and visualized on a computer monitor.

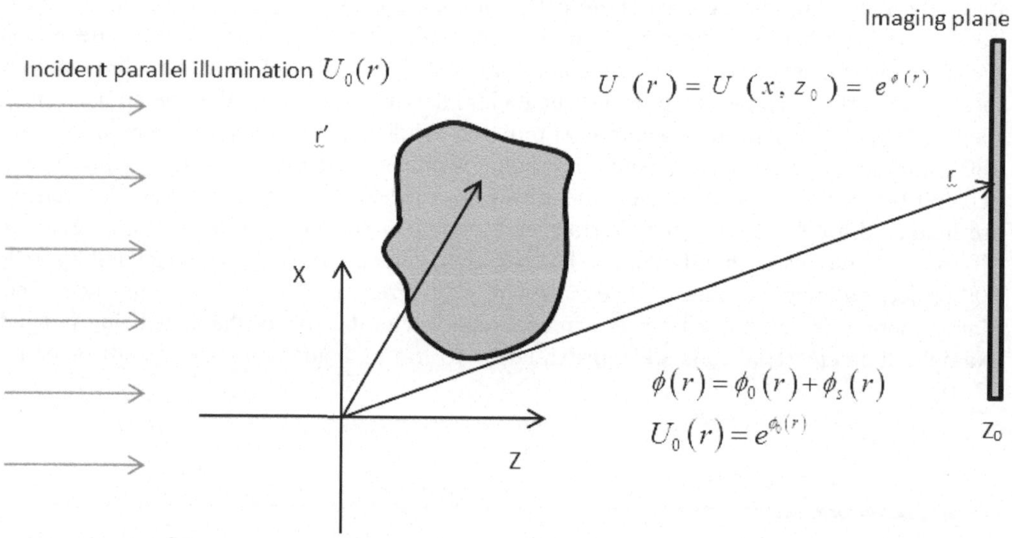

Figure 16.2: Schematic of typical optical imaging. The object is illuminated by a plane wave traveling in the z-direction and the detector array is placed at the imaging plane. The incident field is $U_0(r)$, which can also be expressed as $e^{\phi_0(r)}$ and the scattered field on the imaging plane is $U(r)$, which can also be expressed as $e^{\phi(r)}$. $\phi(r)$ is the sum of $\phi_0(r)$ and $\phi_S(r)$.

Figure 16.2 illustrates a typical optical imaging setup that we will use for the calculation where a plane wave is scattered by an arbitrary object. The scattered field must satisfy wave equation:

$$(\nabla^2 + k^2)\, U(r) = 0 \tag{16.1}$$

We substitute $U(r) = e^{\phi_0(r)+\phi_S(r)}$ into Eq. (16.1) to obtain a solution of

$$\phi_S(r) = \frac{1}{U_0(r)} \iint_{V'} g(r - r')\, U_0(r')\, O(r')\, dr' \tag{16.2}$$

in which

$$O(r) = k_0^2 \left[n^2(r) - 1\right] = k_0^2 \left[(1 + \alpha + i\beta)^2 - 1\right] = k_0^2 \left[(1 + n_\delta(r))^2 - 1\right] \approx 2k_0^2 n_\delta(r) \tag{16.3}$$

The integral in Eq. (16.2) can be represented by $U_B(x, z_0)$ where its Fourier transform is

$$\mathscr{F}\{U_B(x, z_0)\} = U_{BF}(\omega, z_0) = \frac{ie^{i\sqrt{k_0^2-\omega^2}z_0}}{2\sqrt{k_0^2 - \omega^2}} O_F\left(\omega, \sqrt{k_0^2 - \omega^2} - k_0\right) \tag{16.4}$$

which can be approximated by

$$O_F(\omega, 0) \tag{16.5}$$

if $\omega \ll k_0$. Eq. (16.5) is recognized as the Fourier transform of a projection

$$U_B(x, z_0) = \frac{ie^{ik_0 z_0}}{2k_0} \int O(x, z)\, dz = \frac{ie^{ik_0 z_0}}{2k_0} \int 2k_0^2 (\alpha(x, z) + i\beta(x, z))\, dz \tag{16.6}$$

Then substituting Eq. (16.6) into Eq. (16.2), we obtain

$$\phi_S(x, z_0) = \frac{U_B(x, z_0)}{U_0(x, z_0)} = \frac{ie^{ik_0 z_0}}{2k_0 e^{ik_0 z_0}} \int 2k_0^2 (\alpha(x, z) + i\beta(x, z))\, dz = ik_0 \int \alpha(x, z)\, dz - k_0 \int \beta(x, z)\, dz \tag{16.7}$$

Then the ratio between the light intensity on the imaging plane and the incident light is

$$\frac{I_T}{I_0} = \frac{U(x, z_0)\, U^*(x, z_0)}{U_0(x, z_0)\, U_0^*(x, z_0)} = \frac{e^{\phi_0+\phi_S}\left(e^{\phi_0+\phi_S}\right)^*}{e^{\phi_0}\left(e^{\phi_0}\right)^*}$$

$$= \exp\left(ik_0 \int \alpha(x, y)\, dz - k_0 \int \beta(x, y)\, dz\right) \exp\left(-ik_0 \int \alpha(x, y)\, dz - k_0 \int \beta(x, y)\, dz\right)$$

$$= \exp\left(-2k_0 \int \beta(x, y)\, dz\right), \tag{16.8}$$

which is the form of Beer's law. In this derivation, it is assumed that $\omega \ll k_0$, which means that features inside the object should be much larger than the wavelength used. In an optical microscope, the wavelength is about 0.5μm and the features inside cells are smaller than these dimensions this size. As a result, Beer's law may not be suitable to describe the OPTM system.

In absorption OPTM, the incident light is partially coherent, while in fluorescence OPTM the fluorescence signal is incoherent. As a result, these two modes are treated separately. Fig. 16.3 shows 3D imaging of an object in absorption mode using illumination light that is partially coherent. $V(r, z)$ in Fig. 16.3 is called scattering potential [30], which describes the complex refractive index distribution inside the object:

$$n = \alpha + i\beta \tag{16.9}$$

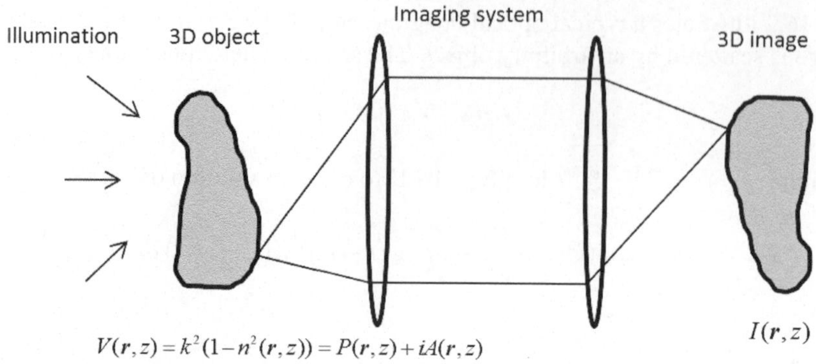

Figure 16.3: 3D imaging of a partially coherently illuminated object in absorption mode.

The real part of scattering potential

$$P = 1-\alpha^2+\beta^2 \tag{16.10}$$

contributes to phase changes from the object, while the imaginary part of scattering potential

$$A = -2\alpha\beta \tag{16.11}$$

is associated with the absorptive part of the object.

The 3D light intensity distribution $I(r,z)$ in the image space can be expressed as [30]:

$$I(\rho,\eta) = B\delta(\rho,\eta)+P(\rho,\eta)T_P(\rho,\eta)+A(\rho,\eta)T_A(\rho,\eta) \tag{16.12}$$

where B corresponds to the background, $P(\rho,\eta)$ is the 3D Fourier transform of $P(\mathbf{r},z)$, $A(\rho,\eta)$ is the 3D Fourier transform of $A(\mathbf{r},z)$, $T_P(\rho,\eta)$ is the transfer function of phase part of the object and $T_A(\rho,\eta)$is the transfer function of absorption part of the object. When a projection is formed by scanning through the object, the contribution of phase part to the projection image is

$$I_{\text{PhaseProjection}}(\mathbf{r}) = \int P(\mathbf{r},z) * T_P(\mathbf{r},z)\,dz \tag{16.13}$$

where the Central Slice Theorem states the Fourier transform of $I_{\text{PhaseProjection}}(\mathbf{r})$ is the multiplication of $P(\rho,\eta)$ and $T_P(\rho,\eta)$:

$$P(\rho,0)T_P(\rho,0) = 0 \tag{16.14}$$

since $T_P(\rho,0)$ is zero when the aperture is circular shape.

As a result, the phase part doesn't contribute to the projection image. The projection image can therefore be written as

$$I(\rho,\eta) = B\delta(\rho,\eta)+A(\rho,\eta)T_A(\rho,\eta) \tag{16.15}$$

Only $A(\mathbf{r},z)$ contributes to the projection image. In experiments, the samples are usually cleared in xylene, which makes α in Eq. (16.12) constant. The only contribution to the projection image is from β, which is the absorption part of complex refractive index of the object.

For fluorescence mode, the fluorescence signal is incoherent, so the image can be described as the convolution of the object and the point spread function (PSF) of the system. This means both absorption and fluorescence images can be considered as a convolution of the object and the PSF. Therefore, the following analysis doesn't distinguish different imaging modes.

Figure 16.4 is a simplified representation of the OPTM technique. X, Y and Z are fixed coordinates in the object space. Z is along the rotation axis of the object, X and Y are in the plane

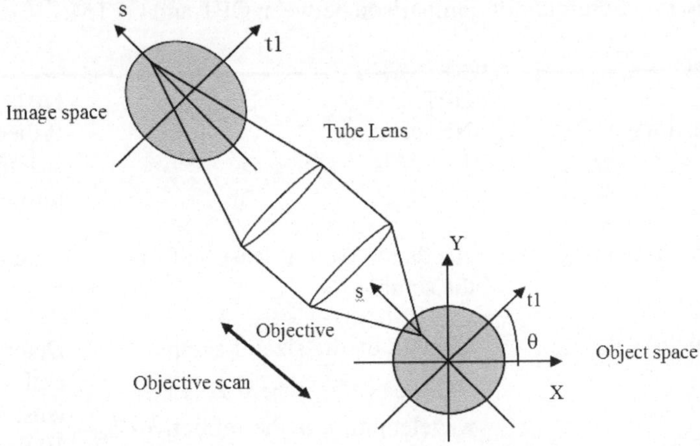

Figure 16.4: Schematic of OPTM when sample is rotated θ degrees.

perpendicular to Z axis. The s-axis is along the optical axis and $\mathbf{t} = (t_1, t_2)$ is in the plane perpendicular to s-axis. Also t_2 and Z are in the same direction. The image of the object $O(\mathbf{t}, s)$ is $I(\mathbf{t}, s) = O(\mathbf{t}, s) * h'(\mathbf{t}, s)$, where $*$ represents convolution operator and $h'(\mathbf{t}, s)$ is the PSF of the objective lens. Projection image $P_\theta(t)$ is obtained by axially scanning the focal plane of the objective through the sample, so $P_\theta(t)$ can be expressed as

$$P_\theta(t) = \int_{-\infty}^{\infty} I(s, \mathbf{t})\, ds = \iiint_{(\mathbf{t}', s')} O(s', \mathbf{t}') \left(\int_{-\infty}^{\infty} h'(s - s', \mathbf{t} - \mathbf{t}')\, ds \right) d\mathbf{t}' ds'$$

$$= \iiint_{(\mathbf{t}', s')} O(s', \mathbf{t}')\, h'_p(\mathbf{t} - \mathbf{t}')\, d\mathbf{t}' ds' = \iint_{\mathbf{t}'} \left(\int_{s'} O(s', \mathbf{t}')\, ds' \right) h'_p(\mathbf{t} - \mathbf{t}')\, d\mathbf{t}'$$

$$= \iint_{\mathbf{t}'} O_P(\mathbf{t}')\, h'_p(\mathbf{t} - \mathbf{t}')\, d\mathbf{t}' = O_P(\mathbf{t}) * h'_p(\mathbf{t}) \tag{16.16}$$

where $O_p\mathbf{t}$ is the projection of the object along optical axis and $h'_p\mathbf{t}$ is the projection of the PSF along the optical axis. Eq. (16.16) shows that the projection image is the convolution of $O_P(\mathbf{t})$ and $h'_p(\mathbf{t})$. The 3D images are reconstructed by performing filtered back-projection to a set of 2D slices perpendicular to rotation axis (Z axis) [28]:

$$O_R(x, y, z) = \int_0^{\pi} \int_{-\infty}^{\infty} S_\theta(w)\, |w|\, e^{j2\pi w t_1}\, dw d\theta \tag{16.17}$$

where

$$S_\theta(w) = \int_{-\infty}^{\infty} P_\theta(t_1, z)\, e^{-j2\pi w t_1}\, dt_1 = \int_{-\infty}^{\infty} O_P(t_1, z) * h'_P(t_1, z)\, e^{-j2\pi w t_1}\, dt_1 \tag{16.18}$$

and $t_1 = x\cos(\theta) + y\sin(e)$.

From Eqs. (16.17) and (16.18) we can see that

$$O_R(x, y, z) = O(x, y, z) * h(x, y, z) \tag{16.19}$$

in which

$$h(x, y, z) = \int_0^{\pi} \int_{-\infty}^{\infty} \left(\int_{-\infty}^{\infty} h'_P(t_1, z)\, e^{-j2\pi w t_1}\, dt_1 \right) |w|\, e^{j2\pi w t_1}\, dw d\theta \tag{16.20}$$

TABLE 16.1: Summary of comparison between OPT and OPTM.

	OPT	OPTM
Projection image formation	No scanning	Projection formed by scanning focal plane through whole sample
Depth of focus of imaging lens	Needs to cover at least half of the sample	Much smaller than size of sample
Resolution	Limited by the size of sample: $r \approx 0.61\sqrt{\frac{\lambda d}{n}}$, where λ is the wavelength, n is the refractive index of environment, d is the size of the sample.	Determined by the lateral resolution of the lens, which can be over 10 times improved [32]

Eq. (16.19) shows that the reconstructed image is the convolution of the original object and new PSF h, which is reconstructed from the projection of the original objective lens PSF.

In conventional optical projection tomography (OPT), the depth of field (DOF) needs to cover at least half of the specimen in order to obtain projection images [31]. As a result, there is a trade-off between image resolution and depth of field. OPTM is a variant of OPT where the projection is obtained by axially scanning the focal plane of high-NA objective lens instead of using depth of field of the objective lens. By using this method, the high NA objective lens can be used to obtain large DOF and high resolution concurrently [32]. The comparison between OPT and OPTM is summarized in Table 16.1.

16.3 Simulation of OPTM Using Individual Microspheres Representing Single Cells

In an effort to better understand image formation in the OPTM, we have developed a complete simulation of the OPTM [33, 34]. Simulating OPTM allows us the opportunity to further assess the accuracy of the reconstructions with a long term goal of understanding how OPTM 3D image grey scale values relate to tissue density. This effort is similar to the one undertaken to produce the Hounsfield units [35] in x-ray CT. X-ray CT's use of the linear approximation and Beer's law make quantitative assessments easier whereas the microscope is hindered not only by numerical aperture and refraction, but also filament intensity variations, ambient light, sample staining variations, and the photon/wave nature of light contribute to this difficult task [36]. OPTM also has mechanical parts that hinder the goal of quantitative reconstructions.

Many groups have used computational modeling to evaluate or enhance diagnostic efficacy of microscopic images. Subramanian et al. utilized a FDTD model to validate scattering coefficients for partial wave spectroscopy (PWS), which correlated small fluctuations in refractive index with pathology [37]. apoglu et al. experimentally validated a model of a partially coherent broadband microscope by analyzing the spectrum observed at the center pixel of two microspheres [38]. Smith-peter et al. analyzed the scattering produced by a biological cell as compared to a tissue phantom illuminated with a focused Gaussian beam [39]. All of these groups recognize that simulations are essential for developing quantitative optical scattering techniques where simulations could lead

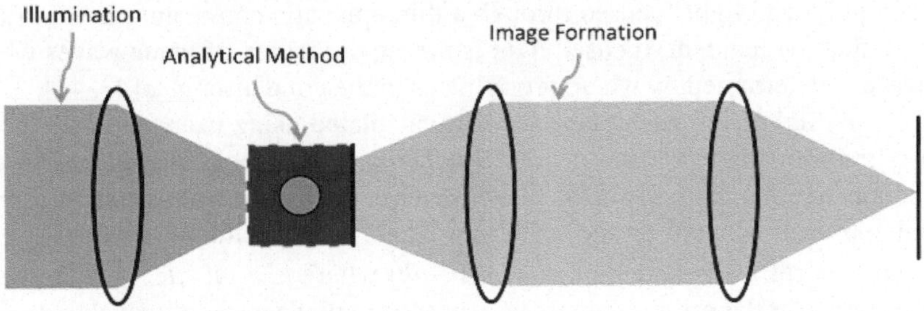

Figure 16.5: Diagram of the near-field Mie theory technique for modeling high NA bright-field, transmission microscopes consisting of illumination, an analytical method, and image formation.

to improved interpretation of light scattering, image reconstruction, and image analysis techniques [40]. For much the same reasons we developed a computational model of the OPTM.

Computational modeling of the OPTM's imaging process is complicated by the use of a high NA condensers and objectives, which preclude the use of most theoretical simplifications, where polarization plays a key role in image formation. For example, Fourier optics techniques, such as Fresnel and Fraunhoffer diffraction, are only valid for paraxial applications [41]. Furthermore, such models ignore the effect of refraction and multiple scattering. We have expanded a high NA model [42] to simulate the OPTM using time-domain [34] and frequency-domain [33] techniques. The time-domain technique utilizes a focused pulse [43] to illuminate a cell in a finite-difference time-domain (FDTD) grid. The scattering calculated in the FDTD grid is subsequently mapped through the objective to the final intensity images. While FDTD has the ability to look at arbitrary objects with many frequencies in a single run, its computational cost is quite high, especially for OPTM applications [33]. The frequency-domain technique combines a matrix formalism with near-field Mie theory to calculate scattering by a microsphere, which is again mapped to the final intensity images. This method is only capable of calculating scattering from a microsphere rather than an arbitrary object, but its computational cost is much more reasonable [33].

The frequency domain methodology is presented as a means to begin evaluation of the various sample, instrument, and reconstruction effects on 3D image formation for the purpose of developing quantitative OPTM. After presenting the theory, the effect of condenser NA and microsphere refractive index are presented as example simulations. Furthermore, other potential simulation applications are explored.

16.3.1 Theory

The OPTM simulation technique is based on high NA image formation theory shown in Figure 16.5, where images are computed in a three-step process. Incident light is defined based on the condenser's NA creating a focused pulse [44]. The focused pulse interacts with the microsphere and the resulting scattered waves are computed on an infinite plane near the objective focal plane [45, 46]. These fields are subsequently mapped through the objective onto the imaging plane. The scattering can be computed in media or free space using arbitrary wavelengths for any desired NA.

16.3.1.1 Illumination

Illumination in a high NA bright-field microscope results in a collection of broadband, focused pulses where the converging nature of the pulses produces a significantly different scattered radiation as compared to plane wave illumination. Light polarized in the x-direction travels down the optical axis interacting with the lens before being diffracted by the exit pupil. The diffraction results in coherent, polarized light focused through a thin aplanatic converging lens [43]. Several groups have shown that the incident, focused light is the superposition of plane waves where the intensity of each wave is determined by where it originates in the condenser NA [43, 44].

The scattered light from each plane wave is calculated using near-field Mie theory [46]. While Mie theory traditionally calculates scattered fields from an x-polarized plane wave propagating in the z-direction, another method allows plane waves to propagate from arbitrary directions [45]. The traditional approach is based on the scattering Bromwich functions with a sphere with a diameter d and a complex refractive index of $m = n(1-ik)$ where $k = \omega(\varepsilon\mu)^{1/2}$ is the wavenumber. The sphere, positioned at the origin, scatters an x-polarized plane wave of wavelength λ traveling along the z-axis. The scattered light can be observed at any arbitrary observation point $\mathbf{r} = (r, \theta, \phi)$. The main equations are presented below, but the readers should refer to [46] for a complete understanding of the mathematical formulation.

The spherical electric fields at observation point $\mathbf{r}$ are:

$$
\begin{aligned}
E_r^s &= E_0 \cos\phi \sum_{n=1}^{\infty} i^{n+1}(-1)^n \frac{2n+1}{n(n+1)} a_n \left[\zeta''_{\mathrm{n}}(kr) + \zeta_n(kr)\right] P_n^1(\cos\theta) \\
E_\theta^s &= \frac{E_0}{kr} \cos\phi \sum_{n=1}^{\infty} i^{n+1}(-1)^n \frac{2n+1}{n(n+1)} \left[a_n \zeta'_{\mathrm{n}}(kr)\, \tau_n(\cos\theta) - i b_n \zeta_n(kr)\, \pi_n(\cos\theta)\right] \\
E_\phi^s &= -\frac{E_0}{kr} \sin\phi \sum_{n=1}^{\infty} i^{n+1}(-1)^n \frac{2n+1}{n(n+1)} \left[a_n \zeta'_{\mathrm{n}}(kr)\, \pi_n(\cos\theta) - i b_n \zeta_n(kr)\, \tau_n(\cos\theta)\right]
\end{aligned}
\tag{16.21}
$$

where E_0 is the intensity of the plane wave, $P_n^1(\cos\theta)$ are the associated Legendre polynomials of the first kind, and $\pi_n(\cos\theta)$ and $\tau_n(\cos\theta)$ are the Legendre functions. The primes indicate the derivative of the function with respect to the value in the parentheses. The $\zeta_n(kr)$ function is a complex combination of spherical Bessel and Hankel functions and $a_n$and b_n are known as the scattering coefficients, dependent on size parameters and half-ordered Bessel functions. The infinite discrete summations are truncated by the Wiscombe's criterion:

$$
n_{max} = \text{round}\left[2 + k_0 r + 4(k_0 r)^{1/3}\right] \tag{16.22}
$$

where the higher order functions are dampened by the $(2n+1)/(n(n+1))$ coefficients reducing their overall contribution.

Rather than altering Mie theory such that it calculates scattering from incident rays propagating from arbitrary directions, the computational plane behind the sphere is altered to include the appropriate yaw, pitch, and roll such that the fields calculated are the correct ones for the desired incident ray. The fields computed on this altered plane are then rotated back such that they are aligned with the original coordinate system. These changes are performed using rotation matrices dependent on the incident direction [45]:

$$
\mathbf{RW}(\theta_i, \phi_i) = \begin{pmatrix} \cos\theta_i \cos^2\phi_i + \sin^2\phi_i & -\sin(\theta_i/2)\, \sin 2\phi_i & -\cos\phi_i \sin\theta_i \\ -\sin(\theta_i/2)\, \sin 2\phi_i & \cos^2\phi_i + \cos\theta_i \sin^2\phi_i & \sin\theta_i \sin\phi_i \\ -\cos\phi_i \sin\theta_i & -\sin\theta_i \sin\phi_i & \cos\theta_i \end{pmatrix} \tag{16.23}
$$

Below the procedure to calculate the scattered light by the microsphere is presented where there are two coordinate systems: the standard coordinates and another coordinate system that aligns with each incident plane wave indicated by a prime. The original observation points on the infinite plane are rotated by the incident ray:

$$
\mathbf{r} = \mathbf{RW}(\theta_i, \phi_i) \cdot \mathbf{r}' \tag{16.24}
$$

to compute near-field Mie theory in the incident plane wave coordinate system (Eq. (16.21)). The spherical Mie theory electric fields are converted into Cartesian coordinates:

$$
E_x^s = \sin\theta\, \cos\phi\, E_r^s + \cos\theta\, \cos\phi\, E_\theta^s - \sin\phi\, E_\phi^s
$$

$$E_y^s = \sin\theta \, \sin\phi \; E_r^s + \cos\theta \, \sin\phi \; E_\theta^s + \cos\phi \; E_\phi^s \tag{16.25}$$
$$E_z^s = \cos\theta \; E_r^s - \sin\phi \; E_\theta^s$$

which are then rotated back to the original Cartesian coordinate system by:

$$\mathbf{E}_s\left(\mathbf{r}'\right) = \mathbf{RW}^{-1}\left(\theta_i, \phi_i\right) \cdot \mathbf{E}_s'\left(\mathbf{r}'\right) 21 \tag{16.26}$$

where $\mathbf{r}' = \mathbf{RW}^{-1}\left(\theta_i, \phi_i\right) \cdot \mathbf{r}$.

The scattered electric fields from each plane wave are integrated as a coherent superposition:

$$\mathbf{E}_c\left(\mathbf{r}_p\right) = B \iint \mathbf{E}_s\left(\mathbf{r}\right) \frac{\sqrt{\cos\theta_i}}{s_z} e^{ikr_p \cos\left(\phi_i - \phi_p\right) \, \sin\theta_i} e^{ikz_p \cos\theta_i} ds_x ds_y \tag{16.27}$$

where B is a complex constant, $\mathbf{E}_s\left(\mathbf{r}\right)$ are the electromagnetic fields calculated from each plane wave incident from $\left(\theta_i, \phi_i\right)$, and the sphere is positioned at $\left(r_p, \theta_p, \phi_p\right)$. The condenser's NA determines the limits of integration. It is important to note that scanning is accomplished in the phase terms of Eq. (16.27) after calculating the scattered fields from each incident ray using Mie theory. Therefore, the scattered fields only have to be calculated once for each incident ray then the sphere can be arbitrarily scanned such that it is fully illuminated. The scattered fields are calculated on a truncated infinite plane, which are mapped to the imaging plane.

16.3.1.2 Image formation

Image formation is treated as a coherent superposition of equivalent magnetic dipoles using the Debye-Wolf integral [42]. The image from each field on the infinite plane is computed separately and subsequently summed to determine the overall electric field at the detector. The *m-theory* of diffraction determines the contribution from each equivalent magnetic dipole across the infinite plane to find the electromagnetic field at any observation point on the infinite half plane extending to $z = \infty$. The electric field at point $\mathbf{P} = \left(x_P, y_P, z_P\right)$ is a result of the superposition of spherical waves from points $\mathbf{Q} = \left(x_Q, y_Q, z_Q\right)$ across surface S_0 through [42]:

$$\mathbf{E}_{\text{img}}\left(x, y\right) = \frac{-jk}{2\pi} \iint_{S_0} \left(\mathbf{r} \times \left(\mathbf{n} \times \mathbf{E}\left(\mathbf{Q}\right)\right)\right) \frac{e^{-jkr}}{r^2} dS \tag{16.28}$$

where $\mathbf{r} = \left(x_P - x_Q, y_P - y_Q, z_P - z_Q\right)$ is a vector pointing from $\mathbf{Q}$ to $\mathbf{P}$. This theory fits in directly with the Debye-Wolf diffraction integral to determine the resulting image at the detector as a result of propagating through the objective. The effect of the objective is incorporated through expansion of generalized Jones matrices used to describe the transformation based on geometric optics simplifications. The electric fields on the image plane for each dipole $\mathbf{p} = \left(p_x, p_y, p_z\right)$ is calculated as though it sits on the optical axis:

$$E_x = p_x \left(I_0^{eq} + I_2^{eq} \cos 2\phi_d \right) + p_y I_2^{eq} \sin 2\phi_d$$
$$E_y = p_y \left(I_0^{eq} - I_2^{eq} \cos 2\phi_d \right) + p_x I_2^{eq} \sin 2\phi_d \tag{16.29}$$
$$E_z = j2 \left(p_x I_1^{eq} \cos\phi_d + p_y I_1^{eq} \sin\phi_d \right)$$

where $\mathbf{r}_d = \left(r_{dt}\cos\phi_d, r_{dt}\sin\phi_d, z_d\right)$ is the field position at the detector and I^{eq} is defined as:

$$I_0^{eq} = \int_0^{\alpha_2} \sqrt{\frac{\cos\theta_2}{\cos\theta_1}} \sin\theta_2 \, \left(\cos\theta_1 + \cos\theta_2 \right) J_0\left(k_d r_{dt} \sin\theta_2 \right) e^{-j\left(k_d z_d \cos\theta_2 - k_1 z_{eq} \cos\theta_1 \right)} \, d\theta_2$$

$$I_1^{eq} = \int_0^{\alpha_2} \sqrt{\frac{\cos\theta_2}{\cos\theta_1}} \sin^2\theta_2 J_1\left(k_d r_{dt} \sin\theta_2 \right) e^{-j\left(k_d z_d \cos\theta_2 - k_1 z_{eq} \cos\theta_1 \right)} d\theta_2 \tag{16.30}$$

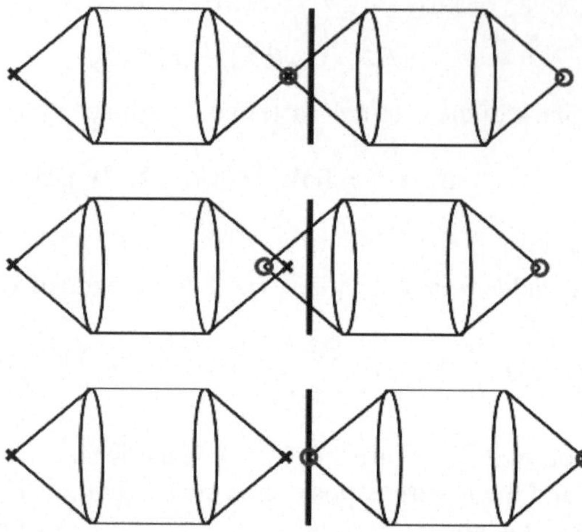

Figure 16.6: Representation of axially scanning the objective in comparison to the condenser illumination. Three different positions of the objective (on the right with focal circles) are shown in relation to the condenser (on the left with focal crosses) and the resampled infinite plane (vertical line). These diagrams show that the near-field scattered light produced by the object would be the same on the resampled infinite plane irrespective of the objective position. The only difference is the distance between the infinite plane and the focus of the objective (i.e., distance between the circle and infinite plane) meaning only the final image formation portion of the algorithm has to be repeated to axially scan through the object.

$$I_2^{eq} = \int_0^{\alpha_2} \sqrt{\frac{\cos\theta_2}{\cos\theta_1}} \sin\theta_2 \,(\cos\theta_1 - \cos\theta_2)\, J_2(k_d r_{dt} \sin\theta_2)\, e^{-j(k_d z_d \cos\theta_2 - k_1 z_{eq} \cos\theta_1)}\, d\theta_2$$

where α_2 is the semiconvergence angle of the detector lens, k_d is the wavenumber on the detector size, k_1 is the wavenumber on the object side, and the magnification β is defined as the ratio of numerical apertures or focal distances. I^{eq} can be pre-computed for each desired focal plane and then the pre-computed values can be interpolated to compute the image of each on-axis dipole.

Once the image for an on-axis dipole is determined, the image position is altered based on the actual position of the dipole and the magnification of the objective lens. The resulting electric fields for each dipole are summed to determine the image found at the detector. This process is defined mathematically as:

$$\mathbf{E}_{\text{img}}(\mathbf{r}_d) = \frac{-jk}{2\pi} \iint_{S_0} \mathbf{E}^{\mathbf{n}\times\mathbf{E}^i(\mathbf{Q})}_{\text{eq,on-axis}}(\mathbf{r}_d + \beta\mathbf{q})\, dS \tag{16.31}$$

where $\mathbf{q}$ is a vector from the intersection of S_0 and the z-axis to the point $\mathbf{Q}$. The total intensity or image at the detector is found from the electric field found at the detector:

$$I(\mathbf{r}_d) = \left|\mathbf{E}_{\text{img}}(\mathbf{r}_d)\right|^2 \tag{16.32}$$

An image at each desired focal plane is a result of summing the contribution from each desired frequency. The process of computing images for each desired focal plane is simplified by altering the relative position of the resampled plane in relation to the focal plane of the objective. This means only the final Debye-Wolf algorithm must be recomputed for each desired focal plane (see Fig. 16.6).

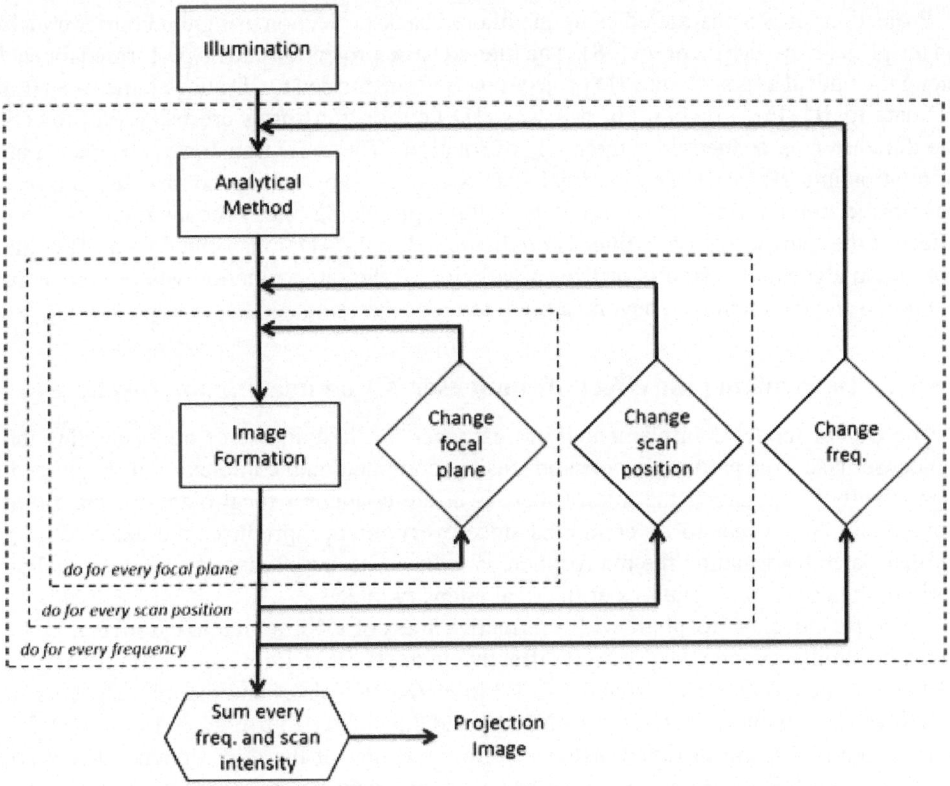

Figure 16.7: Diagram of the process to simulate an OPTM projection image using visual for-loops. The illumination is defined for the desired illumination source and NA, which is incorporated in the analytical method to determine the scattering on an infinite plane near the microsphere. The near-field scattering is used to compute an image at every desired focal plane for all scan positions to illuminate the entire cell. Then the analytical method is performed for another desired frequency and images are computed for all of the same focal planes. Each of these images is finally summed to produce a single projection image. Projection images are acquired for each rotation of the cell and these projections are reconstructed into a three-dimensional image in a final post-processing step (not shown).

16.3.1.3 Simulating a full projection image

The image produced from the description above is from a single focused pulse whose point spread function is potentially not wide enough to illuminate the entire cell. As such, the focused pulse is scanned throughout the imaging plane and the resulting intensity from each scan position is integrated to produce the final image at each focal plane:

$$I_{\text{final}} = \iint I(FP(r,\theta))\, dr d\theta \tag{16.33}$$

where integration is approximated using the extended midpoint.

Figure 16.7 depicts the entire process required to compute a single projection image. A projection is the result of running each method several times to acquire all the required data. All the data is subsequently integrated to produce a single projection image. Projections need to be produced for every desired perspective prior to reconstructing a 3D representation of the microsphere.

Projections are reconstructed using the filtered back-projection using the Fourier transform based on the projection-slice theorem [28]. The filtered back-projection can be performed for each position along the optical axis such that 1D projections are transformed to 2D slices rather than transforming 2D data to 3D (Eq. (16.17)). In this way, 1D Fourier transforms are taken on projections along the dimension associated with the angle of rotation. These 1D transforms are placed at the angle of rotation in a 2D matrix and the final slice is computed by taking the inverse 2D transform. The back-projection by itself acts as a low pass filter, producing blurry reconstructions. To reduce the effect of the transformation, a filter is often applied to the 1D transformed data. The filtered back-projection algorithm currently utilizes a variation of the ramp function where higher frequency is amplified and then removed beyond a point to reduce aliasing.

16.3.2 Determining the effect of condenser NA on imaging microspheres

The OPTM model is implemented in this paper for the purpose of understanding the effect of condenser NA. This particular work reduces the computational complexity of the preceding model significantly by assuming the microsphere is at the condenser focal plane meaning only a single projection image needs to be computed since every rotation produces the exact same projection. Further, laterally scanning the microsphere is reduced because scans at a single radial distance for various angles are pure rotations of the final intensity image.

A 1.5 μm radius microsphere with a refractive index of 1.40, similar to cytoplasm [47], is situated in media similar to optical gel whose refractive index is set at 1.45, similar to that of glycerol [48]. The condenser NA is altered from 0.1 to 1.3 in increments of 0.4 and the microspheres are laterally scanned at increments of 0.15 μm for NA 0.1 and 0.5 and 0.075 μm for NA 0.9 and 1.3. Each scan is extended to 1.8 μm in radial distance from the center of the microsphere. The scattering was calculated for three different wavelengths spanning the 60 nm bandpass filter centered at 588 nm. There was no significant variation between the scattering produced by the upper and lower bounds of the bandpass justifying the limited number of frequencies. Specifically in one test, the two wavelengths produced a Pearson Correlation coefficient above 0.99. This high degree of similarity allowed for a reduction of the computational cost significantly. The wavelengths are 555.3 nm, 581.7 nm, and 610.8 nm chosen to match those used in [34].

The infinite plane used in the resampling is placed at 2.5 μm along the optical axis from the focus of the illumination and the width was set to 24 μm in both lateral directions with a sampling of 100 nm. The objective is constant across all simulations with a 1.3 NA and a 100$\times$ magnification. The detector space has a refractive index of 1.0 and the focal plane is scanned axially through the object from -5 μm to 5 μm at 0.25 μm increments. In the magnified detector space, the images are calculated from -400 μm to 400 μm at 8 μm increments though the units are demagnified for the displayed images. The final intensity images for each focused pulse are loaded into MATLAB® (Mathworks, Natick, MA) and rotated at 5° increments over the entire 360° using *imrotate* function with bicubic interpolation. The projection image is the result of integrating every frequency, focal plane, and scan position (Fig. 16.7). The MATLAB *iradon* function performs reconstructions using the Ram-Lak filter where the simulated projection image is replicated 500 times to mimic acquisition every 0.72° over the entire 360° of rotation.

Axial and lateral cross sections for varying condenser NA are shown in Fig. 16.8 prior to being summed axially to produce projection images. Examination of these results shows it is possible to start to infer which NA should provide the best opportunity for reconstruction. The left column shows the axial scan and the right column shows the in-focus image. Both images are normalized by the maximum intensity values calculated over the entire image stack for each NA.

The 0.1 condenser NA is unable to focus on the sphere where the sphere seems to act more as a focusing agent than the condenser lens producing a hot spot in the axial cross section at 5 μm. The microsphere lensing effect has been well described in the optical trap literature [49] and in some cases groups have actually used microspheres as a lens to measure a rotational diffusion constant

[50, 51]. As in the optical trap work [49], the microsphere's effective focal length was reduced with increasing NA. Additionally, the 0.1 NA results in a shadowing effect behind the microsphere where there is a hole in the intensity at approximately $-4\ \mu$m.

In the 0.5 NA results, the light is much more focused in the position of the microsphere, but again the hot spot is outside the microsphere. The axial length of the sphere appears to extend from approximately $-3.5\ \mu$m to 3.5 μm, which is a direct result of the NA depth of field. The axial cross section using a NA of 0.9 matches more closely to the actual physical size of the 3 μm diameter microsphere, where it appears to extend from approximately $-2\ \mu$m to 2 μm. The hot spot is at the edge of where the sphere should be ending at approximately 1.5 μm. The final row shows the results using a condenser NA of 1.3 where the depth of field of the illumination source has almost no effect on the spreading of the microsphere past its physical dimensions. Additionally, the hot spot is approximately at the center of the microsphere. The 1.3 NA provides the best representation of the physical dimensions of the microsphere in the axial cross section.

The axial stacks of images are summed to produce projection images, which are reconstructed using the filtered back-projection algorithm. Figure 16.8 shows a cross section of the reconstructed images with varying NA. Both the axial and lateral cross sectional reconstructions are the exact same due to the symmetry in the reconstruction, thus the axial cross section is arbitrarily displayed. The 0.1 NA is omitted since the axial stack provides an inability to resemble the microsphere. Rather than displaying the actual reconstructed images, a cross section is presented in Fig. 16.9. The 1.3 NA reconstructed image is also provided in Fig. 16.9 for the reader's curiosity.

FWHM is used as a means to analyze the effect of NA. In most cases, FWHM measures resolution where the smaller the FWHM, the better the resolution. In this particular case, FWHM should be as close to the physical dimensions of the microsphere and not the smallest measurement. The FWHM for NA of 0.5 is 2.36 μm, 2.53 μm for 0.9 NA, and 2.57 μm for 1.3 NA. While increasing NA correlates with better representation of the physical size of the microsphere, there is more energy located outside of the microsphere dimensions in the reconstruction when the projections are based on scanning from $-5\ \mu$m to 5 μm. This effect is a direct result of the axial cross sections shown in Fig. 16.9. The axial cross section computed using a 0.5 NA has a cylindrical shape whereas the axial cross section computed using the NA of 1.3 is more of a cone shape.

In each of the reconstructions, there is a slight increase in intensity at 0 μm, which is explained by the hot spots in the axial cross sections seen in Fig. 16.8. The increase is a result of constructive interference of the waves. Depending on the microsphere size and the wavelengths interrogated, a decrease in intensity can be seen rather than an increase. The decrease is explained by destructive inference. The overall effect of destructive and constructive interference of waves by a microsphere is known as the spot of Arago [52], which helped verify the wave nature of light presented by Fresnel.

In Fig. 16.10, reconstructions with NA of 1.3 are displayed where projections produced by sweeping from $-2\ \mu$m to 2 μm are compared to those produced by sweeping from $-5\ \mu$m to 5 μm. These images show that by limiting the amount of axial information included in the projections there is a major impact on the overall reconstruction where there is less energy outside the microsphere dimensions. The smaller scan distance also minimally reduces the FWHM from 2.57 μm to 2.53 μm, but the difference is inconsequential compared to the reduction in energy outside the sphere. The reduction in information outside the microsphere dimensions suggests that the higher the NA requires more accurate *a priori* information about the axial length of the microsphere in order to produce a more accurate reconstruction.

16.3.3 Potential simulation applications

Mie theory could provide the opportunity to investigate various effects associated with OPTM image formation. Some of the potential effects that could be probed are highlighted in Table 16.2 where they are divided into three categories: sample, instrument, and reconstruction. The effects

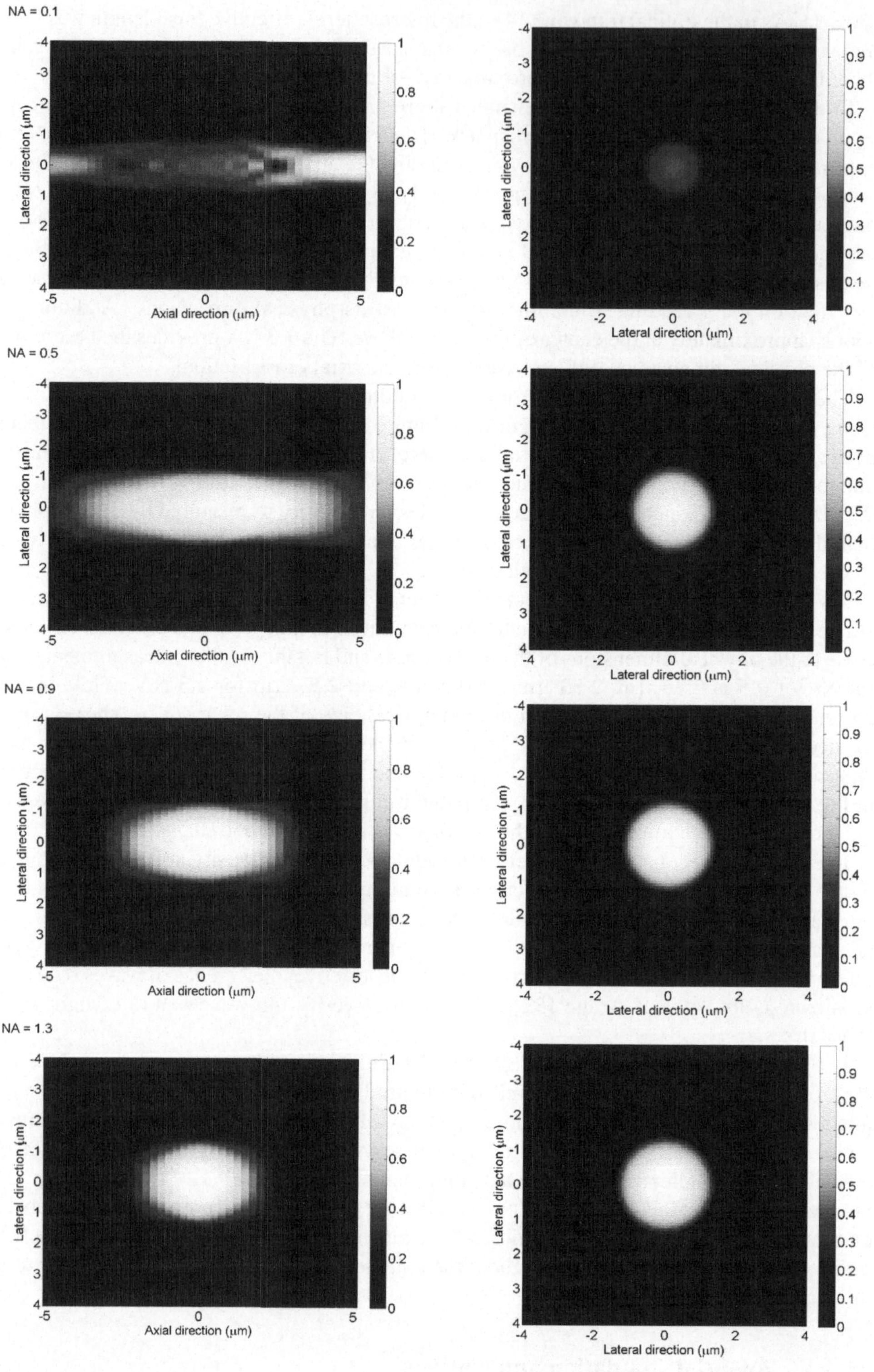

Figure 16.8: Axial cross section (left column) and in-focus image (right column) for varying numerical apertures with a constant microsphere refractive index of 1.40 in media with a refractive index of 1.45. Each set of NA images are normalized by the maximum value calculated in that NA's axial cross section.

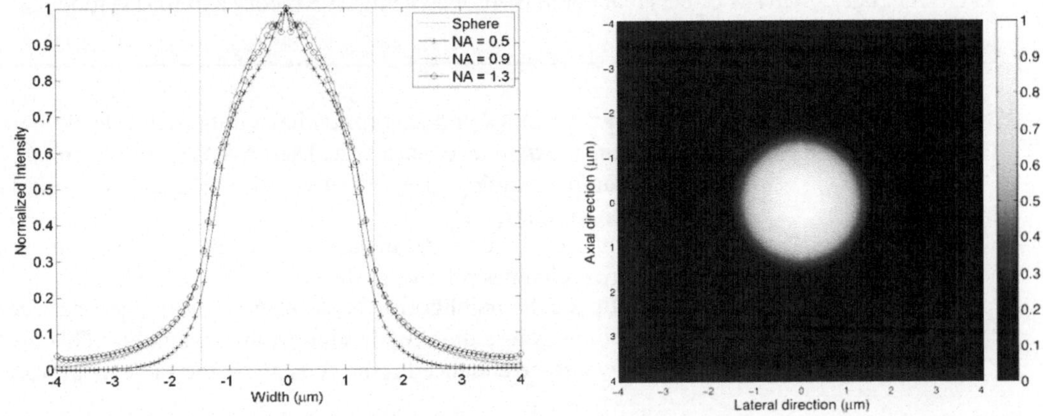

Figure 16.9: Cross sectional reconstruction plot (left) for varying NA for 0.5, 0.9, and 1.3 with a constant microsphere refractive index of 1.4. A 1.3 NA reconstruction (right) is also provided. Each NA intensity plot is individually normalized.

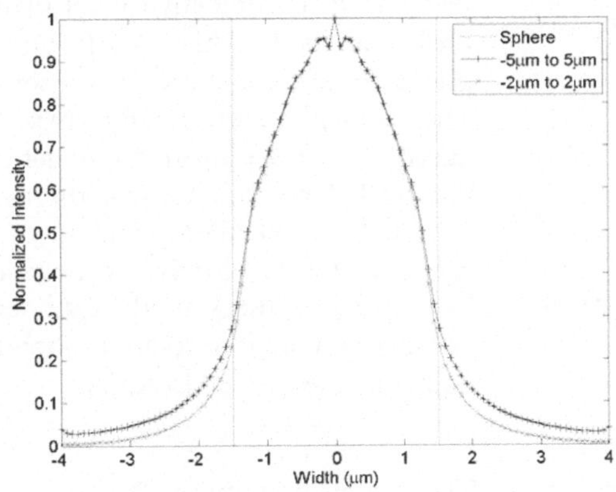

Figure 16.10: Cross sectional reconstruction plot for NA of 1.3 where the projection consists of axial scanning from -5 μm to 5 μm and -2 μm to 2 μm. The microsphere has a refractive index of 1.4. Each plot is individually normalized.

are described without mention of how they would be implemented such that they are fairly intuitive. While Mie theory provides a computationally effective method as compared to FDTD, there is one major tradeoff. It only provides the ability to image microspheres and not arbitrary objects, such as cells. Mie theory has also been developed for cylinders [53] and stratified spheres [54], but analytical methods are not available for arbitrary objects. The stratified sphere and cylinder object types are associated with more sophisticated theory leading to more difficult implementations.

A computationally efficient Mie theory technique is presented to compute near-field scattering from focused illumination. The algorithm utilizes rotation matrices to compute scattering due to plane waves propagating from arbitrary directions. With this framework, we will be able to quantify system parameters and better interpret reconstructions, leading to quantitative microscopy. We hypothesize that if quantitative microscopy is achieved it will improve sensitivity and specificity of early diagnostic tests in both single-cell and tissue analysis.

TABLE 16.2: OPTM effects that could be probed using Mie theory and FDTD models.

Sample Effects	
Refractive index contrast	Refractive index and absorption have important roles in determining the final reconstruction. Their roles are further enhanced by sample staining effects that could be slightly different between samples.
Microsphere location	The microsphere rotates in the micro-capillary such that its axial position changes relative to the condenser focal plane.
Multiple cells (FDTD only [34])	Multiple cells neighboring each other could impact the reconstructions where the illumination would be altered. This problem would be enhanced if the cells are in the same axial plane.
Instrument	
Micro-capillary wobble	The micro-capillary is attached at both ends and further stabilized in the center by coverslips between it and the condenser and objective; however, it is possible that wobbling occurs as it rotates.
Moving condenser focal plane	One potential enhancement is scanning the condenser focal plane with the objective focal plane such that they are completely aligned. This adds to the instrument complexity, but might produce more accurate reconstructions.
Axial scanning	The focal plane of the objective is scanned through the cell based on *a priori* information, but errors might occur such that the focal plane does not scan through the entire cell.
Slow rotation	As rotational speed of the micro-capillary is increased the optical gel/cell mixture may not rotate at the same rate.
Micro-capillary hysteresis	The micro-capillary might experience hysteresis as it rotates causing non-smooth rotation; therefore, rotations could be acquired at unexpected locations.
Reconstruction	
Parallel light approximation	The reconstruction technique utilizes the filtered back-projection based on parallel light propagation. This has yet to be verified using high NA lenses.
Filter used in reconstruction	If the filtered back-projection is the best method for reconstruction, then the filter should be optimized. The work in this paper utilized the ramp filter, while VisionGate utilizes a slight variation of the ramp.
Deconvolution during axial scan	Rather than producing the projection images by optically integrating, equally spaced images could be acquired during scanning through the cell. These images could be individually deconvolved prior to summing them to produce a projection image.

16.4 Multi-Modal Imaging of Isolated Cells for 3D Cytological Analysis

The OPTM technique can be implemented utilizing many different modes of optical microscopy. It can be performed using the original absorption mode with white light and visualized using false

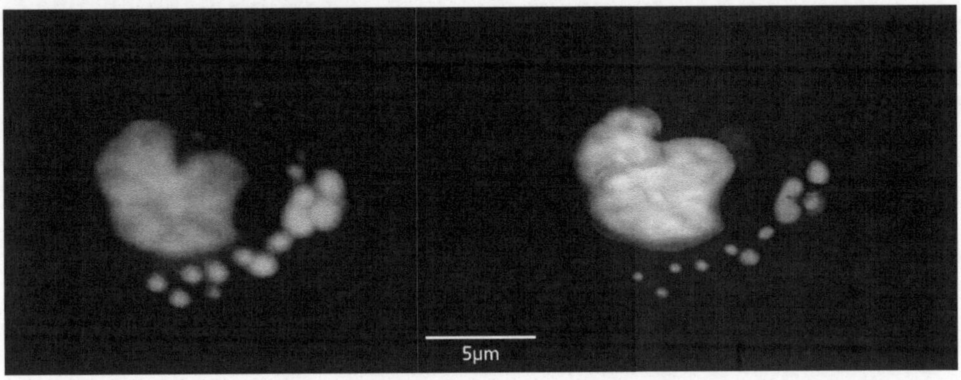

Figure 16.11: (See color insert.) Dual stained alveolar macrophage illustrating color mode imaging using the Cell-CT. On the left, the cell is shown in color mode with a maximum intensity projection. On the right, the cell is volume rendered with color and opacity adjusted to better illustrate cell features of interest. The cytoplasm is represented as a white cloud. The lipid droplets within the cytoplasm show up in bright red. The cell nucleus is imaged with the nuclear envelope and loose chromatin in translucent blue-green. Condensed chromatin within the nucleus was imaged in opaque orange.

coloring [29]. Alternatively absorption can be expanded to examine multi-labeled cells using true color imaging [55]. The Cell-CT can also be configured to image cells twice, once in absorption mode and again in fluorescence mode, providing both biomarker pattern and the morphological structure of a single cell. Below we highlight true-color imaging and dual absorption-fluorescence imaging with verification of isometric spatial resolution in 3D.

16.4.1 Color absorption imaging

The OPTM is capable of performing absorption-based tomography in a color mode. In monochrome mode, white light is filtered at a wavelength that corresponds to the absorption peak for the stain that is used, resulting in maximum contrast in the images. For cells stained with hematoxylin, filtering is done with the passband centered around 588 nm. In color mode, however, specimens are typically stained with more than one dye, with the goal of identifying different structures within the cell by labeling them with different colors [55]. Figure 16.11 shows the cellular contents of a 3D reconstructed alveolar macrophage, a cell type with phagocytotic properties. Alveolar macrophages can be an indicator of gastroesophageal reflux disease. Reflux can cause stomach contents to enter the lungs where they show up as lipid droplets ingested by alveolar macrophages. The cell was dual-stained with hematoxylin and the lipid stain Oil-Red-O and imaged in bright-field/color mode to capture the color of the two stains. The Lipid-laden Macrophage Index is an assay during which a microscopist scores the lipid content of 100 macrophages in a sputum preparation. While normally this is a laborious and inaccurate procedure, the Cell-CT performs the test automatically and with high accuracy.

16.4.2 Dual absorption and fluorescence imaging

The OPTM technique has also been expanded beyond its original absorptive stain implementation to include fluorescence for the purpose of bridging the gap between clinical and research microscopy. This expansion is performed by the integration of epi-illumination fluorescence, which is indicated in Fig. 16.12. Since OPTM can image samples in both absorption and fluorescence

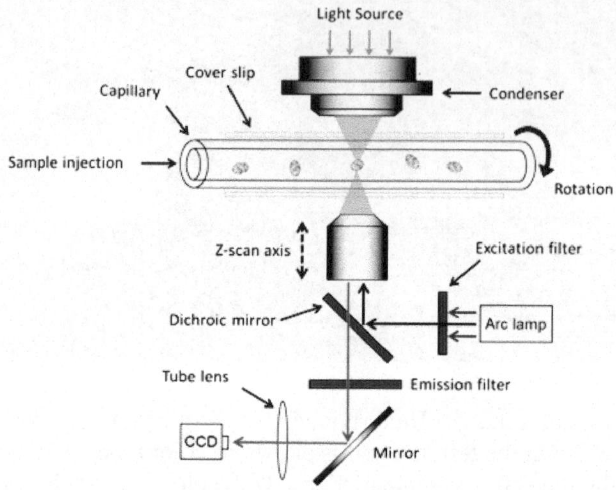

Figure 16.12: Diagram of the dual-mode OPTM incorporating transmitted absorptive imaging using a QTH lamp and an arc lamp for epi-illumination fluorescence mode with standard excitation-emission and beam-splitter filters.

modes, the biomarker pattern and the morphological structure in 3D can be obtained with isometric resolution for the same sample. The quantitative information of the biomarker, such as the concentration and distribution inside the cell, will add more features to the cancer diagnosis, which will consequently improve the sensitivity and specificity of the early cancer diagnosis. At the same time, the gold standards provided by the morphological features can validate the potential of new biomarkers for the diagnosis.

After the cells are chemically fixed and stained, they are injected into the 50 μm inner diameter (ID) capillary tube with index matching gel [29]. The cells are pushed under positive pressure into the optical axis (z-axis in Fig. 16.12) while the capillary tube is being constantly rotated. The objective focal plane is axially scanned while the condenser lens remains stationary. During each axial scan the shutter is open on the camera and the optical projection image is formed at the camera sensor. Currently a series of 500 projection images are acquired over 360° of rotation, while the cell is maintained within the microscope optical axis by fluid pressure control. After a series of absorption projections are acquired, a second rotation of the cell is performed utilizing fluorescence emission tomography. As shown in Fig. 16.12, the fluorescence excitation is added as epi-illumination using a different passband from a second source. Compensation for photobleaching of the fluorescence during the series of emission projections is made in a processing step before 3D reconstruction. This technique calculates the sum of the emission intensities measured by the camera in the first projection and adjusts the subsequent sums of the emission intensities measured in the following projections to correct for photobleaching [56]. Although the two 3D images are acquired in time series (two separate rotations), the absorption image in transmission and the fluorescence image in epi-illumination are in co-registration to within the optical resolution of the Cell-CT instrument [56].

The spatial resolution of the 3D reconstructed images from the multimodal Cell-CT is determined using a high NA objective lens (100×, NA 1.3 Olympus) seated on a piezoelectric positioner (NV40/1CL, Piezosystems Jena). The scanning range was adjusted to transverse the cell nucleus, e.g. 3 μm, 12μm, and 25 μm for sub-wavelength microspheres, A549 lung cancer cells, and Indian muntjac cells arrested in metaphase, respectively. Due to the slow axial scan speed of the objective lens, 500 projections taken at uniform intervals (0.72°) in a full rotation takes about one minute.

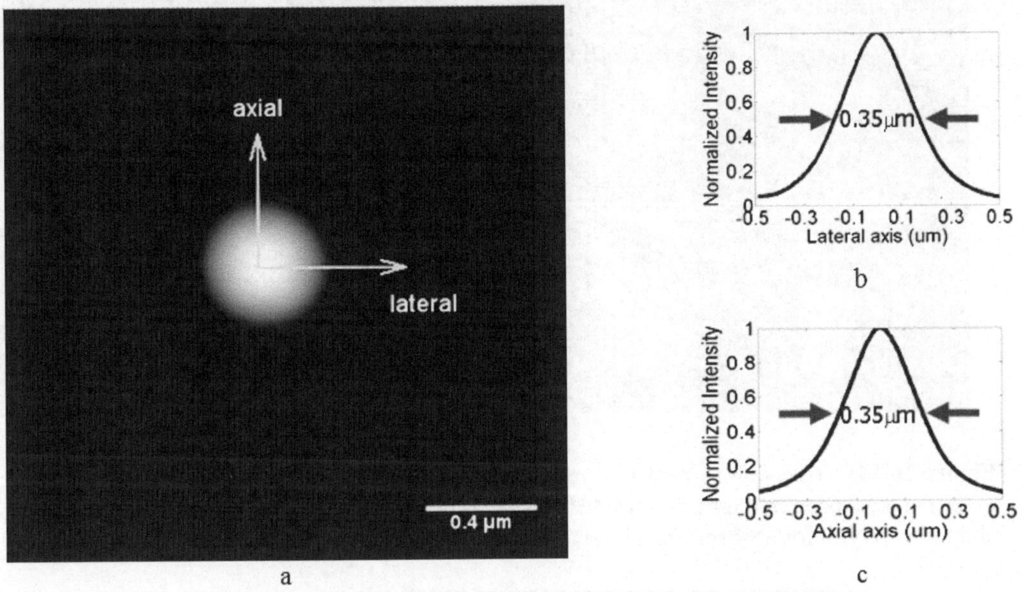

Figure 16.13: Fluorescence microsphere with diameter of 100 nm was imaged using 488 nm of light excitation. Since the size of microsphere is well below the resolution, the reconstructed image of the microsphere is used as a measure of PSF. (a) axial section of PSF; (b) normalized intensity profile along lateral direction; (c) normalized intensity profile along axial direction.

Reconstruction of these projection images using filtered back-projection produces 3D images of 350 nm isometric resolution as shown in Fig. 16.13 for a 100 nm diameter fluorescence microsphere (TransFluorSpheres, Invitrogen). A faster conjugate focal plane method of scanning is now available for acquisition of all 500 projections within a couple of seconds.

To demonstrate co-registration of fluorescence and absorption 3D images, cells from the female Indian muntjac were grown in culture and treated with colchicine (D1925, Sigma) to arrest the cells in metaphase that results in six large chromosomes. Acetic acid methanol (1:3) was used to fix the cells. These cells were then stained with hematoxylin (Gill's Number 1, Electron Microscopy Sciences) for absorption contrast, followed by Sytox Green solution (1/50000 dilution from 5 mM stock, Invitrogen) for fluorescence contrast. Cells were rinsed in HEPES, dehydrated in alcohols, and cleared in xylene before being embedded in optical gel for imaging. The 3D images at 0, 90, 180, and 270 degrees of rotation are shown in Fig. 16.14 which demonstrated co-registration.

OPTM has also been shown to be able to image both cell morphological structure and molecular structure in 3D. In one study, 3D distribution pattern of nuclear protein hnRNP A2/B1 is imaged. hnRNP is found to be overexpressed in Stage I lung cancer cells [57], but not found in normal bronchial epithelium. Lung cancer cell line A549 is used in this experiment. A549 is fixed in formaldehyde and stained with hematoxylin. Then the cells are washed in PBS and incubated with hnRNP A2/B1 primary antibody. Afterwards the cells are incubated with secondary antibody with Alexa Fluor 488. Cells are dehydrated in alcohols, cleared in xylene, and embedded in optical gel for imaging. Figure 16.15 shows the reconstructed images of a A549 cell in absorption and fluorescence.

The Cell-CT can support many different modes of optical microscopy that can be combined with the standard absorbance stain for clinical diagnosis. Gold nanoparticles are useful for single particle and long-exposure images as they do not exhibit photobleaching. A pilot study using A549 cancer cells stained with hematoxylin in transmission and gold nanorods scattering signal in epi-

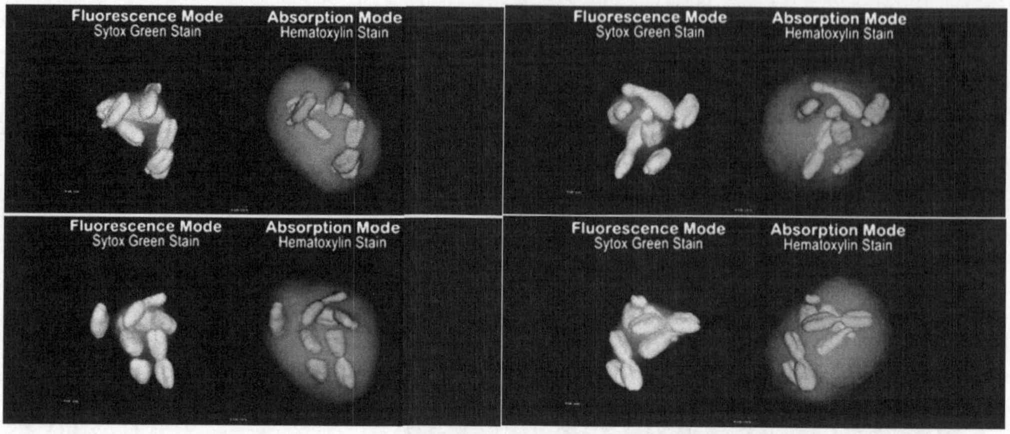

Figure 16.14: (See color insert.) Four perspectives of Indian muntjac cells in fluorescence (left in green) and absorption (right in blue) [56]. The cells are stained with Sytox Green for fluorescence and hematoxylin for absorption. The scale bars indicate 5 μm.

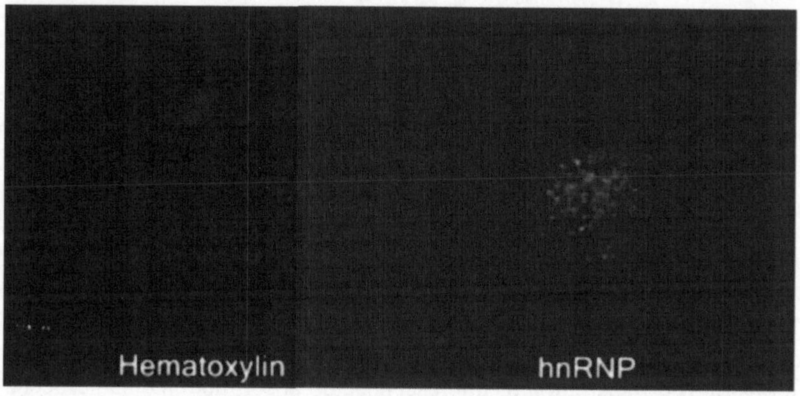

Figure 16.15: (See color insert.) A dual-labeled A549 cell is shown in both absorption (left) and fluorescence (right) mode. Hematoxylin provides contrast in the absorption mode and hnRNP provides contrast in the fluorescence mode.

illumination with polarization filtering [58]. Additional modalities are possible which range from multi-spectral absorption to dark field microscopy [59].

16.4.3 Advanced visualization

3D images resulting from the Cell-CT instrument can be visualized by a cytotechnician or pathologist in similar fashion as a clinical 2D image. However, this image can be taken from any angle or perspective desired by the clinician. Slice thickness can also be chosen to limit the information within the specific perspective. For example, a ciliated columnar cell (Fig. 16.16) is used to demonstrate the use of a thin slice through the strands of cilia that can be used to verify the spatial resolution of the absorbance image. Sweeping a thin slice through a cell can simulate the focus through a cell, but with the advantage that any orientation can be chosen by the clinician to make a diagnosis.

Cells may also be visualized through an erosion process that progressively reveals the cell nuclear

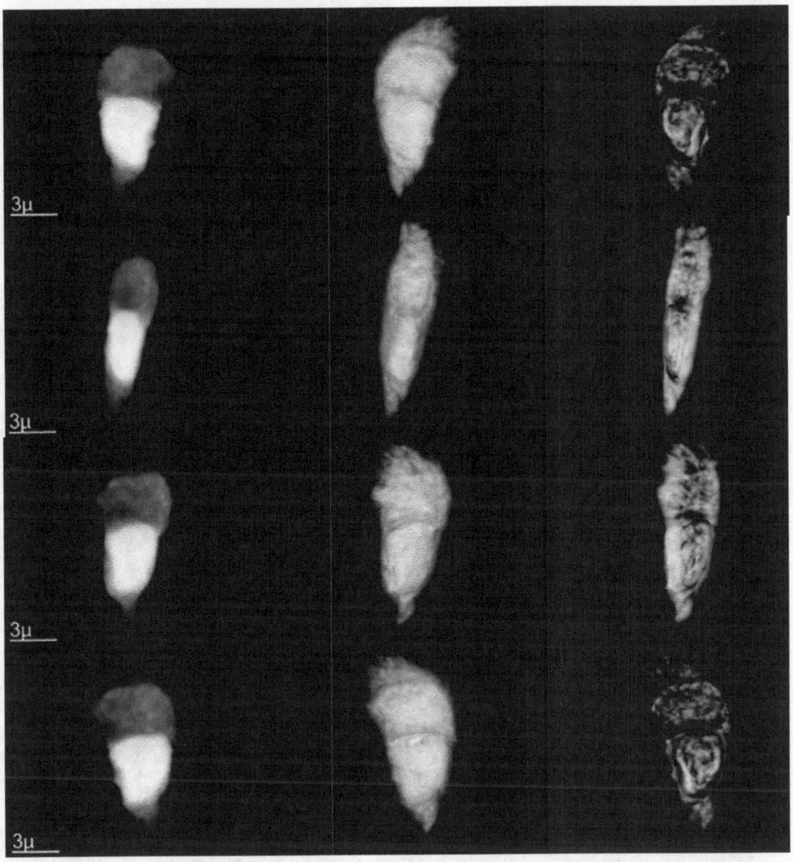

Figure 16.16: (See color insert.) Ciliated columnar epithelial cell viewed from various perspectives. The left column is a maximum intensity representation of the cell, in the middle column is volume rendered with color and opacity adjusted to highlight cell features of interest, and in the right column the colored, volume rendered image is cropped to show internal nuclear structure. Color and opacity adjustment indicates these cellular features: cytoplasm (translucent white), nuclear wall (opaque blue), nucleoplasm (translucent green), and condensed chromatin (opaque red). The cilia filaments at the top of the cell are expected to have a thickness of 200 nm.

contents. In Fig. 16.17, an adenocarcinoma cell is volume rendered with color and opacity adjusted to render various cell components visible. Note the prominent nuclear invagination in the center right of the nucleus. The erosion process shows that this invagination leads into areas within the cell that are devoid of chromatin. Also shown is the prominent conglomeration of condensed chromatin, initially visualized through the green haze of less dense chromatin, and then revealed as an opaque red surface.

Erosion of a volume rendered adenocarcinoma cell where color and opacity have been adjusted to highlight cell structures of interest. Coloring and opacity render the cytoplasm (translucent white), nuclear wall (opaque blue), nucleoplasm (translucent green), and condensed chromatin (opaque red). The cell visualization was further processed to erode the visible aspect of the cell boundary. In the images from top left to bottom right, the threshold for visualization was gradually increased. Thus in the first image one can observe the entire cell and in the final image one sees only the most condensed cell chromatin.

Another way to look at a 3D imaged cell is with a volume sweep-through (Fig. 16.18). The ade-

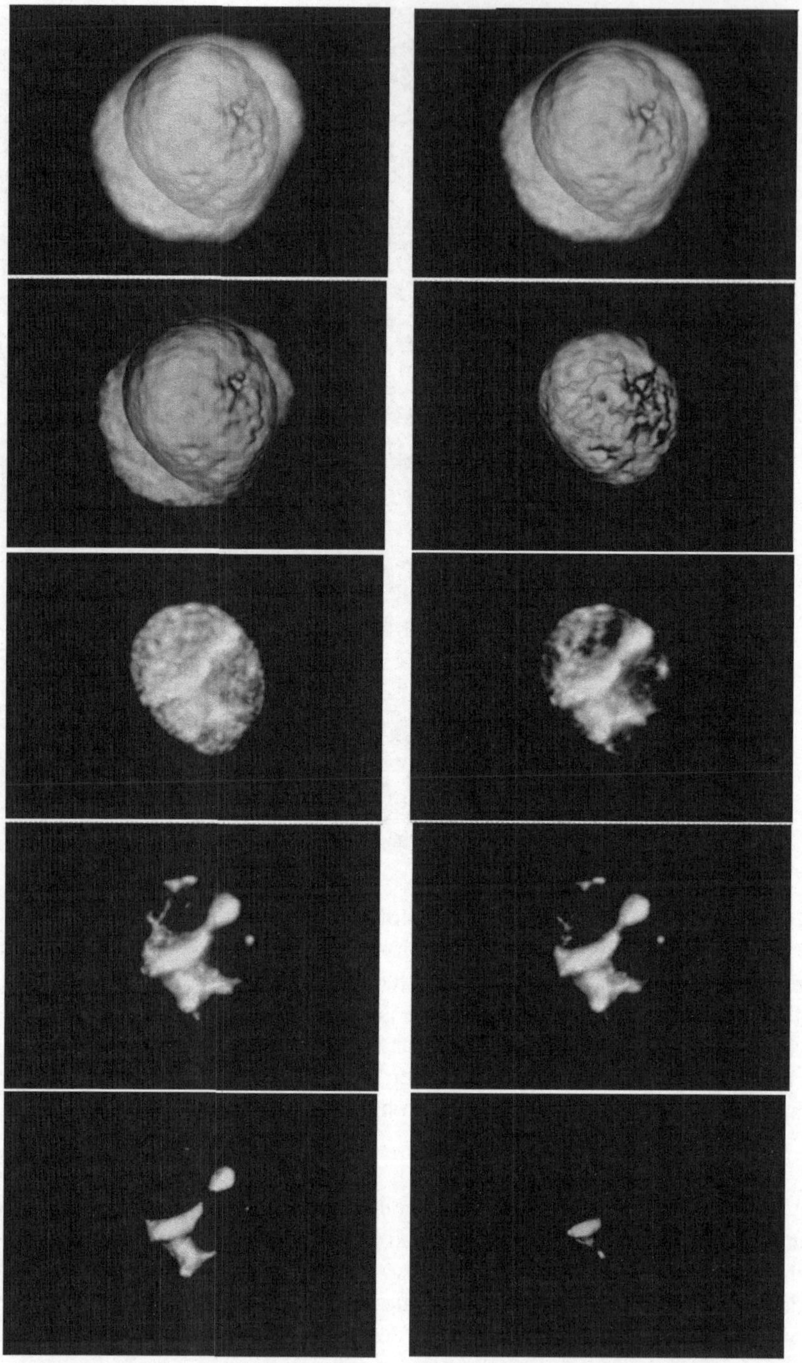

Figure 16.17: (See color insert.) Erosion of a volume rendered adenocarcinoma cell where color and opacity have been adjusted to highlight cell structures of interest. Coloring and opacity render the cytoplasm (translucent white), nuclear wall (opaque blue), nucleoplasm (translucent green), and condensed chromatin (opaque red). The cell visualization was further processed to erode the visible aspect of the cell boundary. In the images from top left to bottom right, the threshold for visualization was gradually increased. Thus in the first image one can observe the entire cell and in the final image one sees only the most condensed cell chromatin.

nocarcinoma cell, in the same orientation as that of Fig. 16.17 was progressively cropped to reveal structures internal to the cell. As the face of the volume rendered cell is cut away, the relationship between the cell invagination and the interior space that is devoid of chromatin is first revealed. As more material is cut away, the condensed chromatin that lies in the posterior portion of the cell is revealed.

The possibility of the Cell-CT to provide high-speed, automated classification of specimens based on 3D imaging represents its most significant potential. 3D imaging represents cells comprehensively thus eliminating slice selection and perspective biases that can result in classification errors so that either disease ridden patients are not detected or normal patients are identified for unnecessary follow-up procedures. Meyer et al. assessed the potential for reducing error rates in specimen classification by imaging a set of normal and abnormal cells in 2D and 3D using OPTM. A set of features was defined for both the 3D images and the 2D images permitting a comparative analysis that is unbiased with respect to the cell population used for study or the features defined. The study shows a dramatic increase in the area the receiver operator curve (ROC) 3D analysis over the 2D analysis [60]. But 3D image analysis opens the potential for a new set of features that can only be assessed in 3D. For example, the invaginations discussed in Figs. 16.17 and 16.18 can only be assessed in 3D. These features have been verified by others, albeit using extremely laborious techniques such as fluorescence recovery after photo-bleaching (FRAP) [61]. An example of a cell imaged with FRAP is shown in Fig. 16.19. The Cell-CT opens the potential for a new wave of cytology, extending the practice into 3D and further improving on the noted study.

Lung cancer remains a leading cause of death despite decades of effort to improve treatments. There are still 160,000 annual lung cancer deaths in the United States alone [62]. While treatment of this deadly disease has escaped the diligent effort of 50 years, nevertheless new evidence proves that screening for lung cancer using X-ray CT promotes a 20% reduction in mortality from the disease when compared with screening based on X-ray alone [63]. While this conclusion puts to rest the debate concerning clinical effectiveness of X-ray CT screening, cost remains troubling [63]. X-ray CT is more sensitive than X-ray and thus the majority of the indications from X-ray CT turn out to be false positive. Debate is now focused on the potential harms and costs of X-ray CT, in the form of increased false positive cases.

In this connection, the Cell-CT could be used along with X-ray CT to reduce false positive results from a pure X-ray CT early detection procedure. One possible detection procedure could rely on sputum cells for evidence of pre-neoplastic cells or cancer cells. Böcking showed that 85.4% of the sputum from cancer bearing hosts have abnormal cells [64] and Neumann *et al.* showed that the cancer cell occurrence rate in sputum is similar irrespective of various diagnostic criteria: squamous carcinoma vs. adenocarcinoma, Stage I versus Stage IV cancer, and others [65]. Based on these findings, the Cell-CT could be used in conjunction with their LuCED® (Lung Cell Evaluation Device) automated classification systems to detect sputum cancer cells [66]. Figure 16.20 shows three cells imaged by the Cell-CT. A normal squamous metaplastic epithelial cell is shown at top. The middle row shows a moderate dysplasia cell and the last shows squamous carcinoma cell. These cells were harvested from sputum. Note the scale bar in Fig. 16.20 allows appreciation of the progression of features from normal to cancer. Also, note that as dysplasia progresses the cytoplasm shrinks, the nucleus enlarges, and the cell chromatin becomes more irregularly distributed throughout the nuclear compartment. This process illustrates basic cytological features that have been known about for 100 years.

Cell and nuclear segmentation and various shape, volume, surface area, and chromatin analyses can be done for each cell [60, 67]. These numbers can be combined with expert assessment of cell type to create a database of features and normal or abnormal cell diagnosis, thus fostering expert based classification. While this effort is still in progress, VisionGate has imaged and classified more than 35,000 cells based on 10-fold cross-validation using the technique of adaptive boosting producing area of ROC measures approaching 0.99. Fully automated classification has the potential to detect abnormal cells in sputum leading to very high overall cancer detection rates. With high

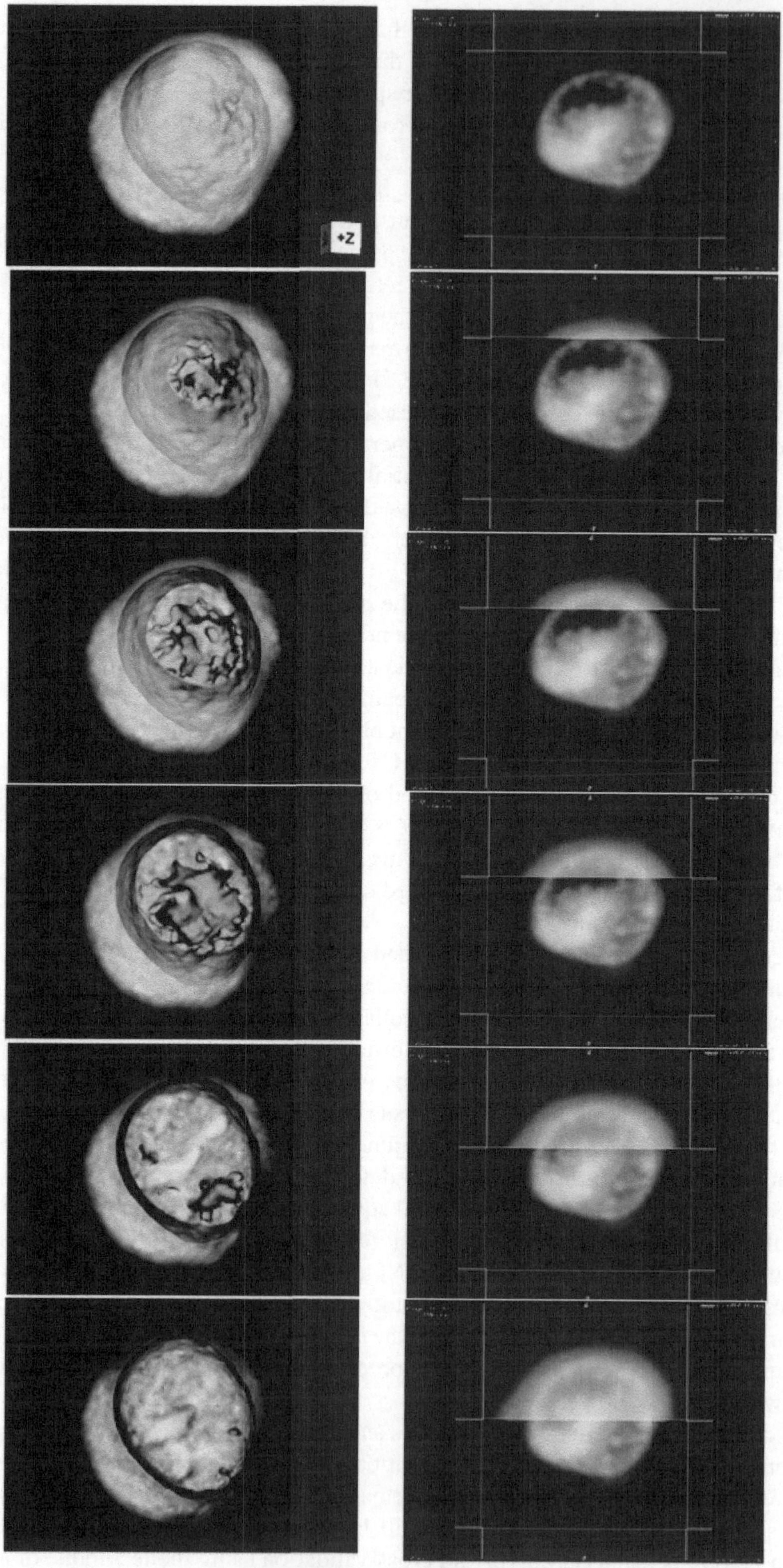

Figure 16.18: (see color insert), caption on next page.

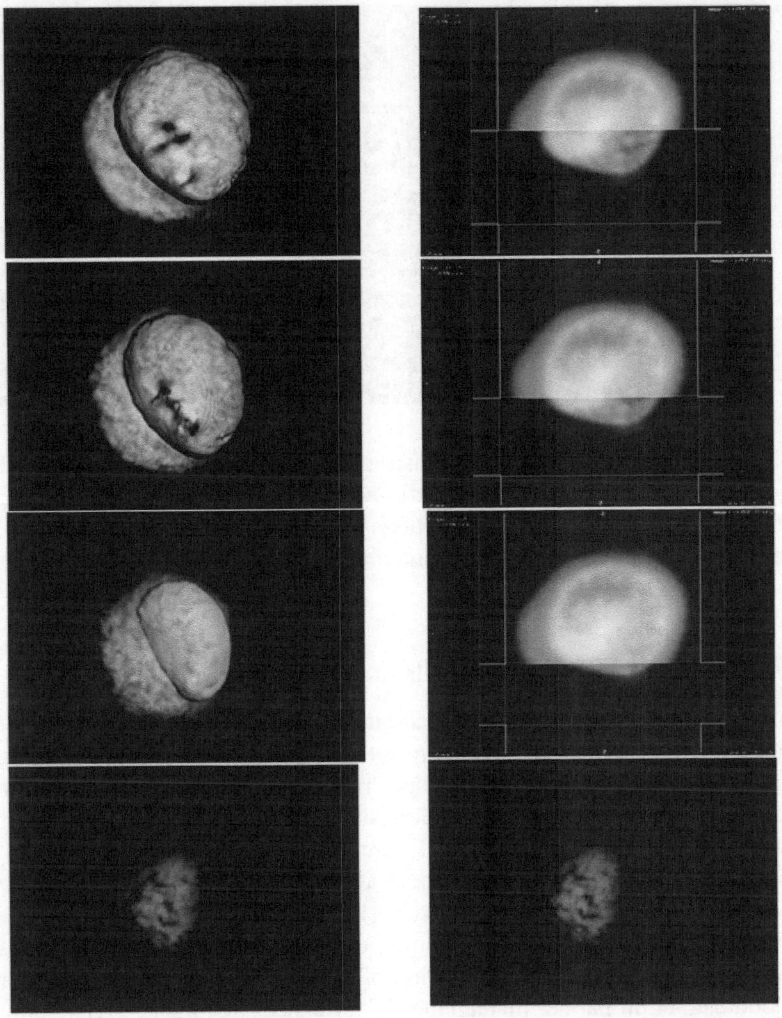

Figure 16.18: (See color insert.) Sweep-through of the adenocarcinoma cell of Fig. 16.17. As with the previous image, the cell was volume rendered with color and opacity adjusted to show the various cell features of interest: cytoplasm (translucent white), nuclear wall (opaque blue), nucleoplasm (translucent green), and condensed chromatin (opaque red). In this sequence the cell is progressively cropped, opening the cell contents for examination. The right images are maximum intensity projections of the cell when viewed through the x-axis. The volume rendered image is shown looking through the z-axis, thus the volume rendered image. The axis of view is indicated by the orientation cube in the first row. Thus, the top line in the maximum intensity images indicates the cropping plane. Low contrast regions on top of the images indicate the part of the cell in the volume rendered image that was cut away.

rates of detection, LuCED may be safely integrated with findings from X-ray CT to remove false-positive findings for possible follow on work [66]. This effort addresses the possible cost aspect of X-ray CT screening alone, making widespread detection a possibility.

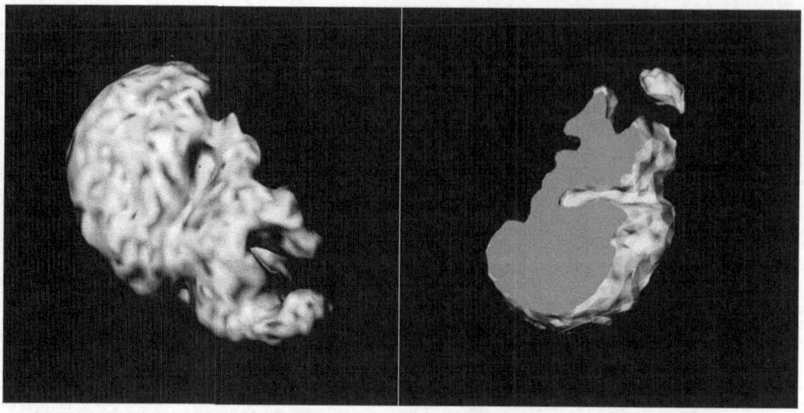

Figure 16.19: (See color insert.) 3D reconstruction of the nucleus of an MDA-MB 231 cell. The left view shows a 3D view of an EGFP-actin-expressing cell and the right column shows a cut away view of the nucleus showing invaginations into the nucleus. This image was provided by Dr. Carolyn Larabell and is similar to one presented in [61].

16.4.4 Future horizons for single cells analysis

The example above illustrates the application of 3D Cell-CT imaging to the detection of lung cancer. The basic methodology of specimen analysis based on absorption imaging and automated classification can be repeated for a host of specimens and analysis objectives. For example, urine could be processed for of evidence of bladder cancer, esophageal swabs could be processed to detect esophageal cancer [68], and the Cell-CT combined with automated cancer cell detection could provide critical feedback in the operating room after a fine needle aspirate specimen has been collected. Specimens could be imaged alive and using deep ultra-violet absorption that can measure the amount of nuclear material without staining or fixing cells. Other applications beyond cancer detection also exist, for example the detection of circulating tumor cells in immuno-magnetically enriched blood can aid in patient management after cancer treatment. Detection of radiation poisoning by examination of erythrocytes in blood can help to scale the threat from a damaged nuclear reactor.

Joint efforts by the UW and VisionGate to promote quantitative feature analysis computed on cells by using validated computational models will aid in the refinement of the Cell-CT optics and allow development of semi-quantitative features, permitting more accurate classifiers with less error in diagnostic specimen analysis. The work reported on is largely based on a manually operated version of the Cell-CT device. For clinical applications, the device has been upgraded to fully automate acquisition such that it is capable of analyzing cells at high speed.

16.5 Preliminary Multi-Cellular Imaging for Future Biopsy Diagnosis Using OPTM

The OPTM has been shown to be a valuable tool for examining internal structures of single cells in 3D. First the device was expanded from absorption to a dual mode device capable of co-registering absorption and fluorescence mode images for quantitative measurement of biomarkers. Recently the OPTM has been extended to perform multi-cell analysis using only absorption contrast

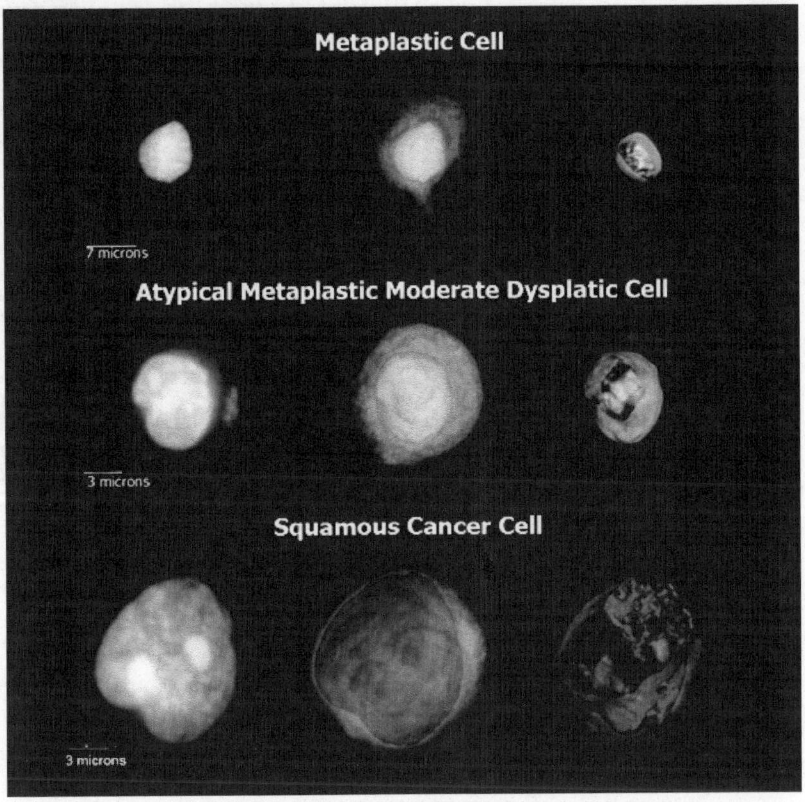

Figure 16.20: (See color insert.) A normal metaplastic epithelial cell (top row), a moderate dysplastic cell (middle row), and a squamous carcinoma cell (bottom row). The left most images show the cell in maximum intensity projection. The middle column shows the volume rendered to include added color and opacity to better visualize cell features: cell cytoplasm (translucent white), nuclear wall (opaque blue), nucleoplasm (translucent green), and condensed chromatin (opaque red). Finally, at right, the cell is cropped to reveal inner nuclear detail. The figure shows the dramatic changes in cell morphology as the cell makes its way through the process of dysplasia and on to adenocarcinoma.

[69]. Average human cells do not exceed 50 μm in diameter. To image these cells, it is sufficient to suspend them inside 50 μm ID capillary tubes. Multi-cellular tissue fragments, such as Fine Needle Aspiration (FNA) biopsies, require the use of larger ID capillary tubes. This increases specimen size to beyond the FOV of the OPTM. In order to image the entire specimen, the power of objective is reduced to increase the FOV. Figure 16.21 illustrates how multiple cells packed inside a 320m ID capillary can be imaged by using a 10× objective [32]. To account for the samples that extend beyond the lateral FOV, the capillary is moved laterally to take multiple images of the specimen (Fig. 16.22). Finally, the images are processed, stitched together (Fig. 16.22), and reconstructed (Fig. 16.23). By using this method, OPTM has the potential to perform analyses on multi-cell biopsy samples [70].

Prior to stitching multiple FOV images together, individual projections are first processed to remove background noise using a background image without any cells. Background pixels can then be identified and removed. This step is critical to ensure successful registration and reconstruction. Sometimes it may not be necessary to remove all of the background. Figure 16.25a shows Fig. 16.21 with its background only partially removed. The capillary tube is visible in the image, and

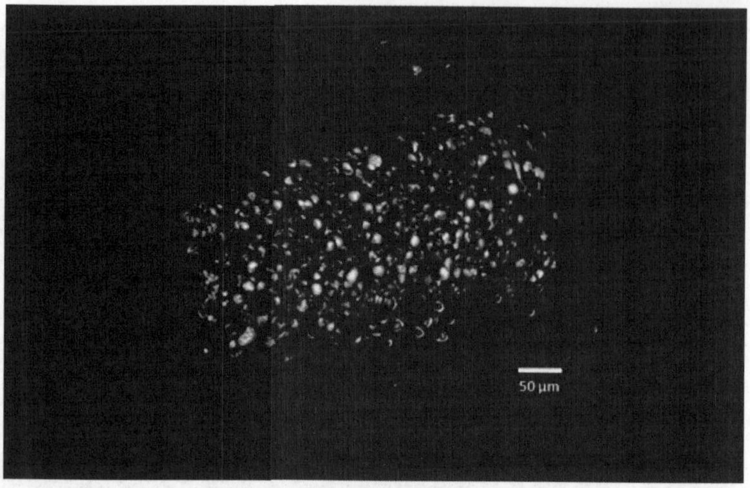

Figure 16.21: 3D reconstruction of one FOV of muntjac cells stained with hematoxylin inside 320 μm ID capillary as seen under 10$\times$ objective. Displayed in VolView 2.0.

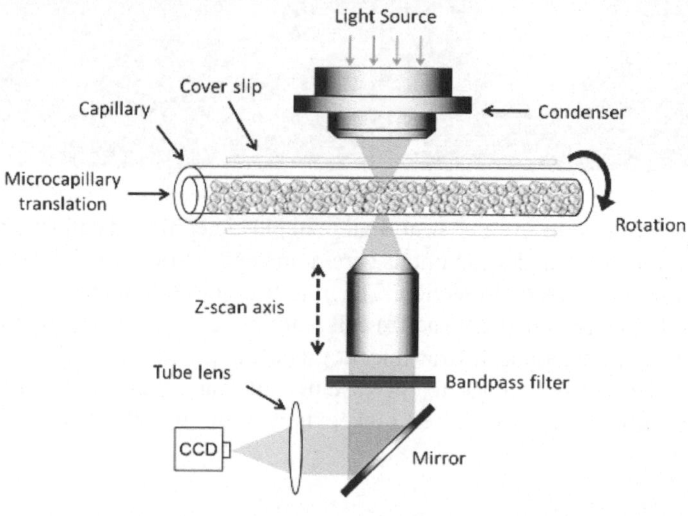

Figure 16.22: Diagram of the OPTM for multi-cell imaging. The micro-capillary tube is rotated to obtain images of different viewing angles. Each FOV is obtained by laterally translating the entire tube. PZT moves the objective lens axially to extend the range of depth of field so high-resolution image can be obtained for larger diameter specimens.

can give users a more intuitive sense of scale. Image registration (aligning two images) is done using phase correlation (PC), a FFT-based cross-correlation method [71]. PC is chosen for its insensitivity to noise and intensity level changes as well as its fast computational speed [72]. Theoretically, the solution to PC is represented by a single peak (Kronecker delta) whose location defines the correct translation vector between two images [71]. The validity of the translation vector is examined by visually inspecting whether the two images align correctly. Using PC, all projections along the same viewing angle are stitched (Fig. 16.22). Lastly, the entire set of stitched projections is used to compute the reconstruction of the specimen with the inverse radon transform.

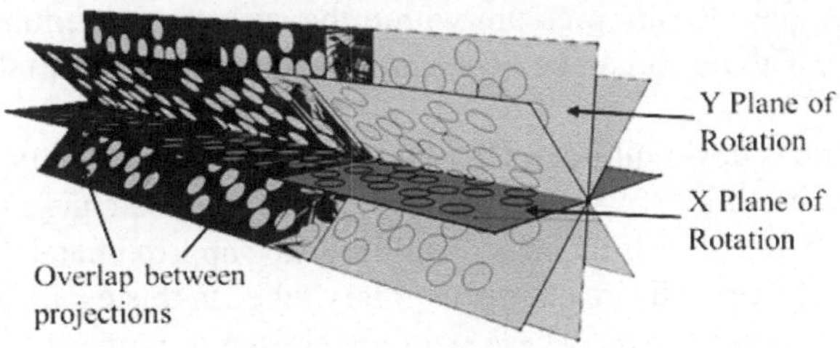

Figure 16.23: Registering each projection plane prior to reconstruction. Projections from four viewing angles (i.e., four projection planes) are illustrated above. Each plane consists of three sets of projections, represented by black, dark gray, and light gray. We register all 2D projections along one viewing angle at a time and repeat for all viewing angles. The offset in all projection planes between sets of projections must be the same, so the resulting registered projection planes will have the same size. This is necessary to perform 3D reconstruction. During implementation, overlapped areas account for approximately 25% of the projection width. Overlap between projections is necessary to implement registration with phase correlation.

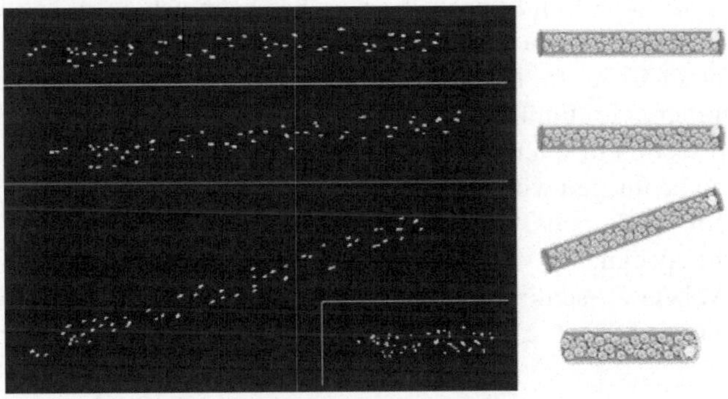

Figure 16.24: 3D visualization of stitched OPTM images of chicken blood nuclei in different orientations rendered using VolView 2.0. Nuclei were stained with hematoxylin and eosin dye and imaged in transmission mode. 62 nuclei in a 50 μm$\times$350 μm capillary are shown. This is used to represent 62 cells in a 250 μm$\times$1750 μm capillary. Cartoons on the right represent the orientation of the images shown on the left. One cell is highlighted for reference. Seven individual sets of projections are stitched together and used for this 3D reconstruction.

16.5.1 Proposed analysis of fine needle aspirates using OPTM

FNA is an established minimally-invasive technique to obtain biopsy specimens. For example, diagnostic samples from thyroid nodules have drastically reduced the need for diagnostic thyroidectomy [73]. In addition, FNAs can be used to diagnose disease of the pancreas, lung, lymph nodes, parotid gland, submandibular gland, and any palpable bumps. The FNA specimen can consist of cells, blood, extracellular fluid, fat, and other biological components. Cells in the aspirate can be sparse and clumped in the presence of these other biological fragments.

Typically, practitioners use 0.41 mm ID (22 G) needle and a 20-mL syringe for FNA [73, 74]. In a study by Glehr et al. the median total number of cells over 15 FNA aspirations was found to be 59,680 cells/mL [73]. In conventional syringes, instability of the internal syringe pressure causes aspirates to backtrack from the needle to inside of the syringe; these aspirates cannot be ejected out for examination. A new FNA device developed by Glehr et al. adds a port to the syringe that stabilizes the internal pressure within the syringe, preventing aspirates from ejecting back into the syringe. The result can be 564% more cells sampled from thyroid nodules, a median of 396,400 cells/mL [73].

Figure 16.24 illustrates how multi-cell OPTM imaging has the capacity to image a higher density of cells that could represent a FNA specimen. In this example, 62 chicken red blood cell nuclei are present along a section of a 50 μm ID micro-capillary tube approximately 350 μm long. These bare nuclei could represent larger cells in a larger capillary tube. In this example, they are about 5 μm in diameter or 1/10 of the capillary ID. These sizes are chosen to represent 25 μm diameter cells in a capillary that is 5 times bigger (250 μm ID and 1750 μm long), which is the size of capillary used for imaging multiple cells with OPTM [69]. Therefore, when scaled up, the specimen in Fig. 16.21 has a density of 721,744 cells/mL. This is more than twice the density of cells obtained by using an advanced FNA syringe (396,400 cells/mL). We conclude that the OPTM has more than enough capacity to image FNA samples.

Assuming a conventional FNA needle biopsy yields a median cell count of approximately 75,000 cells, the length of capillary needed to image all 75,000 cells depends on the anticipated packing density. In Fig. 16.24, cells are sparsely packed, yielding 62 cells/1750 μm. At this density, a 2.1 m section of 250 μm ID capillary would be needed to image all 75,000 cells. At this point, imaging FNA specimen using OPTM becomes impractical unless the cells are flowed through the capillary. However, imaging of more tightly packed nuclei has been achieved, as illustrated in Figs. 16.21 and 16.25 [69]. At this higher packing density, 6 cells (of 25 μm diameter) can be packed into one micrometer section of a 250 μm ID capillary. Therefore 75,000 cells can be packed into a 12.5 mm section of the capillary. Preliminary studies of multi-cell OPTM imaging have shown success in imaging a 15 mm section of the micro-capillary. At these lengths, all cells from a densely packed FNA specimen can be imaged with the OPTM system.

As discussed for single cells, the 3D images generated by the OPTM provides advanced 3D visualization of the specimen, such as being able to display thin slices in any orientation within the capillary. Using VolView visualization software, X-, Y-, and Z-slices through the 3D specimen can be viewed, as shown in Fig. 16.25.

16.5.2 From cytology to histology

Cytology alone often provides insufficient information for tumor diagnosis, resulting in false-negative diagnoses [64, 75–77]. Histological results yield more precise information than cytological diagnoses that analyze isolated cells, smears, and FNAs. The combined cell and tissue samples often improve diagnostic accuracy and can overcome limitations in the amount of information that cytology alone can provide [64, 77, 78]. In some cases, histological tissue samples can show critical information that cannot be obtained from cytology, leading to a change in the diagnostic outcome [75–77]. For example, tissue structure can be apparent, which allows pathologists to identify basement membranes, supporting connective tissue, blood vessels, and the invasive relationship between these structures and tumor cells.

Obtaining a histological tissue specimen often requires the use of core needle biopsy, which is more invasive than FNA. Recent advances in biopsy techniques allow researchers to obtain tissue fragments and cores with increasingly smaller needles [75, 76, 78]. Wittenberg et al. modified standard 22G FNA needles to obtain histological specimens, then processed the samples with standard histological techniques [76]. These techniques include sectioning the specimen into slices for microscopic analysis, which may damage the tissue and compromise the integrity of its biological architecture. Additionally, pathologists do not examine the entire tissue specimen because thin-slice histological analysis results in sampling the specimen. If a method of analyzing whole tissue samples exists, then sampling errors and additional distortion from cutting may be avoided. Using OPTM for histological analysis allows pathologists to examine the entire tissue biopsy specimen. 3D visualization of the specimen would give pathologists a more intuitive view of the tissue archi-

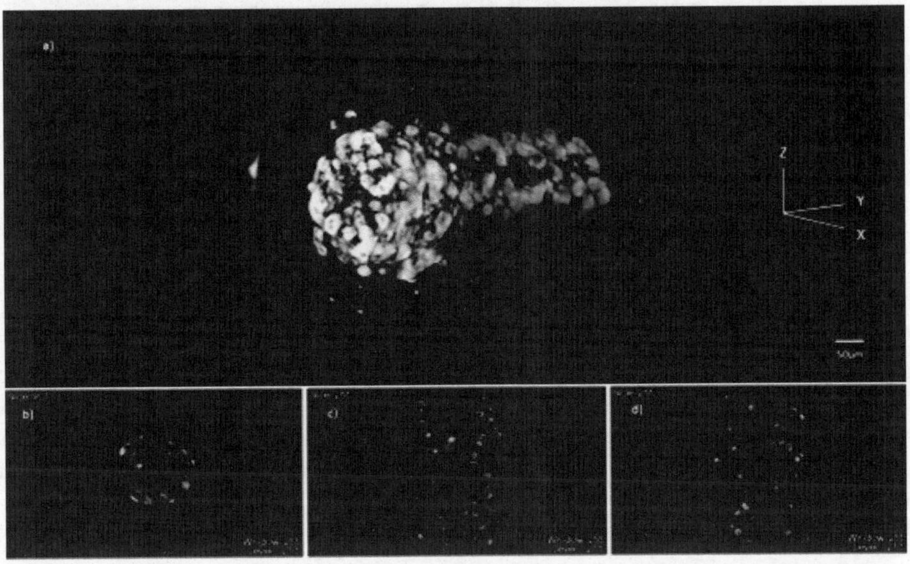

Figure 16.25: 3D reconstruction (a) and slices (b, c, d) of one FOV of muntjac cells stained with hematoxylin inside 320 μm ID capillary as seen under 10× objective. Reconstructions can be rotated to see any orientation. Slices can be obtained along the x-y (b), x-z (c), and y-z (d) planes.

tecture than selected 2D slices can provide. Furthermore, 3D visualization tools are able to show slices of the specimen along any slice planes. Thus, the pathologist has the tools to simulate any orientation of a standard pathological slice, which they are trained to analyze.

OPTM's capability to image tissue is shown in Figs. 16.20 and 16.24; tissue is represented by densely packed cells inside the micro-capillary. Like the FNA samples, tissues also span multiple field of views. This issue is solved by moving the sample laterally and stitching multiple projection images together, a process discussed earlier and illustrated in Fig. 16.21. The challenge in tissue imaging is to minimize the amount of optical scattering that interferes with transmission imaging. Other groups have demonstrated the preservation of high-contrast fluorescence as well as absorption imaging in the presence of optical clearing agents [31]. Unfortunately, the 22G needle produces 0.41 mm thick specimens which may be beyond the 10×–20× extended imaging depth afforded by optical clearing agents [79]. In addition, OPTM imaging of 0.41 mm diameter samples has not been demonstrated. This problem can be solved by using a higher gauge cutting needle to obtain smaller diameter tissue specimens for OPTM imaging. A prototype of a novel biopsy device, the thin-needle core biopsy (TNCB), is able to produce 20 mm length cores of liver tissue that are 0.25 mm in diameter (see Fig. 16.26). A thin-needle core biopsy specimen of this diameter (10-cells across) is expected to be diagnostic, especially when every cell is being imaged in the specimen. This device also has the advantage of reducing invasiveness in biopsy. Compared to typical 1.0-mm diameter samples, 15 times less tissue is extracted from the patient for TNCB specimens. This is highly desirable for biopsies from sensitive organs such as the pancreas, thyroid, and the brain.

In closing, OPTM demonstrates the potential to be a revolutionary tool in clinical pathology. Although many of its applications are still being researched, the results so far are promising. Unlike other 3D imaging microscopes that require fluorescence imaging, OPTM has the ability to perform 3D imaging in multiple modes of transmission (absorptive stains) and reflection (fluorescence). The OPTM is a novel system with the ability to allow clinicians to visualize single cell, multi-cell, and even tissue specimens in 3D as well as in slices; a major advancement over current cytological and histological methods of diagnosis.

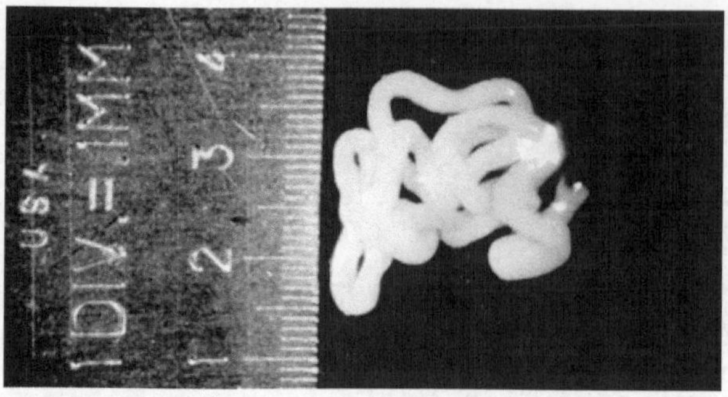

Figure 16.26: Photograph of thin-needle core biopsy (TNCB) taken with a prototype cutting needle device that is able to cut and remove a sample of tissue that is 0.25 mm in diameter and over 20 mm in length. The tissue was cut from fresh chicken liver. To view the TNCB specimen using the OPTM, the additional steps of fixation, staining, and optical clearing are required for 3D visualization.

16.6 Conclusions

The key benefit of OPTM is the submicron isometric resolution of cellular and chromatin structure using a complete range of contrast agents, including the absorbance stains that are used in the vast majority of cancer diagnoses in the world today. Isometric 3D resolution represents the cells comprehensively providing the clinician with complete freedom to select the ideal cutting plane that affords the greatest diagnostic value. Furthermore, the 3D features measured within the volumetric image for disease classifications and computer-aided diagnoses are more sensitive and robust when there is no dependence on 2D slice selection and orientation biases. Classifiers based on current absorption-based morphological features rival the diagnostic ability of a highly trained cyto-technologist or pathologist. These features will no doubt find augmentations as 3D quantitation improves and fluorescence based indications are added, opening a host of new applications.

Questions arise on how new tools and understanding from the research community will be integrated into clinical diagnosis, especially early cancer diagnosis. For example, nanoscale scattering signatures of cells are being measured and correlated to feature sizes below that of conventional optical microscopes, while accurately diagnosing cancer [37, 80–82]. The nanoscale can now be reached with new super-resolution optical microscopes that rely on fluorescence [13–15]. However, a major impediment to translation into clinical practice of pathology is lack of communication between the two communities of researchers and clinicians [1, 4]. The OPTM is expected to play a role in the many steps in this translation process. The first step is to help move conventional cytology and pathology from being reliant on 2D images to visualizing and quantifying features using 3D volumetric images with multimodal contrast mechanisms (absorption, fluorescence, and scattering) [59]. A second step is the development of high throughput cell imaging and multimodal analysis platforms on the OPTM. Since the human observer is expected to be rate limiting in making a diagnosis from a 3D multimodal image, the next step in the translation is expected to be fully automated diagnostic OPTM systems.

Acknowledgments

This work is supported by the National Science Foundation (NSF) grants CBET-1014976 and 1212540, NSF Graduate Research Fellowship grant DGE-0718124, Washington Research Foundation Undergraduate Research Fellowship, and National Institutes of Health BRDG-SPAN grant 1RC3GM093818. Roger A. Schultz and Lisa D. McDaniel at Signature Genomic Laboratories, Spokane, WA provided the Indian muntjac cells. The authors would like to thank Florence W. Patten (VisionGate Inc.) and Melissa P. Upton (Pathology, University of Washington) for insight into the world of cytology and pathology and Anthony Reeves at Cornell University for additional computing resources for simulation of OPTM imaging. Cell-CT is a trademark of VisionGate Inc., (www.visiongate3d.com).

References

[1] D. Zink, A.H. Fischer, and J.A. Nickerson, "Nuclear structure in cancer cells," *Nat. Rev. Cancer* **4** (9), 677–687 (2004).

[2] J.P.A. Baak, *Manual of Quantitative Pathology in Cancer Diagnosis and Prognosis*, Springer-Verlag, Heidelberg, Germany (1991).

[3] B.-M. Ljung, "Techniques of fine-needle aspiration, smear preparation, and principles of interpretation," in *Koss' Diagnostic Cytology and its Histopathologic Bases,* 5 ed., L. G. Koss and M. R. Melamed, eds., Lippincott Williams & Wilkins, Philadelphia (2006), pp. 1056–1080.

[4] L.D. True and C.D. Jordan, "The cancer nuclear microenvironment: Interface between light microscopic cytology and molecular phenotype," *J. Cell. Biochem.* **104** (6), 1994–2003 (2008).

[5] S. Jaffer and I.J. Bleiweiss, "Beyond hematoxylin and eosin—The role of immunohistochemistry in surgical pathology," *Cancer Invest.* **22** (3), 445–465 (2004).

[6] S.J. Jang, J.M. Gardner, and J.Y. Ro, "Diagnostic approach and prognostic factors of cancers," *Adv. Anat. Pathol.* **18** (2), 165–172 (2011).

[7] J.A. Bridge and A.M. Cushman-Vokoun, "Molecular diagnostics of soft tissue tumors," *Arch. Pathol. Lab. Med.* **135** (5), 588–601 (2011).

[8] I. Johnson, and M.T.Z. Spence, *Molecular Probes Handbook, A Guide to Fluorescent Probes and Labeling Technologies,* 11 ed. Carlsbad, CA: Invitrogen Corp (2010).

[9] M. Minsky, "Microscopy Apparatus," U.S. Patent 3 013 467, Dec. 19, 1961.

[10] C.H. Yang and J. Mertz, "Transmission confocal laser scanning microscopy with a virtual pinhole based on nonlinear detection," *Opt. Lett.* **28** (4), 224–226 (2003).

[11] H.U. Dodt and K. Becker, "Confocal microscopy in transmitted light," in *Confocal, Multiphoton, and Nonlinear Microscopic Imaging*, T. Wilson, ed., *Proc. SPIE* **5139**, 79–87 (2003).

[12] Y. Garini, B.J. Vermolen, and I.T. Young, "From micro to nano: Recent advances in high-resolution microscopy," *Curr. Opin. Biotechnol.* **16**, 3–12 (2005).

[13] B. Hein, K.I. Willig, and S.W. Hell, "Stimulated emission depletion (STED) nanoscopy of a fluorescent protein-labeled organelle inside a living cell," *Proc. Nat. Acad. Sci. USA* **105** (38), 14271–14276 (2008).

[14] B. Huang, W. Wang, M. Bates, and X. Zhuang, "Three-dimensional super-resolution imaging by stochastic optical reconstruction microscopy," *Science* **319**(5864), 810–813 (2008).

[15] M.F. Juette, T.J. Gould, M.D. Lessard, M.J. Mlodzianoski, B.S. Nagpure, B.T. Bennett, S.T. Hess, and J. Bewersdorf, "Three-dimensional sub-100 nm resolution fluorescence microscopy of thick samples," *Nat. Methods* **5** (6), 527–529 (2008).

[16] S. Kawata and S. Minami, "The principle and applications of optical microscope tomography," *Acta Histochem. Cytoc.* **19** (1), 73–81 (1986).

[17] V. Lauer, "New approach to optical diffraction tomography yielding a vector equation of diffraction tomography and a novel tomographic microscope," *J. Microsc-Oxford* **205** (2), 165–176 (2002).

[18] S. Kawata, O. Nakamura, and S. Minami, "Optical microscope tomography. I. Support constraint," *J. Opt. Soc. Am. A* **4** (1), 292–297 (1987).

[19] O. Nakamura, S. Kawata, and S. Minami, "Optical microscopye tomography. II. Nonnegative constraint by a gradient-projection method," *J. Opt. Soc. Am. A* **5** (4), 554–561 (1988).

[20] R. Chamgoulov, P. Lane, and C. MacAulay, "Optical computed-tomographic microscope for three-dimensional quantitative histology," *Cell. Oncol.* **26**(5-6), 319–327 (2004).

[21] W. Choi, C. Fang-Yen, K. Badizadegan, S. Oh, N. Lue, R.R. Dasari, and M.S. Feld, "Tomographic phase microscopy," *Nat. Methods* **4** (9), 717–719 (2007).

[22] Y. Sung, W. Choi, C. Fang-Yen, K. Badizadegan, R. R. Dasari, and M. S. Feld, "Optical diffraction tomography for high resolution live cell imaging," *Opt. Exp.* **17** (1), 266–277 (2009).

[23] E. H. Stelzer and S. Lindek, "Fundamental reduction of the observation volume in far-field light microscopy by detection orthogonal to the illumination axis: confocal theta microscopy," *Opt. Commun.* **111**, 536–547 (1994).

[24] S. Kikuchi, K. Sonobe, and N. Ohyama, "Three-dimensional microscopic computed tomography based on generalized Radon transform for optical imaging systems," *Opt. Commun.* **123**, 725–733 (1996).

[25] P. J. Shaw, D. A. Agard, Y. Hiraoka, and J.W. Sedat, "Tilted view reconstruction in optical microscopy - three-dimensional reconstruction of Drosophila melanogaster embryo nuclei," *Biophys. J.* **55** (1), 101–110 (1989).

[26] S. Kikuchi, K. Sonobe, L.S. Sidharta, and N. Ohyama, "Three-dimensional computed tomography for optical microscopes," *Opt. Commun.* **107**, 432–444 (1994).

[27] J. Bradl, B. Rinke, B. Schneider, P. Edelmann, H. Krieger, M. Hausmann, and C. Cremer, "Resolution improvement in 3D microscopy by object tilting," *Microsc. Anal.*, **44** (11), 9–11 (1996).

[28] A. Kak and M. Slaney, *Principles of Computerized Tomographic Imaging*, 1st ed., IEEE Press, New York (1988).

[29] M. Fauver, E. Seibel, J.R. Rahn, M.G. Meyer, F.W. Patten, T. Neumann, and A.C. Nelson, "Three-dimensional imaging of single isolated cell nuclei using optical projection tomography," *Opt. Exp.* **13** (11), 4210–4223 (2005).

[30] N. Streibl, "Three-dimensional imaging by a microscope," *J. Opt. Soc. Am. A* **2** (2), 121–127.

[31] J. Sharpe, U. Ahlgren, P. Perry, B. Hill, A. Ross, J. Hecksher-Sorensen, R. Baldock, and D. Davidson, "Optical projection tomography as a tool for 3D microscopy and gene expression studies," *Science* **296**(5567), 541–545 (2002).

[32] Q. Miao, J. Hayenga, M.G. Meyer, T. Neumann, A.C. Nelson, and E.J. Seibel, "Resolution improvement in optical projection tomography by the focal scanning method," *Opt. Lett.* **35** (2), 3363–3365 (2010).

[33] R.L. Coe and E.J. Seibel, "Computationally efficient method of modeling microsphere near-field scattering illuminated with a focused pulse," in preparation.

[34] R.L. Coe and E.J. Seibel, "Computational modeling of the optical projection tomography microscope using the finite difference time domain method," *J. Opt. Soc. Am. A* **29**(12), (2012).

[35] G.N. Hounsfield, "Computed medical imaging," *Science* **210**, 22–28 (1980).

[36] I.T. Young, "Quantitative microscopy," *IEEE Eng. Med. Biol.*, 59–66 (1996).

[37] H. Subramanian, P. Pradhan, Y. Liu, I. R. Capoglu, J. D. Rogers, H. K. Roy, R. E. Brand, and V. Backman, "Partial-wave microscopic spectroscopy detects subwavelength refractive index fluctuations: an application to cancer diagnosis," *Opt. Lett.* **34** (4), 518–520 (2009).

[38] I.R. Capoglu, C.A. White, J.D. Rogers, H. Subramanian, A. Taflove, and V. Backman, "Numerical simulation of partially coherent broadband optical imaging using the finite-difference time-domain method," *Opt. Lett.* **36** (9), 1596–1598 (2011).

[39] C. Smithpeter, A.K. Dunn, R. Drezek, T. Collier, and R. Richards-Kortum, "Near real time confocal microscopy of cultured amelanotic cells: Sources of signal, contrast agents and limits of contrast," *J. Biomed. Opt.* **3** (4), 429–436.

[40] N.N. Boustany, S.A. Boppart, and V. Backman, "Microscopic imaging and spectroscopy with scattered light," *Annu. Rev. Biomed. Eng.* **12**, 285–314 (2010).

[41] N. Nakajima, "Phase retrieval from a high-numerical-aperture intensity distribution by use of an aperture-array filter," *J. Opt. Soc. Am. A* **26** (10), 2172–2180 (2009).

[42] P. Török, P.R.T. Munro, and E.E. Kriezis, "High numerical aperture vectorial imaging in coherent optical microscopes," *Opt. Exp.* **16** (2), 507–523 (2008).

[43] I.R. Capoglu, A. Taflove, and V. Backman, "Generation of an incident focused light pulse in FDTD," *Opt. Exp.* **16** (23), 19208–19220 (2008).

[44] B. Richards and E. Wolf, "Electromagnetic diffraction in optical systems. II. Structure of the image field in an aplanatic system," *Proc. R. Soc. A* **253** (1274), 358–379 (1959).

[45] P. Torok, P.D. Higdon, R. Juskaitis, and T. Wilson, "Optimising the image contrast of conventional and confocal optical microscopes imaging finite sized spherical gold scatterers," *Opt. Commun.* **155**, 335–341 (1998).

[46] F. Slimani, G. Grehan, G. Gouesbet, and D. Allano, "Near-field Lorenz-Mie theory and its application to microholography," *Appl. Opt.* **23** (22), 4140–4148 (1984).

[47] A. Brunstin and P.F. Mullaney, "Differential light-scattering from spherical mammalian-cells," *Biophys. J.* **14** (6), 439–453 (1974).

[48] N. Martini, J. Bewersdorf, and S.W. Hell, "A new high-aperture glycerol immersion objective lens and its application to 3D-fluorescence microscopy," *J. Microsc-Oxford* **206** (Pt. 2), 146–151 (2002).

[49] T.H. Chow, W.M. Lee, K.M. Tan, B.K. Ng, and C.J.R. Sheppard, "Resolving interparticle position and optical forces along the axial direction using optical coherence gating," *Appl. Phys. Lett.* **97** (23), 231113 (2010).

[50] J.P. Brody and S.R. Quake, "A self-assembled microlensing rotational probe," *Appl. Phys. Lett.* **74** (1), 144–146 (1999).

[51] J.J. Schwartz, S. Stavrakis, and S.R. Quake, "Colloidal lenses allow high-temperature single-molecule imaging and improve fluorophore photostability," *Nat. Nanotechnol.* **5** (2), 127 (2009).

[52] J.E. Harvey and J.L. Forgham, "The spot of Arago: New relevance for an old phenomenon," *Am. J. Phys.* **52** (3), 243–247 (1984).

[53] G. Gouesbet and L. Mees, "Generalized Lorenz–Mie theory for infinitely long elliptical cylinders," *J. Opt. Soc. Am. A* **16** (6), 1333–1341 (1999).

[54] O.B. Toon and T.P. Ackerman, "Algorithms for the calculation of scattering by stratified spheres," *Appl. Opt.* **20** (20), 3657–3660 (1981).

[55] T. Neumann, Q. Miao, J. Yu, M. Fauver, M. Meyer, J. R. Rahn, C.A. Lancaster, E.J. Seibel, and A.C. Nelson, "Simultaneous 3D imaging of morphology and nanoparticle distribution in single cells with the Cell-CT technology," *Engineering in Medicine and Biology Society, 2008. EMBS 2008. 30th Annual International Conference of the IEEE*, 379–381 (2008).

[56] Q. Miao, J.R. Rahn, A. Tourovskaia, M.G. Meyer, T. Neumann, A.C. Nelson, and E.J. Seibel, "Dual-modal three-dimensional imaging of single cells with isometric high resolution using an optical projection tomography microscope," *J. Biomed. Opt.* **14** (6), 064035 (2009).

[57] B. Carpenter, C. MacKay, A. Alnabulsi, M. MacKay, C. Telfer, W.T. Melvin, and G.I. Murray, "The roles of heterogeneous nuclear ribonucleoproteins in tumour development and progression," *Biochim. Biophys. Acta* **1765** (2), 85–100 (2006).

[58] Q. Miao, J. Yu, J.R. Rahn, M.G. Meyer, T. Neumann, A.C. Nelson, and E.J. Seibel, "Dual-mode optical projection tomography microscope using gold nanorods and hematoxylin-stained cancer cells," *Opt. Lett.* **35** (7), 1037–1039 (2010).

[59] Q. Miao, A.P. Reeves, F.W. Patten, and E.J. Seibel, "Multimodal 3D imaging of cells and tissue: Bridging the gap between clinical and research microscopy," *Ann. Biomed. Eng.* **40** (2), 263–276 (2012).

[60] M.G. Meyer, M. Fauver, J.R. Rahn, T. Neumann, and F.W. Patten, "Automated cell analysis in 2D and 3D: A comparative study," *Pattern Recogn.* **42**, 141–146 (2009).

[61] N. Johnson, M. Krebs, R. Boudreau, G. Giorgi, M. LeGros, and C. Larabell, "Actin-filled nuclear invaginations indicate degree of cell de-differentiation," *Differentiation* **71** (7), 414–424 (2003).

[62] A. Jemal, R. Siegel, J. Xu, and E. Ward, "Cancer statistics, 2010," *CA-Cancer J. Clin.* **60** (5), 277–300 (2010).

[63] D.R. Aberle, A.M. Adams, C.D. Berg, W.C. Black, J.D. Clapp, R.M. Fagerstrom, I.F. Gareen, C. Gatsonis, P.M. Marcus, and J.D. Sicks, "Reduced lung-cancer mortality with low-dose computed tomographic screening," *New Engl. J. Med.* **365**, 395–409 (2011).

[64] A. Böcking, "Cytological vs histological evaluation of percutaneous biopsies," *Cardiovasc. Inter. Rad.* **14** (1), 5–12 (1991).

[65] T. Neumann, M.G. Meyer, F.W. Patten, F.L. Johnson, Y.S. Erozan, W. J. Frable, P.K. Gupta, M.B. Zaman, and A.C. Nelson, "Premalignant and malignant cells in sputum from lung cancer patients," *Cancer Cytopathol.* **117** (6), 473–481 (2009).

[66] M.G. Meyer, F.W. Patten, T. Neumann, J.W. Hayenga, D.E. Steinhauer, J.R. Rahn, and A.C. Nelson, "The lung cell evaluation device (luced): early detection of lung cancer in sputum based on 3d morphology," 13th World Conference on Lung Cancer, San Francisco, 2009.

[67] A.P. Reeves, E.J. Seibel, M.G. Meyer, T.V. Apanasovich, and A.M. Biancardi, "Nuclear cytoplasmic cell evaluation from 3D optical CT microscope images," *Proc. SPIE* **8315** (1), 83153C–83156 (2012).

[68] V. Nandakumar, L. Kelbauskas, R. Johnson, and D. Meldrum, "Quantitative characterization of preneoplastic progression using single-cell computed tomography and three-dimensional karyometry," *Cytom. Part A* **79A**, 25–34 (2011).

[69] Q. Miao, J.W. Hayenga, M.G. Meyer, T. Neumann, F.W. Patten, A.C. Nelson, and E.J. Seibel, "High resolution optical projection tomographic microscopy for 3D tissue imaging," *Proc. SPIE* **7904**(2011).

[70] K.F. Chou, Q. Miao, R.L. Coe, and E. J. Seibel, "3D imaging of Fine Needle Aspirates using Optical Projection Tomographic Microscopy," *J. Cytol. Histol.* **S2:001** (2012), accepted for publication.

[71] C.D. Kuglin and D.C. Hines, "The phase correlation image alignment method," *Proc. IEEE 1975 Int. Conf. Cybernet. Society*, 163–165, (1975).

[72] B. Zitová and J. Flusser, "Image registration methods: a survey," *Image Vision Comput* **21** (11), 977–1000 (2003).

[73] M. Glehr, A. Leithner, G. Gruber, P. Wretschitsch, M. Zacherl, T. Kroneis, F. Quehenberger, and R. Windhager, "A new fine-needle aspiration system," *Surg. Innov.* **17** (2), 136–141 (2010).

[74] G. Kocjan, A. Chandra, P. Cross, K. Denton, T. Giles, A. Herbert, P. Smith, D. Remedios, and P. Wilson, "BSCC Code of practice–fine needle aspiration cytology," *Cyotpathology* **20** (5), 283–296 (2009).

[75] R.J. Isler, J.T. Ferrucci, J. Wittenberg, P.R. Mueller, J.F. Simeone, E. vanSonnenberg, and D.A. Hall, "Tissue core biopsy of abdominal tumors with a 22 gauge cutting needle," *Am. J. Roentgenol* **136** (4), 725–728 (1981).

[76] J. Wittenberg, P.R. Mueller, J.T. Ferrucci, J.F. Simeone, E. van Sonnenberg, C.C. Neff, R.A. Palermo, and R.J. Isler, "Percutaneous core biopsy of abdominal tumors using 22 gauge needles: further observations," *Am. J. Roentgenol* **139** (1), 75–80 (1982).

[77] M. Motegi, S. Tanaka, H. Tada, T. Sasaki, A. Hashi, H. Takano, and H. Sasaki, "Comparison of two sampling procedures for diagnosing endometrial carcinoma and hyperplasia: Outpatient tissue biopsy versus cytologic examination," *J. Cytol. Histol.* **2** (3) (2011).

[78] J. Iglesias-Garcia, J.W. Poley, A. Larghi, M. Giovannini, M.C. Petrone, I. Abdulkader, G. Monges, G. Costamagna, P. Arcidiacono, K. Biermann, G. Rindi, C. Dogloni, M. Bruno, and J.E. Dominguesz-Munoz, "Feasibility and yield of a new EUS histology needle: results from a multicenter, pooled, cohort study," *Gastrointest. Endosc.* **73** (6), 1189–1196 (2011).

[79] V.V. Tuchin, *Optical Clearing of Tissues and Blood*, SPIE Press, Bellingham, WA (2006).

[80] P. Wang, R.K. Bista, W.E. Khalbuss, W. Qiu, S. Uttam, K. Staton, L. Zhang, T.A. Brentnall, R.E. Brand, and Y. Liu, "Nanoscale nuclear architecture for cancer diagnosis beyond pathology via spatial-domain low-coherence quantitative phase microscopy," *J. Biomed. Opt.* **15** (6), 066028 (2010).

[81] C. MacAulay, S. Lam, P.W. Payne, J.C. LeRiche, and B. Palcic, "Malignancy-associated changes in bronchial epithelial cells in biopsy specimens," *Anal. Quant. Cytol. Histol.* **17** (1), 55–61 (1995).

[82] N. Anderson, J. Houghton, S. J. Kirk, D. Frank, J. Ranger-Moore, D. S. Alberts, D. Thompson, and P.H. Bartels, "Malignancy-associated changes in lactiferous duct epithelium," *Anal. Quant. Cytol. Histol.* **25** (2), 63–72 (2003).

17

Tissue Optical Clearing

Dan Zhu, Qingming Luo

Britton Chance Center for Biomedical Photonics, Wuhan National Laboratory for Optoelectronics, Huazhong University of Science and Technology, Wuhan, China; Key Laboratory of Biomedical Photonics of Ministry of Education, Huazhong University of Science and Technology, Wuhan, China

Valery V. Tuchin

Saratov State University, Russian Federation; Institute of Precise Mechanics and Control of RAS, Saratov, Russian Federation; University of Oulu, Finland

17.1 Introduction

For the last 20 years, the optical technology for molecular imaging and medical diagnosis with high sensitivity and resolution has been a focus of life science and engineering. Noninvasive lasers or phototherapy have been applied to many branches of medicine, including cosmetic dermatology. However, the limited penetration of visible and near-infrared light caused by the high scattering in turbid biological tissues affects its applicability in preclinical and clinical medicine, and other life science [1].

If the tissue or organisms were transparent, biomedicine would be a breeze. With the ability to see through tissues, scientists could spot the development of tumors more easily in studying animals, biologists could study exactly how an animal's organs developed by observing them as they grow, and neurobiologists could find the neural junction and reveal the secrets of the brain. In brief, the secrets of life would be out there for everyone to see.

It is well known that a transparent adult zebrafish has been created with transgene technique by Richard White, a biologist at the Dana Farber Cancer Institute in Boston, which provides a kind of new animal model for studying cancer pathology and development in real time by using optical imaging *in vivo*. However, the applications of transparent zebrafish cannot resolve all of our problems, so researchers are making strides toward turning human or other animal tissue transparent [1–10]. The body is densely packed with many types of substances, such as bones, vessels, blood cells and many other cell structures and fibers, and light travels through them at different speeds and angles because they have different refractive indices and structures. The result is that light cannot pass through biological tissues in a straight line, much as light doesn't pass through dense fog. To fix this problem, scientists are working on developing ways to block the scattering of tissues. One of the prospective solutions of the problem is a reduction of the light scattering due to the refractive index mismatching of scatters (e.g., collagen, elastin fibers, cells and cell compartments) and the ground material (interstitial fluid and/or cytoplasm) of tissue and blood [6–10].

The tissue optical clearing technique based on immersion of tissues into optical clearing agents (OCAs) with high refractive indices, hyperosmolarity and biocompatibility [3] allows one to effectively control optical properties of tissues, leads to essential reduction of scattering, and therefore enhances the depth to which light penetrates in tissue, and currently attracts great attention [4–13]. This technique, combined with laser speckle imaging [14–15], optical coherence tomography [16–21], fluorescence imaging [22] and laser radiation [23–27], etc. has improved the capabilities of noninvasive optical diagnosis and therapeutic treatments; with nonlinear microscopic imaging or fluorescence imaging, we can enhance imaging depth and obtain microstructure with high resolution [27–37]. Especially when tissue optical clearing technique being applied on investigating the brain [35–36] or central nervous system (CNS) [37], the tissue micro-structural information was obtained with high resolution by using microscopy imaging, which has produced a significant breakthrough in neuroscience.

Here, we will introduce the mechanisms of tissue optical clearing firstly, and then explore how to enhance the tissue optical clearing efficacy and slice tissue with optical clearing technique. Finally, we will pay attention to the safety and the applications *in vivo* of this technique.

17.2 Mechanisms of Tissue Optical Clearing

17.2.1 Optical clearing efficacy of OCAs

Tissues are composed of scattering particles (i.e., cellular organelles, membranes, and fibrils et al.) and background medium (i.e., interstitial fluid and cytoplasm). The former have higher refractive index (1.39–1.47), and the latter have lower refractive index (1.33–1.37). The mismatch of refractive index between the scattering particles and background medium causes the strong scattering of tissue [6–10]. When agents with high refractive index penetrate into tissue, and/or hyperosmolarity agents provide a water flux from tissue, the refractive index of the background medium will increase. The refractive index match in tissue reduces the scattering of tissue, which was regarded as the major mechanism of tissue optical clearing. From this refractive indices matching mechanism of optical clearing, the optical clearing agents (OCAs) with higher refractive indices and/or higher osmolarity (osmolality) would have better optical clearing efficacy on biological tissues. As a matter of fact, the efficacy of optical clearing is not so apparent like refractive index can be measured directly.

Choi et al. [38] defined a parameter, optical clearing potential (OCP), to quantitatively describe the tissue optical clearing efficacy caused by chemical agents. The OCP was defined as:

$$\mathrm{OCP} = \frac{\mu'_{s\,\mathrm{before}}}{\mu'_{s\,\mathrm{after}}} \tag{17.1}$$

where $\mu'_{s\,\mathrm{before}}$ and $\mu'_{s\,\mathrm{after}}$ represent the reduced scattering coefficients of biological tissues investigated before and after OCA application, respectively.

In order to inquire into the dependence of the OCP on the characteristic of OCA, they paid attention to the refractive index and osmolality of each OCA. Table 17.1 summarizes the refractive indices, osmolalities of OCAs, and the corresponding mean OCP values after 20 minute application time of OCA on human skin epidermal side and saline on dermal side. And the mean OCP as a function of OCA's refractive index and osmolarity is shown in Fig. 17.1. It can be found that after

TABLE 17.1: Characteristics of the different optical chemical agents.

Chemical agent	Chemical type	Refractive index	Osmolality (mOsm/kg)	OCP
Saline	Negative control	1.33	280	1.05±0.15
Glycerol	Hydroxy-terminated, positive control	1.47	14550	2.95±0.82
50% TMP	Hydroxy-terminated	1.43	6830	2.19±0.22
100% TMP	Hydroxy-terminated	1.47	13660	2.09±0.71
1,3-butanediol	Hydroxy-terminated	1.44	22050	2.47±0.80
1,4-butanediol	Hydroxy-terminated	1.44	26900	2.95±0.47
Ethylene glycol	Hydroxy-terminated	1.43	22640	2.00±0.60
MPDiol glycol	Hydroxy-terminated	1.44	23640	2.47±0.19
DMSO	Organic solvent	1.47	12900	1.46±0.47
Linoleic acid	Organic acid	1.47	N/A	0.65±0.41
Oleic acid	Organic acid	1.46	N/A	0.67±0.11
P-0062	Hydroxy-terminated prepolymer	1.48	1643	2.15±0.54

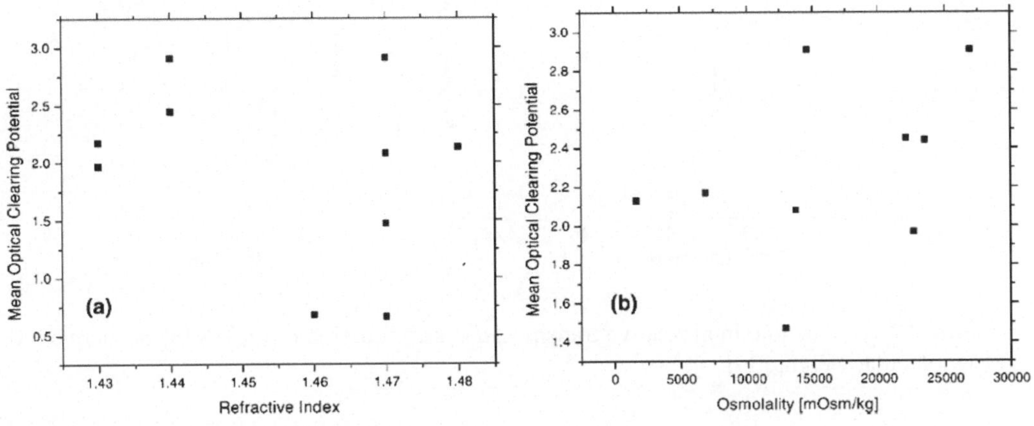

Figure 17.1: Mean OCP as a function of OCA's (a) refractive index and (b) osmolality [38].

OCAs contact with the epidermal side of human dermis *in vitro*, the mean OCP of agents does not correlate with their refractive index nor osmolality. Lipophilic hyperosmotic agents had a mean OCP less than unity.

Considering the optical clearing agents used by Choi et al. [38], they can be sorted into three different groups, i.e., hydroxy-terminated agents, organic solvents, and organic acids. Among the three groups of OCAs, the hydroxy-terminated organic compounds, named alcohols, demonstrated the highest OCP.

Further, Mao et al. focused on six alcohols, i.e., 1-butanol, 1,4-butanediol, 1, 3-propanediol, PEG200, PEG400, glycerol. In order to better stimulate the topical application of OCAs on skin *in*

TABLE 17.2: Characteristics of the different alcohols and saline [39].

Agents	Molecular weight	Refractive index	N (-OH)
1-butanol	74.12	1.40	1
1,4-butanediol	90.12	1.45	2
1,3-propanediol	76.10	1.43	2
PEG200	190–210	1.46	2
PEG400	380–420	1.47	2
glycerol	92.09	1.47 3	
Saline	58.0	1.33	0

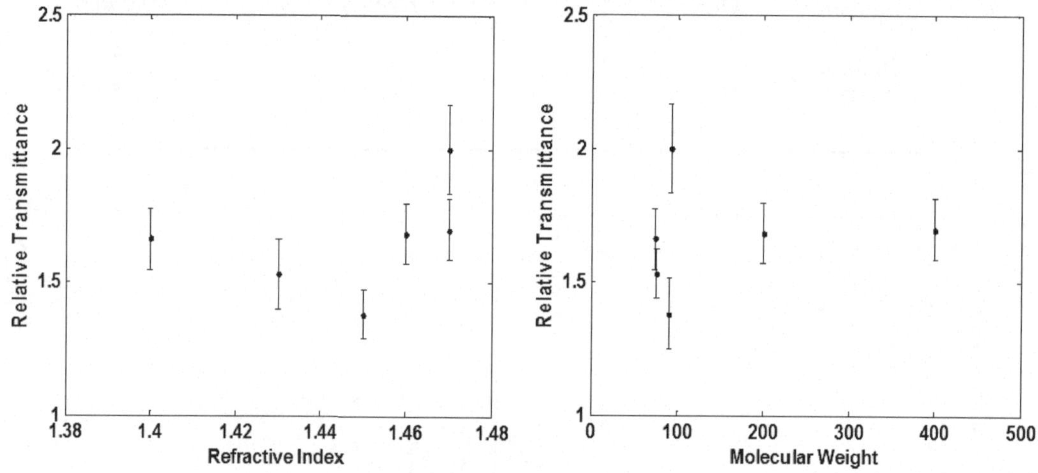

Figure 17.2: The maximal relative transmittance as a function of OCA's (a) refractive index and (b) molecular weight [39].

vivo, OCA was treated to the epidermis and saline to the dermis of porcine skin *in vitro*, and the relative transmittance was used to value the optical clearing effect [39]. The molecular weight and refractive index of the above OCAs and saline are listed in Table 17.2. The correlations between the maximal relative transmittance after 60 min treatment of agents and the refractive index or molecular weight are shown in Fig. 17.2.

The refractive indices of the OCAs used in the work vary from 1.40 to 1.47, while the molecular weight is between 74 and 420. The correlation coefficient between relative transmittance and refractive index is 0.12, and the correlation coefficient between relative transmittance and molecular weight is 0.08, which means neither refractive index nor molecular weight of OCA affects the tissue optical clearing effect directly.

As the scattering of biological tissue is from the mismatch of refractive indices, the higher refractive indices of OCAs should derive higher optical clearing efficacy as better refractive index matching between background medium and solid matter. But both of the above experimental results suggested no direct correlation between refractive index and optical clearing effect. Furthermore, neither osmolality nor molecular weight shows correlation with the optical clearing effect. The limited treatment time of OCAs, which is normally used for optical clearing of living tissues, may be the possible reason for poor correlation, because as it was recently reported that for the total agent-induced mouse brain transparency the treatment may take up to two weeks [36]. Another possibility is from the complexity of the interaction between optical clearing agents and biological tissues, the mechanism of optical clearing might be affected by multiple factors.

17.2.2 Physical mechanism of optical clearing

To further explore the physical mechanism of optical clearing, like the effect of the refractive index increasing of OCA on optical clearing efficacy, tissue phantom may be a good model to block the biological effect of tissues and give a direct answer to the physical mechanism of optical clearing [40]. Among the different types of tissue-simulating phantom, Intralipid, one of the aqueous suspension phantoms, is most suitable in the research. On the one hand, the scattering caused by lipid bilayer vesicles of Intralipid is just close to that by lipid bilayer membrane structures of cells and the scattering property of Intralipid can be predicted based on the distribution of particle sizes [41–44]. On the other hand, when this aqueous suspension phantom is applied to studying the optical clearing effect, the diffuse process of agents can be neglected [45].

Firstly, six different commonly used OCAs, i.e., DMSO, glycerol, 1,4-butanediol, 1,2-propanediol, PEG200, and PEG400, were mixed with 20%-Intralipid. The same total volume of the OCAs or distilled water was added to 20%-Intralipid, so as to keep the concentration of scattering particles of the mixtures constant, as 5%. In order to directly observe the optical clearing of Intralipid caused by OCAs, some photos for background with letters through the normal 5%-Intralipid or its mixture with 50%-OCAs were taken. Figures 17.3a and 17.3b are the photographs of background, and 5% Intralipid solution, and Figs. 17.3c – 17.3h show the photographs of 5%-Intralipid solution and mixtures with 50% OCAs, i.e., 50%-PEG200 (c), -PEG400 (d), -DMSO (e), -glycerol (f), -1,4-butanediol (g), -1,2-propanediol (h). The result shows that 5% Intralipid without any agents conceals the background pattern completely, while all of the mixtures increase the transmittance, and make the background visible in different degree. Here, four kinds of OCAs can keep the solution uniform, and the optical clearing effect decreases gradually in the order of DMSO, glycerol, 1,4-butanediol, 1,2-propanediol. Though PEG200 and PEG400 can also make the solution more transparent, there is some aggregation of particles. This suggests both scattering structure changes

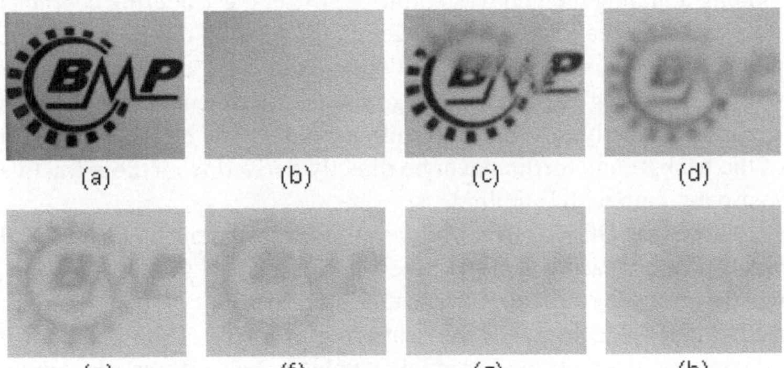

Figure 17.3: The photographic images of OCAs induced optical clearing of Intralipid in the sample cell in Wen's work [40]: background (a), 5%-Intralipid (b), and 5%-Intralipid with 50%-PEG200 (c), -PEG400 (d), -DMSO (e), -glycerol (f), -1,4-butanediol (g), and -1,2-propanediol (h).

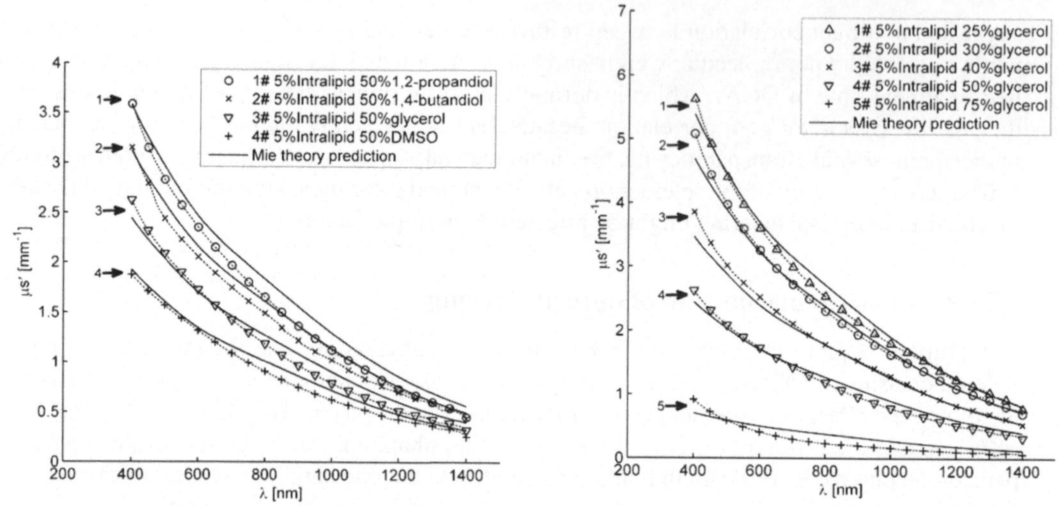

Figure 17.4: The comparison between the theory predicted reduced scattering coefficients and the experimental measured results in Wen's work [40]: (a) 5%-Intralipid with 50%-OCAs (DMSO, glycerol, 1,4-butanediol, and 1,2-propanediol); (b) 5%-Intralipid with 75%-, 50%-, 40%-, 30%-, 25%-glycerol.

and increasing of background refractive index can affect the optical clearing efficacy. For the subgroup of the agents that can keep the scattering structure in the solution, the refractive index of DMSO, glycerol, 1,4-butanediol, 1,2-propanediol decreases gradually and the corresponding optical clearing effect decreases the very same way, which suggested the refractive index matching dominated the optical clearing process.

To make the phantom accessible for theoretical prediction, the particle size distribution of lipid droplets in Intralipid was counted in electron microscope images after the fixing and staining process for the lipid droplets. With the scattering particle size distribution, Mie theory calculation can be used to quantitatively predict the scattering property of Intralipid solution before and after the mixing with OCAs according to their refractive index of the background medium. Meanwhile, the transmittance and reflectance of the solution in a fixed thickness sample cell was measured. Then the inverse adding doubling method was employed to get the scattering coefficients of the Intralipid solution before and after the mixing with different OCAs with different concentration. Figure 17.4 shows the comparison of the theoretical prediction and the experimental measured scattering coefficient. The good matching between the theory and experiment shows the refractive index of the background medium directly can change the efficacy of optical clearing of solution. And the refractive index of the background medium can be directly derived from the refractive index of the OCA used and the mixing ratio with Intralipid.

The results show that OCAs can make Intralipid transparent by changing the structure of the scattering particles or increasing the refractive index of the background medium. If the added OCAs do not change the scattering structure, the scattering coefficient of the mixture is totally determined by the refractive index which makes the scattering property of the phantom be controllable and predicable not only for the scattering coefficient value but also its wavelength dependency.

17.2.3 Dehydration during tissue optical clearing process

Besides the refractive index mismatch of tissue components, the OCA induced tissue dehydration was regarded as an important mechanism of tissue optical clearing [18, 46–54]. A hyperosmotic

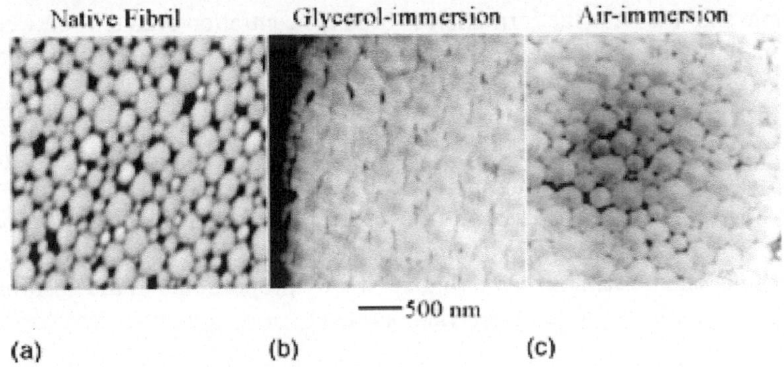

Figure 17.5: TEM images of tail tendon fibrils: native state (a); 20-min glycerol-immersion (b); 2-h air-immersion (c) [50].

OCA provides water flow from the interstitial space out of a tissue, increases the osmolality of interstitial fluid, and draws the water fluid from tissue cell and/or collagen fibers. All these processes reduce the thickness of tissue, make it denser and more OCA coming into tissue, and raise the optical transmittance. Indeed, the dehydration of tissue is commonly happening during the optical clearing process.

When the rat skin tissues after immersion in DMSO and glycerol were compared with the air dried ones, it was found that the air dried rat skin tissues also acquired an enhancement of transmittance like those immersed in OCAs [50]. The described phenomena are quite similar between air dried and OCA immersed, but air drying took a longer time to achieve equally transparency effect. The weight experiments showed that the skin samples after OCA immersion also lost their weight more than intact skin. During the OCAs application by immersion, water is the only fluid coming out of the tissue. Because the exchanges between OCAs and water make OCA fluids into tissue which will increase the weight, the water loss caused by dehydration should be at least greater than the weight increase due OCA flux. The transmission electron microscopy (TEM) can be employed to see the ultrastructure details. As shown in Fig. 17.5, the ultrastructure after the OCA immersion is similar to air drying. Images reveal higher fibril packing density in the glycerol and air-immersed state versus the native state. Volume fraction of tendon fibrils increased from approximately 0.65 to approximately 0.90 due to glycerol- and air-immersion. Measured increase in scattering particle volume fraction corresponds to an approximately 60% decrease in reduced scattering coefficient assuming no change in refractive index ratio between fibrils and surrounding fluid or change in scattering particle size or shape.

The human skin dehydration and hyperosmotic optical clearing agent delivery through epidermis at both intact and perforated (lamp fractional ablation) *stratum corneum* is also described [54]. Accelerated diffusion of water and 88%-glycerol in aqueous solution was found as a result of enhanced epidermal permeability. The dehydration process induced by both stimuli of evaporation (air drying) and osmotic agent action was studied by weight measurements with concurrent monitoring of refractive index alteration of both glycerol solution and water during their interaction with skin samples. The amount of water escaping from skin through the *stratum corneum* due to glycerol action as a hyperosmotic agent and amount of glycerol penetrating through the skin sample were estimated. It was shown with evidence that skin surface fractional microablation reduces the *stratum corneum* barrier function and promotes both enhancement of water escape from skin and penetration of a hyperosmotic agent into skin. The study of the evaporative process allows one to separate the dehydration mechanism of optical clearing from other mechanisms, i.e., refractive index matching by agents or structural modification of collagen. From the practical point of view, free admission of OCAs into skin prevents the formation of high concentration gradients between interstitial liquid and environment solution that decreases the dehydration of tissue and can be considered a positive factor for *in vivo* skin optical clearing, since dehydration relates to decreasing the rate of the fluid exchange process.

The spectroscopy can be employed to further quantitatively analyze the water loss in optical clearing process. Water has strong absorption bands in near infrared region. Xu et al. [46–47] used dual-wavelength analysis method to estimate the water content of skin based on diffuse reflectance spectra over the wavelength range from 800 to 2200 nm. The concentration of analytes in a homogeneous sample without scattering is directly proportional to the absorbance (A_i) at a given wavelength (λ_i) according to the Beer–Lambert law:

$$C = KA_i = K\log(1/R_i) \tag{17.2}$$

In practice, particularly for measurements of biological tissue, the phenomena are far more complicated. This law is no longer applicable because of the interference of analytes other than that under study and, above all, of scattering. The effects of this interference could be partially eliminated by differentiating the apparent absorbance at two wavelengths. For water content prediction, the differentiation of the absorbance at λ_1 = 1100 and λ_2 = 1936 nm was done as follows:

$$C = K(A_1 - A_2) = K\log(R_1/R_2) \tag{17.3}$$

Xu et al. [47] investigated the water content changes of muscle tissues under immersion in 80%-glycerol or 80%-propanediol in 30 min. After immersion, the attenuate coefficients of tissues dramatically decreased in the first 1 min. The decreasing slowed in 1 to 10 min and began to rise again in 10–30 min. The transmission of the tissue sharply increased in the first minute and then slowly increased. By measuring the water content with dual-wavelength method, the water content changes showed good consistency with optical clearing effect, and fast decreased in the first minute and then become slower.

Anyway, the dual-wavelength method for water content prediction is a rapid estimation of water content usually used in food industry [55]. For biological tissue investigation the accuracy cannot be promised and the result is reflecting the relative water content but not the absolute water content. In Yu et al. work [53], a PLS regression model was developed using log 1/*R* spectra within the spectral range from 1100 to 1700 nm. The PLS regression showed good ability of calculating the water content in absolute values. And they compared the reduced changes of scattering coefficients

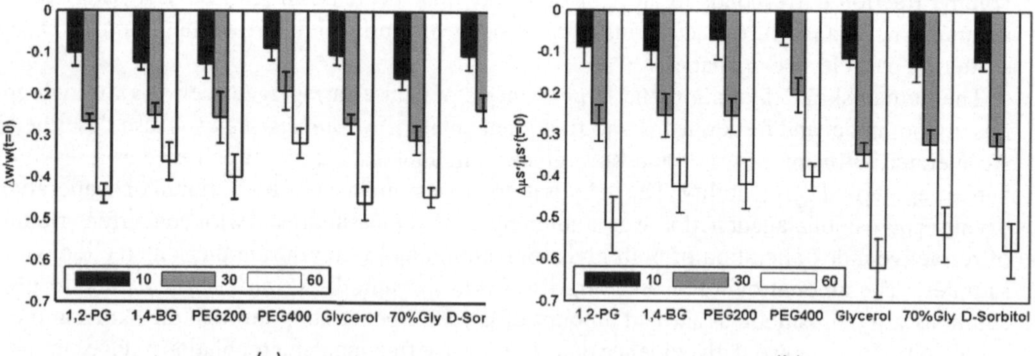

Figure 17.6: Relative reduction of water content (a) and reduced scattering coefficient (b) after 10-, 30-, and 60-min treatment with the OCAs [53].

and changes of water content after six different alcohol OCAs immersion. Figure 17.6 shows the relative changes of reduced scattering coefficient and water content at 10, 30, and 60 min after the application of chemical agents, such as 1,2-propanediol, 1,4-butanediol, PEG200, PEG400, 100%-glycerol, and 70%-glycerol, D-sorbitol. As can be seen from the data, the water content reduces by 46, 41, 45, 44, 36, 39, and 32%, respectively; and the optical clearing effect after a 60-min treatment with the OCAs decreased gradually on the order of glycerol, D-sorbitol, 70%-glycerol, 1,2-propanediol, 1,4-butanediol, PEG200, and PEG400 with the decrease of reduced scattering coefficients by 62, 58, 54, 52, 43, 42, and 40%, respectively. A further statistical analysis was applied to analyze the significant difference between the optical reduced scattering coefficient and the water content induced by each agent. After topical application of glycerol, or D-sorbitol, there is an extremely significant difference ($P < 0.01$) between the relative changes in reduced scattering coefficient and the water content, and there is significant difference ($P < 0.05$) for PEG 400. Whereas, for 1,2- propanediol, 1,4-butanediol, or PEG200, there is no statistical difference between the two sets of data ($P > 0.05$). Hence, it was concluded that dehydration is the main mechanism of skin optical clearing for 1,2-propanediol, 1,4-butanediol, or PEG200 during the 60-min topical treatment, whereas for PEG400, glycerol, or D-sorbitol, some other mechanisms might exist that lead to further clearing besides the dehydration

17.2.4 Molecular mechanism of optical clearing

During the investigation on tissue optical clearing, different OCAs, such as glycerol, polyethylene glycol (PEG), butanediol, TMP, the combined PPG-and PEG-based pre-polymer mixture, sorbitol, xylitol, glucose, dextrose, fructose, sucrose, oleic acid, DMSO and so on, were used [6–13]. These chemical agents can be classified by their chemical structure as alcohols [38–37], sugars [55–56], organic acids [38, 58], and other organic solvents [4, 38, 58]. After having compared the dependence of the optical clearing potential (OCP) on refractive index and osmolality of four different groups of OCAs, i.e., hydroxy-terminated agents, organic solvents, and organic acids, Choi et al. [38] found that the mean agent OCP did not correlate with refractive index or osmolality. Among the three groups of OCAs, the hydroxy-terminated organic compounds, named alcohols, demonstrated the highest OCP (see Fig. 17.7).

Further, studying the efficacy of porcine skin optical clearing *in vitro* caused by six alcohol OCAs, Mao et al. [39] found a rule that the alcohol OCAs that possess more hydroxyl groups have better optical clearing efficacy for porcine skin. According to the number of hydroxyl groups in the chemical structure, they divided the investigated alcohol OCAs into three categories: monohydric alcohols (1-butanol), diatomic alcohols (PEG400, PEG200, 1, 3-propanediol, and 1,4-butanediol), and triatomic alcohols (glycerol). As shown in Fig. 17.8, glycerol, triatomic alcohol, has the greatest optical clearing effect with highest maximal relative transmittance of 2.00; 1-butanol, monohydric alcohol, has the poorest effect with lowest maximal relative transmittance of 1.38; and the four diatomic alcohols are moderate.

The experimental screening of OCAs shows the correlation between the molecular structure and the optical clearing efficacy of OCAs. This kind of correlation reveals that there is some interaction between OCAs and molecules of biological tissues, and the collagen fibers are considered to be the most possible interacting structures of tissue with OCAs.

Collagen fibers have complex self-assemble structures which are the strong scattering sources in biological tissues [59]. Collagen fibers are widely distributed in biological tissues and especially in dermis of skin and cornea of eyes, providing a function of structure supporting. In spite of nearly 30 years' research, there is still not an exact explanation for its complex structure formation. Synthetic collagen-like peptides have been used to demonstrate that self-assembly of collagen I secondary and tertiary structures are driven by specific hydrophobic and electrostatic binding sites. And stability of these structures is enhanced by inductive (electronegativity) effects conferred by hydroxyproline residues. For higher order structures, hydrogen bonding is the primary bonding force between collagen triple helices. OCAs with multiply hydroxyl groups may have strong electronegativity that may screen the hydrogen bones in collagen triple helices that may labilize the higher order structure of collagen to its dissociation. As the screen of hydrogen bones in collagen triple helices is a noncovalent effect, the OCAs effect to the dissociation of collagen can be reversible.

Yeh et al. [60] observed the dissociation of collagen fibers for *in vitro* immersion of tissues in OCAs. Second harmonics generation images of rodent dermis in the presence of 13 M glycerol and upon subsequent rehydration with PBS are shown in Fig. 17.9. Before the glycerol immersion, the fibrous structure of collagen can be clearly seen in the second harmonics generation image

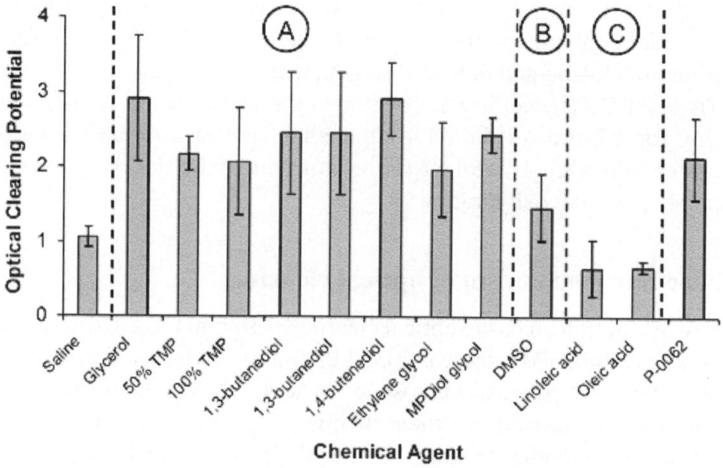

Figure 17.7: OCP of various OCAs under Choi's study [38]. A: hydrophilic hydroxy-terminated chemical agents; (B) hydrophilic organic solvent; (C) lipophilic organic acids; and (D) hydrophilic hydroxyterminated prepolymer.

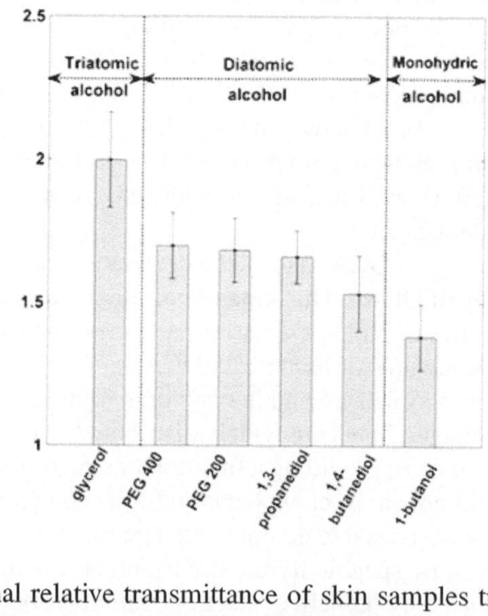

Figure 17.8: The maximal relative transmittance of skin samples treated by three categories of alcohols: triatomic, diatomic, and monohydric alcohols [39].

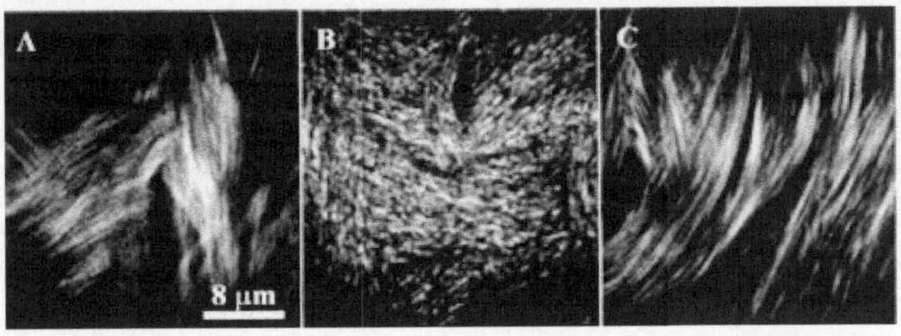

Figure 17.9: Reversible effect of glycerol on rodent dermis. Second harmonics generation images (A) prior to glycerol application; (B) after glycerol application; (C) after rehydration with PBS [60].

(Fig. 17.9A). Following glycerol application, the dermis becomes optically transparent and the fibrous structure unravels into a matted morphology (Fig. 17.9B). Removal of excess glycerol and subsequent application of PBS lead to a recovery of the collagen fibrous structure (Fig. 17.9C).

Molecular dynamics (MD) simulation is a powerful method to analyze the interactions between chemical molecules. Hirshburg et al. [61] began to use MD simulation to explore the hydrogen bonds formation between alcohols and collagen molecules. Figure 17.10 shows the typical hydrogen bond bridges in alcohols. They divided the hydrogen bond bridges formatted between alcohols and collagens into different types. The index of the types is related to the number of carbon atoms of

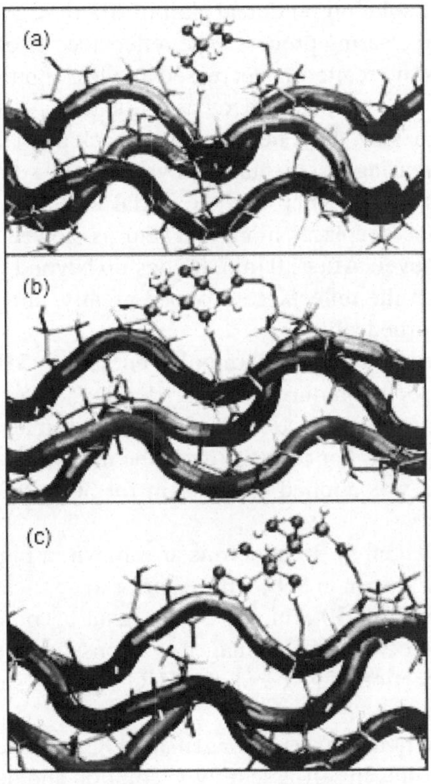

Figure 17.10: Typical hydrogen bond bridges in alcohols. Bridge of –OH groups between one and three carbon positions (type II) in glycerol (a), one and three carbon positions (type II) in xylitol (b), and one and five carbon positions (type IV) in sorbitol (c) [61].

alcohols in a hydrogen bond bridge. Higher bridge types span further across the collagen surface and can potentially disrupt collagen-collagen and collagen-water interactions better than lower bridge types. Thus, alcohols with hydroxyl group pairs with longer distance on carbon chain will have better optical clearing efficacy than alcohols that only have hydroxyl groups next to each other. The simulation results give a good explanation to the fact that 1,3-propanediol was shown to have twice the OCP of 1,2-propanediol even though they had identical molecular weights (76.10 Da), similar refractive index (1.44 versus 1.43), and osmolality (8.3 versus 8.7 Osm/kg) (1,2-propanediol can only form type I bridges, while 1,3-propanediol only forms type II bridges). As the molecular dynamics simulation can reveal the details of interaction between OCAs and tissue structure in the molecular scope, MD stimulation will be a powerful tool in exploring the mechanism of tissue optical clearing and the screening for new high efficacy optical clearing agents.

17.2.5 *In vivo* mechanism of tissue optical clearing

Although plenty of investigations have been performed about the mechanism of optical clearing, all the studies were based on the experiments *in vitro*. In fact, there are big differences between the tissues *in vivo* and *in vitro* in structure and function, and some of the optical clearing agents cannot induce the same optical clearing effect on skin *in vivo* as that *in vitro*. Therefore, it needs to be further discussed whether the mechanism of optical clearing *in vivo* is the same as the results studied *in vitro*.

Wen et al. [62] did some preliminary work on exploring the *in vivo* mechanism of skin optical clearing by glycerol solution. Optical clearing efficacy was achieved by dermal injection of different concentrations of glycerol solution on dorsal skin of SD rats. A VIS-NIR fiber spectrometer was used to monitor the optical clearing process. The reflectance of optical clearing dropped during the optical clearing process as the scattering decreased and less light was reflected from skin.

After injection of glycerol, reflectance decreases due to the reduction of scattering in the region of 400-900 nm. As time goes by, the reflectance goes back up. The result shows, for 20%-glycerol, after the injection the decreasing of reflectance is very small. After 5 min, it returns to initial level. After 30 min, it increases to be higher than the initial level as swelling. For 30%-glycerol, after the injection the reflectance decreases more and returns slower. After 10 min, the reflectance is still lower than the initial level. After 30 min, it goes up beyond the original reflectance. For 75%-glycerol, after the injection the reflectance dropped greatly, about 70%, and the spectrum lost its shape. After 30 min, it returned a little.

It has been demonstrated that second harmonic generation (SHG) imaging can be used in monitoring collagen fibers dissociation during optical clearing. The rat skin was cut down in size of 5 mm $\times$ 5 mm at 10 min after the injection of glycerol and imaged at approximately 30 μm from dermal side on the SHG system. For control group, the normal rat skin was also imaged under SHG system and 13 M glycerol was applied on the skin for 30 min *in vitro* to see the collagen fibers dissociation in SHG images.

The SHG images of collagen fibers in dermis are shown in Fig. 17.11. For *in vitro* experiment, collagen fibers can be clearly seen in SHG images prior to application of glycerol. After immersing the sample in 13 M glycerol for 30 min, the SHG signal becomes much weaker and the bundled pattern can no longer be observed in SHG images as a consequence of collagen dissociation. For the skin cut in 10 min after injection of glycerol, the SHG signal is strong and no collagen dissociation is observed.

It is supposed the interaction between collagen and OCAs screens non-covalent attractive forces resulting in inhibition of collagen self-assembly in solution and destabilization of high-order structures in skin [60-61]. The change in collagen structure and size can lead to a substantial reduction in tissue light scattering. Therefore, they concluded the collagen dissociation is an important mechanism in optical clearing. However, the dissociation of collagen hasn't been found in these SHG images of *in vivo* injection of glycerol. This is mainly caused by the difference between *in vivo*

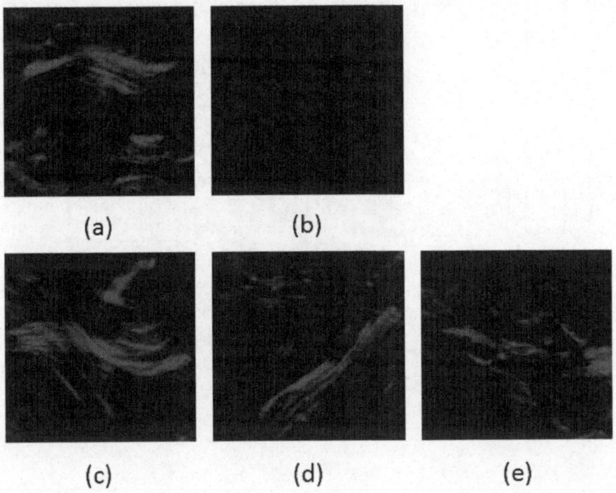

Figure 17.11: Second harmonic generation images of normal skin sample (a), the skin sample immersed in 13 M glycerol for 30 min (b) and skin samples cut in 10 min after injection of: 20%-glycerol (c); 30%-glycerol (d); 75%-glycerol (e) [62].

and *in vitro* investigation, because the metabolism may take away the OCA and decrease local concentration of glycerol. Anyway, it is still an early stage of *in vivo* investigation for optical clearing mechanism. It has a long way to go on the development of the theory for optical clearing. But for further consideration, the research of this mechanism is the basis for the development of the optical clearing technique. So the investigation of this mechanism should be an important focus of optical clearing study.

17.3 Enhancement Method of Tissue Optical Clearing

The tissue optical clearing efficacy depends on the immersion of tissue into OCAs, the longer the tissue immerses, the more transparent the tissue becomes [39]. Therefore, the treated process usually needs to last a longer time; for instance, it needs two weeks for the mouse brain to become transparent when immersed into an innovative agent called Sca*l*e developed by Miyawaki's group [36].

Comparing with other soft tissues, skin optical clearing might be more difficult by topical treatment of OCA. It is the reason that the barrier function of stratum corneum (SC) restricts the penetration of optical clearing agents (OCAs) into dermis [63–64]. For *in vivo* applications of optical clearing technique, the direct exposure of skin dermis to OCAs makes OCAs penetrate into dermis much more easily. However, OCAs at low concentration cannot make skin optical clearing, while OCAs at high concentration could induce edema, suppuration, or even scarring [5, 65]. In order to develop effective and safe ways to breach the SC integrity and accelerate the permeability of OCAs into dermis, many methods have been proposed, including physical enhancement [19, 64, 66–67, 72–79], chemistry penetration enhancer [63, 80–90], and their combination [87, 91–92].

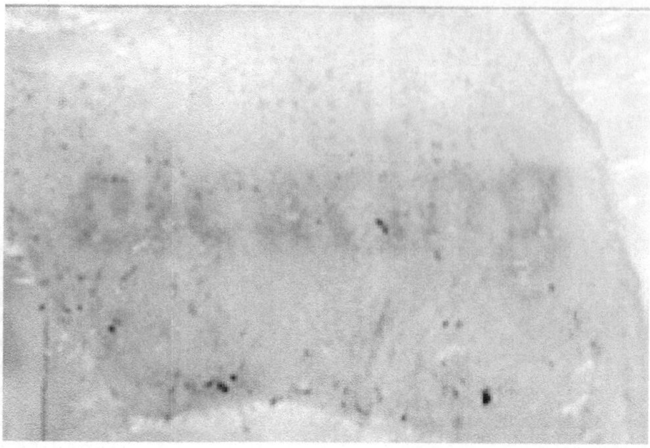

Figure 17.12: Photographic image of rat skin sample treated by two light pulses and 40%-glucose for 60 min [67].

17.3.1 Physical enhancement

Laser and Intense Pulsed Light (IPL) have been used as common tools for clinical cosmetic therapy [68], and also have been used to effectively improve drug or OCAs transepidermal delivery [64, 66–71]. Stumpp et al. [66] used a 980 nm diode laser to irradiate hamster and rat skin with artificial absorption substrates on the surface. The laser irradiation was strongly absorbed and provided precise heating to breach the SC diffusion barrier. After successful removal of the absorption substrates, glycerol was applied to the skin surface. Optical coherence tomography (OCT) was used simultaneously to image the treated area to record the optical tissue properties for 30–45 min. Results indicated that there was an improvement of up to 42% deeper into skin for the ability to measure an OCT signal.

A flashlamp (intense pulsed light, 650–1200 nm, 525–1200 nm, 470–1400 nm) system with the help of an island damage mask was also used to destruct the skin integrity [67]. In the study, the mask with a pattern of carbon-black absorbing centers was applied to the skin surface to absorb light strongly and to create a lattice of islets of damage. Fresh rat skin, farm pig and Yucatan pig skin *ex vivo*, and human skin samples *ex vivo* and *in vivo* were used to verify the optical clearing efficacy of glycerol at different concentration, 40%-glucose as well as 60%-propylene glycol. Transmittance was measured dynamically to record the clearing process. After 1–1.5 hrs of OCAs application, a lattice of islands of limited thermal damage produced on skin surface allowed for substantially enhanced penetration rate of topically applied OCAs, and enhanced optical transmittance (Fig. 17.12). The fractional laser microablation of skin surface by 2940-nm erbium laser pulses with the energy from 0.5 to 3.0 J (Palomar Lux2940, Palomar Medical Technologies Inc.) and the ultrasonic treatment may have a good impact of OCA delivery, including agent delivering by micro-nanoparticle containers [68].

Further, different light sources at different dose and pulse modes were applied to irradiate rat skin *in vivo*, and glycerol was subsequently applied to the dorsal skin [64]. Reflectance of the treated skin area was detected to evaluate optical clearing efficacy. Results showed that the relative decrease of reflectance for irradiated skin samples was eight to nine times more than that of non-irradiated skin samples. *In vitro* study also proved that laser irradiation was able to increase light penetration depth, as Fig. 17.13 shows. This study certified both Q-switched and long pulsed Nd:YAG laser (1,064 nm) irradiation could improve skin permeability effectively and facilitate OCA transepidermal delivery.

In addition to laser irradiation, other mechanical options were also utilized to breach the SC barrier function, including ultrasound application [73–75], tape stripping [24], sandpaper grinding

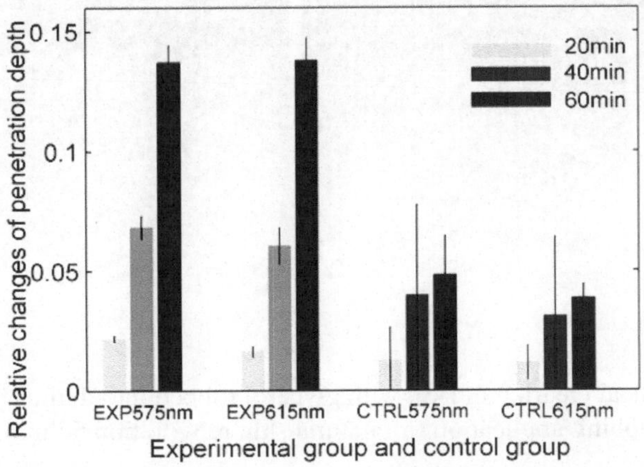

Figure 17.13: Relative increase rate of the light penetration depth for laser irradiated (EXP) and non-irradiated (CTRL) skin samples after glycerol treatment for 20, 40 and 60 min [64].

[76], and microneedle rolling [77–78].

Xu et al. [73] successfully enhanced OCAs to permeate into skin dermis by ultrasound with a frequency of 1 MHz. Ultrasound treatment was performed for about 15 min on *in vitro* fresh porcine skin to which was applied alcohol solution, and then the skin sample was occluded with the OCAs on the surface for 60 minutes. The ultrasound was performed in a pulsed mode and at a low frequency to minimize thermal effects. The OCAs used include glycerol, propylene glycol, butanediol, butanol, polyethylene glycol (PEG200, PEG400). Light transmittance was measured as well as OCT imaging was also taken. Compared with OCA application alone, the light transmittance of ultrasound-OCA treated skin samples increased by 31–57%, and the light penetration depth for OCT imaging was also significantly increased, as Fig. 17.14 shows.

Abrasion of the skin SC by gentle rubbing with a piece of sandpaper was capable of enhancing the

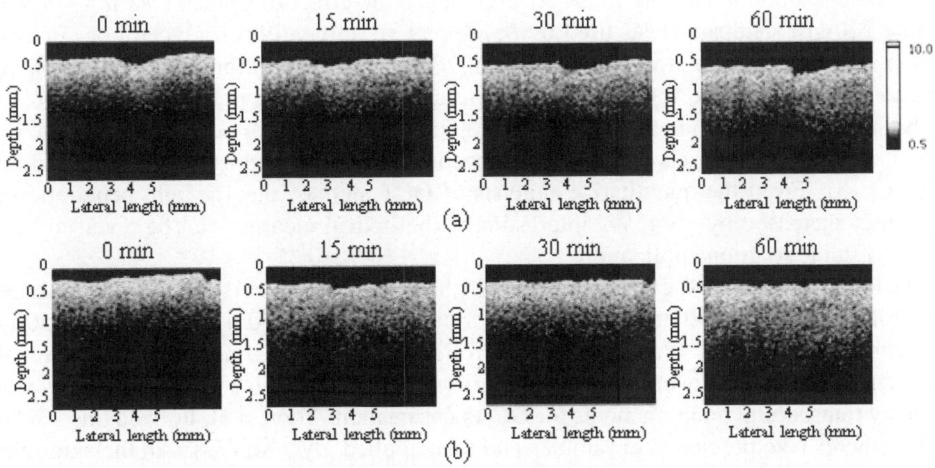

Figure 17.14: OCT images of *in vitro* porcine skin at 0, 15, 30, and 60 min after topical application of OCA (a) and OCA with assistance of 15-min ultrasound application (b) [73].

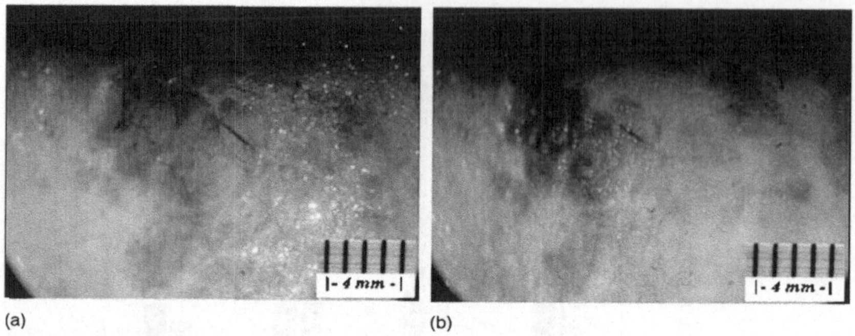

Figure 17.15: Optical clearing of skin with glycerol rubbed into dermis by grit sandpaper: 8 min after glycerol and rubbing application (a); natural skin rehydration 50 min after glycerol removing (b) [76].

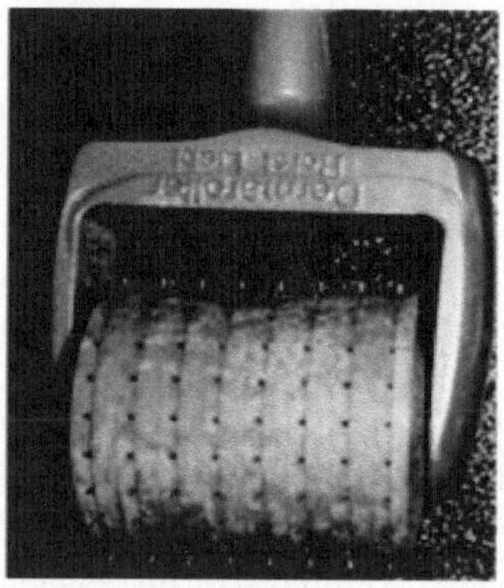

Figure 17.16: Image of a microneedle roller.

percutaneous amount and rate of OCAs and induce the effect of optical clearing efficacy. A piece of fine 220-grit sandpaper was used by Stumpp et al. to gently rub glycerol or dextrose solution into *in vivo* hamster skin after hair depilation [76]. The manual rubbing with OCAs on skin surface was continued for two to four minutes in different directions and performed gently to avoid injury to the skin. In a few minutes after the rubbing, the skin became optically cleared little by little and subcutaneous blood vessels could be visualized and the surrounding tissue remained opaque (see Fig. 17.15). From the quantitative analysis of OCT signals, the 1/e light penetration depth was obviously increased by 36-43%. Interestingly, the optical clearing can be reversed by phosphate buffered saline solution application.

The integrity of skin SC can be directly breached by a mechanical tool called a microneedle roller. The roller usually has 192 needles on a cylindrical surface, with 70 μm diameter and 500 μm height for each needle, as Fig. 17.16 shows. The roller rolling for 50 times each in horizontal, vertical, and diagonal directions over the skin epidermis is able to result in a micro-hole array which serves as many transdermal microchannels for OCAs permeation. Yoon et al. utilized this kind of roller to roll on the *ex vivo* porcine skin samples and then applied glycerol [77]. All the skin samples were placed over a customized modulation transfer function target (MTFT) to acquire cross-polarized images. The contrast and relative contrast of the MTFT were quantitatively calculated to evaluate the enhanced efficacy of the microneedle roller in skin optical clearing. They found the contrast was increased by approximately two-fold for the microneedle roller treated samples compared with the

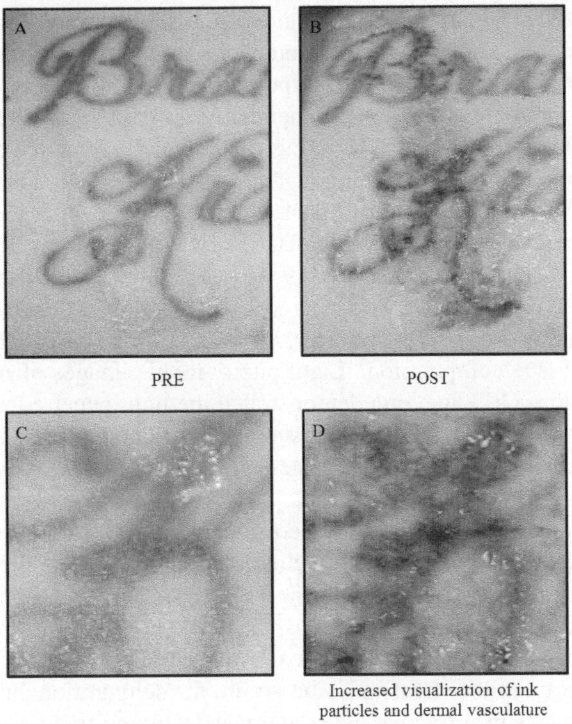

Figure 17.17: Photographs of tattoos pre- (A and C) and post-glycerol (B and D) application [79]. As in B and D, the ink was much more intensified and vasculature was visualized.

control samples 30 min after glycerol application.

Since ultrasound or microneedle roller treatment of skin samples alone could enhance OCAs transepidermal delivery, what would be the combination effect of ultrasound and microneedle? Yoon et al. [78] utilized the combined treatment of *ex vivo* porcine skin samples and then applied 70%-glycerol. The transmittance and reflectance spectra were measured to obtain the reduced scattering coefficients. And diffuse reflectance images were also obtained. As reported, the glycerol transepidermal diffusion rate of skin samples treated by the combination method was approximately 2.3-fold higher than that of samples treated by microneedle roller alone.

Breaching the SC integrity by mechanical methods is an effective way to promote OCAs transepidermal delivery; total or partial ablation of the SC is an additional way to facilitate the OCAs permeation [54, 68]. Tape stripping is a common method used to remove the SC [24]. Tape stripping was usually performed gently and repeated for about 30 strippings to make the skin surface glisten but not damaged. In addition, medical grade cyanoacrylate adhesive bonded on the slide surface was also used to remove the SC [79]. The slide with cyanoacrylate was applied to skin with moderate pressure for appropriate 3 min and then released, keeping for two more minutes. When the slide was peeled, the SC was successfully adhered to the substrate and removed from skin. This process should be repeated for a few times to make the skin glisten. OCAs were subsequently applied to the treated skin area by a low pressure transdermal application device which also infiltrated the OCAs permeation. Tattoos in the skin dermis with removed *stratum corneum* (SC) were much more clearly seen than those with non-removed SC (Fig. 17.17).

The OCT imaging also revealed that the radiation was able to reach deeper regions. For laser tattoo removal, the contrast ratio of the tattoo images and ratio of light absorbed fractions in tattoo area with and without skin optical clearing are important characteristics showing efficiency of laser treatment [21, 80, 81]. Usually increased scattering at shorter wavelengths leads to an increase in the fluence levels required to provide sufficient energy to the tattoo pigment layer. This often leads to undesirable results including scarring, hypopigmentation, hyperpigmentation, depigmentation, pigment darkening, or allergic reactions. Beneficially, at tissue optical clearing the incident density of laser energy for tattoo removal can be reduced in dependence on the tattoo localization depth on 50%-60% in blue-green, on 30%-40% in red, and 10%-20% in NIR spectral range [24, 80, 81].

One of the mechanisms of skin optical clearing is tissue dehydration. A mechanical facility called two tissue optical clearing devices (TOCD) was invented by Rylander et al. to displace water in tissue and reduce light scattering [19, 82]. The TOCD consisted of an array of pins fixed on the inner chamber surface and two brims to interface with skin surface. When the device was connected to a vacuum pump ($\sim$ 750 mm Hg), the brims formed an airtight seal and the pins induced spatially localized tissue compression. Light photographic images of *in vivo* human skin showed localized compression. OCT imaging demonstrated the light penetration depth at spatial positions was increased up to three-fold and the contrast of the epidermal-dermal junction was also increased. OCT M-Scans of *ex vivo* porcine skin revealed an increase for the average group refractive index indicating a decrease in water contents.

Tissue mechanical compression is an effective technology for its reversible optical clearing [8]. Recent studies were directed to apply this technology to OCT, where the penetration depth and image contrast are limited due to high scattering [19, 83–86]. Using a hemispherically tipped glass rod 20 mm long with a 3-mm tip diameter as a probe for localized skin compression and concurrent OCT imaging via this glass rod at a mean wavelength of 1310 nm, the authors of [85] have demonstrated that for similar effective tissue strain, air dehydration and mechanical compression produce similar changes in refractive index and water volume fraction. These data directly prove the concept that mechanical compression may cause local water removal within compressed regions of the tissue [8], i.e., the localized mechanical compression of skin decreases tissue thickness and water content and increases refractive index and OCT signal intensity.

Due to different mechanical properties and water content of epithelial and stromal layers the compression-induced changes in scattering properties of these two layers are different. Thus better contrasting of these layers in OCT images is expected, which was experimentally proved for human rectum *ex vivo* [21]. The same group has reported recent studies on mechanical compression of human skin *in vivo* [84]. The probe was pressed onto human skin with the pressure varying from 0.07 to 0.35 N/mm^2 during 10–15 min while the OCT images of the skin were acquired continuously at a rate of 1 image every 5 s. The temporal dependences of OCT image contrast for the epidermis-dermis junction measured at low and high pressures for volunteers of different ages were associated with different dynamics of water inflow, in particular connected with the different balance of free and bounded water for the young and aged skin and different elasticity of the skin of the various age groups [84].

17.3.2 Chemical penetration enhancer

In addition to physical methods, chemical penetration enhancers used in medicine and cosmetic have also been introduced into skin optical clearing technique, such as Azone [87-88], Oleic acid [58, 89], DMSO [47, 90–92], Thiazone [63, 93–95], and propylene glycol (PG) [96] to accelerate permeability of OCAs into skin to improve the skin optical clearing efficacy.

Xu et al. [88] evaluated the effect of Azone as a penetration enhancer to elevate the OCAs permeation. Glycerol at different concentrations and PG were mixed with Azone, respectively. 60 min after the skin samples treated by PG-Azone or glycerol-Azone mixture, the light transmittance at 1276 nm was increased by 37.3 and 41.1%, respectively; diffuse reflectance at 1066 nm was decreased by 20.6 and 29.3%, respectively. Compared with the optical clearing effect of 80% glycerol, the effect for 40%-glycerol-Azone or 40%-PG-Azone mixture was analogous, which indicated that OCAs permeation was markedly enhanced by Azone.

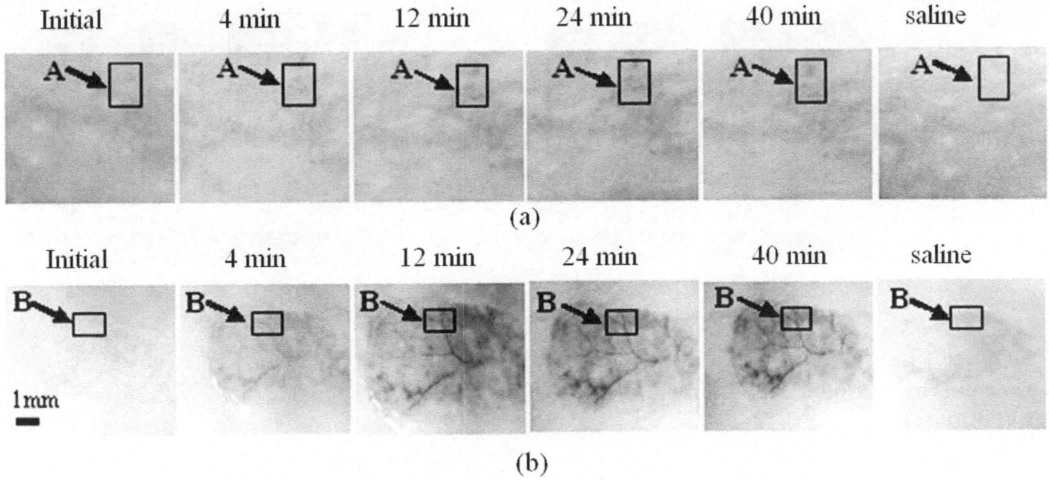

Figure 17.18: Visibility of subcutaneous blood vessels of *in vivo* rat skin before and after treatment with PEG400 (a) and PEG400-Thiazone mixture (b) [63].

Oleic acid (OA) is a mono-unsaturated fatty acid and has also been widely used as a kind of safe transdermal enhancer in the field of drug delivery. In the field of skin optical clearing, the synergistic effect of OA as a promoter to facilitate OCAs permeation into skin tissue has been studied. The mixture of OA-PG and DMSO-PG were respectively applied to fresh porcine skin *in vitro*. From the results of near infrared spectroscopy, mass loss measured and skin permeability assessment, it was speculated that OA had a similar enhancing effect as DMSO did. OA has been considered to be a safe enhancer, so it could also be an optimal enhancer for skin optical clearing [58,89].

Dimethyl sulfoxside (DMSO) was used not only as hyperosmotic agent to induce optical clearing efficacy but also as an OCAs penetration enhancer [47, 58, 90–92]. Previous studies have showed that the mixed solution of glycerol and DMSO was able to play a synergistic effect on optical clearing of gastric and skin tissue, due to the carrier effect of DMSO. However, DMSO possesses potential toxicity and possible side effects to *in vivo* skin, which limits its usage to improve *in vivo* skin optical clearing.

Thiazone, as an innovative penetration enhancer in the fields of pharmaceutical industry and cosmetics, has a skin penetration effect 2.99 times that of Azone [97]. It was first introduced into the investigation of skin optical clearing by Mao et al. [93] and then its use gradually increased [94-95]. Compared with DMSO, Azone or PG, it was found that Thiazone possessed the highest penetration enhancing effect for *in vitro* skin [96]. Taking both the enhancing effect and clinical safety into account, Thiazone may be a better enhancer than DMSO for skin optical clearing. For *in vivo* study, Thiazone also revealed the best enhancing ability to enhance OCA to permeate into skin and made the subcutaneous blood vessels clearly visible after treatment for 12 min and the transparent efficacy of skin will be lasting. After 40-min treatment of the mixture, the saline solution was applied to the area of interest. Immediately, the skin recovered to the initial state, as Fig. 17.18 shows [63].

17.3.3 Combination of physical and chemical enhancement

A solo physical breaching or chemical enhancer was effective to induce skin optical clearing efficacy. Their combination would show much greater potential to overcome the SC barrier function and facilitate OCAs penetration into deep skin [98–99].

Ultrasound [sonophoresis (SP)] has been proved to be effective to destruct the tight junction of the SC "brick-wall" structure and increase OCAs permeation. Sodium lauryl sulfate (SLS) is a

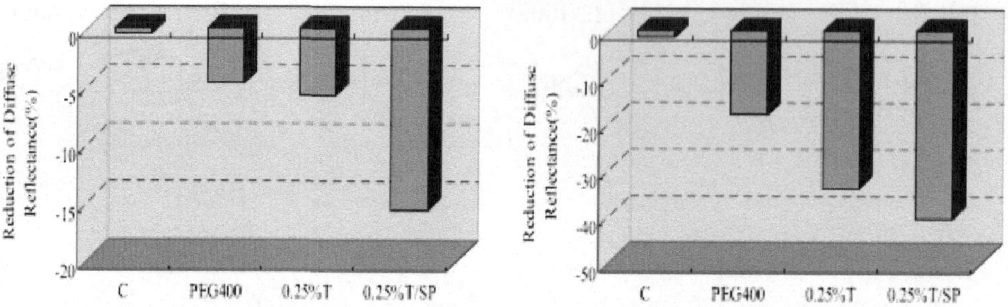

Figure 17.19: Reduction in diffuse reflectance at 540 nm for human skin tissues after 10 (a) and 60 min (b) treatment with nothing (C), pure PEG400, 0.25%-Thiazone (T), and 0.25%-Thiazone/SP (T/SP) [99].

surfactant and often used as penetration enhancer in pharmaceutical and cosmetic products. The combined utilization of ultrasound and SLS was performed on *in vitro* porcine skin and the synergistic enhanced effect on OCAs permeation was investigated [98].

Once the solutions (60%-glycerol (Gly), Gly/SLS) were respectively applied to skin samples, ultrasound at 0.75 W over the 3-cm probe was performed on the samples for a period of 15 min. Light transmittance and imaging depth of OCT were recorded. Results showed that OCA/SP/SLS treatment exhibited a most effective enhancement in increasing light transmittance and improving OCT imaging depth. Moreover, the combination of SP and SLS was able to reduce the treated time compared with SP solo-treatment. Ultrasound treatment was also utilized to combine with

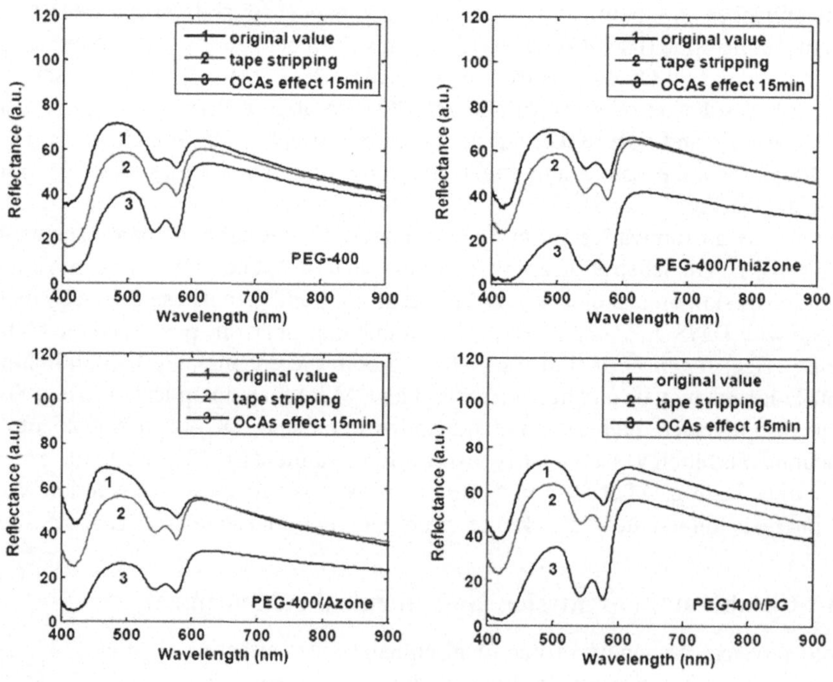

Figure 17.20: Diffuse reflectance of *in vivo* rat skin before and after treatment of tape stripping and chemical enhancer/OCA solution [95].

Thiazone (T) to enhance PEG400 penetrate into skin [99]. The mixed solution of PEG400/0.25%-T was applied to the surface of *in vitro* porcine skin samples or *in vivo* human skin. It is shown in Fig. 17.19 that the diffuse reflectance decreased by approximately 33.7, 3.3- and 2.7-fold in T/SP compared with that of the samples in Control, PEG400 and T, respectively. At the 60 min, the decrease in diffuse reflectance of samples in T/SP is about 2.2- and 1.2-fold compared with that of the samples in PEG400 and Thaizone, respectively, at 540 nm. And the OCT imaging depth increased 41.3%, which was of a significant difference compared with control samples.

The associative action of tape stripping with chemical enhancers, i.e., Thiazone, Azone and PG, had performed over *in vivo* rat dorsal skins [95]. Tape stripping was implemented onto the epithelium surface for about three to four times to loosen the skin SC and then a mixed solution of enhancer/PEG400 was applied to the stripped skin area. Diffuse reflectance was measured, as Fig. 17.20 shows, chemical enhancers combined with physical stripping method was able to facilitate more PEG400 penetrate into skin and decreased the reflectance. The changes caused by the four kinds of agents vary; the largest changes in reflectance were induced by PEG-400/Thiazone, and then, PEG-400/Azone second, PEG-400/PG third, and pure PEG-400.

17.4 Slicing Tissue with Optical Clearing Technique

With the development of the tissue optical clearing technique, this technique is now playing an important role in the biomedical field for obtaining high resolution microstructures.

17.4.1 Optical clearing technique for improving imaging depth of microscopy

Various high resolution optical imaging methods have greatly impacted biomedical research. However, due to the strong scattering of biological tissue, the penetration depth of light in tissue is very limited. As a result, the imaging depth and contrast of these techniques are usually restricted. Fortunately, the development of the tissue optical clearing technique provides a new opportunity for expanding the application of these optical imaging methods.

According to the previous studies, the tissue optical clearing technique has been used to improve the imaging depth and contrast of many optical imaging methods, including Optical Coherence Tomography [16–21, 50, 82–84, 100–112], confocal microscopy [33, 113], Raman micro spectroscopy [114–116], Infrared Fourier spectroscopy [90], fluorescence and bioluminescence imaging [22, 31, 117–119], two-photon microscopy [29], second harmonic generation imaging [28, 120–121], laser speckle contrast imaging [14–15, 122], and polarization imaging [8, 120, 123], and some positive results have been attained. Among these, the combination of optical clearing and optical microscopy, has attracted more and more attention [29–30, 32–37, 113, 124–127]. In this section, we will review some exciting studies on the enhancement of optical microscopy with optical clearing.

Actually, protein solutions with high refraction were suggested long ago in cell microscopy to improve intracellular imaging [128]. The cedar-wood oil or vaseline oil has been traditionally used in classical microscopy to enhance the match of refractive index, and thus improve the imaging quality [129]. However, the tremendous potential application of this technology on the enhancement in imaging depth and contrast of optical microscopy was not regarded until Tuchin's and Welsh's groups proposed to control tissue optical properties using immersion agents [3, 4]. One of the inspiring researches that related to this application was performed by Cicchi et al. [29]. In their study, the *ex vivo* human skin (150 μm thick) was immersed in 0.5 ml of an optical clearing agent (glycerol, propylene glycol, or glucose) and then imaged with two-photon microscopy. The typical result is shown in Fig. 17.21. After the application of the optical clearing agent, the images showed sig-

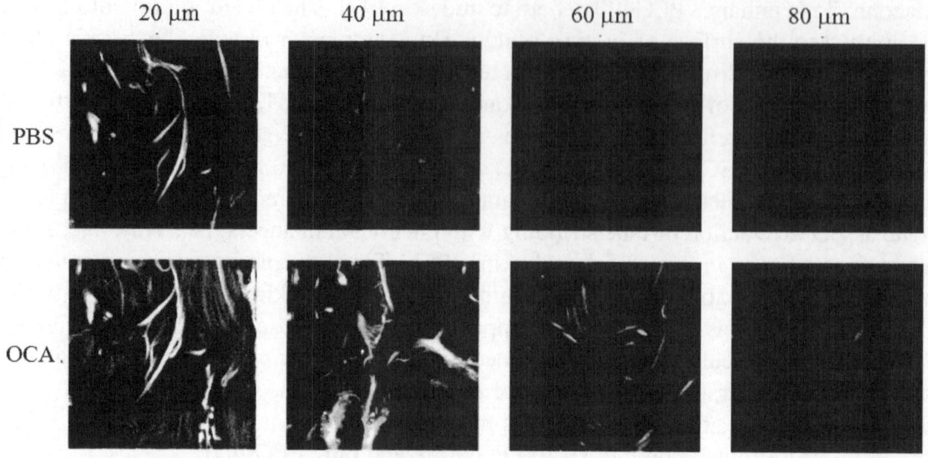

Figure 17.21: Images of *ex vivo* human skin tissue sample immersed in PBS (upper) and after immersion in glycerol (lower) for 7 min obtained with two-photon microscopy [29].

nificant enhancement in the image contrast and penetration depth (from 40 μm to 80 μm) compared with PBS. And this study provides an option for the applications of two-photon microscopy or other nonlinear optical biopsies in deep tissue imaging.

17.4.2 Three-dimensional reconstruction of tissue microstructures

Noting that the tissue optical clearing technique could significantly improve the penetration depth and image contrast of optical microscopy, some groups tried to combine these two techniques for the three-dimensional reconstruction of microstructures of biological tissues [32–37].

In 2002, Chiang's group developed a new optical clearing agent called FocusClear [130], which is better than 80%-glycerol-saline. By direct immersion of 500 μm tissue in their solution, the biological structures, including animal and plant cells, biological organisms, and biological compounds and devices, became more transparent.

After the invention of this FocusClear solution, Chiang's group carried out a series of researches and obtained a lot of exciting results [32–33]. By applying the optical clearing solution, they were able to achieve integrated three-dimensional visualization of microstructure and vascular network of various biological tissues. In 2010, they reported the three-dimensional reconstruction of the ileal and islet microstructure and vascular network successively [32–33]. In the two reports, with cardiac perfusion of a kind of lipophilic dye DiD (1,1'-dioctadecyl-3,3,3',3'- tetramethylindodicarbocyanine perchlorate), the mouse blood vessels were labeled. And then after 4%-paraformaldehyde-fixed and labeled, the ileum or islet tissue sample was immersed in the FocusClear solution for clearing and imaged with confocal microscopy. By the combination of fluorescent labeling, optical clearing and confocal microscopy, the microstructure and vascular network was able to be visualized with subcellular-level resolution. Some typical results are shown in Fig. 17.22 and Fig. 17.23. Compared with the microtome-based tissue imaging, the optical clearing method can reduce the light scattering in mouse tissue and thus yields continuous optical sections. The microstructure reconstructed by this method is more integrated.

Dickie et al. [30] also developed a method for three-dimensional *in situ* visualization of microvasculature of whole-mount tissue which could also be compatible with other labeling techniques, and found that the tissue samples could be visualized to a depth of up to 1500 μm. In their study, after

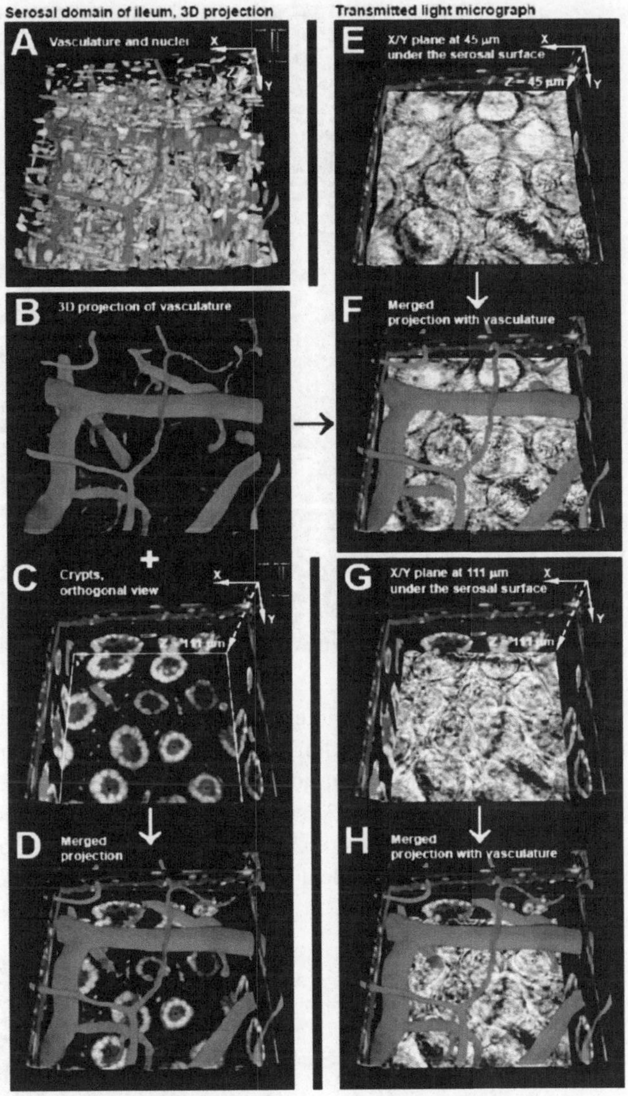

Figure 17.22: (See color insert.) Three-dimension images of the ileal vascular network at the serosal domain. (A) Merged stereo projection of vascular (cyan) and nuclei (gray). (B-D) Separate and merged projections of the three-dimensional vascular network and the microstructure of the ileal crypts illustrated by the orthogonal slices (nuclei: red; GFP: green). (E-H) Merged projections of 3D vascular network and orthogonal views of the combined fluorescent and transmitted light micrographs. In (E, F) and (G, H), the focal planes of the transmitted light images were at the depth of 45 μm and 111 μm from the serosal surface, respectively [32].

labeling of the luminal surfaces of endothelial cells by fluorescently conjugated lectin and filling of the microvascular with carbon or fluorescent nanoparticles/Mercox, the thick tissue samples, i.e., brain, adipose tissue (epididymal fat pad), skeletal muscle (gastrocnemius) obtained from adult mice were then cleared by running through a series of 3:1, 1:1 and 1:3 (v/v) MeOH:BABB (a mixture solution of benzyl alcohol and benzyl benzoate with a volume ratio of 1:2) and 100% BABB until the tissue sample was transparent. After that, the cleared tissue was imaged by a laser scanning

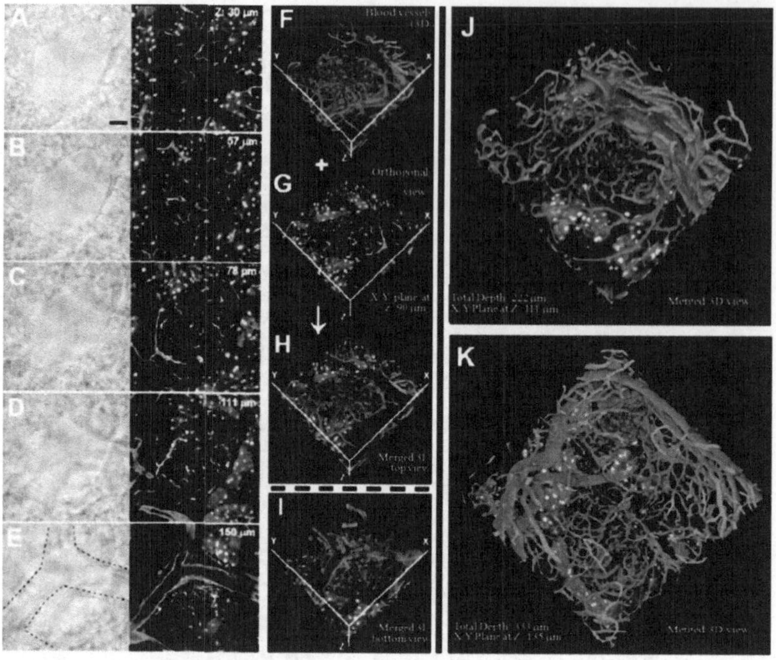

Figure 17.23: (See color insert.) Three-dimensional images of islet vascular in the mouse pancreas. (A)–(E) Images of transmitted light (left) and fluorescence (right) at different depths in the pancreatic tissue specimen. (Vascular: cyan; nuclei: red). (F)–(I) Separate and merged stereo images of blood vessels and the islet/pancreatic structure. (H) and (I) Projections from the top and bottom halves of the imaged area. Dimensions of the scanned volume: 369 μm (x) $\times$369 μm (y) $\times$ 225 μm (z, depth). (J) and (K) Two typical three-dimensional projections of the islet vascular network [33].

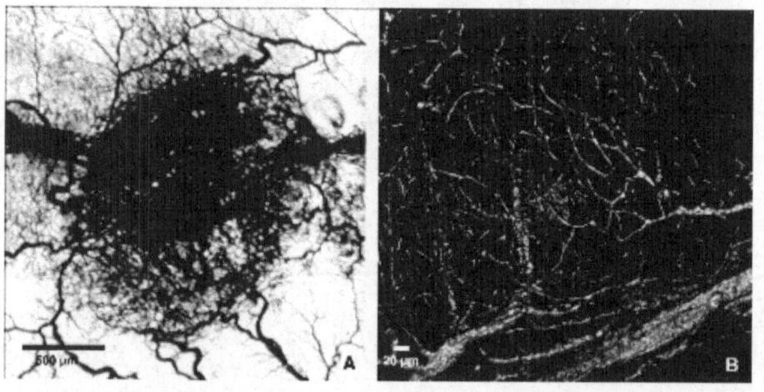

Figure 17.24: (A) Three-dimensional images of cleared, carbon perfused, orthotopically implanted intracranial tumor obtained with light microscopy at a low magnification. (B) Higher magnification three-dimensional images of carbon perfused brain vasculature obtained with confocal microscopy [30].

confocal microscope. If other interested structures need to be labeled, the related protocols could be conducted before the tissue sample was cleared. With this method, the group was able to visualize the microvasculature of various normal and tumor tissue samples to a depth of up to 1500 μm within a three-dimensional context. Figure 17.24 shows an example of their results. The method developed in this study would be of great significance for the research of tumor vascular and other tissues.

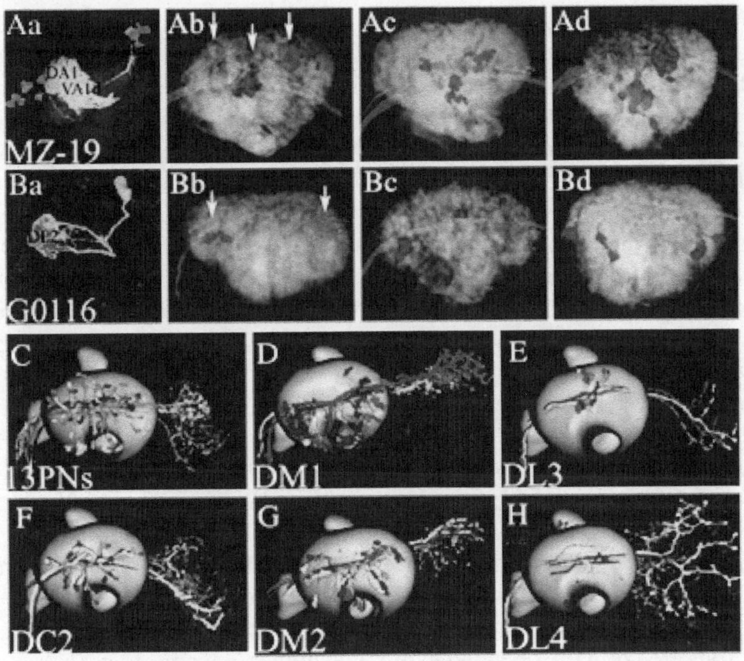

Figure 17.25: (See color insert.) Projection patterns of projection neurons (PNs) in Calyx and lateral horn. (A) Confocal images of GAL4-Mz19 expression pattern. (Aa) DA1 is innervated by dendrites of seven lateral PNs, and VA1d in the antenna lobe (AL) is innervated by six dorsal PNs. (Ab–Ad) Stereotyped spatial distributions of PN axon terminals obtained from three representative flies. The arrows indicate three clusters (arrows) at the medial calyx forming by PN axon terminals. (B) Confocal images of GAL4-G0116 expression pattern. (Ba) DL2 is innervated by dendrites of two dorsal PNs. (Bb–Bd) Stereotyped spatial distribution of bilateral clusters of axon terminals (arrows) in the calyx obtained from three representative flies. The AL and calyx are stained by DiD. (C) Simultaneous visualization of 13 PNs (indicated by 13 different colors) which is allowed by mushroom body warping, each PN innervates a different AL glomerulus. (D–H) The alignment of PNs innervating the same AL glomerulus from five different flies (indicated by five different colors). (Aa) and (Ba), anterior view; all others, posterior view [34].

17.4.3 Optical clearing technique for 3D reconstructions of neuronal networks

Neuroscience research has been a hot topic in the life science field. Techniques like computer tomography or magnetic resonance imaging (MRI) do not yield cellular resolution, and mechanical slicing procedures are not only likely to lose some important information, but also need a long time to get the ultra-structure of whole brain. The development of optical imaging method provides a good tool for exploring microstructure and function of neuronal networks [34–37]. Optical clearing agent reduced the scattering in tissue by refractive uniformity and enhanced the light penetration depth. Subcellular imaging can be achieved for thick tissue. It is useful for light microscopy–based connectomics of cellular networks in brain and other tissues which will contribute to the discovery of new biological principles in connectomics and circuit genetics [34–37].

Chiang's group performed some studies in this area with their invented FocusClear solution [34]. In their study, the paraformaldehyde-fixed and labeled fly brains were cleared in the FocusClear solution for about 5 min. After that, the brain samples were immersed in a drop of MountClear (CelExplorer, Taiwan) for confocal imaging. By some processing techniques, they were able to gain the map of olfactory representation in the drosophila mushroom body, and found that the olfactory coding at the antenna lobe (AL) was likely to be decoded in the mushroom body and then transferred via distinct lobes to separate higher brain centers. Figure 17.25 shows an example of a dual stereotypy which reveals the projection pattern of projection neurons. Without doubt, the combination of optical clearing and optical microscopy would contribute to the research of neuroscience significantly.

However, FocusClear solution can make transparent only the tissues with thickness under 500 μm. For the intact mouse brain, this depth is not enough to complete the 3D reconstructions of neuronal networks. Dodt et al. [35] modified ultramicroscopy (Fig. 17.26a) by combining it with an optical clearing method they developed to obtain three-dimensional reconstructions of neuronal networks in the whole mouse brain. Brain samples were dehydrated in a 30%-, 50%-, 70%-, 80%-, 96%- and twice in 100%-ethanol for 1 d respectively, and the brains were rinsed in 100%-hexane for 1 h. Then they were transferred into a clearing solution of benzyl-alcohol and benzyl-benzoate for at least 2 d (Fig. 17.26b).

Anatomical details of the whole brain were obtained by imaging both the GFP and autofluorescence signal of GFP mice using ultramicroscopy, as shown in Fig. 17.26c. Excised hippocampi were visualized with the labeled cell bodies in detail as shown in Fig. 17.26d. Three-dimensional reconstructions of the dendritic networks were obtained from the optical sections which are shown in Fig. 17.26e. Individual dendritic spines were legible using a 20× objective (NA, 0.4) with a correction collar as shown in Fig. 17.26f. This is most remarkable, as confocal images of spine bearing neurons are normally obtained with much higher NA objectives (NA >1.2).

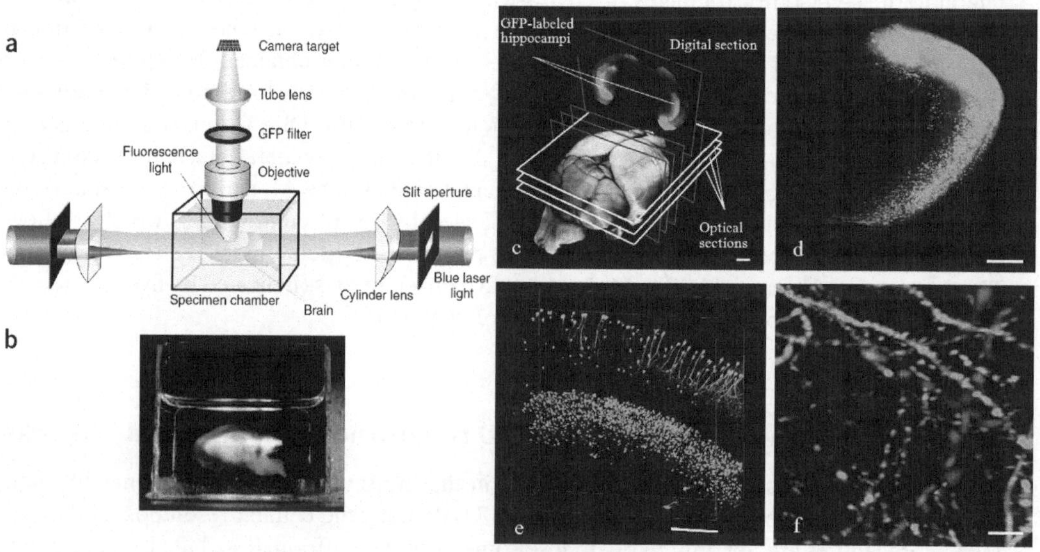

Figure 17.26: (See color insert.) Brain imaging. (a) Principle of ultramicroscopy. (b) A photo of intact mouse brain in optical clearing agent. (c) Reconstruction of a whole mouse brain from 550 optical sections. Scale bars represent 1 mm. (d) Reconstruction of excised hippocampus from 410 optical sections. Scale bars represent 500 mm. (e) Three-dimensional reconstruction of part of a whole hippocampus using 132 optical sections. Scale bars represent 200 mm. (f) Three-dimensional reconstruction of dendritic spines of CA1 pyramidal neurons obtained with a higher resolution objective (20x; NA, 0.4). Scale bars represent 5 mm [35].

Unfortunately, the optical clearing method proposed by Dodt et al. diminished EGFP fluorescence intensity over time [35]. In order to overcome this disadvantage, they developed recently a tetrahydrofuran (THF)-based clearing technique that makes the adult spinal cord and brainstem of rodents transparent and, thereby, amenable to deep tissue fluorescence imaging (see Fig. 17.27). Using this method, they determined the trajectories of regenerating sensory axons and found that

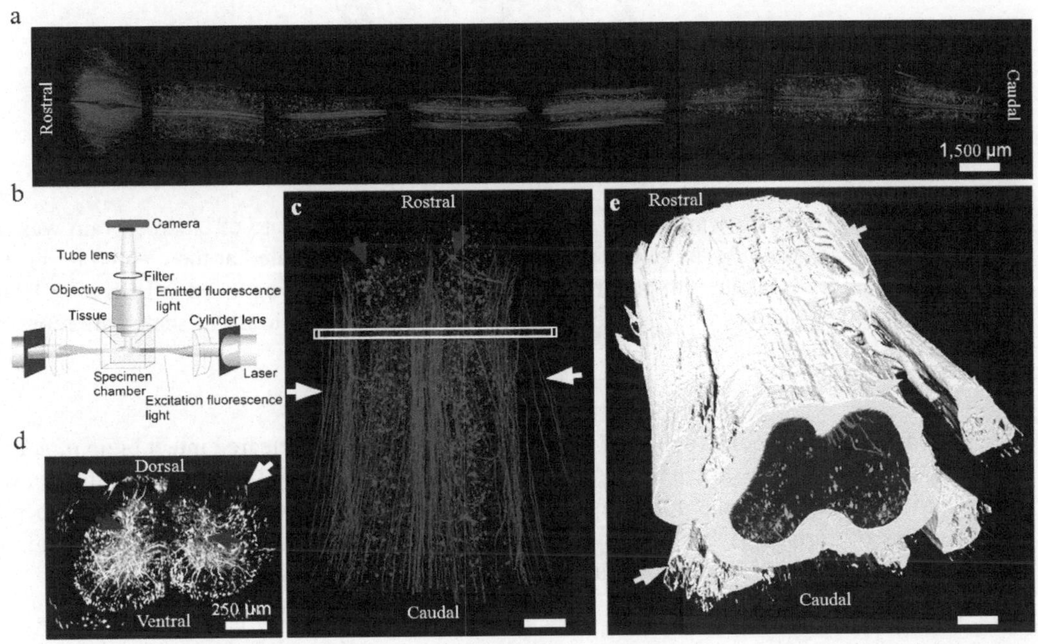

Figure 17.27: (See color insert.) The spinal cord imaging of GFP-M mice. (a) Entire spinal cord of a GFP-M mouse cut into 3- to 4-mm-long segments, cleared and imaged with ultramicroscopy. (b) Principle of ultramicroscopy. (c) A spinal cord segment (length 4 mm, T12 to L2 spine level) of a GFP-M mouse scanned with ultramicroscopy shown in a horizontal view. (d) Cross-view projection (50-μm thickness) of the indicated region in c. White arrows in c, d mark individual axons in the white matter; red arrows mark cell bodies in the gray matter. (e) Traced white and gray matter boundaries and axon bundles (yellow arrows) [37].

growth-competent axons as well as axons that have been considered to be growth incompetent show regenerative features. The results suggest that visualizing cells in unsectioned central nervous system (CNS) tissue holds promise for assessing experimental therapies in spinal cord injury and other neurological pathologies.

Hama et al. [36] imaged intact fixed mouse brain using Sca*l*e, an aqueous reagent which consists mainly of urea, glycerol and Triton X-100, to achieve comprehensive and high-resolution three-dimensional reconstructions of brain [36]. This aqueous reagent could render biological samples optically transparent and completely preserves fluorescent signals in the clarified structures that can be beyond the current imaging depth limit.

Intact fixed mouse brain was immersed in the most effective solution named Sca*l*eA2 for > 2 weeks. Cleared brain was placed above a patterned background as shown in Fig. 17.28a or by irradiation with 532-nm laser beam as shown in Fig. 17.28b. Whole mouse embryos were also cleared by Sca*l*eA2 shown in Fig. 17.28c.

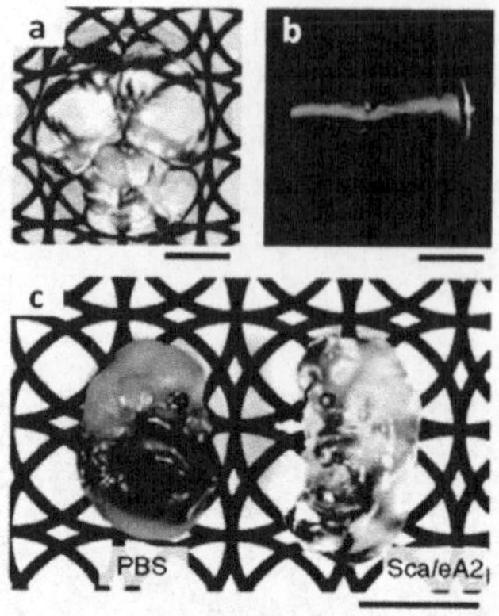

Figure 17.28: Tissue clearing performance of Sca*l*eA2. (a) A photo of cleared brain was taken with patterned background. (b) A 1-mW, 532-nm laser beam irradiated at the cleared brain. (c) A photo of two embryos taken with patterned background. Left, embryo placed in PBS after fixation. Right, embryo incubated in Sca*l*eA2 solution for 2 weeks after fixation. All scale bars represent 5 mm [36].

Three-dimensional reconstruction of neuronal networks from the cleared intact brain of a YFP-H mouse using TPEFM was shown in Fig. 17.29a. The three-dimensional architectures of brain which is from the pial surface to the dorsal tip of the CA1 region are shown in Fig. 17.29b. Subcellular architectures of cortical layer V/VI pyramidal neurons such as individual dendritic spines were legible in an expanded view as shown in Fig. 17.29c.

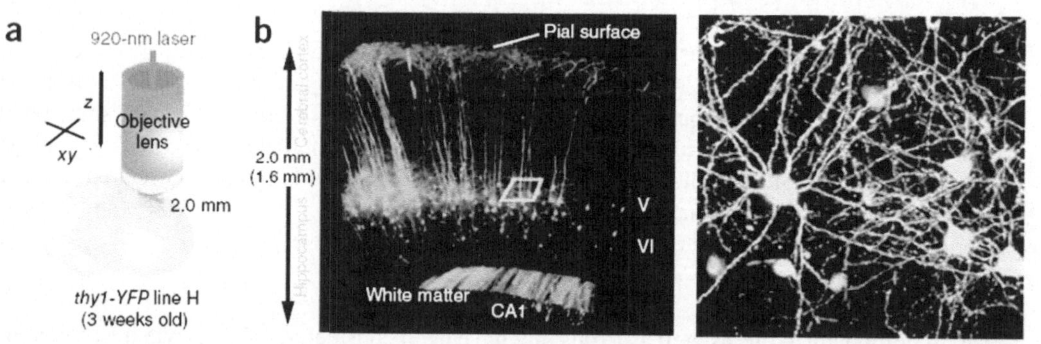

Figure 17.29: Three-dimensional reconstructions of Sca*l*eA2-treated brain of YFP-H mice. (a) The experimental setup for TPEFM imaging. (b) Reconstruction of Sca*l*eA2-treated brain in the cerebral cortex and hippocampus of YFP-H mice. (c) An expanded view at a depth of 0.9 mm (a yellow box in b). Scale bars represent 50 mm [36].

In order to investigate the vascular niche for neural stem cells (NSCs) in the subgranular zone (SGZ) of the dentate gyrus in the hippocampus, Hama et al. explored the utility of Sca*l*e for imaging of those discrete cell populations and quantitative measurement of their geometric properties.

After subsequent fixation, an excised hippocampus of an adult transgenic mouse (7 weeks old) was treated with Sca*l*eA2 for 2 d for TPEFM imaging as shown in Fig. 17.30a. NSCs were labeled

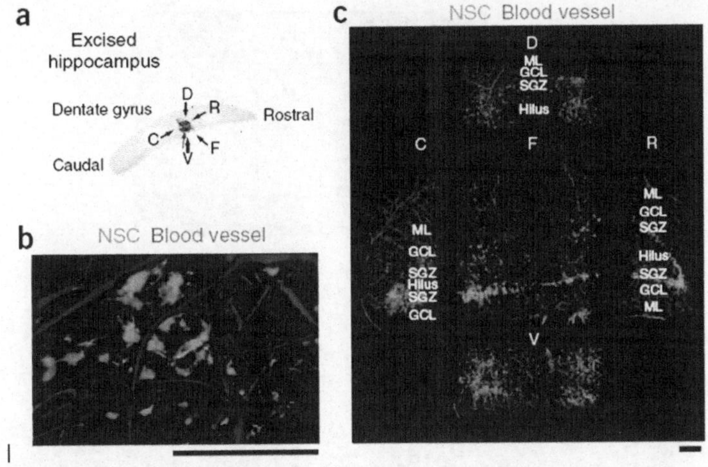

Figure 17.30: (See color insert.) Blood vessels and neural stem cells (NSCs) nuclei in the subgranular zone (SGZ) of adult mice. (a) Schematic diagram of TPEFM imaging for cleared excised hippocampus. (b) An expanded view of NSCs (green) and blood vessels (red) in the SGZ. (c) Distribution of NSCs and blood vessels in the hippocampus. Scale bars represent 500 mm [36].

with GFP, and blood vessels with Texas Red. A nation sight of NSCs was found exclusively in the SGZ. Plenty of them made considerable interface with blood vessels through their radial glia-like processes as shown in Fig. 17.30b. The three-dimensional architectures of NSCs and blood vessels in the hippocampus were created from five different angles as shown in Fig. 17.30c. Along the longitudinal axis of the hippocampus, the density of NSCs varied substantially which is obvious in the image. This result suggests that the activity of hippocampal neurogenics cannot be evaluated by the number of NSCs in a single section.

In addition, the optical clearing technique is helpful for some other labeling techniques such as Fucci technique and immunohistochemistry. Hama et al. employed Sca*l*eU2, composed of 4 M urea, 30%-glycerol, and 0.1%-Triton X-100, to analyze cell-cycle profiles of mouse embryogenesis in transgenic mouse that expresses the Fucci probe, which provides a comprehensive perspective of proliferation versus differentiation in the developing brain [36].

In any case optical clearing technique solves the problem of low optical depth for imaging to a certain extent. It is significantly important for three-dimensional reconstructions of tissue and organ which will contribute to the discovery of new biological principles in connectomics and circuit genetics. The application prospects of optical clearing technique will be bright in the future.

17.5 *In Vivo* Application of Tissue Optical Clearing Technique

The tissue optical clearing technique is not only applied to *in vitro* imaging, but also shows enormous potential for *in vivo* optical imaging, diagnosis and therapy. It is noted that before the optical clearing method is applied *in vivo*, it is necessary to investigate the safety of optical clearing agents to these tissues. Here, the effects of optical clearing agents on morphology, microstructure and function of tissue will be reviewed. Finally, the *in vivo* imaging and therapy will also be introduced.

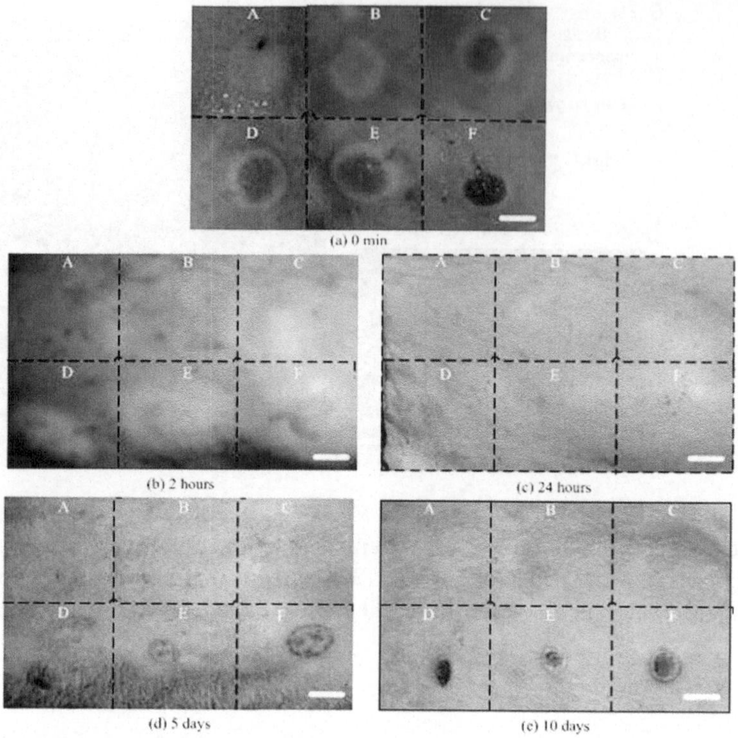

Figure 17.31: Photographic images of rat skin after dermal injection of saline (A), 20%-glycerol (B), 30%-glycerol (C), 40%-glycerol (D), 50%-glycerol (E), 75%-glycerol (F), respectively (Bar=5 mm) [65].

17.5.1 Effects of optical clearing agents on morphology of skin

Among the investigation of tissue optical clearing, glycerol is one of the most common OCA of skin, but its optical clearing efficacy is not very high for topical treatment of *in vivo* skin. So it is usually adopted by dermal injection of glycerol to avoid the *stratum corneum* barrier. In the case of high concentration solutions, it did a lot of harm to biological tissue, even stopping blood flow and obstructing the blood vessel [17]; whereas low concentration solutions do not have optical clearing effect. Therefore, it is necessary to discuss the moderate concentration of glycerol as for *in vivo* application [65]. Mao et al. observed the dynamical changes in morphology of local skin during 2 weeks after dermal injection of glycerol.

The influences of glycerol on morphological changes of rat skin *in vivo* were investigated by dermal injection of 0.05 ml 75%-, 50%-, 40%-, 30%-, and 20%-glycerol and saline solution. The skin morphological changes had been observed for 2 weeks and photographic images of the area of interest were taken. Figure 17.31 shows the typical results. It can be seen that the glycerol solution with high concentrations (40%, 50%, and 75%) would lead to the necrosis of local skin, which was irreversible after a 2-week recovery. And the glycerol solution with lower concentrations (20% and 30%) did not cause damage to skin.

In the above study, the optical clearing agents were dermal injected to the dorsal skin *in vivo*. Actually, in practical applications, the optical clearing agents are usually applied by topical application. In this way, the doses of optical clearing agents that penetrate into skin are very small, and the effects of optical clearing agents on skin would be reduced.

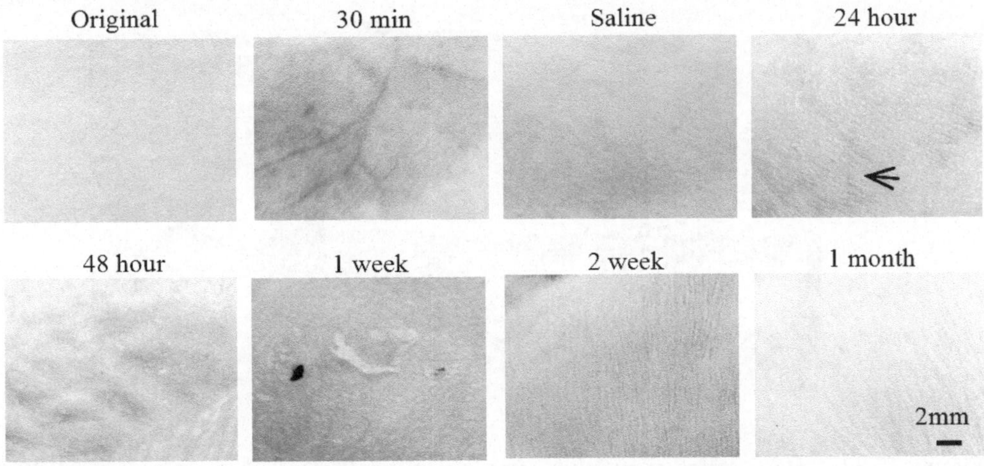

Figure 17.32: Morphological changes of rat skin before and after topical application of the mixture of PEG400 and Thiazone [131].

Thiazone, a chemical penetration enhancer, can facilitate the permeability of optical clearing agents. Zhu et al. topically treated the mixture of PEG400 and Thiazone on the epidermis of rat skin and observed the dermal blood vessels and obtained the blood flow [63]. Further, they made some investigations on the safety of skin after the topical application of the optical clearing agents, and the typical results are shown in Fig. 17.32. The mixture of PEG400 and Thiazone was topically applied on the dorsal rat skin, and the morphological photos were recorded for a month. The results indicated that, the subcutaneous blood vessels could be observed directly after the application of the mixture solution for 30 min, and the treatment of saline solution could make the skin recover to turbid state. After 48 hours, the skin area was wrinkled and hardened; some inflammation might occur inside the skin. However, after 2 weeks' recovery, the hair growth and skin morphology were not influenced by the optical clearing agent at all [131].

In the above investigations, the effects of optical clearing agents on skin are different. Presumably when the agents are topically applied to skin, the dosage that penetrates into the skin is very low. In this condition, the effects of these agents are negligible. Thus, we can conclude that there are no long-term effects on morphology of skin by topical application of optical clearing agents.

17.5.2 Effects of optical clearing agents on microstructure of skin

Further, effects of optical clearing agents on the microstructure of skin are investigated after topical application of the mixture of PEG400 and Thiazone. The typical results are shown in Figs. 17.33 and 17.34. It can be seen that after topical application of the mixture for 30 min, the epidermis of skin became extremely thin, the *stratum corneum* was destroyed and the arrangement of subepidermal collagen became loose. Then, after a 48-hour recovery, some degree of inflammation occurred inside the epidermis of skin, but the collagen arrangement became dense again. After 1 week, the skin began to rebuild; some vacuoles occurred in the epidermal layer of skin which may be due to superficial edema. However, after 2 weeks, the skin recovered to its initial state, and the development of skin was not affected by the optical clearing agent [131].

In conclusion, topical application of optical clearing agents may cause some degree of inflammation to skin in a short time; however, after a long-term recovery, the morphology and microstructure of skin are not affected by the optical clearing agents at all. In addition, direct application of optical clearing agents to blood vessels would decrease the blood flow or even block the blood vessels, and

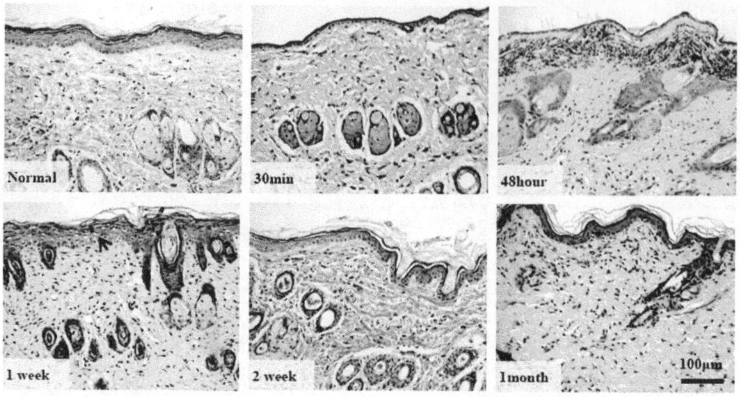

Figure 17.33: H&E stains of rat skin after topical application of the mixture of PEG400 and Thiazone. Arrow—the area where a vacuole exists [131].

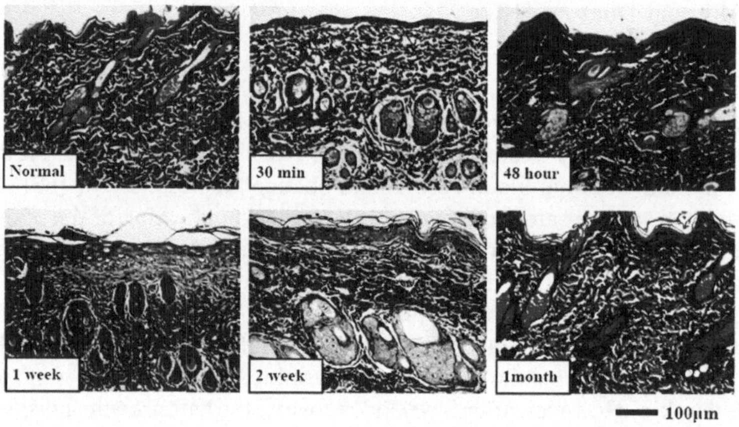

Figure 17.34: Masson stains of rat skin after topical application of the mixture of PEG400 and Thiazone [131].

the long-term recovery is defined by OCA washing out and metabolic activity (toxicity) of the agent [132]. In future studies, the metabolic toxicity of optical clearing agents to the organ systems of the body should be considered, and the body growth condition should also be put into issue.

17.5.3 Effects of optical clearing agents on blood vessels and blood flow

One of the primary objectives for tissue optical clearing is to observe the blood vessels and blood flow non-invasively. Thus, apart from skin, it is necessary to investigate whether the action of optical clearing agents would induce some damage to the blood vessels. In 2003, G. Vargas et al. investigated the effects of hyperosmotic agents on morphological changes of blood vessels [17]. The glycerol solutions with different concentrations (100% and 75%) were directly applied on the subdermal side of hamster dorsal skin *in vivo*, and then a set of photographic images were taken at different treatment times to see the morphological changes of blood vessels. The results demonstrated that the application of glycerol might induce occlusion of blood vessels, and the morphological changes in blood vessels could be reversed by using phosphate-buffered saline. Some typical results of 100%-glycerol are shown in Fig. 17.35.

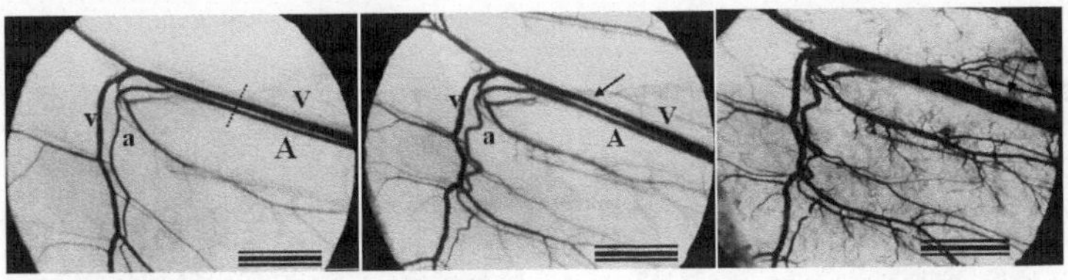

Figure 17.35: Morphological changes of subdermal blood vessels in the hamster dorsal skin flap window before (a) and after the application of 100% glycerol solution to subdermal skin for 0 min (b), 10 min (c), 15 min (d) and 20 min (e), respectively; (f) Blood vessels after the application of phosphate-buffered saline for 5 min. c-focal constriction, * areas of darkening (occluded). Scale bar = 0.25 cm [17].

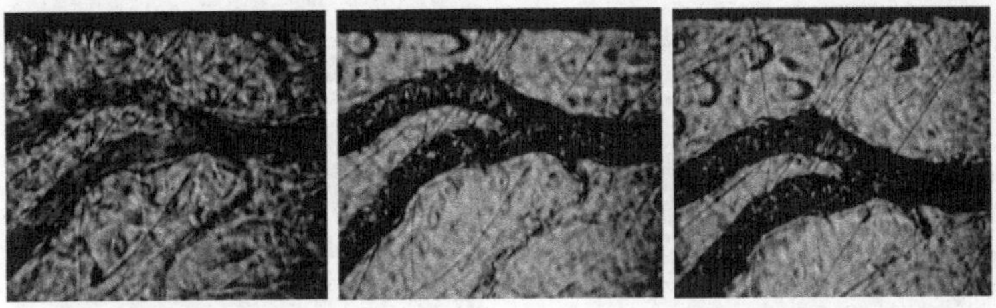

Figure 17.36: Images before (a) and after the application of 40%-glucose solution to microvessels of rat mesentery for 30 sec (b) and 5 min (c), respectively [132].

Galanzha et al. [132] also paid some attention to the biocompatibility of optical clearing agents. In their study, the rat mesentery was used as the animal model. 10 μl of glucose (20%, 25%, 30%, 35% and 40%) and glycerol (75%) were directly applied to the interested microvessels, and then the region of interest was captured by a digital video camera and analyzed to measure the diameter and blood flow velocity of the microvessels. They found that the application of glycerol and glucose solution would induce short-term slowing down and local stasis of the microvessels, and some degree of dilation also occurred during the treatment time. In addition, lower concentrations of solution would cause less change in microcirculation. Figure 17.36 shows the typical results of 40%-glucose.

Cheng et al. [133] investigated the effect of hyperosmotic chemical agents on *in vivo* cerebral blood flow. After removing the rabbit skull and a small area of *dura mater*, the glycerol solution was directly applied near the exposed area, and the cerebral blood flow in the exposed area was monitored by Laser Speckle Imaging. The results demonstrated that, at the initial state, the application of glycerol solution would induce the decrease of blood flow by 20–30%, and the *dura mater* would become clear, however, after a very short time ($\sim$70s), the blood flow velocity would begin to increase and the *dura mater* become turbid again due to wash out of glycerol from the target space (as shown in Fig. 17.37). Therefore, the challenges for the design of an optical clearing technique for application *in vivo* were not only the clearing effects and the duration of the action of the chemical agents but also the influence of the glycerol on the tissue's normal physiological function.

However, the above studies only paid attention to the short-term effects of various optical clearing agents on the blood vessels and blood flow. Perhaps these effects might continue or change with the treating time lasting. Thus, research on the long-term effects of optical clearing agents on blood vessels is needed. Zhu et al. [134] investigated the short-term and long-term effects of glycerol and glucose on blood vessels in chick chorioallantoic membrane (CAM). 10 μl or 40 μl warm glycerol

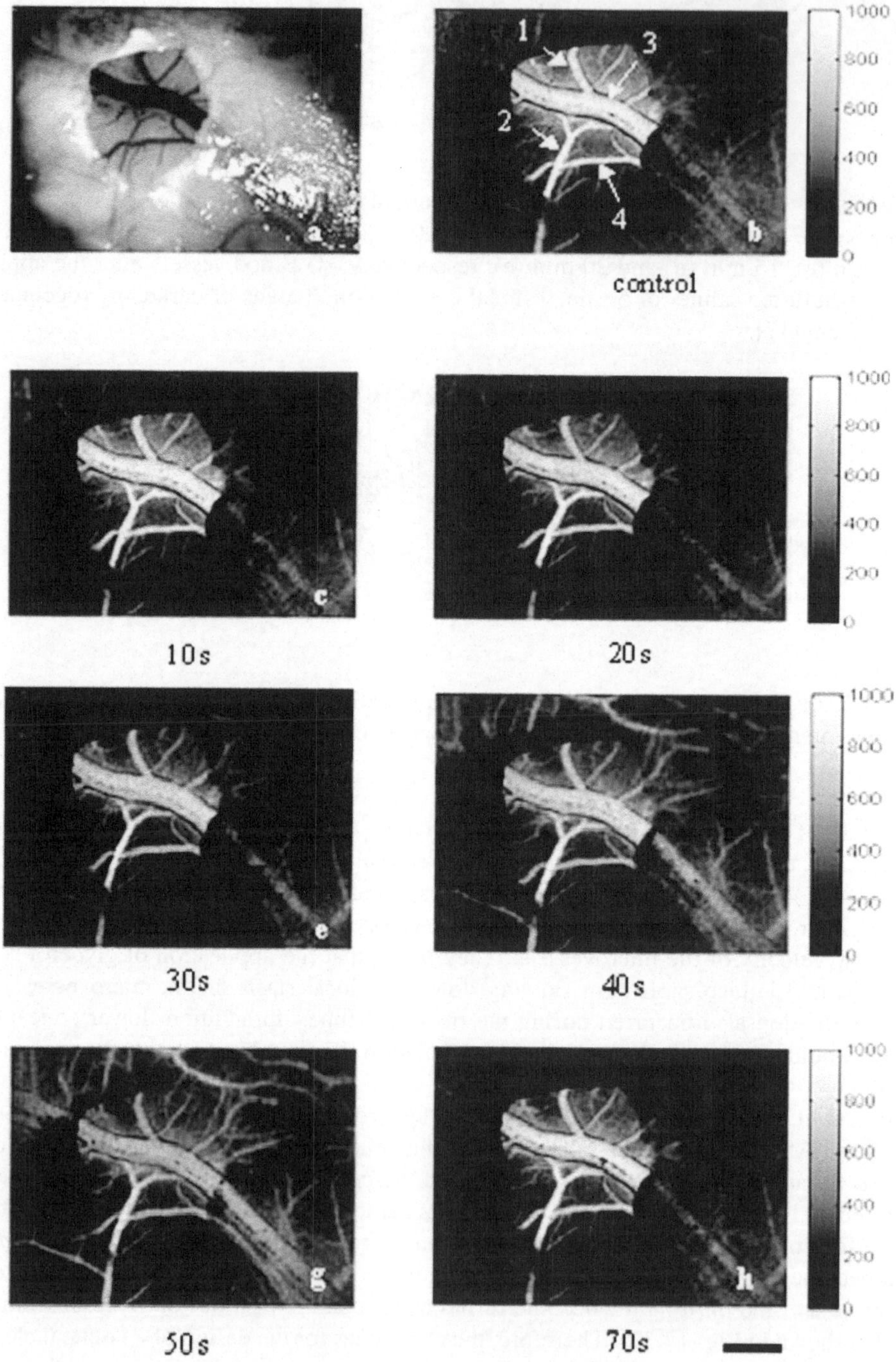

Figure 17.37: Effects of glycerol on cerebral blood flow: white-light images of the area of interest (a); speckle velocity images before the application of glycerol solution (control) (b); speckle velocity images after the application of glycerol for 10–70 s, respectively (c–h) [133].

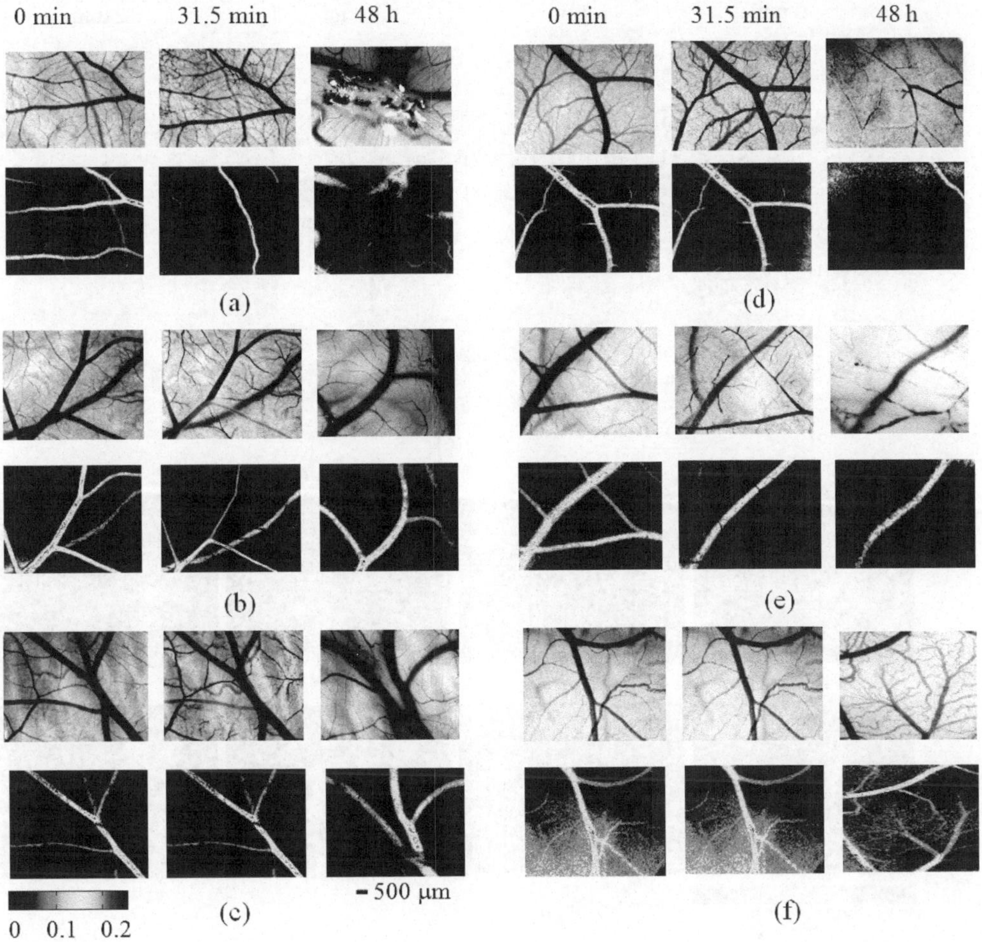

Figure 17.38: (See color insert.) White-light (top row) and speckle velocity (bottom row) images before, 31.5 min after and 2 days after the application of different agents (40 μl): (a) 100%-glycerol, (b) 50%-glycerol, (c) 25%-glycerol, (d) 40%-glucose, (e) 20%-glucose, and (f) saline [134].

(100%, 50% and 25%) and glucose (40% and 20%) was dropped on the blood vessels, and the region of interest was imaged by the laser speckle imaging system for 30 min. Moreover, the area of interest was imaged again 1 day and 2 days later. They found that the action of hyperosmotic agents would decrease the local blood flow and even block the blood vessels. Long-term observations demonstrated that the developments of most blood vessels were stunted. In addition, the effects were also related to the dosage of the agents, including concentration and volume. The effects would increase with the dosage of agents. Some typical results are showed in Fig. 17.38.

In conclusion, direct application of optical clearing agents would decrease the blood flow velocity or even block the blood vessels in a short time. Long-term observations indicate that the agents stunt the development of blood vessels in the CAMs. Short-term effects of glycerol are very strong and are confined to a local region. The blood flow can be recovered to different extents if the blood vessel is not blocked completely. In contrast, long-term effects of glucose are more serious than short-term effects. The effects will be decreased with the dose of the agents.

Mao et al. directly applied 30%-glycerol on the dermal blood vessels of rat skin flap window, and the changes in blood flow were observed by Laser Speckle Contrast Imaging system. They found

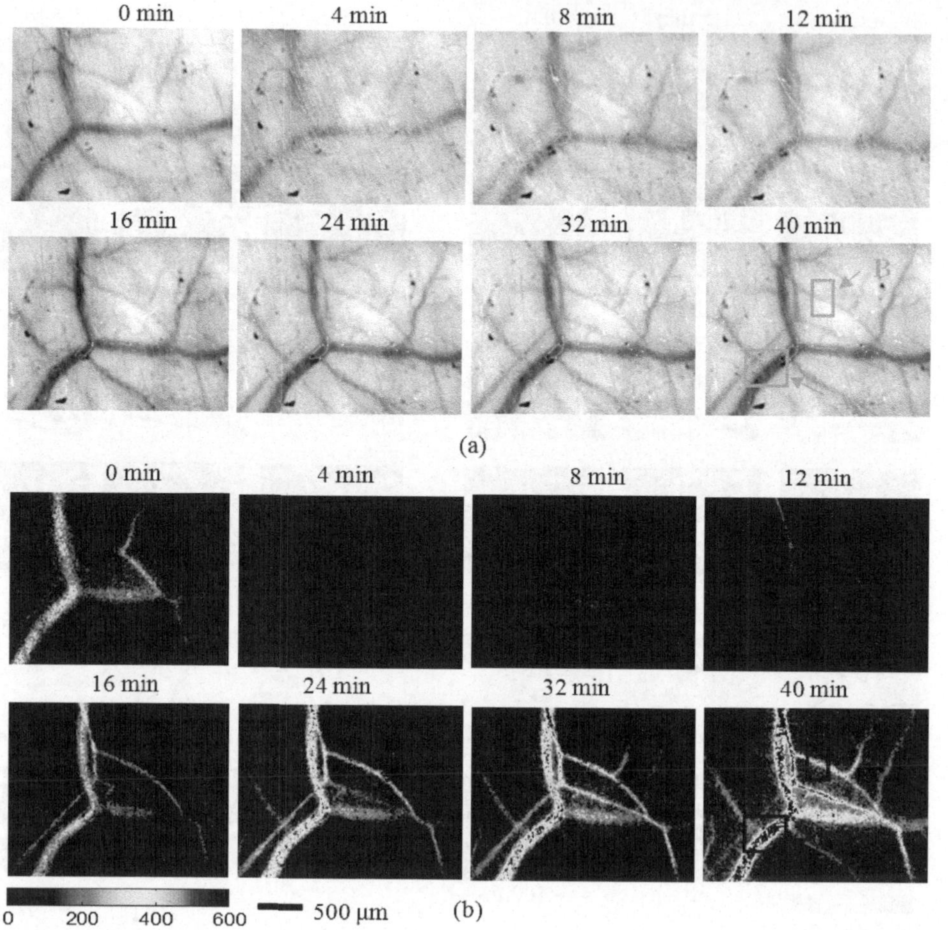

Figure 17.39: White-light images (a) and speckle velocity images (b) before and after the application of 30%-glycerol to dermal blood vessels [135].

that the flow velocity decreased in the beginning and began to recover from 16 min (as shown in Fig. 17.39). Thus, it can be concluded that, in a short time, the application of glycerol does not affect the blood flow of skin flap window [135].

17.5.4 High-resolution imaging dermal blood flow through the intact rat skin

Apart from the contributions to optical microscopy and microstructure reconstruction, the optical clearing methods can also help to noninvasively (or at least invasively) acquire the *in vivo* rat skin microcirculation information.

Impairment of skin microcirculation is one of the main features in advanced clinical stages of peripheral vascular disease. Recently, some noninvasive methods have been available to investigate skin microcirculation in clinical settings as well as improve disease management, i.e., capillaroscopy allows the investigation of skin capillary morphology and density, laser Doppler flowmetry allows real-time assessment of perfusion of skin volume, and transcutaneous measurement of oxygen tension provides continuous information about skin oxygenation [136]. However, none of them can provide structural and functional information of dermal vessels simultaneously with high resolu-

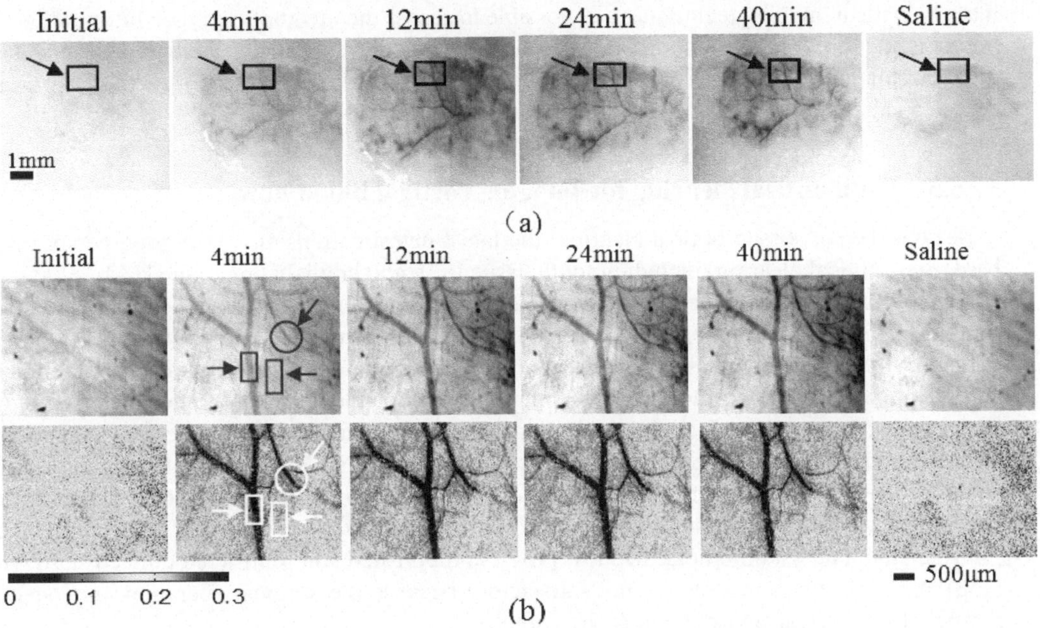

Figure 17.40: (a) Photographic images of rat skin *in vivo* before and after treatment with the mixture of PEG400 and Thiazone. (b) White-light (top row) and temporal contrast images (bottom row) of rectangle areas in (a) after treatment with the mixture of PEG400 and Thiazone [63].

tion. In contrast, laser speckle contrast imaging (LSCI), a full-field optical technique, can produce a two-dimensional map of blood flow with high spatial-temporal resolution [137–143], which plays an important role in studying cerebral blood flow [140], mesentery microcirculation [143], etc. Unfortunately, it suffers from a limited penetration depth of light in turbid tissues, as the previous investigations were restricted within the imaging of blood flow in transparent tissues.

Zhu et al. [63] developed an optical clearing method to make the skin transparent and to image the dermal blood flow trough intact skin. After having topically applied a mixture of PEG400 and Thiazone to rat dorsal skin *in vivo*, some large vessels through the intact skin can be seen in Fig. 17.40a. At the beginning, the dermal blood vessel is invisible to the naked eye. After having topically applied the mixture of PEG400 and Thiazone on the rat skin for 4 min, we can observe some large vessels through the intact skin. Up to 12 min, even the small branch vessels can be distinguished clearly, just as the region in the rectangle shows. Moreover, this situation will be allowed to continue. After 40-min treatment of the mixture, the saline solution was applied onto the area of interest. Immediately, the skin is recovered to the initial state and the blood vessels are out of view. Figure 17.40b show the magnified image in Fig. 17.40a and the corresponding speckle temporal contrast image constructed by calculating the speckle temporal contrast.

The photographic images in the top row show the visual optical clearing process of skin, and the temporal contrast maps in the bottom row are quite consistent with the photographs shown in the top row. The image quality becomes better by topical application of the mixture, and more details of the dermal blood vessels can be seen. The temporal contrast maps demonstrate that the topical application of the mixture can decrease the temporal contrast of the vessels, which provides better visualization of the blood flow. The treatment of saline can make the dermal vessels invisible very quickly, and then the contrast can be recovered.

This optical clearing method enables us to observe dermal blood vessels and image dermal blood flow through intact rat skin by the LSCI technique. Furthermore, by combining this method with the intrinsic optical imaging technique, it is possible to access the metabolic oxygen information of skin microcirculation. It is very important to diagnose peripheral vascular disease based on subcutaneous microcirculation. Also, with certain techniques, the pharmacological effect of some kind of vascular drugs can also be evaluated.

17.5.5 Skull optical clearing for imaging cortical blood flow

Besides the soft tissue optical clearing, the latest investigations also give good perspectives for hard tissue optical clearing, including tooth tissue [83], and cranial bone tissue [144-145].

Optical imaging techniques have provided potential power to investigate cortical structure and function *in vivo*. For instance, Laser Speckle Imaging has been widely applied to map the changes in cortical blood flow, which has provided valuable insight into many aspects of cortical function [146–147]. Applications of two-photon microscopy imaging have contributed to our understanding of a broad array of neurobiological phenomena, including the dynamics of single channels in individual synapses and the functional organization of cortical maps [148]. However, the high scattering of the skull becomes a barrier to cortical optical neuro-imaging *in vivo*. In order to solve this problem, the craniotomy was applied to establish cranial windows [149–153], i.e, removed skull, cranial window [150–151], thinned skull cranial window [152], and polished and reinforced thinned skull window [153] et al., but these models are not satisfactory because the surgical operation may change the normal physiological environment of the cortex.

The tissue optical clearing technique based on immersion of tissues into optical clearing agents is highly promising to help us to get the high resolution imaging of the cortex. Common optical clearing agents of soft tissue, glycerol or propylene glycerol (PG) were applied to immerse the skull *in vitro*, and showed reduction of the scattering of the skull [144]. Recently, an innovative skull optical clearing solution (SOCS) was invented to make mice skull transparent quickly [145]. This solution is composed of various biocompatibility agents, whose main components include laurinol, weak alkaline substances, EDTA, dimethyl sulfoxide, sorbitol, alcohol, and glucose. After treatment with SOCS, the typical white-light images of skull samples are shown in Fig. 17.41. The results show that the turbid skull completely conceals the USAF target; 25 min after being treated with SOCS, the target can be visible clearly through the treated skull.

For quantitative comparison, the resolutions through the skull after treatment with glycerol, PG or SOCS were calculated using the USAF target, and the results are summarized in Table 17.3. It can be found that after being treated with glycerol or PG, the measured resolution through the skull increases with treatment time, but the results for 24 hours are still worse than that after treatment with SOCS for 25 min. And the optimal resolution, from the saturation concentration (60%) of

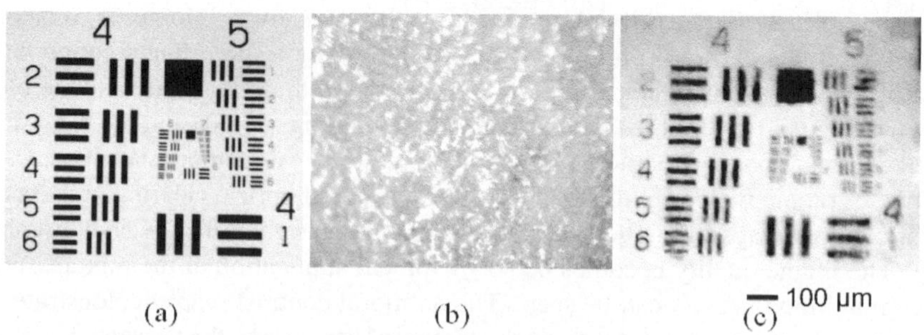

Figure 17.41: (a) White-light images of SOCS-induced optical clearing of *in vitro* skull. (a) Image of the central region of a 1951 USAF target; (b)-(c) Images of the USAF target through the *in vitro* skull before and 25 min after treatment with SOCS, respectively [145].

TABLE 17.3: Resolution through *in vitro* skull after treatment with different solutions for different time.

Solution		Glycerol	PG	SOCS
Resolution (μm)	25 min	>62.6	>62.6	8.4±0.5
	1 hour	>62.6	>62.6	
	24 hour	33.7±2.2	33.7±2.2	

laurinol, can achieve 8.4 μm, which closes to the CCD pixel size (6.45 μm × 6.45 μm).

In order to inquire the SOCS induced optical clearing efficacy of skull *in vivo*, the initial white-light image was taken by the CCD camera as the control. After the SOCS was topically treated on mice skull for 25 min, and a craniotomy was performed to remove some parts of the treated skull, the white-light images were acquired, respectively. Figure 17.42 (a), (b) and (c) show typical white-light images of the intact skull, the treated skull and removed skull rectangle area A, and Figure 17.42 (d), (e) and (f) are the magnified images of the rectangle area A in Figure 17.42 (a), (b) and (c). It can be seen that the intact skull is almost turbid, and the cortical blood vessels are hard to distinguish. After treatment with SOCS, the skull becomes transparent, and the cortical micro-vessels can be observed clearly. Through the exposed cortex and the transparent skull after being treated with SOCS for 25 min, the minimum resolution diameter (MRD) of micro-vessel is 12.8±0.9 μm and 14.4±0.8 μm, respectively.

Figure 17.43 (a), (b), and (c) show the speckle contrast images of cortical blood flow through the intact skull, transparent skull and exposed cortex, which correspond to the same area shown in Figure 17.42 (d), (e), and (f). The darker the region, the faster the blood flows, and the wider the dark region, the larger the diameter of vessel. It can be seen that the blood flow of a few large vessels can be measured hazily through the intact skull, while the blood flow distribution of cortical micro-

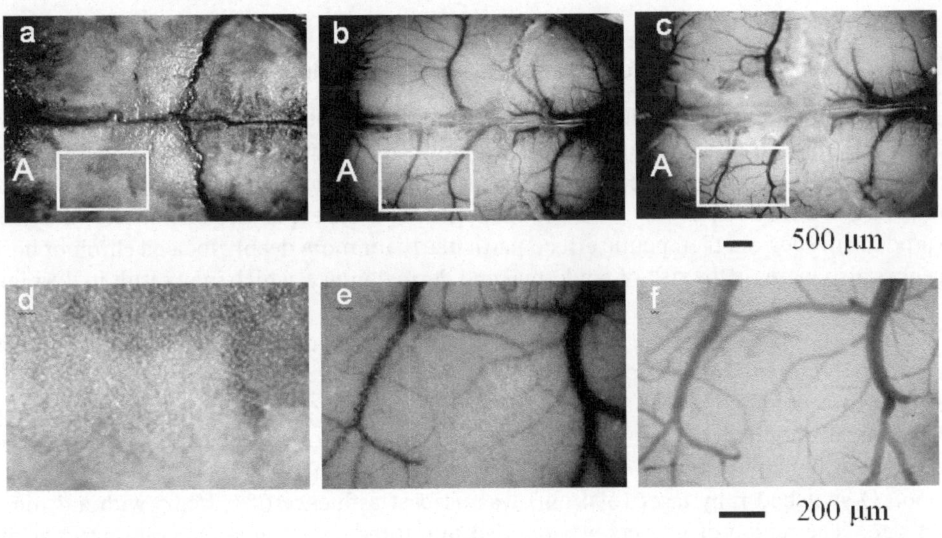

Figure 17.42: Typical white-light images obtained from intact skull (a), the transparent skull after SOCS treatment for 25 min without (b) and with exposed cortex of rectangle area A (c). (d), (e) and (f) are the corresponding magnified images of the rectangle area A shown in (a), (b) and (c) [145].

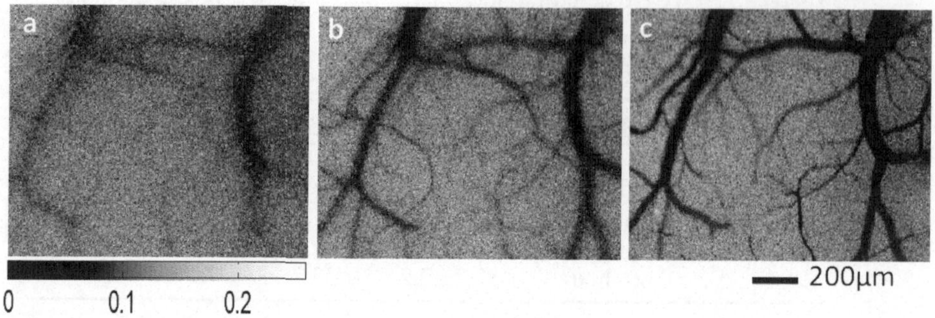

Figure 17.43: Laser speckle temporal contrast images. (a)–(c) demonstrate the speckle contrast images corresponding to the area in Figure 17.42 (d)–(f), respectively [145].

vessels in details can be distinguished clearly through the transparent skull and exposed cortex. Comparing Figure 17.43(a) with Figure 17.43(b), the obtained blood flow distribution of larger vessels in the cortex through the intact skull is consistent with that through the transparent skull, which indicates that the SOCS has no obvious influence on the cortical blood flow. Comparing Figure 17.43(b) with Figure 17.43(c), the distribution of blood flow of micro-vessels through the transparent skull and the exposed cortex are totally the same. The obtained image contrast through the transparent skull is much better than that through the intact skull, but is not obviously different from the exposed cortex.

Therefore, it can be concluded that the skull optical clearing method provides an innovative transparent cranial window for accessing high resolution cortical structural and functional information, which can avoid the limitations of the craniotomy based cranial window. We believe that combining the transparent cranial window with the multi-photon microscopy or other optical imaging techniques will help us to study cortex neural activity *in vivo*, which is very beneficial for neuroscience research.

17.5.6 Therapeutic applications of tissue optical clearing

Human skin is a complex and highly scattering medium at visible and near-infrared wavelengths due to variations in refractive indices of different constituents. In light-based therapeutics, dermal scattering diminishes the depth of light penetration and attenuates the effective fluence that reaches to the targeted chromophores. Even though higher radiant exposures or fluencies may be required to produce the desired therapeutic effect, particularly for more deeply located chromophores, higher fluences also increase the risk of epidermal and dermal injury, which may result in dyspigmentation and scarring.

Khan et al. reported that the use of hyperosmotic optical clearing agents, which were composed of a pre-polymer mixture of polypropylene glycol and polyethylene glycol, PPG:PEG, can permit the laser to penetrate intact human skin and temporarily alter local optical properties *in vivo* [23]. They topically applied the clearing agent (PPG:PEG) prior to Q-switched 532 nm and 694 nm laser treatment of human skin *in vivo* from a 40-year-old man (SPT IV) for a 15-year-old India ink arm tattoo. Q-switched ruby laser (694 nm) was used at a fluence of 6 J/cm^2 with a 4 mm diameter spot size. The region of interest was divided into three areas: area (1) control, no agent or laser treatment; (2) laser alone; (3) skin pre-treated with optical clearing agent (2 hours under occlusion) followed by laser treatment (Fig. 17.44A). No post-operative wound care was provided for any areas. One day post-treatment, the patient developed several hemorrhagic blisters on area 2 while area 3 showed only minimal erythema (Fig. 17.44B). At 1 month follow-up, significant clearing of

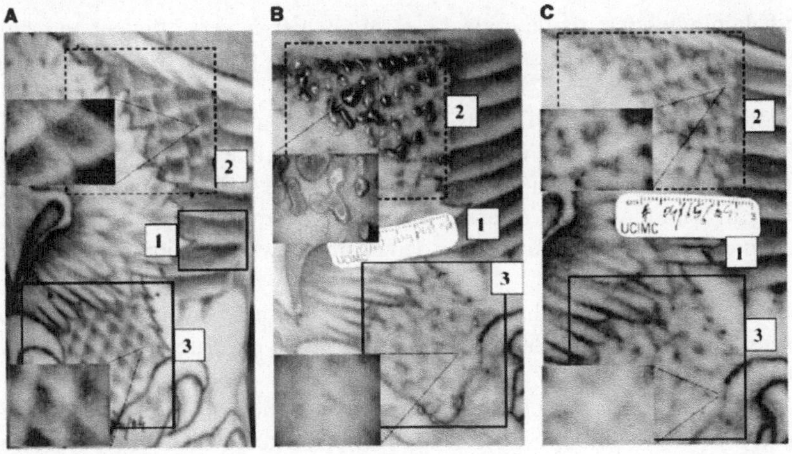

Figure 17.44: A–C: Gross and close-up digital images of a 15-year-old tattoo before and after laser treatment. A: Before treatment (area 1) control, no agent or laser treatment; (area 2) laser alone; (area 3) topical application of clearing agent followed by laser treatment. Insets represent cross-polarized close-up views (4×) of areas 2 and 3. B: One day post-treatment. Insets represent linear-polarized close-up views (4×) of the surface topography of areas 2 and 3. Of note is the extensive blistering in area 2. C: One month after single laser treatment. Insets represent cross-polarized close-up views (4×) of areas 2 and 3. Note the significant clearing of the tattoo ink in the area pretreated with optical clearing agent [23].

tattoo in area 3 was observed as opposed to only minimal clearing in area 2 (Fig. 17.44C).

The results demonstrate that topically applied clearing agents (PPG:PEG) allow more photons to reach the target as well as reduce the back scattered light. Higher fluences for deeper dermal targets can be used much more safely and effectively without damaging the epidermis, especially when treating patients with darker skin types. PPG:PEG is safe, effective, and well tolerated for optical clearing of human skin. Prospective, comparative, and controlled clinical studies should be further performed so that the role of topically applied optical clearing agents in light-based therapeutics can be fully understood.

Other positive examples of optical clearing technique application to precise laser ophthalmic surgery using femtosecond lasers are described in [154–155].

17.6 Conclusion

In this review we have demonstrated some facilities of optical clearing (OC) technology in tissue and whole organism optical sectioning. Advantages and drawbacks of the method were underlined. Evidently, to apply this technology for a particular task in medicine or developmental biology all advantages and disadvantages should be accounted for. However, a few particular areas of medicine can be demonstrated for a wider application of OC. For example, it may help to provide more effective skin and mucosal tumor imaging [112] and immediately more precise laser disruption of pathological abnormalities. The possibility to image even deeper structures of sentinel lymph nodes at the single cell level, follow-up photoacoustic detection and photothermal purging of metastasis targeted by nanoparticles, was recently demostrated with the help of OC [156].

In ophthalmology sclera tissue optical clearing, which is very efficient and simple to do *in vivo* [157], also can be effectively used for laser therapy and precise tissue dissection and removal of small abnormalities [154–155].

In developmental biology OCT holds great promise as a routine research tool for 3-D analysis of mammalian embryos, especially with usage of biocompatible OCAs. It was already shown in fixed tissues of mouse embryos that 25%-glycerol enhanced the OCT signal by 25% at the depth of about 200 to 500 μm with the optical clearing rate of 27 μm/min [103]. *In vivo* optical clearing of rat newborn in propylene glycol solution was demonstrated with the aim to study vessel network using optical imaging [158].

Another large field of OC technology application is drug delivery monitoring, including optical glucose sensing [5, 9–14, 19, 159–160], which is based on drug or glucose metabolic impact on tissue optical properties.

In this review we mostly concentrated on soft tissue optical clearing. In addition, hard tissue optical clearing, especially skull optical clearing, was presented, which will replace current transparent cranial window based on craniotomy [144–145].

Acknowledgments

We would like to thank Ekaterina Galanzha, Alexey Bashkatov, and Elina Genina from Saratov State University for collaboration; the PhD students Xiang Wen, Jing Wang, Caihua Liu and Yang Zhang in Britton Chance Center for Biomedical Photonics, for collecting and sorting materials, which helped quicken the draft. This work was supported by the grants of the National Major Scientific Research Program of China (No. 2011CB910401), the National Nature Science Foundation of China (Nos. 30770552, 81171376, 91232710), the Foundation for Innovative Research Groups of the NFSC (No. 61121004), NSFC-RFBR for international cooperation (Nos. 30911120074, 812111313), the Research Fund for the Doctoral Program of Higher Education of China (No. 20110142110073) and 111 Project of Ministry of Education and State Administration of Foreign Experts Affairs of China. This work was also supported in part by RFBR grants 11-02-00560-a, 11-02-12248-ofi-m, 12-02-92610-KO_a, and 13-02-91176-NSFC_a; 224014 PHOTONICS4LIFE of FP7-ICT-2007-2; 1.4.09 of RF Ministry of Education and Science; RF Governmental contracts 02.740.11.0770, 02.740.11.0879, 11.519.11.2035, 14.B37.21.0728, 14.B37.21.0563, and 14.512.11.0022; FiDiPro, TEKES Program (40111/11), Finland; SCOPES EC, Uzb/Switz/RF, Swiss NSF, IZ74ZO 137423/1; RF President's grant "Scientific Schools," 1177.2012.2.

References

[1] M. Wenne, "The most transparent research," *Nat. Med.* **15** (10), 1106–1109 (2009).

[2] E. Gratton, "Deeper tissue imaging with total detection," *Science* **331**(6020), 1016–1017 (2011).

[3] V.V. Tuchin, I.L. Maksimova, D.A. Zimnyakov, I.L. Kon, A.H. Mavlutov, and A.A. Mishin, "Light propagation in tissues with controlled optical properties," *J. Biomed. Opt.* **2**, 401–417 (1997).

[4] G. Vargas, E.K. Chan, J.K. Barton, H.G. Rylander, and A.J. Welch, "Use of an agent to reduce scattering in skin," *Lasers Surg. Med.* **24** (2), 133–141 (1999).

[5] G. Vargas, *Reduction of Light Scattering in Biological Tissue: Implications for Optical Diagnostics and Therapeutics*, Austin: The University of Texas (2001).

[6] V.V. Tuchin, "Optical clearing of tissues and blood using the immersion method," *J. Phys. D: Appl. Phys.* **38**, 2497–2518 (2005).

[7] V.V. Tuchin, "Optical immersion as a new tool to control optical properties of tissues and blood," *Laser Phys.* **15**, 1109–1136 (2005).

[8] V.V. Tuchin, *Optical Clearing of Tissues and Blood*, PM154, SPIE Press, Bellingham, WA, 2006.

[9] V.V. Tuchin, "A clear vision for laser diagnostics (review)," *IEEE J. Sel. Top. Quantum Electron* **13**, 1621–1628 (2007).

[10] E.A. Genina, A.N. Bashkatov, and V.V. Tuchin, Tissue optical immersion clearing, *Expert Rev. Med. Devices* **7** (6), 825–842 (2010).

[11] E.A. Genina, A.N. Bashkatov, K.V. Larin, and V.V. Tuchin, "Light–tissue interaction at optical clearing" *in Laser Imaging and Manipulation in Cell Biology*, F.S. Pavone (ed.), WILEY-VCH Verlag GmbH & Co. KGaA, Weinheim (2010).

[12] V.V. Tuchin, R.K. Wang, and A.T. Yeh (eds.), "Special section on optical clearing of tissues and cells," *J. Biomed. Opt.***13**, 021101-021114 (2008).

[13] V.V. Tuchin, M.Leahy, and D. Zhu (eds.), "Special issue on optical clearing for biomedical imaging in the study of tissues and biological fluids," *J. Innov. Opt. Health Sci.* **3** (3), 147–219 (2010).

[14] C. Ayata, A.K. Dunn, Y. Gursoy-Özdemir, Z. Huang, D.A. Boas, and M.A. Moskowitz, "Laser speckle flowmetry for the study of cerebrovascular physiology in normal and ischemic mouse cortex," *J. Cereb. Blood Flow Metab.* **24**, 744–755 (2004).

[15] J. Wang, D. Zhu, M. Chen, and X. Liu, "Assessment of optical clearing induced improvement of laser speckle contrast imaging," *J. Innovat. Opt. Health Sci.* **3** (3), 159–167 (2010).

[16] R.K. Wang, X. Xu, V.V. Tuchin, and J.B. Elder, "Concurrent enhancement of imaging depth and contrast for optical coherence tomography by hyperosmotic agents," *J. Opt. Soc. Am. B* **18** (7), 948–953 (2001).

[17] G. Vargas, A. Readinger, S.S. Dosier, and A.J. Welch, "Morphological changes in blood vessels produced by hyperosmotic agents and measured by optical coherence tomography," *Photochem. Photobiol.* **77**, 541–549 (2003).

[18] Y. He, and R.K. Wang, "Dynamic optical clearing effect of tissue impregnated with hyperosmotic agents and studied with optical coherence tomography," *J. Biomed. Opt.* **9** (1), 200–206 (2004).

[19] C. Drew, T.E. Milner, and C.G. Rylander, "Mechanical tissue optical clearing devices: evaluation of enhanced light penetration in skin using optical coherence tomography," *J. Biomed. Opt.* **14** (6), 064019 (2009).

[20] X. Guo, Z. Guo, H. Wei, H. Yang, Y. He, S. Xie, G. Wu, H. Zhong, L. Li, and Q. Zhao, "In vivo quantification of propylene glycol, glucose and glycerol diffusion in human skin with optical coherence tomography," *Laser Phys.* **20** (9), 1849–1855 (2010).

[21] P.D. Agrba, M.Y. Kirillin, A.I. Abelevich, E.V. Zagaynova, and V.A. Kamensky, "Compression as a method for increasing the informativity of optical coherence tomography of biotissues," *Opt. Spectrosc.* **107** (6) 853–858 (2009).

[22] K. Moulton, F. Lovell, E. Williams, P. Ryan, D.C. Lay Jr., D. Jansen, and S. Willard, "Use of glycerol as an optical clearing agent for enhancing photonic transference and detection of salmonella typhimurium through porcine skin," *J. Biomed. Opt.* **11**, 054027 (2006).

[23] M.H. Khan, S. Chess, B. Choi, K.M. Kelly, and J.S. Nelson, "Can topically applied optical clearing agents increase the epidermal damage threshold and enhance therapeutic efficacy," *Lasers Surg. Med.* **35**, 93–95 (2004).

[24] R.J. McNichols, M.A. Fox, A. Gowda, S. Tuya, B. Bell, and M. Motamedi, "Temporary dermal scatter reduction: quantitative assessment and implications for improved laser tattoo removal," *Lasers Surg. Med.* **36**, 289–296 (2005).

[25] G. Vargas, J.K. Barton, and A.J. Welch, "Use of hyperosmotic chemical agent to improve the laser treatment of cutaneous vascular lesions," *J. Biomed. Opt.* **13** (2), 021114 (2008).

[26] C.M. Cilip, A.E. Ross, J.P. Jarow, and N.M. Fried, "Application of an optical clearing agent during noninvasive laser coagulation of the canine vas deferens," *J. Biomed. Opt.* **15** (4), 048001 (2010).

[27] M.H. Khan, B. Choi, S. Chess, K.M. Kelly, J. McCullough, and J.S. Nelson, "Optical clearing of *in vivo* human skin: implications for light-based diagnostic imaging and therapeutics," *Lasers Surg. Med.* **34**, 83–85 (2004).

[28] S. Plotnikov, V. Juneja, A.B. Isaacson, W.A. Mohler, and P.J. Campagnola, "Optical clearing for improved contrast in second harmonic generation imaging of skeletal muscle," *Biophys. J.* **90** (1), 328–339 (2006).

[29] R. Cicchi, F.S. Pavone, D. Massi, and D.D. Sampson, "Contrast and depth enhancement in two-photon microscopy of human skin ex vivo by use of optical clearing agents," *Opt. Express* **13** (7), 2337–2344 (2005).

[30] R. Dickie, R.M. Bachoo, M.A. Rupnick, S.M. Dallabrida, G.M. DeLoid, J. Lai, R.A. DePinho, and R.A. Rogers, "Three-dimensional visualization of microvessel architecture of whole-mount tissue by confocal microscopy," *Microvasc. Res.* **72**(1-2), 20–26 (2006).

[31] E.D. Jansen, P.M. Pickett, M.A. Mackanos, and J. Virostko, "Effect of optical tissue clearing on spatial resolution and sensitivity of bioluminescence imaging," *J. Biomed. Opt.* **11** (4), 041119 (2006).

[32] Y. Fu, and S. Tang, "Optical clearing facilitates integrated 3D visualization of mouse ileal microstructure and vascular network with high definition," *Microvasc. Res.* **80**, 512–521 (2010).

[33] Y.Y. Fu, C.H. Lu, C.W. Lin, J.H. Juang, G. Enikolopov, E. Sibley, A.S. Chiang, and S.C. Tang, "Three-dimensional optical method for integrated visualization of mouse islet microstructure and vascular network with subcellular-level resolution," *J. Biomed. Opt.* **15** (4), 046018 (2010).

[34] H.H. Lin, J.S.Y. Lai, A.L. Chin, Y.C. Chen, and A.S. Chiang, "A map of olfactory representation in the drosophila mushroom body," *Cell* **128**, 1205–1217 (2007).

[35] H.U. Dodt, U. Leischner, A. Schierloh, N. Jährling, C.P. Mauch, K. Deininger, J.M. Deussing, M. Eder, W. Zieglgnsberger, and K. Becker, "Ultramicroscopy: three-dimensional visualization of neuronal networks in the whole mouse brain," *Nat. Methods* **4** (4), 331–336 (2007).

[36] H. Hama, H. Kurokawa, H. Kawano, R. Ando, T. Shimogori, H. Noda, K. Fukami, A. Sakaue-Sawano, and A. Miyawaki, "Sca*l*e: a chemical approach for fluorescence imaging and reconstruction of transparent mouse brain," *Nat. Neurosci.* **14**, 1481–1488 (2011).

[37] A. Ertürk, C.P. Mauch, F. Hellal, F. Förstner, T. Keck, K. Becker, N. Jährling, H. Steffens, M. Richter, M. Hübener, E. Kramer, F. Kirchhoff, H.U. Dodt, and F. Bradke, "Three-dimensional imaging of the unsectioned adult spinal cord to assess axon regeneration and glial responses after injury," *Nat. Med.* **18**, 166–171 (2012).

[38] B. Choi, L. Tsu, E. Chen, T.S. Ishak, S.M. Iskandar, S. Chess, and J.S. Nelson, "Determination of chemical agent optical clearing potential using in vitro human skin," *Lasers Surg. Med.* **36**, 72–75 (2005).

[39] Z. Mao, D. Zhu, Y. Hu, X. Wen, and Z. Han, "Influence of alcohols on the optical clearing effect of skin *in vitro*," *J. Biomed. Opt.* **13** (2), 021104 (2008).

[40] X. Wen, V.V. Tuchin, Q. Luo, and D. Zhu, "Control the scattering of Intralipid by using optical clearing agents," *Phys. Med. Biol.* **54**, 6917–6930 (2009).

[41] O.O. Abugo, Z. Gryczynski, and J.R. Lakowicz, "Modulation sensing of fluorophores in tissue: a new approach to drug compliance monitoring," *J. Biomed. Opt.* **4**, 429–442 (1999).

[42] H.J.van Staveren, C.J. Moes, J.van Marle, S.A. Prahl, and M.J.C.van Gemert, "Light scattering in Intralipid-10% in the wavelength range of 400–1100 nm," *Appl. Opt.* **30**, 4507–4514 (1991).

[43] B. Guo, Y. Wang, Y. Wang, and H. Le, "Mid-infrared laser measurements of aqueous glucose," *J. Biomed. Opt.* **12**, 024005 (2007).

[44] K.J. Jeon, I.D. Hwang, S. Hahn, and G. Yoon, "Comparison between transmittance and reflectance measurements in glucose determination using near infrared spectroscopy," *J. Biomed. Opt.* **11**, 014022-7 (2006).

[45] M. Kinnunen, and R. Myllylä, "Application of optical coherence tomography, pulsed photoacoustic technique, and time-of-flight technique to detect changes in the scattering properties of a tissue-simulating phantom," *J. Biomed. Opt.***13**, 024005 (2008).

[46] X. Xu, and R.K. Wang, "The role of water desorption on optical clearing of biotissue: studied with near infrared reflectance spectroscopy," *Med. Phys.* **30** (6), 1246–1253 (2003).

[47] X. Xu, and R.K. Wang, "Synergistic effect of hyperosmotic agents of dimethyl sulfoxide and glycerol on optical clearing of gastric tissue studied with near infrared spectroscopy," *Phys. Med. Biol.* **49**, 457–468 (2004).

[48] R.K. Wang, "Role of mass diffusion and water desorption on optical clearing of biological tissue immersed with the hyperosmotic agents," *Proc. SPIE* **5330**, 160–166 (2004).

[49] R.K. Wang, Y. He, and V.V. Tuchin, "Effect of dehydration on optical clearing and OCT imaging contrast after impregnation of biological tissue with biochemical agents," *Proc. SPIE* **5316**, 119–127 (2004).

[50] C.G. Rylander, O.F. Stumpp, T.E. Milner, N.J. Kemp, J.M. Mendenhall, K.R. Diller, and A.J. Welch, "Dehydration mechanism of optical clearing in tissue," *J. Biomed. Opt.* **11** (4), 041117 (2006).

[51] L. Oliveira, A. Lage, M.P. Clemente, and V.V. Tuchin, "Rat muscle opacity decrease due to the osmosis of a simple mixture," *J. Biomed. Opt.* **15** (5), 055004 (2010).

[52] Y. Tanaka, A. Kubotaa, M. Yamatob, T. Okanob, and K. Nishida, "Irreversible optical clearing of sclera by dehydration and cross-linking," *Biomaterials* **32** (4), 1080–1090 (2011).

[53] T. Yu, X. Wen, V.V. Tuchin, Q. Luo, and D. Zhu, "Quantitative analysis of dehydration in porcine skin for assessing mechanism of optical clearing," *J. Biomed. Opt.* **16** (9), 095002 (2011).

[54] E.A. Genina, A.N. Bashkatov, A.A. Korobko, E.A. Zubkova, V.V. Tuchin, I.V. Yaroslavsky, and G.B. Altshuler, "Optical clearing of human skin: comparative study of permeability and dehydration of intact and photothermally perforated skin," *J. Biomed. Opt.* **13** (2), 021102 (2008).

[55] B.G. Osborne, *Near Infrared Spectroscopy in Food Analysis*, Longman Scientific and Technical, New York (1986).

[56] J. Hirshburg, B. Choi, J.S. Nelson, and A.T. Yeh, "Correlation between collagen solubility and skin optical clearing using sugars," *Lasers Surg. Med.* **39**, 140–144 (2007).

[57] J. Hirshburg, B. Choi, J.S. Nelson, and A.T. Yeh, "Collagen solubility correlates with skin optical clearing," *J. Biomed. Opt.* **11** (4), 040501 (2006).

[58] J. Jiang, and R.K. Wang, "Comparing the synergistic effects of oleic acid and dimethyl sulfoxide as vehicles for optical clearing of skin tissue *in vitro*," *Phys. Med. Biol.* **49**, 5283–5294 (2004).

[59] A.T. Yeh, and J. Hirshburg, "Molecular interactions of exogenous chemical agents with collagen implications for tissue optical clearing," *J. Biomed. Opt.* **11** (1), 014003 (2006).

[60] A.T. Yeh, B. Choi, J.S. Nelson, and B.J. Tromberg, "Reversible dissociation of collagen in tissues," *J. Invest. Dermatol.* **121** (6), 1332–1335 (2003).

[61] J.M. Hirshburg, K.M. Ravikumar, W. Hwang, and A.T. Yeh, "Molecular basis for optical clearing of collagenous tissues," *J. Biomed. Opt.* **15** (5), 055002 (2010).

[62] X. Wen, Z. Mao, Z. Han, V.V. Tuchin, and D. Zhu, "*In vivo* skin optical clearing by glycerol solutions: mechanism," *J. Biophotonics*, **3** (1), 44–52 (2010).

[63] D. Zhu, J. Wang, Z. Zhi, X. Wen, and Q. Luo, "Imaging dermal blood flow through the intact rat skin with an optical clearing method," *J. Biomed. Opt.* **15** (2), 026008 (2010).

[64] C. Liu, Z. Zhi, V.V. Tuchin, Q. Luo, and D. Zhu, "Enhancement of skin optical clearing efficacy using photo-irradiation," *Lasers Surg. Med.* **42** (2), 132–140 (2010).

[65] Z. Mao, Z. Han, X. Wen, Q. Luo, and D. Zhu, "Influence of glycerol with different concentration on skin optical clearing and morphological changes in vivo," *Proc. SPIE* **7278**, 72781T (2008).

[66] O. Stumpp, A. Welch, T.E. Milner, and J. Neev, "Enhancement of transepidermal skin clearing agent delivery using a 980 nm diode laser," *Lasers Surg. Med.* **37** (4), 278–285 (2005).

[67] V.V. Tuchin, G.B. Altshuler, A.A. Gavrilova, A.B. Pravdin, D. Tabatadze, J. Childs, and I.V. Yaroslavsky, "Optical clearing of skin using flashlamp-induced enhancement of epidermal permeability," *Lasers Surg. Med.* **38** (9), 824–836 (2006).

[68] E.A. Genina, L.E. Dolotov, A.N. Bashkatov, G.S. Terentyuk, G.N. Maslyakova, E.A. Zubkina, V.V. Tuchin, I.V. Yaroslavsky, G.B. Altshuler, "Fractional laser microablation of skin aimed at enhancing its permeability for nanoparticles," *Quant. Electr.* **41** (5) 396–401 (2011).

[69] E.V. Ross, "Laser versus intense pulsed light: Competing technologies in dermatology," *Lasers Surg. Med.* **38**, 261–272 (2006).

[70] A. Fujiwara, T. Hinokitani, K. Goto, and T. Arai, "Partial ablation of porcine stratum corneum by argon-fluoride excimer laser to enhance transdermal drug permeability," *Lasers Med. Sci.* **19**, 210–217 (2005).

[71] C. Gómez, A. Costela, I. Garca-Moreno, F. Llanes, J.M. Teijn, and D. Blanco, "Laser treatments on skin enhancing and controlling transdermal delivery of 5-Fluorouracil," *Lasers Surg. Med.* **40**, 6–12 (2008).

[72] J.S. Nelson, J.L. McCullough, T.C. Glenn, W.H. Wright, L.H. Liaw, and S.L. Jacques, "Mid-infrared laser ablation of stratum corneum enhances *in vitro* percutaneous transport of drugs," *J. Invest. Dermatol.* **97**, 874–879 (1991).

[73] X. Xu, Q. Zhu, and C. Sun, "Assessment of the effects of ultrasound-mediated alcohols on skin optical clearing," *J. Biomed. Opt.* **14** (3), 034042 (2009).

[74] H. Zhong, Z. Guo, H. Wei, Z. Zhang, H. Yang, and S. Xie, "Reflectance spectroscopy study of low-frequency ultrasound and glycerol on skin optical clearing," *Spectroscopy and Spectral Anal.* **29** (12), 3190–3194 (2009).

[75] H. Zhong, Z. Guo, H. Wei, C. Zeng, H. Xiong, Y. He, and S. Liu, "In vitro study of ultrasound and different-concentration glycerol-induced changes in human skin optical attenuation assessed with optical coherence tomography," *J. Biomed. Opt.* **15** (3), 036012 (2010).

[76] O. Stumpp, B. Chen, and B. Welch, "Using sandpaper for noninvasive transepidermal optical skin clearing agent delivery," *J. Biomed. Opt.* **11** (4), 041118 (2006).

[77] J. Yoon, T. Son, E.H. Choi, B. Choi, J.S. Nelson, and B. Jung, "Enhancement of optical skin clearing efficacy using a microneedle roller," *J. Biomed. Opt.* **13** (2), 021103 (2008).

[78] J. Yoon, D. Park, T. Son, J. Seo, J.S. Nelson, and B. Jung, "A physical method to enhance transdermal delivery of a tissue optical clearing agent: combination of microneedling and sonophoresis," *Lasers Surg. Med.* **42** (5), 412–417 (2010).

[79] A.M. Fox, D.G. Diven, K. Sra, A. Boretsky, T. Poonawalla, A. Readinger, M. Motamedi, and R.J. McNichols, "Dermal scatter reduction in human skin: a method using controlled application of glycerol," *Lasers Surg. Med.* **41**, 251–255 (2009).

[80] E.A. Genina, A.N. Bashkatov, V.V. Tuchin, G.B. Altshuler, and I.V. Yaroslavsky, "Possibility of increasing the efficiency of laser-induced tattoo removal by optical skin clearing," *Quant. Electr.* **38** (6), 580–587 (2008).

[81] A.N. Bashkatov, E.A. Genina, V.V. Tuchin, and G.B. Altshuler, "Skin optical clearing for improvement of laser tattoo removal," *Laser Physics* **19** (6), 1312–1322 (2009).

[82] C.G. Rylander, T.E. Milner, S.A. Baranov, and J.S. Nelson, "Mechanical tissue optical clearing devices: enhancement of light penetration in *ex vivo* porcine skin and adipose tissue," *Lasers Surg. Med.* **40**, 688–694 (2008).

[83] K.V. Larin, M.G. Ghosn, A.N. Bashkatov, E.A. Genina, N.A. Trunina, and V.V. Tuchin, "Optical clearing for OCT image enhancement and in-depth monitoring of molecular diffusion," *IEEE J. Select. Tops. Quant. Electr.* **18** (2012).

[84] M.Y. Kirillin, P.D. Agrba, and V.A. Kamensky, "*In vivo* study of the effect of mechanical compression on formation of OCT images of human skin," *J. Biophotonics* **3**, 752–758 (2010).

[85] A.A. Gurjarpadhye, W.C. Vogt, Y. Liu, and C.G. Rylander, "Effect of localized mechanical indentation on skin water content evaluated using OCT," *Int. J. Biomed. Imaging* 2011, 817250 (2011).

[86] E.K. Chan, B. Sorg, D. Protsenko, M. O'Neil, M. Motamedi, and A.J. Welch, "Effects of compression on soft tissue optical properties," *IEEE J. Sel. Tops. Quant. Electron.* **2** (4), 943–950 (1996).

[87] J.W. Wiechers and R.A. de Zeeuw, "Transdermal drug delivery: efficacy and potential applications of the penetration enhancer Azone," *Drug Design and Delivery* **6** (2), 87–100 (1990).

[88] X. Xu, and Q. Zhu, "Evaluation of skin optical clearing enhancement with Azone as a penetration enhancer," *Opt. Commun.* **279**, 223–228 (2007).

[89] J. Jiang, and R.K. Wang, "How different molarities of oleic acid as enhancer exert its effect on optical clearing of skin tissue in vitro," *J. X-ray Sci. Technol.* **13** (3), 149–159 (2005).

[90] J. Jiang, M. Boese, P. Turner, and R.K. Wang, "Penetration kinetics of dimethyl sulphoxide and glycerol in dynamic optical clearing of porcine skin tissue in vitro studied by Fourier transform infrared spectroscopic imaging," *J. Biomed. Opt.* **13** (2), 021105 (2008).

[91] A.K. Bui, R.A. McClure, J. Chang, C. Stoianovici, J. Hirshburg, A.T. Yeh, and B. Choi, "Revisiting optical clearing with dimethyl sulfoxide (DMSO)," *Lasers Surg. Med.* **41** (2),142–148 (2009).

[92] M. Zimmerley, R.A. McClure, B. Choi, and E.O. Potma, "Following dimethyl sulfoxide skin optical clearing dynamics with quantitative nonlinear multimodal microscopy," *Appl. Opt.* **48** (10), D79–D87 (2009).

[93] Z. Mao, Y. Hu, Y. Zheng, W. Lu, Q. Luo, and D. Zhu, "Experimental study on influence of thiazone on optical clearing of piglet skin *in vitro*," *Acta Optical Sinica* **27** (3), 526–530, 2007(in Chinese).

[94] J. Jiang, W. Chen, R.K. Wang, and K. Xu, "Availability of thiazone as an enhancer for optical clearing of skin tissue *in vitro*," *Proc. SPIE* **6858**, 1–8 (2008).

[95] J. Wang, X. Zhou, S. Duan, Z. Chen, and D. Zhu, "Improvement of *in vivo* rat skin optical clearing with chemical penetration enhancers," *Proc. SPIE* **7883**, 78830Y-1(2011).

[96] Z. Zhi, Z. Han, Q. Luo, and D. Zhu, "Improve optical clearing skin *in vitro* with propylene glycol as a penetration enhancer," *J. Innovat. Opt. Health Sci.* **2** (3), 269–278 (2009).

[97] L. Xiong, "A new skin penetration promoter: Thiazone," *Fine Spec. Chem.* **12**, 9–11 (2004) (in Chinese).

[98] X. Xu, Q. Zhu, and C. Sun, "Combined effect of ultrasound-SLS on skin optical clearing," *IEEE Photonic Tech. L.* **20** (24), 2117– 2119(2008).

[99] H. Zhong, Z. Guo, H. Wei, L. Guo, C. Wang, Y. He, H. Xiong, and S. Liu, "Synergistic effect of ultrasound and thiazone–PEG 400 on human skin optical clearing *in vivo*," *Photochem. Photobiol.* **86**, 732–737 (2010).

[100] M.G. Ghosn, V.V. Tuchin, and K.V. Larin, "Depth-resolved monitoring of drug diffusion in tissues using optical coherence tomography," *Opt. Lett.* **31** (15), 2314–2316, 2006.

[101] M.G. Ghosn, V.V. Tuchin, and K.V. Larin, "Non-destructive quantification of analytes diffusion in cornea and sclera by using optical coherence tomography, *Invest. Ophthal. Visual Sci.* (IOVS) **48** (6), 2726–2733 (2007).

[102] M.G. Ghosn, E.F. Carbajal, N. Befrui, V.V. Tuchin, and K.V. Larin, "Differential permeability rate and percent clearing of glucose in different regions in rabbit sclera," *J. Biomed. Opt.* **13**, 021110-1–6 (2008).

[103] I.V. Larina, E.F. Carbajal, V.V. Tuchin, M.E. Dickinson, and K.V. Larin, "Enhanced OCT imaging of embryonic tissue with optical clearing," *Laser Phys. Lett.* **5** (6), 476–479 (2008).

[104] M.G. Ghosn, N. Sudheendran, M. Wendt, A. Glasser, V.V. Tuchin, and K.V. Larin, "Monitoring of glucose permeability in monkey skin *in vivo* using optical coherence tomography," *J. Biophotonics* **3** (1-2), 25–33 (2010).

[105] N. Sudheendran, M. Mohamed, M.G. Ghosn, V.V. Tuchin, and K.V. Larin, "Assessment of tissue optical clearing as a function of glucose concentration using optical coherence tomography," *J. Innov. Opt. Health Sci.* **3** (3), 169–176 (2010).

[106] S.G. Proskurin and I.V. Meglinski, "Optical coherence tomography imaging depth enhancement by superficial skin optical clearing," *Laser Phys. Lett.* **4** (11), 824–826 (2007).

[107] M. Kinnunen, R. Myllylä and S. Vainio, "Detecting glucose-induced changes in in *vitro* and *in vivo* experiments with optical coherence tomography," *J. Biomed. Opt.* **13** (2), 021111 (2008).

[108] M. Bonesi, S.G. Proskurin, and I.V. Meglinski, "Imaging of subcutaneous blood vessels and flow velocity profiles by optical coherence tomography," *Laser Phys.* **20** (4), 891–899 (2010).

[109] Z. Zhu, G. Wu, H. Wei, H. Yang, Y. He, S. Xie, Q. Zhao, and X. Guo, "Investigation of the permeability and optical clearing ability of different analytes in human normal and cancerous breast tissues by spectral domain OCT," *J. Biophotonics* **5**, 1–8 (2012).

[110] J. Wang, Y. Liang, S. Zhang, Y. Zhou, H. Ni, and Y. Li, "Evaluation of optical clearing with the combined liquid paraffin and glycerol mixture," *Biomed. Opt. Express.* **2** (8), 2329–2338 (2011).

[111] X. Guo, Z.Guo, H. Wei, H. Yang, Y. He, S. Xie, G. Wu, X. Deng, Q. Zhao, and L. Li, "*In vivo* comparison of the optical clearing efficacy of optical clearing agents in human skin by quantifying permeability using optical coherence tomography," *Photochem. Photobiol.* **87** (3), 734–740 (2011).

[112] Q.L. Zhao, J.L. Si, Z.Y. Guo, H.J. Wei, H.Q. Yang, G.Y. Wu, S.S. Xie, X.Y. Li, X. Guo, H.Q. Zhong, and L.Q. Li, "Quantifying glucose permeability and enhanced light penetration in *ex vivo* human normal and cancerous esophagus tissues with optical coherence tomography," *Laser Phys. Lett.* **8** (1), 71–77 (2011).

[113] I.V. Meglinski, A.N. Bashkatov, E.A. Genina, D.Y. Churmakov, and V.V. Tuchin, "The enhancement of confocal images of tissues at bulk optical immersion," *Laser. Phys.* **13** (1), 65–69 (2003).

[114] P.J. Caspers, A.C. Williams, E.A. Carter, H.G.M. Edwards, B.W. Barry, H.A. Bruining and G.J. Puppels, "Monitoring the penetration enhancer dimethyl sulfoxide in human stratum corneum *in vivo* by confocal Raman spectroscopy," *Pharmaceut. Res.* **19** (10), 1577–1580 (2002).

[115] M.V. Schulmerich, J.H. Cole, K.A. Dooley, M.D. Morris, J.M. Kreider, and S.A. Goldstein, "Optical clearing in transcutaneous Raman spectroscopy of murine cortical bone tissue," *J. Biomed. Opt.* **13** (2), 021108 (2008).

[116] D. Huang, W. Zhang, H. Zhong, H. Xiong, X. Guo, and Z. Guo, "Optical clearing of porcine skin tissue *in vitro* studied by Raman microspectroscopy," *J. Biomed. Opt.* **17** (1), 015004 (2012).

[117] Y. He, R.K. Wang, and D. Xing, "Enhanced sensitivity and spatial resolution for *in vivo* imaging with low-level light-emitting probes by use of biocompatible chemical agents," *Opt. Lett.* **28** (21), 2076–2078 (2003).

[118] A. Matsui, S.J. Lomnes and J.V. Frangioni, "Optical clearing of the skin for near-infrared fluorescence image-guided surgery," *J. Biomed. Opt.* **14** (2), 024019 (2009).

[119] E.V. Migacheva, A.B. Pravdin and V.V. Tuchin, "Alterations in autofluorescence signal from rat skin *ex vivo* under optical immersion clearing," *J. Innov. Opt. Health Sci.* **3** (3), 147–152 (2010).

[120] T. Yasui, Y. Tohno, and T. Araki, "Characterization of collagen orientation in human dermis by two-dimensional second-harmonic-generation polarimetry," *J. Biomed. Opt.* **9** (2), 259–264 (2004).

[121] R. LaComb, O. Nadiarnykh, S. Carey, and P.J. Campagnola, "Quantitative second harmonic generation imaging and modeling of the optical clearing mechanism in striated muscle and tendon," *J. Biomed. Opt.* **13** (2), 021109 (2008).

[122] M.A. Vilensky, D.N. Agafonov, D.A. Zimnyakov, V.V. Tuchin, and R.A. Zdrazhevskii, "Speckle-correlation analysis of the microcapillary blood circulation in nail bed," *Quant. Electr.* **41** (4), 324–328 (2011).

[123] C. Macdonald and I. Meglinski, "Backscattering of circular polarized light from a disperse random medium influenced by optical clearing," *Laser Phys. Lett.*, 8 (4), 324–328 (2011).

[124] S. Tanev, V.V. Tuchin, and P. Paddon, "Cell membrane and gold nanoparticles effects on optical immersion experiments with normal and cancerous cells: FDTD modeling," *J. Biomed. Opt.* **11** (6), 025606-1–6 (2006).

[125] S. Tanev, V. Tuchin, P. Cheben, P. Bock, J. Schmid, S. Janz, D. Xu, J. Lapointe, A. Densmore, and J. Pond, "Advances in the FDTD design and modeling of nano- and bio-photonics applications," *Photon Nanostruct: Fundam. Appl.* (2011);

[126] C.E. Rommel, C. Dierker, L. Schmidt, S. Przibilla, G. von Bally, B. Kemper, and J. Schnekenburger, "Contrast-enhanced digital holographic imaging of cellular structures by manipulating the intracellular refractive index," *J. Biomed. Opt.* **15** (4), 041509-1–10 (2010).

[127] V.V. Tuchin (ed.), *Advanced Optical Cytometry: Methods and Disease Diagnoses*, Wiley-VCH Verlag GmbH & Co. KGaA, Weinheim, 2011

[128] R. Barer, K.F.A. Ross, and S. Tkaczyk, "Refractometry of living cells," *Nature* **171**(4356), 720–724 (1953).

[129] W. Redisch, E.J. Messina, G. Hughes, and C. Mcewen, "Capillaroscopic observations in rheumatic diseases," *Ann. Rheum. Dis.* **29**, 244–253 (1970).

[130] A.S. Chiang, "Aqueous tissue clearing solution," US Patent 6472216B1 (2002).

[131] J. Wang and D. Zhu, "Preliminary investigations of rat skin after topical application of optical clearing agent," *Proc. SPIE* **7999**, 79990G (2011).

[132] E.I. Galanzha, V.V. Tuchin, A.V. Solovieva, T.V. Stepanova, Q. Luo, and H. Cheng, "Skin backreflectance and microvascular system functioning at the action of osmotic agents," *J. Phys. D: Appl. Phys.* **36** (14), 1739–1746 (2003).

[133] H. Cheng, Q. Luo, S. Zeng, S. Chen, W. Luo, and H. Gong, "Hyperosmotic chemical agent's effect on in vivo cerebral blood flow revealed by laser speckle," *Appl. Opt.* **43** (31), 5772–5777 (2004).

[134] D. Zhu, J. Zhang, H. Cui, Z. Mao, P. Li, and Q. Luo, "Short-term and long-term effects of optical clearing agents on blood vessels in chick chorioallantoic membrane," *J. Biomed. Opt.* **13** (2), 021106 (2008).

[135] Z. Mao, X. Wen, J. Wang, and D. Zhu, "The biocompatibility of the dermal injection of glycerol *in vivo* to achieve optical clearing," *Proc. SPIE* **7519**, 75191N (2009).

[136] M. Rossi and A. Carpi, "Skin microcirculation in peripheral arterial obliterative disease," *Biomed. Pharmacother.* **58**, 427–431 (2004).

[137] J.D. Briers and S. Webster, "Laser speckle contrast analysis (LASCA): a non-scanning, full-field technique for monitoring capillary blood flow," *J. Biomed. Opt.* **1**, 174–179 (1996).

[138] J.D. Briers, G. Richards, and X.W. He, "Capillary blood flow monitoring using laser speckle contrast analysis (LASCA)," *J. Biomed. Opt.* **4** (1), 164–175 (1999).

[139] J.D. Briers, "Laser Doppler, speckle and related techniques for blood perfusion mapping and imaging," *Physiol. Meas.* **22**, R35–R66 (2001).

[140] S. Liu, P. Li, and Q. Luo, "Fast blood flow visualization of high-resolution laser speckle imaging data using graphics processing unit," *Opt. Express* **16** (19), 14321–14329 (2008).

[141] H. Cheng, Q. Luo, S. Zeng, S. Cheng, J. Cen, and H. Gong, "Modified laser speckle imaging method with improved spatial resolution," *J. Biom. Opt.* **8**, 559–564 (2003).

[142] P. Li, S. Ni, L. Zhang, S. Zeng, and Q. Luo, "Imaging cerebral blood flow through the intact rat skull," *Opt. Lett.* **31**, 1824–1826 (2006).

[143] D. Zhu, W. Lu, Y. Weng, H. Cui, and Q. Luo, "Monitoring thermal induced changes in tumor blood flow and micro-vessels with laser speckle contrast imaging," *Appl. Opt.* **46**, 1911–1917 (2007).

[144] E.A. Genina, A.N. Bashkatov, and V.V. Tuchin, "Optical clearing of cranial bone," *Adv. Opt. Technol.* 267867-1–8 (2008).

[145] J. Wang, Y. Zhang, T.H. Xu, Q.M. Luo, and D. Zhu, "An innovative transparent cranial window based on skull optical clearing," *Laser Phys. Lett.* **9** (6), 469–473 (2012).

[146] P. Li, S. Ni, L. Zhang, S. Zeng, and Q. Luo, "Imaging cerebral blood flow through the intact rat skull with temporal laser speckle imaging," *Opt. Lett.* **31** (12), 1824–1826 (2006).

[147] D. A. Boas, and A. K. Dunn, "Laser speckle contrast imaging in biomedical optics," *J. Biomed. Opt.* **15** (1), 011109 (2010).

[148] K. Svoboda, and R. Yasuda, "Principles of two-photon excitation microscopy and its applications to neuroscience," *Neuron* **50** (6), 823–839 (2006).

[149] H. T. Xu, F. Pan, G. Yang, and W. B. Gan, "Choice of cranial window type for in vivo imaging affects dendritic spine turnover in the cortex," *Nat. Neurosci.* **10** (5), 549–551 (2007).

[150] W. A. Lee, J. L. Chen, H. Huang, J. H. Leslie, Y. Amitai, P. T. So, and E. Nedivi, "A dynamic zone defines interneuron remodeling in the adult neocortex," *Proc. Natl. Acad. Sci.* **105** (50), 19968–19973 (2008).

[151] A. Holtmaat, T. Bonhoeffer, D. K. Chow, J. Chuckowree, V. De Paola, S. B. Hofer, M. Hubener, T. Keck, G. Knott, W. C. A. Lee, R. Mostany, T. D. Mrsic-Flogel, E. Nedivi, C. Portera-Cailliau, K. Svoboda, J. T. Trachtenberg, and L. Wilbrecht, "Long-term, high-resolution imaging in the mouse neocortex through a chronic cranial window," *Nat. Protoc.* **4** (8), 1128–1144 (2009).

[152] J. Grutzendler, N. Kasthuri, and W.B. Gan, "Long-term dendritic spine stability in the adult cortex," *Nature* **420**(6917), 812–816 (2002).

[153] P.J. Drew, A.Y. Shih, J.D. Driscoll, P.M. Knutsen, P. Blinder, D. Davalos, K. Akassoglou, P.S. Tsai, and D. Kleinfeld, "Chronic optical access through a polished and reinforced thinned skull," *Nat. Methods* **7** (12), 981–984 (2010).

[154] Z.S. Sacks, R.M. Kurtz, T. Juhasz, and G.A. Mourau, "High precision subsurface photodisruption in human sclera," *J. Biomed. Opt.* **7** (3), 442–450 (2002).

[155] A.A. Alekhin, A.A. Ionin, S.E. Kozhushko, I.M. Kourylyova, S.I. Kudryashov, K.K. Kuz'min, V.G. Likhvansteva, M.V. Samoylov, L.V. Seleznev, D.V. Sinitsyn, and S.D. Zakharov, "*In vitro* femtosecond laser subsurface micro-disruption inside human cornea and pre-cleared sclera," *Laser Phys. Lett.* **7** (6), 463–466 (2010).

[156] E.I. Galanzha, M.S. Kokoska, E.V. Shashkov, J.-W. Kim, V.V. Tuchin, and V.P. Zharov, "*In vivo* fiber photoacoustic detection and photothermal purging of metastasis targeted by nanoparticles in sentinel lymph nodes at single cell level," *J. Biophotonics*, **2**, 528–539 (2009).

[157] E.A. Genina, A.N. Bashkatov, Yu. P. Sinichkin, V.V. Tuchin, "Optical clearing of the eye sclera *in vivo* caused by glucose," *Quant. Electr.* **36** (12), 1119–1124 (2006).

[158] E. Galanzha, V. Tuchin, and V. Zharov, "Optical clearing in small animals: an application for *in vivo* lymph flow cytometry," *Lasers Surg. Med.* **19** Suppl., 10 (2007).

[159] V.V. Tuchin (ed.), *Handbook of Optical Sensing of Glucose in Biological Fluids and Tissues*, CRC Press, Taylor & Francis Group, London, 2009.

[160] E.A. Genina, A.N. Bashkatov, V.V. Tuchin, M.G. Ghosn, K.V. Larin, and T.G. Kamenskikh, "Cortexin diffusion in human eye sclera," *Quant. Electron.* **41** (5), 407–413 (2011).

Index